# Lecture Notes in Computer Science 8149

*Commenced Publication in 1973*
Founding and Former Series Editors:
Gerhard Goos, Juris Hartmanis, and Jan van Leeuwen

Kensaku Mori   Ichiro Sakuma
Yoshinobu Sato   Christian Barillot
Nassir Navab (Eds.)

# Medical Image Computing and Computer-Assisted Intervention – MICCAI 2013

16th International Conference
Nagoya, Japan, September 22-26, 2013
Proceedings, Part I

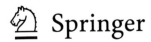 Springer

Volume Editors

Kensaku Mori
Nagoya University, Japan
kensaku@is.nagoya-u.ac.jp

Yoshinobu Sato
Osaka University, Japan
yoshi@image.med.osaka-u.ac.jp

Nassir Navab
Technical University of Munich
Germany
nassir.navab@tum.de

Ichiro Sakuma
University of Tokyo, Japan
sakuma@bmpe.t.u-tokyo.ac.jp

Christian Barillot
IRISA, Rennes, France
christian.barillot@irisa.fr

ISSN 0302-9743                          e-ISSN 1611-3349
ISBN 978-3-642-40810-6                  e-ISBN 978-3-642-40811-3
DOI 10.1007/978-3-642-40811-3
Springer Heidelberg New York Dordrecht London

Library of Congress Control Number: 2013946897

CR Subject Classification (1998): I.4, I.5, I.3.5-8, I.2.9-10, J.3, I.6

LNCS Sublibrary: SL 6 – Image Processing, Computer Vision, Pattern Recognition, and Graphics

*Typesetting:* Camera-ready by author, data conversion by Scientific Publishing Services, Chennai, India

Printed on acid-free paper

Springer is part of Springer Science+Business Media (www.springer.com)

# Preface

The 16th International Conference on Medical Image Computing and Computer Assisted Intervention, MICCAI 2013, was held in Nagoya, Japan during September 22–26, 2013 at Toyoda Auditorium, Nagoya University. The conference was held on a university campus, unlike the past three conferences. Toyoda Auditorium is memorable for all Nagoya University students, because entrance and graduation ceremonies are held in it during cherry-blossom season. Since MICCAI is the premier conference in the field of medical image computing and computer assisted surgery, it was our great honor to host it. Nagoya University has more than 50 years of history in medical image processing, which was initiated by Prof. Jun-ichiro Toriwaki. Nagoya also is famous for transportation and aerospace industries that utilize many robotics technologies. These robots are also manufactured in the Nagoya area and have become indispensable in current medical interventions.

This is the second time that the MICCAI conference has been held in Japan; the 5th MICCAI was held in Tokyo in 2002, which was the first MICCAI in Asia or Oceania. In MICCAI 2002, 184 papers were accepted among 321 submissions, and the conference included five satellite half-day tutorials. Since then, MICCAI has become a much larger event and typically includes 250 accepted papers from 800 submissions and 30 satellite events. At MICCAI 2013, 262 papers were accepted from 798 submissions; 34 satellite events (workshops, challenges, tutorials) were accepted.

The Program Committee (PC) of MICCAI 2013 was comprised of 101 members coordinated by a program chair and two program co-chairs from three countries. Each of the 798 papers was assigned to one primary and two secondary PC members. The primary member knew the identity of the authors, but the secondary ones did not. Each PC member had five to ten papers as the primary member and another ten to twenty as the secondary member, according to their expertise and the subject matter of the paper. The primary PC member assigned three or more external reviewers to each paper. 835 external reviewers provided 2794 reviews (359 words on average per review): 3.5 reviews per paper. At this stage, 76 papers, which failed to receive sufficient support from the external reviews, were rejected without further consideration. The authors of the remaining 722 papers were given the opportunity to rebut the anonymous reviews, based on which discussions among the reviewers took place. Finally, two secondary members independently provided meta-reviews by taking all input (the reviews, rebuttal, discussion, and the paper itself) into account to make an acceptance or rejection recommendation. For a few papers that had only two external reviews, the secondary members provided detailed reviews in addition to the meta-reviews.

A two-day PC meeting was held in Tokyo with 32 of its members. Prior to the meeting, the initial acceptance of 198 papers was decided, because they were ranked high by the external reviewers as well as two secondary PC members. 362 papers were rejected because they did not receive enough support from the reviewers or the two secondary members. Each of the remaining 162 borderline papers was considered in the following three-phase decision process.

- First stage: Six groups of five or six PC members ranked the 162 papers to select the best 36 papers for acceptance and rejected the lowest 72 papers.
- Second stage: A different set of groups selected the best 18 papers for acceptance from the remaining 54 papers and rejected 18 papers.
- Third stage: The program chair and the co-chairs selected an additional ten papers from the remaining 18 papers by considering the topics, the institutional variety, and the quality.

262 papers were finally accepted, for a 32.8% acceptance rate. The PC members also selected a set of papers suitable for oral presentation, from which the program chair and co-chairs finally decided a list of 37 oral papers by taking the variety of topics as well as the suitability for oral presentation into account. During all the review processes, possible conflicts of interests were carefully monitored and avoided as far as possible. The geographic and keyword distributions of the accepted papers are summarized in the figures.

All accepted papers were presented during three poster sessions. Oral papers were further presented during six single-track plenary oral sessions. We are greatly indebted to the reviewers and the PC members for their extraordinary efforts of careful evaluations of the submissions within a very short time frame.

In addition to the three days of the MICCAI main conference, the annual MICCAI event hosted satellite workshops, tutorials, and challenges that were organized on the day before and after the main conference. This year's call for submissions for workshops and tutorials recorded 30 workshop / challenge proposals (including four half-day proposals) and seven tutorial proposals (also including four half-day proposals). These proposals were independently reviewed by the workshop, tutorial and challenge chair teams, headed by Hongen Liao (Tsinghua University), Pierre Jannin (University of Rennes 1), Simon Warfield (Harvard Medical School), and Akinobu Shimizu (Tokyo University of Agriculture and Technology).

In the review process for the proposals for these events, we emphasized the following points. The workshop proposals were reviewed under criteria that addressed whether the workshop emphasized an open problem addressed in the MICCAI community. Tutorial proposals were reviewed based on whether they provided educational material for training new professionals in the field, including students, clinicians, and new researchers. Also, we emphasized tutorials that focused on existing sub-disciplines of MICCAI with known material, approaches, and open problems. Challenge proposals were reviewed based on whether they were interactive and encouraged problem solving. Although all of the workshop proposals were very strong, the workshop chairs selected 22 workshops (including three half-day workshops), six tutorials (including four half-day tutorials), and six challenges (including one half-day challenge and one challenge included in the workshop). We thank the workshop, tutorial, and challenge chairs for their hard work organizing such a comprehensive and unique program.

The highlights of the MICCAI 2013 events were the keynote lectures by Dr. Atsushi Miyawaki (Riken) and Prof. Toshio Fukuda (Meijo University). Dr. Miyawaki's talk focused on new imaging technology that enables us to cruise inside a cell. Prof. Fukuda discussed simulation-based medicine for intravascular surgery. We believe these two talks provided deep insights into new technologies and highlighted the future and emerging trends in these areas.

A public lecture, which was held on the day before MICCAI's main conference, widely introduced MICCAI to the public. Three distinctive guest speakers show the state-of-the-art technologies in the MICCAI field. Prof. Koji Ikuta presented exciting nano-robotics technologies. Prof. Yoshihiro Muragaki presented technologies for advanced intelligent operating theaters. Prof. Hidefumi Kobatake demonstrated the technologies and medical applications of computational anatomy. This wonderful public lecture was managed by Prof. Ken Masamune (The University of Tokyo.)

The First International Workshop on Medical Imaging and Computer-assisted Intervention (MICI Workshop) was independently organized just after the PC meeting at The University of Tokyo under the support. This workshop shared knowledge among the public audience and PC members who are experts in the MICCAI field.

MICCAI 2013 would not have been possible without the efforts of many people behind the scenes. We thank the Organizing, Executive, and Local Executive Committee members. The Scientific Council of Japan provided great assistance organizing this conference in Japan. The Japan Society of Computer Aided Surgery (JSCAS), headed by Prof. Masaki Kitajima (International University of Wealth and Health), also helped organize it. Prof. Takeyoshi Dohi (Tokyo Denki University) supervised a successful MICCAI meeting as a founders of the MICCAI Society and the general chair of MICCAI 2002. We also thank Prof. Etsuko Kobayashi (The University of Tokyo) and Prof. Takayuki Kitasaka (Aichi Institute of Technology) for handling the financial issues. Dr. Toshiyuki Okada (Osaka University) efficiently organized the review process and compiled the proceedings. Prof. Masahiro Oda (Nagoya University) solved facility management problems. Dr. Takehiro Ando and Dr. Junchen Wang made local arrangements for the PC meeting. Prof. Daniel Rueckert (Imperial College) helped us from the preparation of MICCAI 2013 proposal to actual conference management.

We also thank the MICCAI Secretaries, Janette Wallace, Jackie Williams, and Johanne Langford of the team from Canada. We communicated with them by e-mail around midnight every day (the time difference between Nagoya and Toronto is 11 hours) for advice regarding the conference organization. Without their help, the MICCAI 2013 conference would not have been successful. We thank the MICCAI Board headed by Prof. James Duncan (Yale University) and Prof. Alison Noble (University of Oxford) for trusting us with the organization of the MICCAI 2013 conference. They gave us a lot of freedom and advice.

We also thank our secretaries, Mizuru Suzuki, Kengo Suzuki, and Emi Tanahashi (Inter Group Corp.) for their hard work handling so many requests from attendees. We say a special thanks to Rie Ohashi (Nagoya University), Ai Okano (The University of Tokyo), and Naho Obata (The University of Tokyo). The original MICCAI 2013 logos and banners were sketched by the following four students of the Aichi Institute of Technology: Miki Takahashi, Kaori Suzuki, Hikaru Sekiguchi, and Yuiko Kori.

We appreciate the financial support from the Nagoya Convention and Visitors Bureau, The Murata Science Foundation, and the Daiko Foundation. We are deeply grateful to Nagoya University for allowing us to use the Toyoda Auditorium for MICCAI 2013.

We also deeply thank our sponsors and exhibitors for their financial support.

Our initial proposal for MICCAI 2013 was accepted during MICCAI 2010 in Beijing. Six months later, a huge earthquake devastated North East Japan. Thousands of people lost their lives. We encountered many difficult situations, including the threat of radiation from the Fukushima Nuclear Power Plant. Many people from countries all over the world helped Japan and offered assistance. We are deeply grateful.

The next MICCAI conference will be held during September 14–18, 2014 in Boston, which is the one of the most beautiful cities in the world. It hosted the 1st MICCAI conference in 1998. We are looking forward to seeing all of you in Boston in 2014!

September 2013

Kensaku Mori
Ichiro Sakuma
Yoshinobu Sato
Christian Barillot
Nassir Navab

# Accepted MICCAI 2013 Papers

## Biomedical Keyword

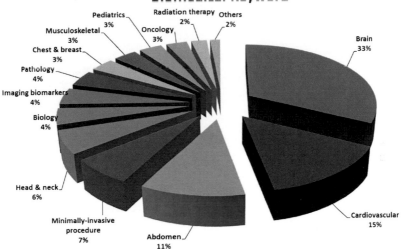

- Pediatrics 3%
- Radiation therapy 2%
- Others 2%
- Musculoskeletal 3%
- Oncology 3%
- Chest & breast 3%
- Pathology 4%
- Imaging biomarkers 4%
- Biology 4%
- Head & neck 6%
- Minimally-invasive procedure 7%
- Abdomen 11%
- Brain 33%
- Cardiovascular 15%

## Technical Keyword

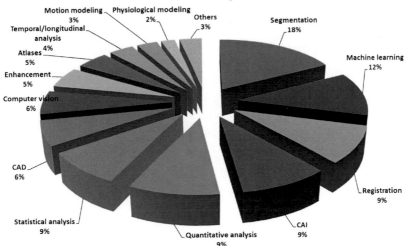

- Motion modeling 3%
- Physiological modeling 2%
- Others 3%
- Temporal/longitudinal analysis 4%
- Atlases 5%
- Enhancement 5%
- Computer vision 6%
- CAD 6%
- Statistical analysis 9%
- Quantitative analysis 9%
- CAI 9%
- Registration 9%
- Machine learning 12%
- Segmentation 18%

## Imaging Modality Keyword

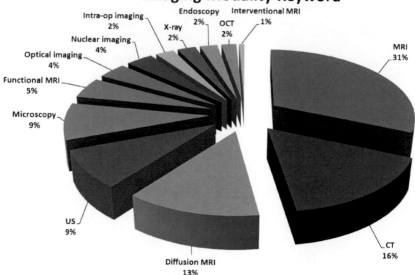

## Country of First Author

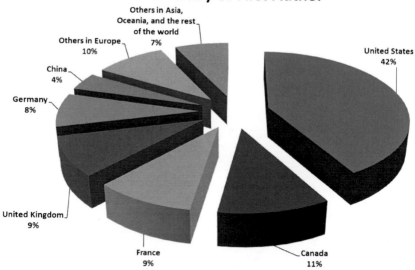

# Organization

## General Chair and Co-chair

| | |
|---|---|
| Kensaku Mori | Nagoya University, Japan |
| Ichiro Sakuma | The University of Tokyo, Japan |

## Program Chair and Co-chairs

| | |
|---|---|
| Yoshinobu Sato | Osaka University, Japan |
| Christian Barillot | INSERM, France |
| Nassir Navab | TU Munich, Germany |

## Workshop Chair and Co-chairs

| | |
|---|---|
| Hongen Liao | Tsinghua University, China |
| Simon Warfield | Harvard Medical School, USA |
| Pierre Jannin | University of Rennes 1, France |
| Akinobu Shimizu | Tokyo University of Agriculture and Technology, Japan |

## Organizers

MICCAI 2013 Organizing Committee
Japan Society of Computer Aided Surgery
Scientific Council of Japan

## Co-organizers

Information and Communications Headquarters, Nagoya University
Graduate School of Information Science, Nagoya University

## MICCAI Society, Board of Directors

| | |
|---|---|
| Alison Noble (President) | University of Oxford, United Kingdom |
| Sebastien Ourselin (Treasurer) | University College London, United Kingdom |
| Wiro Niessen (Exec. Director) | Erasmus MC - University Medical Centre, The Netherlands |
| Gabor Fichtinger (Secretary) | Queen's University, Canada |
| Stephen Aylward | Kitware, Inc., USA |

Nicholas Ayache                 INRIA, France
Polina Golland                  MIT, USA
David Hawkes                    University College London, United Kingdom
Kensaku Mori                    Nagoya University, Japan
Xavier Pennec                   INRIA, France
Josien Pluim                    University Medical Center Utrecht,
                                   The Netherlands
Daniel Rueckert                 Imperial College London, United Kingdom
Dinggang Shen                   UNC, USA

## Consultants to Board

Alan Colchester                 University of Kent, United Kingdom
Terry Peters                    University of Western Ontario, London,
                                   Canada
Richard Robb                    Mayo Clinic College of Medicine, USA

## Executive Officers

President:                      Alison Noble, United Kingdom
Executive Director              Wiro Niessen, The Netherlands
Secretary                       Gabor Fichtinger, Canada
Treasurer                       Sebastien Ourselin, United Kingdom
Elections Officer               Richard Robb, USA
Awards Coordinator              Gabor Fichtinger, Canada

## Non-executive Officers

Society Secretariat             Janette Wallace, Canada
Recording Secretary             Jackie Williams, Canada
Fellow Nomination
   Coordinator                  Terry Peters, Canada

## Student Board Members

President                       Hakim Achterberg, The Netherlands
Website Officer                 Katherine Gray, United Kingdom
Treasurer                       Sinara Vijayan, Norway
Profession Events Officer       Maxime Taquet, Belgium
Student Communication
   and Social Events Officer    Kristin McLeod, France

# MICCAI 2013 Program Committee

| | |
|---|---|
| Purang Abolmaesumi | University of British Columbia, Canada |
| Burak Acar | Boğaziçi University, Turkey |
| Daniel Alexander | University College London, UK |
| Stephen Aylward | Kitware, USA |
| Wolfgang Birkfellner | Medical University of Vienna, Austria |
| Albert C. S. Chung | HKUST, Hong Kong |
| Ela Claridge | University of Birmingham, UK |
| D. Louis Collins | McGill University, Canada |
| Dorin Comaniciu | Siemens, USA |
| Tim Cootes | University of Manchester, UK |
| Stephane Cotin | Inria, France |
| Antonio Criminisi | Microsoft Research, UK |
| Christos Davatzikos | University of Pennsylvania, USA |
| Benoit Dawant | Vanderbilt University, USA |
| Marleen de Bruijne | Erasmus MC & University of Copenhagen, The Netherlands & Denmark |
| Hervé Delingette | Inria, France |
| Rachid Deriche | Inria, France |
| James S Duncan | Yale University, USA |
| Philip Edwards | Imperial College London, UK |
| Randy Ellis | Queen's University, Canada |
| Gabor Fichtinger | Queen's University, Canada |
| P. Thomas Fletcher | University of Utah, USA |
| Alejandro Frangi | University of Sheffield, UK |
| James Gee | University of Pennsylvania, USA |
| Guido Gerig | University of Utah, USA |
| Ben Glocker | Microsoft Research, UK |
| Leo Grady | HeartFlow, USA |
| Hayit Greenspan | Tel Aviv University, Israel |
| Alexander Hammers | Neurodis Foundation, France |
| Nobuhiko Hata | Harvard Medical School, USA |
| David Hawkes | University College London, UK |
| Tobias Heimann | Siemens, Germany |
| Joachim Hornegger | University of Erlangen-Nuremberg, Germany |
| Ameet Jain | Philips, USA |
| Pierre Jannin | Inserm, France |
| Tianzi Jiang | Chinese Academy of Sciences, China |
| Marie-Pierre Jolly | Siemens, USA |
| Leo Joskowicz | Hebrew University of Jerusalem, Israel |
| Ioannis Kakadiaris | University of Houston, USA |
| Nico Karssemeijer | Radboud University, The Netherlands |
| Ron Kikinis | Harvard Medical School, USA |
| Rasmus Larsen | Technical University of Denmark, Denmark |
| Shuo Li | GE Healthcare, Canada |

| | |
|---|---|
| Hongen Liao | Tsinghua University, China |
| Marius George Linguraru | Children's National Medical Center, USA |
| Tianming Liu | University of Georgia, USA |
| Cristian Lorenz | Philips, Germany |
| Anant Madabhushi | Case Western Reserve University, USA |
| Frederik Maes | KU Leuven, Belgium |
| Jean-Francois Mangin | CEA, France |
| Anne Martel | University of Toronto, Canada |
| Ken Masamune | University of Tokyo, Japan |
| Yoshitaka Masutani | University of Tokyo, Japan |
| Dimitris Metaxas | Rutgers University, USA |
| Mehdi Moradi | University of British Columbia, Canada |
| Mads Nielsen | University of Copenhagen, Denmark |
| Poul Nielsen | University of Auckland, New Zealand |
| Wiro Niessen | Erasmus MC & TU Delft, The Netherlands |
| Alison Noble | Oxford University, UK |
| Sebastien Ourselin | University College London, UK |
| Nicolas Padoy | University of Strasbourg, France |
| Nikos Paragios | Centale & Ponts-Paris Tech, France |
| Xavier Pennec | Inria, France |
| Terry M Peters | Roberts Research Institute, Canada |
| Josien Pluim | UMC Utrecht, The Netherlands |
| Kilian Pohl | University of Pennsylvania, USA |
| Torsten Rohlfing | SRI International, USA |
| François Rousseau | CNRS, France |
| Daniel Rueckert | Imperial College London, UK |
| Mert Rory Sabuncu | Harvard Medical School, USA |
| Tim Salcudean | University of British Columbia, Canada |
| Julia A. Schnabel | Oxford University, UK |
| Dinggang Shen | University of North Carolina, USA |
| Akinobu Shimizu | Tokyo University of A & T, Japan |
| Kaleem Siddiqi | McGill University, Canada |
| Lawrence Staib | Yale University, USA |
| Danail Stoyanov | University College London, UK |
| Colin Studholme | Washington, USA |
| Martin Styner | University of North Carolina, USA |
| Chris Taylor | University of Manchester, UK |
| Russell Taylor | Johns Hopkins University, USA |
| Bertrand Thirion | Inria, France |
| Paul Thompson | UCLA, USA |
| Jocelyne Troccaz | CNRS, France |
| Regis Vaillant | GE Healthcare, France |
| Bram van Ginneken | Radboud University, The Netherlands |
| Koen Van Leemput | Harvard Medical School, USA |
| Baba Vemuri | University of Florida, USA |
| Ragini Verma | University of Pennsylvania, USA |

| | |
|---|---|
| Rene Vidal | Johns Hopkins University, USA |
| Christian Wachinger | MIT, USA |
| Simon Warfield | Harvard Medical School, USA |
| Jürgen Weese | Philips, Germany |
| Wolfgang Wein | TU Munich, Germany |
| William Wells | Harvard Medical School, USA |
| Carl-Fredrik Westin | Harvard Medical School, USA |
| Guang Zhong Yang | Imperial College London, UK |
| Ziv Yaniv | Children's National Medical Center, USA |
| Alistair Young | University of Auckland, New Zealand |
| Guoyan Zheng | University of Bern, Switzerland |
| Darko Zikic | Microsoft Research, UK |

## MICCAI 2013 Organizing Committee

Kensaku Mori
Ichiro Sakuma
Yoshinobu Sato
Yen-Wei Chen
Kiyoyuki Chinzei
Takeyoshi Dohi
Masakatsu G. Fujie
Hiroshi Fujita
Hidemi Goto
Hideaki Haneishi
Yoshinori Hasegawa
Makoto Hashizume
Hidekata Hontani
Koji Ikuta
Atsushi Imiya
Hiroshi Iseki
Shoji Kido
Masaki Kitajima
Takayuki Kitasaka
Hidefumi Kobatake
Etsuko Kobayashi

Yasuhiro Kodera
Hongen Liao
Ken Masamune
Yoshitaka Masutani
Yoshito Mekada
Mamoru Mitsuishi
Ken'ichi Morooka
Yoshihiro Muragaki
Shinji Naganawa
Masato Nagino
Toshiya Nakaguchi
Yoshikazu Nakajima
Ryoichi Nakamura
Shigeru Nawano
Noboru Niki
Atsushi Nishikawa
Makoto Nokata
Akinobu Shimizu
Toru Tamaki
Morimasa Tomikawa
Toshihiko Wakabayashi

## MICCAI 2013 Executive Committee

Kensaku Mori
Ichiro Sakuma
Yoshinobu Sato
Takehiro Ando
Jumpei Arata

Yuichiro Hayashi
Shingo Iwano
Yasukazu Kajita
Takayuki Kitasaka
Etsuko Kobayashi

Hongen Liao
Ken Masamune
Yoshito Mekada
Shinji Mizuno
Ryoichi Nakamura
Yukitaka Nimura

Masahiro Oda
Toshiyuki Okada
Jun Okamoto
Shinya Onogi
Takashi Suzuki
Junchen Wang

## MICCAI 2013 Local Executive Committee

Kensaku Mori
Yuichiro Hayashi
Takayuki Kitasaka
Xiongbiao Luo
Yoshito Mekada
Shinji Mizuno
Yoshihiko Nakamura

Yukitaka Nimura
Masahiro Oda
Daniel Rueckert
Kengo Suzuki
Mizuru Suzuki
Emi Tanahashi

## MICCAI 2013 Reviewers

Abugharbieh, Rafeef
Achterberg, Hakim
Acosta-Tamayo, Oscar
Adluru, Nagesh
Afacan, Onur
Afsari, Bijan
Aganj, Iman
Ahmadi, Seyed-Ahmad
Aja-Fernández, Santiago
Akhondi-Asl, Alireza
Alam, Kaisar
Alander, Jarmo
Alexander, Andrew
Ali, Sahirzeeshan
Alic, Lejla
Aljabar, Paul
Allan, Maximilian
An, Jungha
Andres, Bjoern
Angelini, Elsa
Angelopoulou, Elli
Antony, Bhavna
Anwander, Alfred
Arbel, Tal

Arimura, Hidetaka
Ashburner, John
Assemlal, Haz-Edine
Atasoy, Selen
Atkins, Stella
Aubert-Broche, Berengere
Audette, Michel
Auzias, Guillaume
Avants, Brian
Awate, Suyash
Axel, Leon
Ayad, Maria
Bach Cuadra, Meritxell
Baka, Nora
Baldock, Richard
Baloch, Sajjad
Barbu, Adrian
Barmpoutis, Angelos
Barratt, Dean
Bartoli, Adrien
Basavanhally, Ajay
Batmanghelich, Nematollah
Batmanghelich, Kayhan
Bauer, Stefan

Baumann, Michael
Becker, Tim
Beichel, Reinhard
Bekkers, Erik
Ben Ayed, Ismail
Bergeles, Christos
Berger, Marie-Odile
Bergmeir, Christoph
Bernal, Jorge Luis
Bernardis, Elena
Betrouni, Nacim
Bhatia, Kanwal
Bhotika, Rahul
Biesdorf, Andreas
Bilgic, Berkin
Bismuth, Vincent
Blaschko, Matthew
Bloy, Luke
Blum, Tobias
Boctor, Emad
Bodenstedt, Sebastian
Bogunovic, Hrvoje
Boisvert, Jonathan
Boroczky, Lilla
Bosch, Johan
Bouarfa, Loubna
Bouix, Sylvain
Bourgeat, Pierrick
Brady, Michael
Bria, Alessandro
Brost, Alexander
Buelow, Thomas
Butakoff, Constantine
Caan, Matthan
Cahill, Nathan
Cai, Weidong
Camara, Oscar
Cao, Kunlin
Cardenes, Ruben
Cardoso, Manuel Jorge
Carmichael, Owen
Caruyer, Emmanuel
Castañeda, Victor
Castro-Gonzalez, Carlos
Cater, John

Cattin, Philippe C.
Cebral, Juan
Celebi, M. Emre
Cetingul, Hasan Ertan
Chakravarty, M. Mallar
Chan, Raymond
Chefd'hotel, Christophe
Chen, Ting
Chen, Chao
Chen, George
Chen, Xinjian
Chen, Elvis C. S.
Chen, Thomas Kuiran
Chen, Terrence
Cheng, Jian
Cheriet, Farida
Chinzei, Kiyoyuki
Chitphakdithai, Nicha
Chou, Yiyu
Chowdhury, Ananda
Christensen, Gary
Chung, Moo
Cifor, Amalia
Cimen, Serkan
Cinquin, Philippe
Ciuciu, Philippe
Clarkson, Matthew
Clarysse, Patrick
Clouchoux, Cédric
Cobzas, Dana
Colliot, Olivier
Commowick, Olivier
Cook, Philip
Corso, Jason
Costa, Maria
Coulon, Olivier
Counsell, Serena J.
Coupe, Pierrick
Cowan, Brett
Crimi, Alessandro
Crum, William
Cui, Xinyi
Cuingnet, Remi
Daducci, Alessandro
Daga, Pankaj

Dahl, Anders L.
Darkner, Sune
Dauguet, Julien
David, Liu
De Craene, Mathieu
De Raedt, Sepp
Dehghan, Ehsan
Deligianni, Fani
Delong, Andrew
Demiralp, Cagatay
Demirci, Stefanie
Deng, Xiang
Dequidt, Jeremie
Descoteaux, Maxime
Desvignes, Michel
Dibella, Edward
Diciotti, Stefano
Dijkstra, Jouke
Dimaio, Simon
Ding, Kai
Donner, René
Douiri, Abdel
Dowling, Jason
Doyle, Scott
Drechsler, Klaus
Du, Yuhui
Duan, Qi
Duchateau, Nicolas
Duchesnay, Edouard
Duchesne, Simon
Dufour, Pascal
Duriez, Christian
Durrleman, Stanley
Dzyubachyk, Oleh
Ecabert, Olivier
Egger, Jan
Ehrhardt, Jan
El-Baz, Ayman
Elen, An
Elliott, Colm
Elson, Daniel
Ennis, Daniel
Enquobahrie, Andinet
Erdt, Marius
Eskildsen, Simon

Eslami, Abouzar
Essert, Caroline
Fahmi, Rachid
Fallavollita, Pascal
Fan, Yong
Farag, Aly
Fedorov, Andriy
Fei, Baowei
Fenster, Aaron
Figl, Michael
Figueroa, C. Alberto
Fishbaugh, James
Fitzpatrick, J Michael
Florack, Luc
Fogtmann, Mads
Fonov, Vladimir
Forestier, Germain
Foroughi, Pezhman
Fouard, Celine
Freiman, Moti
Freysinger, Wolfgang
Friman, Ola
Fripp, Jurgen
Frouin, Vincent
Fua, Pascal
Funka-Lea, Gareth
Fuster, Andrea
Gangeh, Mehrdad
Ganz, Melanie
Gao, Mingchen
Gao, Wei
Gao, Yaozong
Garcia-Lorenzo, Daniel
Garyfallidis, Eleftherios
Gaser, Christian
Georgescu, Bogdan
Ghanbari, Yasser
Gholipour, Ali
Ghosh, Aurobrata
Giannarou, Stamatia
Gibson, Eli
Giger, Maryellen
Gilles, Benjamin
Gilson, Wesley
Ginsburg, Shoshana

Gobbi, David
Goh, Alvina
Goksel, Orcun
Gonzalez Ballester, Miguel Angel
Gooya, Ali
Gorospe, Giann
Graham, Jim
Gramfort, Alexandre
Gray, Katherine
Grbic, Sasa
Guerrero, Julian
Guetter, Christoph
Gulsun, Mehmet Akif
Gupta, Aditya
Gur, Yaniv
Gutman, Boris
Guye, Maxime
Hacihaliloglu, Ilker
Haeck, Tom
Haeffele, Ben
Hager, Gregory D
Hahn, Horst
Hajnal, Joseph
Haldar, Justin
Hamamci, Andac
Hamarneh, Ghassan
Hamm, Jihun
Hanaoka, Shouhei
Haneishi, Hideaki
Hanson, Dennis
Hao, Xiang
Harders, Matthias
Hatt, Chuck
Haynor, David
He, Huiguang
Heckemann, Rolf
Heese, Harald
Heinrich, Mattias Paul
Heldmann, Stefan
Hernandez, Monica
Hinkle, Jacob
Hipwell, John
Hirano, Yasushi
Holmes, David
Hong, Jaesung

Hong, Byung-Woo
Honnorat, Nicolas
Hontani, Hidekata
Howe, Robert
Hu, Mingxing
Hu, Zhihong
Hu, Yipeng
Huang, Heng
Huang, Xiaolei
Huang, Junzhou
Huisman, Henkjan
Hyde, Damon
Iglesias, Juan Eugenio
Ingalhalikar, Madhura
Ionasec, Razvan
Isgum, Ivana
Jagadeesan, Jayender
Jain, Aastha
Jain, Saurabh
Janoos, Firdaus
Janowczyk, Andrew
Jbabdi, Saad
Jian, Bing
Jiang, Yifeng
Johnson, Hans
Jomier, Julien
Jordan, Petr
Joshi, Anand
Joshi, Sarang
Joung, Sanghyun
Kabus, Sven
Kachelrieß, Marc
Kaden, Enrico
Kadoury, Samuel
Kahl, Fredrik
Kainmueller, Dagmar
Kang, Xin
Kapoor, Ankur
Kapur, Tina
Karamalis, Athanasios
Karimaghaloo, Zahra
Kataoka, Hiroyuki
Katouzian, Amin
Kazanzides, Peter
Keeve, Erwin

Kerckhoffs, Roy
Kerrien, Erwan
Khalvati, Farzad
Khan, Ali R.
Khurd, Parmeshwar
Kim, Minjeong
Kim, Boklye
Kim, Kio
Kindlmann, Gordon
Kirchberg, Klaus
Kirisli, Hortense
Kitasaka, Takayuki
Klein, Martina
Klein, Tassilo
Klein, Stefan
Klinder, Tobias
Koay, Cheng
Kobayashi, Yo
Kohlberger, Timo
Komodakis, Nikos
Konukoglu, Ender
Krieger, Axel
Krissian, Karl
Kruggel, Frithjof
Kumar, Rajesh
Kumar, Ankur
Kumar, Ritwik
Kunz, Manuela
Kurkure, Uday
Kwok, Ka-Wai
Kwon, Dongjin
Ladikos, Alexander
Lalys, Florent
Landman, Bennett
Langs, Georg
Lapeer, Rudy
Laporte, Catherine
Lartizien, Carole
Lasser, Tobias
Lasso, Andras
Lauze, Francois
Law, Max W.K.
Lecoeur, Jeremy
Ledesma-Carbayo, Maria-J
Ledig, Christian

Lee, George
Lee, Tim
Lee, Su-Lin
Lee, Junghoon
Lefèvre, Julien
Lekadir, Karim
Lelieveldt, Boudewijn
Lenglet, Christophe
Lensu, Lasse
Lepore, Natasha
Leung, Kelvin
Li, Chunming
Li, Ying
Li, Hongsheng
Li, Ming
Li, Yang
Li, Kaiming
Li, Fuhai
Li, Bo
Li, Gang
Liao, Shu
Liao, Rui
Liao, Jun
Lin, Ming
Linte, Cristian
Litjens, Geert
Liu, Huafeng
Liu, Sidong
Liu, Xiaoxiao
Liu, Jianfei
Liu, Xiaofeng
Liu, Manhua
Liu, Meizhu
Lo, Pechin
Loew, Murray
Lombaert, Herve
Loog, Marco
Lorenzi, Marco
Lu, Le
Lu, Xiaoguang
Lu, Chao
Luboz, Vincent
Lucas, Blake
Lueth, Tim
Lui, Lok Ming

Luo, Xiongbiao
Lézoray, Olivier
Ma, Burton
Machiraju, Raghu
Mackay, Alex
Maddah, Mahnaz
Maduskar, Pragnya
Magee, Derek
Mahdavi, Seyedeh Sara
Maier-Hein (né Fritzsche), Klaus H.
Maier-Hein, Lena
Major, David
Majumdar, Angshul
Makram-Ebeid, Sherif
Malandain, Gregoire
Manduca, Armando
Manjon, Jose V.
Manniesing, Rashindra
Mansi, Tommaso
Marchal, Maud
Mariottini, Gian Luca
Marrakchi-Kacem, Linda
Marsland, Stephen
Martin-Fernandez, Marcos
Martinez-Perez, Elena
Martí, Robert
Mateus, Diana
Matsumiya, Kiyoshi
Mattes, Julian
Maurel, Pierre
Mcclelland, Jamie
Mccormick, Matthew
Medrano-Gracia, Pau
Mehrabian, Hatef
Meier, Dominik
Meinzer, Hans-Peter
Melbourne, Andrew
Menze, Bjoern
Merlet, Sylvain
Mertzanidou, Thomy
Metz, Coert
Meyer, Chuck
Meyer, Francois
Michailovich, Oleg
Michel, Fabrice

Miga, Michael
Miller, James
Miller, Karol
Mirota, Daniel
Modat, Marc
Modersitzki, Jan
Mohamed, Ashraf
Momayyez, Parya
Montiel, J.M. Martiínez
Montillo, Albert
Morooka, Ken'ichi
Mory, Benoit
Mountney, Peter
Mousavi, Zahra
Mousavi, Parvin
Mozer, Pierre
Mueller, Susanne
Murgasova, Maria
Murphy, Keelin
Mylonas, George
Müller, Henning
Nageotte, Florent
Najman, Laurent
Napel, Sandy
Nappi, Janne
Narayana, Ponnada
Natarajan, Shyam
Negahdar, Mohammadreza
Neumuth, Thomas
Ng, Bernard
Niaf, Emilie
Nichols, Thomas
Nickisch, Hannes
Nicolau, Stephane
Nie, Jingxin
Niederer, Steven
Niethammer, Marc
Nikou, Christophoros
Nir, Guy
Noble, Jack
Noblet, Vincent
Nolte, Lutz
Nordsletten, David
Novak, Carol
O'Donnell, Thomas

O'Donnell, Lauren
Oda, Masahiro
Oguz, Ipek
Okada, Toshiyuki
Okada, Kazunori
Okur, Aslı
Olabarriaga, Silvia
Oliver, Arnau
Onogi, Shinya
Oost, Elco
Oshinski, John
Otake, Yoshito
Ou, Yangming
Ozarslan, Evren
Padfield, Dirk
Palaniappan, Kannappan
Pallavaram, Srivatsan
Panagiotaki, Eleftheria
Paniagua, Beatriz
Papademetris, Xenios
Papadopoulo, Theo
Parisot, Sarah
Park, Jinhyeong
Park, Mi-Ae
Passat, Nicolas
Patriciu, Alexandru
Paul, Perrine
Paulsen, Rasmus
Pauly, Olivier
Payne, Christopher
Pearlman, Paul
Pedemonte, Stefano
Penney, Graeme
Pernus, Franjo
Peter, Loic
Peterlik, Igor
Peters, Jochen
Petersen, Jens
Petitjean, Caroline
Peyrat, Jean-Marc
Pham, Dzung
Pike, Bruce
Pitiot, Alain
Piuze, Emmanuel
Pizer, Stephen

Platel, Bram
Poignet, Philippe
Poline, Jean-Baptiste
Polzehl, Joerg
Poot, Dirk
Pop, Mihaela
Poynton, Clare
Pozo, Jose Maria
Prasad, Gautam
Prastawa, Marcel
Pratt, Philip
Prevost, Raphael
Prevrhal, Sven
Prince, Jerry
Punithakumar, Kumaradevan
Qazi, Arish A.
Qian, Zhen
Qiu, Anqi
Quellec, Gwenole
Qureshi, Hammad
Radeva, Petia
Radulescu, Emil
Rahmatullah, Bahbibi
Rajagopalan, Vidya
Rajpoot, Nasir
Ramezani, Mahdi
Rangarajan, Anand
Raniga, Parnesh
Rao, Anil
Rasoulian, Abtin
Rathi, Yogesh
Ray, Nilanjan
Redouté, Jérôme
Reichl, Tobias
Reinertsen, Ingerid
Reisert, Marco
Reiter, Austin
Rettmann, Maryam
Reuter, Martin
Reyes-Aldasoro, Constantino
Reyes, Mauricio
Rhode, Kawal
Ribbens, Annemie
Richa, Rogério
Riddell, Cyrill

Riklin Raviv, Tammy
Risser, Laurent
Rit, Simon
Rittscher, Jens
Rivaz, Hassan
Riviere, Denis
Riviere, Cameron
Robinson, Emma
Roche, Alexis
Roehl, Sebastian
Rohling, Robert
Rohr, Karl
Ropinski, Timo
Roth, Holger
Rothgang, Eva
Roux, Ludovic
Roysam, Badrinath
Rueda, Sylvia
Russakoff, Daniel
Rusu, Mirabela
Saalbach, Axel
Sadeghi-Naini, Ali
Salvado, Olivier
San Jose Estepar, Raul
Sanchez, Clarisa
Sarrut, David
Savadjiev, Peter
Schaap, Michiel
Scherrer, Benoit
Schneider, Caitlin
Schultz, Thomas
Schweikard, Achim
Seiler, Christof
Sermesant, Maxime
Seshamani, Sharmishtaa
Shah, Shishir
Shamir, Reuben R
Shekhovtsov, Alexander
Shen, Tian
Shen, Li
Shi, Yundi
Shi, Feng
Shi, Kuangyu
Shi, Wenzhe
Shi, Yonggang

Shi, Pengcheng
Shi, Yonghong
Simpson, Amber
Simpson, Ivor
Singanamalli, Asha
Singh, Nikhil
Singh, Vikas
Sinkus, Ralph
Slabaugh, Greg
Smal, Ihor
Smeets, Dirk
Sofka, Michal
Soler, Luc
Sommer, Stefan
Song, Xubo
Song, Gang
Sotiras, Aristeidis
Sparks, Rachel
Sporring, Jon
Staring, Marius
Staroswiecki, Ernesto
Stauder, Ralf
Stehle, Thomas
Stewart, James
Stolka, Philipp
Styles, Iain
Subramanian, Navneeth
Suetens, Paul
Suinesiaputra, Avan
Suk, Heung-Il
Summers, Ronald
Sundar, Hari
Suzuki, Kenji
Swanson, Kristin
Syeda-Mahmood, Tanveer
Sznitman, Raphael
Sørensen, Lauge
Tahmasebi, Amir
Taimouri, Vahid
Talbot, Hugues
Tan, Tao
Tanner, Christine
Tao, Xiaodong
Taquet, Maxime
Taron, Maxime

Tasdizen, Tolga
Taylor, Zeike
Thielemans, Kris
Thienphrapa, Paul
Thiriet, Marc
Thompson, Chris
Tiwari, Pallavi
Toews, Matthew
Tohka, Jussi
Tokuda, Junichi
Tomas Fernandez, Xavier
Tosun, Duygu
Toth, Robert
Totz, Johannes
Toussaint, Nicolas
Tristán-Vega, Antonio
Tsoumpas, Charalampos
Tu, Zhuowen
Tunc, Birkan
Turkheimer, Federico
Tustison, Nicholas
Twining, Carole
Türetken, Engin
Ukwatta, Eranga
Ullrich, Sebastian
Unal, Gozde
Unay, Devrim
Ungi, Tamas
Uzunbas, Mustafa
Van Assen, Hans
Van Der Laak, Jeroen
Van Rikxoort, Eva
Van Stralen, Marijn
Van Vliet, Lucas J.
Van Walsum, Theo
Vannier, Michael
Varoquaux, Gael
Veenland, Jifke
Venkataraman, Archana
Vercauteren, Tom
Veta, Mtiko
Vialard, Francois-Xavier
Vidal, Camille
Vignon, Francois
Villard, Pierre-Frederic

Visentini-Scarzanella, Marco
Visvikis, Dimitris
Viswanath, Satish
Vitanovski, Dime
Vogel, Jakob
Vogelstein, Joshua
Voigt, Ingmar
Von Berg, Jens
Voros, Sandrine
Vos, Frans
Vos, Pieter
Vosburgh, Kirby
Vrooman, Henri
Vrtovec, Tomaz
Waechter-Stehle, Irina
Waelkens, Paulo
Wahle, Andreas
Wan, Tao
Wang, Haibo
Wang, Zhijie
Wang, Li
Wang, Qian
Wang, Song
Wang, Lichao
Wang, Liansheng
Wang, Yalin
Wang, Chaohui
Wang, Lejing
Wang, Peng
Wang, Zhimin
Wang, Hongzhi
Ward, Aaron
Wassermann, Demian
Weber, Frank Michael
Wee, Chong-Yaw
Wei, Liu
Weller, Daniel
Wels, Michael
Werner, Rene
Wesarg, Stefan
Whitaker, Ross
Whittingstall, Kevin
Wiemker, Rafael
Wiles, Andrew
Witz, Jean-François

Wolf, Ivo
Wolz, Robin
Wright, Graham
Wu, Xiaodong
Wu, Guorong
Wuensche, Burkhard
Wörz, Stefan
Xie, Yuchen
Xie, Hua
Xie, Jun
Xiong, Guanglei
Xu, Lei
Xu, Sheng
Xu, Rui
Xu, Jun
Xue, Zhong
Yamashita, Hiromasa
Yan, Pingkun
Yang, Lin
Yankam Njiwa, Josiane A.
Yao, Jianhua
Yap, Pew-Thian
Yaqub, Mohammad
Ye, Dong Hye
Yendiki, Anastasia
Yeniaras, Erol
Yeo, B.T. Thomas
Yigitsoy, Mehmet
Yin, Zhaozheng
Yoo, Terry
Yoshida, Hiro
Young, Jonathan
Yushkevich, Paul
Zagorchev, Lyubomir

Zaidi, Habib
Zappella, Luca
Zawadzki, Robert
Zeng, Wei
Zerubia, Josiane
Zhan, Liang
Zhan, Yiqiang
Zhang, Jingya
Zhang, Shaoting
Zhang, Li
Zhang, Daoqiang
Zhang, Weidong
Zhang, Pei
Zhang, Hui
Zhao, Tao
Zhao, Qian
Zheng, Yefeng
Zheng, Yuanjie
Zhong, Hua
Zhou, X. Sean
Zhou, S. Kevin
Zhou, Yan
Zhou, Kevin
Zhou, Luping
Zhou, Jinghao
Zhu, Hongtu
Zhu, Ning
Zhu, Dajiang
Zhuang, Xiahai
Zollei, Lilla
Zosso, Dominique
Zuluaga, Maria A.
Zwiggelaar, Reyer

# Awards Presented at MICCAI 2012, Nice, France

*MICCAI Society Enduring Impact Award*: The Enduring Impact Award is the highest award of the MICCAI Society. It is a career award for continued excellence in the MICCAI research field. The 2012 Enduring Impact Award was presented to *Jerry Prince*, Johns Hopkins University, USA.

*MICCAI Society Fellowships*: MICCAI Fellowships are bestowed annually on a small number of senior members of the society in recognition of substantial scientific contributions to the MICCAI research field and service to the MICCAI community. In 2012, fellowships were awarded to:

- *Alison Noble* (Oxford University, UK)
- *Wiro Niessen* (Erasumus Medical Centre, The Netherlands)
- *Nassir Navab* (Technical University of Munich, Germany)

*Medical Image Analysis Journal Award Sponsored by Elsevier*: *Benoit Scherrer*, for his paper entitled "Super-Resolution Reconstruction to Increase the Spatial Resolution of Diffusion Weighted Images from Orthogonal Anisotropic Acquisitions", authored by Benoit Scherrer, Ali Gholipour and Simon K. Warfield.

*Best Paper in Computer-Assisted Intervention Systems and Medical Robotics*: *Benjamin Bejar* for his paper entitled "Surgical Gesture Classification from Video Data", authored by Benjamin Bejar, Luca Zappella, Rene Vidal.

*Young Scientist Publication Impact Award Sponsored by Kitware Inc.*: MICCAI papers by a young scientist from the past 5 years were eligible for this award. It is made to a researcher whose work had an impact on the MICCAI field in terms of citations, secondary citations, subsequent publications, h-index. The 2012 Young Scientist Publication Impact Award was given to *Caroline Brun*: "A Tensor-Based Morphometry Study of Genetic Influences on Brain Structure using a New Fluid Registration Method" authored by C. Brun, N. Lepore, X. Pennec, Y.-Y. Chou, K. McMahon, G.I. de Zubicaray, M. Meredith, M.J. Wright, A.D. Lee, M. Barysheva, A.W. Toga, P.M. Thompson.

*MICCAI Young Scientist Awards*: The Young Scientist Awards are stimulation prizes awarded for the best first authors of MICCAI contributions in distinct subject areas. The nominees had to be full-time students at a recognized university at, or within, two years prior to submission. The 2012 MICCAI Young Scientist Awards were given to:

- *Hang Su* for his paper entitled: "Phase Contrast Image Restoration Via Dictionary Representation of Diffraction Patterns", authored by Hang Su, Zhaozheng Yin, Takeo Kanade, and Seungil Huh

– *Eli Gibson*, for his paper entitled: "Registration Accuracy: How Good is Good Enough? A Statistical Power Calculation Incorporating Image Registration Uncertainty", authored by Eli Gibson, Aaron Fenster and Aaron D. Ward
– *Stephanie Marchesseau* for her paper entitled: "Cardiac Mechanical Parameter Calibration Based on the Unscented Transform", authored by Stephanie Marchesseau, Herve Delingette, Maxime Sermesant, Kawal Rhode, Simon G. Duckett, C. Aldo Rinaldi, Reza Razavi, and Nicholas Ayache
– *Roland Kwitt* for his paper entitled: "Recognition in Ultrasound Videos: Where am I?", authored by Roland Kwitt, Nuno Vasconcelos, Sharif Razzaque, and Stephen Aylward
– *Robin Wolz*, for his paper entitled: "Multi-Organ Abdominal CT Segmentation Using Hierarchically Weighted Subject-Specific Atlases", authored by Robin Wolz, Chengwen Chu, Kazunari Misawa, Kensaku Mori, Daniel Rueckert

# Table of Contents – Part I

## Physiological Modeling and Computer-Assisted Intervention

## Brain Imaging

## Imaging, Reconstruction, and Enhancement I

## Registration I

# Machine Learning, Statistical Modeling, and Atlases I

# Computer-Aided Diagnosis and Imaging Biomarkers I

## Intraoperative Guidance and Robotics I

## Microscope, Optical Imaging, and Histology I

## Cardiology I

# Vasculatures and Tubular Structures I

# Brain Imaging and Basic Techniques

## Diffusion MRI I

## Brain Segmentation and Atlases I

# Table of Contents – Part II

## Motion Modeling and Compensation

## Segmentation I

# Machine Learning, Statistical Modeling, and Atlases II

# Computer-Aided Diagnosis and Imaging Biomarkers II

## Physiological Modeling, Simulation, and Planning I

## Microscope, Optical Imaging, and Histology II

## Cardiology II

# Vasculatures and Tubular Structures II

# Brain Segmentation and Atlases II

## Functional MRI and Neuroscience Applications I

# Table of Contents – Part III

## Image Reconstruction and Motion Modeling

## Machine Learning in Medical Image Computing

# Imaging, Reconstruction, and Enhancement II

## Registration II

## Segmentation II

## Physiological Modeling, Simulation, and Planning II

## Intraoperative Guidance and Robotics II

## Microscope, Optical Imaging, and Histology III

## Diffusion MRI II

# Brain Segmentation and Atlases III

# Functional MRI and Neuroscience Applications II

# Fast Data-Driven Calibration of a Cardiac Electrophysiology Model from Images and ECG

Oliver Zettinig[1,2], Tommaso Mansi[1], Bogdan Georgescu[1], Elham Kayvanpour[3],
Farbod Sedaghat-Hamedani[3], Ali Amr[3], Jan Haas[3], Henning Steen[3],
Benjamin Meder[3], Hugo Katus[3], Nassir Navab[2], Ali Kamen[1],
and Dorin Comaniciu[1]

[1] Siemens Corporation, Corporate Technology, Imaging and Computer Vision,
Princeton, NJ, USA
[2] Computer Aided Medical Procedures, Technische Universität München, Germany
[3] University Hospital Heidelberg, Department of Internal Medicine III - Cardiology,
Angiology and Pneumology, Heidelberg, Germany

**Abstract.** Recent advances in computational electrophysiology (EP) models make them attractive for clinical use. We propose a novel data-driven approach to calibrate an EP model from standard 12-lead electrocardiograms (ECG), which are in contrast to invasive or dense body surface measurements widely available in clinical routine. With focus on cardiac depolarization, we first propose an efficient forward model of ECG by coupling a mono-domain, Lattice-Boltzmann model of cardiac EP to a boundary element formulation of body surface potentials. We then estimate a polynomial regression to predict myocardium, left ventricle and right ventricle endocardium electrical diffusion from QRS duration and ECG electrical axis. Training was performed on 4,200 ECG simulations, calculated in $\approx 3\,s$ each, using different diffusion parameters on 13 patient geometries. This allowed quantifying diffusion uncertainty for given ECG parameters due to the ill-posed nature of the ECG problem. We show that our method is able to predict myocardium diffusion within the uncertainty range, yielding a prediction error of less than $5\,ms$ for QRS duration and $2°$ for electrical axis. Prediction results compared favorably with those obtained with a standard optimization procedure, while being 60 times faster. Our data-driven model can thus constitute an efficient preliminary step prior to more refined EP personalization.

## 1 Introduction

With the improvement in patient care after myocardium infarction or cardiomyopathies, the prevalence of cardiac rhythm disorders has increased significantly [1]. Electrocardiography (ECG) is the preferred tool to assess arrhythmias, conduction abnormalities and the effects of treatments on the electrical activity of the heart. However, with the development of non-invasive treatments, more detailed and predictive electrophysiology (EP) assessment is necessary [1].

The last decade has seen tremendous progress in computational modeling of cardiac EP [2]. Recent numerical methods are enabling near real-time EP computation [3,4]. To be applied in clinical practice, these models need to be

K. Mori et al. (Eds.): MICCAI 2013, Part I, LNCS 8149, pp. 1–8, 2013.

adjusted to capture patient physiology. Current approaches use inverse problem methods to estimate electrical diffusivity or action potential duration from invasive endocardial mapping [5] or body surface mapping (BSM) [6,7]. However, these methods are computationally demanding as they require hundreds of forward model runs. Another limitation is the lack of availability of these diagnostic modalities: invasive measurements are often avoided, whereas BSM is still not widely available. Methods based on standard ECG would therefore constitute good alternatives when comprehensive EP information is not available.

At the same time, efficient machine learning algorithms have been developed for medical applications. First applied for anatomy detection and segmentation [8], applications for model personalization are now being investigated. In [9], the authors derived a surrogate EP model based on polynomial chaos theory to personalize an Eikonal model and quantify parameter uncertainty. Statistical learning has also been employed to back-project BSM potentials onto the epicardium [10]. Provided the parameter space is sufficiently sampled, statistical learning can constitute an efficient approach for model personalization.

In this context, we propose a novel method to calibrate a cardiac EP model based on commonly available 12-lead ECG measurements. As a first step, we focus on cardiac depolarization and aim at estimating ventricular electrical diffusion only, the other EP parameters being fixed to their nominal values. To be able to scan the parameter space, we introduce a novel ECG model based on a mono-domain, Lattice-Boltzmann EP model. Then, we use a data-driven approach to estimate a polynomial regression whose predictors are standard ECG parameters (QRS duration, electrical axis) and responses are myocardium diffusivity parameters (Sec. 2). Thanks to the computational efficiency of our framework, we show in Sec. 3 that our approach is able to reach the intrinsic uncertainty of the problem, which could be quantitatively estimated from 4,200 forward simulations. The proposed method also compared favorably with NEWUOA [5], a standard inverse problem algorithm, and yielded promising results on three patient data. As discussed in Sec. 4, our data-driven approach may constitute a preliminary calibration step for patient-specific EP modeling.

## 2      Method

### 2.1      Fast Forward Model of Cardiac ECG

**Patient-Specific Model of Cardiac Anatomy.** The first step of our approach consists in segmenting the heart geometry from clinical images (Fig. 1). A robust, data-guided machine learning algorithm is employed to automatically segment cardiac chambers and epicardium from cine MRI images [8]. Next, the biventricular myocardium domain at end-diastasis is mapped onto a Cartesian grid and represented as a level-set. Finally, fiber architecture is calculated by following a rule-based approach [3]: Below the basal plane, fiber elevation angles vary linearly from epi- ($-70°$) to endocardium ($+70°$), which are then extrapolated up to the valves based on geodesic distance (Fig. 2b). The heart is registered to a torso atlas using Procrustes analysis. The entire pipeline is fully automatic but under expert guidance to allow manual corrections.

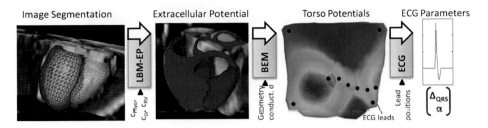

**Fig. 1.** Steps of proposed forward model of ECG. *See text for details.*

**Lattice-Boltzmann Model of Myocardium Transmembrane Potentials.**
As the proposed data-driven model relies on global ECG information, simplified mono-domain EP methods can be employed, since they have been shown to preserve the essential ECG features well [11,12]. In this work, the trans-membrane potential (TMP) $v(t) \in [-70\,mV, 30\,mV]$ is calculated according to the Mitchell-Schaeffer model (see [3,13] and references therein):

$$\frac{\partial v}{\partial t} = \frac{h(t)v^2(1-v)}{\tau_{in}} - \frac{v}{\tau_{out}} + c\nabla \cdot D\nabla v \qquad (1)$$

$h(t)$ is a gating variable that models the state of the ion channels ($dh/dt = (1-h)/\tau_{open}$ if $v < v_{gate}$, $dh/dt = -h/\tau_{close}$ otherwise). $c$ is the tissue diffusivity whose anisotropy is captured by the tensor $D$. The $\tau$'s and $v_{gate}$ are parameters that control the dynamics of the action potential. This complex PDE is solved using the LBM-EP method [3], an efficient Lattice-Boltzmann algorithm. Five domains are considered: left and right ventricular septum, used to pace the heart to mimic the His bundle; left and right endocardia with fast electrical diffusivity, $c_{LV}$ and $c_{RV}$, to mimic the Purkinje network; and the myocardium, with slower diffusivity $c_{Myo}$ (Fig. 2b).

**Boundary Element Model of Torso Potentials.** Torso potentials are calculated in three steps. First, extra-cellular potentials are estimated from the TMP by using the elliptic formulation proposed in [12], where the diffusion anisotropy ratio $c_i(\mathbf{x})/c_e(\mathbf{x}) = \lambda$ is assumed constant ($\mathbf{x}$ is the spatial position, $c_i$ and $c_e$ are the intra-cellular and extra-cellular diffusion coefficients respectively). With that hypothesis, the extra-cellular potential $\phi_e$ writes:

$$\phi_e(\mathbf{x}, t) = \frac{\lambda}{1+\lambda} \frac{1}{|\Omega|} \int_\Omega (v(\mathbf{y}, t) - v(\mathbf{x}, t))d\mathbf{y} \qquad (2)$$

$\Omega$ is the entire myocardium domain. Second, $\phi_e$ is mapped back to the epicardium surface mesh $S_H$ using tri-linear interpolation. Finally, the extra-cellular potentials are projected onto the torso surface $S_B$ using a boundary element method (BEM) [14]. The potential $\phi(\mathbf{x})$ at any point $\mathbf{x}$ of the thoracic domain writes, in virtue of Green's second identity,

$$\phi(\mathbf{x}) = \frac{1}{4\pi} \int_{S_B} \phi_B \frac{\mathbf{r} \cdot \mathbf{n}}{||\mathbf{r}||^3} dS_B - \frac{1}{4\pi} \int_{S_H} \left[ \phi_e \frac{\mathbf{r} \cdot \mathbf{n}}{||\mathbf{r}||^3} + \frac{\nabla\phi_e \cdot \mathbf{n}}{||\mathbf{r}||} \right] dS_H \qquad (3)$$

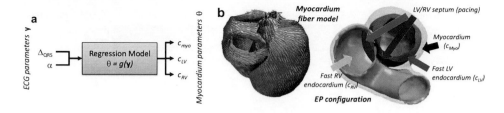

**Fig. 2. a)** Schematic diagram of the data-driven backward ECG model. **b)** Myocardium fiber model in one patient and EP configuration. *See text for details.*

where $\mathbf{r}$ is the vector defined by $\mathbf{x}$ and the integration point. By discretizing $S_B$ and $S_H$ into triangulations, the linear systems $P_{BB}\,\phi_B + P_{BH}\,\phi_e + G_{BH}\,\Gamma_H = 0$ and $P_{HB}\,\phi_B + P_{HH}\,\phi_e + G_{HH}\,\Gamma_H = 0$ can be constructed. The matrices P and G contain coefficients depending entirely on the geometry, and can therefore be precomputed, while the matrix $\Gamma_H$ collects the gradients $\nabla\phi_H$. Finally, $\phi$ on the body is given by $\phi_B = \left(P_{BB} - G_{BH}G_{HH}^{-1}P_{HB}\right)^{-1}\left(G_{BH}G_{HH}^{-1}P_{HH} - P_{BH}\right)\phi_e$.

**ECG Calculation.** We finally compute the standard Einthoven, Goldberger and Wilson leads, and derive the QRS duration $\Delta_{QRS}$ and mean electrical axis angle $\alpha$ automatically. The QRS complex is detected as in [15] by convolving the squared derivative of each limb lead $y_f(t) = [d/dt\,y(t)]^2$ with a sliding average kernel (window size $24\,ms$) for increased robustness. A threshold value of $0.8\,mV^2ms^{-2}$ has proven to be sufficient for detecting $\Delta_{QRS}$. The electrical axis is computed based on the leads I and II: $\alpha = \arctan((2h_{II} - h_I)/(\sqrt{3}h_I))$, where the $h_i$'s are the sum of R and S peak amplitudes in the respective leads.

## 2.2   Data-Driven Estimation of Myocardium EP Diffusion

The forward ECG model can be seen as a dynamic system $\mathbf{y} = f(\theta)$. In this work, the free parameters $\theta$ are the diffusivity values, $\theta = (c_{Myo}, c_{LV}, c_{RV})$, whereas the outputs $\mathbf{y}$ are the ECG parameters, $\mathbf{y} = (\Delta_{QRS}, \alpha)$, which are often available from ECG traces (Fig. 2). Calibrating the EP model thus consists in evaluating a function $g(\mathbf{y})$ that approximates the inverse problem $\theta = g(\mathbf{y}) \approx f^{-1}(\mathbf{y})$.

$\Delta_{QRS}$ and $\alpha$ can vary significantly within the population, even in normal subjects, due to heart morphology, position, and other factors not directly related to myocardium diffusivity. To cope with these variabilities, we normalize $\Delta_{QRS}$ and $\alpha$ by scouting the space of possible values by means of three forward simulations: one with normal diffusivity parameters ($F_1$: $c_{LV} = c_{RV} = 16,000\,mm^2/s$, $c_{Myo} = 6,000\,mm^2/s$), one with low LV diffusivity (LBBB-like scenario, $F_2$: $c_{LV} = 1,200\,mm^2/s$, $c_{RV} = 16,000\,mm^2/s$, $c_{Myo} = 1,000\,mm^2/s$) and one with low RV diffusivity (RBBB-like scenario, $F_3$, the other way round). The normalized parameters are then defined by $\overline{\Delta_{QRS}} = \Delta_{QRS}/\Delta_{QRS_{F_1}}$ and $\overline{\alpha} = (\alpha - \alpha_{F_2})/(\alpha_{F_3} - \alpha_{F_2})$. By doing so, the ECG parameters are relative to a nominal, patient-specific simulation, which intrinsically considers patient geometry features. Finally, we learn the model $\theta = g(\overline{\Delta_{QRS}}, \overline{\alpha})$ by using multivariate polynomial regression method of degree seven [16], which offered a good

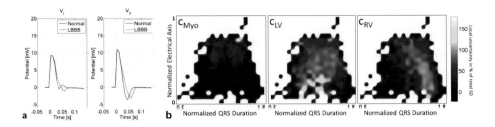

**Fig. 3. a)** QRS complex in simulated limb ECG leads $V_I$ and $V_{II}$ in normal and left bundle branch block physiology (LBBB). Our model was able to capture longer QRS due to delayed depolarization in LBBB. **b)** Estimated diffusion standard deviation (SD) in % of total SD for known electrical axis and QRS duration. The highest uncertainty is found in the healthy range of parameters (center of plots).

compromise between prediction accuracy and generalization (no significant differences in performance could be distinguished with orders varying from 4 to 9). In this work, one regression function is learned for each diffusivity parameter independently, $\mathbf{g} = (g_{Myo}, g_{LV}, g_{RV})$. We also investigated multivariate regression splines (MARS) and gradient boosting, which yielded very similar results. After having trained $\mathbf{g}$, the diffusivity parameters are estimated from the measured and normalized ECG features: $(c_{\hat{M}yo}, c_{\hat{L}V}, c_{\hat{R}V}) = \mathbf{g}(\overline{\Delta_{QRS}}, \overline{\alpha})$.

## 3   Experiments and Results

### 3.1   Forward ECG Model Evaluation and Uncertainty Analysis

**Experimental Protocol.** Thirteen dilated cardiomyopathy (DCM) patients were used, for which an anatomical model was automatically created based on cine MRI images. Then, a total of 4,200 EP simulations were generated on a $1.5\,mm$ isotropic Cartesian grid with diffusivity coefficients uniformly sampled between $1,000\,mm^2/s$ and $16,000\,mm^2/s$ under the constraints $c_{Myo} \le c_{LV}$ and $c_{Myo} \le c_{RV}$. Electrode positions were chosen to coincide with appropriate vertex positions. Implemented on GPU (NVIDIA GeForce GTX 580), the model could compute the ECG of one cardiac cycle in $\approx 3\,s$.

**Forward Model Evaluation.** Normal EP was modeled in one dataset with $c_{LV} = c_{RV} = 16,000\,mm^2/s$, $c_{Myo} = 1,000\,mm^2/s$ (Fig. 1, second panel). A left bundle branch block (LBBB) scenario was mimicked by setting $c_{LV} = 5,000\,mm^2/s$. As one can see from Fig. 3a, R and S wave trends were qualitatively realistic. In particular, the model was able to capture prolonged QRS due to the slow conduction in the LBBB case. As our model concentrates on the ventricular EP only, calculated ECG did not incorporate P waves. Missing Q waves could also be explained by the absence of His bundle excitation in our EP model, as the whole septum area is triggered (Sec. 2.1). Experiments with different fiber angles ($-50/50°$, $-70/70°$, $-90/90°$) showed that the QRS duration remains constant and the electrical axis stays in the diagnostically same range for pathological configurations $F_2$ and $F_3$ with a standard deviation of $15.8°$.

**Uncertainty Analysis.** Based on the 4,200 simulations, we analyzed the intrinsic uncertainty of the ECG inverse problem, i.e. the uncertainty in cardiac diffusion parameters given $\Delta_{QRS}$ and $\alpha$. For that study, normalized values (Sec. 2.2) were used to minimize the effects of geometry. Each $(\Delta_{QRS}, \alpha)$ pairs were grouped in $20 \times 20$ bins. For each bin, the standard deviation (SD) of $c_{Myo}, c_{LV}$ and $c_{RV}$ was calculated. Total SD over the entire dataset was $2,146\,mm^2/s$, $4,142\,mm^2/s$ and $4,123\,mm^2/s$ respectively. Fig. 3b reports the local SD per bin in % of the total SD. The local SD is on average 20%, 52% and 40% of the total SD for $c_{Myo}, c_{LV}$ and $c_{RV}$ respectively, with up to 150% of variation. Interestingly, similar variations were obtained patient-wise. These results clearly reflect the ill-posed nature of the ECG inverse problem under our forward model and constitute first estimates of the optimal bound in accuracy for any inverse problem to estimate myocardium diffusion that rely on $\Delta_{QRS}$ and $\alpha$ only. The uncertainty may decrease if more ECG parameters are considered.

## 3.2    Evaluation of the Data-Driven Calibration Model

**Evaluation on Synthetic Data.** Our model was evaluated using leave-one-patient-out cross-validation. On average, $c_{Myo}$ could be estimated within 23% of the total SD, while $c_{LV}$ and $c_{RV}$ were predicted within 56% and 55% respectively, i.e. up to the intrinsic uncertainty of the problem. Without normalization, errors were betwen 114% and 440% of the total SD. The proposed model-based normalization procedure was thus able to compensate for inter-patient geometry variability. To evaluate the accuracy of the regression model in the observable space of ECG parameters, $\Delta_{QRS}$ and $\alpha$ computed by the calibrated forward model were compared with the known ground truth. As illustrated in Fig. 4a-b, an average error of $4.9 \pm 5.5\,ms$ for $\Delta_{QRS}$ (mean $\pm$ SD) and $1.6 \pm 1.7°$ for $\alpha$ was obtained. These errors were in the range of clinical variability. Moreover, calibrated simulations were significantly (t-test p-value $< 0.001$) more precise than those obtained with nominal diffusivity values ($\Delta_{QRS}$ error: $19.8 \pm 14.3\,ms$, $\alpha$ error: $4.3 \pm 3.4°$). Additionally, while our prediction was on average centered around the ground truth QRS duration (average bias: $+0.5\,ms$), the $\Delta_{QRS}$ calculated with default parameters was $19.0\,ms$ too short. This result was expected since the default parameters correspond to healthy physiology whereas conduction abnormalities cause prolonged QRS durations. Using our calibration technique may thus be preferable to using nominal parameters when only ECG is available.

**Comparison with NEWUOA.** We compared the performance of the regression model with those obtained with NEWUOA [5], a gradient-free inverse problem method. The cost function was defined as $f(\Delta^i_{QRS}, \alpha^i) = (\Delta^{known}_{QRS} - \Delta^i_{QRS})^2 + \lambda(\alpha^{known} - \alpha^i)^2$ with $\lambda = 0.1$ to account for the different orders of magnitude between ECG parameters. Similarly to our regression model, tissue diffusivities $c_{Myo}, c_{LV}$ and $c_{RV}$ could be estimated within 23%, 64% and 54% of the total SD, respectively, which was also close to the limit of data uncertainty. Errors in $\Delta_{QRS}$ and $\alpha$ calculated using the NEWUOA-personalized forward model were on average $8.7 \pm 11.1\,ms$ (significantly biased compared to our approach) and $-0.2 \pm 7.6°$ respectively. From a computational point of view, NEWUOA took about $10\,min$

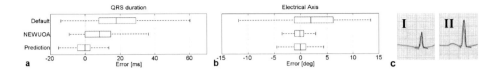

**Fig. 4. a, b)** QRS duration and electrical axis error distributions for ECG simulations with nominal (top), NEWUOA-predicted (center) and regression-predicted (bottom) diffusivity parameters. Our approach yielded more accurate predictions. **c)** Measured (*black*) and simulated (*blue*) $V_I$ and $V_{II}$ leads after model calibration for one patient.

to converge, while our approach required only $10\,s$ to calculate the three forward simulations for the normalization. Hence, our approach not only yielded more predictive calibrations but was also $60\times$ more efficient.

**Evaluation on Real Cases.** The method was finally evaluated on four DCM patients for which clinical ECG was available. Diffusivity parameters were estimated based on measured QRS duration and electrical axis angle using the trained regression model. For one patient, myocardium diffusivity could not be calibrated as the measured electrical axis ($\alpha = -63°$) was outside the range of the training set. However, for the three other patients, plausible diffusion coefficients could be estimated ($2426 - 7584\,mm^2/s$ for $c_{Myo}$, and $6691 - 12532\,mm^2/s$ for $c_{LV}$ and $c_{RV}$). We then calculated the ECG using the calibrated forward model, yielding a promising average error of $0.35 \pm 0.28\,ms$ for $\Delta_{QRS}$ and $15.6° \pm 9.6°$ for $\alpha$ respectively. Fig. 4c illustrates the calculated ECG overlaid on top of the real ECG for one patient, showing promising agreement.

## 4    Conclusion and Future Work

In this paper, we have shown that the calibration of patient-specific cardiac electrophysiology models is possible from standard 12-lead ECG measurements. By learning a data-driven regression model from simulated ECG signals, we were able to predict diffusivity parameters for various regions of the myocardium, up to the limit of the underlying uncertainty due to the intrinsic ill-posedness of the inverse ECG problem. We could also, for the first time to the best of our knowledge, quantify the uncertainty in estimated myocardium diffusion when only ECG data is employed, under the assumptions of our forward model. Experiments with synthetic ECG data and four patients showed promising results, with significant improvement with respect to nominal diffusivity values and better predictive power compared to NEWUOA calibration. Thus, our method can provide good preliminary personalization, prior to more refined estimation if invasive or BSM measurements are available. Future extensions of our framework include the analysis of the entire ECG trace, improved capture of geometrical features, refinement of the forward model to include more sophisticated activation patterns and other parameters of the EP model, and non-linear manifold learning to improve the performances on unseen data. In addition, an electromechanical model of the heart currently under development will help us in quantifying the error introduced by assuming a static myocardium.

# References

1. Marcus, G.M., Keung, E., Scheinman, M.M.: The year in review of cardiac electrophysiology. JACC 61(7), 772–782 (2013)
2. Clayton, R.H., Bernus, O., Cherry, E.M., Dierckx, H., Fenton, F.H., Mirabella, L., Panfilov, A.V., Sachse, F.B., Seemann, G., Zhang, H.: Models of cardiac tissue electrophysiology: Progress, challenges and open questions. PBMB 104(1), 22–48 (2011)
3. Rapaka, S., Mansi, T., Georgescu, B., Pop, M., Wright, G.A., Kamen, A., Comaniciu, D.: LBM-EP: Lattice-Boltzmann method for fast cardiac electrophysiology simulation from 3D images. In: Ayache, N., Delingette, H., Golland, P., Mori, K. (eds.) MICCAI 2012, Part II. LNCS, vol. 7511, pp. 33–40. Springer, Heidelberg (2012)
4. Talbot, H., Marchesseau, S., Duriez, C., Sermesant, M., Cotin, S., Delingette, H.: Towards an interactive electromechanical model of the heart. Int. Focus 3(2) (2013)
5. Relan, J., Chinchapatnam, P., Sermesant, M., Rhode, K., Ginks, M., Delingette, H., Rinaldi, C.A., Razavi, R., Ayache, N.: Coupled personalization of cardiac electrophysiology models for prediction of ischaemic ventricular tachycardia. Int. Focus 1(3), 396–407 (2011)
6. Dössel, O., Krueger, M., Weber, F., Schilling, C., Schulze, W., Seemann, G.: A framework for personalization of computational models of the human atria. In: IEEE Proc. EMBC 2011, pp. 4324–4328 (2011)
7. Wang, L., Wong, K.C., Zhang, H., Liu, H., Shi, P.: Noninvasive computational imaging of cardiac electrophysiology for 3-d infarct. IEEE TBE 58(4), 1033 (2011)
8. Zheng, Y., Barbu, A., Georgescu, B., Scheuering, M., Comaniciu, D.: Four-chamber heart modeling and automatic segmentation for 3-D cardiac CT volumes using marginal space learning and steerable features. IEEE TMI 27(11), 1668–1681 (2008)
9. Konukoglu, E., Relan, J., Cilingir, U., Menze, B.H., Chinchapatnam, P., Jadidi, A., Cochet, H., Hocini, M., Delingette, H., Jaïs, P., Haïssaguerre, M., Ayache, N., Sermesant, M.: Efficient probabilistic model personalization integrating uncertainty on data and parameters: Application to Eikonal-diffusion models in cardiac electrophysiology. PBMB 107(1), 134–146 (2011)
10. Jiang, M., Lv, J., Wang, C., Huang, W., Xia, L., Shou, G.: A hybrid model of maximum margin clustering method and support vector regression for solving the inverse ECG problem. Computing in Cardiology 2011, 457–460 (2011)
11. Boulakia, M., Cazeau, S., Fernández, M.A., Gerbeau, J.-F., Zemzemi, N.: Mathematical modeling of electrocardiograms: a numerical study. Ann. Biomed. Eng. 38(3), 1071–1097 (2010)
12. Chhay, M., Coudière, Y., Turpault, R.: How to compute the extracellular potential in electrocardiology from an extended monodomain model. RR-7916, INRIA (2012)
13. Mitchell, C., Schaeffer, D.: A two-current model for the dynamics of cardiac membrane. Bull. Math. Biol. 65(5), 767–793 (2003)
14. Shou, G., Xia, L., Jiang, M., Wei, Q., Liu, F., Crozier, S.: Solving the ECG forward problem by means of standard H- and H-hierarchical adaptive linear boundary element method. IEEE TBE 56(5), 1454–1464 (2009)
15. Kohler, B.U., Hennig, C., Orglmeister, R.: The principles of software QRS detection. IEEE Engineering in Medicine and Biology Magazine 21(1), 42–57 (2002)
16. Friedman, J., Hastie, T., Tibshirani, R.: The Elements of Statistical Learning: Data Mining, Inference, and Prediction. Springer (2009)

# Toward Online Modeling for Lesion Visualization and Monitoring in Cardiac Ablation Therapy

Cristian A. Linte, Jon J. Camp, David R. Holmes III,
Maryam E. Rettmann, and Richard A. Robb

Biomedical Imaging Resource, Mayo Clinic, Rochester, MN, USA
{linte.cristian,robb.richard}@mayo.edu

**Abstract.** Despite extensive efforts to enhance catheter navigation, limited research has been done to visualize and monitor the tissue lesions created during ablation in the attempt to provide feedback for effective therapy. We propose a technique to visualize the temperature distribution and extent of induced tissue injury via an image-based model that uses physiological tissue parameters and relies on heat transfer principles to characterize lesion progression in near real time. The model was evaluated both numerically and experimentally using *ex vivo* bovine muscle samples while emulating a clinically relevant ablation protocol. Results show agreement to within $5°C$ between the model-predicted and experimentally measured end-ablation tissue temperatures, as well as comparable predicted and observed lesion characteristics. The model yields temperature and lesion updates in near real-time, thus providing reasonably accurate and sufficiently fast monitoring for effective therapy.

## 1  Introduction

Catheter ablation entails the navigation of a percutaneously inserted catheter into the heart and delivery of radio-frequency (RF) energy to induce local tissue necrosis to electrically isolate regions that generate or propagate arrhythmia. Cardiac ablation procedures are conducted under image guidance, where medical imaging, typically X-ray fluoroscopy, is used to guide the catheter to the intracardiac targets [1]. Reported ventures into the treatment of cardiac arrhythmia have been somewhat discouraging, with a fairly high number of patients requiring revisions [2]. We have identified two significant factors that have hampered the success of catheter ablation therapy: inadequate visualization inside the beating heart for accurate targeting of the arrhythmic sites; and lack of effective feedback (i.e., lesion size and tissue injury) on the ablation process.

Visualization in traditional ablation procedures has been impeded by the inherent limitations of X-ray fluoroscopy, mainly arising due to poor visualization of the endocardial surface and requisite catheter contact. Our prior research has addressed the limitations of traditional guidance [3], by developing a novel prototype system for advanced visualization for image-guided cardiac ablation. This platform incorporates pre-operative, patient-specific cardiac models, electro-physiology data acquired via commercial navigation systems, tracked US imaging, and tracking of the ablation catheter.

K. Mori et al. (Eds.): MICCAI 2013, Part I, LNCS 8149, pp. 9–17, 2013.

The other critical factor to successful ablation, which we address here, is intra-operative feedback on the quality of the delivered lesions. While several groups have developed mathematical and physiological models [1] to investigate lesion development in response to RF energy delivery [4,5] for cardiac ablation, to our knowledge, little effort has been channeled toward the integration of such models into the clinical workflow, to visualize and monitor tissue injury, and avoid incomplete electrical pathway isolation during ablation. The slow progress has primarily been attributed to the challenge of developing sufficiently fast ablation models capable of computing temperature distribution and lesion progression in real time [6].

To complement our navigation platform with simultaneous online therapy monitoring [7,8], here we propose a fast and reasonably accurate surrogate ablation model that provides estimates of temperature distribution, tissue damage and lesion progression. The cardiologist will have access to a dynamic visual display of "ablation lesion maps" consisting of sequentially created lesions, rather than just a glyph indicating the catheter location, which can be used to guide the delivery of subsequent lesions to ensure suppression of arrhythmia.

## 2    Materials and Methods

### 2.1    Ablation Model

The tissue response to RF energy can be approximated with sufficient accuracy by a coupled resistive - conductive heat transfer process [1]. The proposed surrogate ablation model incorporates a resistive component occurring at the electrode-tissue interface, and a conductive component responsible for the energy diffusion into the tissue. The heat transfer equilibrium equation the tissue during ablation is governed by the bioheat equation [9]:

$$\rho \cdot c \cdot \frac{\partial T}{\partial t} \; = \; \nabla \cdot (k \nabla T) \; + \; q \; - \; Q_p \; + \; Q_m \tag{1}$$

where $\rho$ is the density $(kg/m^3)$, $c$ is the specific heat $(J/kg \cdot K)$, $k$ is the thermal conductivity $(W/m \cdot K)$; $Q_p$ is the perfusion heat loss $(W/m^3)$ — typically neglected for cardiac ablation [10], $Q_m$ is the metabolic heat generation $(W/m^3)$, which was shown to be insignificant [11,12], and, lastly, $q$ is the heat source $(W/m^3)$, representing the energy deposited into the tissue within a small radius around the electrode and approximated by a purely resistive, quasi-static Joule heating.

**Model Formulation and Image-Based Implementation:** The ablation electrode is represented by a virtual construct based on the physical properties of the electrode, and its interaction with the tissue is defined by means of voxel occupancy in the image volume. The delivered power is absorbed within the first 1-1.5 mm from the electrode surface. During clinical procedures, energy is gradually delivered to the tissue up to a set level (30-50W), then modulated to maintain the electrode temperature at a preset value [13] (typically

60°C - 90°C). The temperature control is modeled according to the gradient between the preset target and the dynamically updated electrode-tissue interface temperature, and modulates power delivery to maintain the target temperature. Tissue voxels remote from the catheter receive energy via heat conduction, modeled as isotropic diffusion. Tissue thermal conductivity has been traditionally treated as a constant parameter with a nominal value of $0.51 - 0.59\ W/m \cdot K$ for myocardium [14], while the other physiological parameters used in the model are assigned literature-suggested values [15]: as follows ($\rho_{blood} = 1000 kg/m^3$, $\rho_{tissue} = 1070 kg/m^3$, $c_{blood} = 4180 J/kg \cdot K$, and $c_{tissue} = 3500 J/kg \cdot K$). The endocardial blood flow is modeled by maintaining the blood pool voxels at 37°C.

Our proposed ablation model follows an image-based implementation, using an anatomical 3D image (i.e., a patient-specific cardiac CT or MR) labeled as blood and tissue compartments, with assigned physiological parameters. The following *image volumes* are used to predict tissue temperature, extent of tissue damage, and lesion progression during ablation: a *conductivity volume* is generated by assigning each image compartment (i.e., tissue and blood pool) the appropriate conductivity values; an image volume of the tissue region is initialized to 37°C and labeled as the initial tissue *temperature volume*; a tissue *exposure volume* is generated based on the cumulative "exposure" (i.e., area under the temperature-time curve explained later) of each voxel in the tissue *temperature volume*; lastly, a tissue *lesion volume* is generated by digitally marking voxels in the tissue *exposure volume* as either irreversible lesion if exposed to 55°C or above for at least 5 s, or reversible lesion penumbra otherwise.

**Tissue Damage and Lesion Characterization:** Modeling studies have used the 50°C isotherm to assess tissue damage reversibility — tissue rendered non-viable after ablation could be defined by the volume enclosed by the 50°C isothermal surface [16]. However, since tissue damage is a function of temperature and time [6], we define *cumulative exposure* as a measure of induced tissue injury.

Cumulative exposure is the area under the temperature-time curve calculated on a voxel-basis over the duration of the ablation: $E = \int_{0}^{t_{cell-death}} T(t)\ dt + \int_{t_{cell-death}}^{t_{max}} T(t)\ dt$, where $t_{cell-death}$ is the time at which a voxel has reached the cell-death temperature ($T_{cell-death} = 55°C$). The former term represents the voxel exposure prior to reaching cell-death temperature (i.e., reversible damage and lesion penumbra), while the latter term represents the voxel exposure beyond cell-death temperature for 5 s or longer (i.e., irreversible damage and core lesion).

A more traditional approach for quantifying tissue injury follows an Arrhenius relationship [17]: $\Omega(t) = \int_{0}^{t} P \cdot e^{\frac{-\Delta E}{R \cdot T}}\ dt$, where $T$ is the voxel tissue temperature (K), $R$ is the universal gas constant, and P ($s^{-1}$) and $\Delta E$ ($J/mole$) are tissue specific kinetic coefficients evaluated experimentally [18] and validated against RF ablation experiments [12]. Tissue damage accumulates linearly with time and hyperbolically with temperature, rendering tissue injury as reversible for $\Omega < 0.5$, and irreversible for $\Omega > 1.0$. As demonstrated in section **3**, both the Arrhenius and the 50°C isotherm tissue injury criteria yield consistent results with our proposed exposure criterion, yet at a higher computational expense.

## 2.2   Numerical Model Evaluation

We conducted numerical experiments to assess model behaviour in response to several parameters, including tissue damage criteria, electrode-tissue contact, and also simulated a cooled vs. dry electrode ablation, as shown in section **3**.

## 2.3   *Ex vivo* **Experimental Evaluation**

To validate our model we conducted a series of *ex vivo* ablation experiments. Bovine muscle samples (1-cm thick) were submerged in a 0.9% saline bath. Endocardial blood flow was mimicked using an immersion circulator (6 L/min flow-rate) that maintained the saline at 36±0.5°C. A RF power generator (Boston Scientific, Natick, MA) was used to deliver energy via a non-cooled 9F 4 mm electrode. The catheter was depressed into the tissue by 1.5 mm, to achieve firm hemispherical contact. The generator was operated in temperature-control mode at 90°C target temperature and 40W maximum power level. Direct tissue temperature measurements, considered as ground truth, were recorded using focal 0.8 mm dia. fiberoptic temperature probes inserted at specific tissue locations.

## 3   Model Evaluation and Results

**Tissue Damage Criteria:** We compared the extent of injury characterized according to our tissue exposure formulation (irreversible damage above 55°C for 5s or longer), to the Arrhenius (irreversible for $\Omega > 1.0$), and 50°C isotherm damage criteria. As shown in **Fig. 1**, the size of the irreversibly-damaged region predicted by the voxel exposure criterion is within 1 mm diameter difference from the region predicted by the Arrhenius and 50°C isotherm criteria.

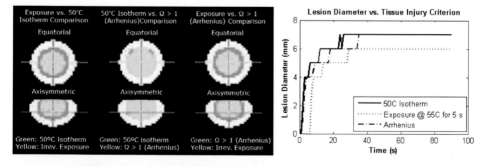

**Fig. 1.** Comparison of the irreversible region assessed according to the three injury criteria. Irreversible lesion diameter predicted by the injury criteria: the voxel exposure criterion leads to lesion diameter within 1 mm of that assessed according to the Arrhenius and 50°C isotherm injury criteria.

**Electrode-Tissue Contact:** The extent of electrode-tissue contact is a direct indicator of the lesion size [19]. We address electrode-tissue contact by modeling three different cases of electrode penetration depth, and asses the outcome according to the achieved lesion dimension as illustrated in **Fig. 2**.

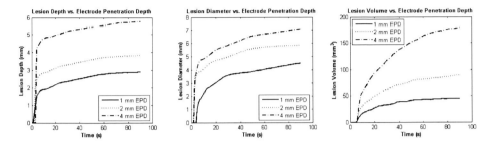

**Fig. 2.** Model-predicted lesion depth, diameter and volume as a result of increasing electrode-penetration depth (1, 2 and 4 mm). Observed trends (larger lesions with deeper penetration) are consistent with previous simulation results reported in [20].

**Cooled vs. Dry Electrode Ablation:** In addition to modeling traditional ablation catheters with no active cooling, we employed the approximation adopted in [21,22] to model a cooled ablation procedure and assessed its effects by characterizing the resulting lesion. Cooling was modeled by setting a lower temperature boundary condition at the electrode surface equal to the temperature of the cooling fluid. This first order approximation will be improved by allowing heat exchange between the electrode and tissue. **Fig. 3** shows the model-predicted tissue temperature at the end of 90-second ablation procedures, with no electrode

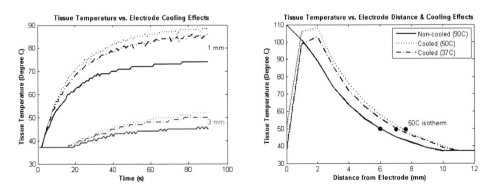

**Fig. 3.** End-ablation tissue temperature at 1 and 3 mm from electrode tip during a non-cooled, 90°C temperature-controlled ablation, as well as two cooled ablations at 50°C and 37°C. Cooling leads to the shift of the 50°C isotherm from ∼ 6 mm to ∼ 8 mm. These findings agree with [22] — electrode cooling shifts the hot spots away from the electrode resulting in deeper lesions.

**Table. 1.** Model-predicted and experimentally measured tissue tissue temperature distribution during 60 s ablation at 90° C

| Time Stamp (sec) | Proximal Lesion Location Measured Temp. (°C) | Predicted Temp. (°C) | Distal Lesion Location Measured Temp. (°C) | Predicted Temp. (°C) |
|---|---|---|---|---|
| 11.2 | 68.9 ± 4.9 | 63.8 | 37.2 ± 1.7 | 37.1 |
| 19.6 | 73.0 ± 5.2 | 70.7 | 39.0 ± 1.6 | 37.9 |
| 30.8 | 76.2 ± 4.8 | 74.9 | 39.8 ± 2.3 | 38.7 |
| 39.2 | 77.4 ± 5.3 | 77.2 | 40.6 ± 2.6 | 40.3 |
| 50.4 | 78.7 ± 5.4 | 78.8 | 40.9 ± 3.2 | 41.2 |
| 58.8 | 79.1 ± 4.9 | 78.9 | 41.5 ± 3.4 | 42.3 |

**Table. 2.** Model-predicted lesion characterization parameters during 60 s ablation at 90° C

| Time Stamp (sec) | Lesion Volume (mm³) | Maximum Lesion Dia. (mm) | Surface Lesion Dia. (mm) | Surface Exposure Dia. (mm) |
|---|---|---|---|---|
| 5 | 30.2 | 3.8 | 4.0 | 7.6 |
| 10 | 44.1 | 4.2 | 4.5 | 8.3 |
| 20 | 63.1 | 4.8 | 4.8 | 8.6 |
| 30 | 77.5 | 5.2 | 4.9 | 9.0 |
| 40 | 84.5 | 5.6 | 4.9 | 9.1 |
| 60 | 96.0 | 5.8 | 5.0 | 9.4 |

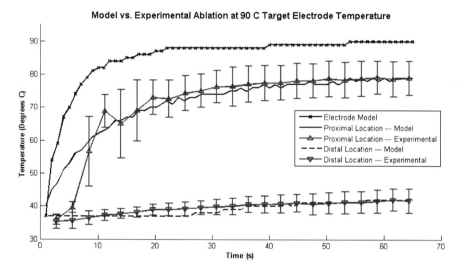

**Fig. 4.** Time-varying temperature plots of the electrode model, as well as model-predicted and experimentally-measured (Mean ± Std. Dev.) temperatures at the proximal and distal locations

cooling (90°C ablation), and two cooled ablations at 50°C and 37°C. The cooling effect led to higher tissue temperatures at both locations, and contributed to the shift of the temperature distribution deeper within the tissue.

**Experimental Model Evaluation:** Four fiberoptic temperature probes were inserted into the tissue samples in a symmetric pattern relative to the ablation electrode at specified radial distance (R) and depth (D); two probes measured tissue temperature at 2.5 mm R x 3 mm D from the electrode (proximal location), and two probes measured temperature at 5 mm R x 3 mm D (distal location). Measurements were recorded simultaneously from all temperature probes and experiments were repeated three times on fresh tissue samples.

Table 1 and **Fig. 4** summarizes the tissue temperature distribution at the two lesion locations, showing agreement within 5°C between the model-predicted and experimentally recorded temperatures.

The modeled lesions were characterized according to lesion volume, maximum diameter, surface lesion diameter, and surface exposure diameter, summarized in **Table 2**. After the experiments, the samples were analyzed according to the diameter and depth of the region marked by tissue discolouration, also known to correspond with the volume enclosed by 50°C isothermal surface [6]. The lesion measurements predicted by the model were consistent with those observed in the digital images of the post-ablation samples (**Fig. 5**).

**Fig. 5** also shows 2D cross-sectional renderings of the model-generated lesion at 5, 10, 30, and 60 s during the ablation. The irreversibly damaged tissue region appears brighter and is surrounded by the lesion penumbra.

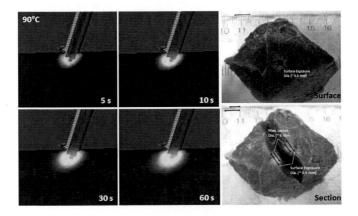

**Fig. 5.** Cross-sectional rendering of the model-predicted tissue damage at four time points during 90°C ablation. Note the irreversibly damaged region appearing bright and surrounded by the lesion penumbra. Post-ablation digital images of a typical sample following 90°C ablation: a surface exposure diameter of ∼ 9 mm and a maximum lesion diameter of ∼ 6 mm shown in the section, both consistent with the model-predicted dimensions.

## 4    Discussion

We describe the development, implementation, and evaluation of an image-based ablation model designed to assist with procedure guidance and provide visualization and monitoring of lesion progression during RF ablation. Given the real-time guidance requirement and the understanding of clinically acceptable accuracy, this model is not intended to provide the computational rigor of previously developed finite element models of tissue ablation; it is rather a "surrogate" model that demonstrates effective and fast extension of a theoretical model into a practical tool, designed for efficient intra-operative integration with our navigation platform for image-guided cardiac ablation therapy.

We explored the effect of electrode penetration depth as a contact surrogate, electrode cooling, and also compared our exposure tissue injury criterion to two other criteria explored in the literature. Numerical experiments confirmed previous findings, while the experimental studies also demonstrated agreement within 5°C between the model-predicted and experimentally measured temperature profiles. Lastly, the predicted and observed lesion patterns were also in agreement, suggesting sufficiently accurate modeling of the ablation process.

In its current form, the model is implemented using a 0.5 mm isotropic image substrate, which is inline with the typical resolution of clinical-quality acquired images, as well as the 1.0-2.0 mm accuracy of the magnetic tracking system used to identify the position and pose of the ablation catheter.

The proposed model was implemented on a standard desktop PC (Intel Core2 Quad 2.5 GHz, 8 GB DDR2 RAM) and provided near real-time updates of the tissue temperature distribution and lesion progression. modeling a 60s ablation cycle in ~ 1 minute The computational efficiency can be further improved via parallel multi-thread computing and GPU implementation, enabling lesion monitoring with minimal workflow latency.

Once integrated within the prototype guidance and navigation platform for left atrial ablation therapy, the thermal model will provide the cardiologist with online visualization and monitoring of the changes induced in the tissue during RF energy delivery. In addition to the catheter navigation information available from the image guidance environment (i.e., the tracked catheter tip dictates the location where the ablation lesion should be displayed), the physiological changes occurring in the tissue will be displayed by means of temperature colour maps superimposed on the pre-operative anatomical model, thereby providing improved guidance for the delivery of subsequent lesions.

## 5    Conclusions and Future Work

Given the support provided by new methodologies of planning, simulation and training, the proposed ablation model demonstrates effective and fast extension of a theoretical model into a practical tool that will allow for quantitative monitoring of individual ablation therapy with integrated guidance [8,23].

Knowledge of the true ablation sites and their characterization as necrotic or endemic via DCE-MRI [24] is of significant importance for the *in vivo* validation of the thermal model. As such, future efforts will focus on estimating electrode-tissue interaction and contact using the system-integrated real-time US imaging, as well as evaluating the predicted lesions and guidance abilities of the enhanced system *in vivo* against post-procedural assessment of lesion development as characterized using delayed contrast-enhanced (DCE)-MR imaging, as well as post-mortem using tissue staining techniques.

## References

1. Haemmerich, D.: Crit. Rev. Biomed. Eng. 38(1), 53–63 (2010)
2. Pappone, C., et al.: Circ. 102, 2619–2628 (2000)
3. Rettmann, M.E., et al.: Comput. Methods Programs Biomed. 95, 95–104 (2009)

 4. Pearce, J.A.: Crit. Rev. Biomed. Eng. 38(1), 1–20 (2010)
 5. Payne, S.J., et al.: Crit. Rev. Biomed Eng. 38(1), 21–30 (2010)
 6. Berjano, E.J.: Biomed. Eng. Online. 18, 5–24 (2006)
 7. Johnson, P.C., et al.: Ann. Biomed. Eng. 30, 1152–1161 (2002)
 8. Villard, C., et al.: Comput. Methods Biomech. Biomed. Engin. 8, 215–227 (2005)
 9. Pennes, H.H.: J. Appl. Physiol. 85, 5–34 (1948)
10. Haines, D.E., et al.: Pacing Clin. Electrophysiol. 12, 962–976 (1989)
11. Chang, I.A., et al.: Biomed. Eng. Online. 3, 1–19 (2004)
12. Labonté, S.: IEEE Trans. Biomed. Eng. 41, 108–115 (1994)
13. Jain, M.K., et al.: IEEE Trans. Biomed. Eng. 46, 1405–1412 (1999)
14. Holmes, K.R.: http://www.ece.utexas.edu/~valvano/research/Thermal.pdf
15. Shahidi, A.V., et al.: IEEE Trans. Biomed. Eng. 41, 963–968 (1994)
16. Panescu, D., et al.: IEEE Trans. Biomed. Eng. 42, 879–890 (1995)
17. Diller, K.R., et al.: Ann. NY Acad. Sci. 888, 153–165 (1999)
18. Pearce, J.A., et al.: Proc. IEEE Eng. Med. Biol. Conf., 256–258 (1998)
19. Yokoyama, K., et al.: Circ. Arrhythm. Electrophisiol. 1(5), 354–362 (2008)
20. Jain, M.K., et al.: Proc. IEEE Eng. Med. Biol. Conf., 245–247 (1998)
21. Berjano, E.J., et al.: Proc. IEEE Eng. Med. Biol. Cong., 2496–2498 (1997)
22. Jain, M.K., et al.: Proc. IEEE Eng. Med. Biol. Conf., 273–274 (1995)
23. Banovac, F., et al.: Med. Phys. 32(5), 2698–2705 (2005)
24. Knowles, B.R., et al.: IEEE Trans. Biomed. Eng. 57, 1467–1475 (2010)

# Prediction of Cranio-Maxillofacial Surgical Planning Using an Inverse Soft Tissue Modelling Approach

Kamal Shahim[1], Philipp Jürgens[2], Philippe C. Cattin[3], Lutz-P. Nolte[1],
and Mauricio Reyes[1]

[1] Institute for Surgical Technology and Biomechanics, University of Bern, Bern, Switzerland
{kamal.shahim,lutz.nolte,mauricio.reyes}@istb.unibe.ch
[2] Department of Cranio-Maxillofacial Surgery, University of Basel, Basel, Switzerland
pjuergens@uhbs.ch
[3] Medical Image Analysis Center (MIAC), University of Basel, Basel, Switzerland
philippe.cattin@unibas.ch

**Abstract.** In cranio-maxillofacial surgery, the determination of a proper surgical plan is an important step to attain a desired aesthetic facial profile and a complete denture closure. In the present paper, we propose an efficient modeling approach to predict the surgical planning on the basis of the desired facial appearance and optimal occlusion. To evaluate the proposed planning approach, the predicted osteotomy plan of six clinical cases that underwent CMF surgery were compared to the real clinical plan. Thereafter, simulated soft-tissue outcomes were compared using the predicted and real clinical plan. This preliminary retrospective comparison of both osteotomy planning and facial outlook shows a good agreement and thereby demonstrates the potential application of the proposed approach in cranio-maxillofacial surgical planning prediction.

**Keywords:** surgical planning prediction, soft-tissue simulation, mass-tensor modeling, cranio-maxillofacial surgery.

## 1 Introduction

Soft tissue simulation approaches are used in CMF surgery to predict the post-operative facial appearance of patients undergoing orthognathic surgeries. Besides functional improvements (chewing, swallowing, breathing etc.), the aesthetic enhancement is of major concern in affected patients, as they want to know before surgery how they will look like post-operatively. The current simulation approaches for soft tissue deformations following CMF surgery show good results in terms of accuracy and compliance to the clinical workflow [1-3]. In these approaches, the goal is to use a biomechanical model to predict how the patient's facial soft tissues will deform given an osteotomic surgical plan. The simulation is then capable of providing the surgeon with a post-operative scenario, from which adaptations or changes to the surgical plan can be performed in order to prepare the patient for the changes in his/her appearance. An alternative way would be the virtual creation of a facial outlook according to the desires of the patient and surgeon recommendations, from

K. Mori et al. (Eds.): MICCAI 2013, Part I, LNCS 8149, pp. 18–25, 2013.

which the surgical plan could be derived. In this paper we present an approach to predict the surgical plan necessary to attain a desired post-operative patient's facial outcome and an optimal occlusion between mandibular sections. The method features an inverse modeling paradigm used to predict the displacement of bony structures from the desired post-operative outcome. We present preliminary results on six patient cases undergoing different types of orthognathic surgery, demonstrating the ability of the method to predict the surgical plan needed to attain the post-operative scenario.

## 2    Method

In this section the workflow for the surgical plan prediction is presented. An overview of the proposed pipeline is presented in **Fig. 1**. First, the pre-operative tissue model and information (i.e. typical osteotomy segments, muscle prediction, and mechanical information) are built from the pre-operative CT scan, as proposed in [3]. Based on this model, the desired post-operative outlook can then be derived by means of a Computer Aided Design (CAD) tool that allows the surgeon to deform the pre-operative model. We use the resulting surface-to-surface displacement as boundary condition of a biomechanical model [3], which allows us to compute the deformation of the internal soft tissues in contact with the bone segments (called hereafter inverse soft tissue deformation). In the last step, an iterative surface-to-surface rigid registration with occlusion (denture equilibration) and collision constraints is used to compute the final predicted planning by registering the bony segments to the internal soft tissues. Below, we explain in more detail the inverse soft tissue deformation and final estimation of the osteotomy plan.

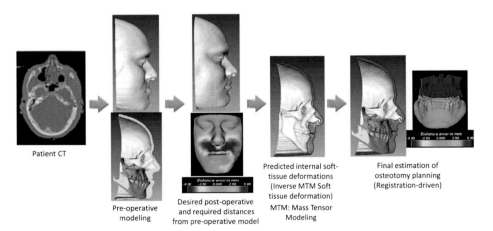

Patient CT

Pre-operative modeling

Desired post-operative and required distances from pre-operative model

Predicted internal soft-tissue deformations (Inverse MTM Soft tissue deformation) MTM: Mass Tensor Modeling

Final estimation of osteotomy planning (Registration-driven)

**Fig. 1.** Illustration of the proposed concept for patient-specific CMF surgical plan prediction. The required displacement boundary conditions over the pre-operative skin surface are obtained based on the comparison with the desired facial outlook. Using MTM modeling, the deformations of internal soft tissues are computed, from which the final estimation of the planning is obtained from an occlusion-constrained registration-driven approach.

## 2.1    Soft Tissue Simulation

**Pre-operative Tissue and Bone Modeling**
Following the approach presented in [3], we derive from the pre-operative CT scan, a pre-operative model of the patient that includes soft tissues (external and internal), bone tissues (skull, maxilla, and mandible), and predicted facial muscles. Osteotomy segments are derived from the surgeon, and mechanical information (material properties and boundary conditions) is set following [3, 4]. As an example, **Fig. 4** shows the pre-operative models of six patients that underwent CMF surgery. Note that for visualization purposes the predicted facial muscles are not visualized, but used in the simulations.

**Boundary Conditions for Inverse Soft Tissue Modeling**
From the pre-operative model, the desired outlook can be generated by means of CAD software, or any other surface deformation based approach that enables "sculpturing" of the pre-operative model. The resulting displacements starting from the pre-operative to the desired outlook model are regarded as displacement boundary conditions (see **Fig. 2**a). This information enables the connection between the desired outlook, the biomechanically driven estimation of internal soft tissue deformations and the final prediction of the surgical plan. In addition, as proposed in [3], sliding contact is defined on the teeth area in order to improve the simulation accuracy in the error-sensitive region (see **Fig. 2**b). The most posterior plane of the volumetric soft-tissue model is assumed fixed (**Fig. 2**c). The remaining points are considered free to move.

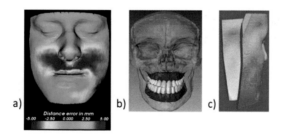

**Fig. 2.** Three types of boundary conditions defined on the patient model a) surface skin displacement b) sliding sections illustrated with different colours c) fixed points

**Biomechanical Simulation Using Mass Tensor Modeling (MTM)**
In order to compute the deformation of internal soft tissues in contact with the bone segments, we used the defined boundary conditions and Mass Tensor Modeling (MTM) simulation [3, 4]. By using MTM in a reverse way, we are able to derive deformations of the internal soft tissues. As facial soft tissues follow an elastic behavior, we are able to seemingly invert boundary conditions of the simulation so to derive bone segment displacements from the displacements of the external soft tissues.

## 2.2    Osteotomy Planning Prediction by Constrained Surface Registration

In the last step, the final planning is derived by surface-to-surface registration. Since surface points in the deformed internal soft tissue are in contact with maxilla and mandible segments, we use an Iterative Closest Point (ICP) based registration method to recover the displacements of the bone segments. In order to consider proper occlusion for denture equilibration and collision for realistic surface matching, we extended the constrained ICP approach presented in [5] to consider deviations from a perfect occlusion as well as collision amongst maxilla, mandible, and internal soft tissues. We modeled occlusion by measuring the misalignment between the maxilla and mandibular dental arches through manually selecting anatomically corresponding points (at least three) on each arc (e.g. tip of the vestibular cuspid on the first upper premolar and contact point on first and second lower premolar), as proposed in [6]. The registration process then aims at minimizing the surface distance errors $e^{upper}$, $e^{lower}$, and $e^{arch}$, for maxilla, mandible, and denture arches, respectively, with penalizations $W_x^{(\cdot)} = \gamma^{(\cdot)}\|e_x^{(\cdot)}\|$ if point $x$ infringes collision, and $W_x^{(\cdot)} = 1$, otherwise. Weights $\gamma^{(\cdot)}$ are set to weigh the amount of collision penalization and are set empirically [5]. Weights $\alpha$ and $\beta$ are used to weigh the balance between occlusion and desired outlook. Collision is computed as in [5].

$$argmin\ \alpha \left( \sum_i W_i^{upper}\|e_i^{upper}\|^2 + \sum_j W_j^{lower}\|e_j^{lower}\|^2 \right) + \beta \sum_k W_k^{arch}\|e_k^{arch}\|^2 \tag{1}$$

To find the set of rigid transformations for the bone segments that minimize (1), we used alternating optimization heuristics considering the desired outlook components and occlusion. As example, **Fig. 3** (a-c) shows the displacement of bone segments for case number five. See **Fig. 3** (d) as example of recovered occlusion.

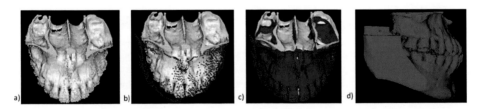

**Fig. 3.** Example of bone segment displacements obtained using the constrained ICP registration. Yellow points (a) are the pre-operative tissue points in the vicinity of the bone surface. Red points in (b) are the deformed internal tissue points after inverse soft tissue modeling. White and red bone segments in (c) correspond to the pre-operative and final predicted segments, respectively. (d) An example of recovered occlusion in patient no. 5.

# 3    Results

## 3.1    Clinical Data and Evaluation Procedure

To evaluate the proposed approach six patient datasets that underwent different types of CMF surgery were analyzed retrospectively. For each case, pre- and post-operative CT scans were available as well as the surgical plan.

In order to evaluate the ability of the method to predict the surgical plan based on a given facial outcome, we took advantage of the retrospective data and considered the real post-operative outlook as the desired outlook, and the actual surgical plan as ground truth. For each case, occlusion and compliance to the desired outlook was set equally (i.e. $\alpha = \beta = 0.5$ in Eq. (1)).

For each case, pre-operative models were created and osteotomy segments reproduced based on the type of CMF surgery chosen by the surgeon [3]. **Fig. 4** shows for each case the pre-, and post-operative bone segments (white and green, respectively) as well as the pre-operative patient face.

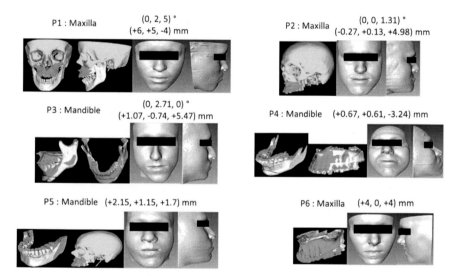

**Fig. 4.** Osteotomy segments for the six clinical cases that underwent different types of CMF surgery. For each case pre- and post-operative situations are displayed in white and green, respectively. The pre-operative patient face is shown next to the surgical plan. The amount of rotation (axial, sagittal, coronal) and translation (horizontal, vertical, anterior-posterior) are presented on top for the respective segment.

## 3.2    Comparison of Predicted and Actual CMF Surgical Plan

In order to assess the accuracy of the proposed method, the predicted segments for each patient were compared with the respective actual post-operative segments. For each patient the pre-operative, predicted, and actual post-operative osteotomy segment are shown with white, orange and green color in **Fig. 5**, respectively. Using the protocol described in [3], distance measurements between corresponding points of the predicted and the actual post-operative segments were quantified and are shown as color-coded images on the rightmost column in **Fig. 5**. The predicted segments present a good similarity to the actual post-operative segments except for case number five, where despite of the agreement in rotation for the mandible segment, the inverse modelling predicted a different advancement of mandible, which was found to be due to the occlusion constraints. After inspection of the post-operative segments and discussion with the surgeon, the proposed predicted planning was regarded as an improvement over the actual executed plan as shown in **Fig. 3** (d). Complete processing time was below 10 mins on each case compared to hours needed for the current clinical workflow.

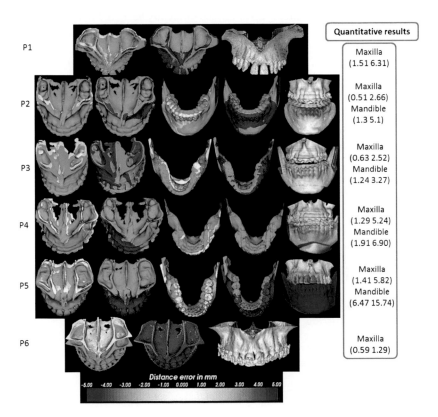

**Fig. 5.** Predicted (orange color), actual post-operative (green color), and pre-operative segments (white color) for the respective patients. The quantitative results (distance errors) from the post-operative segments are shown as color-coded images on the predicted model on the rightmost column with the (median maximum) error values in mm indicated for the respective segments. The blue color means the proposed approach falls posteriorly than the real post-operative segment.

### 3.3 Soft Tissue Prediction

As an additional evaluation, simulated soft-tissue outcomes were compared using the predicted and real clinical plan. We remark that in this case the real post-operative outcome was not used for comparison in order to remove from the evaluation the implicit error of the MTM simulation, which can favorably compensate for errors in the predicted surgical plan or add error to the evaluation of the surgical plan prediction. Distance measurements between corresponding points of the simulated and the post-operative surface skin were quantified based on the method presented in [3], and are displayed for all cases in **Fig. 6** using a color-coded map, where the red color means the simulated skin surface falls posteriorly to the post-operative surface mesh, and blue indicates that the simulation lies anteriorly to the post-operative skin surface. The white color is associated with the range [-2,2] mm, the clinically accepted range where simulation errors are not recognizable by the human eye [7]. The facial simulation results using the predicted and actual planed approach are in close agreement, except for case number five where the predicted plan for the mandible section is different from the actual one due to the ability of the approach to propose a better occlusion.

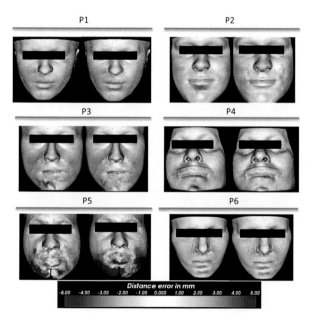

**Fig. 6.** Color-map comparison of distance errors between simulation results using the predicted (left column) and actual (right column) osteotomy planning in six patients. Please note that the red colour indicates posterior position of simulation compared to the post-operative.

## 4 Conclusion

In this paper we have presented an approach to predict a CMF surgical plan based on the desired post-operative facial outlook. The proposed approach employs a fast biomechanical model to derive from the desired facial outlook, the deformation of internal soft tissues, which is followed by constrained surface registration between bone segments and internal soft tissues. The proposed registration component considers collision and occlusion constraints, and its formulation allows us to derive in a straightforward manner different levels of interplay between quality of occlusion and compliance to the desired outlook (i.e. constraints relaxation). Furthermore, and in regards to a biomechanical simulation that would model the entire ensemble of bone and soft tissues, the proposed approach avoids known issues of layer detachment and convergence related to the high elasticity transition present at the interface of bone and soft tissue materials. Preliminary results on a prospective set of clinical cases showed in five out of six cases a high level of agreement to the actual surgical plan, and one case where the proposed approach was confirmed to improve the actual executed plan. Our method differs in concept with reference [3] and is like an inverse simulation accounting for optimal occlusion and non-collision and desired facial outlook. The desired outlook can be easily defined by the surgeon using a CAD software [8]. In the presented paper, we did not use any CAD system, instead and for validation purposes, we considered the post-operative profile as the desired outlook.

**Acknowledgment.** This work was funded by the Swiss National Center of Competence in Research Computer Aided and Image Guided Medical Interventions (Co-Me).

# References

1. Mollemans, W., Schutyser, F., Nadjmi, N., Maes, F., Suetens, P.: Predicting soft tissue deformations for a maxillofacial surgery planning system: From computational strategies to a complete clinical validation. Medical Image Analysis 11, 282–301 (2007)
2. Marchetti, C., Bianchi, A., Muyldermans, L., Di Martino, M., Lancellotti, L., Sarti, A.: Validation of new soft tissue software in orthognathic surgery planning. International Journal of Oral and Maxillofacial Surgery 40, 26–32 (2011)
3. Kim, H., Jürgens, P., Weber, S., Nolte, L.-P., Reyes, M.: A new soft-tissue simulation strategy for cranio-maxillofacial surgery using facial muscle template model. Progress in Biophysics and Molecular Biology 103, 284–291 (2010)
4. Cotin, S., Delingette, H., Ayache, N.: A hybrid elastic model for real-time cutting, deformations, and force feedback for surgery training and simulation. The Visual Computer 16, 437–452 (2000)
5. Kozic, N., Weber, S., Büchler, P., Lutz, C., Reimers, N., González Ballester, M.Á., Reyes, M.: Optimisation of orthopaedic implant design using statistical shape space analysis based on level sets. Medical Image Analysis 14, 265–275
6. Nadjmi, N., Mollemans, W., Daelemans, A., Van Hemelen, G., Schutyser, F., Bergé, S.: Virtual occlusion in planning orthognathic surgical procedures. International Journal of Oral and Maxillofacial Surgery 39, 457–462 (2010)
7. Xia, J.J., Gateno, J., Teichgraeber, J.F., Christensen, A.M., Lasky, R.E., Lemoine, J.J., Liebschner, M.A.K.: Accuracy of the Computer-Aided Surgical Simulation (CASS) System in the Treatment of Patients With Complex Craniomaxillofacial Deformity: A Pilot Study. Journal of Oral and Maxillofacial Surgery 65, 248–254 (2007)
8. Oliveira-Santos, T., Baumberger, C., Constantinescu, M., Olariu, R., Nolte, L.-P., Alaraibi, S., Reyes, M.: 3D Face Reconstruction from 2D Pictures: First Results of a Web-Based Computer Aided System for Aesthetic Procedures. Annals of Biomedical Engineering 41, 952–966

# String Motif-Based Description of Tool Motion for Detecting Skill and Gestures in Robotic Surgery

Narges Ahmidi[1], Yixin Gao[1], Benjamín Béjar[2], S. Swaroop Vedula[1],
Sanjeev Khudanpur[1,3], René Vidal[1,2,3], and Gregory D. Hager[1]

[1] Department of Computer Science
[2] Department of Biomedical Engineering
[3] Department of Electrical and Computer Engineering,
Johns Hopkins University, Baltimore, MD 21218, USA

**Abstract.** The growing availability of data from robotic and laparoscopic surgery has created new opportunities to investigate the modeling and assessment of surgical technical performance and skill. However, previously published methods for modeling and assessment have not proven to scale well to large and diverse data sets. In this paper, we describe a new approach for simultaneous detection of gestures and skill that can be generalized to different surgical tasks. It consists of two parts: (1) descriptive curve coding (DCC), which transforms the surgical tool motion trajectory into a coded string using accumulated Frenet frames, and (2) common string model (CSM), a classification model using a similarity metric computed from longest common string motifs. We apply DCC-CSM method to detect surgical gestures and skill levels in two kinematic datasets (collected from the da Vinci surgical robot). DCC-CSM method classifies gestures and skill with 87.81% and 91.12% accuracy, respectively.

**Keywords:** surgical motion, descriptive models, gesture and skill classification, geometry, descriptive curve coding, robotic surgery.

## 1 Introduction

Methods that are currently used to assess acquisition and maintenance of surgical skill in the training laboratory and operating room suffer from significant shortcomings [1]. Existing methods are focused on either subjective global evaluation of performance or unstructured, descriptive feedback [1,2]. Some evaluation metrics such as total task completion time and path length reasonably correlate with surgical skill but are not instructive, i.e. they provide limited information to the trainee on whether and how to improve their performance in different stages of the task. On the other hand, unstructured, descriptive feedback typically requires the presence of a senior surgeon and is inefficient [1,2].

The advent of robotic surgery has created new opportunities to automate objective assessment of skill acquisition by surgical trainees. Because surgeons may exhibit different levels of skill at various stages of the task, automated skill assessment requires the detection of gestures that are being performed. Prior approaches to

K. Mori et al. (Eds.): MICCAI 2013, Part I, LNCS 8149, pp. 26–33, 2013.

automatically detect surgical skill and gestures have significant performance and utility limitations (Table 1) [3-9]. For example, Hidden Markov Models (HMMs) and other statistical methods such as Linear Dynamical Systems (LDS) were used to detect surgical gestures with reasonable accuracy (around 85%). Our objective in this paper is to present and evaluate a general approach for signal representation, called Descriptive Curve Coding (DCC) using accumulated Frenet frames (AFF) followed by analysis of string motifs, which can be used to simultaneously identify both surgical skill and gestures using kinematic data describing surgical motion.

## 2     Experiment Setup

We used two datasets to develop and validate our methods. The first dataset (DS-I) has been described in detail elsewhere [5,9]. It contains 39 trials of a four-throw continuous suturing task (performed by 8 surgeons in multiple sessions) on a bench-top model using the da Vinci surgical robot (Intuitive Surgical, Inc., Sunnyvale, California). The second dataset (DS-II), with 110 trials, was collected from 18 surgeons performing interrupted suturing followed by either a square knot or a surgeon's knot using the da Vinci surgical robot [10]. The operators performed multiple sessions over several days, repeating the suture/knot-tying task three times in each session. The surgical task in DS-II is more complex compared to that in DS-I.

The data from each task was manually segmented, i.e., the start and the end of every gesture in a task were annotated, by watching the endoscopic-video recordings. The gesture labels were specified by an experienced surgical educator, and manually assigned by two researchers in our lab (88% average chance-corrected-agreement between annotators). We used 10 gestures from DS-I (total of 787 sample gestures) under the same experiment setup explained in [5]. We used seven gestures from DS-II: grab needle, grab suture, grab suture-tail, pull needle, pull suture, rotate suture once, rotate suture twice. Because kinematic data does not contain information about the surgical environment (e.g., object being held), we combined the gestures into three context-free groups: grab (722 samples; average duration of 2 sec), pull (431 samples; average duration of 1.3 sec), and rotate (137 samples; duration of 3.8 sec).

Our ground truth for skill assessment consisted of Global Rating Scores (GRS) assigned based on the Objective Structured Assessment of Technical Skills (OSATS) approach [11]. An experienced surgical educator, who was masked to the identity of the operator, assigned the scores by watching video recordings of operators performing the tasks. The OSATS approach is comprised of six elements; each one scored using a Likert scale ranging from 1 to 5. In practice, a single GRS is assigned for the entire task, whereas automated assessment can be continuous over the task (i.e., assigns a skill level to each gesture in a task).

We considered trials for which an operator was assigned a score of 3 on at most two items and a score 4 or 5 on the other items on the GRS as being at "expert" skill level; trials with a score less than 3 on all items on the GRS as being at "novice" skill level; and trials that fell in between the expert and novice categories as being at "intermediate" skill level. DS-II contains 30 novice-level trials, 37 intermediate-level trials, and 43 expert-level trials.

# 3    Methodology

Our approach is comprised of three steps (Fig. 1): feature extraction (signal representation through AFF and DCC), training (string-motif-based model, metrics, and classification), and finally evaluation of the classification on a test dataset.

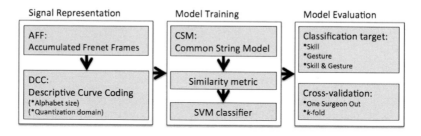

**Fig. 1.** Three steps comprising our approach for gesture/skill classification

## 3.1    Accumulated Frenet Frames (AFF)

In [4], we introduced the idea of DCC using Frenet Frames (FF), which assign a local coordinate system to each point of a trajectory, based on the local curvature. The coding system defined on FFs is coordinate-independent and thus independent of the surgical setup. However, FFs alone do not adequately represent the curvature of some smooth trajectories, as explained below. Therefore, we introduce AFF, which accumulates changes in direction of the motion trajectory over short spatial or temporal windows and thus is more sensitive to gradual changes.

The tool tip movement is represented by a sequence of local frames (Fig. 2a). Each frame is comprised of three orthogonal unit vectors: $\vec{v_i}$ follows the tangent of the curve $(\vec{w_i})$, $\vec{u_i}$ is the normal vector following the concavity of the curve, and $\vec{n_i}$ is the binormal vector formed as the cross-product of $\vec{v_i}$ and $\vec{u_i}$. In the original FF, $\vec{v_i}$ directly followed the tangent vector, whereas in AFF, it follows the last considerable change of direction (defined in 3.2). The AFF accumulates small changes of direction until they are large enough to update the frame orientation.

## 3.2    Descriptive Curve Coding (DCC)

DCC transforms the time series of AFF into a coded string representation of tool motion by mapping each motion to a small set of canonical directions. Let $S = \{0, 1, \ldots, n\}$ be the index set of vectors comprising the coding alphabet. The following equation is used to generate an alphabet representing direction changes of $\pi/2^p$:

$$[\vec{x}]_p = [\vec{x}]_{p-1} \cup \left[ (\overrightarrow{x_i + x_j}) / \left\| \overrightarrow{x_i + x_j} \right\| \mid |\vec{x_i} \otimes \vec{x_j}| \neq 0; \ \vec{x_i}, \vec{x_j} \in [\vec{x}]_{p-1} \right]$$

$$[\vec{x}]_1 = [\vec{0}, \ \vec{v_i}, \ \vec{v_i} \otimes \vec{u_i}, \ \vec{u_i} \otimes \vec{v_i}, \ \vec{u_i}, \ \overrightarrow{-u_i}, \ \overrightarrow{-v_i}]$$

For example, Figure 2a shows a set of vectors encoding direction as cardinal directions (the base case of equation above, p=1). [x]₁ contains six orthogonal vectors indicating the possible changes of direction plus no-motion (DCC7): '$x_0$: no-motion', '$x_1$: forward', '$x_2$: left', '$x_3$: right', '$x_4$: down', '$x_5$: up', '$x_6$: backward'. $[x]_2$ defines a 19-element alphabet (DCC19), which includes all bisectors of DCC7 vectors. Fig. 3 illustrates differences in representation between FF and AFF and between DCC7 and DCC19. The representation by AFF is closer to the original shape than the representation by FF (Fig. 3). In addition, using a larger alphabet size (DCC19 vs. DCC7) results in signal representations that are closer to the original shapes.

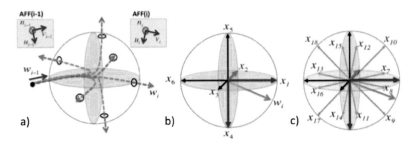

**Fig. 2.** Possible changes in the direction of the motion trajectory at a given point: a) the change of direction of the motion trajectory between $w_i$ (current window) and $w_{i-1}$ (previous window) is encoded using a set of predefined possible vectors $[x]$. b) seven element alphabet when changes larger than $\pi/4$ are of interest (DCC7), or c) nineteen element alphabet when changes larger than $\pi/8$ are of interest (DCC19).

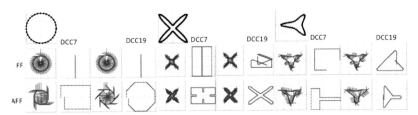

**Fig. 3.** First row: the original shape. Even columns show the representation of the curve after coding by DCC7 or DCC19, respectively. Odd columns show $u$ (red) and $v$ (blue) vectors of either FF (second row) or AFF (third row) along the curve. Using AFF with DCC19 clearly provides the most detailed approximation to the original shape.

### 3.3    Common String Model (CSM)

DCC encodes each motion trajectory j as a string $T_j$ of length m. We hypothesize that within this string, there are recurring string patterns (string motifs) that correlate with the gesture being performed, and the skill with which it is being performed. Thus, within a training set $\{T_j\}$, we apply an algorithm to extract the 'Longest Common String' (LCS) for each pair of strings $< T_x, T_y >$ using the dynamic time warping approach. LCS returns three values: the longest common motifs (C), number of joint occurrences (N), and the set of motif locations in each training string (O). The collection of triples $< C, N, O >$ computed by applying LCS to each pair of strings in

$\{T_j\}$ forms the dictionary D. For example, if LCS finds a common motif C between $T_x$ and $T_y$ and the motif C occurs at elements $X, Z$ in $T_x$ and element Y in $T_y$, the entry in the dictionary would be:

$$LCS(T_x, T_y) = < C, N_{xy} = 3, \qquad O_{xy} = \{X, Y, Z\} >$$

If C is found in other pairs of strings, for example in $< T_h, T_q >$, then we update the dictionary entry for C by summing $N_{xy}$ and $N_{hq}$, and merging the sets $O_{xy}$ and $O_{hq}$.

## 3.4    Similarity Metric and Classifier

We used the following equation to measure the pseudo-similarity value between a given string $T_y$ and a dictionary D:

$$Similarity\,(T_y, D) = \frac{1}{d} * \sum_{C_i \in D \cap T_y} (\log(P_i) + w_1 * \log(|C_i|) + w_2 * \log(A_i))$$

$$A_i = \frac{1}{1 + \sum_{J \in O}|Y - J|}$$

where $C_i$ represents each of the $d$ motifs found in both $T_y$ and CSM. $P_i$ is the frequency of motif $C_i$ appearing in the model and $|C_i|$ represents the length of the motif $C_i$. $A_i$ is a measure of the mis-alignment between the location of $C_i$ in $T_y$ (denoted as Y) and the location of $C_i$ in the training samples (J). The weight factors $w_1$ and $w_2$ are learned using a gradient descent algorithm to optimize the performance of the metric for a given classification problem as explained below. The similarity metric tends to assign higher values to test strings with longer matching motifs with the model. However, it also applies a misalignment penalty for motifs that do not occur during corresponding segments of the surgical task.

## 3.5    Training

For a given classification problem, a dictionary is computed for each class of interest. For a given set of weights the pseudo-similarity provides a value determining the affinity of a given test string to each dictionary. A Support Vector Machine (SVM) classifier is trained using a feature vector S (comprised of pseudo-similarities), and the performance is tabulated. The weights, $w_1$ and $w_2$, are optimized to maximize the classifier's performance by tuning the pseudo-similarity to be as discriminative as possible for a given task.

## 4    Evaluation and Results

We analyzed DS-I for gesture classification and DS-II for both gesture and skill classification. For gesture classification in both DS-I and DS-II, we apply three methods assuming that the boundaries are known (from manual annotation): HMM [9], LDS [5], and DCC-CSM. The HMM method was configured as a 3-state, 3-mixtures (3S3M), and a 3-state, 1-mixture (3S1M), along with 9-dimensional linear discriminant analysis (LDA). The LDS algorithm used Martin and Frobenius distance metrics, and nearest neighbor (NN) and SVM as classifiers. We tried different orders for the dynamical models (range from 3 to 15) and reported the best results obtained. We also examine the performance of DCC-CSM under varying conditions – using two types of "windows" for encoding the motion trajectory (with resolutions of either 0.25mm in the spatial domain or 25ms in the temporal domain), and using alphabets of two sizes (DCC7 and DCC19).

For our evaluations, we used three validation methods – leave-one-session-out ("SO"), leave-one-user-out ("UO"), and $k$-fold cross-validation (leave 20% out). For our analyses using DS-I, we under-sampled gesture classes to include 43 samples (median of class size) to create balanced (B) training datasets. We also report results of our analyses on DS-I using unbalanced (UB) training datasets (except DCC-CSM). Tables 2 to 5 include both macro- and micro- averages of correct classification.

We investigated the following using DCC-CSM on DS-II: gesture classification for a known skill level, skill classification for a known gesture, and simultaneous gesture and skill classification (assuming neither is known). For simultaneous classification of gesture and skill, we trained nine models (3 gestures times 3 skill levels). The model that is most similar to the test sample represents both gesture and skill.

**Table 1.** Gesture detection performance with unknown boundaries – micro averages of correct frames- reported in the literature for various algorithms using dataset DS-I. *=one-trial-out.

| Suturing task | HMM- 3S3M | S-LDS [9] | HMM-HLDA [9] | FA-HMM [9] | SHMM [6] |
|---|---|---|---|---|---|
| SO | 72%* | 80.79% | 74.13% | 78.27% | 81.1% |
| UO | 69% | 67.1% | N/A | 57.2% | 67.8% |

**Table 2.** Gesture classification performance, assuming known boundaries, macro (top number) and micro (bottom number) averages, percentage of correct segments on DS-I (chance=10%)

| Suturing task | | HMM 3S3M | HMM 3S1M | LDS NN Mar | LDS NN Fro | LDS SVM Mar | LDS SVM Fro | DCC7, spatial | DCC7, temporal | DCC19, spatial | DCC19, temporal |
|---|---|---|---|---|---|---|---|---|---|---|---|
| SO | B | 67.49 | 85.98 | 66.97 | 74.59 | 72.46 | 82.53 | - | - | - | - |
|  |  | 71.69 | 87.12 | 74.60 | 80.00 | 80.12 | 87.69 | | | | |
|  | UB | 68.43 | 88.72 | 67.10 | 74.29 | 64.88 | 80.23 | 79.92 | 86.79 | 82.92 | 77.88 |
|  |  | 73.68 | 91.81 | 82.22 | 83.65 | 81.62 | 90.01 | 80.10 | 85.26 | 81.39 | 83.23 |
| UO | B | 49.54 | 59.61 | 54.77 | 58.41 | 62.16 | 68.07 | - | - | - | - |
|  |  | 56.45 | 64.04 | 63.28 | 65.66 | 69.35 | 75.76 | | | | |
|  | UB | 48.67 | 63.49 | 55.77 | 56.98 | 59.63 | 69.82 | 74.70 | 75.88 | 79.65 | 72.28 |
|  |  | 57.08 | 71.60 | 69.02 | 70.10 | 75.41 | 81.39 | 78.18 | 79.92 | 78.56 | 80.81 |

On DS-I, previous algorithms for gesture classification, assuming unknown boundaries, achieved a classification accuracy of up to 81% (Table 1). In contrast, assuming known boundaries, most variants of HMM, LDS, and DCC-CSM methods achieved comparable or better gesture classification accuracies on the same dataset (Table 2). Specifically, HMM with the simpler model (3S1M), LDS (SVM Fro), and DCC7 (temporal) appear to perform better than the other methods we evaluated. Since DCC-CSM memorizes the performed pattern, its performance decreases significantly with smaller classes. Those insignificant performances were excluded from Table 2.

On DS-II, DCC-CSM methods (DCC7, temporal) classified gestures more accurately than HMM and LDS methods within nearly all skill levels (Table 3). All methods were sensitive to training with data leaving-one-user-out.

Our findings on gesture classification using DS-I are not directly comparable to those using DS-II. However, the near perfect gesture classification by DCC-CSM methods on DS-II suggests that these methods are sensitive to size of the training sample. DCC-CSM methods using temporal windows were more accurate than those using spatial windows. We believe that the differential performance between temporal and spatial windows is because the former captures change over time, which is a component of velocity of the motion trajectory. DCC19 was not consistently more accurate than DCC7, as we anticipated this maybe because DCC19 yields shorter strings than DCC7 that are then commonly seen for each gesture.

**Table 3.** Gesture classification performance (with known skill level), macro (top number) and micro (bottom number) averages, percentage of correct segments on DS-II (chance=33%).

| Evaluation method | Known skill level | HMM 3S3M | HMM 3S1M | NN Mar | NN Fro | SVM Mar | SVM Fro | DCC7 spatial | DCC7 temporal | DCC19 spatial | DCC19 temporal |
|---|---|---|---|---|---|---|---|---|---|---|---|
| k-fold | Novice | 59.98 61.35 | 73.05 75.78 | 70.97 69.92 | 70.82 71.18 | 71.93 75.27 | 74.78 78.75 | 90.77 91.83 | 96.94 98.35 | 75.77 75.85 | 79.87 80.89 |
| | Inter | 70.31 67.81 | 81.14 83.46 | 71.45 72.03 | 71.80 71.99 | 71.12 74.38 | 76.63 78.10 | 76.62 83.78 | 98.81 99.25 | 92.14 91.17 | 82.74 83.80 |
| | Expert | 69.41 69.13 | 80.26 81.96 | 66.44 66.76 | 69.91 68.54 | 63.64 70.00 | 67.34 71.74 | 87.78 91.38 | 94.81 95.90 | 86.14 87.46 | 88.35 92.15 |
| UO | Novice | 53.89 55.73 | 64.17 63.93 | 64.15 67.08 | 64.56 65.70 | 66.53 71.14 | 75.42 74.78 | 69.38 67.99 | 74.18 83.39 | 47.32 55.40 | 85.33 89.58 |
| | Inter | 75.17 68.63 | 74.02 78.63 | 69.28 69.87 | 66.95 69.48 | 70.19 73.18 | 72.90 76.01 | 63.88 54.91 | 70.03 74.07 | 70.94 70.18 | 74.23 75.76 |
| | Expert | 52.95 59.62 | 71.14 76.05 | 57.72 60.60 | 61.29 64.92 | 53.13 62.08 | 64.96 72.38 | 57.06 45.71 | 88.32 89.73 | 71.66 78.57 | 75.52 78.08 |

DCC-CSM methods achieved nearly 98% skill classification accuracy for the "pull" gesture (Table 4). DCC-CSM methods simultaneously classified both gesture and skill with nearly 97% accuracy (k-fold; Table 5), which was sensitive to training with data leaving out one user.

**Table 4.** Skill classification performance (with known performed gesture), macro/micro averages on DS-II (chance=33%)

| Evaluation method | Known gesture | DCC7 spatial | DCC7 temporal | DCC19 spatial | DCC19 temporal |
|---|---|---|---|---|---|
| k-fold | grab | 90.85 91.14 | 84.78 86.16 | 88.26 89.10 | 82.74 83.45 |
| | pull | 90.20 90.00 | 97.85 97.86 | 90.66 90.68 | 96.85 96.85 |
| | rotate | 90.25 91.60 | 93.13 93.60 | 88.64 89.00 | 95.23 95.80 |
| UO | grab | 63.17 64.22 | 91.88 91.45 | 40.41 42.44 | 78.60 78.73 |
| | pull | 72.52 73.20 | 86.26 86.71 | 68.45 70.10 | 71.29 71.10 |
| | rotate | 85.29 85.87 | 75.39 76.09 | 72.02 71.74 | 74.76 75.00 |

**Table 5.** Simultaneous gesture and skill classification performance (with no prior knowledge) on DS-II (chance=11%)

| Evaluation method | DCC7 spatial | DCC7 temporal | DCC19 spatial | DCC19 temporal |
|---|---|---|---|---|
| k-fold | 94.98 96.62 | 84.78 96.92 | 88.48 91.37 | 92.41 91.37 |
| UO | 66.05 67.47 | 70.91 78.35 | 47.46 50.30 | 58.83 68.64 |

## 5    Conclusion

We evaluated DCC-CSM methods, and compared them with existing HMM and LDS methods, for detection of surgical gestures and skill on two datasets using two cross-validation approaches. DCC-CSM methods were at least as accurate or were more accurate than HMM and LDS methods under most experimental conditions on both datasets. Whereas HMM and LDS methods relied on a detailed kinematic representation of surgical tool motion, DCC-CSM methods used only position and orientation of the tool-tip. DCC-CSM methods offer a way to seamlessly classify both gesture and skill. The sensitivity of DCC-CSM methods to detect various surgical gestures, in other datasets, using alternate similarity metrics and different methods to assign the ground-truth for skill has yet to be evaluated.

**Acknowledgment.** This work was funded by NSF CDI-0941362 and CPS CNS-0931805. Any opinions, findings, conclusions or recommendations expressed in this material are those of the authors and do not necessarily reflect the views of the National Science Foundation. Benjamín Béjar was supported in part by the Talentia Fellowships Program of the Andalusian Regional Ministry of Economy, Innovation and Science. The authors would like to thank Dr. Grace Chen for scoring the surgeries and Anand Malpani, Lingling Tao and George Chen for assistance in data annotation.

# References

1. Bell, R.H.: Why Johnny cannot operate. Surgery 146, 533–542 (2009)
2. Gearhart, S.L., Wang, M.H., Gilson, M.M., Chen, B., Kern, D.E.: Teaching and assessing technical proficiency in surgical subspecialty fellowships. Journal of Surgical Education 69, 521–528 (2012)
3. Reiley, C.E., Lin, H.C., Yuh, D.D., Hager, G.D.: A Review of Methods for Objective Surgical Skill Evaluation. Surgical Endoscopy 25, 356–366 (2011)
4. Ahmidi, N., Hager, G.D., Ishii, L., Gallia, G.L., Ishii, M.: Robotic Path Planning for Surgeon Skill Evaluation in Minimally-Invasive Sinus Surgery. In: Ayache, N., Delingette, H., Golland, P., Mori, K. (eds.) MICCAI 2012, Part I. LNCS, vol. 7510, pp. 471–478. Springer, Heidelberg (2012)
5. Zappella, L., Béjar, B., Hager, G., Vidal, R.: Surgical gesture classification from video and kinematic data. Medical Image Analysis (2013)
6. Tao, L., Elhamifar, E., Khudanpur, S., Hager, G.D., Vidal, R.: Sparse Hidden Markov Models for Surgical Gesture Classification and Skill Evaluation. In: Abolmaesumi, P., Joskowicz, L., Navab, N., Jannin, P. (eds.) IPCAI 2012. LNCS, vol. 7330, pp. 167–177. Springer, Heidelberg (2012)
7. Rosen, J., Solazzo, M., Hannaford, B., Sinanan, M.: Task decomposition of laparoscopic surgery for objective evaluation of surgical residents' learning curve using hidden Markov model. Computer Aided Surgery 7(1), 49–61 (2002)
8. Dosis, A., Bello, F., Gillies, D., Undre, S., Aggarwal, R., Darzi, A.: Laparoscopic task recognition using hidden Markov models. Studies in Health Technology and Informatics 111, 115–122 (2005)
9. Varadarajan, B.: Learning and inference algorithms for dynamical system models of dexterous motion. PhD thesis, Johns Hopkins University (2011)
10. Kumar, R., Jog, A., Vagvolgyi, B., Nguyen, H., Hager, G.D., Chen, C.C.G.: Objective measures for longitudinal assessment of robotic surgery training. The Journal of Thoracic and Cardiovascular Surgery 143(3), 528–534 (2012)
11. Martin, J.A., Regehr, G., Reznick, R., MacRae, H., Murnaghan, J., Hutchison, C., Brown, M.: Objective Structured Assessment of Technical Skill for Surgical Residents. British Journal of Surgery 84, 273–278 (1997)

# Global Registration of Ultrasound to MRI Using the LC² Metric for Enabling Neurosurgical Guidance

Wolfgang Wein[1], Alexander Ladikos[1], Bernhard Fuerst[2], Amit Shah[2], Kanishka Sharma[2], and Nassir Navab[2]

[1] ImFusion GmbH, München, Germany
[2] Computer Aided Medical Procedures, Technische Universität München, Germany

**Abstract.** Automatic and robust registration of pre-operative magnetic resonance imaging (MRI) and intra-operative ultrasound (US) is essential to neurosurgery. We reformulate and extend an approach which uses a Linear Correlation of Linear Combination (LC²)-based similarity metric, yielding a novel algorithm which allows for fully automatic US-MRI registration in the matter of seconds. It is invariant with respect to the unknown and locally varying relationship between US image intensities and both MRI intensity and its gradient. The overall method based on this both recovers global rigid alignment, as well as the parameters of a free-form-deformation (FFD) model. The algorithm is evaluated on 14 clinical neurosurgical cases with tumors, with an average landmark-based error of $2.52\,mm$ for the rigid transformation. In addition, we systematically study the accuracy, precision, and capture range of the algorithm, as well as its sensitivity to different choices of parameters.

## 1 Introduction

Modern neurosurgery heavily relies on both pre-operative and interventional medical imaging, in particular MRI and US. MRI provides a good visualization of tumors, a relatively large field of view and good reproducibility. Its use as intra-operative imaging modality is possible [8], however with limited accessibility to the patient and high workflow complexity. On the other hand, US is inexpensive and easy to use, but imaging quality is reduced, fewer anatomical details are visible and, in general, US is operator-dependent and harder to interpret. Also, the field of view is limited and direction dependent. The combination of both modalities would allow to integrate high-contrast pre-operative MRI data into the interventional suite. Therefore, quick, robust and automatic alignment of MRI and US images is of high importance. In contrast to MRI, ultrasound provides real-time 2D images, which, when tracking the ultrasound transducer, can be interpreted in 3D space. This has been used in the past decades for brain examinations, for instance to localize tumors, determine their tissue and boundary properties, and detect brain shift.

Registering US and MRI images is a complex and still not satisfactorily solved problem, mostly because the nature of the represented information is completely

K. Mori et al. (Eds.): MICCAI 2013, Part I, LNCS 8149, pp. 34–41, 2013.

different for both modalities. MRI intensities are correlated to relaxation times, which in turn depend on the tissue type and hydrogen concentration, while US images are a representation of acoustic impedance transitions. Those in turn can be both reflections on large structures (hence correlating to some extent to the gradient of MRI), or reflections from the tissue inhomogeneities that cause the characteristic brightness and texture of certain tissue types (in that case correlating to the MRI intensities directly). As an additional challenge, US exhibits various direction-dependent artifacts.

Therefore, the basic and well known off-the-shelf registration approaches are known to fail, which includes registration using cost functions based on sum of squared distances, mutual information [4] or correlation ratio [12]. A method which uses a measure based on 3D gradient orientations in both US and MRI is presented in [3], however such an approach discards valuable MRI intensity information and hence requires either optimal data or close initialization. Many of the best existing approaches transform MRI and/or US intensities under application- and organ-specific considerations, in order to make them easily comparable. This is done, for example, for liver vasculature in [9], with significant effort due to learning-based pre-processing. Similarly, pseudo-US images may be generated using segmented structures from MRI [1,2,5,6]. In light of the modality-specific considerations, the most promising general strategy for robust US-MRI registration, without relying on application-specific pre-processing or segmentation, is to compare US to both the MRI intensity and its gradient, as pioneered in [12], where a global polynomial intensity relationship is fitted during registration. The alternating optimization of the rigid pose and the polynomial coefficients, as well as the fact that it is a global mapping, limit the convergence range. Higher-dimensional Mutual Information ($\alpha$-MI) is theoretically suited to assess US-MRI alignment based on both intensity and gradient information (in fact, an arbitrary number of features may be used). However, current approaches are neither practical in terms of implementation effort nor computation time [11]. Powerful tools for image registration are similarity measures which are invariant to local changes, such as local normalized cross-correlation (invariant wrt. local brightness and contrast). In [13] the similarity measure Linear Correlation of Linear Combination ($LC^2$) is presented, which exhibits local invariance to how much two channels of information contribute to an ultrasound image. The entire method has been specially designed for US-CT registration, where a strong correlation between X-ray attenuation coefficients and acoustic impedance is known, which allows a simulation of ultrasound effects from CT. These incorporate estimates of the acoustic attenuation, multiple reflections, and shadowing, which can not directly be estimated from MRI.

In this paper, we adapt the $LC^2$ formulation for the registration of interventional US to (pre-operative) MRI, and extend it to non-linear deformations. It results in a globally convergent, robust new algorithm, which we evaluate on a database of 14 patients with ground-truth information.

## 2   Method

**Similarity Measure:** Instead of correlating US intensities with two channels of simulated information from CT as in [13], we use $LC^2$ to correlate US with both the MRI intensity values $p$ and its spatial gradient magnitude $g = |\nabla p|$. The local $LC^2$ value is computed for each pixel $\mathbf{x_i}$ in each ultrasound image, considering a neighborhood $\Omega(\mathbf{x_i})$ of $m$ pixels. For each patch of $m$ pixels, the contribution of MRI intensity values $p$ and gradient magnitudes $g$ are unknown. Therefore, we define an intensity function $f(\mathbf{x_i})$ as a function of the transformed MRI intensities $p_i = p(T(\mathbf{x_i}))$ and gradients $g_i = g(T(\mathbf{x_i})) = |\nabla p_i|$ as:

$$f(\mathbf{x_i}) = \alpha p_i + \beta g_i + \gamma, \tag{1}$$

where $y_i = \{\alpha, \beta, \gamma\}$ denotes the unknown parameters of the influence of the MRI intensities and gradients within $\Omega(\mathbf{x_i})$. They can be estimated by minimizing the difference of the intensity function and the ultrasound image intensity $u_i$:

$$\left\| M \begin{pmatrix} \alpha \\ \beta \\ \gamma \end{pmatrix} - \begin{pmatrix} u_1 \\ \vdots \\ u_m \end{pmatrix} \right\|^2 \quad \text{where } M = \begin{pmatrix} p_1 & g_1 & 1 \\ \vdots & \vdots & \vdots \\ p_m & g_m & 1 \end{pmatrix}, \tag{2}$$

which can be solved using ordinary least squares with the pseudo-inverse of M. This results in a parameter triple $y_i$ for each pixel $\mathbf{x_i}$, which is only depending on the neighborhood $\Omega(\mathbf{x_i})$ and therefore compensating for changing influences of tissue interfaces or organ-internal intensities. The local similarity is then:

$$S(u, M) = 1 - \frac{\sum_{\mathbf{x_i}} |u(\mathbf{x_i}) - My|^2}{\sum_{\mathbf{x_i}} Var(u(\mathbf{x_i}))} \tag{3}$$

The overall similarity is the weighted sum of eq. 3 with the local variance of the US image. This suppresses regions without structural appearance, therefore allowing to cope with ultrasonic occlusions implicitly, without the need to simulate them.

**Computation:** We compute $LC^2$ on the original 2D US image slices located in 3D-space through the tracking data, as opposed to using a 3D compounded volume. This has four main advantages:

1. An unnecessary resampling step of the ultrasound image data, which may degrade its quality, is avoided.
2. Registration can start as soon as the first US frames are available, catering to real-time applications in the operating room.
3. One may also optimize the US probe calibration parameters or further parameters expressing e.g. tracking system errors.
4. Image information within slices is inherently more consistent, because all scan-lines of an image are acquired within a short duration and void of tracking errors.

Extracting the MRI intensity and gradient at the presumed location in the 3D volume is performed on the GPU using its hardware tri-linear interpolation. We then compute eq. 3 using a multi-core recursive filtering strategy; however a GPU implementation is equally possible. The MRI image data is used in full resolution (typically iso-tropic voxel size of $0.5mm$). The higher-resolution US frames are down-sampled such that their pixel size is smaller than twice the voxel size (assuring that tri-linear interpolation never discards MRI voxel information within the oblique US planes). Similarly, US frames are skipped such that no overlapping planes occur, with average spacing between the image centers < $1.5mm$ (mostly yielding smaller spacing in the area of interest).

**Optimization of Rigid Transformation:** Due to the least-squares fitting in eq. 2 which is computed for every US image pixel, an analytic derivative of $LC^2$ is difficult to compute. Therefore we use Bound Optimization by Quadratic Approximation (BOBYQA) [10], which internally creates own derivative approximations, resulting in fewer evaluations than most other direct search methods. While we recommend and use this optimizer throughout this paper, clinical requirements on capture range may necessitate other techniques. In particular, global optimization strategies may be chosen that perform a more thorough search within specified bounds.

**Deformable Registration:** The optimizer first seeks the 6 rigid transformation parameters as described above. Successively, we use a free-form deformation model with cubic splines, which is applied in the same GPU kernel which extracts MRI intensity/gradient information. More specifically, $2x2x4$ control points are placed within the bounding box of the rigidly registered ultrasound sweep. The 3-displacement vectors are then optimized for all control points using BOBYQA.

## 3    Experiments and Results

### 3.1    Clinical Data

To evaluate our method and compare the results to other publications, we used a publicly available database containing Brain Images with Tumors for Evaluation from Montreal Neurological Institute (MNI BITE) [7], with pre-operative T1-weighted MRI and pre-resection 3D freehand US from 14 patients. Initial transformations and corresponding landmarks for each US-MRI pair are included. Therefore we can provide ground truth evaluations, and denote the average Euclidean distance of the landmarks as Fiducial Registration Error (FRE).

### 3.2    Registration Results

Tab. 1 depicts the results of our algorithm for all 14 data sets.[1] Our rigid registration yields almost exactly the same FRE values as [3], which suggests that both methods achieve the correct optimum transformation. The errors in [11] are

---

[1] Computation times measured with Intel i7-3770 CPU and NVIDIA GTX 570 GPU.

**Table 1.** Overview of clinical data [7], previous published results [3,11], and results using our method for rigid and deformable registration including computation times

| Dataset Overview and Related Methods | | | | | | | | | | | | | | |
|---|---|---|---|---|---|---|---|---|---|---|---|---|---|---|
| Patient Number | 1 | 2 | 3 | 4 | 5 | 6 | 7 | 8 | 9 | 10 | 11 | 12 | 13 | 14 | mean |
| Number of Tags | 37 | 35 | 40 | 32 | 31 | 37 | 19 | 23 | 21 | 25 | 25 | 21 | 23 | 23 | - |
| Initial FRE $(mm)$ | 4.93 | 6.30 | 9.38 | 3.93 | 2.62 | 2.30 | 3.04 | 3.75 | 5.09 | 2.99 | 1.52 | 3.70 | 5.15 | 3.77 | 4.18±5.20 |
| US Spacing $(mm)$ | 0.24 | 0.42 | 0.23 | 0.20 | 0.25 | 0.17 | 0.24 | 0.18 | 0.18 | 0.22 | 0.16 | 0.18 | 0.21 | 0.19 | 0.22±0.20 |
| FRE in [3] $(mm)$ | 4.89 | 1.79 | 2.73 | 1.68 | 2.12 | 1.81 | 2.51 | 2.63 | 2.7 | 1.95 | 1.56 | 2.64 | 3.47 | 2.94 | 2.53±0.87 |
| FRE in [11] $(mm)$ | - | 2.05 | 2.76 | 1.92 | 2.71 | 1.89 | 2.05 | 2.89 | 2.93 | 2.75 | 1.28 | 2.67 | 2.82 | 2.34 | 2.57±0.82 |

| Registration Results using $LC^2$ | | | | | | | | | | | | | | |
|---|---|---|---|---|---|---|---|---|---|---|---|---|---|---|
| FRE Rigid $(mm)$ | 4.82 | 1.73 | 2.76 | 1.96 | 2.14 | 1.94 | 2.33 | 2.87 | 2.81 | 2.06 | 2.18 | 2.67 | 3.58 | 2.48 | 2.52 ±0.87 |
| Precision $(mm)$ | 0.01 | 0.01 | 0.01 | 0.01 | 0.02 | 0.01 | 0.05 | 0.30 | 0.02 | 0.00 | 0.03 | 0.15 | 0.05 | 0.04 | 0.05 ±0.08 |
| Time Rigid $(sec)$ | 5.9 | 8.3 | 11.1 | 5.7 | 7.1 | 8.2 | 18.2 | 8.6 | 6.0 | 23.4 | 17.3 | 25.8 | 8.1 | 7.0 | 11.5 ±6.8 |
| FRE Def. $(mm)$ | 4.95 | 1.64 | 2.43 | 1.91 | 2.26 | 2.2 | 2.52 | 3.64 | 2.65 | 2.09 | 1.76 | 2.45 | 3.71 | 2.76 | 2.64 ±0.9 |
| Time Def. $(sec)$ | 158 | 141 | 279 | 92 | 133 | 166 | 563 | 312 | 76 | 675 | 597 | 93 | 106 | 282 | 262 ±204 |

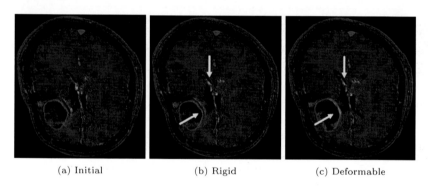

(a) Initial      (b) Rigid      (c) Deformable

**Fig. 1.** Registration result of patient 6, with US superimposed on an axial MRI slice

slightly higher (with computation times of several hours per data set), which indicates that applying their proposed deformable registration to the mostly rigid[2] data does not provide much benefit. Similarly, our deformable registration can further improve on the FRE value only in a few of the cases. We believe that the change of landmark errors induced by deformable registration lies within the range of the fiducial localization error (FLE) of the data, especially since some of the landmarks are located along boundaries, not only 3D-corner structures. Fig. 1 depicts the registration results on patient 6. It can be seen that the visual alignment is significantly improved after deformable registration.

### 3.3   Accuracy, Precision and Capture Range

While some initial errors are significantly away from the correct optimum (e.g. patients 2 and 3), an analysis about the suitability of our algorithm to reach the optimum under all conditions is required. Randomized trials were

---

[2] The pre-resection ultrasound has been acquired before opening the dura.

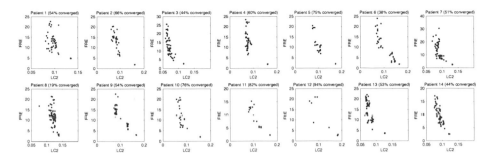

**Fig. 2.** Random study results of all patients. The converged results are clustered in the lower right corner (highlighted in blue, outliers red).

executed on all data sets, repeating the rigid registration for randomly displaced starting positions ($\pm 10mm/^\circ$ in all 6 parameters). Comparing the final FRE against the $LC^2$ metric, we discovered that the best pose is always perfectly separated by a significantly higher similarity. This proves that our method allows for global registration; the results for all patients are shown in Fig. 2, including the percentage of converged executions. The mean value of the converged results is the *accuracy*, its standard deviation the *precision*, and the range of initial FRE values from which all executions converge with a smaller than desired number of outliers is the *capture range*. The outlier behavior is also visualized in figure 4(a), where their number is plotted against the initial FRE for some patients. For an initial FRE $< 8mm$ a single local optimization with BOBYQA is sufficient.

Unfortunately, precision and capture range are often not reported in the literature. Since the gradient orientation alignment (GOA) method [3] yields similar FRE values, we implemented it and re-ran the aforementioned randomized trials with it. We obtain $> 90\%$ outliers; further investigation into the cost function properties revealed that only a minor local optimum is present, see Fig. 3(b) for an example. A possible explanation is, that without further heuristics the GOA method would line up strong gradients from e.g. dura mater or skull; besides, using only gradients larger than a threshold limits the image content considered, preventing a smooth similarity increase. While we believe these to be general issues, it has to be acknowledged that better results may be obtained by changing certain implementation details such as resolution, smoothing and interpolation.

### 3.4    Parameter Sensitivity

To investigate the sensitivity of our method to the choice of parameters, we computed accuracy and precision for different $LC^2$ patch sizes, and number of US frames used (i.e. spacing in between), see Fig. 4. The registration results are similar for patch sizes 2-24, therefore our method is rather insensitive to the choice of this parameter. For all other results presented, we used a value of 9 (hence $m = (2 * 9 + 1)^2 = 361$). Overly large patches result in a global mapping of MRI intensity and gradient, removing the main advantage of $LC^2$ over other methods (robustness wrt. local changes of intensity-gradient relationship). Consistently good results are obtained with an average spacing $< 5\,mm$.

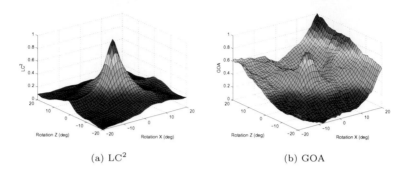

(a) LC$^2$                    (b) GOA

**Fig. 3.** Plots of different cost functions for two rotation parameters on patient 2

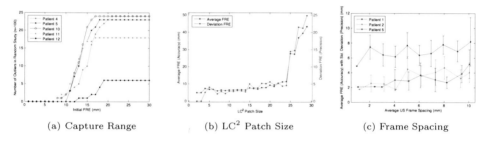

(a) Capture Range          (b) LC$^2$ Patch Size          (c) Frame Spacing

**Fig. 4.** Relationship between initial FRE and outliers (a); dependency of accuracy on LC$^2$ patch size (b) and US frame spacing (c)

For deformable registration, we chose $< 1.5\,mm$ to make sure we are not missing even smallest structures. Last but not least, we have investigated the effect of using the dot product of the MRI gradient $g$ with the US beam direction, instead of $g$ directly. This reduces the influence of vertical gradients, similar to the US simulation in [13]. Interestingly, this results in $10 - 25\%$ more outliers (the cost function becomes more non-linear due to the added directional dependance).

## 4    Conclusion

We have introduced an algorithm based on the LC$^2$ similarity metric, which can rigidly register US-MRI data within a few seconds, and non-linearly within a few minutes. Apart from its efficiency and global convergence, its main strength lies in its simplicity. As opposed to previous works involving the simulation of US imaging, we actually refrain from using the US beam direction and attenuation (which is more difficult with MRI as opposed to CT), and directly compare the MRI intensity and 3D gradient magnitude to US. This smoothens the topology of the cost function, while LC$^2$ at the same time locally picks the most suited structures. We have shown that the cost function allows for global registration, thoroughly evaluating our method on all 14 patients of an US-MRI image database. We obtain superior results both in terms of computation time and robustness with respect to previously proposed methods on the same data.

**Acknowledgments.** The authors affiliated with Technische Universität München are partially supported by the EU 7th Framework Program (FP7/2007-2013 and FP7/ICT-2009-6) under Grant Agreements No. 256984 (EndoTOFPET-US) and No. 270460 (ACTIVE) and by a Marie Curie Early Initial Training Network Fellowship under contract number (PITN-GA-2011-289355-PicoSEC-MCNet).

# References

1. Comeau, R.M., Sadikot, A.F., Fenster, A., Peters, T.M.: Intraoperative Ultrasound for Guidance and Tissue Shift Correction in Image-Guided Neurosurgery. Medical Physics 27, 787 (2000)
2. Coupé, P., Hellier, P., Morandi, X., Barillot, C.: 3D Rigid Registration of Intraoperative Ultrasound and Preoperative MR Brain Images Based on Hyperechogenic Structures. Journal of Biomedical Imaging 2012, 1 (2012)
3. De Nigris, D., Collins, D.L., Arbel, T.: Fast and Robust Registration Based on Gradient Orientations: Case Study Matching Intra-Operative Ultrasound to Pre-Operative MRI in Neurosurgery. In: Abolmaesumi, P., Joskowicz, L., Navab, N., Jannin, P. (eds.) IPCAI 2012. LNCS, vol. 7330, pp. 125–134. Springer, Heidelberg (2012)
4. Huang, X., Hill, N., Ren, J., Guiraudon, G., Boughner, D., Peters, T.: Dynamic 3D Ultrasound and MR Image Registration of the Beating Heart. In: Medical Image Computing and Computer-Assisted Intervention 2005, pp. 171–178 (2005)
5. King, A., Rhode, K., Ma, Y., Yao, C., Jansen, C., Razavi, R., Penney, G.: Registering Preprocedure Volumetric Images With Intraprocedure 3-D Ultrasound Using an Ultrasound Imaging Model. IEEE Trans. Med. Imag. 29(3), 924–937 (2010)
6. Kuklisova-Murgasova, M., Cifor, A., Napolitano, R., Papageorghiou, A., Quaghebeur, G., Noble, J.A., Schnabel, J.A.: Registration of 3D Fetal Brain US and MRI. In: Ayache, N., Delingette, H., Golland, P., Mori, K. (eds.) MICCAI 2012, Part II. LNCS, vol. 7511, pp. 667–674. Springer, Heidelberg (2012)
7. Mercier, L., Del Maestro, R., Petrecca, K., Araujo, D., Haegelen, C., Collins, D.: Online Database of Clinical MR and Ultrasound Images of Brain Tumors. Medical Physics 39, 3253 (2012)
8. Moriarty, T., Kikinis, R., Jolesz, F., Black, P., Alexander, E.: Magnetic resonance imaging therapy. Intraoperative MR imaging. Neurosurg. Clin. N Am. 7, 323–331 (1996)
9. Penney, G., Blackall, J., Hamady, M., Sabharwal, T., Adam, A., Hawkes, D., et al.: Registration of Freehand 3D Ultrasound and Magnetic Resonance Liver Images. Medical Image Analysis 8(1), 81–91 (2004)
10. Powell, M.J.: The BOBYQA Algorithm for Bound Constrained Optimization without Derivatives. Cambridge Report NA2009/06, University of Cambridge (2009)
11. Rivaz, H., Collins, D.L.: Self-similarity Weighted Mutual Information: A New Non-rigid Image Registration Metric. In: Ayache, N., Delingette, H., Golland, P., Mori, K. (eds.) MICCAI 2012, Part III. LNCS, vol. 7512, pp. 91–98. Springer, Heidelberg (2012)
12. Roche, A., Pennec, X., Malandain, G., Ayache, N.: Rigid Registration of 3-D Ultrasound with MR Images: A New Approach Combining Intensity and Gradient Information. IEEE Transactions on Medical Imaging 20(10), 1038–1049 (2001)
13. Wein, W., Brunke, S., Khamene, A., Callstrom, M., Navab, N.: Automatic CT-Ultrasound Registration for Diagnostic Imaging and Image-Guided Intervention. Medical Image Analysis 12(5), 577 (2008)

# Real-Time Dense Stereo Reconstruction Using Convex Optimisation with a Cost-Volume for Image-Guided Robotic Surgery[*]

Ping-Lin Chang[1], Danail Stoyanov[3], Andrew J. Davison[1],
and Philip "Eddie" Edwards[1,2]

[1] Department of Computing
[2] Department of Surgery and Cancer
Imperial College London, United Kingdom
{p.chang10,a.davison,eddie.edwards}@imperial.ac.uk
[3] Centre for Medical Image Computing and Department of Computer Science
University College London, United Kingdom
danail.stoyanov@ucl.ac.uk

**Abstract.** Reconstructing the depth of stereo-endoscopic scenes is an important step in providing accurate guidance in robotic-assisted minimally invasive surgery. Stereo reconstruction has been studied for decades but remains a challenge in endoscopic imaging. Current approaches can easily fail to reconstruct an accurate and smooth 3D model due to textureless tissue appearance in the real surgical scene and occlusion by instruments. To tackle these problems, we propose a dense stereo reconstruction algorithm using convex optimisation with a cost-volume to efficiently and effectively reconstruct a smooth model while maintaining depth discontinuity. The proposed approach has been validated by quantitative evaluation using simulation and real phantom data with known ground truth. We also report qualitative results from real surgical images. The algorithm outperforms state of the art methods and can be easily parallelised to run in real-time on recent graphics hardware.

## 1 Introduction

An important challenge in robotic-assisted laparoscopic surgery is the 3D reconstruction of the observed surgical site. The recovered 3D scene can provide a rich source of information for visualisation and interaction, enabling vision-based camera tracking and registration to a preoperative model for surgical navigation [2, 6, 7]. With the da Vinci surgical system the presence of a stereoscopic laparoscope means that computational stereo is a practical and feasible approach to *in vivo* reconstruction [3, 15]. However, surgical scenes are challenging for 3D reconstruction algorithms because of texture-poor appearance, occlusions, specular reflection and discontinuities due to instruments.

[*] This research is partly supported by ERC Starting Grant 210346, CRUK grant A8087/C24250 and The Royal Academy of Engineering/EPSRC Research Fellowship.

Reconstruction of the stereo-endoscopic view for surgical navigation has been an active area of research for over a decade [6,7]. Much of the prior work has focused on beating heart surgery [3,5,9,15], where the reconstructed heart surface could be used for motion stabilisation or registration to a preoperative model. To achieve smooth and robust stereo reconstruction, methods have been proposed that use a parametric surface description [5] to overcome texture homogeneity. Alternatively region growing starting from sparse features has been reported [15] and thin-plate spline interpolation of robust features [9]. A sophisticated framework which uses a hybrid CPU-GPU algorithm to fuse temporal reconstruction into a global model has been proposed [10]. In all cases the aim is to approach real-time reconstruction, and to this end GPU implementations and parallelisation are necessary.

In this paper, we build on recent advances in computer vision and the use of variational techniques to efficiently and effectively reconstruct stereo-endoscopic scenes using stereo image pairs. This is achieved by constructing a cost-volume with a reliable data term and performing convex optimisation to solve a Huber-$L^1$ model. The proposed algorithm can also be effectively parallelised on the GPU for real-time performance. Compared with the state of the art, the proposed approach yields more accurate reconstruction in empirical studies. We illustrate this with extensive validation using synthetic and phantom data with known ground truth and qualitative results from *in vivo* robotic surgery sequences.

## 2   Proposed Approach

The first step of the proposed algorithm is to construct a 3D cost-volume using a pixel-wise data term with respect to the disparities. An efficient convex optimisation for solving a Huber-$L^1$ model is then performed by decoupling the model into a Huber-$L^2$ model and the cost-volume, which can be resolved by a primal-dual algorithm and exhaustive search alternately.

### 2.1   Cost-Volume Construction

In definition, a cost-volume $C : \Omega_C \to \mathbf{R}$, where $\Omega_C \subseteq \mathbf{R}^3$, is a discrete function which maps a 3-vector to a cost value. In rectified stereo matching the cost-volume is also called the disparity space image (DSI) [12] which is defined as

$$C\big(\mathbf{x}, \mathbf{u}(\mathbf{x})\big) = \rho\big(I_l(\mathbf{x}), I_r(\mathbf{x}')\big). \tag{1}$$

The stereo images are assumed to be undistorted and rectified in advance. Functions $I_l$ and $I_r : \Omega_I \to \mathbf{R}^3$ are the left and right colour image and $\Omega_I \subseteq \mathbf{R}^2$. As per convention, the Eq. 1 takes the left image as reference and stereo matching is performed in the right image, and thus $\mathbf{x} = (x, y)^\top$ and $\mathbf{x}' = (x - \mathbf{u}(\mathbf{x}), y)^\top$. The function $\mathbf{u} : \Omega_I \to \mathcal{D}$ maps a pixel location to a set of discrete integer disparities within a range $\mathcal{D} = [d_{min}, d_{max}]$. The cost-volume $C$ is then constructed using all of the disparities for each pixel in the image domain $\Omega_I$. The size of the cost-volume is therefore $|\Omega_I| \times |\mathcal{D}|$. Note that the resolution of the disparity $|\mathcal{D}|$, $d_{min}$ and $d_{max}$ are dependent on scenes and camera profiles.

**Robust Data-Fidelity Term.** In a pure vision-based reconstruction problem, the function $\rho$ in the Eq. 1 can be an arbitrary photometric measure which defines the data-fidelity term. The data fidelity is essential since the later convex optimisation significantly relies on it.

We illustrate the effects of different measures with a simulation stereo pair generated by a textured cone model as shown in Fig. 1a. Raw reconstruction is achieved using a winner-takes-all scheme which extracts the disparity pixel-wise according to the minimum cost. The simplest absolute difference (AD) measure gives a very noisy raw reconstruction as shown in Fig. 1b. To reduce the noise, one may adopt the sum of absolute differences (SAD) or sum of squared differences (SSD) which aggregate costs locally. Alternatively, applying more sophisticated edge-preserving local filtering can yield an even better result [8, 10]. Fig. 1c shows the result after bilateral filtering (BF) is applied to Fig. 1b. However, our empirical studies have shown that if the original measure is error-prone, the later aggregation in the cost-volume space can increase the error, which results in poor data-fidelity. This commonly happens in textureless regions, half-occluded areas and where the illumination changes.

In contrast, zero-mean normalised cross-correlation (ZNCC) implicitly performs the aggregation using a window patch, so correlation is calculated over a pixel neighbourhood. This results in a measure more tolerant to different camera gain or bias and can also provide better fidelity in textureless regions. Fig. 1d shows the raw reconstruction using ZNCC. In this work we therefore use ZNCC as the data term measure to construct the cost-volume.

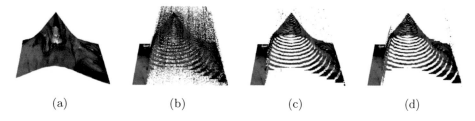

(a)                (b)                (c)                (d)

**Fig. 1.** The raw reconstruction results using a winner-takes-all scheme with the cost-volume. (a) The simulated ground truth textured model. (b) The raw reconstruction using AD. (c) The result after applying BF to (b). (d) The raw reconstruction using ZNCC.

## 2.2   Huber-$L^1$ Convex Optimisation with the Cost-Volume

Starting with the coarse reconstruction, the unknown disparity function $\mathbf{u}$ is further optimised by solving a Huber-$L^1$ variational energy functional which takes the cost-volume as data term and an image-driven weighted Huber-norm as a regulariser term. This is defined as

$$E(\mathbf{u}) = \int_{\Omega_I} \left\{ w(\mathbf{x}) \|\nabla \mathbf{u}(\mathbf{x})\|_{\varepsilon} + \lambda C(\mathbf{x}, \mathbf{u}(\mathbf{x})) \right\} \, \mathrm{d}\mathbf{x}, \tag{2}$$

where

$$\| \cdot \|_\varepsilon = \begin{cases} \frac{\| \cdot \|_2^2}{2\varepsilon} & \text{if } \| \cdot \|_2 \leq \varepsilon \\ \| \cdot \|_1 - \frac{\varepsilon}{2} & \text{otherwise.} \end{cases} \quad (3)$$

The Huber-norm $\| \cdot \|_\varepsilon$ allows the regulariser to constrain the gradient of disparity to a $L^2$ norm within a range $\varepsilon$ and out of that range a $L^1$ norm forming a total variation (TV) model so that $\varepsilon$ can adjust the degree of undesired staircasing effect and is normally set to 0.01 [16]. The effect of the regulariser is adjusted by $\lambda$. To design an image-driven anisotropic regulariser which can maintain disparity discontinuity across image edges, the function $w$ is defined as:

$$w(\mathbf{x}) = \exp(-\alpha \|\nabla I(\mathbf{x})\|_2). \quad (4)$$

Specifically, where a region has high edge magnitude, the output of this weighting function becomes low, which reduces the effect of the regulariser. We can flexibly adjust the support of the exponential function by setting variable $\alpha$.

Since Eq. 2 is non-convex in the data term and only convex in the regulariser term, to discover the global minimum, conventional approaches for optical flow or variational reconstruction algorithm resort to coarse-to-fine scheme [16]. This requires a good initial state for the global minimum to be found. In addition, reconstruction of coarser layers can lose details in the scene. By contrast, having a cost-volume helps us to avoid the expensive warping scheme. Following a recent large displacement optical flow algorithm [13], we decouple the data term and regulariser term by an auxiliary function $\mathbf{a} : \Omega_I \to \mathcal{D}$ to form a new energy functional:

$$E(\mathbf{u}, \mathbf{a}) = \int_{\Omega_I} \left\{ w(\mathbf{x}) \|\nabla \mathbf{u}(\mathbf{x})\|_\varepsilon + Q(\mathbf{u}(\mathbf{x}), \mathbf{a}(\mathbf{x})) + \lambda C(\mathbf{x}, \mathbf{a}(\mathbf{x})) \right\} d\mathbf{x}, \quad (5)$$

where

$$Q(\mathbf{u}(\mathbf{x}), \mathbf{a}(\mathbf{x})) = \frac{1}{2\theta} (\mathbf{u}(\mathbf{x}) - \mathbf{a}(\mathbf{x}))^2. \quad (6)$$

The first part $w(\mathbf{x}) \|\nabla \mathbf{u}(\mathbf{x})\|_\varepsilon + Q(\mathbf{u}(\mathbf{x}), \mathbf{a}(\mathbf{x}))$ is actually a Huber-$L^2$ model [1] which is similar to TV-$L^2$ Rudin-Osher-Fatemi model [11] and its global minimum can be found by using an efficient primal-dual algorithm [1,4] for solving the $\mathbf{u}$. Given a temporary solution $\mathbf{u}$, the global minimum of the later part $Q(\mathbf{u}(\mathbf{x}), \mathbf{a}(\mathbf{x})) + \lambda C(\mathbf{x}, \mathbf{a}(\mathbf{x}))$ can be simply found by performing an exhaustive search on $\mathbf{a}(\mathbf{x})$ among the disparities in the cost-volume. $\theta$ should be set as a small number to ensure $\mathbf{a}(\mathbf{x}) \simeq \mathbf{u}(\mathbf{x})$ when the algorithm converges.

The primal-dual algorithm works in continuous space so can directly achieve sub-pixel accuracy. Furthermore, the rate of convergence is $O(n)$ [1] which means we need only a few iterations to finish the process. This yields a very efficient and effective convex optimisation in contrast to a traditional global method such as the graph cuts. Following the cone model example in Fig. 1, Fig. 2 shows the convergence curves of the Huber-$L^1$ convex optimisation using different measures. ZNCC requires much fewer iterations to converge. The reconstruction result is

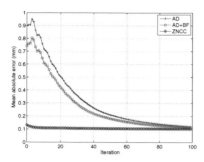 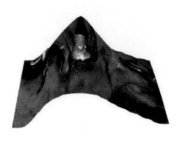

**Fig. 2.** Left: Convergence of the primal-dual algorithm using different measures as data term. The mean absolute error is calculated by comparing the reconstructed depth with the ground truth depth. Right: The result after the Huber-$L^1$ convex optimisation.

also shown in Fig. 2. One can observe the point cloud is now much smoother and the staircasing effect due to the discrete cost-volume has been largely eradicated.

## 3    Empirical Studies

All experiments are conducted on a workstation equipped with 3.1 GHz quad cores CPU and one NVIDIA GeForce GTX 670 graphics card with 2 GB global memory. To maximally exploit the power of parallel computation, all the calculations including the cost-volume construction and the convex optimisation are implemented in CUDA. Currently the proposed reconstruction approach is able to run at 20 fps with the resolution $|\mathbf{\Omega}_I| = 360 \times 288$ and $|\mathcal{D}| = 32$.

We first conduct a noise study to evaluate the robustness for different measures. The proposed approach is then quantitatively evaluated using a cardiac phantom dataset with an independent ground truth. Images in real robot-assisted laparoscopic prostatectomy are reconstructed for qualitative evaluation. In all experiments, only the disparity range $\mathcal{D}$ is dynamic and the rest of parameters for the convex optimisation are set as constants $\{\epsilon, \alpha, \theta, \lambda\} = \{0.01, 0.5, 0.1, 50\}$. The convex optimisation is finished in 150 iterations or if the energy function appears to have converged.

### 3.1    Noise Study

To investigate the robustness of different data terms, we intentionally add white noise to the stereo images of the cone model shown in Fig. 1a. In this experiment the disparity range is set as $\mathcal{D} = [50, 80]$. The resulting reconstruction mean absolute errors (MAE) under different noise variance are reported in Table 1. The results show that there is not much difference between different measures when the image is clean. However, when the noise level becomes large, the measure using simplest pixel-to-pixel AD degrades significantly. In contrast, AD+BF and ZNCC, which perform local cost aggregation, remain accurate in the presence of noise. ZNCC has the best performance in all cases.

**Table 1.** Under different degrees of noise $\sigma$, the reconstruction MAE (mm) compared with the ground truth after the convex optimisation using different data-fidelity terms for the stereo pair of the cone model

|        | $\sigma = 0$ | $\sigma = 0.01$ | $\sigma = 0.015$ | $\sigma = 0.02$ |
|:------:|:------------:|:---------------:|:----------------:|:---------------:|
| AD     | 0.121        | 0.623           | 0.877            | 2.035           |
| AD+BF  | 0.121        | 0.189           | 0.798            | 1.521           |
| ZNCC   | **0.102**    | **0.185**       | **0.661**        | **1.487**       |

## 3.2   Cardiac Phantom Experiment

The proposed algorithm is quantitatively evaluated by two cardiac datasets collected from [14] which have an associated registered CT model as ground truth as shown in Fig. 3. It should be noted that the ground truth is generated by a 3D/2D point-based registration algorithm, which will inevitably introduce some errors.

Before doing the reconstruction, the stereo image pair are rectified by the provided camera calibration. We further remove the black background by setting an intensity threshold, since such a background does not occur in real surgical images and also it may cause bias when comparing different algorithms. The disparity images are cropped by 15 pixels at the image borders when doing the statistics. In this experiment the disparity range is set as $\mathcal{D} = [0, 30]$.

In Table 2, the MAE and root mean square error (RMSE) to the ground truth point are reported for different real-time dense algorithms using a single stereo pair. The corresponding standard deviation among all frames is also reported. The reconstruction results for a single frame are shown in Fig. 3.

Structure propagation using sparse feature points (SPFP) [15] is a real-time quasi-dense method and fast cost-volume filtering (FCVF) [8] is a local edge-preserving filtering method. A recent real-time dense reconstruction using temporal information (DRTI) algorithm [10] that produces highly accurate reconstruction is also compared, and we compare results of MAE with the best results quoted in their paper. It is evident that our algorithm outperforms the others.

**Table 2.** Statistics of different algorithms with respect to MAE, RMSE and the percentage of reconstructed points compared with the ground truth

|          |           | Proposed Approach | SPFP [15]        | FCVF [8]         | DRTI [10] |
|:--------:|:---------:|:-----------------:|:----------------:|:----------------:|:---------:|
| Cardiac1 | MAE(mm)   | $1.24 \pm 0.89$   | $2.36 \pm 0.92$  | $4.87 \pm 0.87$  | 1.45      |
|          | RMSE(mm)  | $1.85 \pm 0.82$   | $3.876 \pm 0.87$ | $8.24 \pm 0.92$  | N/A       |
|          | Density(%)| 100               | 92               | 100              | N/A       |
| Cardiac2 | MAE(mm)   | $1.47 \pm 1.23$   | $3.20 \pm 1.15$  | $5.37 \pm 1.53$  | 1.53      |
|          | RMSE(mm)  | $2.658 \pm 1.47$  | $4.85 \pm 1.82$  | $7.73 \pm 1.56$  | N/A       |
|          | Density(%)| 100               | 90               | 100              | N/A       |

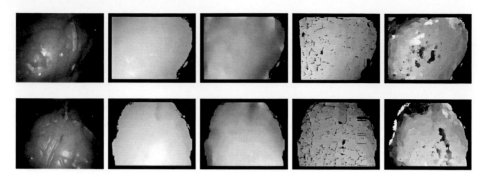

**Fig. 3.** The cardiac phantoms datasets. The disparity maps showing the reconstruction results from left to right: Ground truth, the proposed approach, SPFP [15] and FCVF [8].

### 3.3   Qualitative Evaluation in *in vivo* Images

To qualitatively evaluate the performance of the proposed approach on *in vivo* images, endoscopic stereo images from real robot-assisted laparoscopic prostatectomy are reconstructed as shown in Fig. 4 and in an accompanying video[1]. The overall geometry is well captured. Specular highlights may still cause some mis-matching, which can be resolved by fusing temporal models, and we will investigate this idea as part of our future work.

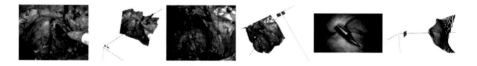

**Fig. 4.** Qualitative evaluation of the reconstruction results using the proposed approach. The images are obtained from stereo endoscopic camera in real robot-assisted surgery. We recommend to view these images on-screen and zoomed in.

## 4   Conclusions

In this paper, we have proposed an efficient and effective dense stereo reconstruction method using convex optimisation with a cost-volume. Empirical studies have shown that our reconstruction results outperform the current state of the art methods for endoscopic images and can also run in real-time on the GPU. This is a significant advancement towards improved vision-based tracking of the endoscope and is an important step towards providing image guidance to endoscopic procedures. In our future work, we will be developing dense camera tracking techniques and will extend the current algorithm to fuse a sequence of video images. This will improve the reconstructed model and provide more advanced means for tackling the occlusion at instrument-tissue boundaries.

---

[1] http://www.doc.ic.ac.uk/~pc3509

# References

1. Chambolle, A., Pock, T.: A first-order primal-dual algorithm for convex problems with applications to imaging. Journal of Mathematical Imaging and Vision 40(1), 120–145 (2011) 45
2. Chang, P.-L., Chen, D., Cohen, D., Edwards, P.E.: 2D/3D registration of a preoperative model with endoscopic video using colour-consistency. In: Linte, C.A., Moore, J.T., Chen, E.C.S., Holmes III, D.R. (eds.) AE CAI 2011. LNCS, vol. 7264, pp. 1–12. Springer, Heidelberg (2012) 42
3. Devernay, F., Mourgues, F., Coste-Maniere, E.: Towards endoscopic augmented reality for robotically assisted minimally invasive cardiac surgery. In: International Workshop on Medical Imaging and Augmented Reality, pp. 16–20 (2001) 42, 43
4. Handa, A., Newcombe, R.A., Angeli, A., Davison, A.J.: Applications of legendre-fenchel transformation to computer vision problems. Tech. Rep. DTR11-7, Department of Computing at Imperial College London (2011) 45
5. Lau, W.W., Ramey, N.A., Corso, J.J., Thakor, N.V., Hager, G.D.: Stereo-based endoscopic tracking of cardiac surface deformation. In: Barillot, C., Haynor, D.R., Hellier, P. (eds.) MICCAI 2004. LNCS, vol. 3217, pp. 494–501. Springer, Heidelberg (2004) 43
6. Mirota, D.J., Ishii, M., Hager, G.D.: Vision-based navigation in image-guided interventions. Annual Review of Biomedical Engineering 13, 297–319 (2011) 42, 43
7. Mountney, P., Stoyanov, D., Yang, G.-Z.: Three-dimensional tissue deformation recovery and tracking. IEEE Signal Processsing Magazine 27(4), 14–24 (2010) 42, 43
8. Rhemann, C., Hosni, A., Bleyer, M., Rother, C., Gelautz, M.: Fast cost-volume filtering for visual correspondence and beyond. In: IEEE Conference on Computer Vision and Pattern Recognition (CVPR), pp. 3017–3024 (2011) 44, 47, 48
9. Richa, R., Bo, A.P.L., Poignet, P.: Towards robust 3D visual tracking for motion compensation in beating heart surgery. Medical Image Analysis 15(3), 302–315 (2011) 43
10. Rohl, S., Bodenstedt, S., Suwelack, S., Dillmann, R., Speidel, S., Kenngott, H., Muller-Stich, B.P.: Dense GPU-enhanced surface reconstruction from stereo endoscopic images for intraoperative registration. Medical Physics 39(3), 1632–1645 (2012) 43, 44, 47
11. Rudin, L., Osher, S., Fatemi, E.: Nonlinear total variation based noise removal algorithms. Physica D: Nonlinear Phenomena 60(1-4), 259–268 (1992) 45
12. Scharstein, D., Szeliski, R.: A taxonomy and evaluation of dense two-frame stereo correspondence algorithms. International Journal of Computer Vision (1), 131–140 (2002) 43
13. Steinbrucker, F., Pock, T., Cremers, D.: Large displacement optical flow computation without warping. In: IEEE International Conference on Computer Vision (ICCV), pp. 1609–1614 (2009) 45
14. Stoyanov, D.: Stereoscopic scene flow for robotic assisted minimally invasive surgery. In: Ayache, N., Delingette, H., Golland, P., Mori, K. (eds.) MICCAI 2012, Part I. LNCS, vol. 7510, pp. 479–486. Springer, Heidelberg (2012) 47
15. Stoyanov, D., Scarzanella, M.V., Pratt, P., Yang, G.-Z.: Real-time stereo reconstruction in robotically assisted minimally invasive surgery. In: Jiang, T., Navab, N., Pluim, J.P.W., Viergever, M.A. (eds.) MICCAI 2010, Part I. LNCS, vol. 6361, pp. 275–282. Springer, Heidelberg (2010) 42, 43, 47, 48
16. Werlberger, M., Trobin, W., Pock, T., Wedel, A., Cremers, D., Bischof, H.: Anisotropic Huber-L1 Optical Flow. In: British Machine Vision Conference (BMVC), pp. 108.1–108.11 (2009) 45

# Combining Surface and Fiber Geometry: An Integrated Approach to Brain Morphology

Peter Savadjiev[1,2], Yogesh Rathi[2], Sylvain Bouix[2], Alex R. Smith[3],
Robert T. Schultz[4], Ragini Verma[3], and Carl-Fredrik Westin[1]

[1] Laboratory for Mathematics in Imaging and
[2] Psychiatry Neuroimaging Laboratory
Brigham and Women's Hospital, Harvard Medical School, Boston, MA, USA
[3] Section of Biomedical Image Analysis, Dept. of Radiology,
University of Pennsylvania, Philadelphia, PA, USA
[4] Children's Hospital of Philadelphia, Philadelphia, PA, USA

**Abstract.** Despite the fact that several theories link cortical development and function to the development of white matter and its geometrical structure, the relationship between gray and white matter morphology has not been widely researched. In this paper, we propose a novel framework for investigating this relationship. Given a set of fiber tracts which connect to a particular cortical region, the key idea is to compute two scalar fields that represent geometrical characteristics of the white matter and of the surface of the cortical region. The distributions of these scalar values are then linked via Mutual Information, which results in a quantitative marker that can be used in the study of normal and pathological brain structure and development. We apply this framework to a population study on autism spectrum disorder in children.

## 1 Introduction

The shape of brain structures is an important feature thought to reflect various neurodevelopmental processes, which makes it of particular interest in neuroscience. A large body of neuroimaging literature has been devoted to studying the geometry of the brain's cortical surface, in terms of measures such as curvature, area, thickness, gyrification (e.g., [1]). However, the relationship between gray and white matter morphology has not been extensively studied, despite the fact that several theories link cortical development and function to the development of white matter and its geometrical structure (e.g., [2]). In fact, most *in vivo* neuroimaging investigations of white matter have focused on voxel-based diffusion tensor imaging (DTI) measures such as fractional anisotropy (FA), mean, radial and axial diffusivities. As this type of information is of very different nature (i.e. non-geometrical), it is not clear how to combine such DTI-based findings on the white matter (WM), with morphological findings in the gray matter (GM).

Possibly as a result of this discrepancy, the problem of mapping white matter properties onto cortical geometry has not been widely investigated. In [3], tractography information is used to help determine corresponding points on the

K. Mori et al. (Eds.): MICCAI 2013, Part I, LNCS 8149, pp. 50–57, 2013.

cortical surface of different subjects. More recently, [4] define correspondence between WM tracts and GM locations by extending the tract in a straight line from the tip of the tract to the boundary of the cortex. This approach is rather heuristic, and does not take into account the complex cerebral cortex structure which often causes axons to bend when they enter the gray matter.

In this paper, we introduce a novel framework to associate geometrical information from the white matter and the cortical surface without such severe restrictions. To quantify cortical surface geometry, standard features from the differential geometry of surfaces exist and have been widely used in the medical image community. Such features include functions of the surface's principal curvatures, e.g. the mean and Gaussian curvatures, or the shape index and curvedness [1]. However, a lot less work has been done on the geometry of white matter fibers. In the diffusion MRI community, the *sub-voxel* geometry of fibers has been defined based for example on the diffusion-weighted signal, e.g. [5], or based on neighborhood regularization, e.g. [6]. However, for the purposes of the present work, we need larger scale *macrostructural* white matter geometry features, i.e. in features that span more than a single voxel. A method that provides such features is that of [7], where fiber geometry is computed based on the differential geometry of curve sets. By measuring the variation of a curve's tangent vector in all directions orthogonal to the curve, this method provides a quantitative measure of fiber dispersion, or spread.

While it may be self-evident that the geometry of the white matter and that of the gray matter must somehow be related, it is not currently known whether a precise relationship actually exists, or what its formulation is. One could attempt to provide an explicit model for this relationship via formulas linking cortical folding with the spread and curvature of white matter fibers. However, such an approach would require extensive knowledge of brain tissue biomechanics and is essentially impossible with current neuroimaging technology.

In this work, we propose a simpler approach based on information theory. Given a set of fiber tracts which connect to a particular cortical region of interest (ROI), we first compute a scalar field over the fiber tracts, and separately a second scalar field over the cortical region. These two scalar fields represent a geometric characteristic of the white matter and of the gray matter, respectively. Then, we capture the relationship between them through the Mutual Information function. This type of approach is general, in that it can be applied with any scalar characteristics of the gray and the white matter. It also avoids the need to specify one-to-one correspondences between individual fibers and specific points on the cortex, as such correspondences are inherently unstable and depend on various parameters and tractography algorithm specifics.

We illustrate our approach with a small-scale study on autism. We focused our experiments specifically on the *pars orbitalis* region of the inferior frontal gyrus (IFG), a region that has been involved in semantic processing of language. We chose this region as the IFG and the *pars orbitalis* have been previously implicated in autism (e.g., [8]) and other neurodevelopmental disorders.

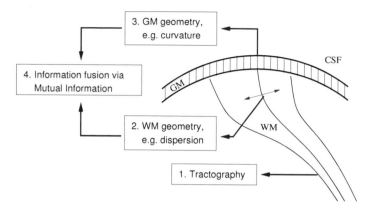

**Fig. 1.** A schematic illustration of the four steps in our pipeline

## 2    Methods

Our approach is summarized with the following four steps:

1) Perform tractography to define the white matter tracts of interest.

2) Compute the geometry of these tracts.

3) Compute the geometry of the cortical regions they connect to.

4) Quantify the relationship between the geometry of white matter and that of gray matter.

As detailed below, Step 1) is performed with the multi-fiber tracking algorithm of [9], and is used as in [7]. Step 2) implements the geometry method of [7], while steps 3) and 4) are the contribution of the present paper, and are described in more detail. Fig. 1 summarizes these steps.

### 2.1    Geometry Computation (Steps 1-3)

Following the work of [7], we first computed whole-brain tractography using the HARDI multi-fiber tractography method of [9]. This tractography algorithm is robust to partial volume effects and to complex fiber configurations. The next step was done with the help of FreeSurfer (http://surfer.nmr.mgh.harvard.edu), a freely available software tool. We extracted the interhemispheric tracts connecting the *pars orbitalis* area of the inferior frontal gyrus of both hemispheres, using the FreeSurfer cortical parcellation of these areas as extraction masks.

Once the tracts were extracted, we computed the *Total Dispersion* ($TD$) measure of [7]. Given a set of curves that represent white matter fibers, and a tangent vector $E_T$ at each point along each curve, we measure the rate of change of $E_T$ in 20 directions uniformly distributed on the unit circle, in the plane orthogonal to $E_T$. At each point along each curve, this samples the "dispersion distribution function" (DDF) of [7], a function that represents the amount of fibre dispersion in each direction orthogonal to the fibre. The $TD$ measure at each point is then defined as the average value of the DDF. As the DDF can be computed at a

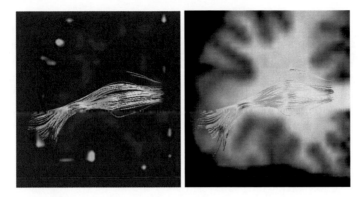

**Fig. 2.** A zoom-in on an anterior coronal view of the right hemisphere with fibers connecting the *pars orbitalis*. The fibers are colored by $TD$, such that low $TD$ values are indicated with red/yellow, and high values with green/blue. Please keep in mind that fiber dispersion is a 3D phenomenon. Left: a volume rendering of the mean curvature of the GM/WM boundary surface, such that blue/purple intensities denote the curvature sign and magnitude. Right: the T1 image, shown for anatomical reference.

variety of spatial scales [7], we used an empirically selected scale parameter value $S = 10$mm.

In addition to performing cortical surface parcellation, the FreeSurfer tool also extracts the GM/WM boundary surface. This surface is represented as a mesh, with the principal curvatures calculated at each vertex. At each vertex in the *pars orbitalis* cortical region, we computed the mean curvature $Cm$, defined as the mean of the surface's two principal curvatures $\kappa_1$ and $\kappa_2$. Note that while the FreeSurfer parcellation was registered to the diffusion MRI space to allow for cortical ROIs to be used as extraction masks for the tractography, all surface curvature computations are performed in the original FreeSurfer space, to avoid the introduction of registration artifacts.

As an illustration, we show in Fig. 2 the fibers connecting to the *pars orbitalis* region in the right hemisphere, colored by the $TD$ value at each point. Note the 'bottleneck' with low $TD$ (yellow/red), and the fibers' dispersion towards the cortex (green/blue). We overlay these fibers onto a volume representing the mean curvature of the GM/WM boundary surface. To create this visualization, the mean curvature values were rasterized into a 3D volume with the mri_surf2vol utility (part of the FreeSurfer toolkit). The resulting volume was then registered to the diffusion MRI space (which gives a thickness to the surface as a by-product). As an anatomical reference, we also show the fibers over the T1 image.

## 2.2 Fusion of WM and GM Geometry Information via Mutual Information (Step 4)

The above preprocessing steps give, at each point along the fiber tract of interest, a scalar quantifying the dispersion of the tract at that point. In addition, at each point on the cortical surface ROI, we have a scalar quantifying the mean curvature (or possibly another feature) of the surface at that point. The probability density functions (pdf) of these values can then be estimated, and the relationship between them captured via a quantity known as *Mutual Information* (MI) [10]. The MI between two random variables measures the amount of information they share. The higher the MI value, the more 'dependent' the variables are, i.e. the more knowledge we gain of one by knowing the value of the other. MI should not be confused with the correlation between two variables, which measures the strength of the linear relationship between them. MI is much more general, as it does not assume any particular form for the relationship between the two variables. MI has been widely used in medical imaging, in particular for image registration (e.g., [11]). Here, the use of MI allows us to combine information between geometrical measures on the white matter and on the gray matter.

The Mutual Information of two continuous random variables $X$ and $Y$ is defined as follows [10]:

$$M(X;Y) = \int_Y \int_X p(x,y) \log \left( \frac{p(x,y)}{p(x)p(y)} \right) dxdy, \tag{1}$$

where $p(x,y)$ is the joint probability density function of $X$ and $Y$, and $p(x)$ and $p(y)$ are their respective marginal probability densities. In our implementation, to compute $M$ we used the MILCA estimator [12], which is available online. This is a robust estimator which does *not* require *a priori* knowledge of the joint density of the two variables. This is in contrast to MI computations typical to the image registration literature, which usually require explicit correspondence between two images to compute their pixel-based joint density. In our work, we do not compute MI between two images. Rather, we use kernel density estimation [13] to compute one probability density estimate for $Cm$ over the cortical area and another one for $TD$ over the connecting white matter tract. We treat these two density estimates as two one-dimensional signals, and we then use the method of [12] to compute MI between them. Because of this, explicit pointwise correspondence between white matter and cortical locations is not required.

## 3      Experiments

### 3.1      Subjects and Data Acquisition

We illustrate our method with a small-scale study on autism. Autism has been characterized as a disorder in which the brain undergoes an early period of overgrowth, from birth to approximately age 4. This early period of excessive growth is thought to be followed by abnormally slow or even arrested growth [14]. Based on this knowledge, we hypothesize that our MI based measure will reveal a difference in the trajectory of brain development with age. Of course, the main purpose of this study is to illustrate the method, and not to make any conclusive clinical claims about autism. The study is only preliminary, as it uses a relatively small number of subjects, and is focused on a single cortical region.

Diffusion and structural MRI data were acquired from 15 healthy male controls (HC, age range: 6.4 - 13.9 years, mean: 10.3, std dev: 2.4) and 14 male autism spectrum disorder patients (ASD, age range: 6.4 - 13.3 years, mean: 10.0, std dev: 2.1).

All imaging was performed using a Siemens 3T Verio$^{TM}$ scanner with a 32 channel head coil. Structural images were acquired on all subjects using an MP-RAGE imaging sequence (TR/TE/TI − 19s/2.54ms/.9s, 0.8mm in plane resolution, 0.9mm slice thickness). In addition, A HARDI acquisition was also performed using a monopolar Stejskal-Tanner diffusion weighted spin-echo, echo-planar imaging sequence with the following parameters: TR/TE=14.8s/110ms, b=3000s/mm$^2$, 2mm isotropic resolution, and 64 gradient directions as well as two b0 images. The DW-MRI images for both acquisitions of each subject were then filtered using a joint linear minimum mean squared error filter for removal of Rician noise. Eddy Current Correction was then performed using registration of each DWI volume to the unweighted b0 image.

### 3.2 Results

To test our hypothesis, we computed the correlations between subject age and $\tilde{M} \equiv M(Cm, TD)$. The correlations in the left hemisphere were not significant, so we focus on the right hemisphere. In the HC group, we obtained a significant Pearson correlation coefficient (p=0.0403). However, due to the presence of apparent outliers, we also computed the correlation using a robust linear regression method, as implemented with the 'robustfit' Matlab routine. This robust correlation was more significant (p=0.00022). As for the ASD group, we did not obtain a significant correlation (p=0.95 for the Pearson correlation, p=0.98 for the robust correlation), which may indicate a pathology-based alteration of the normal course of brain development. These results are shown in Fig. 3, and appear to fall in line with the notion that autism may be characterized by early brain overgrowth (till about age 4), followed by a reduced or arrested brain growth [14]. Our regression results suggest that at age 6, ASD children have a higher $\tilde{M}$ value than healthy controls. This value doesn't appear to change at later age in ASD children, while there is a steady change in healthy controls. Again, this study is based on a single cortical region (previously implicated in ASD), thus a more global analysis is needed prior to making strong clinical claims. Nevertheless, our results illustrate potential applications of the method.

## 4   Summary and Discussion

We introduced the motivation and groundwork for a novel analysis of the relationship between white matter geometry and cortical surface geometry. This relationship could be informative in many contexts in neuroscience, such as the study of neurodevelopment or the progression of atrophy in neurodegenerative diseases. Our proposed approach is relatively simple, yet we showed it holds a potential for discovering pathology-based differences. Our preliminary results suggest that normal age-related changes in the brain may be altered by ASD

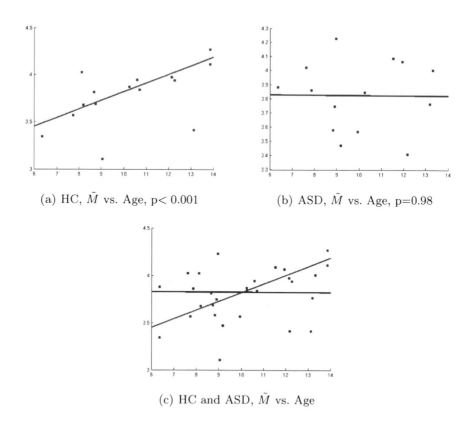

(a) HC, $\tilde{M}$ vs. Age, p< 0.001          (b) ASD, $\tilde{M}$ vs. Age, p=0.98

(c) HC and ASD, $\tilde{M}$ vs. Age

**Fig. 3.**    Correlation in the Right hemisphere between Age (x-axis) and $\tilde{M} = M(Cm, TD)$. Top row: Control (HC) subjects (Left). ASD subjects (Right). Bottom row: Both groups shown in the same plot. The lines indicate the fit obtained by robust correlation for each group, with the corresponding p-values indicated.

pathology. It is particularly interesting that in controls, we find significant correlations in the right hemisphere (as opposed to the left), as previous work on lateralization has implicated the right hemisphere in autism (e.g., [15]).

The basic framework described in this paper can be extended in several ways. First of all, metrics other than Mutual Information can be used, such as kernel-based methods [16]. Methods based on machine learning can also be applied to 'learn' the relationship between the two types of geometry. In future work, we will perform an investigation over a parcellation of the entire cerebral cortex, which will then be incorporated into a network analysis framework in order to detect global patterns of change. Finally, a promising application area of our methods lies in longitudinal studies.

**Acknowledgements.** Work supported by NIH grants R01 MH092862, R01 MH074794, R01 MH082918, R01 MH097979, P41 RR013218, P41 EB015902, Pennsylvania Department of Health grants SAP 4100042728, SAP 4100047863, and Swedish Research Council (VR) grant 2012-3682.

# References

1. Awate, S.P., Yushkevich, P.A., Song, Z., Licht, D.J., Gee, J.C.: Cerebral cortical folding analysis with multivariate modeling and testing: Studies on gender differences and neonatal development. NeuroImage 53(2), 450–459 (2010)
2. Van Essen, D.C.: A tension-based theory of morphogenesis and compact wiring in the central nervous system. Nature 385, 313–318 (1997)
3. Oguz, I., Niethammer, M., Cates, J., Whitaker, R., Fletcher, T., Vachet, C., Styner, M.: Cortical correspondence with probabilistic fiber connectivity. In: Prince, J.L., Pham, D.L., Myers, K.J. (eds.) IPMI 2009. LNCS, vol. 5636, pp. 651–663. Springer, Heidelberg (2009)
4. Tozer, D.J., Chard, D.T., Bodini, B., Ciccarelli, O., Miller, D.H., Thompson, A.J., Wheeler-Kingshott, C.A.M.: Linking white matter tracts to associated cortical grey matter: A tract extension methodology. NeuroImage 59(4), 3094–3102 (2012)
5. Kaden, E., Knösche, T.R., Anwander, A.: Parametric spherical deconvolution: Inferring anatomical connectivity using diffusion MR imaging. NeuroImage 37, 474–488 (2007)
6. Savadjiev, P., Campbell, J.S.W., Descoteaux, M., Deriche, R., Pike, G.B., Siddiqi, K.: Labeling of ambiguous sub-voxel fibre bundle configurations in high angular resolution diffusion MRI. NeuroImage 41(1), 58–68 (2008)
7. Savadjiev, P., Rathi, Y., Bouix, S., Verma, R., Westin, C.F.: Multi-scale characterization of white matter tract geometry. In: Ayache, N., Delingette, H., Golland, P., Mori, K. (eds.) MICCAI 2012, Part III. LNCS, vol. 7512, pp. 34–41. Springer, Heidelberg (2012)
8. Raznahan, A., Toro, R., Proitsi, P., Powell, J., Paus, T., Bolton, P.F., Murphy, D.G.M.: A functional polymorphism of the brain derived neurotrophic factor gene and cortical anatomy in ASD. J. Neurodev. Disord. 1(3), 215–223 (2009)
9. Malcolm, J.G., Shenton, M.E., Rathi, Y.: Filtered multi-tensor tractography. IEEE Trans. on Medical Imaging 29, 1664–1675 (2010)
10. Cover, T.M., Thomas, J.A.: Elements of Information Theory. Wiley, NYC (1991)
11. Wells III, W.M., Viola, P., Atsumi, H., Nakajima, S., Kikinis, R.: Multi-modal volume registration by maximization of mutual information. Med. Image Anal. 1(1), 35–51 (1996)
12. Kraskov, A., Stögbauer, H., Grassberger, P.: Estimating mutual information. Physical review. E, Statistical, Nonlinear, and Soft Matter Physics 69(6 pt. 2) (2004)
13. Bowman, A.W., Azzalini, A.: Applied Smoothing Techniques for Data Analysis. Oxford University Press, New York (1997)
14. Courchesne, E.: Brain development in autism: early overgrowth followed by premature arrest of growth. Mental Retardation and Developmental Disabilities Research Reviews 10, 106–111 (2004)
15. Tager-Flusberg, H., Joseph, R.M.: Identifying neurocognitive phenotypes in autism. Phil. Trans. Royal Soc. London B: Biol. Sci. 358(1430), 303–314 (2003)
16. Gretton, A., Bousquet, O., Smola, A.J., Schölkopf, B.: Measuring statistical dependence with Hilbert-Schmidt norms. In: Jain, S., Simon, H.U., Tomita, E. (eds.) ALT 2005. LNCS (LNAI), vol. 3734, pp. 63–77. Springer, Heidelberg (2005)

# Multi-atlas Based Simultaneous Labeling of Longitudinal Dynamic Cortical Surfaces in Infants

Gang Li, Li Wang, Feng Shi, Weili Lin, and Dinggang Shen

Department of Radiology and BRIC, University of North Carolina at Chapel Hill, NC, USA

**Abstract.** Accurate and consistent labeling of longitudinal cortical surfaces is essential to understand the early dynamic development of cortical structure and function in both normal and abnormal infant brains. In this paper, we propose a novel method for simultaneous, consistent, and unbiased labeling of longitudinal dynamic cortical surfaces in the infant brain MR images. The proposed method is formulated as minimization of an energy function, which includes the data fitting, spatial smoothness and temporal consistency terms. Specifically, in the spirit of multi-atlas based label fusion, the data fitting term is designed to integrate adaptive contributions from multi-atlas surfaces, according to the similarity of their local cortical folding with that of the subject surface. The spatial smoothness term is designed to adaptively encourage label smoothness based on the local folding geometries, i.e., also allowing label discontinuity at sulcal bottoms, where the cytoarchitecturally and functionally distinct cortical regions are often divided. The temporal consistency term is further designed to encourage the label consistency between temporal corresponding vertices with similar local cortical folding. Finally, the entire energy function is efficiently minimized by a graph cuts method. The proposed method has been successfully applied to the labeling of longitudinal cortical surfaces of 13 infants, each with 6 serial images scanned from birth to 2 years of age. Both qualitative and quantitative evaluation results demonstrate the validity of the proposed method.

**Keywords:** Infant cortical surface, longitudinal cortical surface labeling.

## 1 Introduction

The human cerebral cortex develops dynamically in the first 2 years of life [1], with all primary and secondary cortical folding being well established at term birth [2]. Accurate and consistent labeling of longitudinal dynamic infant cortical surfaces into regions of interest (ROIs) is essential to understand postnatal development of cortical structure and function in both normal and abnormal infant brains. Many methods have been developed for the labeling of a single cortical surface. However, applying these methods to each longitudinal cortical surface independently is likely to generate longitudinally-inconsistent labeling results, especially in the ambiguous cortical regions, thus leading to inaccurate cortex development measurements. One strategy to ensure the longitudinal consistent labeling is to first label the cortical surface of a selected time point (usually the first or the last time point), and then propagate the labeling

K. Mori et al. (Eds.): MICCAI 2013, Part I, LNCS 8149, pp. 58–65, 2013.

result to other time points. However, the surface labeling results by this strategy could be biased by the selected time point, in addition to the potential propagation of labeling errors. Accordingly, efforts have been made towards unbiased and consistent labeling of longitudinal cortical surfaces. For example, in the longitudinal pipeline of FreeSurfer, a within-subject template is first built by rigidly aligning all longitudinal images of a subject to a median image, and then the cortical surfaces of the within-subject template are reconstructed and labeled. These labeled cortical surfaces will be rigidly transformed back to the space of each longitudinal image as initialization and further deformed independently to refine the labeling results [3]. Although this independent refinement may be suitable for the adults with small longitudinal changes, it becomes problematic when applied to the infants with dynamic longitudinal changes.

In this paper, we propose a novel method for simultaneous, consistent, and unbiased labeling of longitudinal dynamic cortical surfaces in serial infant brain MR images. The proposed method is formulated as minimization of an energy function, which includes the data fitting, spatial smoothness, and temporal consistency terms. The data fitting term is designed to integrate adaptive contributions from multiple atlas surfaces, according to the similarities of their local cortical folding with the subject surface. The spatial smoothness term is also designed to adaptively encourage label smoothness based on the local folding geometries. The temporal consistency term is further designed to adaptively encourage longitudinal label consistency based on the temporal similarities of local cortical folding. The energy function is efficiently minimized by the alpha-expansion graph cuts method [4]. The proposed method has been successfully applied to labeling of longitudinal cortical surfaces of 13 infants, each with 6 serial images in the first 2 years of life. Both qualitative and quantitative evaluation results demonstrate the accuracy and consistency of the proposed method.

## 2 Methods

### 2.1 Dataset and Image Preprocessing

Serial T1, T2, and diffusion-weighted MR images of 13 healthy infants (9 males/4 females) were acquired at every 3 months from 2 weeks to 1.5 years of age, using a Siemens 3T head-only MR scanner. T1 images (160 axial slices) were acquired with the following imaging parameters: TR/TE = 1900/4.38ms, flip angle = 7, resolution = $1 \times 1 \times 1$ mm$^3$. T2 images (70 axial slices) were acquired with the imaging parameters: TR/TE = 7380/119ms, flip angle = 150, resolution = $1.25 \times 1.25 \times 1.95$ mm$^3$. Diffusion-weighted images (DWI) (60 axial slices) were acquired with the parameters: TR/TE = 7680/82 ms, resolution = $2 \times 2 \times 2$ mm$^3$, 42 non-collinear diffusion gradients, and diffusion weighting $b$ =1000s/mm$^2$. Distortion correction of DWI was also performed. T2 images and fractional anisotropy (FA) images, derived from DWI, were rigidly aligned onto their T1 images and further resampled to $1 \times 1 \times 1$ mm$^3$. For each set of aligned T1, T2, and FA images, non-cerebral tissues were removed. Then, all longitudinal images of the same infant were rigidly aligned. Brain tissue was segmented by a 4D level-set method by integration of the complementary information of T1, T2 and FA images [5]. After tissue segmentation, non-cortical structures were masked and filled, and each brain was separated into left and right hemispheres.

Then, the inner cortical surface (the interface between white matter (WM) and gray matter (GM)) of each hemisphere was reconstructed by correcting topological defects and tessellating WM as a triangular mesh [1]. The inner cortical surface was further inflated and mapped to a standard sphere [6]. All longitudinal cortical surfaces of the same infant were group-wisely aligned to establish within-subject correspondences using Spherical Demons [7]. **Fig. 1(a)** shows the longitudinal inner surfaces of a representative infant, color-coded by the mean curvatures. **Fig. 1(b)** shows group-wisely aligned longitudinal spherical surfaces of the infant, again color-coded by the mean curvatures. As can be seen, all primary and secondary cortical folding are well established at term birth. Moreover, the longitudinal cortical folding are quite stable during postnatal development and thus are well aligned by group-wise surface registration.

The publically available 39 cortical surfaces with manual parcellation based on sulcal bottoms by experts [7, 8] were adopted as multi-atlas surfaces. Information on image acquisition and demographics can be found in [8]. To warp atlas surfaces to subject surfaces, all atlas surfaces were first group-wisely aligned using Spherical Demons [7]. Then each longitudinal surface of the subject was aligned onto the group-wisely aligned atlas surfaces [7]. Finally, the deformation field from each atlas surface to the subject surface was computed by concatenating the deformation field from this atlas surface to the group-wisely aligned atlas surfaces and the deformation field from the group-wisely aligned atlas surfaces to the subject surface. Accordingly, each atlas surface can be warped to each subject surface. Note that the group-wise alignment is only required to perform one time, and can be used for all subjects, thus

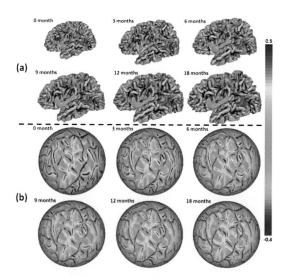

**Fig. 1.** (a) Longitudinal inner cortical surfaces of a representative infant, color-coded by the mean curvatures. (b) Group-wisely aligned longitudinal spherical surfaces of the infant, color-coded again by the mean curvatures. Red colors indicate sulci and blue colors indicate gyri.

this strategy is computationally much more efficient than the conventional way of pair-wise registration between each atlas surface and each longitudinal surface of the subject. On the other hand, due to the inter-individual variability of the cortical folding patterns and also the regularization constraints in the registration, a subject surface and each warped atlas surface might not have the maximum similarity of their local cortical folding. This issue will be taken care for surface labeling in the **section 2.2**.

## 2.2    Simultaneous Labeling of Longitudinal Cortical Surfaces

The proposed method for simultaneous, consistent, and unbiased labeling of longitudinal cortical surfaces in the infant is formulated as an energy minimization problem:

$$E = E_d + \alpha_s E_s + \alpha_t E_t \qquad (1)$$

where $E_d$ is the data fitting term, $E_s$ is the spatial smoothness term, and $E_t$ is temporal consistency term. $\alpha_s$ and $\alpha_t$ are the weighting parameters.

**Data Fitting Term.** To define the data fitting term, we take advantage of multi-atlas based methods, which account for atlas-subject variability [9]. Given $K$ atlas surfaces with each having $L$ labels, the data fitting term is defined as:

$$E_d = \sum_x -log P_x(l_x) \qquad (2)$$

where $P_x(l_x)$ indicates the probability of assigning a label $l_x \in \{1, ..., L\}$ to a vertex $x$ in a subject surface. The label probability at a vertex is computed based on the shape information of labels in the atlas surfaces, as well as the differences of local cortical folding between the subject surface and atlas surfaces. The latter is defined based on the average absolute difference of mean curvatures in local surface patches:

$$D\big(S(x), S(x_k)\big) = \frac{1}{|\Omega_S|}\sum_{y \in \Omega_S}|H(y) - H(y_k)| \qquad (3)$$

where $D(\cdot,\cdot)$ is the cortical folding difference between two surface patches, and $S(\cdot)$ is a local surface patch, defined as a circular region $\Omega_S$ on the spherical surface with the radius of $2.5mm$ (set experimentally) surrounding a center vertex. $|\Omega_S|$ is the number of vertices in the surface patch. $x_k$ is the corresponding point in atlas surface $k$, for the vertex $x$ in a subject surface. $y$ is a vertex in the subject surface patch, and $y_k$ is its corresponding point in the atlas surface $k$. $H(\cdot)$ is the mean curvature.

   To use the shape information of labels in atlas surfaces, we adopt the logarithm of odds model [9] based on the signed geodesic distance map on the original cortical surface, computed by the fast marching method on triangular meshes. Denoting $d_{k,l_x}(\cdot)$ as the signed geodesic distance map of label $l_x$ in the atlas surface $k$ that has been warped to the subject surface, and also setting the inside of the label being positive values, the label probability of the vertex $x$ is finally defined as:

$$P_x(l_x) = \frac{1}{K}\sum_{k=1}^{K} \exp\big(-\gamma D\big(S(x), S(x_k')\big)\big) * \frac{1}{Z_k(x_k')}\exp\big(\beta d_{k,l_x}(x_k')\big) \qquad (4)$$

where $Z_k(x_k') = \sum_{l=1}^{L} \exp(\beta d_{k,l}(x_k'))$ is the partition function for atlas surface $k$. The first term in **Eq. (4)** is the weight of the atlas surface $k$, and the second term in

**Eq. (4)** is the probability of observing label $l_x$ at subject vertex $x$ based on the atlas surface $k$. Positive parameters $\beta$ and $\gamma$ are experimentally set as 1.0 and 2.0, respectively. $x'_k$ could be the corresponding point $x_k$ in the atlas surface $k$ for the subject vertex $x$ determined by surface registration. However, it might not achieve the maximum similarity of local cortical folding due to registration errors. Therefore, after surface registration, a better corresponding point $x'_k$ in the atlas surface $k$ for the subject vertex $x$ can be further determined by local searching for the most similar surface patch: $x'_k = \arg\min D(S(x), S(x^*_k))$, $x^*_k \in N(x)$. $N(\cdot)$ is the search range, defined as a circular region on the spherical surface with the radius of $2.5mm$ surrounding the vertex $x$.

**Spatial Smoothness Term.** The spatial smoothness term represents the sum of the costs of labeling a pair of spatial neighboring vertices in a subject surface:

$$E_s = \Sigma_{\{x,y\} \in N_s} V^s_{x,y}(l_x, l_y) \tag{5}$$

where $N_s$ is the set of the one-ring neighboring vertex pairs in a cortical surface. $V^s_{x,y}$ indicates the cost of labeling a pair of spatial neighboring vertices $x$ and $y$ as $l_x$ and $l_y$, respectively. The costs of discontinuous labeling are set as small values at highly bended cortical regions, e.g. sulcal bottoms, where the cytoarchitecturally and functionally distinct cortical regions are often divided, similarly as done by the manual labels in atlas surfaces by experts [8]. The costs of discontinuous labeling are set as large values at other regions, i.e. flat cortical regions. $V^s_{x,y}(l_x, l_y)$ is thus defined as:

$$V^s_{x,y}(l_x, l_y) = \frac{(1+\mathbf{n}(x)\cdot\mathbf{n}(y))}{2} * \frac{(e^{-|H(x)|}+e^{-|H(y)|})}{2} * (1 - \delta(|l_x - l_y|)) \tag{6}$$

where $\mathbf{n}$ is the normal direction and $\delta$ is the Dirac delta function. If $l_x = l_y$, $\delta(|l_x - l_y|) = 1$; otherwise, $\delta(|l_x - l_y|) = 0$. Therefore, $V^s_{x,y}(l_x, l_y)$ is 0, if $l_x = l_y$. At highly bended cortical regions, e.g. sulcal bottoms, $x$ and $y$ belonging to different regions generally have quite different normal directions and also large magnitudes of mean curvatures, therefore, both the first and second terms in **Eq. (6)** are small values; while $x$ and $y$ in the same region generally have the similar normal direction but large magnitudes of mean curvatures, only the second term in **Eq. (6)** is a small value. If $x$ and $y$ are at other cortical regions, i.e. flat cortical regions, their normal directions will be quite similar and their magnitudes of mean curvatures are close to 0, thereby, both the first and second terms in **Eq. (6)** are close to 1.

**Temporal Consistency Term.** The temporal consistency term represents the sum of the costs of labeling a pair of temporal corresponding vertices between a pair of longitudinal cortical surfaces:

$$E_t = \Sigma_{\{x,y\} \in N_t} V^t_{x,y}(l_x, l_y) = \Sigma_{\{x,y\} \in N_t} \exp\left(-\gamma D(S(x), S(y))\right)(1 - \delta(|l_x - l_y|)) \tag{7}$$

where $N_t$ is the set of temporal corresponding vertex pairs, and defined in any two longitudinal surfaces in a subject. $V^t_{x,y}$ indicates the cost of labeling a pair of temporal corresponding vertices $x$ and $y$ as $l_x$ and $l_y$, respectively. The cost of discontinuous labeling of a pair of temporal corresponding vertices is set based on their local cortical folding similarity. To avoid bias and reduce computational cost in conventional pair-wise registration, temporal correspondences are determined by group-wise registration of all longitudinal surfaces of the same infant as mentioned in **section 2.1**.

Finally, the multi-label alpha-expansion graph cuts method [4] is adopted to minimize the above defined energy function. Specifically, longitudinal surfaces are represented as an undirected weighted graph $\mathcal{G} = (\mathcal{V}, \mathcal{E})$, where $\mathcal{V}$ is the set of nodes, including all vertices on the longitudinal surfaces and the terminals represented by labels. $\mathcal{E} = \mathcal{E}_N \cup \mathcal{E}_T$ is the collection of edges, where $\mathcal{E}_N$ is the edges formed by spatial neighboring and temporal corresponding vertices, called n-links, and $\mathcal{E}_T$ is the edges formed by vertices to terminals, called t-links. In this graph, $D_x$ describes the edge weight of t-links, and $V^s_{x,y}$ and $V^t_{x,y}$ describe the edge weights of n-links. For more details of the graph cuts method, please refer to [4].

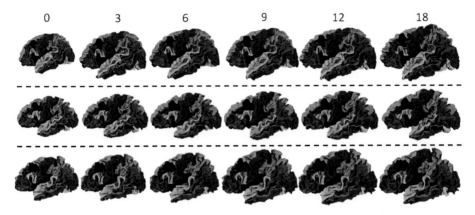

**Fig. 2.** Longitudinal cortical surface labeling results in 3 representative infant subjects, each with 6 longitudinal cortical surfaces at 0, 3, 6, 9, 12 and 18 months

## 3    Results

The proposed method has been applied to the labeling of longitudinal cortical surface in 13 healthy infants, each with serial images acquired at 0, 3, 6, 9, 12 and 18 months. Parameters $\alpha_s$ and $\alpha_t$ in **Eq. (1)** are both set as 0.15 in all experiments. Our method takes around 10 minutes (for energy computation and minimization) to label all longitudinal cortical surfaces for each subject on a PC with Intel Xeon 2.26GHz CPU and 4GB memory. **Fig. 2** shows longitudinal surface labeling results on left hemispheres of 3 typical subjects by the proposed method. As can be seen, the labeling results are visually quite reasonable and consistent. **Fig. 3** shows close-up views of representative longitudinal surface labeling results by the proposed method, and also FreeSurfer [3, 8] where the same atlases were used to train the classifiers. As can be observed, the proposed method achieves longitudinally more consistent results than FreeSurfer.

To quantitatively evaluate the accuracy of the longitudinal cortical surface labeling results, we have an expert manually annotate the precentral gyrus (PreCG) and superior temporal gyrus (STG) in the first and last time-point cortical surfaces of the left hemisphere in each of the 13 subjects, according to the mean-curvature based cortical surface labeling protocol in [8]. We calculate the Dice coefficients between automatic and manual labeling regions. **Fig. 4** shows the Dice coefficients of PreCG and STG on the 13 subjects by 3 different methods. The average Dice coefficients for PreCG/STG are 0.941/0.939 (proposed method), 0.932/0.930 (proposed method without temporal constraint (by setting $\alpha_t$ as 0)), and 0.918/0.914 (FreeSurfer), respectively. As can be seen, the proposed method achieves the highest Dice coefficient.

To further demonstrate the consistency of the longitudinal surface labeling results, **Fig. 5(a)** shows label boundaries of the aligned longitudinal spherical surfaces of a typical subject by the proposed method and FreeSurfer. As can be seen, the proposed method achieves temporally more consistent labeling boundaries than FreeSurfer. To quantitatively evaluate the consistency, we compute the average value of mean symmetric distance of boundaries [8] for labeled regions between each pair of aligned longitudinal surfaces in each of 13 infants, as shown in **Fig. 5(b)**. The average boundary distance by 3 methods are 0.52±0.002mm (proposed method), 0.75±0.03mm (proposed method without temporal constraint), and 0.90±0.03mm (FreeSurfer), respectively. The proposed method achieves the lowest boundary distance.

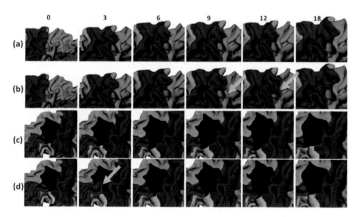

**Fig. 3.** Close-up views of representative longitudinal cortical surface labeling results. (a) and (c) Results by the proposed method. (b) and (d) Results by FreeSurfer. Yellow arrows indicate several regions with longitudinally-inconsistent labels by FreeSurfer.

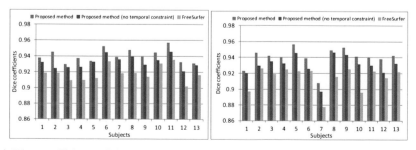

**Fig. 4.** Dice coefficients of precentral (left) and superior temporal (right) gyri by the proposed method, the proposed method without temporal constraint, and FreeSurfer on 13 subjects

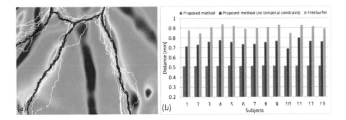

**Fig. 5.** (a) Label boundaries of all aligned longitudinal surfaces of a typical subject, overlaid on the mean spherical surface that is color-coded by the average mean curvatures. Red curves are the results by the proposed method, and white curves are the results by FreeSurfer. (b) Average boundary distance of all labels between every pair of aligned longitudinal surfaces in each of 13 infants by the proposed method (with and without temporal constraint) and FreeSurfer.

## 4    Discussion and Conclusion

This paper presented a novel method for consistent labeling of longitudinal dynamic infant cortical surface using multi-atlas surfaces. The preliminary results on 13 infants demonstrated its promising performance. Our main contributions are: first, we proposed a data fitting term based on the shape information adaptively derived from atlas surfaces; second, we proposed a spatial smoothness term adaptive to the cortical folding geometries and also a temporal consistency term adaptive to the temporal similarities of the cortical folding. Our future work includes parameter optimization, more validation, and application to a large-scale dataset for early brain development study.

## References

1. Li, G., Nie, J., Wang, L., et al.: Mapping Region-Specific Longitudinal Cortical Surface Expansion from Birth to 2 Years of Age. Cereb. Cortex. (2012)
2. Hill, J., Dierker, D., Neil, J., et al.: A surface-based analysis of hemispheric asymmetries and folding of cerebral cortex in term-born human infants. J. Neurosci. 30, 2268–2276 (2010)
3. Reuter, M., Schmansky, N.J., Rosas, H.D., Fischl, B.: Within-subject template estimation for unbiased longitudinal image analysis. Neuroimage 61, 1402–1418 (2012)
4. Boykov, Y., Kolmogorov, V.: An experimental comparison of min-cut/max-flow algorithms for energy minimization in vision. IEEE Trans. PAMI 26, 1124–1137 (2004)
5. Dai, Y., Shi, F., Wang, L., Wu, G., Shen, D.: iBEAT: A Toolbox for Infant Brain Magnetic Resonance Image Processing. Neuroinformatics (2012)
6. Fischl, B., Sereno, M.I., Dale, A.M.: Cortical surface-based analysis. II: Inflation, flattening, and a surface-based coordinate system. Neuroimage 9, 195–207 (1999)
7. Yeo, B.T., Sabuncu, M.R., Vercauteren, T., et al.: Spherical demons: fast diffeomorphic landmark-free surface registration. IEEE Trans. Med. Imaging 29, 650–668 (2010)
8. Desikan, R.S., Segonne, F., Fischl, B., et al.: An automated labeling system for subdividing the human cerebral cortex on MRI scans into gyral based regions of interest. Neuroimage 31, 968–980 (2006)
9. Sabuncu, M.R., Yeo, B.T., Van Leemput, K., et al.: A generative model for image segmentation based on label fusion. IEEE Trans. Med. Imaging 29, 1714–1729 (2010)

# Identifying Group-Wise Consistent White Matter Landmarks via Novel Fiber Shape Descriptor

Hanbo Chen[1], Tuo Zhang[1,2], and Tianming Liu[1]

[1] Department of Computer Science and Bioimaging Research Center,
The University of Georgia, Athens, GA, USA
[2] School of Automation, Northwestern Polytechnical University, Xi'an, China

**Abstract.** Identification of common and corresponding white matter (WM) regions of interest (ROI) across human brains has attracted growing interest because it not only facilitates comparison among individuals and populations, but also enables the assessment of structural/functional connectivity in populations. However, due to the complexity and variability of the WM structure and a lack of effective white matter streamline descriptors, establishing accurate correspondences of WM ROIs across individuals and populations has been a challenging open problem. In this paper, a novel fiber shape descriptor which can facilitate quantitative measurement of fiber bundle profile including connection complexity and similarity has been proposed. A novel framework was then developed using the descriptor to identify group-wise consistent connection hubs in WM regions as landmarks. 12 group-wise consistent WM landmarks have been identified in our experiment. These WM landmarks are found highly reproducible across individuals and accurately predictable on new individual subjects by our fiber shape descriptor. Therefore, these landmarks, as well as proposed fiber shape descriptor has shown great potential to human brain mapping.

**Keywords:** White Matter Landmark, DTI, Group-wise Consistency, Fiber Shape Descriptor.

## 1   Introduction

Identification of common and corresponding white matter (WM) regions of interest (ROIs) across human brains has attracted growing interest not only in that it facilitates comparison among individuals and populations, but also because it makes it possible to assess structural/functional connectivity in populations [1]. One mainstream of previous methods developed in the field so far largely relies on building white matter atlases via registration methods [2, 3] to establish correspondence across subjects. Alternatively, voxel based or fiber tract based features have been newly applied to identify WM ROIs. For instance, in [4], FOD (fiber orientation distribution) has been applied to identify pathologies. In [5], group-wise shape analysis based on fiber tracts has been performed to study WM. In [6], an effective fiber bundle shape descriptor called trace-map has been developed. Base on the trace-map feature [6], a map of discrete cortical landmarks named DICCCOL [7] that possess group-wise consistent white matter fiber connection patterns across individuals has been identified.

K. Mori et al. (Eds.): MICCAI 2013, Part I, LNCS 8149, pp. 66–73, 2013.

However, identifying reliable WM landmarks is still a challenging open problem due to the complexity and variability of the brain structure and a lack of effective white matter streamline descriptors [1]. For instance, the accuracy and reliability of registration based method are limited due to the substantial variability in brain anatomy and structure between individuals. As for most voxel based methods, they are based on local information and have difficulty in establishing between-subject correspondences. In [7], the authors successfully solved the above mentioned issues by introducing an effective fiber bundle shape descriptor of trace map [6]. However, since those identified DICCCOL landmarks locate on cortical surface, the remarkable cortical folding pattern variation may be a major barrier to further improvement.

Motivated by the achievements and the challenges in [6], we developed a novel shape descriptor to characterize the connection patterns of a fiber bundle. Instead of focusing on the shape of streamline fibers as in [6], our descriptor centers on the global connection pattern of fibers. In particular, our proposed descriptor is based on probability density which enables the measurement of directional statistic features. Based on this descriptor, an effective searching/optimization framework is designed to identify WM landmarks that: 1) are highly connected hubs in the brain; 2) are reproducible across individuals. The reason we aim to identify hubs as landmarks lies in that the human brain networks have been shown to be a small-world network [8]. In such network, hubs are more robust, consistent, and could be used to identify subnodes. Thus, by identifying hubs in WM, those landmarks can be potentially used as initial points to establish correspondences across individuals, which will bring great potential to the study of human brain mapping, such as WM landmark-guided image registration. In comparison to existing model-driven WM landmark identification methods [2, 3], the major novelty of our work is that it is data-driven and thus can better handle the complexity and variability of the WM architecture.

## 2    Methods

In this paper, brain ROI is defined as a sphere in the space. To identify WM landmarks with abovementioned properties from ROIs, first, we borrowed the idea from [6] and defined a novel spherical probabilistic distribution based connection map feature vector to describe the fiber profile (Fig. 1(b)). Then, the connection pattern complexities of ROIs are measured to identify WM landmarks (Fig. 1(c-d)). Finally, the locations of landmarks are iteratively optimized in each subject's own space to increase group-wise consistency of these landmarks' connection profiles (Fig. 1 (e)). The computational pipeline of the proposed framework is summarized in Fig. 1.

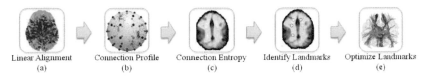

Linear Alignment        Connection Profile        Connection Entropy        Identify Landmarks        Optimize Landmarks
(a)                          (b)                          (c)                          (d)                          (e)

**Fig. 1.** Illustration of the computational pipeline, consisting of 5 steps

## 2.1    ROI Connection Map

First, definitions of several key concepts and terms are given.

*ROI fiber bundle*: An ROI is defined as a sphere with a predefined radius (5mm in this paper). The fiber streamlines passing through this sphere is viewed as the fiber bundle of the corresponding ROI.

*Fiber principal orientation*: For each fiber, its principal orientation is described by a norm vector $v$ which is the first principal component of the points $X$ along the fiber such that:

$$\max( \sum_{x_i \in X} (v \cdot (x_i - \overline{x}))^2 \mid |v| = 1) \tag{1}$$

where $\overline{x}$ is the center of the points in $X$.

*Fiber connection profile*: For a bundle of fibers, by projecting the principal orientation $v$ of each fiber to a unit sphere, the connection profile of this fiber bundle can be represented and interpreted by the points distributed on the sphere. As illustrated in Fig. 2(a-b), the complex fiber bundle connection pattern is mapped to the surface of a sphere without the loss of global information and could be further reduced in dimension via directional statistics method. Notably, as fiber is non-directional connection, both its principal direction $v$ and the opposite direction $-v$ will be projected to the sphere.

*Connection map*: The probability density of orientation vector on the sphere is applied to describe the connection map of fiber bundles. Specifically, the sphere is subdivided into 48 equal sized pixels as defined in the HEALPix [9]. The number of points within each pixel out of the total number of points is calculated as the probability density. In this way, the fiber connection profile is represented by a connection map with a vector of 48 numbers such that:

$$P(V) = \{P_1(V), P_2(V), \cdots, P_{48}(V)\} \tag{2}$$

$$P_k(V) = \frac{\|V \cap R_k\|}{\|V\|} \quad (k = 1 \cdots 48) \tag{3}$$

where $R_k$ is the area covered by pixel $k$, and $\|V\|$ is the number of points on the unit sphere. The advantage of this representation is the capability of representing complex fiber bundle connection pattern with a simple one dimensional feature vector without the loss of major information. As shown in Fig. 2, the connection maps are similar for the fiber bundles sharing similar shapes. For the bundles with different shapes, the connection maps would be distinct. Notably, this representation may have difficulty in distinguishing the fiber bundles with similar shapes but connecting in the opposite direction, or the fiber bundles with similar orientations but different lengths (e.g. the anterior thalamic projection V.S. the inferior fronto-occipital and uncinate fasciculus). These issues could potentially be solved by defining fiber connection direction and introducing multiple spherical shells for fiber bundles with different lengths.

*Connection entropy*: As the HEALPix pixels [9] are the squares evenly distributed on the sphere with equal size, the entropy of orientation vectors $V$ distributed on the sphere could be directly obtained from $P(V)$:

$$H(V) = \sum_{i=1 \cdots 48} -P_i(V) \log_{48} P_i(V) \tag{4}$$

*Connection similarity*: The similarity between two connection maps is measured by cosine similarity:

$$S(P(V_i), P(V_j)) = \frac{P(V_i) \cdot P(V_j)}{\|P(V_i)\| \cdot \|P(V_j)\|} \tag{5}$$

Both connection entropy and similarity are values between 0 and 1. As shown in Fig. 2, higher connection entropy indicates higher connection pattern complexity, and higher similarity value indicates higher similarity between fiber bundles.

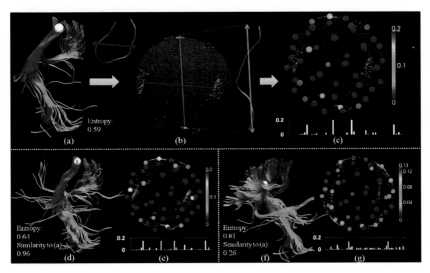

**Fig. 2.** Illustration of ROI connection profile. (a), (d), (f): DTI-derived fibers connected to an ROI. The ROI is defined by a sphere in space (white bubble). (b) Illustration of projecting fibers' orientations to a sphere to obtain connection profile. The white dots are the projection points of fibers. The red and blue lines indicate the main orientation of the corresponding fibers and their projections on the unit sphere. (c), (e), (g): The probabilistic distributions of connection profiles of the fiber bundles shown on their left. The center of each sampling pixel is shown and color-coded by the probability density. Corresponding connection map feature vector is shown at the bottom by histogram.

## 2.2    Identify, Optimize and Predict WM Landmarks

To identify the group-wise consistent WM landmarks that play the hub roles, we need to find the ROIs that maximize the connection entropy (meaning more diverse connections) and cross-subject connection similarity (meaning group-wise consistency) at the same time. The optimization is thus designed to maximize the energy function (equivalent to minimizing the distance function) described below:

$$E(X) = \sum_{x_i \in X} (E_{int}(x_i) + \lambda E_{ext}(x_i)) \tag{6}$$

$$E_{int}(x_i) = \sum_{j=1\cdots n} H(V(F(x_i^j))) \tag{7}$$

$$E_{ext}(x_i, \overline{X}) = \sum_{j=1\cdots n} S(V(F(x_i^j)), \overline{V(F(X))}) \tag{8}$$

where $X$ is the set of a landmark in all subjects. $E_{int}(x_i)$ is the internal energy function of connection entropy. $E_{ext}(x_i)$ is the external energy function of connection similarity. $\lambda$ is the tradeoff (empirically set to 1 in this paper). $F(x_i^j)$ is the fiber bundle passing through the landmark $x_i$ of subject $j$.

The landmark searching framework follows the pipeline shown in Fig. 1. First, the subjects are initially aligned to the same space by linear registration (FSL FLIRT [10]). Then, taking each voxel in the space as the center of an ROI, the connection map entropy of fiber bundles passing through each ROI is computed for each subject. By averaging these connection entropy images, a group-wise connection entropy map is obtained (Fig. 3(a)). Distinguishable regions with high average connection entropy values in this map are visually identified as the initial landmarks. Due to the individual variability and misalignment, the fiber profiles of these initial landmarks could be different. To solve this problem, the landmarks' locations are optimized iteratively with random walks in each subject to maximize the energy function in Eq. (6) as described in Algorithm 1. After optimization, the converged landmarks are then used as template for prediction on new individual brains. The prediction process used a similar framework as optimization. First, the brain of new subject with DTI data is registered to the template space. Then, the space around the initial location of each landmark is searched for the point that maximizes external energy $E_{ext}(x^*, \overline{X}_{template})$ defined in Eq. (8) to guarantee the similarity with template.

| | |
|---|---|
| Input: | Initial Landmarks **X**, Streamline Fibers **F** |
| 1 | For landmark i |
| 2 |     For subject j |
| 3 |         For k=1...N |
| 4 |             Generate random vector $v_{random}$ |
| 5 |             If $E(x_{ij}+v_{random})>E(x_{ij})$ |
| 6 |                 $x_{ij}=x_{ij}+v_{random}$ |
| 7 |     Re-do step 2 to 6 if location of $x_i$ changed |

**Algorithm 1.**

## 3    Experiment Results

Two sets of data are applied. One is acquired from 18 healthy young adults who are equally distributed as training subjects and prediction testing subjects. The parameters are: matrix size $128\times128$, 60 slices, image resolution $2\times2\times2mm^3$ isotropic, TR=15s, ASSET=2, 3 B0 images, 30 optimized gradient directions, b-value=1000. Another dataset publicly released by Human Connectome Project (HCP)[11] contains DTI data of 64 healthy subjects. This dataset is applied to test prediction of trained landmarks. The DTI data preprocessing was performed via FSL [10] which includes eddy current correction, skull removal, computing FA image, tissue segmentation, and linear registration. Fiber tracking was performed via MedINRIA [12] using streamline model and then registered to the same space.

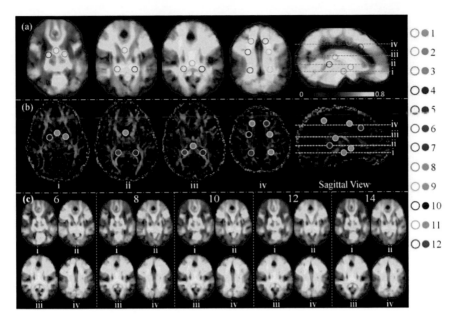

**Fig. 3.** Visualization of average entropy map and the location of 12 landmarks. The location of each landmark is indicated by colored ring/bubble. The location of each axial plan is illustrated by dash line in the sagittal view on the right. (a) Average entropy map of 9 randomly pick subjects. (b) Slices of RGB color-coded principal diffusion tensor direction of template subject volume with corresponding view to (a). (c) Average entropy map of randomly picked subjects with different numbers (6/8/10/12/14). The view is the same as (a).

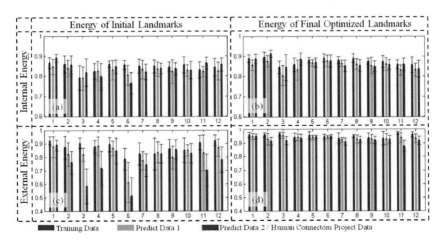

**Fig. 4.** Average internal and external energy of each landmark in different dataset

After preprocessing, entropy map is computed for randomly picked subjects with different subject numbers (6/8/9/10/12/14). The result is similar and consistent between different groups with different sizes Fig. 3(a,c). Thus we randomly picked 9 subjects for training. Finally, 12 landmarks with high connection entropy were visually identified and then automatically optimized as shown in Fig. 3(a-b). Taking the training subjects as the template, these 12 landmarks are predicted on other 9 subjects as well as 64 subjects from HCP data for validation. The average internal energies and external energies are shown in Fig. 4. For training data, both internal and external energies are relatively high, which indicates that these landmarks are consistent connection hubs in brain WM. For prediction data, compared with initial landmarks (obtained via linear registration), the energies of finally optimized landmarks are much higher, which suggests that these landmarks are very reproducible in new subjects and could be predicted with our proposed framework.

To further examine anatomical meaning of these landmarks, we randomly picked one training subject and one prediction subject to visualize major pathways passing these landmarks (Fig. 5). By observation, all these landmarks locate at the intersection point or the connection concentration regions of major fiber pathways. For instance, landmark 3 and 4 are close to the thalamus of each brain spheres, and the fiber tracts such as thalamic radiations, corticopontine tract and corticalspinal tract concentrate around this region. For landmark 5 and 6, the fiber pathways from different lobes intersect at this region, e.g. corpus callosum, posterior thalamic radiation, superior longitudinal fasciculus, and superior longitudinal fasciculus, and stria terminalis/fornix. The pathways that go through these landmarks will be further examined in our future work.

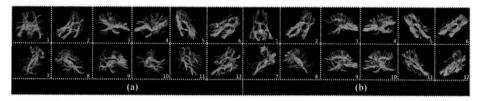

**Fig. 5.** Visualization of fiber bundle of 12 landmarks of (a) a training subject and (b) a testing subject. The landmarks are represented by white bubbles in each sub-figure. The IDs of the landmarks are listed on the right-bottom corner.

## 4      Conclusion and Discussion

A novel fiber shape descriptor has been proposed to characterize the connection patterns of a fiber bundle. The advantage of this descriptor lies in that: (1) it is based on orientation probability density distribution, thus enabling direct calculation of directional statistic features such as similarity or entropy; (2) it can be efficiently calculated with a decision tree which makes it fast to compute. Our validation experiment suggests that this descriptor can quantitatively measure the similarity and connection complexity of fiber bundles with high accuracy. Based on proposed descriptor, a novel computational framework has been developed to identify and predict landmarks that are group-wise consistent connection hubs in WM region. Finally, 12 landmarks with dense connection and high reproducibility across individuals are identified and validated. The major novelty and contribution of WM landmark discovery framework lies in its data-driven nature that can better handle the complexity and variability of the WM structures, in comparison to existing model-driven methods.

In the future, these WM landmarks will be used as initial points to establish cross-individual correspondences for brain image registration. Also, a hierarchical brain connection map will be built based on these WM landmarks to facilitate brain structural/functional connection studies in population. For instance, with each individual, we will first recognize their WM landmarks and then the consistent cortical regions that are connected to these landmarks. Afterward, the sub-connected regions between these consistent cortical regions could be recognized iteratively to populate the landmarks on the cortical brain with consistent connectomes. Finally, it is noted that future applications of the proposed fiber shape descriptor is not limited to the frame work introduced. It has broader potential to be applied in fiber shape related clustering problems such as connection based cortical segmentation optimization [13] or diffusion tensor image based functional ROIs prediction [14].

**Acknowledgements.** Data were provided [in part] by the Human Connectome Project, WU-Minn Consortium (Principal Investigators: David Van Essen and Kamil Ugurbil; 1U54MH091657) funded by the 16 NIH Institutes and Centers that support the NIH Blueprint for Neuroscience Research; and by the McDonnell Center for Systems Neuroscience at Washington University.

# References

1. Derrfuss, J., Mar, R.A.: Lost in localization: the need for a universal coordinate database. NeuroImage 48, 1–7 (2009)
2. Mori, S., et al.: Stereotaxic white matter atlas based on diffusion tensor imaging in an ICBM template. NeuroImage 40, 570–582 (2008)
3. Yap, P.-T., Wu, G., Zhu, H., Lin, W., Shen, D.: TIMER: tensor image morphing for elastic registration. NeuroImage 47, 549–563 (2009)
4. Bloy, L., Ingalhalikar, M., Eavani, H., Roberts, T.P.L., Schultz, R.T., Verma, R.: HARDI based pattern classifiers for the identification of white matter pathologies. In: Fichtinger, G., Martel, A., Peters, T., et al. (eds.) MICCAI 2011, Part II. LNCS, vol. 6892, pp. 234–241. Springer, Heidelberg (2011)
5. O'Donnell, L.J., Westin, C.-F., Golby, A.J.: Tract-based morphometry for white matter group analysis. NeuroImage 45, 832–844 (2009)
6. Zhu, D., Zhang, D., Faraco, C., Li, K., Deng, F., Chen, H., Jiang, X., Guo, L., Miller, L.S., Liu, T.: Discovering dense and consistent landmarks in the brain. In: Székely, G., Hahn, H.K., et al. (eds.) IPMI 2011. LNCS, vol. 6801, pp. 97–110. Springer, Heidelberg (2011)
7. Zhu, D., et al.: DICCCOL: Dense Individualized and Common Connectivity-Based Cortical Landmarks. Cerebral Cortex. (2012)
8. Bullmore, E., Sporns, O.: Complex brain networks: graph theoretical analysis of structural and functional systems. Nature Reviews. Neuroscience 10, 186–198 (2009)
9. Gorski, K.M., et al.: HEALPix: A Framework for High-Resolution Discretization and Fast Analysis of Data Distributed on the Sphere. The Astrophysical Journal 622, 759–771 (2005)
10. Jenkinson, M., et al.: FSL. NeuroImage 62, 782–790 (2012)
11. Van Essen, D.C., et al.: The Human Connectome Project: a data acquisition perspective. NeuroImage 62, 2222–2231 (2012)
12. Toussaint, N., Souplet, J., Fillard, P.: MedINRIA: Medical image navigation and research tool by INRIA. In: MICCAI. pp. 1–8 (2007)
13. Clarkson, M.J., Malone, I.B., Modat, M., Leung, K.K., Ryan, N., Alexander, D.C., Fox, N.C., Ourselin, S.: A framework for using diffusion weighted imaging to improve cortical parcellation. In: Jiang, T., Navab, N., Pluim, J.P.W., Viergever, M.A., et al. (eds.) MICCAI 2010, Part I. LNCS, vol. 6361, pp. 534–541. Springer, Heidelberg (2010)
14. Zhang, T., et al.: Predicting functional cortical ROIs via DTI-derived fiber shape models. Cerebral Cortex. 22, 854–864 (2012)

# The Importance of Being Dispersed:
# A Ranking of Diffusion MRI Models for Fibre Dispersion Using *In Vivo* Human Brain Data

Uran Ferizi[1,2], Torben Schneider[2], Maira Tariq[1],
Claudia A.M. Wheeler-Kingshott[2], Hui Zhang[1], and Daniel C. Alexander[1]

[1] CMIC, Dept. Computer Science and Dept. Medical Physics and Bioengineering,
University College London, United Kingdom
[2] NMR Research Unit, Department of Neuroinflammation, Institute of Neurology,
University College London, United Kingdom
uran.ferizi.10@ucl.ac.uk

**Abstract.** In this work we compare parametric diffusion MRI models which explicitly seek to explain fibre dispersion in nervous tissue. These models aim at providing more specific biomarkers of disease by disentangling these structural contributions to the signal. Some models are drawn from recent work in the field; others have been constructed from combinations of existing compartments that aim to capture both intracellular and extracellular diffusion. To test these models we use a rich dataset acquired *in vivo* on the corpus callosum of a human brain, and then compare the models via the Bayesian Information Criteria. We test this ranking via bootstrapping on the data sets, and cross-validate across unseen parts of the protocol. We find that models that capture fibre dispersion are preferred. The results show the importance of modelling dispersion, even in apparently coherent fibres.

## 1 Introduction

Diffusion MRI probes the tissue microstructure, by measuring the water dispersion in biological tissue. This technique is often applied in the brain, especially where parallel fibres restrict the water mobility anisotropically, thus providing putative measures of white matter integrity and connectivity.

Currently, the standard model for imaging diffusion in tissue is the diffusion tensor (DT) [1], which assumes a trivariate Gaussian dispersion pattern. Derived indices, e.g. mean diffusivity or fractional anisotropy, can correlate with major tissue damage, but lack the sensitivity and the specificity to provide indices such as axon radius, density, orientation and permeability. Stanisz et al. [2] pioneered a multi-compartment representation of separate diffusive processes in nervous tissue. The Ball-and-Stick model, by Behrens et al. [3] is the simplest possible two-compartment model with restricted axonal diffusion and isotropic extra-axonal diffusion. A recent class of parametric models has emerged to describe data better by additionally accounting for fibre directional incoherence, which is abundant in the brain, even at a sub-voxel level.

K. Mori et al. (Eds.): MICCAI 2013, Part I, LNCS 8149, pp. 74–81, 2013.

Ball-and-Sticks [3] can have more-than-one intracellular diffusion compartments. Zhang et al. [4] constructed NODDI to describe fibres with an explicit orientation dispersion index derived from a Watson distribution and tests the model with *in-vivo* human whole-brain data. Sotiropoulos et al. [5] design Ball-and-Rackets to describe fibre fanning through a Bingham distribution by extending the Ball-and-Sticks model [3]. The Bingham distribution extends the Watson distribution to account for asymmetric/anisotropic dispersion. This model is then applied to post-mortem macaque monkey brain data.

In this work, similar to the taxonomy provided in Panagiotaki et al. [6], we construct models that combine Ball (for isotropic diffusion), Zeppelin (for 2D anisotropic diffusion) or Tensor (for 3D anisotropic diffusion) for extracellular diffusion, with various models for intracellular diffusion: two-Sticks, a Watson or Bingham distribution of Sticks. We also add a further compartment for isotropically restricted diffusion: Dot (a zero radius sphere) or CSF. We then fit these models to a very rich dataset and, in addition to the fitting quality, we take into account the model complexity by using the Bayesian Information Criterion in order to discover which models explain the data best. Lastly, to validate the *BIC* ranking, we test the models through both bootstrapping on the data sets and prediction of unseen parts of the protocol.

## 2   Methods

This section first describes the models, then the data acquisition and the preprocessing done to obtain a set of measurements for fitting the models. Lastly, we detail the fitting procedure and the criterion applied to compare the models.

### 2.1   Models

**Generic Model:** The signal for a model with two or more types of compartments can be expressed as: $S = S_0 \left\{ \sum f_{ic}^k S_{ic}^k + f_{rc} S_{rc} + (1 - f_{rc} - \sum f_{ic}^k) S_{ec} \right\}$, where $f_{ic}$ is the weight of the intracellular signal compartment $S^{ic}$, $f_{rc}$ is the weight of the isotropically restricted signal compartment $S_{rc}$, $S_{ec}$ is the extracellular signal compartment, and $k$ is the compartment index.

**Extracellular Compartments:** The compartments used to capture signal outside the axons and the isotropically restricted compartments are the Tensor, the Zeppelin, the Zeppelin with tortuosity and the Ball. *Tensor* signal is modelled through the DT, as $S = \exp[\lambda_1(e_1 e_1^t) + \lambda_2(e_2 e_2^t) + \lambda_3(e_3 e_3^t)]$, where $e_1$, $e_2$ and $e_3$ are the three characteristic vectors that define the 3D orientation of the Tensor and, along those directions, $\lambda_1$, $\lambda_2$ and $\lambda_3$ give the size of the tensor (or "apparent diffusivity"). The *Zeppelin* is a special case of the Tensor where $\lambda_2 = \lambda_3$. We follow Szafer et al. [7] to express the *Zeppelin with tortuosity*, which has the radial diffusivity expressed in terms of the axial one, $\lambda_2 = \lambda_1 f_{ic}$. Further, setting all three eigenvalues the same makes a *Ball*, where $\lambda_1 = \lambda_2 = \lambda_3$.

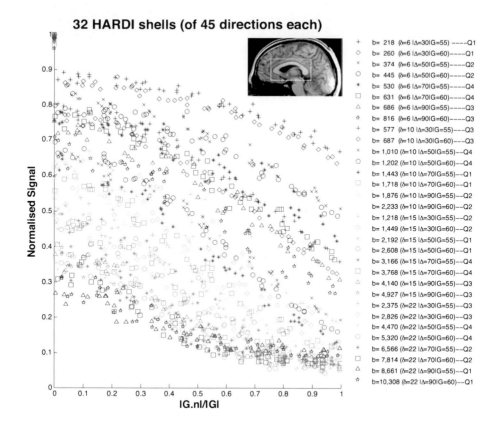

**Fig. 1.** The $2°$ data set. The legend gives b-value ($\delta \mid \Delta \mid |\mathbf{G}|$) in units of s/mm$^2$(ms|ms|mT/m); Q1-Q4 on the right define the four quarters of the full protocol used in the cross-validation. The insert picture is of a sagittal slice of the brain; boxed is the scanned volume, encompassing the corpus callosum. $\mathbf{G}$ is the applied gradient vector and $\mathbf{n}$ is the fibre direction; the x-axis gives the absolute value of the cosine of the angle between the applied gradient and fibre direction: to the left, the gradient is perpendicular to the fibres; to the right, parallel.

**Intracellular Compartments:** Sticks are used to represent the axonal diffusion, via either a discrete set of Sticks [3] (we pick two) or an underlying Bingham/Watson fibre orientation distribution [4,5]. The *Bingham* distribution is $f(\mathbf{n}|\kappa_1, \kappa_2, \boldsymbol{\mu}_1, \boldsymbol{\mu}_2) = [{}_1F_1(\frac{1}{2}, \frac{3}{2}, \kappa_1, \kappa_2)]^{-1}\exp[\kappa_1(\boldsymbol{\mu}_1 \cdot \mathbf{n})^2 + \kappa_2(\boldsymbol{\mu}_2 \cdot \mathbf{n})^2]$, where $\kappa_1$ and $\kappa_2$ are the concentration parameters, such that $\kappa_1 \geq \kappa_2 \geq 0$; the mutually orthogonal vectors $\boldsymbol{\mu}_1$ and $\boldsymbol{\mu}_2$ indicate the orientation axes of fibre dispersion. This is similar to a bivariate Gaussian distribution with elliptical contours on the sphere. The denominator, ${}_1F_1$, is a confluent hypergeometric function of first kind [8]. The *Watson* distribution is a special case of the Bingham distribution, where there is only one $\kappa$ and $\boldsymbol{\mu}$ ($\kappa_2 = 0$); this corresponds to circular contours on the sphere.

## 2.2 Data Acquisition and Preprocessing

We use a PGSE sequence on a 3T Phillips scanner, with cardiac gating and TR=4s. The full protocol uses 32 HARDI shells. Each shell has a unique set of 45 directions, randomly rotated to enhance the angular resolution. The protocol has a wide range of achievable b-values, 218 to 10,308 s/mm$^2$, combining $\delta = \{6, 10, 15, 22\}$ms, $\Delta = \{30, 50, 70, 90\}$ms, $|\mathbf{G}| = \{55, 60\}$mT/m, and three interwoven b=0 acquisitions.

The data is acquired in two separate non-stop sessions, each lasting about 4.5hrs (the "2x4hr" dataset). The field-of-view is centred on the mid-sagittal slice of the corpus callosum (CC), where we assume coherently oriented CC fibres are perpendicular to the image plane. There are nine 4mm-thick sagittal slices, the image size is 64 x 64 and the in-plane resolution is 2mm x 2mm.

After manually registering all DW images to the unweighted image of the b=1,202s/mm$^2$ shell, using only image translations, we fit the DT to this b=1,202 shell to select a set of voxels with coherently oriented fibres. Voxels with FA>0.6 and principal eigenvector within $\eta=2°$ of the assumed fibre direction are retained. There are 24 voxels remaining, all in 2 slices close to the mid-sagittal plane, and mostly in the genu. A similar procedure is performed with $\eta=5°$, which leaves 66 voxels, and deviation 10° which leaves 99 voxels, in both cases across the genu and mid-body.

Before fitting the models, the signal of each DW slice is normalised by the b=0 images with the same echo time (TE). A single dataset is then created by averaging the voxels selected above. Fig.1 shows the signal from the 2° dataset, containing 1,536=32*(3+45) measurements.

## 2.3 Model Fitting and Selection

We use the open source Camino toolkit [10] to fit the models. Each model is fitted 250 times, using the Levenberg-Marquardt algorithm with a perturbed starting point from initial estimates drawn from the DT, to extract the parameters that produce the minimum objective function. The fitting uses an offset-Gaussian noise model to construct the objective $LSE = \sum_{i=1}^{N} \frac{1}{\sigma^2}(\tilde{S}_i - \sqrt{S_i^2 + \sigma^2})^2$, where $N$ is the number of measurements, $\tilde{S}_i$ is the $i$-th measured signal, $S_i$ its prediction from the model; $\sigma^2$ is the signal variance, which we estimate *a priori* from the b=0 images (this corresponds to an SNR of around 20). This objective function accounts for bias introduced by the Rician noise inherent in the MRI data in a way that is more numerically stable and computationally efficient than a full Rician log-likelihood objective function.

For model selection, we use the $BIC = -2\log(L) + K\log(N)$ where $L$ is the likelihood of model parameters given the data, $N$ is the number of measurements and $K$ is the number of free parameters. We evaluate the $BIC$ for each fitted model and then rank all models from lowest $BIC$ (best) to highest (worst).

**Table 1.** Various model parameters from different data sets of angular thresholds of 2°, 5° and 10°. The models are ordered top-down by the $BIC$ score of 2° data set. Here, we also include the estimates (shown in bold) from the best model of a previous ranking of non-dispersive parametric models [9]. [Note: Zepp=Zeppelin; ZepT=Zeppelin with tortuosity;Tens=Tensor; St=Stick; Bing=Bingham; Wat=Watson].

| Param. | Models | BIC 2x4_2 | 2x4_5 | 2x4_10 | Intra.1 Vol.Fr. 2x4_2 | 2x4_5 | 2x4_10 | Extra. Vol.Fr. 2x4_2 | 2x4_5 | 2x4_10 | CSF/Dot Vol.Fr. 2x4_2 | 2x4_5 | 2x4_10 | Axial Diff. 2x4_2 | 2x4_5 | 2x4_10 | Radial Diff. 2x4_2 | 2x4_5 | 2x4_10 | Kappa 2x4_2 | 2x4_5 | 2x4_10 |
|---|---|---|---|---|---|---|---|---|---|---|---|---|---|---|---|---|---|---|---|---|---|---|
| 10 | Zepp.Bing.CSF. | 513 | 380 | 359 | 0.56 | 0.59 | 0.60 | 0.29 | 0.30 | 0.31 | 0.15 | 0.11 | 0.09 | 2.0 | 1.9 | 1.9 | 0.5 | 0.6 | 0.7 | 6.9 | 7.1 | 6.5 |
| 9 | ZepT.Bing.CSF. | 516 | 377 | 356 | 0.59 | 0.59 | 0.60 | 0.28 | 0.30 | 0.31 | 0.13 | 0.11 | 0.09 | 2.0 | 1.9 | 1.9 | 0.6 | 0.7 | 0.7 | 7.0 | 7.1 | 6.5 |
| 12 | Tens.Bing.CSF. | 516 | 383 | 362 | 0.56 | 0.59 | 0.60 | 0.29 | 0.30 | 0.31 | 0.15 | 0.11 | 0.09 | 2.0 | 1.9 | 1.9 | 0.6 | 0.7 | 0.8 | 8.1 | 8.0 | 7.3 |
| 10 | Tens.Wat.CSF. | 519 | 392 | 369 | 0.55 | 0.59 | 0.60 | 0.29 | 0.29 | 0.30 | 0.16 | 0.12 | 0.10 | 2.0 | 1.9 | 1.9 | 0.5 | 0.7 | 0.7 | 5.4 | 5.5 | 5.3 |
| 8 | Zepp.Wat.CSF. | 531 | 401 | 373 | 0.56 | 0.59 | 0.60 | 0.29 | 0.30 | 0.31 | 0.15 | 0.11 | 0.09 | 2.0 | 1.9 | 1.9 | 0.5 | 0.6 | 0.7 | 5.6 | 5.6 | 5.4 |
| 7 | ZepT.Wat.CSF. | 533 | 398 | 369 | 0.59 | 0.60 | 0.60 | 0.28 | 0.30 | 0.31 | 0.13 | 0.11 | 0.09 | 2.0 | 1.9 | 1.9 | 0.6 | 0.6 | 0.7 | 5.8 | 5.6 | 5.4 |
| 9 | ZepT.Bing.Dot | 542 | 367 | 342 | 0.53 | 0.52 | 0.52 | 0.43 | 0.44 | 0.44 | 0.03 | 0.04 | 0.04 | 2.1 | 2.0 | 2.0 | 0.9 | 0.9 | 0.9 | 9.4 | 10.4 | 9.3 |
| 10 | Zepp.Bing.Dot | 544 | 366 | 340 | 0.50 | 0.48 | 0.48 | 0.45 | 0.47 | 0.47 | 0.04 | 0.05 | 0.05 | 2.1 | 2.0 | 2.0 | 0.9 | 0.8 | 0.8 | 10.3 | 12.0 | 11.0 |
| 12 | Tens.Bing.Dot | 548 | 371 | 345 | 0.51 | 0.49 | 0.48 | 0.45 | 0.46 | 0.47 | 0.04 | 0.05 | 0.05 | 2.1 | 2.0 | 2.0 | 1.0 | 0.9 | 0.9 | 10.7 | 12.5 | 11.5 |
| 10 | Tens.Wat.Dot | 557 | 385 | 355 | 0.49 | 0.47 | 0.47 | 0.46 | 0.48 | 0.48 | 0.04 | 0.05 | 0.05 | 2.1 | 2.0 | 2.0 | 1.0 | 0.9 | 0.9 | 8.1 | 8.7 | 8.2 |
| 9 | Zepp.Bing. | 559 | 398 | 370 | 0.64 | 0.65 | 0.64 | 0.36 | 0.35 | 0.36 | | | | 2.2 | 2.1 | 2.0 | 1.0 | 1.0 | 1.0 | 6.6 | 6.7 | 6.2 |
| 7 | ZepT.Wat.Dot | 559 | 390 | 357 | 0.53 | 0.52 | 0.52 | 0.44 | 0.44 | 0.44 | 0.03 | 0.04 | 0.04 | 2.1 | 2.0 | 2.0 | 1.0 | 0.9 | 0.9 | 7.4 | 7.7 | 7.2 |
| 8 | Zepp.Wat.Dot | 561 | 389 | 356 | 0.50 | 0.48 | 0.48 | 0.46 | 0.47 | 0.47 | 0.04 | 0.05 | 0.05 | 2.1 | 2.0 | 2.0 | 0.9 | 0.8 | 0.8 | 8.0 | 8.6 | 8.2 |
| 11 | Tens.Bing. | 561 | 399 | 372 | 0.65 | 0.65 | 0.65 | 0.35 | 0.35 | 0.35 | | | | 2.2 | 2.1 | 2.1 | 1.2 | 1.1 | 1.1 | 7.2 | 7.4 | 6.8 |
| 9 | Tens.Wat. | 575 | 418 | 384 | 0.64 | 0.65 | 0.65 | 0.36 | 0.35 | 0.35 | | | | 2.2 | 2.1 | 2.1 | 1.1 | 1.1 | 1.0 | 5.5 | 5.5 | 5.3 |
| 8 | ZepT.Bing. | 576 | 416 | 385 | 0.62 | 0.62 | 0.62 | 0.38 | 0.38 | 0.38 | | | | 2.2 | 2.1 | 2.1 | 0.8 | 0.8 | 0.8 | 6.5 | 6.5 | 6.0 |
| 7 | Zepp.Wat. | 576 | 419 | 383 | 0.64 | 0.65 | 0.65 | 0.36 | 0.35 | 0.35 | | | | 2.2 | 2.1 | 2.1 | 1.0 | 1.0 | 1.0 | 5.6 | 5.5 | 5.3 |
| 6 | ZepT.Wat. | 593 | 437 | 398 | 0.62 | 0.63 | 0.63 | 0.38 | 0.37 | 0.37 | | | | 2.2 | 2.1 | 2.1 | 0.8 | 0.8 | 0.8 | 5.4 | 5.3 | 5.1 |
| 12 | Tens.St.St.Dot | 652 | 464 | 439 | 0.23 | 0.22 | 0.21 | 0.56 | 0.56 | 0.56 | 0.07 | 0.07 | 0.08 | 2.0 | 1.9 | 1.9 | 0.8 | 0.8 | 0.8 | | | |
| 10 | Zepp.St.St.Dot | 658 | 464 | 437 | 0.23 | 0.22 | 0.21 | 0.56 | 0.56 | 0.56 | 0.07 | 0.07 | 0.08 | 2.0 | 1.9 | 1.9 | 0.8 | 0.7 | 0.7 | | | |
| 12 | Tens.St.St.CSF. | 674 | 562 | 557 | 0.22 | 0.24 | 0.23 | 0.41 | 0.41 | 0.42 | 0.21 | 0.18 | 0.17 | 1.5 | 1.5 | 1.4 | 0.5 | 0.5 | 0.5 | | | |
| 10 | Zepp.St.St.CSF. | 692 | 570 | 565 | 0.23 | 0.25 | 0.24 | 0.41 | 0.41 | 0.42 | 0.21 | 0.18 | 0.17 | 1.5 | 1.4 | 1.4 | 0.4 | 0.4 | 0.5 | | | |
| 8 | Ball.Bing. | 729 | 590 | 583 | 0.72 | 0.71 | 0.71 | 0.28 | 0.29 | 0.29 | | | | 2.2 | 2.1 | 2.1 | | | | 6.0 | 6.2 | 5.9 |
| 9 | Ball.Bing.Dot | 732 | 593 | 586 | 0.72 | 0.71 | 0.71 | 0.28 | 0.29 | 0.29 | 0.00 | 0.00 | 0.00 | 2.2 | 2.1 | 2.1 | | | | 6.0 | 6.2 | 5.9 |
| 9 | Ball.Bing.CSF. | 732 | 593 | 586 | 0.72 | 0.71 | 0.71 | 0.28 | 0.29 | 0.29 | 0.00 | 0.00 | 0.00 | 2.2 | 2.1 | 2.1 | | | | 6.0 | 6.2 | 5.9 |
| 6 | Ball.Wat. | 745 | 610 | 596 | 0.72 | 0.72 | 0.71 | 0.28 | 0.28 | 0.29 | | | | 2.2 | 2.1 | 2.1 | | | | 5.2 | 5.3 | 5.2 |
| 7 | Ball.Wat.CSF. | 748 | 613 | 599 | 0.72 | 0.72 | 0.71 | 0.28 | 0.28 | 0.29 | 0.00 | 0.00 | 0.00 | 2.2 | 2.1 | 2.1 | | | | 5.2 | 5.3 | 5.2 |
| 7 | Ball.Wat.Dot | 748 | 613 | 599 | 0.72 | 0.72 | 0.71 | 0.28 | 0.28 | 0.29 | 0.00 | 0.00 | 0.00 | 2.2 | 2.1 | 2.1 | | | | 5.2 | 5.3 | 5.2 |
| 7 | **Zepp.St.Dot** | **784** | **597** | **570** | **0.29** | **0.30** | **0.29** | **0.62** | **0.62** | **0.62** | **0.09** | **0.09** | **0.09** | **1.9** | **1.9** | **1.8** | **0.7** | **0.7** | **0.7** | | | |
| 10 | Tens.Cyl.CSF. | 832 | 735 | 739 | 0.29 | 0.31 | 0.31 | 0.47 | 0.47 | 0.48 | 0.24 | 0.22 | 0.21 | 1.3 | 1.3 | 1.3 | 0.3 | 0.4 | 0.4 | | | |
| 9 | ZepT.St.St.Dot | 843 | 652 | 640 | 0.33 | 0.33 | 0.32 | 0.50 | 0.50 | 0.50 | 0.05 | 0.05 | 0.05 | 1.8 | 1.7 | 1.7 | 1.1 | 1.1 | 1.1 | | | |
| 11 | Tens.St.St. | 859 | 687 | 666 | 0.28 | 0.28 | 0.27 | 0.52 | 0.51 | 0.52 | | | | 1.7 | 1.6 | 1.6 | 0.9 | 0.9 | 0.9 | | | |
| 9 | Zepp.St.St. | 874 | 695 | 674 | 0.29 | 0.28 | 0.27 | 0.52 | 0.51 | 0.52 | | | | 1.6 | 1.6 | 1.6 | 0.8 | 0.8 | 0.8 | | | |
| 9 | ZepT.St.St.CSF. | 881 | 718 | 712 | 0.35 | 0.35 | 0.34 | 0.39 | 0.41 | 0.43 | 0.12 | 0.10 | 0.08 | 1.5 | 1.5 | 1.4 | 0.9 | 0.9 | 0.9 | | | |
| 8 | ZepT.St.St. | 895 | 713 | 696 | 0.32 | 0.31 | 0.30 | 0.50 | 0.49 | 0.50 | | | | 1.6 | 1.6 | 1.5 | 1.0 | 1.0 | 1.0 | | | |
| 8 | Ball.St.St. | 1,161 | 978 | 965 | 0.28 | 0.27 | 0.27 | 0.46 | 0.46 | 0.46 | | | | 1.5 | 1.5 | 1.5 | | | | | | |
| 9 | Ball.St.St.Dot | 1,162 | 977 | 965 | 0.24 | 0.26 | 0.25 | 0.47 | 0.46 | 0.47 | 0.02 | 0.02 | 0.02 | 1.6 | 1.5 | 1.5 | | | | | | |
| 9 | Ball.St.St.CSF. | 1,164 | 981 | 969 | 0.28 | 0.27 | 0.26 | 0.46 | 0.46 | 0.46 | 0.00 | 0.00 | 0.00 | 1.5 | 1.5 | 1.5 | | | | | | |

## 3   Results

Table 1 lists main parameter estimates across all three datasets (with $\eta=2°$, 5° and 10°). We have also included the best model from a previous ranking of non-dispersive parametric models [9], and a similar model with CSF instead of Dot. Four groups can be distinguished:

i) all combinations that include an anisotropic extracellular compartment and a Bingham/Watson intracellular compartment;

ii) models similar to (i) but instead using two-Sticks for their intracellular compartment, excluding models that use tortuosity or those without a spherically restricted compartment;

iii) all models incorporating an isotropic extracellular compartment with a Bingham/Watson intracellular compartment; and

iv) all exceptions to two-Sticks models in (ii).

The models that include a Bingham/Watson distribution outperform two-Sticks ones not simply because of their good quality of fit to the data but also reduced complexity.

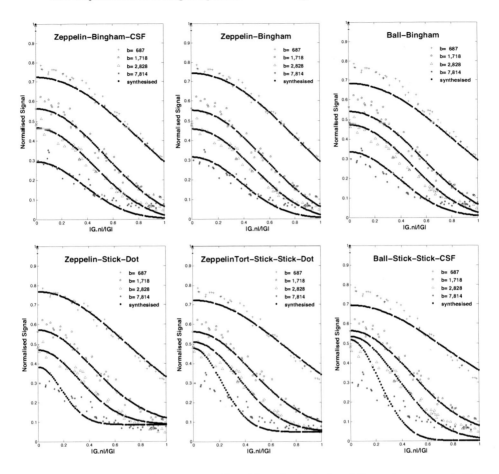

**Fig. 2.** A comparison of raw vs. predicted/synthesised signal from six representative models. The models are ordered in decreasing ranking left-right, top-bottom.

Within group (i), CSF models perform best for $\eta=2°$ but, as $\eta$ increases, Dot models are best. In this group, models using tortuosity produce similar estimates to those of the unconstrained Zeppelin, suggesting that meaningful constraints on the model parameters simplify the problem at little cost to fitting quality.

Across angular thresholds, the axial diffusivity is about $2x10^{-9}$ $mm^2/s$, and the radial diffusivity is around one-quarter of this in models with CSF, but one-half in others; this is to be expected as the CSF compartment has a fixed diffusivity of $3x10^{-9}$ $mm^2/s$ and higher volume fraction than Dot.

As $\eta$ increases from $2°$ to $5°$, all models reflect the signal improvement from averaging across more voxels (24 vs. 66, resp.) through decreasing $BIC$ and increasing fibre incoherence $\kappa$; however, at $10°$ (with 99 voxels averaged), the fitting improves slightly, but $\kappa$ reflects the increased fibre coherence through decreasing $\kappa$.

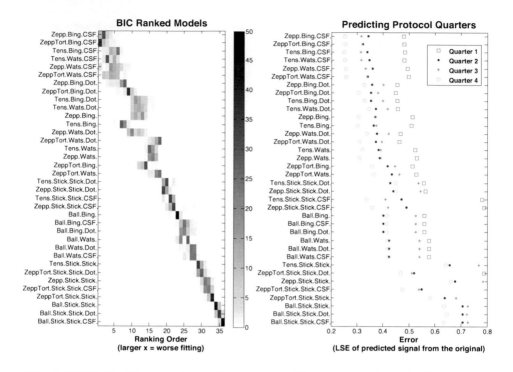

**Fig. 3.** LEFT: Positional variance diagrams over 100 bootstraps from the 2° data sets. The frequency of x-axis ranking is given by the shade of grey.
RIGHT: The accuracy of predicting unseen quarters of the protocol using parameters fitted to data from the remaining three-quarters. The ranking is as in Table 1.

Fig.2 shows the fit of some representative models to the data, to illustrate the difference between the actual signal and that generated from the model.

Fig.3 shows on the left the positional variance diagram for the *BIC* ranking through classical bootstrap. Each bootstrap data set is constructed through a random selection in each shell of the same number of data points, with replacement. The group structure remains unchanged, though there are minor variations within each group.

On the right of Fig.3, the relative performance of each model in reproducing unseen parts of the dataset is shown. We divide the data into four quarters, by randomly assigning low and high $\Delta$s into four groups. Then, we choose signal coming from three-quarters of the dataset to fit our models to and, from the parameter estimates drawn from these quarters, synthesise signal for the missing part. Next, we evaluate the sum of squared differences *LSE* compared to that unseen quarter. This provides an alternative model selection routine, to confirm and validate the ranking by *BIC* and, broadly speaking, the trends in both techniques agree.

## 4    Discussion

In this preliminary work, we have shown the advantage of dispersion models in describing data even in a homogeneous region of the brain such the CC.
In such structure, where a multitude of function specific fibre tracts bundle together, there is inhomogeneity that can produce a dispersion pattern, which is something that these models may reflect. In particular, the single mode orientation distributions (Watson/Bingham) outperform two discrete orientations (two-Sticks). As in previous work, an anisotropic extracellular compartment benefits the fitting, as does the addition of an isotropically restricted compartment.

We acknowledge that averaging voxels across parts of the CC and minor misalignments during image registration may exaggerate the dispersion, so this will be our future work. Testing the models voxel-by-voxel will help us see how consistent the model selection is within regions. We also intend to extend the investigation to other white matter structures that have greater dispersion.

**Acknowledgements.** EPSRC support this work through grants EP/E007748 and EP/I027084/01. We thank the MS Society of Great Britain for supporting the NMR unit. This work was supported by National Institute of Health Research and UCLH.

## References

1. Basser, P.J., Mattiello, J., LeBihan, D.: Estimation of the effective self-diffusion tensor from the NMR spin echo. J. Magn. Reson. B. 103, 247–254 (1994)
2. Stanisz, G.J., Szafer, A., Wright, G.A., Henkelman, M.: An analytical model of restricted diffusion in bovine optic nerve. Magn. Reson. Med. 37, 103–111 (1997)
3. Behrens, T.E., Woolrich, M.W., Jenkinson, M., Johansen-Berg, H., Nunes, R.G., Clare, S., Matthews, P.M., Brady, J.M., Smith, J.M.: Characterization and propagation of uncertainty in diffusion-weighted MR imaging. Magn. Reson. Med. 50, 1077–1088 (2003)
4. Zhang, H., Schneider, T., Wheeler-Kingshott, C.A.M., Alexander, D.C.: Practical in vivo neurite orientation dispersion and density imaging of the human brain. NeuroImage 61, 1000–1016 (2012)
5. Sotiropoulos, S., Behrens, T.E., Jbabdi, S.: Ball and Rackets: Inferring Fibre Fanning from Diffusion-weighted MRI. NeuroImage 60, 1412–1425 (2012)
6. Panagiotaki, E., Schneider, T., Siow, B., Hall, M.G., Lythgoe, M.F., Alexander, D.C.: Compartment models of the diffusion MR signal in brain white matter: A taxonomy and comparison. Neuroimage 59, 2241–2254 (2012)
7. Szafer, A., Zhong, J.H., Gore, J.C.: Theoretical model for water diffusion in tissues. Magn. Reson. Med. 33, 697–712 (1995)
8. Mardia, K.V., Jupp, P.E.: Distributions on spheres. Directional Stats., 159–192 (2000)
9. Ferizi, U., Schneider, T., Panagiotaki, E., Nedjati-Gilani, G., Zhang, H., Wheeler-Kingshott, C.A.M., Alexander, D.C.: Ranking Diffusion MRI Models with In Vivo Human Brain Data. In: 10th IEEE International Symposium on Biomedical Imaging (2013)
10. Cook, P.A., Bai, Y., Nedjati-Gilani, S., Seunarine, K.K., Hall, M.G., Parker, G.J., Alexander, D.C.: Camino: Open-source diffusion-MRI reconstruction and processing. In: 14th Scientific Meeting of the ISMRM 2759 (2006)

# Estimating Constrained Multi-fiber Diffusion MR Volumes by Orientation Clustering

Ryan P. Cabeen[1], Mark E. Bastin[2], and David H. Laidlaw[1]

[1] Computer Science Department, Brown University, Providence, RI, USA
{cabeen,dhl}@cs.brown.edu
[2] Centre for Clinical Brain Sciences, University of Edinburgh, Edinburgh, UK
Mark.Bastin@ed.ac.uk

**Abstract.** Diffusion MRI is a valuable tool for mapping tissue microstructure; however, multi-fiber models present challenges to image analysis operations. In this paper, we present a method for estimating models for such operations by clustering fiber orientations. Our approach is applied to ball-and-stick diffusion models, which include an isotropic tensor and multiple sticks encoding fiber volume and orientation. We consider operations which can be generalized to a weighted combination of fibers and present a method for representing such combinations with a mixture-of-Watsons model, learning its parameters by Expectation Maximization. We evaluate this approach with two experiments. First, we show it is effective for filtering in the presence of synthetic noise. Second, we demonstrate interpolation and averaging by construction of a tractography atlas, showing improved reconstruction of white matter pathways. These experiments indicate that our method is useful in estimating multi-fiber ball-and-stick diffusion volumes resulting from a range of image analysis operations.

**Keywords:** diffusion imaging, tractography, atlasing, multi-fiber models, white matter, ball-and-stick, filtering, interpolation.

## 1 Introduction

Diffusion magnetic resonance imaging enables quantitative mapping of tissue microstructure properties. This modality is especially valuable for studying white matter in the human brain, as water molecule diffusion models enable both local measurement of fiber integrity as well as more global reconstruction of white matter structure through tractography. While these are rich sources of information, multi-direction diffusion models pose a challenge for common operations, such as filtering, interpolation, and averaging. This is due to the directional nature of fiber models and the correspondence problem of matching fibers between voxels [1]. This is a major concern for atlas-based neuroimaging studies, where these operations are used to spatially normalize a population and perform statistical analysis.

Our contribution is the presentation and evaluation of an approach for filtering, interpolating, and averaging ball-and-stick fiber models, a multi-compartment

K. Mori et al. (Eds.): MICCAI 2013, Part I, LNCS 8149, pp. 82–89, 2013.

water diffusion model that has relatively few parameters and is commonly used for tractography [2]. Our approach bears most similarity to a method for interpolating multi-tensor models by Taquet, et al. [3]. While the ball-and-stick model consists of tensor compartments, they are not positive definite, so the Gaussian mixture simplification approach proposed in that work is not well defined for this constrained model. Instead, we employ the mixture-of-Watsons model proposed for fiber modeling by Rathi el al [4], present an efficient Expectation Maximization algorithm for learning its parameters from weighted samples, and evaluate its applications with two experiments. The Watson distribution has been notably used to model fibers in several other works, including characterizing orientation error [5], performing filtered tractography [6], statistical testing [7], and atlas space averaging [8].

In the following section, we first review the ball-and-stick diffusion model, then show how mixture-of-Watsons clustering can be used to estimate multi-fiber volumes, followed by a description of an Expectation Maximization algorithm to efficiently learn the model parameters. We then present results from two experiments: the first tests the performance of mixture-of-Watsons filtering in the presence of synthetic noise, comparing to the heuristic discussed by Taquet, et al. [3]; the second demonstrates the construction and virtual dissection of a tractography atlas, comparing it to the single tensor and heuristic reconstructions. We end with a discussion and concluding remarks.

## 2   Methods

### 2.1   Diffusion Model

A common multi-fiber model consists of a linear combination of tensors. The predicted signal $S_i$ of the $i$-th volume for such a model is:

$$S_i = S_0 \sum_{j=0}^{M} f_j \exp\left(-b_i \boldsymbol{g}_i^T \mathbf{D}_j \boldsymbol{g}_i\right) \tag{1}$$

given M fiber compartments, gradient encoding direction $\boldsymbol{g}_i$, b-value $b_i$, unweighted signal $S_0$, fiber volume fraction $0 \leq f_j \leq 1$, and $\sum_{j=0}^{M} f_k = 1$. In this paper, we consider the ball-and-stick variety of this model, which is constrained to have a completely isotropic first component $\mathbf{D}_0 = \operatorname{diag}(d, d, d)$ and completely anisotropic subsequent components $\mathbf{D}_j = d\boldsymbol{v}_j \boldsymbol{v}_j^T$, given diffusivity $d$ and fiber orientation $\boldsymbol{v}_j$. The anisotropic tensor is given by the outer-product of the fiber orientation vector, whose eigenvalues are $\{1, 0, 0\}$. It should be noted that this tensor is not positive definite, thus Riemannian tensor manifold methods and the Burg matrix divergence [3] are not well defined.

### 2.2   Mixture-of-Watson Estimation

In this section, we describe our method for estimating ball-and-stick models with mixture-of-Watson clustering. We take an approach similar to [3] and consider operations which can be generalized as weighted combinations of fiber compartments. Examples include per-voxel averaging across a population, trilinear interpolation, and Gaussian filtering. For simplicity, we use set notation to represent combinations of fibers. A single voxel model can be described by a volume-weighted combination $S_i = \bigcup_j^{N_i} (f_{ij}, v_{ij})$, and a weighted combination of all grouped voxel models $G$ can then be defined by the combination of those voxel-wise models, where each resulting weight is the product of the voxel volume fraction $f_{ij}$ and the per-model weight $s_i$:

$$G = \bigcup_i^M (s_i, S_i) = \bigcup_i^M \bigcup_j^{N_i} (s_i f_{ij}, v_{ij}) = \bigcup_k^K (w_k, v_k) \qquad (2)$$

where $K = \sum_i^M N_i$, and $k$ indexes $(i, j)$, i.e. $w_k = s_i f_{ij}$ and $v_k = v_{ij}$.

This weighted combination alone offers one solution to operations such as averaging and interpolating, but the result is overly complex. Taquet, et al. [3] have proposed Gaussian mixture simplification as an approach to reduce this complexity for the case of multi-tensor models; however, this method is not well-defined for the stick models, as previously explained. Our approach offers a similar clustering-based solution by modeling the distribution of fibers by a mixture-of-Watsons, which was suggested for multi-fiber modeling [4]. The Watson distribution [9] is a model for directional statistics that was proposed for single fiber modeling by Cook, et al. [5] and bears similarity to a Gaussian distribution. The space of directions can be modeled as points on the $S^2$ with antipodal equivalence, i.e. $\{v \in \mathbb{R}^3 : ||v|| = 1 \text{ and } v \sim -v\}$. Its probability density, given concentration $\kappa$ is then:

$$W(v; \theta) = A(\kappa) \exp\left(\kappa \left(\mu^T v\right)^2\right) \qquad (3)$$

for model parameters $\theta = (\mu, \kappa)$ and normalization constant $A(\kappa) = M(\frac{1}{2}, \frac{3}{2}, \kappa)^{-1}$ given by the confluent hyper-geometric function, sometimes known as $_1F_1$ or the Kummer function. The density of the set of fibers $G$ can then be modeled by a mixture of $C$ Watson distributions:

$$p(v; \Theta) = \sum_{c=1}^C \alpha_c W(v; \theta_c) \qquad (4)$$

given mixture model parameters $\Theta = (\alpha_1, \theta_1, ..., \alpha_C, \theta_C)$ and $\sum \alpha_c = 1$. The number of components $C$ controls the resulting complexity and may be chosen by some method of model selection, which is not explored here. We use a weighted samples version of the Expectation Maximization algorithm presented by Sra, et al. [10] to learn the parameters. The assignment and update steps are described as follows.

**E-Step:** Assign responsibility of each component $c$ for each fiber $k$

$$\pi_{kc} = p(c|\boldsymbol{v}_k, \Theta) = \frac{\alpha_c W(\boldsymbol{v}_k|\theta_c)}{\sum_c^C \alpha_c W(\boldsymbol{v}_k|\theta_c)} \tag{5}$$

**M-Step:** Update the model parameters for each component $c$

$$\alpha_c = \frac{\sum_k^K w_k \pi_{kc}}{\sum_k^K w_k} \tag{6}$$

$$\boldsymbol{\mu}_c = \frac{\sum_k^K w_k \pi_{kc} \boldsymbol{v}_k \boldsymbol{v}_k^T \boldsymbol{\mu}_c}{||\sum_k^K w_k \pi_{kc} \boldsymbol{v}_k \boldsymbol{v}_k^T \boldsymbol{\mu}_c||} \tag{7}$$

$$\kappa_c = \frac{\sum_k^K w_k \pi_{kc}}{\sum_k^K w_k \pi_{kc} \left(1 - (\boldsymbol{\mu}_c^T \boldsymbol{v}_k)^2\right)} \tag{8}$$

where $\kappa$ and $A(\kappa) = \frac{\kappa}{\pi \exp(\kappa)}$ are found similarly to Schwartzman, et al. [7]. This process can also be adapted to a "k-means" algorithm, similar to diametrical clustering, with hard assignment in the E-step and fixed parameters in the M-step. The k-means approach is initialized from a set of randomly selected fibers, and the Expectation Maxmization-approach is initialized with the k-means solution. The resulting clustering is then used to estimate a simpler fiber model $\hat{G} = \bigcup_c^C (\alpha_c, \boldsymbol{\mu}_c)$, by assigning the mixing parameters to volume fractions and component means to fiber orientations. We compare to a "heuristic" method described in [3]. This heuristic makes a simplifying assumption that fiber compartments are matched across voxels by volume-fraction rank, as opposed to the proposed matching defined by clustering. For example, when averaging two-direction models, the smaller volume compartments would be averaged separately from the larger volume compartments.

## 3   Experiments and Results

### 3.1   Data Acquisition and Processing

Diffusion volumes were acquired from 80 healthy volunteers uniformly distributed in age from 25 to 64 years with 39 male subjects following an IRB-approved protocol. Imaging was conducted on a GE 1.5T scanner with a voxel size of 2mm x 2mm x 2mm, matrix size 128x128, and 72 contiguous axial slices. For each subject, a total of 71 volumes were acquired, with seven $T_2$-weighted volumes (b-value 0 s/mm$^2$) and 64 diffusion-weighted volumes (b-value 1000s/mm$^2$) and distinct gradient encoding directions. All diffusion MRI data were corrected for motion and eddy current artifacts by affine registration to the first $T_2$-weighted volume using FSL Flirt (http://www.fmrib.ox.ac.uk) with a mutual information cost function. The gradient encoding directions were rotated to account for the alignment, and non-brain tissue was removed using FSL Bet. Single tensor models were fit using FSL DTIfit, and two-direction ball-and-stick diffusion models were fit using FSL Xfibres. All subjects were mapped to a population-specific template by tensor registration using DTI-TK [11].

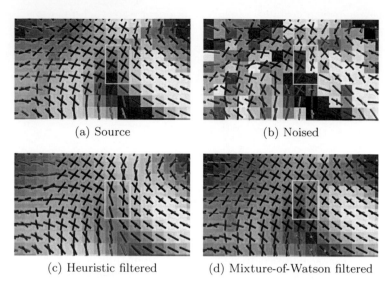

(a) Source          (b) Noised

(c) Heuristic filtered      (d) Mixture-of-Watson filtered

**Fig. 1.** Gaussian filtering of noisy fibers and the results of the heuristic and mixture-of-Watson filtering. Voxels with particularly poor heuristic performance are highlighted in yellow.

### 3.2 Filtering Experiment

In our first experiment, we tested the effect of Gaussian filtering in the presence of noise for a single subject. We introduced varying levels of Gaussian noise in the volume fractions and orientations ($\Delta\sigma_f = 0.01$ and $\Delta\sigma_v = 0.05$), followed by renormalization. We then filtered with weights defined by a Gaussian kernel ($\sigma = 2$mm, 5 voxel support) with the heuristic, k-means, and Expectation Maximization approaches. We computed the error $E$ between the source and each of the noised and filtered volumes at each noise level:

$$E(A, B) = \min\left(D(A_0, B_0) + D(A_1, B_1), D(A_0, B_1) + D(A_1, B_0)\right) \quad (9)$$

$$D(x, y) = \frac{(f_x + f_y)}{2} \frac{180}{\pi} \arccos\left(|\boldsymbol{v}_x^T \boldsymbol{v}_y|\right) \quad (10)$$

given a pair of two fiber voxel models $A = \{A_0, A_1\}$ and $B = \{B_0, B_1\}$, where $D$ is the volume-weighted angular difference between a pair of compartments. Fig. 1 shows an example slice accompanied by the noised and filtered fibers. We found the heuristic approach failed to restore some crossings where fibers had roughly equal volume, as highlighted in Fig. 1. We found the proposed approach to have lower error than the heuristic approach across all noise levels, with the Expectation Maximization approach outperforming the k-means approach, as shown in Fig. 2. Our serial implementation ran in five minutes on an Intel i5 2.6 GHz machine with 8GB of RAM and typically converged in fewer than 10 iterations.

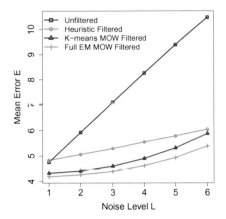

**Fig. 2.** The mean error as a function of noise level and type of filtering. Shown is the error for unfiltered (red square), heuristic (green circle), k-means (blue triangle), and full Expectation Maximization mixture-of-Watsons (orange cross) filtered volumes.

### 3.3 Atlasing Experiment

In our second experiment, we constructed a tractography atlas from the 80 subject population. Volumes were resampled into atlas space using both heuristic and mixture-of-Watsons interpolation with reorientation by finite strain rotation $\mathbf{J}/\sqrt{\mathbf{JJ}^T}$ [11]. Both cases used the same spatial transform computed with DTI-TK. Following this, the co-registered fibers were averaged using each method. Results are shown in Fig. 3. In our implementation, the interpolation took five minutes per subject, and population averaging took five minutes in total.

Deterministic streamline tractography was performed with both interpolation approaches with weights chosen by trilinear interpolation. Single tensor tracking was also performed for comparison. Multiple directions were included similarly to [1]. Termination criteria were a volume fraction of 0.10 and angle of 35°. Other tracking parameters include step size of 1.5mm, one seed per voxel, and Runge-Kutta integration. Our serial tracking implementation took 10 minutes for the given parameters.

Major bundles were manually segmented using slice-based masks in TrackVis (www.trackvis.org), and included the corpus callosum, corona radiata, interior fronto-occipital fasciculus (IFOF), uncinate fasciculus, interior longitudinal fasciculus, and several portions of the superior longitudinal fasciculs (SLF). We compared the mean length and number of curves in each tract. We found close agreement among methods except the following. The two dorsal portions of the SLF were not present in the single tensor atlas, and the heuristic SLF had 50% fewer curves and 40% shorter length than the mixture-of-Watsons SLF. The mixture-of-Watsons IFOF had 50% fewer curves but equal length to both other methods. The corpus callosum in the single tensor was similar to the heuristic reconstruction, but the mixture-of-Watsons reconstruction contained numerous anatomically plausible crossing fibers. These results are illustrated in Fig. 3.

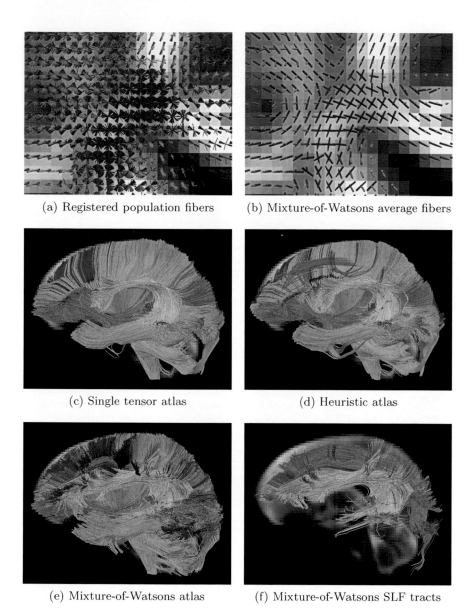

(a) Registered population fibers     (b) Mixture-of-Watsons average fibers

(c) Single tensor atlas     (d) Heuristic atlas

(e) Mixture-of-Watsons atlas     (f) Mixture-of-Watsons SLF tracts

**Fig. 3.** Construction and virtual dissection of atlas space tractography using the single tensor, heuristic, and mixture-of-Watsons estimation methods. Shown are examples of co-registered multi-fiber models (a) and their mixture-of-Watsons average (b). Also shown are tracks derived from a single tensor model (c), multi-fiber heuristic (d), and multi-fiber mixture-of-Watsons (e) approaches. The most significant strengths of the proposed method were in the superior longitudinal fasciculus, shown in (f), and corpus callosum (not shown). All cases used spatial transforms computed with DTI-TK from an 80 subject normal population.

## 4   Discussion and Conclusions

We presented a method for performing filtering, interpolation, and averaging of multi-fiber ball-and-stick diffusion models using mixture-of-Watsons clustering. We found the presented Expectation Maximization algorithm to efficiently learn the mixture model parameters, and our experiments to demonstrate the value of the approach in several common volume analysis applications. Our first experiment suggests that the filtering method reduces error introduced by orientation noise. Our second experiment showed that our approach allows the reconstruction of white matter pathways across a large population, and the method improved the reconstruction of several major bundles, including the superior longitudinal fasciculus and corpus callosum. Notable limitations are that the diffusivity is not handled, the number of mixture components must be specified explicitly, and other reorientation strategies have not been explored. In conclusion, we find our approach to be an efficient and effective way to estimate multi-fiber ball-and-stick diffusion volumes resulting from a number of image analysis operations.

## References

1. Bergmann, O., Kindlmann, G., Peled, S., Westin, C.F.: Two-tensor fiber tractography. In: 4th IEEE International Symposium on Biomedical Imaging: From Nano to Macro, ISBI 2007, pp. 796–799. IEEE (2007)
2. Behrens, T., Berg, H.J., Jbabdi, S., Rushworth, M., Woolrich, M.: Probabilistic diffusion tractography with multiple fibre orientations: What can we gain? Neuroimage 34(1), 144–155 (2007)
3. Taquet, M., Scherrer, B., Benjamin, C., Prabhu, S., Macq, B., Warfield, S.K.: Interpolating multi-fiber models by Gaussian mixture simplification. In: 2012 9th IEEE International Symposium on Biomedical Imaging (ISBI), pp. 928–931. IEEE (2012)
4. Rathi, Y., Michailovich, O., Shenton, M.E., Bouix, S.: Directional functions for orientation distribution estimation. Medical Image Analysis 13(3), 432–444 (2009)
5. Cook, P.A., Alexander, D.C., Parker, G.J.: Modelling noise-induced fibre-orientation error in Diffusion-Tensor MRI. In: 2004 IEEE International Symposium on Biomedical Imaging: Nano to Macro, pp. 332–335. IEEE (2004)
6. Malcolm, J.G., Michailovich, O., Bouix, S., Westin, C.F., Shenton, M.E., Rathi, Y.: A filtered approach to neural tractography using the Watson directional function. Medical Image Analysis 14(1), 58 (2010)
7. Schwartzman, A., Dougherty, R.F., Taylor, J.E.: Cross-subject comparison of principal diffusion direction maps. Mag. Res. Medicine 53(6), 1423–1431 (2005)
8. Yap, P.T., Gilmore, J.H., Lin, W., Shen, D.: Poptract: population-based tractography. IEEE Transactions on Medical Imaging 30(10), 1829–1840 (2011)
9. Watson, G.S.: Distributions on the circle and sphere. Journal of Applied Probability, 265–280 (1982)
10. Sra, S., Jain, P., Dhillon, I.: Modeling data using directional distributions: Part II. Technical Report TR-07-05, Department of Computer Science, University of Texas at Austin, Austin, Texas (2007)
11. Zhang, H., Yushkevich, P.A., Alexander, D.C., Gee, J.C., et al.: Deformable registration of Diffusion Tensor MR images with explicit orientation optimization. Medical Image Analysis 10(5), 764–785 (2006)

# Connectivity Subnetwork Learning
# for Pathology and Developmental Variations

Yasser Ghanbari[1], Alex R. Smith[1], Robert T. Schultz[2], and Ragini Verma[1,*]

[1] Section of Biomedical Image Analysis, University of Pennsylvania, Philadelphia, PA
{Yasser.Ghanbari,Alex.Smith,Ragini.Verma}@uphs.upenn.edu
[2] Center for Autism Research, Children's Hospital of Philadelphia, Philadelphia, PA
schultzrt@mail.chop.edu

**Abstract.** Network representation of brain connectivity has provided a novel means of investigating brain changes arising from pathology, development or aging. The high dimensionality of these networks demands methods that are not only able to extract the patterns that highlight these sources of variation, but describe them individually. In this paper, we present a unified framework for learning subnetwork patterns of connectivity by their projective non-negative decomposition into a reconstructive basis set, as well as, additional basis sets representing development and group discrimination. In order to obtain these components, we exploit the geometrical distribution of the population in the connectivity space by using a graph-theoretical scheme that imposes locality-preserving properties. In addition, the projection of the subject networks into the basis set provides a low dimensional representation of it, that teases apart the different sources of variation in the sample, facilitating variation-specific statistical analysis. The proposed framework is applied to a study of diffusion-based connectivity in subjects with autism.

**Keywords:** Connectivity analysis, non-negative matrix factorization, locality preserving projections, graph embedding, population difference.

## 1 Introduction

Analysis of brain connectivity networks created from DTI, MEG/EEG, or fMRI data has provided a novel insight into brain changes arising from pathology, development or aging [1, 2]. The high dimensionality of these networks has necessitated the development of methods that can extract the connectivity patterns of the population and separate components pertaining to each source of variation. In this paper, we provide such a method of extracting the basis of patterns using a locality-preserving basis learning, which helps provide a low dimensional representation of the subject networks that can then be used to study group differences, or train pathology specific or developmental biomarkers. Traditional analysis techniques, such as PCA and ICA, provide dimensionality reduction in

---

* Authors acknowledge support from grants NIH-MH092862 (PI: R. Verma), Pennsylvania Department of Health (SAP#4100042728, SAP#4100047863, PI: R. Schultz).

K. Mori et al. (Eds.): MICCAI 2013, Part I, LNCS 8149, pp. 90–97, 2013.

brain network investigations [3] but may lack the physiological interpretability of non-negative connectivity matrices. Recently, non-negative matrix factorization (NMF) methods [4] have provided interpretable sparse bases characterizing multivariate data [5–8]. The non-negativity constraints, facilitate interpretability of the components as sparse connectivity matrices [6], but are unable to separate patterns that represent the different sources of variability in the population.

This paper presents a framework for learning sparse subnetwork patterns of non-negative connectivity matrices by their projective non-negative decomposition into sets of i) *discriminative* or pathology-specific, ii) *developmental* (age related), and iii) *reconstructive* components. The decomposition maintains the interpretation of each component as a connectivity matrix and their associated coefficients as the weight of the subnetwork, while providing a succinct low dimensional representation of the population amenable to statistical analysis.

While the method is generalizable to any type of non-negative connectivity matrix, we have demonstrated the applicability of the framework to DTI-based structural connectivity networks for a population of subjects with autism spectrum disorder (ASD). Our method is able to extract components that describe the underlying patterns of pathology related variability, as well as patterns of developmental (age) variation. In addition, the corresponding low dimensional representation of the subjects in these basis components is able to identify group differences in pathology, and quantify the age related variations.

## 2   Methods

The connectivity network of each subject can be modeled as a linear combination of several components that act as the building blocks of the brain network system [6]. Due to their symmetry, the upper triangular elements of a connectivity matrix are represented by $x_i$ for the subject $i$. To compute the $r$ connectivity components whose mixture constructs the original non-negative connectivity matrices, a matrix factorization is used as $X \approx W\Phi$, where columns of $X = [x_1, x_2, \ldots, x_n] \in \mathbb{R}^{m \times n}$, i.e. $x_i$, represent the connectivity matrices, and columns of $W = [w_1, w_2, \ldots, w_r] \in \mathbb{R}^{m \times r}$, i.e. $w_j$, are representative of the normalized basis connectivity components. These components $w_j$ are then mixed by each column of the loading matrix $\Phi = [\varphi_1, \varphi_2, \ldots, \varphi_n] \in \mathbb{R}^{r \times n}$ to approximate the corresponding column of $X$ [8].

### 2.1   Projective Non-negative Basis Learning

Inspired by [6], we assume that $\Phi$ is the projection of $X$ onto $W$, i.e. $\Phi = W^T X$. The projective properties of the NMF coefficients ($\Phi$) help imbibe orthogonality properties into components [8]. Hence, the reconstruction of original non-negative connectivity matrices can be obtained by minimizing the cost function $F_1(W) = \|X - WW^T X\|_F^2$ with respect to $W \geq 0$. This can be denoted by

$$\min_{W \geq 0} F_1(W) = \min_{W \geq 0} trace\left\{ \left(X - WW^T X\right) \left(X - WW^T X\right)^T \right\}. \quad (1)$$

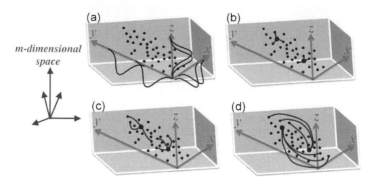

**Fig. 1.** Illustration of a two-group $m$-dimensional points lying on a 3-D manifold, shown as a cube in the $m$-dimensional space. (a) Point distributions when projected into $\vec{x}$, $\vec{y}$ or $\vec{z}$. (b) The 3-nearest-neighbor graph $\hat{G}$ of two selected magnified points. (c) The graph $\check{G}$ with edges connecting points whose subjects are of similar ages. (d) The 3-farthest-point graph $\tilde{G}$ of the same two points.

## 2.2   Locality Preserving Bases with Graph Embedding

We split the set of $r$ components into three subsets $W = [\hat{W}, \check{W}, \tilde{W}]$ where $\hat{W} = [w_1, \ldots, w_q]$ are the *discriminative* basis components, $\check{W} = [w_{q+1}, \ldots, w_{q+p}]$ are the *developmental* basis components, and $\tilde{W} = [w_{q+p+1}, \ldots, w_r]$ is the complementary space containing the *reconstructive* basis components which minimizes the reconstruction error together with $\hat{W}$ and $\check{W}$. Thus, the coefficient matrices are also split into $\hat{\Phi} = \hat{W}^T X$, $\check{\Phi} = \check{W}^T X$, and $\tilde{\Phi} = \tilde{W}^T X$. A proper modeling of such intent would provide at most $q$ of those bases which are likeliest to provide population discrimination to belong to $\hat{W}$, and $p$ of those which are likeliest to account for the developmental variations in $\check{W}$.

To clarify our mathematical modeling, suppose that the $m$-dimensional connectivity points $(x_i)$ of two groups lie on a 3-D manifold, as illustrated in Fig. 1(a), and are to be projected into an $r = 3$ dimensional subspace with $q = 1$ discriminative (say $\vec{y}$), $p = 1$ developmental (say $\vec{z}$), and $r - q - p = 1$ reconstructive components (say $\vec{x}$). In order to achieve this, we construct three separate graphs made up of these $m$-dimensional points as their vertices. The first graph is an intrinsic $k$-nearest-neighbor graph [5, 9] which connects point $i$ to $j$ if point $j$ is among the $k$ nearest neighbors of point $i$ (as illustrated in Fig. 1(b)). This graph is used for obtaining the discriminative component $\hat{W}$. The second graph connects point $i$ to point $j$ if point $j$ is among the $k$ farthest points to point $i$ (illustrated in Fig. 1(d)), which is used for obtaining the reconstructive component $\tilde{W}$. The third graph, used for obtaining the developmental component $\check{W}$, connects point $i$ to $j$ if subject $j$'s age is among the $k$ nearest ages to subject $i$, irrespective of the two points' distance (illustrated in Fig. 1(c)).

There are a variety of approaches that can characterize separability of multivariate data-points. Most of such techniques can be unified in the framework of graph embedding [5, 9]. Let $G = \{X, S\}$ be an undirected weighted graph of $n$ vertices, i.e. data points $\boldsymbol{x}_i$, with a symmetric matrix $\boldsymbol{S} \in \mathbb{R}^{n \times n}$ with non-negative elements, within the range of 0 to 1, corresponding to the edge weight of the graph. The Laplacian matrix $\boldsymbol{L}$ of the graph is then defined by $\boldsymbol{L} = \boldsymbol{D} - \boldsymbol{S}$ where $\boldsymbol{D}$ is a diagonal matrix with $D_{ii} = \sum_{j=1}^{n} S_{ij}$ [9].

In order for the bases in $\hat{\boldsymbol{W}}$ to provide discriminatory information, we would like the resulting coefficients $(\hat{\boldsymbol{\varphi}}_i)$ of nearby $\boldsymbol{x}_i$ points to stay close to each other to group together when projected into $\hat{\boldsymbol{W}}$. This can be obtained by minimizing

$$\min_{\boldsymbol{W} \geq 0} F_2(\boldsymbol{W}) = \min_{\hat{\boldsymbol{W}} \geq 0} \sum_{i=1}^{n} \sum_{j=1}^{n} \|\hat{\boldsymbol{\varphi}}_i - \hat{\boldsymbol{\varphi}}_j\|^2 \hat{S}_{ij} = \min_{\hat{\boldsymbol{W}} \geq 0} trace \left\{ \hat{\boldsymbol{\Phi}} \hat{\boldsymbol{L}} \hat{\boldsymbol{\Phi}}^T \right\}, \quad (2)$$

where $\hat{\boldsymbol{S}} = [\hat{S}_{ij}]$ is the similarity matrix composed of the edge weights in the $k$-nearest-neighbor graph $\hat{G} = \{\boldsymbol{X}, \hat{\boldsymbol{S}}\}$ of the $m$-dimensional points $\boldsymbol{x}_i$, as illustrated in Fig. 1(b). According to the equation (2), if data-points $\boldsymbol{x}_i$ and $\boldsymbol{x}_j$ are close, their edge weight $S_{ij}$ will be large, and therefore, the cost function $F_2(\hat{\boldsymbol{W}})$ gets minimized only if the corresponding coefficients $\hat{\boldsymbol{\varphi}}_i$ and $\hat{\boldsymbol{\varphi}}_j$ remain close.

Similarly, in order to capture the connectivity space of developmental variations, we form a developmental graph $\breve{G} = \{\boldsymbol{X}, \breve{\boldsymbol{S}}\}$, as in Fig. 1(c), in which $\boldsymbol{x}_i$ is connected with an edge to $\boldsymbol{x}_j$ if subject $i$ is within the $k$ nearest age to subject $j$, and vice versa. Therefore, the space of developmental variations, $\breve{\boldsymbol{W}}$, grouping the coefficients $(\breve{\boldsymbol{\varphi}}_i)$ of subjects with similar ages, is computed by minimizing $F_3(\boldsymbol{W}) = \sum_{i=1}^{n} \sum_{j=1}^{n} \|\breve{\boldsymbol{\varphi}}_i - \breve{\boldsymbol{\varphi}}_j\|^2 \breve{S}_{ij} = trace \left\{ \breve{\boldsymbol{\Phi}} \breve{\boldsymbol{L}} \breve{\boldsymbol{\Phi}}^T \right\}$ when $\breve{\boldsymbol{W}} \geq 0$.

As explained earlier, we exploit the graph of $k$-farthest points $\tilde{G} = \{\boldsymbol{X}, \tilde{\boldsymbol{S}}\}$ (as illustrated in Fig. 1(d)), to impose the representative coefficients $(\tilde{\boldsymbol{\varphi}}_i)$ of the farthest points to remain as close as possible in the lower dimensional space when projected into the reconstructive set $\tilde{\boldsymbol{W}}$. This is performed by minimizing $F_4(\boldsymbol{W}) = \sum_{i=1}^{n} \sum_{j=1}^{n} \|\tilde{\boldsymbol{\varphi}}_i - \tilde{\boldsymbol{\varphi}}_j\|^2 \tilde{S}_{ij} = trace \left\{ \tilde{\boldsymbol{\Phi}} \tilde{\boldsymbol{L}} \tilde{\boldsymbol{\Phi}}^T \right\}$ subject to $\tilde{\boldsymbol{W}} \geq 0$.

### 2.3   Objective Function and Optimization Solution

To achieve the above objectives, and according to the projective properties of the model, i.e. $\boldsymbol{\Phi} = \boldsymbol{W}^T \boldsymbol{X}$, the final objective function is modeled to minimize

$$F(\boldsymbol{W}) = trace \left\{ \left( \boldsymbol{X} - \boldsymbol{W} \boldsymbol{W}^T \boldsymbol{X} \right) \left( \boldsymbol{X} - \boldsymbol{W} \boldsymbol{W}^T \boldsymbol{X} \right)^T \right\} +$$
$$\lambda \left( trace \left\{ \hat{\boldsymbol{W}}^T \boldsymbol{X} \hat{\boldsymbol{L}} \boldsymbol{X}^T \hat{\boldsymbol{W}} \right\} + trace \left\{ \breve{\boldsymbol{W}}^T \boldsymbol{X} \breve{\boldsymbol{L}} \boldsymbol{X}^T \breve{\boldsymbol{W}} \right\} + trace \left\{ \tilde{\boldsymbol{W}}^T \boldsymbol{X} \tilde{\boldsymbol{L}} \boldsymbol{X}^T \tilde{\boldsymbol{W}} \right\} \right), \quad (3)$$

where $\lambda$ is a tunable parameter to balance the two terms of reconstruction error norm and graph embedding. To minimize (3) with $\boldsymbol{W} \geq 0$, we use a gradient descent approach, updating $W_{ij} = W_{ij} - \eta_{ij} \frac{\partial F}{\partial W_{ij}}$ with step-sizes $\eta_{ij} \geq 0$, where

$$\frac{\partial F}{\partial W} = -4\left(XX^TW\right) + 2\left(WW^TXX^TW\right) + 2\left(XX^TWW^TW\right)$$
$$+ \lambda \left[2X\hat{L}X^T\hat{W}, \; 2X\check{L}X^T\check{W}, \; 2X\tilde{L}X^T\tilde{W}\right]. \quad (4)$$

Regarding that $\hat{L} = \hat{D} - \hat{S}$, $\check{L} = \check{D} - \check{S}$ and $\tilde{L} = \tilde{D} - \tilde{S}$, and the fact that both $D$ and $S$ have non-negative elements, our non-negativity constraint is guaranteed by positive initialization of $W$ and applying the step-size $\eta_{ij} = \dfrac{\frac{1}{2}W_{ij}}{\left(WW^TXX^TW + XX^TWW^TW + \lambda\left[X\hat{D}X^T\hat{W}, X\check{D}X^T\check{W}, X\tilde{D}X^T\tilde{W}\right]\right)_{ij}}$. This results in the following multiplicative updating solution

$$W_{ij} = W_{ij} \frac{\left(2XX^TW + \lambda\left[X\hat{S}X^T\hat{W}, \; X\check{S}X^T\check{W}, \; X\tilde{S}X^T\tilde{W}\right]\right)_{ij}}{\left(WW^TXX^TW + XX^TWW^TW + \lambda\left[X\hat{D}X^T\hat{W}, X\check{D}X^T\check{W}, X\tilde{D}X^T\tilde{W}\right]\right)_{ij}}.$$
$$(5)$$

For the stability of convergence, at each iteration, each column of $W$ is normalized by $w_i = \frac{w_i}{\|w_i\|_2}$. Starting with initial random positive elements on $W$, the iterative procedure will converge to the desired $W = [\hat{W}, \check{W}, \tilde{W}] \geq 0$.

## 3    Results

The proposed method provides a framework for extracting three sets of network components from the population. The discriminatory and developmental set of components are expected to show localized sparse sub-networks which mostly capture the changes related to pathology and developmental variations. The reconstructive basis set consists of global networks of dominant connectivity patterns. The number of bases is population dependent; however, we show that even with relatively small numbers, we can obtain stable group differences.

**Dataset Demographics and Connectivity Measures.** We study the applicability of our method on a dataset of DTI connectivity matrices computed for a population of ASD subjects and typically developing controls (TDCs). Our dataset consisted of 83 male children, 24 ASD and 59 TDCs, aged 6-18 years (mean=12.9yrs, SD=3.0 in ASD, and mean=11.6yrs, SD=3.2 in TDC, no significant group difference in age). DTI was acquired for each subject (Siemens 3T Verio, 32 channel head coil, single shot spin echo sequence, TR/TE = 11000/76 ms, b = 1000 s/mm$^2$, 30 gradient directions). 79 ROIs from the Desikan atlas were extracted to represent the nodes of the structural network. Probabilistic tractography [10] was performed from each of these regions with 5000 streamline fibers sampled per voxel, resulting in a $79 \times 79$ matrix of weighted connectivity values, where each element represents the conditional probability of a pathway between regions, normalized by the active surface area of the seed ROI.

**Connectivity Component Analysis.** The $79 \times 79$ connectivity matrix of each subject was vectorized to its $m = 3081$ upper triangular elements. To compute the components, we set $\lambda = 1$ and used $k = 3$ to construct the three graphs, and correspondingly calculated their graph edge weights ($S$) using a Gaussian kernel [9]. We used $q = 4$ discriminative, $p = 2$ developmental, and 6 reconstructive components (we suggest the number of reconstructive components be equal to the total of other components). The iterative procedure of equation (5) yielded components shown in Fig. 2. The connectivity components shown were sparse and thresholded for binary visualization to show the dominant edges. Also, in regards to the orthogonality of the discriminative and developmental components, the non-orthogonality between any two of these components was measured by computing their inner products (or angle) which were all less than 0.04 (between 88 and 90 degrees), in a scale of 0 (90-degree) to 1 (0-degree).

The vectorized connectivity of each subject was projected into the discriminative and developmental components to obtain the coefficients for subsequent statistical t-test to validate the discriminative bases and compare between the ASD and TDC groups. We divided the 83 subjects into three closely-balanced age groups of 6–10 (age group I, 25 subjects), 10–13.5 (age group II, 28 subjects), and 13.5–18 years old (age group III, 30 subjects). A t-test was performed between the coefficients of the subjects in these age groups to validate the ability of the developmental components in capturing the effect of age. We then correlated the coefficients of all subjects with their age. Results are given in Table 1.

It is observed that the discriminatory and developmental bases obtained are quite sparse with localized patterns as expected, while the reconstructive network

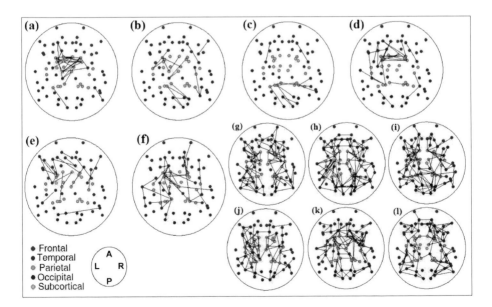

**Fig. 2.** The $r=12$ connectivity basis components learned by the proposed method. (a)–(d) are the $q=4$ discriminative bases, (e)–(f) are the $p=2$ developmental components, and (g)–(l) compose the set of the 6 reconstructive bases.

**Table 1.** Statistical group analysis of the coefficients of the ASD-TDC bases

| Component label | ASD-TDC group $t(p)$–values | Age group II vs. group I $t(p)$–values | Age group III vs. group II $t(p)$–values | Basis coeffs' correlation with age |
|---|---|---|---|---|
| a | -3.2 (0.002) | -1.6 (0.1) | -0.7 (0.5) | -0.24 |
| b | -1.2 (0.2) | -0.6 (0.6) | -0.3 (0.8) | -0.14 |
| c | +0.5 (0.6) | -1.5 (0.1) | -1.3 (0.2) | -0.32 |
| d | -2.3 (0.02) | -2.1 (0.04) | -2.3 (0.02) | -0.48 |
| e | +0.7 (0.5) | +1.9 (0.06) | +3.0 (0.004) | +0.55 |
| f | -3.1 (0.004) | -4.0 (0.0002) | -1.7 (0.09) | -0.54 |

components are globally connected. Table 1 shows the results of group-wise and age-based statistics on the coefficients of discriminatory (a-d) and developmental (e-f) components. Group-based analysis shows that the discriminative basis (a) is able to differentiate ASD and TDC groups with a high statistical significance ($p = 0.002$). Inspection of this component in Fig. 2 shows distinct connectivity deficiencies in the thalamic network, and inter-hemispheric subcortical connections in children with ASD. The low correlation with age of this component (column 5, table 1) is indicative of the fact that this component concentrates on the pathology-related patterns in the data. The developmental basis (e) does not show any group related differences, but has a high positive correlation with age. It demonstrates significant age increase ($p = 0.004$) between the second and third age ranges (age>10). Its positive correlation with age suggests that the connections between (mainly) left frontal and its nearby frontal, temporal, and subcortical regions significantly develop with age (correlation=+0.55), likely capturing ongoing maturation of language and executive functioning. The second developmental basis (f) shows an independent sub-network that diminishes (based on its negative correlation=-0.54 with age) significantly with development, especially during the younger ages (age<13.5, $p = 0.0002$). The behavior of the two components (e) and (f) are opposite with respect to age, as indicated by the sign of the correlation. Of interest is the discriminative component (d), that shows the second highest group difference, with several frontal regions compromised. However, this component also shows a relatively high correlation with age. The analysis of the components shows that our method is able to extract components that capture the changes due to pathology (a) and age (e); there are components such as (d) and (f) that are representative of changes in both. This may be an indication of those aspects of pathology that are linked with age and cannot be completely separated, yet help in providing a comprehensive picture of the pattern of changes in the population.

Our experiments have shown that the reconstructive components do not show any significant age-group differences or age correlation, but two mild significances (components h and j, $p > 0.01$) in ASD-TDC group difference; while interesting, for the purposes of the paper we have concentrated on the discriminative and developmental components. Also, we have observed that the average of the reconstructive coefficients are an order of magnitude larger than the discriminative and developmental basis coefficients. Thus, due to their relatively small coefficients, the discriminatory and developmental bases do not play a significant role in the reconstruction, and therefore, would not have been captured by solving only for the reconstruction components as has been done in the literature. However, the graph-embedded modeling proposed in this work has been able to extract them from the connectivity matrices of the two populations and comprehensively capture the pathology and age specific changes, which were the two major sources of variation in this population.

## 4    Conclusion

We have presented a novel technique for simultaneously extracting the discriminatory and developmental sub-networks of a population via graph embedding. Our method consists of an NMF basis learning scheme with locality preserving properties, and provides group-discriminatory as well as developmental network components. Application to a dataset of ASD subjects provided a discriminatory basis which revealed significant inter-hemisphere subcortical connectivity deficiencies. The developmental bases captured subnetworks which changed with age. The framework is generalizable to non-negative functional networks, as well as to modeling and identifying other forms of variation in the population.

## References

1. Vissers, M., et al.: Brain connectivity and high functioning autism: a promising path of research that needs refined models, methodological convergence, and stronger behavioral links. Neurosci. Biobehav. Rev. 36(1), 604–625 (2012)
2. Dennis, E.L., Jahanshad, N., et al.: Development of brain structural connectivity between ages 12 and 30: A 4-tesla diffusion imaging study in 439 adolescents and adults. Neuroimage 64, 671–684 (2013)
3. Calhoun, V., et al.: Modulation of temporally coherent brain networks estimated using ica at rest and during cognitive tasks. Hum. Brain Mapp. 29(7), 828–838 (2008)
4. Lee, D.D., Seung, H.S.: Learning the parts of objects by non-negative matrix factorization. Nature 401(6755), 788–791 (1999)
5. Yan, S., et al.: Graph embedding and extensions: a general framework for dimensionality reduction. IEEE Trans. Patt. Anal. Mach. Intell. 29(1), 40–51 (2007)
6. Ghanbari, Y., Bloy, L., Batmanghelich, K., Roberts, T.P.L., Verma, R.: Dominant component analysis of electrophysiological connectivity networks. In: Ayache, N., Delingette, H., Golland, P., Mori, K. (eds.) MICCAI 2012, Part III. LNCS, vol. 7512, pp. 231–238. Springer, Heidelberg (2012)
7. Berry, M.W., et al.: Algorithms and applications for approximate nonnegative matrix factorization. Comput. Stat. Data Anal. 52, 155–173 (2007)
8. Yang, Z., Oja, E.: Linear and nonlinear projective nonnegative matrix factorization. IEEE Trans. Neural Netw. 21(5), 1734–1749 (2010)
9. He, X., Niyogi, P.: Locality preserving projections. In: Advances in neural information processing systems (NIPS), vol. 16, pp. 153–160 (2004)
10. Behrens, T., et al.: Non-invasive mapping of connections between human thalamus and cortex using diffusion imaging. Nat. Neurosci. 6(7), 750–757 (2003)

# Detecting Epileptic Regions Based on Global Brain Connectivity Patterns

Andrew Sweet[1], Archana Venkataraman[1], Steven M. Stufflebeam[2],
Hesheng Liu[2], Naoro Tanaka[2], Joseph Madsen[3], and Polina Golland[1]

[1] MIT Computer Science and Artificial Intelligence Laboratory, Cambridge, MA
[2] Athinoula A. Martinos Center for Biomedical Imaging, Boston, MA
[3] Boston Children's Hospital, Boston, MA

**Abstract.** We present a method to detect epileptic regions based on functional connectivity differences between individual epilepsy patients and a healthy population. Our model assumes that the global functional characteristics of these differences are shared across patients, but it allows for the epileptic regions to vary between individuals. We evaluate the detection performance against intracranial EEG observations and compare our approach with two baseline methods that use standard statistics. The baseline techniques are sensitive to the choice of thresholds, whereas our algorithm automatically estimates the appropriate model parameters and compares favorably with the best baseline results. This suggests the promise of our approach for pre-surgical planning in epilepsy.

## 1 Introduction

Focal epilepsy is a chronic neurological disorder, in which seizures are triggered by a few isolated regions before spreading to the rest of the brain [1]. In cases where anticonvulsant medication fails to mitigate these seizures, surgical resection of the epileptic regions may be prescribed. Accurate localization of these regions is crucial to minimize the size of the excision, and hence, to limit potential damage to brain function. For some patients, localization is achieved using intracranial electroencephalography (iEEG), in which electrodes are implanted directly onto the cortical surface. Unfortunately, iEEG is highly invasive and only provides limited coverage of the cortex.

Recently, it has been suggested that epilepsy is associated with functional disorganization during and between seizures [2]. Resting state functional MRI (rsfMRI) can help quantify this disorganization since temporal correlations in rsfMRI reflect the intrinsic functional connectivity of the brain [3]. rsfMRI is particularly attractive for epilepsy because it is non-invasive and provides full coverage of the cortex. Prior empirical studies have revealed abnormal functional connectivity in focal epilepsy patients [4], which may roughly correspond to epileptic regions [5]. However, these analyses focused on pre-defined brain networks and produced results that are sensitive to user-specified parameters. Here, we demonstrate a novel method that automatically identifies epileptic regions based on global functional connectivity patterns.

K. Mori et al. (Eds.): MICCAI 2013, Part I, LNCS 8149, pp. 98–105, 2013.
© Springer-Verlag Berlin Heidelberg 2013

Most prior work in connectivity analysis is motivated by population studies and is ill suited to epilepsy. For example, univariate tests and random effects analysis are commonly used to identify statistical differences between a clinical population and normal controls [6]. In contrast to population studies, we cannot assume that the abnormal regions are common across patients. Furthermore, connectivity analysis typically yields discriminative *connections* and provides little insight into the associated region proportion. Therefore, even patient-specific connectivity analysis is not suitable for this application [7]. One solution is to aggregate population differences across connections into information about regions [8]. However, this approach still assumes a consistent set of abnormal regions for the clinical population. In contrast, our method detects abnormal regions within a heterogeneous patient group.

We demonstrate our algorithm on a case study of six epilepsy patients. Our results correspond well with the epileptic regions localized via iEEG.

## 2    Extracting Diseased Regions from Connectivity

Fig. 1 illustrates our assumptions about the relationship between the diseased brain regions and the observed abnormalities in functional networks. Our model operates on a parcellation of the brain into regions that are consistently defined across subjects. In this work, we subdivide the cortical surface into 50-100mm$^2$ patches, which are comparable in size to the coverage of a single iEEG electrode. Optimizing the parcellation to maximize detection accuracy is a non-trivial problem that we leave for future work.

We assume that epileptic regions are the foci of abnormal neural communications in the brain. Hence, they are associated with the greatest deviations from the functional connectivity template of a control population. Below we formalize the random variables in our model and summarize the corresponding inference algorithm to fit the model to the data. We then describe how to evaluate the the detection performance of our method.

**Diseased Regions.** The binary vector $R^m = [R_1^m, \ldots, R_N^m]$ indicates the state, healthy ($R_i^m = 0$) or diseased ($R_i^m = 1$), for each region $i \in \{1, \ldots, N\}$ in patient $m$, $\forall m = 1, \ldots, M$. We assume an *i.i.d.* Bernoulli prior for $R_i^m$ with the unknown parameter $\pi^r$ shared across regions and patients, i.e., $P(R_i^m = 1) = \pi^r$.

**Latent Connectivity.** The labels $R^m$ imply a graph of abnormal functional connectivity, which emanates from diseased regions based on a simple set of rules: (1) a connection between two diseased regions is always abnormal, (2) a connection between two healthy regions is always healthy, and (3) a connection between a healthy and a diseased region is abnormal with probability $\eta$. We use latent functional connectivity variables $F_{ij}$ and $\bar{F}_{ij}^m$ to model the neural synchrony between regions $i$ and $j$ in the control population and in patient $m$, respectively. Formally, the latent functional connectivity template $F_{ij}$ of the control population is a tri-state random variable drawn from a multinomial distribution

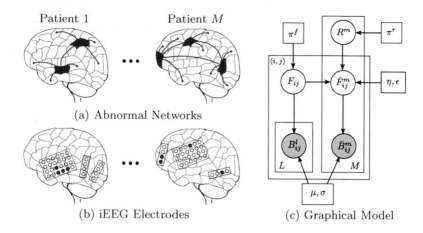

(a) Abnormal Networks

(b) iEEG Electrodes          (c) Graphical Model

**Fig. 1.** (a) Latent network model of diseased regions in a heterogeneous population. The red nodes are diseased regions and are unique for each patient; red edges correspond to abnormal functional connections emanating from the diseased regions. (b) Electrode arrays are placed on the surface of each patient's brain. Red circles denote electrodes that exhibit abnormal activity. (c) Graphical representation of our generative model. Vector $R^m$ specifies diseased regions in patient $m$. $F_{ij}$ and $\bar{F}_{ij}^m$ represent the latent functional connectivity between regions $i$ and $j$ in the control population and in the $m^{th}$ patient, respectively. $B_{ij}^l$ and $\bar{B}_{ij}^m$ are the observed time course correlations in control subject $l$ and epilepsy patient $m$, respectively. Boxes denote non-random parameters; circles indicate random variables; shaded variables are observed.

with parameter $\pi^f$. These states represent little or no functional co-activation ($F_{ij} = 0$), positive functional synchrony ($F_{ij} = 1$), and negative functional synchrony ($F_{ij} = -1$). For notational convenience, we represent $F_{ij}$ as a length-three indicator vector $[F_{ij,-1} \quad F_{ij0} \quad F_{ij1}]$ with exactly one of its elements equal to one, i.e., $P(F_{ijk} = 1) = \pi_k^f$.

Ideally, $\bar{F}_{ij}^m \neq F_{ij}$ for abnormal connections and $\bar{F}_{ij}^m = F_{ij}$ for healthy connections. To account for noise and subject variability, we assume that the latent connectivity can deviate from the above rules with probability $\epsilon$:

$$P(\bar{F}_{ij}^m | F_{ij}, R_i, R_j) = \begin{cases} (1-\epsilon)^{F_{ij}^T \bar{F}_{ij}^m} \left(\frac{\epsilon}{2}\right)^{1-F_{ij}^T \bar{F}_{ij}^m}, & R_i^m = R_j^m = 0, \\ \epsilon^{F_{ij}^T \bar{F}_{ij}^m} \left(\frac{1-\epsilon}{2}\right)^{1-F_{ij}^T \bar{F}_{ij}^m}, & R_i^m = R_j^m = 1, \\ \epsilon_1^{F_{ij}^T \bar{F}_{ij}^m} \left(\frac{1-\epsilon_1}{2}\right)^{1-F_{ij}^T \bar{F}_{ij}^m}, & R_i^m \neq R_j^m, \end{cases} \quad (1)$$

such that $\epsilon_1 = \eta\epsilon + (1-\eta)(1-\epsilon)$. The first condition in Eq. (1) states that if both regions are healthy ($R_i^m = R_j^m = 0$), then the edge $\langle i, j \rangle$ is healthy and the functional connectivity of patient $m$ is equal to that of the control population with probability $1 - \epsilon$, and it differs with probability $\epsilon$. The second term is similarly obtained by replacing $\epsilon$ with $1 - \epsilon$. The probability $\epsilon_1$ in the third condition reflects the coupling between $\eta$ and $\epsilon$ when the region labels differ.

Although we specify separate region and connectivity variables for each patient, the parameters $\{\pi^r, \eta, \epsilon\}$ associated with the disease are shared across the patient group. Under this assumption, the characteristics of change are common across patients, but the disease is localized to a different subset of regions in each individual. Our model can also be applied to a single patient.

**Data Likelihood.** The rsfMRI correlation $B_{ij}^l$ is a noisy observation of the functional connectivity template $F_{ij}$, i.e., $P(B_{ij}^l | F_{ijk} = 1; \{\mu, \sigma^2\}) = \mathcal{N}(B_{ij}^l; \mu_k, \sigma_k^2)$, where $\mathcal{N}(\cdot; \mu, \sigma^2)$ is a Gaussian distribution with mean $\mu$ and variance $\sigma^2$. We fix $\mu_0 = 0$ to center the parameter estimates. The likelihood of $\bar{B}_{ij}^m$ has the same functional form and parameter values, but uses the latent functional connectivity $\bar{F}_{ij}^m$ of patient $m$ instead of the control template $F_{ij}$.

**Approximate Inference.** We combine the prior and likelihood terms to obtain the full probability distribution for the generative model in Fig. 1(c). Our goal is to estimate the region labels $\{R^m\}$ from the observed rsfMRI correlations $\{B, \bar{B}\}$. To improve robustness of the estimation, we marginalize out the latent functional connectivity $\bar{F}^m$ for all patients $m = 1, \ldots, M$.

The resulting expressions are heavily coupled across patients and across pairwise connections. Therefore, we use a fully factorized variational approximation (mean-field) to the posterior distribution of the remaining latent variables $\{R^m, F\}$ for maximum likelihood estimation of the parameters $\Theta = \{\pi, \epsilon, \eta, \mu, \sigma^2\}$. We emphasize that both the posterior distributions of the latent variables and the non-random model parameters $\Theta$ are estimated directly from the data.

The marginal posterior probability $\hat{p}_i^m = P(R_i^m = 1 | B, \bar{B}; \hat{\Theta})$ quantifies how likely region $i$ in patient $m$ is to be diseased given the observed connectivity data $\{B, \bar{B}\}$ and the parameter estimates $\hat{\Theta}$.

**Baseline Methods.** Our generative framework automatically infers the region labels based on global connectivity patterns. To evaluate the accuracy and stability of our approach, we consider two baseline methods that also translate connection information into region properties.

The first method counts the number of connections that differ from a control population. Formally, we quantify the deviation associated with connection $\langle i, j \rangle$ in patient $m$ via the z-statistic $z_{ij}^m = (\bar{B}_{ij}^m - m_{ij})/s_{ij}$, where $m_{ij}$ and $s_{ij}$ are the mean and standard deviation of the corresponding rsfMRI correlations $\{B_{ij}^l : l = 1 \ldots L\}$ within the healthy population. The *connectivity* statistic summarizes the deviations associated with region $i$ in patient $m$ as the proportion of significantly different connections: $\hat{z}_i^m(\alpha) = \frac{1}{N-1} \sum_{j \neq i} \mathbb{1}(|z_{ij}^m| > \alpha)$, where $\alpha$ is a user-specified significance threshold and $\mathbb{1}(\cdot)$ is a function that is equal to 1 if its argument is true and is 0 otherwise. The absolute value accommodates both positive and negative correlation differences.

The second method computes the degree $d_i^m$ of region $i$ in patient $m$ by counting the number of connections with rsfMRI correlation above a user-specified threshold $\beta$, i.e., $d_i^m = \sum_{j \neq i} \mathbb{1}(\bar{B}_{ij}^m > \beta)$. The associated *degree* statistic $\bar{z}_i^m(\beta)$ quantifies how abnormal the degree of a node is relative to the null distribution estimated from the normal population. This statistic is closely related to the approach of [5], which, to the best of our knowledge, is the only existing method to localize epileptic regions based on whole-brain rsfMRI connectivity analysis.

***Model Evaluation.*** The iEEG electrode labels indicate one of three possible scenarios: abnormal activity as a seizure begins (*ictal*), abnormal activity between seizures (*interictal*), and no abnormal activity. Our goal is to identify the ictal areas that correspond to epileptic regions while simultaneously avoiding detection in the areas of normal activity.

As the iEEG electrodes lie on the surface of the brain, the cortical origin of the abnormal activity measured at each electrode is uncertain. This uncertainty is exacerbated by potential misalignment and significant brain shift due to the required craniotomy. Therefore, quantifying the agreement between the electrode labels and the diseased regions identified by the methods is not necessarily helpful. Instead, we qualitatively evaluate the performance of each method by visual comparison. We deem successful detections to be those that overlap with or are immediately adjacent to the ictal areas. We emphasize that the electrode grids cover only a fraction of the cortical surface; we cannot draw conclusions about any detections outside of this coverage.

## 3   Experimental Results

We have performed extensive simulations on synthetic data, in which the observations are sampled from our model. The experiments demonstrate that our inference algorithm recovers the true region labels for a wide range of model initializations. We omit these results here and instead focus on the clinical findings.

***Data and Pre-processing.*** We illustrate our method on a clinical study of six focal epilepsy patients. For each patient, the data includes an anatomical scan (MPRAGE, TE=3.44ms, FOV=256mm × 256mm, res=1mm$^3$), a between-seizure rsfMRI scan (EPI, 152-456 vols, TR=5s, TE=30ms, res=2mm$^3$), a CT volume acquired after iEEG electrode implantation (res=0.5 × 0.5 × 2.5-5mm), and the iEEG electrode labels. Anatomical and rsfMRI scans were acquired for 38 control subjects using the same imaging protocols.

We uniformly subdivide the Freesurfer cortical surface template [9] into $N = 1153$ regions and non-linearly register the resulting parcellation to the MNI152 template [10]. Our rsfMRI processing pipeline includes motion correction via rigid registration, slice timing correction and spatial normalization to the MNI152 template. We then spatially smooth each volume using a 6mm Gaussian kernel, temporally low-pass filter the time courses and remove global contributions from the white matter, ventricles and the whole brain. The rsfMRI observation $B_{ij}^l$ is computed as the Pearson correlation coefficient between the mean time courses of region $i$ and region $j$ in subject $l$.

The CT volume is rigidly registered to the MPRAGE volume using FSL [10]. While the registration is mostly accurate, the electrodes appear within the cortical surface due to brain shift during implantation. We correct for brain shift

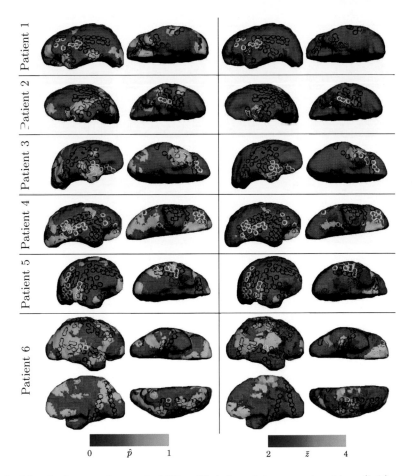

**Fig. 2.** Marginal posterior probability $\hat{p}_i^m$ inferred by our algorithm (left) and the degree statistic $\bar{z}_i^m$ (right), projected to the smoothed pial surface of each patient. The correlation threshold is set to $\beta = 0.5$. iEEG electrodes are shown as circles with colors denoting expert labels: normal activity (black), interictal abnormal activity (yellow) and ictal abnormal activity (red). Only views with electrode coverage are shown.

by projecting each electrode center onto its closest vertex on the smoothed pial surface [9]. For evaluation, we project the baseline and model results onto the smoothed pial surface by associating each vertex with the maximum value along its normal, up to 20mm inside the cortex. This is because abnormal activity measured on the brain surface can originate from within the cortical ribbon.

***Detecting Epileptic Regions.*** Fig. 2 visualizes the marginal posterior probability $\hat{p}_i^m$ obtained by our method, with the degree statistic $\bar{z}_i^m$ as a baseline result. We set the correlation threshold at $\beta = 0.5$, which yields qualitatively similar results to those presented in [5]. We display only the regions for which $\bar{z}_i^m > 2$, which roughly corresponds to an uncorrected p-value of $p < 0.05$.

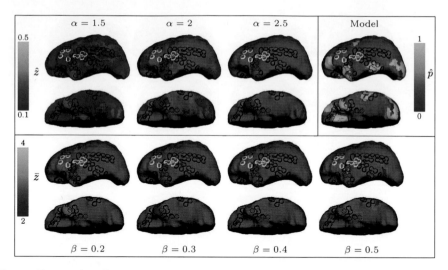

**Fig. 3.** Region localization for Patient 1 when sweeping the significance threshold $\alpha$ for the connectivity statistic $\hat{z}_i^m$ (top left) and the correlation threshold $\beta$ for the degree statistic $\bar{z}_i^m$ (bottom). The model results are presented for comparison (top right). iEEG electrodes are shown as circles with colors denoting expert labels: normal activity (black), interictal abnormal activity (yellow) and ictal abnormal activity (red).

Our algorithm identifies a much richer set of abnormal regions than the degree statistic $\bar{z}_i^m$. This translates to better detection of the ictal areas in Patient 1, Patient 4 and Patient 6. Our model also localizes many of the interictal areas in Patient 3, Patient 4 and Patient 5. While not strictly epileptic, interictal regions can develop after surgery to trigger seizures in the future [1]. In general, our algorithm avoids regions with normal activity. It also detects regions where there is no electrode coverage. Although we can only speculate about whether these regions are epileptic, they may be good candidate locations for electrode placement in pre-surgical planning. Patient 6 is the most difficult case as evidenced by the widespread electrode coverage. Here, both baseline methods fail to detect the frontal areas; instead, they favor regions with no electrode coverage. In contrast, our model correctly identifies all the ictal regions.

Optimizing the threshold $\alpha$ of the connectivity statistic against the iEEG electrode labels leads to a similar detection accuracy to that of our method but with more false detections in the areas of normal activity (not shown). The optimal parameter value varies across subjects, which highlights the challenge of using standard hypothesis testing in this application.

***Parameter Sweep.*** Fig. 3 illustrates how varying the user-defined threshold parameters in the baseline methods affects the results. Although the connectivity statistic $\hat{z}_i^m$ can identify the ictal regions, the results are sensitive to the threshold $\alpha$. In contrast, the degree statistic $\bar{z}_i^m$ marginally detects the ictal regions for any threshold $\beta$. Lowering $\beta$ would include more regions, but it does not make sense to use such a low correlation threshold to identify functional connections.

In contrast to the baseline methods, our algorithm is completely data-driven and automatically selects the appropriate parameter values. Empirically, we observe a sensitivity to threshold values for all six patients.

# 4   Conclusions

We have proposed a novel generative framework for epilepsy based on refMRI correlations. Our model assumes that epileptic foci induce a network of abnormal functional connectivity in the brain. The resulting algorithm consistently detects regions in the immediate vicinity of the ictal spiking areas, as localized by iEEG. Future directions include applying the method to a larger patient cohort and evaluating the effects of region size on the detection performance. Small patches can better localize the epileptic regions but are susceptible to inter-subject variability and registration errors. Conversely, large patches mitigate these issues but may smooth away focal effects. Overall, our results illustrate the promise of our approach for pre-surgical planning in epilepsy.

**Acknowledgments.** This work was supported in part by the National Alliance for Medical Image Computing (NIH NIBIB NAMIC U54-EB005149), the Neuroimaging Analysis Center (NIH NCRR NAC P41-RR13218 and NIH NIBIB NAC P41-EB-015902), the NSF CAREER Grant 0642971 and the MIT Lincoln Lab Collaboration.

# References

1. Lüders, H., et al.: The Epileptogenic Zone: General Principles. Epileptic Disorders: International Epilepsy Journal with Videotape 8(suppl. 2) , S1–S9 (2006)
2. Kramer, M., et al.: Epilepsy as a Disorder of Cortical Network Organization. The Neuroscientist 18(4), 360–372 (2012)
3. Fox, M., Raichle, M.: Spontaneous Fluctuations in Brain Activity Observed with Functional Magnetic Resonance Imaging. Nature 8, 700–711 (2007)
4. Luo, C., et al.: Disrupted Functional Brain Connectivity in Partial Epilepsy: a Resting-State fMRI Study. PloS one 7(1), e28196 (2011)
5. Stufflebeam, S., et al.: Localization of Focal Epileptic Discharges using Functional Connectivity Magnetic Resonance Imaging. Journal of Neurosurgery, 1–5 (2011)
6. Greicius, M.D., et al.: Resting-State Functional Connectivity in Major Depression: Abnormally Increased Contributions from Subgenual Cingulate Cortex and Thalamus. Biological Psychiatry 62, 429–437 (2007)
7. Varoquaux, G., Baronnet, F., Kleinschmidt, A., Fillard, P., Thirion, B.: Detection of Brain Functional-connectivity Difference in Post-stroke Patients using Group-level Covariance Modeling. In: Jiang, T., Navab, N., Pluim, J.P.W., Viergever, M.A. (eds.) MICCAI 2010, Part I. LNCS, vol. 6361, pp. 200–208. Springer, Heidelberg (2010)
8. Venkataraman, A., Kubicki, M., Golland, P.: From Brain Connectivity Models to Identifying Foci of a Neurological Disorder. In: Ayache, N., Delingette, H., Golland, P., Mori, K. (eds.) MICCAI 2012, Part I. LNCS, vol. 7510, pp. 715–722. Springer, Heidelberg (2012)
9. Fischl, B.: FreeSurfer. NeuroImage 62, 774–781 (2012)
10. Smith, S., et al.: Advances in Functional and Structural MR Image Analysis and Implementation as FSL. NeuroImage 23(51), 208–219 (2004)

# Joint Intensity Inhomogeneity Correction for Whole-Body MR Data*

Oleh Dzyubachyk[1], Rob J. van der Geest[1], Marius Staring[1], Peter Börnert[1,2],
Monique Reijnierse[1], Johan L. Bloem[1], and Boudewijn P.F. Lelieveldt[1,3]

[1] Department of Radiology, Leiden University Medical Center,
Leiden, The Netherlands
[2] Philips Research Laboratories, Hamburg, Germany
[3] Intelligent Systems Department, Delft University of Technology,
Delft, The Netherlands

**Abstract.** Whole-body MR receives increasing interest as potential alternative to many conventional diagnostic methods. Typical whole-body MR scans contain multiple data channels and are acquired in a multi-station manner. Quantification of such data typically requires correction of two types of artefacts: different intensity scaling on each acquired image stack, and intensity inhomogeneity (bias) within each stack. In this work, we present an all-in-one method that is able to correct for both mentioned types of acquisition artefacts. The most important properties of our method are: 1) All the processing is performed jointly on all available data channels, which is necessary for preserving the relation between them, and 2) It allows easy incorporation of additional knowledge for estimation of the bias field. Performed validation on two types of whole-body MR data confirmed superior performance of our approach in comparison with state-of-the-art bias removal methods.

**Keywords:** Whole-body MRI, multi-spectral MRI, multi-station acquisition, intensity inhomogeneity correction, intensity standardization.

## 1 Introduction

Whole-body (WB) MR has become a subject of intensive research for having a large potential in being an alternative to other imaging modalities with high anatomical detail. Nowadays, it has found clinical application in, among others, oncology, e.g. in assessment of multiple myeloma (MM), or cardiology, e.g. in obesity studies [1].

WB MR acquisitions are typically performed in multiple stages [2], a restriction imposed by the limited field of view of the MR scanner. For further processing, all the separately acquired image stacks need to be combined into a single volume. Such reconstructed volumes typically exhibit two types of irregularity:

---

* This research was supported by the Dutch Technology Foundation STW (Stichting Technische Wetenschappen) via grant 10894.

K. Mori et al. (Eds.): MICCAI 2013, Part I, LNCS 8149, pp. 106–113, 2013.

intensity inhomogeneity (bias) within each stack and a different dynamic intensity range for each station [3]. Both inhomogeneities cause significant problems for further image processing, thus robust removal of these artifacts would be highly desired.

A number of methods has been developed during last years for correction of both types of intensity inhomogeneity. An extensive review of the bias correction methods can be found in [4]. For dealing with the second type of intensity inhomogeneity, several specialized methods have been developed [3].

Here we present a novel all-in-one method for volume reconstruction from multi-station multi-spectral WB MR data. The developed method performs correction of both types of intensity inhomogeneity. The main methodological contribution of this work is two-fold: 1) We extend the Coherent Local Intensity Clustering (CLIC) framework [5] to the multi-spectral data case with joint estimation of the bias field for all data channels (Section 2.2), that allows preserving relation between them; and 2) Two novel optimization constraints (Section 2.4) were added to the model for improved estimation of the bias field. The following section describes our method and its novel parts in full detail.

## 2    Method

Our method is based on the CLIC framework, which was extended in several parts to cope with the complexity of our data. More precisely, the following modifications were developed in comparison with the original method:

- All the processing is performed jointly on all available data channels. This is important for preserving correspondence between these channels.
- We consider the bias field $b$ to be additive, which is achieved by applying the logarithmic transformation to the general MR acquisition model

$$I = J + b + n_{bio}, \tag{1}$$

  where $I$ and $J$ are logarithms of the measured and the true signal correspondingly, and $n_{bio}$ is the "biological noise". Additive bias model is more appropriate when the tissue-related bias is more prominent than the hardware-related one, and drastically simplifies solving the constrained optimization model.
- The possibilistic clustering [6] is used instead of the probabilistic one.
- The scaled Mahalanobis distance [6] is used instead of the Euclidean one.
- The centers $c_i$ and the fuzzy covariance matrices $\Sigma_i$ [7] of each cluster $i = \overline{1, N}$ are kept fixed to the values estimated from the data's intensity histogram; see Section 2.3.

Here we formulate our model assuming WB MR data with two channels, but all the methods can be directly extended to the three and more channels case.

### 2.1    Inter-station Intensity Calibration

Inter-station data calibration is applied for equalization of the intensity of different stacks within the same scan. Depending on the anatomical region to which the acquired image stack corresponds, its intensity distribution can vary considerably from that of other stacks. The equalization is performed according to the approach described by Jäger and Hornegger [3]: each joint intensity histogram $H_i$ is registered to the histogram $H_{\text{ref}}$ of a reference station, and the calculated deformation fields are used for performing the intensity mapping. For performing all the registrations, we used the software tool "elastix" [8].

## 2.2   Joint Multi-spectral Bias Correction via Possibilistic Clustering

The CLIC framework estimates the bias field and the tissue probability maps based on two core assumptions: 1) The object consists of a finite number of tissue classes $N$, each of them having a constant true intensity value $c_i$ ($i = \overline{1, N}$); and 2) The estimated bias field $b$ is slowly varying.

These assumptions allow to partition the entire image domain $\Omega$ into disjoint tissue regions $\Omega_i$ ($i = \overline{1, N}$) via fuzzy classification [9]. The tissue classification and the bias field estimation is formulated as a single optimization problem. For the case of an additive bias field (1), this requires minimization of the following energy functional

$$J(U, \mathbf{c}, b) \triangleq \int \sum_{i=1}^{N} \int u_i^q(\mathbf{y}) K(\mathbf{x} - \mathbf{y}) \left| I(\mathbf{y}) - b(\mathbf{x}) - c_i \right|^2 d\mathbf{y} d\mathbf{x}, \qquad (2)$$

where $c_i$ is the center of the cluster $i = \overline{1, N}$, and $u_i$ is the membership probability function of the corresponding tissue; $\mathbf{x}$ and $\mathbf{y}$ are Cartesian coordinates on $\Omega$; $q \geq 1$ is a scalar; and $K$ is truncated Gaussian kernel.

The energy (2) is convex with respect to the variables $b$, $\mathbf{c}$ and $U$, thus the model unknowns can easily be determined by differentiation with respect to the corresponding variables. For joint bias correction on two channels, the energy functional (2) for the vector image intensity $\mathbf{I} = (I_1, I_2)$, bias field $\mathbf{b} = (b_1, b_2)$, and centers $\mathbf{c}_i = (c_{1,i}, c_{2,i})$ of each cluster $i = \overline{1, N}$ can be written as

$$J(U, \mathbf{c}, \mathbf{b}) = \int \sum_{i=1}^{N} u_i^q(\mathbf{y}) d_i(\mathbf{y}; \mathbf{c}, \mathbf{b}) d\mathbf{y}, \qquad (3)$$

where

$$d_i(\mathbf{y}; \mathbf{c}, \mathbf{b}) = \int K(\mathbf{x} - \mathbf{y}) d\mathbf{x} \left[ s_{11,i} \left( I_1(\mathbf{y}) - b_1(\mathbf{x}) - c_{1,i} \right)^2 + (s_{12,i} + s_{21,i}) \times \right.$$

$$\left. (I_1(\mathbf{y}) - b_1(\mathbf{x}) - c_{1,i}) (I_2(\mathbf{y}) - b_2(\mathbf{x}) - c_{2,i}) + s_{22,i} \left( I_2(\mathbf{y}) - b_2(\mathbf{x}) - c_{2,i} \right)^2 \right],$$

and [6]

$$\begin{pmatrix} s_{11,i} & s_{12,i} \\ s_{21,i} & s_{22,i} \end{pmatrix} = (\Sigma_i^{\text{new}})^{-1} |\Sigma_i^{\text{new}}|^{1/n_d}.$$

Here we use an improved estimate $\Sigma_i^{\text{new}}$ [7] of the covariance matrix $\Sigma_i$, and $n_d$ is the data dimensionality (in our case $n_d = 3$).

Within the possibilistic clustering framework, the class membership functions are given by the following expression [6]

$$\widehat{u}_i = \left[ 1 + \left( \frac{d_i(\mathbf{I})}{\eta_i} \right)^{\frac{1}{q-1}} \right]^{-1} , \qquad i = \overline{1, N}, \qquad (4)$$

where $\eta_i$ is the bandwidth of each cluster. Our definition of this parameter is given in Section 2.3. Differentiation of (3) with respect to $\mathbf{b}$ gives us a following linear system of equations for calculating the bias field, whose solution can be written as

$$\widehat{b}_{s,k} = T_s^{(3-k)} Q_s^{(k)} - T_s^{(3)} Q_s^{(3-k)}, \quad k = \overline{1, 2}, \qquad (5)$$

where the variables $P_s^{(1:3)}$, $Q_s^{(1:2)}$, and $T_s^{(1:3)}$ are defined in the Appendix. The values of $u_i$ ($i = \overline{1, N}$) and $\mathbf{b}$ are iteratively updated till convergence by using expressions given in equations (4) and (5).

### 2.3   Algorithm Initialization

Our algorithm is initialized by estimating the mean $c_i$, the covariance $\Sigma_i$, and the bandwidth $\eta_i = \int_{R_i} d_i(\mathbf{x}) d\mathbf{x}$ of each cluster $i = \overline{1, N}$ from segmented joint histogram. Based on the typical appearance of the joint histograms, we identify $N$ as the number of present clusters. Consequently, the joint histogram is automatically segmented using a region-growing-type algorithm into $N$ regions $R_i$ corresponding to each of the observed clusters.

### 2.4   Constrained Optimization

*Overlap Constraint.* Multi-station MR data is typically acquired with relatively large overlap between the neighboring stations. The real image intensities in the overlap region of each pair of neighboring stations should be approximately equal

$$J(\mathbf{x}) = J\left(D_s(\mathbf{x})\right), \qquad \mathbf{x} \in O_s^{(2)}, \quad s = \overline{1, N_s - 1}. \qquad (6)$$

This property can be used to further improve the quality of bias correction. Here index $s$ denotes the image stack; $N_s$ is the total number of stations in the data set; $O_s^{(1)}$ and $O_s^{(2)}$ are respectively the overlap regions of stack $S_s$ with the previous and the next stacks; and $D_s(\mathbf{x})$ is the function that maps $O_s^{(2)}$ onto $O_{s+1}^{(1)}$. Providing such extra knowledge into the system is especially important as the regions adjacent to the boundary are the most prone to geometric distortions.

Condition (6) is incorporated into our model as an optimization constraint

$$\mathcal{J}_{constr}^{overlap} = \mathcal{J} + \sum_{s=1}^{N_s-1} \boldsymbol{\lambda}_s \left[ (K * \mathbf{I}_s - \mathbf{b}_s) - (K * \mathbf{I}_{s+1} - \mathbf{b}_{s+1}) (D_s) ) \right], \qquad (7)$$

where $\boldsymbol{\lambda}_s = (\lambda_{s,1}, \lambda_{s,2})$ ($s = \overline{1, N_s - 1}$) is the vector of Lagrange multipliers [10] for both image channels for $\mathbf{x} \in O_s^{(2)}$. The full derivation of the equivalents of equations (5) for the constrained optimization case is presented in the Appendix.

*Linearity Constraint.* For the two-point Dixon imaging, each voxel belongs to one of the following classes: background (air), water, or fat. In order to better preserve the relation between the last two classes, we introduce the following constraint for $\mathbf{x} \in \{\mathbf{x} : \text{argmax}_i(\mathbf{u}_i(\mathbf{x})) \in \{i_w, i_f\}\}$:

$$\mathcal{J}_{constr}^{linear} = \mathcal{J} + \sum_{s=1}^{N_s} \lambda_s \sum_{k=1}^{2} (-1)^{3-k} a_{3-k} \left[ (K * \mathbf{I}_{s,k} - \mathbf{b}_{s,k}) - c_{i_w,k} \right], \qquad (8)$$

where $\mathbf{a} = \mathbf{c}_{i_w} - \mathbf{c}_{i_f}$, and $i_w$ and $i_f$ denote correspondingly the background, the water, and the fat class. Such constraint imposes a linear relation between the two foreground classes (water and fat). Final expressions for the Lagrangian multiplier $\lambda$ and the bias field $\mathbf{b}$ for the described constrained optimization problem are given in the Appendix.

## 2.5   Intensity Standardization and Volume Reconstruction

Inter-scan intensity standardization is applied when the analysis involves multiple different scans, e.g. for baseline–follow-up comparisons. In this case, WB volumes belonging to different patients or follow-up scans of the same patient require prior intensity calibration. We achieve this by registering joint histograms of the complete body volumes, using a similar approach to the one described in Section 2.1.

Finally, all the separately acquired image stacks are reconstructed into a single volume using the geometric information recorded by the scanner. Since the data is acquired with some overlap between the neighboring stations, the information from both stacks has to be combined in the overlap region. The combined image is constructed by using the image blending method [11].

## 3   Experiments and Results

In this section, we apply the described method to two large sets of WB MR data: multiple myeloma patients data set, and two-point water-fat Dixon data set. Bias correction performance of our method was validated by comparing it to that of the two state-of-the art methods: N4 [12] and the original CLIC algorithm [5].

*MM Patients Data Set.* The MM patients data set consisted of 24 WB volumes of 8 patients, and was acquired on a commercial human WB 1.5T MR Philips Intera system. Each WB volume had both a $T_1$-weighted ($T_1W$) and a Short Tau Inversion Recovery (STIR) or $T_2$-STIR sequence. Number of scans per patient varied from 1 to 4, with approximately six month interval between the follow-up scans. 3D image stacks with coronal slice direction were acquired with the overlap approximately equal to 5% of the total volume of the two stacks. For improved estimation of the bias field in the overlap area, the overlap optimization constraint introduced in Section 2.4 was used. Processing time on a typical volume of size $1500 \times 500 \times 50$ voxels was around 20 minutes.

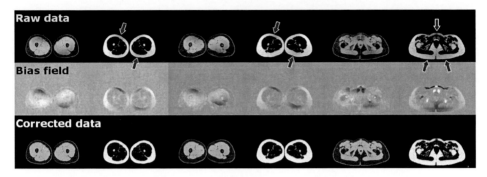

**Fig. 1.** Result of bias correction on a two-point Dixon data set. The areas of the most significant quality improvement are indicated by the arrows. The estimated inhomogeneity field is in nice agreement with characteristic RF wave propagation problems known in quadrature body coil transmission at 3T.

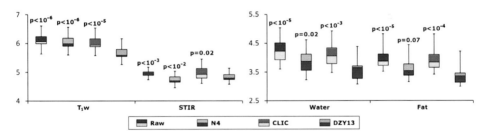

**Fig. 2.** Bias correction performance of our method on the MM patients data set (left) and the two-point Dixon data set (right). The histogram entropy of the raw data and that corrected by three methods: N4, CLIC, and the presented method (labeled as DZY13), is shown. Lower histogram entropy indicates better bias correction. Statistical significance was calculated using the paired Kolmogorov-Smirnov test with the DZY13 method as the reference.

*Two-point Dixon Data Set.* For two-point Dixon data, in vivo experiments were conducted on 8 healthy adults using a 3.0T clinical Philips Achieva Tx scanner. For simplicity and patient comfort reasons, the body coil was used for RF transmission and reception in the quadrature mode. 3D multi-station spoiled gradient echo (FFE) imaging was performed using a dual-echo-Dixon imaging sequence [13] with alternating readout gradients for water-fat separation. Bias correction on this data set was performed by using the algorithm described in Section 2, with the linearity optimization constraint. Processing time for both typical volume sizes $256 \times 256 \times 1520$ voxels and $336 \times 336 \times 960$ voxels was around 30 minutes.

A typical result of performing bias correction by our method is shown in Figure 1. The histogram entropy [4], which is widely applied for measuring the quality of bias correction when a ground truth is not available, was used for quantitative evaluation. The results with respect to the entropy intensity histogram of the raw images and the images corrected by our algorithm and two reference methods N4 and CLIC are shown in Figure 2. This analysis clearly indicates large quality improvement of the data corrected by our method, and its better performance in comparison with the reference state-of-the-art bias removal algorithms.

## 4    Conclusions

In this paper, we have presented a new algorithm for reconstruction of a complete volume from multiple separately acquired stations in multi-spectral WB MR data. Our method performs reconstruction of two types of intensity inhomogeneity, and combines all the acquired stations into a single volume. Among the novelties introduced in our algorithm compared to established methodology, the most important two are: 1) The joint processing (bias correction, calibration, standardization, etc.) on all available data channels; and 2) Integration of optimization constraints for improved estimation of the bias field. The described algorithm is applied to two different types of WB MR data, resulting in considerable quality improvement of the volumes reconstruction.

## References

1. Kullberg, J., Angelhed, J.E., Lönn, L., Brandberg, J., Ahlström, H., Frimmel, H., Johansson, L.: Whole-body T1 mapping improves the definition of adipose tissue: Consequences for automated image analysis. J. Magn. Reson. Im. 24(2), 394–401 (2006)
2. Börnert, P., Aldefeld, B.: Principles of whole-body continuously-moving-table MRI. J. Magn. Reson. Im. 28(1), 1–12 (2008)
3. Jäger, F., Hornegger, J.: Nonrigid registration of joint histograms for intensity standardization in magnetic resonance imaging. IEEE Trans. Med. Imag. 28(1), 137–150 (2009)
4. Belaroussi, B., Milles, J., Carme, S., Zhu, Y.M., Benoit-Cattin, H.: Intensity nonuniformity correction in MRI: Existing methods and their validation. Med. Image Anal. 10(2), 234–246 (2006)
5. Li, C., Xu, C., Anderson, A.W., Gore, J.C.: MRI tissue classification and bias field estimation based on coherent local intensity clustering: A unified energy minimization framework. In: Prince, J.L., Pham, D.L., Myers, K.J. (eds.) IPMI 2009. LNCS, vol. 5636, pp. 288–299. Springer, Heidelberg (2009)
6. Krishnapuram, R., Keller, J.M.: A possibilistic approach to clustering. IEEE Trans. Fuz. Sys. 1(2), 98–110 (1993)
7. Babuška, R., van der Veen, P., Kaymak, U.: Improved covariance estimation for Gustafson-Kessel clustering. In: Proc. 2002 IEEE Int. Conf. Fuz. Sys (FUZZ-IEEE 2002), Honolulu, Hawaii, USA, vol. 2, pp. 1081–1085 (2002)
8. Klein, S., Staring, M., Murphy, K., Viergever, M., Pluim, J.: elastix: a toolbox for intensity-based medical image registration. IEEE Trans. Med. Imag. 29(1), 196–205 (2010)
9. Bezdek, J., Pal, S.: Fuzzy Models for Pattern Recognition, 1st edn. IEEE Press (1992)

10. Bertsekas, D.P.: Constrained Optimization and Lagrange Multiplier Methods, 1st edn. Optimization and Neural Computation Series. Athena Scientific (1996)
11. Burt, P.J., Adelson, E.H.: A multiresolution spline with application to image mosaics. ACM Trans. Graph. 2, 217–236 (1983)
12. Tustison, N., Gee, J.: N4ITK: Nick's N3 ITK implementation for MRI bias field correction. Insight J. (January-June 2009)
13. Eggers, H., Brendel, B., Duijndam, A., Herigault, G.: Dual-echo Dixon imaging with flexible choice of echo times. Magn. Reson. Med. 65(1), 96–107 (2011)

# Appendix

We introduce the following notation for $k = \overline{1,2}$ and $l = \overline{1,3}$

$$P_s^{(k)} = 2K * \sum_{i=1}^{N} u_{i,s}^q s_{kk,i}, \qquad P_s^{(3)} = K * \sum_{i=1}^{N} u_{i,s}^q (s_{12,i} + s_{21,i}),$$

$$Q_s^{(k)} = K * \sum_{i=1}^{N} u_{i,s}^q \left[ 2(I_{s,k} - c_{i,k})s_{kk,i} + (I_{s,3-k} - c_{i,3-k})(s_{12,i} + s_{21,i}) \right],$$

$$T_s^{(l)} = \frac{P_s^{(l)}}{P_s^{(1)} P_s^{(2)} - \left( P_s^{(3)} \right)^2}, \qquad R_s^{(k)} = K * I_{s,k} - T_s^{(3-k)} Q_s^{(k)} + T_s^{(3)} Q_s^{(3-k)},$$

Using the optimization constraint (7), the following equivalent of the expression (5) can be derived for $k = \overline{1,2}$

$$\widehat{b}_{s,k}^{(c)} = \widehat{b}_{s,k} + T_s^{(3)} \left( \lambda_{s-1,3-k}(D_s^{-1}) + \lambda_{s,3-k} \right) - T_s^{(3-k)} \left( \lambda_{s-1,k}(D_s^{-1}) + \lambda_{s,k} \right), \quad (9)$$

where $D_s^{-1}(\mathbf{x})$ denotes the inverse mapping of $O_{s+1}^{(1)}$ onto $O_s^{(2)}$.

Combining (9) with the constraint (7), we obtain a linear system of equations for calculating the Lagrange multipliers $\boldsymbol{\lambda}$. Its solution for $k = \overline{1,2}$ is given by

$$\lambda_{s,k} = \frac{V_s^{(k)} W_s^{(k)} - V_s^{(3)} W_s^{(3-k)}}{V_s^{(1)} V_s^{(2)} - \left( V_s^{(3)} \right)^2}, \quad V_s^{(l)} = T_s^{(l)} + T_{s+1}^{(l)}(D_s), \quad W_s^{(k)} = R_s^{(k)} - R_{s+1}^{(k)}(D_s).$$

Substituting this solution into (9) gives us the resulting expressions for $\mathbf{b}$.

For the case of the optimization constraint (8), the following expression for the bias field $\widehat{\mathbf{b}}^{(c)}$ is obtained

$$\widehat{b}_{s,k}^{(c)} = \widehat{b}_{s,k} + (-1)^{3-k} \lambda_s (a_{3-k} T_s^{(3-k)} + a_k T_s^{(3)}), \qquad k = \overline{1,2}. \quad (10)$$

Substituting the latter into the constraint (8) gives us

$$\lambda_{s,k} = \frac{a_2(K * I_{s,1} - \widehat{b}_{s,1} - c_{1,i_w}) - a_1(K * I_{s,2} - \widehat{b}_{s,2} - c_{2,i_w})}{a_1^2 T_s^{(1)} + a_2^2 T_s^{(2)} + 2a_1 a_2 T_s^{(3)}}, \qquad k = \overline{1,2}.$$

This solution, together with (10), gives us the final expression for the bias $\mathbf{b}$.

# Tissue-Specific Sparse Deconvolution for Low-Dose CT Perfusion

Ruogu Fang[1], Tsuhan Chen[1], and Pina C. Sanelli[2,3]

[1] Department of Electrical and Computer Engineering, Cornell University, Ithaca, NY, USA
[2] Department of Radiology, Weill Cornell Medical College, New York, NY, USA
[3] Department of Public Health, Weill Cornell Medical College, New York, NY, USA

**Abstract.** Sparse perfusion deconvolution has been recently proposed to effectively improve the image quality and diagnostic accuracy of low-dose perfusion CT by extracting the complementary information from the high-dose perfusion maps to restore the low-dose using a joint spatio-temporal model. However the low-contrast tissue classes where infarct core and ischemic penumbra usually occur in cerebral perfusion CT tend to be over-smoothed, leading to loss of essential biomarkers. In this paper, we extend this line of work by introducing tissue-specific sparse deconvolution to preserve the subtle perfusion information in the low-contrast tissue classes by learning tissue-specific dictionaries for each tissue class, and restore the low-dose perfusion maps by joining the tissue segments reconstructed from the corresponding dictionaries. Extensive validation on clinical datasets of patients with cerebrovascular disease demonstrates the superior performance of our proposed method with the advantage of better differentiation between abnormal and normal tissue in these patients.

## 1 Introduction

Computed tomography perfusion (CTP) [1] has been more commonly used in patients with cerebrovascular diseases to characterize tissue perfusion. Specifically, in acute stroke patients, detection of ischemic regions has been a main focus in the literature. The associated excessive radiation exposure of CTP has aroused great concern due to over-dosage leading to biological effects including hair loss, skin burn and increased cancer risk [2]. Even currently recommended CTP scanning parameters still contribute to increased lifetime cancer risk. Sparse perfusion deconvolution (SPD) [3][4] is a recently proposed method for low-dose CTP deconvolution. Different from previous methods [5][6], whose image prior has been based on some simplifying assumptions, SPD is a data-driven method that restores the input low-dose perfusion map using a spatio-temporal model. The model is regularized by a sparse combination of atoms from a global dictionary learned from the high-dose perfusion maps. In this way, spatial priors are incorporated on-the-fly. SPD is able to remove the noise and can preserve the vascular structure and contrast in low-dose perfusion maps.

Theoretically, a global dictionary is able to capture sufficient image information for different tissue classes, given abundant training data from each class. Learned global dictionaries have been applied to various domains including image super-resolution [7] and deformable shape modeling [8]. However empirically the optimization procedure

K. Mori et al. (Eds.): MICCAI 2013, Part I, LNCS 8149, pp. 114–121, 2013.

which minimizes the overall reconstruction error, tends to favor high-contrast patches to the low-contrast ones in both the learning and reconstruction procedures. For medical images, the subtle variations and changes embedded in the low-contrast tissue classes such as white matter can be crucial for disease detection and diagnosis [9].

In this paper, we propose a tissue-specific sparse deconvolution method to address the limitations above. Our method starts from segmenting the brain into different tissue classes. A modified version of automated model-based tissue classification [10] is employed to segment the brain tissue classes. Then tissue-specific dictionaries are learned from the training segments of each class. Finally we use weighted sparse deconvolution method to restore each tissue class and stitch them together. The extensive experiments demonstrate the superior performance of our method. It is important to note that all the preprocessing methods to denoise the dynamic CT data can be complimented with our proposed deconvolution algorithm to achieve better performance.

Our main contribution is two-fold: (1) Tissue-specific dictionaries for each tissue class are employed in place of the global dictionary to capture the low-contrast tissue class and delicate structural details. (2) Weighted sparse deconvolution based on the probability of the tissue classification is proposed for a unified reconstruction of the low-dose perfusion maps. In vivo brain acute stroke and aneurysmal SAH patients data, we demonstrate the superiority of our proposed method in CBF estimation that leads to better separation between normal and ischemic tissue.

## 2 Tissue-Specific Approach to Sparse Deconvolution

### 2.1 Tissue Classification

We first classify the voxels in the dynamic brain CTP data into four tissue classes: vessel, gray matter (GM), white matter (WM) and cerebrospinal fluid (CSF). Since computational efficiency is very important in our framework for real-time clinical diagnosis, we choose a simple yet effective segmentation approach by adapting a tissue classification algorithm for MRI [10]. We first compute the median value for each voxel along the temporal axis since different tissue classes have different contrast perfusion characteristics. Expectation-maximization segmentation is employed on the median map to obtain probability maps of GM, WM and CSF, while contexture information is incorporated by a Markov Random Field (MRF). The reason for choosing median map as a robust measurement of the tissue contrast in CTP is because of its higher tissue contrast compared to other statistics in our experiments. Vessel is segmented by thresholding the original CBF value. The vessel voxels in other tissue probability maps are set to zero to guarantee mutually occlusive segmentations. Tissue probability maps on a representative dataset are shown in Fig. 1. The following reconstruction does not heavily depend on the segmentation accuracy, since each tissue dictionary is learned from over 10,000 patches and represents dominant patterns in the training patches.

### 2.2 Tissue-Specific Dictionary Learning

Based on the tissue classification from the previous section, we obtain $M$ sets $S_m$ of training patches, $m = Vessel, GM, WM, CSF$, by classifying a patch $y$ from a

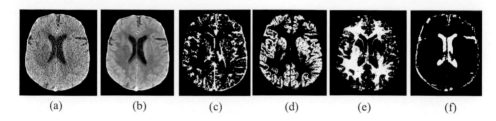

(a)        (b)        (c)        (d)        (e)        (f)

**Fig. 1.** Brain tissue classification by the automatic algorithm on the median map. (a) A slice in the enhanced CTP data (b) Median map. Probability maps of (c) Vessel (d) Gray matter (e) White matter (f) CSF.

---

**Algorithm 1.** The framework of online dictionary learning in mini-batch mode.

---

**Input:** Initialized dictionary $D_0 \in \mathbf{R}^{n \times k}$, input data $y_i \in \mathbf{R}^n$, number of iterations $T$, regularization parameter $\lambda \in R$.

**Output:** Learned dictionary $D_T$.

$A_0 = 0$, $B_0 = 0$.

**for** $t = 1 \rightarrow T$ **do**

    Randomly draw a set from $Y$: $y_{t,1}, y_{t,2}, \ldots, y_{t,\tau}$.

    **for** $i = 1 \rightarrow \tau$ **do**

        **Sparse coding:** $\alpha_{t,i} = \arg\min_{\alpha \in \mathbf{R}^k} \frac{1}{2}\|y_{t,i} - D_{t-1}\alpha\|_2^2 + \lambda\|\alpha\|_1$.

    **end for**

    $A_t = \beta A_{t-1} + \sum_{i=1}^{\tau} \alpha_{t,i}\alpha_{t,i}^T$, $B_t = \beta B_{t-1} + \sum_{i=1}^{\tau} y_{t,i}\alpha_{t,i}^T$,

    where $\beta = \frac{\theta + 1 - \tau}{\theta + 1}$, and $\theta = t\tau$ if $t < \tau$, $\theta = \tau^2 + t - \tau$ otherwise.

    **Dictionary update:** Compute $D_t$, so that:

    $\arg\min_D \frac{1}{t}\sigma_{i=1}^{t}\frac{1}{2}\|y_i - D\alpha_i\|_2^2 + \lambda\|\alpha_i\|_1 = \arg\min_D \frac{1}{t}(\frac{1}{2}Tr(D^T D A_t) - Tr(D^T B_t))$.

**end for**

---

training image to class $i$ if more than 50% of voxels in the patch $y$ belongs to class $i$. Voxels from other classes are then removed from the patch.

To learn the tissue-specific dictionary $\mathbf{D}^m$, $m = Vessel, GM, WM, CSF$, we use the recently developed online learning algorithm [11] which is able to update the dictionary with every batch of new training samples and avoids the time-consuming reconstruction of the entire dictionary when new samples come. Given a set of high-dose CBF patches $Y^m = \{y_i^m\}_{i=1}^{N}$ for a specific tissue type $m$, each as a column vector of size $N$. $\alpha_i$ in $R^K$ is a sparse vector to make $\mathbf{D}\alpha_i$ an approximation to $y_i^m$ with certain error tolerance. $A^m = [\alpha_1, \ldots, \alpha_N]$. We seek the dictionary $\mathbf{D}^m$ in $\mathbf{R}^{N \times K}$ in that minimizes

$$\min_{\mathbf{D}^m, \mathbf{A}^m} \sum_{i=1}^{N} \|y_i^m - \mathbf{D}^m\alpha_i\|_2 + \mu_2\|\alpha_i\|_1 \tag{1}$$

The framework of online dictionary learning is depicted in Algorithm 1. The dictionary is updated efficiently using block-coordinate descent based on stochastic approximation. Because it only exploits a small batch of newly coming data in the dictionary update step, it is therefore much faster than K-SVD or other off-line learning algorithms.

Since computational efficiency is very important in our framework, we can efficiently update the tissue-specific dictionaries with newly coming data using online learning. Moreover online learning also does not require the loading of all data at the same time, which is unfeasible in clinical practice, and results in less memory cost.

### 2.3 Weighted Sparse Deconvolution

Let's assume dynamic CTP data $C$ in $R^{N \times T}$ composed of $N$ tissue enhancement curves (TEC) at voxels of interest (VOI) $[x, y, z]^T$ and $T$ time points. The residue impulse function (RIF) is represented by $R$ in $R^{N \times T}$, indicating the delaying of the remaining contrast tracer in the VOI. $f$ in $R^N$ is the CBF map to be estimated and $D$ is the learned dictionary. The deconvolution step in SPD algorithm computes the CBF map of low-dose CTP data using both temporal convolution model and tissue-specific dictionary-based spatial regularization by solving:

$$J = \mu_1 \|C^m - C_a R^m\|_2^2 + \|f^m - D^m \alpha\|_2^2 + \mu_2 \|\alpha\|_1 \tag{2}$$

where $C^m$, $R^m$, $D^m$ and $f^m$ are the corresponding TEC, RIF, dictionary and CBF for tissue class $m$ for a patch of size $N \times N$. The final global CBF parametric map is generated by averaging the areas of neighboring patches with overlap of one pixel.

Eq. (2) is solved by an EM style algorithm with iterative employment of two processes: 1) sparse coding process which minimizes with respect to $\alpha$ with $f$ fixed, 2) quadratic solver which efficiently minimizes this simplified linear inverse problem, as in [4]. Two procedures are iteratively employed to obtain $f^m$ and $\alpha^m$ for each tissue type. Proper initialization in Eq. (2) with the output of cTSVD poses the optimization at a good start point and is supposed to mitigate local minima. We also observe our results are quite stable with respect to the training dataset.

The probability map of each tissue class is obtained by employing the model-based segmentation algorithm [10] on the median map of the low-dose CTP data. For every tissue class $m$, a tissue-specific patch $\hat{f}_i^m$ is reconstructed using the corresponding tissue-specific dictionary of tissue class $m$. The patch $\hat{f}_i^m$ is then weighted by the probability map of class $m$ for patch $f_i$ and all probability-weighted tissue-specific patches are summed together to obtain the final reconstruction.

Using tissue-specific dictionaries to enhance low-dose CTP maps, SPD obtains three additional advantages: 1) Segmentation information is incorporated into the dictionary learning and reconstruction. 2) Each tissue type has sufficient atoms in the tissue-specific dictionary to reconstruct. 3) Tissue specific parameter settings can be employed according to the spatial smoothness of each tissue class.

## 3 Experiments

To evaluate the performance of the proposed tissue-specific sparse deconvolution (TS-SPD) method, we apply it to a cerebrovascular disease dataset of 20 cases CTP scanned at tube current 190mA from our medical institute. Out of 20 subjects, 10 are used as training and validation (6 with CTP deficits in the brain and 4 normal), and the remaining 10 are used for testing purpose (5 with CTP deficits and 5 normal). For all experiments of SPD, the dictionary used are of size $64 \times 256$ designed to handle perfusion image patches of $8 \times 8$ pixels with 256 atoms in the dictionary. We download the online dictionary learning for sparse representation code from the authors' website[1], and the model-based brain segmentation code[2]. The optimal parameters are obtained empirically from the training and validation dataset are: $\mu_1 = 0.01, 0.02, 0.04, 0.08$ and $\mu_2 = 0.2, 0.4, 0.8, 1$ for vessel, GM, WM and CSF. The threshold for vessel segmentation is 70 mL/100g/min on the CBF map, as found to be the optimal value in our empirical experiments.

Since repetitive scanning of the same patient at different radiation doses is unethical, correlated Gaussian noise is added to the high-dose CTP data to simulate low-dose CTP data at $I$ mA following the practice in [12]: $I = (K^2 \cdot I_0)/(K^2 + \sigma_a^2 \cdot I_0)$, where $\sigma_a$ is the standard deviation of the added noise, $I_0 = 190$mA is the tube current at high-dose, $K = 103.09$mA$^{\frac{1}{2}}$ is a constant. Low tube current of 15.6 mA was simulated by adding correlated Gaussian noise with standard deviation of 25. CBF maps computed from CTP data obtained at high tube current of 190 mA were regarded as the reference standard. We present both the visual and quantitative results to demonstrate performance of the proposed method, with the comparison to cTSVD [13] and KSVD-SPD [3].

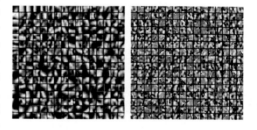

**Fig. 2.** Left: Global dictionaries learned using K-SVD. Right: Tissue-specific dictionary for white matter. The global dictionary is dominated by high-contrast, edge-like atoms, while the tissue-specific dictionary for WM has more low-contrast, fine structured atoms, as highlighted by red boxes.

**Tissue-Specific Dictionaries:** Figure 2 shows the globally learned dictionary using K-SVD and the tissue-specific dictionary for white matter. The global dictionary is trained on a dataset of 40,000 $8 \times 8$ patches of high-dose CBF perfusion maps randomly sampled from 10 training subjects and initialized with the redundant DCT dictionary. Each tissue-specific dictionary is trained using 10,000 $8 \times 8$ patches of the corresponding tissue category from the same training subjects. We could observe from the global dictionary that high-contrast patches with edges and corners dominate the dictionary atoms. In comparison, the tissue-specific dictionary for white matter preserves the texture and image characteristics for this tissue class.

**CBF Perfusion Map:** We then compare three methods by visually observing the estimated CBF perfusion maps of two patients. As shown in Figs. 3, among the three low-dose CBF maps, the CBF maps generated using our proposed TS-SPD algorithm recovers the information of high-dose CBF maps from the low-dose CTP data with best overall performance. The arteries and veins as well as the micro-vessels are better

---

[1] http://spams-devel.gforge.inria.fr/
[2] http://sourceforge.net/projects/niftyseg/

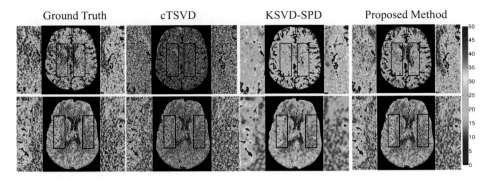

Ground Truth          cTSVD          KSVD-SPD          Proposed Method

**Fig. 3.** CBF maps and zoomed-in regions. A 63-year-old female with acute stroke has an ischemic region in the right hemisphere of the brain (1st row) and a 35-year-old female with left middle cerebral artery (LMCA) perfusion deficit caused by aneurysmal SAH (2nd row). (Note representations in medical images display the sides of the images in reverse order) LMCA and RMCA are enlarged for comparison next to each image. The low-contrast tissue classes in the LMCA and RMCA regions are highly noisy in cTSVD images, and are over-smoothed by KSVD-SPD, while TS-SPD preserves the subtle variations and are closest to the ground truth.

**Table 1.** Quantitative comparison of PSNR (dB) in CBF maps at low-dose are reported for 10 CTP cases by cTSVD, KSVD-SPD and our TS-SPD. Stroke and SAH indicate the two subjects in Fig. 3 respectively. The best performance is in bold-face type.

| PSNR | Brain | | | GM | | | WM | | |
|---|---|---|---|---|---|---|---|---|---|
| | Stroke | SAH | All data | Stroke | SAH | All data | Stroke | SAH | All data |
| cTSVD | 43.51 | 34.87 | 33.57 | 12.81 | 15.94 | 15.91 | 19.99 | 18.65 | 17.82 |
| KSVD-SPD | 45.80 | 37.11 | 34.91 | 17.53 | 18.08 | 17.88 | 22.80 | 19.75 | 19.41 |
| TS-SPD | **47.84** | **38.38** | **36.65** | **18.92** | **19.66** | **19.91** | **25.02** | **22.56** | **22.28** |

defined, while the delicate structures of the white matter and CSF are preserved. While the noise is greatly suppressed in the low-dose CBF maps for both enhancement algorithms, KSVD-SPD tends to smooth the image too much, especially the non-vessel structures. Our TS-SPD algorithm overcomes these drawbacks and preserves both the vessel boundaries and the low-contrast structures of WM and CSF with tissue-specific dictionaries and adaptive parameter settings for each tissue class.

**Asymmetry:** To visualize the asymmetry in the left and right middle cerebral artery in Fig. 3, we compute the intensity difference maps between LMCA and RMCA for three methods, as shown in Fig. 4. The intensity difference map of cTSVD is too noisy to identify the asymmetry of LMCA and RMCA vessel structures, while KSVD-SPD blurs the details of the vessel structure. The proposed method generates the different map with better contrast and spatial resolution for diagnosis of asymmetry in LMCA and RMCA.

**Quantitative Comparisons:** We report the PSNR (peak signal-to-noise-ratio) values for two cases in Fig. 3 and all testing subjects on the whole brain, GM and WM in Table 1. The GM and WM are the tissue regions in the brain affected by stroke and other

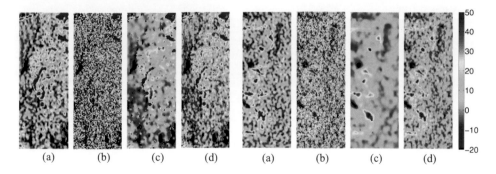

**Fig. 4.** Zoomed-in regions of the intensity difference maps between LMCA and RMCA of the acute stroke (left) and SAH (right) patients estimated by (a) Ground truth (b) cTSVD (c) KSVD-SPD (d) Proposed TS-SPD. Arteries are delineated in red, CSF in blue.

ischemic processes. The proposed method again achieves the highest PSNR (usually 2∼3 dB higher) in all cases, allowing for better discrimination ability of these brain regions, by preserving the tissue structures for differentiation of infarct core and ischemic penumbra in specific regions of the brain assisting neuroradiologists in diagnosis.

**Ischemic Voxels Clustering:** We also perform the clustering experiment as in [3] by aggregating all voxels (within VOI) from the normal hemisphere into a single "normal" cluster and the pathologic hemisphere into an "abnormal" cluster. To quantify the separability between normal and ischemic CBF values, we define the distance between these two clusters as: $d = (m_1 - m_2)/\sqrt{\sigma_1^2/n_1 + \sigma_2^2/n_2}$, where $m_1$, $m_2$ are the means, and $\sigma_1$ and $\sigma_2$ are the standard deviations of CBF in the normal and ischemic clusters, $n_1$ and $n_2$ are the number of normal voxels ischemic voxels, respectively. We hypothesized that our TS-SPD algorithm to produce larger distance $d$, that is, to more definitely differentiate between normal and ischemic tissues. Table 2 shows the distance between normal and abnormal clusters for the two cases in Fig. 3 and all subjects with CTP deficits. TS-SPD separates the two clusters with greatest distance. One-tail paired t-test yields $p = 0.051$ between cTSVD and KSVD-SPD, and $p = 0.015$ between KSVD-SPD and TS-SPD.

**Table 2.** Quantitative comparison of the normalized distance between ischemic and normal tissue clusters. The best performance of each column is in bold-face type. (Unit: mL/100g/min)

| Method | Stroke | SAH | All data |
|--------|--------|-------|----------|
| cTSVD | 42.71 | 46.03 | 49.91±5.12 |
| KSVD-SPD | 57.19 | 53.96 | 55.62±3.91 |
| TS-SPD | **63.25** | **56.64** | **59.60±3.82** |

## 4  Conclusion

In this paper, we have proposed a novel tissue-specific dictionary learning and deconvolution approach for CBF perfusion map enhancement in low-dose cerebral CTP.

We take advantage of the distinctive image information of each tissue category available in the high-dose CBF maps to recover the missing texture and structural information in the low-dose CBF maps. This is achieved by performing a spatio-temporal sparse deconvolution based on tissue-specific dictionaries learned from high-dose CBF map segmentation. Our method consistently outperforms the state-of-art methods, especially in GM and WM where the cerebrovascular disease diagnoses mostly rely. In the future, we will evaluate the feasibility of applying our method in clinical practice using CTP acquired at low radiation dose in patients with cerebrovascular disease.

# References

1. Miles, K.A., Griffiths, M.R.: Perfusion CT: a worthwhile enhancement? British Journal of Radiology 76(904), 220–231 (2003)
2. Wintermark, M., Lev, M.: Fda investigates the safety of brain perfusion CT. American Journal of Neuroradiology 31(1), 2–3 (2010)
3. Fang, R., Chen, T., Sanelli, P.C.: Sparsity-based deconvolution of low-dose perfusion CT using learned dictionaries. In: Ayache, N., Delingette, H., Golland, P., Mori, K. (eds.) MICCAI 2012, Part I. LNCS, vol. 7510, pp. 272–280. Springer, Heidelberg (2012)
4. Fang, R., Chen, T., Sanelli, P.C.: Towards robust deconvolution of low-dose perfusion CT: Sparse perfusion deconvolution using online dictionary learning. Medical Image Analysis (2013)
5. He, L., Orten, B., Do, S., Karl, W., Kambadakone, A., Sahani, D., Pien, H.: A spatio-temporal deconvolution method to improve perfusion CT quantification. IEEE Transactions on Medical Imaging 29(5), 1182–1191 (2010)
6. Calamante, F., Gadian, D., Connelly, A.: Quantification of bolus-tracking MRI: Improved characterization of the tissue residue function using Tikhonov regularization. Magnetic Resonance in Medicine 50(6), 1237–1247 (2003)
7. Yang, J., Wright, J., Huang, T., Ma, Y.: Image super-resolution as sparse representation of raw image patches. In: IEEE Conference on Computer Vision and Pattern Recognition, CVPR 2008, pp. 1–8. IEEE (2008)
8. Zhang, S., Zhan, Y., Metaxas, D.: Deformable segmentation via sparse representation and dictionary learning. Medical Image Analysis (2012)
9. Hoeffner, E., Case, I., Jain, R., Gujar, S., Shah, G., Deveikis, J., Carlos, R., Thompson, B., Harrigan, M., Mukherji, S.: Cerebral perfusion CT: Technique and clinical applications. Radiology 231(3), 632–644 (2004)
10. Van Leemput, K., Maes, F., Vandermeulen, D., Suetens, P.: Automated model-based tissue classification of MR images of the brain. IEEE Transactions on Medical Imaging 18(10), 897–908 (1999)
11. Mairal, J., Bach, F., Ponce, J., Sapiro, G.: Online dictionary learning for sparse coding. In: Proceedings of the 26th Annual International Conference on Machine Learning, pp. 689–696. ACM (2009)
12. Britten, A., Crotty, M., Kiremidjian, H., Grundy, A., Adam, E.: The addition of computer simulated noise to investigate radiation dose and image quality in images with spatial correlation of statistical noise: an example application to X-ray CT of the brain. British Journal of Radiology 77(916), 323–328 (2004)
13. Wittsack, H., Wohlschläger, A., Ritzl, E., Kleiser, R., Cohnen, M., Seitz, R., Mödder, U.: CT-perfusion imaging of the human brain: advanced deconvolution analysis using circulant singular value decomposition. Computerized Medical Imaging and Graphics 32(1), 67–77 (2008)

# Learning the Manifold of Quality Ultrasound Acquisition

Noha El-Zehiry[1], Michelle Yan[1], Sara Good[2], Tong Fang[1], S. Kevin Zhou[1], and Leo Grady[1,*]

[1] Siemens Corporation, Corporate Technology
[2] Siemens Healthcare

**Abstract.** Ultrasound acquisition is a challenging task that requires simultaneous adjustment of several acquisition parameters (the depth, the focus, the frequency and its operation mode). If the acquisition parameters are not properly chosen, the resulting image will have a poor quality and will degrade the patient diagnosis and treatment workflow. Several hardware-based systems for autotuning the acquisition parameters have been previously proposed, but these solutions were largely abandoned because they failed to properly account for tissue inhomogeneity and other patient-specific characteristics. Consequently, in routine practice the clinician either uses population-based parameter presets or manually adjusts the acquisition parameters for each patient during the scan. In this paper, we revisit the problem of autotuning the acquisition parameters by taking a completely novel approach and producing a solution based on image analytics. Our solution is inspired by the autofocus capability of conventional digital cameras, but is significantly more challenging because the number of acquisition parameters is large and the determination of "good quality" images is more difficult to assess. Surprisingly, we show that the set of acquisition parameters which produce images that are favored by clinicians comprise a 1D manifold, allowing for a real-time optimization to maximize image quality. We demonstrate our method for acquisition parameter autotuning on several live patients, showing that our system can start with a poor initial set of parameters and automatically optimize the parameters to produce high quality images.

## 1   Introduction

Ultrasound imaging requires the adjustment of multiple parameters, e.g. the depth, focus, the frequency and the frequency operation mode (general or Tissue Harmonics Imaging (THI)). The correct choice of parameters has a great impact on the quality of the output image and, in practice, the default parameters recommended by the manufacturer do not always produce a good quality image, The acquisition of a good quality image is a very challenging task especially for difficult patients who have large body habitus. In particular, an abdominal scan involves multiple organs at different depths, is strongly affected by body habitus and requires significant manual tuning (20-45 minutes on average). Previous efforts to

---

* Leo Grady is currently the VP of research and development at HeartFlow Inc.

K. Mori et al. (Eds.): MICCAI 2013, Part I, LNCS 8149, pp. 122–130, 2013.

produce a good quality image have focused on the hardware aspect of the acquisition by designing probes that have the potential to provide better images [1,2,3]. For example, a curvilinear probe enables larger tissue penetration at the expense of the anatomic image resolution, while a linear array probe provides fine details but can only scan superficial structures. Other hardware solutions include introducing new materials to the sensors used in the transducer [4] and adaptive beamforming with its variations [5,6,7] Image analysis approches focus on postprocessing to enhance the image after the acquisition is complete (e.g. [8]). Postprocessing methods transform the acquired data rather than improve the acquisition.

We revisit the problem of autotuning the acquisition parameters by presenting a novel software-only approach based on image analytics and inspired by the autofocus system in a conventional digital camera. However, tuning the acquisition parameters of an ultrasound device is significantly more challenging than conventional camera autofocus due to the larger number of parameters and the challenge in measuring the quality of an ultrasound image. In contrast, autofocus in a digital camera optimizes a simple measure of image sharpness over just one parameter (focal length). The key contribution of our work is to learn a low-dimensional manifold on which lie all acquisition parameters that result in sonographer preferred images. We then train a machine learning system to model the image quality assessment given be experts and show how to efficiently optimize the image quality over the low-dimensional manifold of sonographer preferred acquisition parameters.

## 2   Methods

Our method for automatic tuning the ultrasound acquisition parameters is inspired by the autofocus in a digital camera. The autofocus in digital cameras works by optimizing the focal length to obtain the image with the best contrast. In ultrasound acquisition, we aim at developing an *ultrasound autotuning* in a similar manner, except that ultrasound acquisition is significantly more challenging since it requires optimization of several parameters instead of just focal length. The second major challenge is that the quality of the ultrasound image, unlike the optical image captured with the autofocus of a conventional digital camera, cannot be simply assessed by measuring the contrast. In this section we present the formulation of the autotuning problem for ultrasound and we will keep the parallel analogy to the autofocus in digital cameras to enhance the exposition of our solution.

Let the configuration of ultrasound parameters consisting of the depth, focus, frequency and operation mode (THI or GEN) be denoted as $x$ and the image acquired with $x$ be denoted as $I(x)$. Assume that the quality of the image can be represented by a function $Q(I(x))$. The autotuning problem is described as

$$\max_x \ Q(I(x)). \tag{1}$$

In the autofocus for digital cameras, $x$ is simply the focal length and $Q(I(x))$ is the image contrast. In ultrasound autotuning, there are two challenges that we must address in the paper: First, the development of a quality measure $\mathcal{Q}(I(x))$ for the ultrasound image. Second, the solution of (1) , i.e., finding the optimal parameter configuration $x$ the provides an image $I(x)$ with the maximum quality.

## 2.1  Image Quality Assessment

The assessment of ultrasound image quality is a perceptual characteristic that is difficult to model with an explicit formula, since it depends on several factors such as brightness, sharpness, contrast, resolution, and whether the organ of interest is in focus or not. In the absence of an explicit formula for $\mathcal{Q}(I(x))$, we propose to sample a range of images $I(x)$ and learn the $\mathcal{Q}(I(x))$ mapping for perceptual quality. We train a Support Vector Machine (SVM) regressor based on a set of biologically-inspired features [9,10]. The feature extraction scheme uses a hierarchical approach that consists of four layers of computational units, building an increasingly complex and invariant feature representation by alternating between simple $S$ layers and complex $C$ layers. We have chosen this hierarchical model as it emulates the object recognition in the human visual cortex. The training images were collected from 9 different subjects and we tested on 4 different subjects that were never scanned in the training phase. The data set consists of abdominal scans of seven different organs for each subject: aorta, liver, right kidney, left kidney, pancreas, spleen and gall bladder. A total of 192 images were used in the training. A sonographer provided a grade for each image. The convention used for the grading as suggested by the expert clinician is as follows: Grades 1-6 are given to a poor quality image that cannot be used for diagnosis and treatment. Grades 7-8 are given to to minimally acceptable images Grades 9-10 are given to images for which no further improvement is possible. The variability between 9-10 reflects the variability in an expert's preference. For each input image, we used the feature extraction in [9] and calculated a total of 4075 features. We have performed a Sequential Minimum Optimization (SMO) regression with a normalized polynomial kernel and a reduced feature set that has 10 features.

## 2.2  Optimization

The second challenge in designing the *ultrasound autotuning* is the optimization of the image quality or choosing the parameter configuration that produces the best quality image. For digital cameras, a gradient search is sufficient to solve the problem because it is a 1D search for the optimal focal length and hence can be done efficiently. However, ultrasound autotuning is more challenging than autofocusing a digital camera because ultrasound autotuning requires optimization over several parameters. A naive solution  would be to do a grid search for the parameter configuration that optimizes the image quality. However, this is very computationally expensive and cannot be performed in real-time acquisition systems. A key insight of our paper is that the known relationship of the acquisition parameters can be exploited to perform a search over a lower-dimensional space of virtual parameters. As an example of this relationship between acquisition parameters, the physics of ultrasound dictates that a deeper focal depth should require a lower frequency. To perform a dimensionality reduction on our space of acquisition parameters, we employ manifold learning. Specifically, we applied manifold learning to determine if a lower dimensional manifold contains all configurations of acquisition parameters that produce large $\mathcal{Q}(I(X))$. Training data were collected from 9 different subjects. For each subject, 7 different organs were scanned. We obtained a total of 32 "good" configurations that produce images with grade 9 or 10 as judged by an expert. We applied *diffusion maps* manifold learning [11] on the 32 configurations to learn the intrinsic dimensionality of the acquisition parameters.

Although we suspected that the relationship between parameters would lead to a lower-dimensional manifold, we were surprised to find that **the manifold of configuration parameters leading to a good image is one-dimensional**, the manifold is depicted in Figure 1(a). This one-dimensional manifold of good parameters means that any good quality ultrasound image can be determined by optimizing a single virtual parameter. Consequently, we can perform the parameter optimization very quickly by projecting the input parameter configuration to the manifold of good parameter configurations (using k-nearest neighbors) and then optimizing the configuration parameter by a simple gradient ascent (relative to $\mathcal{Q}(I(X))$) along the manifold surface. The algorithm is shown in Algorithm 1.

## 3    Experimental Results

The objective of our experiments is two fold: First, to test the quality score produced by our system against the quality score assigned by an expert. Second,

---

**Input**: Default acquisition parameters  $x$ and the learned manifold pairs $(x, y)$. $y$ is
    the representation of $x$ on the learned 1D manifold
**Output**:  Parameter configuration that produces the best quality image

---

INITIALIZE $x_i$ to $x$ and calculate $\mathcal{Q}(I(x_i))$
**while** $\mathcal{Q}(I(x_i + 1)) > \mathcal{Q}(I(x_i))$ **do**

  1. Project the set of parameters $x_i$ to the lower dimensional manifold using an interpolation of the $k$NN with $k = 5$, to obtain lower dimensional configuration $y$.
  2. Find $y_m$ the closest point to $y$ on the manifold.
  3. Take a small step $t$ along the manifold  to obtain the new low-d parameters $y_{i+1}$.
  4. From the database of pairings $(x, y)$, obtain the back projection $x_{i+1}$ that corresponds to the adjusted low-d parameters $y_{i+1}$. $x_{i+1}$ is the new set of parameters in the original parameter space.
  5. Acquire a new image $I(x_{i+1})$ and calculate $\mathcal{Q}(I(x_{i+1}))$

**end**
**if** $\mathcal{Q}(I(x_{i+1})) < \mathcal{Q}(I(x_i))$ *and direction of movement has never been changed* **then**
 |  Change the movement direction and GOTO 1.
**else**
 |  Terminate
**end**

---

**Algorithm 1.** Steps for automated tuning of ultrasound acquisition

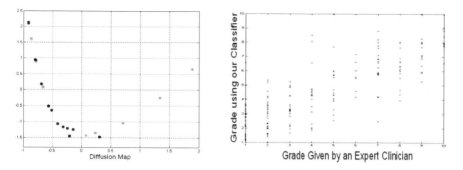

**Fig. 1.** Left: Manifold of parameters producing good images. Different colors indicate different organs. Right: Correlation between the expert's grade and our system.

to test, on live patients, whether our ultrasound autotuning system succeeds to provide a parameter configuration that produces a good quality image. Our experiments are performed using a Siemens S2000 Ultrasound scanner.

### 3.1 Quality Assessment Evaluation

For the testing of the quality assessment, we have used 280 images that were not used in training. Figure 1(b) depicts a scatter plot of the grades given by the expert clinician and the grades obtained by our system for the training data set. The correlation coefficient on the ratings was 0.82 and the average error on the training set was 1.3 (in units of 1-10 scale).

### 3.2 Live Ultrasound Acquisition with Our Autotuning System

We tested our autotuning system with a live ultrasound acquisition where the expert clinician starts with default preset parameters that usually yields bad/moderate image quality and our system generates the new set of parameters to acquire a second image. The clinician is asked to rate the output image and evaluate whether or not this image can be used in the clinic. If the expert clinician rates the image acquired with the new parameters as a bad image, we re-adjust the parameters based on a small step along the manifold shown in Figure 1 (a) and we repeat this process until a good quality image is reached or no further improvement can be made. We chose to run the testing on abdomen scans because each of the seven organs is scanned with a different set of parameters. Manually changing the parameters when moving from one organ to another is very tedious and requires 20-45 minutes per scan. Replacing the manual acquisition tuning with an automatic tuning would provide a great benefit to the workflow.

Figure 2 shows the detailed steps of one of our experiments. In this experiment, we aim at scanning the aorta. We started from the abdomen default set of parameters. The default parameters generated a poor quality image as judged by the expert (grade = 2). Our system applied Algorithm 1 to autotune the parameters until termination. In Figure 2 the top left corner of each image has

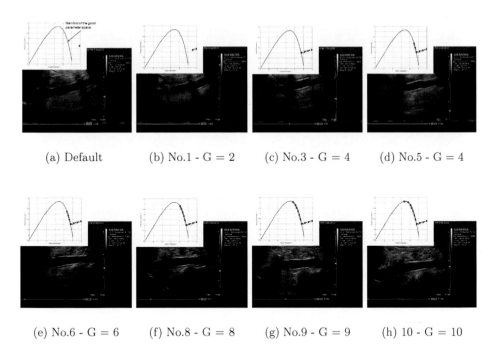

(a) Default          (b) No.1 - G = 2          (c) No.3 - G = 4          (d) No.5 - G = 4

(e) No.6 - G = 6          (f) No.8 - G = 8          (g) No.9 - G = 9          (h) 10 - G = 10

**Fig. 2.** Autotuning of the acquisition parameters for an aorta scan. The first image is acquired with the Siemens abdomen default preset (Frequency = THI/H 5MHz, depth = 16cm and focus = 10cm). The last image is acquired using the auto tuned parameters (Frequency = THI/ H 6MHz, depth =11cm and focus = 6cm).
Note: We are only showing 7 iterations out of 10 due to space limitation.

a schematic diagram that illustrates the idea of the parameter adjustment along the manifold, each red circle represents the projection of the acquisition parameters to the 1D manifold and the arrows represent the movement towards/along the manifold of the good parameter space depicted by the blue curve in the figure. The caption of each subfigure shows the iteration number and the grade (G) given by the expert.

Figure 3 shows a sample of our results for different subjects and different organs. The examples of this figure reveal different aspects of strength for our autotuning algorithm. These images are acquired from three different subjects with varying body mass indices (the subject in the first row has the lowest body mass index and the subject in the third row has the highest body mass index) which reflects that our algorithm works equally well for these challenging image acquisition scenarios. The first example in the figure tests whether the algorithm is capable of providing a good set of parameters if the starting set deviates from the manufacturer recommendation. The starting set of parameters were recommended by the clinician. The clinician's recommendation is generally based on the gender, race and body mass index of the patient. We have performed 5 acquisitions with a clinician's recommended parameter initializations and in all

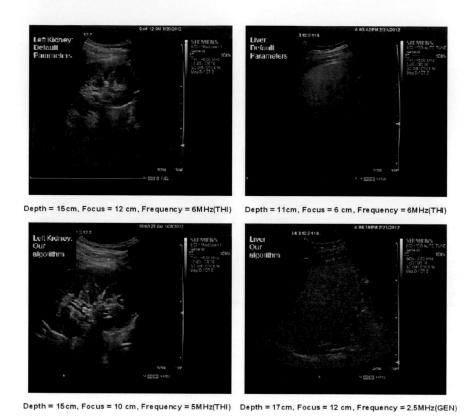

Depth = 15cm, Focus = 12 cm, Frequency = 6MHz(THI)    Depth = 11cm, Focus = 6 cm, Frequency = 6MHz(THI)

Depth = 15cm, Focus = 10 cm, Frequency = 5MHz(THI)    Depth = 17cm, Focus = 12 cm, Frequency = 2.5MHz(GEN)

**Fig. 3.** Sample results for the autotuning system. Row 1: Left kidney. Row 2: Liver.

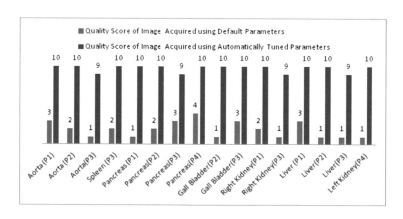

**Fig. 4.** Quantitative Assessment. Results for 16 different scans spanning four different patients and seven different organs.

cases our system autotunes the parameters to produce a good quality image as judged by the expert. The kidney image obtained by the autotuned parameters was graded 10 by the expert clinician. The example in the second row shows the scan of a fatty liver which is very challenging as it requires very deep penetration. The figure depicts that our algorithm was capable of producing the correct frequency, depth and focus for imaging.

Figure 4 shows a summary of the quantitative assessment of our algorithm. The testing scan were performed on four different patients (denoted as P1, P2, P3 and P4) that were not scanned in the training phase. Due to limited scanner time, we could not scan the seven organs for each subject, however, we managed to test 16 different scenarios. In all of our experiments, the algorithm provided a set of parameters that yielded a good quality image rated 9 or 10 by an expert. The summary is given by the bar chart depicted in Figure 4.

## 4   Conclusion and Future Work

In contrast to previous work on the topic of ultrasound acquisition autotuning which employed hardware solutions, we proposed a novel software-only solution that learns the manifold of the set of ultrasound acquisition parameters which produce high-quality images. Our experiments show the surprising fact that this set lies on a 1D manifold. We demonstrated the excellent performance of our system and its capability to produce a good quality image (100% accuracy) in live ultrasound acquisition experiments. Comparison to hardware-based solutions was not presented due to the lack of access to such hardware systems. The future work will focus on the improvement of the quality assessment performance to reach higher correlation between the expert clinician's grade and the grade obtained by our system. We also plan to run a large scale study that contains more data to validate our manifold.

## References

1. Smith, S., Goldberg, R.: Multilayer piezoelectric ceramics for two-dimensional transducers. IEEE Trans. on Ultrasonics, Ferroelectrics and Frequency Control (1994)
2. Mooney, M., Wilson, M.: Linear array transducers with improved image quality for vascular ultrasonic imaging. Hewlett-Packard Journal (1994)
3. Dhanaliwala, A.H., Hossack, J., Mauldin, W.: Assessing and improving acoustic radiation force image quality using a 1.5-d transducer design. IEEE Trans. Ultrasonics, Ferroelectrics and Frequency Control (2012)
4. Zhu, J.: A holey-structured metamaterial for acoustic deep-subwavelength imaging. Nature Physics (2010)
5. Asl, B.M.: Minimum variance beamforming combined with adaptive coherence weighting applied to medical ultrasound imaging. IEEE Trans. Ultrasonics, Ferroelectrics and Frequency Control (2009)
6. Xu, M., Chen, Y., Ding, M., Ming, Y.: Adaptive minimum variance beamforming combined with phase coherence imaging for ultrasound imaging. SPIE Medical Imaging (2012)

7. Nilsen, C.I., Hafizovic, I.: Beamspace adaptive beamforming for ultrasound imaging. IEEE Trans. Ultrasonics, Ferroelectrics and Frequency Control (2009)
8. Su, Y., Wang, H., Wang, Y., et al.: Speckle reduction approach for breast ultrasound image and its application to breast cancer diagnosis. European J. of Radiology (2010)
9. Serre, T., Wolf, L., Bileschi, S., Riesenhuber, M., Poggio, T.: Robust object recognition with cortex-like mechanisms. IEEE PAMI 29, 411–426 (2007)
10. Mutch, J., Lowe, D.G.: Object class recognition and localization using sparse features with limited receptive fields. IJCV 80(1), 45–57 (2008)
11. Coifman, R., Lafon, S.: Diffusion maps. Applied and Computational Harmonic Analysis 21, 5–30 (2006)

# Example-Based Restoration of High-Resolution Magnetic Resonance Image Acquisitions

Ender Konukoglu, Andre van der Kouwe, Mert Rory Sabuncu, and Bruce Fischl

Martinos Center for Biomedical Imaging, MGH, Harvard Medical School, USA

**Abstract.** Increasing scan resolution in magnetic resonance imaging is possible with advances in acquisition technology. The increase in resolution, however, comes at the expense of severe image noise. The current approach is to acquire multiple images and average them to restore the lost quality. This approach is expensive as it requires a large number of acquisitions to achieve quality comparable to lower resolution images. We propose an image restoration method for reducing the number of required acquisitions. The method leverages a high-quality lower-resolution image of the same subject and a database of pairs of high-quality low/high-resolution images acquired from different individuals. Experimental results show that the proposed method decreases noise levels and improves contrast differences between fine-scale structures, yielding high signal-to-noise ratio (SNR) and contrast-to-noise ratio (CNR). Comparisons with the current standard method of averaging approach and state-of-the-art non-local means denoising demonstrate the method's advantages.

## 1 Introduction

Resolution in medical imaging sets a fundamental limit on the scale of structures that can be visualized. Increasing resolution yields numerous benefits for both basic research and clinical applications. In magnetic resonance imaging (MRI), higher field strengths and array receive coils allow acquisition of increased resolution. This increase, however, comes at the expense of lower signal-to-noise ratio (SNR) and lower contrast-to-noise ratio (CNR). Scientists currently acquire multiple high-resolution (high-res) images of the same structure and average them to recover the SNR(CNR) lost by the increased resolution. This approach comes at an extremely steep price: doubling the resolution requires scanning 64 times as long to achieve comparable SNR for 3D encoded acquisitions. Obtaining high quality images with reduced scan time is a necessary step to make higher-resolution imaging feasible for clinical practice and available for a larger number of research studies. We believe that image restoration can provide a viable alternative to acquiring a large number of scans.

Restoration (denoising) is an active field of research in both computer vision and MRI literature. The most popular approaches that have been applied to MRI are based on Gaussian filtering[1], wavelet decompositions[14], anisotropic diffusion[9,11], non-parametric estimation[2] and non-local means[8,3,5,13]. While these are successful in denoising MRI, they do not take into account the specific aspects of high-res acquisition. As a result, although they are able

K. Mori et al. (Eds.): MICCAI 2013, Part I, LNCS 8149, pp. 131–138, 2013.

to increase the SNR, they are not effective in restoring the contrast between fine-scale anatomical details in the presence of severe noise.

High-res acquisitions in MRI are particularly difficult for restoration. The noise levels often severely distort the appearance of fine-scale structures, whose restoration based only on a small number of acquisitions is challenging (see Fig.1). Conversely, problem specific aspects related to high-res acquisition can help restoration. First, high-quality low-resolution (low-res) images (e.g. 1 $mm^3$) can be acquired rapidly. These provide coarse level prior information for restoration. However, low-res does not provide enough information for restoring fine scale structures. Second, similarity of anatomy across individuals can complement the short-comings of low-res acquisitions as prior information. Previously acquired high-quality low/high-res image pairs of different subjects provide empirical prior that can help link different resolutions and guide restoration.

This article presents a restoration method that aims to reduce the number of acquisitions required to obtain a high-quality high-res MRI. It integrates low-res acquisition and a training database of pairs of high-quality low/high-res images in a probabilistic formulation. This method shares similarities with dictionary-based methods for denoising, such as [7,12]. However, the proposed method does not learn a dictionary to integrate the database into the restoration. Instead, it builds on a patch-based synthesis framework, which has been successfully used in super-resolution [15], image analogies [10] and synthesis [16]. Experimental results on five subjects demonstrate the capabilities of the method for achieving noise levels that would normally require more acquisitions. The proposed method improves SNR and CNR, revealing fine-scale structures. Comparisons with the state-of-the-art non-local means denoising algorithm illustrate the advantages of the proposed method for restoring high-res MRI.

## 2    Restoration Method

We model an MRI image, $I$, as a mapping from space to intensity values, i.e., $I : \Omega \to \mathbb{R}$, where $\Omega \subset \mathbb{N}^3$ is a discrete domain. A high-res MRI acquisition, $\tilde{H}_m$, is a noisy version of an ideal noise-free high-res image $H$. The current approach for restoring $H$ from a set $\{\tilde{H}_m\}_{m=1}^M$ is the point-wise averaging $\mathbf{x} \in \Omega$: $\hat{H}(\mathbf{x}) = \sum_m \tilde{H}_m(\mathbf{x})/M$, which requires $M$ to be as high as 7 or 8 to overcome the severe noise levels, for e.g. 0.5 $mm$ resolution. Following, we present a restoration method that aims to reduce the required $M$.

**Probabilistic Model:** The inputs of the proposed method are: i) the high-res acquisitions, $\{\tilde{H}_m\}_{m=1}^M$; ii) the corresponding high-SNR low-res image, $L$, registered and up-sampled with tri-linear interpolation to the same grid as $\tilde{H}_m$'s; and iii) a *training* database of coupled high-SNR low/high-res images $\{(L_q, H_q)\}_{q=1}^Q$, previously acquired, from different subjects. The goal of the algorithm is to estimate the high-SNR high-res image $H$, denoted by $\hat{H}$.

The proposed method works on image patches. A patch of size $d \in \mathbb{N}$ in an image $I$ at location $\mathbf{x}$ is the set of intensities over the neighborhood voxels, i.e., $I^d(\mathbf{x}) \triangleq \{I(\mathbf{y}) : \mathbf{y} \in W^d(\mathbf{x})\}$, where $W^d(\mathbf{x}) \triangleq \{\mathbf{y} : \|\mathbf{x} - \mathbf{y}\|_\infty \leq d\}$ is the neighborhood of $\mathbf{x}$. For instance, $W^1(\mathbf{x})$ is the set that includes $\mathbf{x}$ and its 26 immediate neighbors, and $I^1(\mathbf{x})$ are the set of intensities within $W^1(\mathbf{x})$.

We estimate each patch in $\hat{H}$ by maximizing the posterior probability:

$$
\hat{H}^d(\mathbf{x}) = \underset{H^d(\mathbf{x})}{\operatorname{argmax}}\, p(H^d(\mathbf{x})|L^d(\mathbf{x}), \{\tilde{H}^d_m(\mathbf{x})\}) = \underset{H^d(\mathbf{x})}{\operatorname{argmax}}\, p(H^d(\mathbf{x}), L^d(\mathbf{x}), \{\tilde{H}^d_m(\mathbf{x})\})
$$

$$
= \underset{H^d(\mathbf{x})}{\operatorname{argmax}}\, p(L^d(\mathbf{x}), H^d(\mathbf{x})) \prod_m p(\tilde{H}^d_m(\mathbf{x})|H^d(\mathbf{x})\}) \tag{1}
$$

To reach (1), we assumed (i) $p(\tilde{H}^d_m(\mathbf{x})|H^d(\mathbf{x}), L^d(\mathbf{x})\}) = p(\tilde{H}^d_m(\mathbf{x})|H^d(\mathbf{x})\})$, i.e., in the presence of $H$, image $L$ provides no additional information about each $H_m$; and (ii) $p(\{\tilde{H}^d_m(\mathbf{x})\}|H^d(\mathbf{x})\}) = \prod_m p(\tilde{H}^d_m(\mathbf{x})|H^d(\mathbf{x})\})$, i.e., each low-SNR image $H_m$ is conditionally independent given $H$.

We further assume the following Gaussian noise model: $p(\tilde{H}^d_m(\mathbf{x})|H^d(\mathbf{x})\}) = \mathcal{N}\left(H^d(\mathbf{x}), \sigma_n \mathbf{I}\right)$, where $\mathcal{N}(\cdot, \cdot)$ represents the normal distribution and $\mathbf{I}$ is the identity matrix. The reasons for this choice are two-folds. First, empirically we observed that the noise distribution for each high-res acquisition can be well approximated with a Gaussian (see Fig. 1). Second, point-wise averaging is the solution of the model that ignores $p\left(L^d(\mathbf{x}), H^d(\mathbf{x})\right)$ in Equation 1. This second point links the proposed method to the current practice.

The key component of the proposed method is $p(L^d(\mathbf{x}), H^d(\mathbf{x}))$. There are multiple ways of defining this term. One could, for example, use a parametric form that models subsampling. Without anatomically informed priors, however, this approach would fail to model structures that are only visible at high-res. As a result, unless these structures are prominent in the noisy acquisitions, they cannot be restored. For brain MRI, an alternative approach is to leverage the anatomical similarities between individuals by using available training datasets. Here, we take this approach and use the training database $\{(L_q, H_q)\}_{q=1}^{Q}$ to estimate the joint distribution $p(L^d(\mathbf{x}), H^d(\mathbf{x}))$ using a non-parametric model:

$$
p\left(L^d(\mathbf{x}), H^d(\mathbf{x})\right) = \frac{1}{Q|W^D(\mathbf{x})|} \sum_{q=1}^{Q} \sum_{y \in W^D(\mathbf{x})} \mathbf{K}_{\Sigma}\left(L^d(\mathbf{x}), L^d_q(\mathbf{y})\right) \mathbf{K}_{\Sigma}\left(H^d(\mathbf{x}), H^d_q(\mathbf{y})\right) \tag{2}
$$

where $W^D(\mathbf{x})$ is the $D$-neighborhood of $\mathbf{x}$, $|\cdot|$ denotes set cardinality, $\mathbf{K}_{\Sigma}(I, J) = \exp\left\{-\frac{1}{2}(I - J)^T \Sigma^{-1}(I - J)\right\}/\sqrt{2\pi\det(\Sigma)}$, $\Sigma(\mathbf{x}_1, \mathbf{x}_2) = \sigma^2 \exp\left\{-\|\mathbf{x}_1 - \mathbf{x}_2\|_2^2/\alpha^2\right\}$ and $\det(\cdot)$ is the matrix determinant. $\Sigma$ models the spatial correlation in the residuals and has two global parameters, $\sigma$ and $\alpha$. More refined parameterizations can also be used, for example by assigning locally varying parameters. In that case, however, the estimation of the parameters becomes more challenging. In Eq. 2, the summation over the voxel index $\mathbf{y}$ allows us to consider patches at voxels other than $\mathbf{x}$. This enriches the training data used for voxel $\mathbf{x}$ and models misalignments between the subjects.

**Optimization:** To solve Eq. 1 with the definition of Eq. 2, one can use numerical methods such as Expectation Maximization. This, however, becomes computationally intractable because a separate iterative optimization needs to be run at each voxel $\mathbf{x}$, and the summation over all training patches can be expensive when the training dataset is large (e.g. when $D$ is large). As a first order approximation we propose to use

$$p\left(L^d(\mathbf{x}), H^d(\mathbf{x})\right) \approx \max_{q,\mathbf{y} \in W^D(\mathbf{x})} \mathbf{K}_{\Sigma}\left(L^d(\mathbf{x}), L_q^d(\mathbf{y})\right) \mathbf{K}_{\Sigma}\left(H^d(\mathbf{x}), H_q^d(\mathbf{y})\right). \quad (3)$$

This type of approximation can be justified when the dimensionality of the problem is high and the training samples are sparse. In Eq. 3, in the same spirit as k-means clustering, the new image is associated with the closest training patch and the probability value is computed solely based on this association. The main advantage of adopting Eq. 3 is that it converts the problem given in Eq. 1 to

$$\operatorname*{argmax}_{H^d(\mathbf{x})} \left\{ \max_{q,\mathbf{y} \in W^D(\mathbf{x})} \mathbf{K}_{\Sigma}\left(L^d(\mathbf{x}), L_q^d(\mathbf{y})\right) \mathbf{K}_{\Sigma}\left(H^d(\mathbf{x}), H_q^d(\mathbf{y})\right) \prod_m p(\tilde{H}_m^d(\mathbf{x}) | H^d(\mathbf{x}))\right\},$$
$$(4)$$

which can be solved efficiently. We observe that for a fixed $q$ and $\mathbf{y}$, the outer optimization of Eq. 4 yields a closed-form solution:

$$\hat{H}_{q,\mathbf{y}}^d(\mathbf{x}) = \left(\frac{M}{\sigma_n^2}\mathbf{I} + \Sigma^{-1}\right)^{-1} \left(\frac{1}{\sigma_n^2}\mathbf{I}\sum_{m=1}^M \tilde{H}_m^d(\mathbf{x}) + \Sigma^{-1}H_q^d(\mathbf{y})\right). \quad (5)$$

This reduces the problem in Eq. 4 to solving:

$$\operatorname*{argmax}_{q,\mathbf{y}} \mathbf{K}_{\Sigma}\left(L^d(\mathbf{x}), L_q^d(\mathbf{y})\right) \mathbf{K}_{\Sigma}\left(\hat{H}_{q,y}^d(\mathbf{x}), H_q^d(\mathbf{y})\right) \prod_m p\left(\tilde{H}_m^d(\mathbf{x}) | \hat{H}_{q,\mathbf{y}}^d(\mathbf{x})\right).$$

Combining the last two terms and Eq. 5, we can rewrite this as:

$$q^*, \mathbf{y}^* = \operatorname*{argmax}_{q,\mathbf{y}} \mathbf{K}_{\Sigma}\left(L^d(\mathbf{x}), L_q^d(\mathbf{y})\right) \mathbf{K}_{\Sigma+\mathbf{I}\sigma_n^2/M}\left(\frac{1}{M}\sum_m^M H_m^d(\mathbf{x}), H_q^d(\mathbf{y})\right) \quad (6)$$

and the final estimate is given as $\hat{H}^d(\mathbf{x}) = \hat{H}_{q^*,\mathbf{y}^*}^d(\mathbf{x})$.

Equation 6 can be solved using the powerful patch-matching procedure borrowing ideas from patch-based segmentation systems [6]. Following the brain-specific strategy as given in [6] we linearly align the new subject data $L$, $\{\tilde{H}_m\}$ with each training subject $\{(L_q, H_q)\}$ via affine registration, and perform exhaustive search over a restricted spatial neighborhood, $W^D(\mathbf{x})$. The cost of searching over $W^D(\mathbf{x})$ can be reduced by employing a multi-resolution grid pyramid.

The presented method restores $\hat{H}^d(\mathbf{x})$ for each $\mathbf{x}$ independently. $\hat{H}^d(\mathbf{x})$ contains the intensity estimates for $\mathbf{x}$ and all its neighbors in $W^d(\mathbf{x})$. We compute the final estimate $\hat{H}(\mathbf{x})$ by averaging the estimates from all the patches containing $\mathbf{x}$. The interactions between neighboring voxels could alternatively be modeled as a prior distribution over $H$. This, however, would remove the possibility of solving each $H^d(\mathbf{x})$ independently, which enables parallelization.

**Variation on the Model:** A variation of the presented model is to remove the dependence on $L^d(\mathbf{x})$ and only model $p(H^d(\mathbf{x}), \{\tilde{H}_m^d(\mathbf{x})\})$. This case corresponds to only using the high-res acquisitions and the high-res images in the database to restore $H$. In this case, most of the derivations follow suit and the restoration process reduces to solving $q^*, \mathbf{y}^* = \text{argmax}_{q,\mathbf{y}} \, \mathbf{K}_{\boldsymbol{\Sigma}+\mathbf{I}\sigma_n^2/M} \left( \frac{1}{M} \sum_m^M H_m^d(\mathbf{x}), H_q^d(\mathbf{y}) \right)$, where the restored image patch is computed as $\hat{H}^d(\mathbf{x}) = \hat{H}_{q^*,\mathbf{y}^*}^d(\mathbf{x})$.

**Setting the Parameters:** The probabilistic model has five free parameters, $\sigma_n$, $\sigma$, $\alpha$, $d$ and $D$. The first three we set using heuristic strategies. We first assume the noise variance $\sigma_n$ is constant across subjects, i.e., the noise properties remain similar across images. Thus we can directly estimate $\sigma_n$ on the training dataset, where each $H_q$ is associated with multiple low-quality acquisitions $\{\tilde{H}_{q,m}\}$. We estimate $\sigma_n$ as the square root of the mean square difference between $H_q$ and $\{\tilde{H}_{q,m}\}$ on the training dataset. $\sigma$ and $\alpha$ values define the influence domain of each kernel in the non-parametric distribution in Eq. 2. For a given subject, we estimate these parameters based on the high-SNR low-res images $L^d(\mathbf{x})$ and $\{L_q^d(\mathbf{x})\}$. We first compute the following empirical covariance matrix $S = \frac{1}{N} \sum_{\mathbf{x}_n} \left( L^d(\mathbf{x}_n) - L_{q_n^*}^d(\mathbf{y}_n^*) \right) \left( L^d(\mathbf{x}_n) - L_{q_n^*}^d(\mathbf{y}_n^*) \right)^T$, where $(q_n^*, \mathbf{y}_n^*) = \text{argmax}_{q,\mathbf{y}} \left\| L^d(\mathbf{x}) - L_q^d(\mathbf{y}) \right\|_2$, using $N$ randomly selected voxels $\mathbf{x}_n \in \Omega$. We then determine $\sigma$ and $\alpha$ by minimizing the square difference between $\boldsymbol{\Sigma}(\cdot, \cdot)$ and the sample covariance $S$. $d$ and $D$ are set empirically.

## 3   Experiments

We tested the proposed restoration method on a dataset of five subjects. For each subject, seven high-res T1w images at a resolution of $(500\mu m)^3$ and one low-res T1w image at the resolution of $1 \ mm^3$ were acquired on a 3T Siemens Trio scanner with a 3D encoded MPRAGE using a 32-channel receive coil. The protocol took 7 minutes to acquire each high-res image and 3.5 minutes to acquire the low-res images. Fig. 1-(a-c) show, for a subject, the low-res image, a high-res acquisition and the average high-res image, respectively. Fig. 1-d plots the histogram of the difference between each high-res acquisition shown in (c) and the average of seven shown in (b), "the noise distribution", along with the best fitting Gaussian distribution in red.

We performed leave-one-out experiments, where for each test case the images of the remaining subjects were used to construct the corresponding training database. We used two different ways to construct the training database high-res images: i) by averaging the seven high-res acqusitions (set1) and ii) by first averaging then denoising the average image by the non-local means (NLM) algorithm as proposed in [5] (set2). For each test case, we performed seven restorations, where for each restoration we assumed a different number, $M$, of high-res low-SNR scans. The restoration quality is quantified using two measures, SNR and CNR, which are computed based on the claustrum: a fine scale structure that is only visible in the high-res. Two regions-of-interests were drawn on the

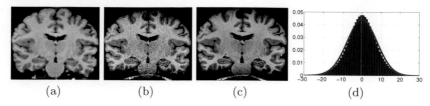

(a)                    (b)                    (c)                    (d)

**Fig. 1.** (a) T1w image at 1 $mm^3$ resolution (b) T1w image at $(500\ \mu m)^3$ acquisition (c) Average of seven $(500\ \mu m)^3$ images (d) Histogram of the difference between (b) and (c), and overlayed is the best fit Gaussian distribution to the histogram

average of seven high-res acquisitions, one within the claustrum and another within the external capsule, which borders the claustrum (see Fig. 3-a). SNR was computed as the ratio of the average intensity value to the standard deviation within the claustrum ROI. CNR was computed as the absolute difference of mean intensities of the two ROIs divided by the combined standard deviation.

We tested three variants of the proposed model: (i) "model HL" uses both $L$ and $\tilde{H}_m$ for the test images and set1 type training database, (ii) "model H" uses only $\tilde{H}_m$ and set1 type database, and (iii) "model HLD" uses both $L$ and $\tilde{H}_m$ and set2 type database. We used a patch size of $d = 1$ and ran patch-matching in a multi-resolution pyramid of three levels at resolutions $(2\ mm)^3$, $1\ mm^3$ and $(500\ \mu m)^3$ with a search neighborhood of $D = 8\ mm, 4\ mm, 2\ mm$, respectively. We compared the restoration quality of the proposed method with four benchmark methods: (i) the point-wise averaging, (ii) block-wise NLM [5] (NLMBO), (iii) oracle-based DCT filter [13] (ODCT) and (iv) pre-filtered rotationally invariant NLM [13] (PRINLM) all applied to the point-wise averaging result[1] The noise level estimations for the latter three methods were performed using the method proposed in [4] and all the parameters were set as suggested in [13].

Fig. 2 plots the results with respect to $M$ (and acquisition times corresponding to each $M$ in paranthesis). The bars correspond to average values obtained over five test cases and the errorbars are the standard errors. In terms of SNR, model HLD achieved the highest values for all $M$. The highest CNR values were obtained by HLD for $M < 4$ and NLMBO for $M \geq 3$. The high CNR and SNR values achieved by the models HL and HLD demonstrate that the proposed approach can drastically reduce noise and improve contrast simultaneously. The differences between models H and HL show that the integration of the low-res image is advantageous. Considering acquisition times, the proposed methods, in particular model HLD, provides substantial benefits for low $M$.

Fig. 3 displays visual results from two subjects: (a) slices of high-res images and the ROIs (blue = claustrum, red = external capsule) and (b) restoration results of NLMBO, HL and HLD for $M = 1, 3$. These images demonstrate that depending on the noise level NLM might not be enough. The proposed models HL and HLD are able restore the image even in high noise levels. e.g. $M = 1$.

---

[1] The implementations for (ii-iv) are from
http://personales.upv.es/jmanjon/denoising/prinlm.html

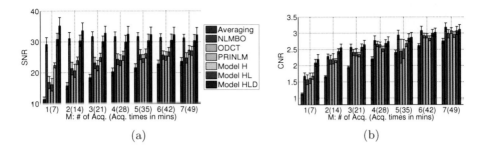

(a)                                                              (b)

**Fig. 2.** Quantitative restoration results vs. number of acquisitions and acquisition times in minutes: (a) SNR at the ROI drawn on the claustrum, see Fig. 3, (b) CNR computed between the claustrum and the external capsule. The bars are mean statistics over 5 subjects and errorbars are standard errors.

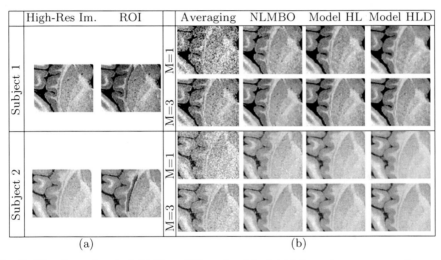

**Fig. 3.** Visual results: (a-left) Two different subjects' high-res images zoomed around the claustrum (left). (a-right) ROIs (blue = claustrum, red = external capsule). (b) Restored images: (left to right) averaging, NLMBO and the proposed models.

## 4    Conclusions

In this work we proposed a restoration method for improving the quality of high-res MRI acquisitions. Our experiments demonstrate that the method is able to reduce the severe noise levels and improve the contrast between neighboring fine-scale structures. The method achieves this by leveraging low-res images and a training database, which provides an empirical prior on the appearance of structures at different resolutions. The preliminary results are promising and suggest the possibility of reducing the number of acquisitions needed to obtain high-quality high-res MRI at higher-field strengths.

**Acknowledgements.** Support for this research was provided in part by the NIH (P41-RR14075, U24RR021382, R01EB006758, AG022381, 5R01AG008122-22, RC1AT005728-01, R01NS052585-01, 1R21NS072652-01, 1R01NS070963, 1S10RR023401, 1S10RR019307, 1S10RR023043, R21MH096559, R01HD071664, R33DA026104, 1K25EB013649-01), BrightFocus Alzheimer's pilot grant (AHAF-A2012333), The Autism & Dyslexia Project funded by the Ellison Medical Foundation, and by the NIH Blueprint for Neuroscience Research (5U01-MH093765), part of the multi-institutional Human Connectome Project. BF has a financial interest in CorticoMetrics, which are reviewed by MGH and Partner's HealthCare.

# References

1. Ashburner, J., Friston, K.J.: Voxel-based morphometry the methods. Neuroimage 11(6), 805–821 (2000)
2. Awate, S.P., Whitaker, R.T.: Feature-preserving mri denoising: A nonparametric empirical bayes approach. IEEE TMI 26(9), 1242–1255 (2007)
3. Buades, A., Coll, B., Morel, J.M.: A non-local algorithm for image denoising. In: CVPR, vol. 2, pp. 60–65. IEEE (2005)
4. Coupé, P., Manjón, J.V., Gedamu, E., Arnold, D.L., Robles, M., Collins, D.L., et al.: Robust rician noise estimation for mr images. Med. Image Anal. 14(4), 483–493 (2010)
5. Coupé, P., et al.: An optimized blockwise nonlocal means denoising filter for 3-d magnetic resonance images. IEEE TMI 27(4), 425–441 (2008)
6. Coupé, P., et al.: Patch-based segmentation using expert priors: Application to hippocampus and ventricle segmentation. Neuroimage 54(2), 940–954 (2011)
7. Elad, M., Aharon, M.: Image denoising via sparse and redundant representations over learned dictionaries. IEEE TIP 15(12), 3736–3745 (2006)
8. Fischl, B., Schwartz, E.L.: Adaptive nonlocal filtering: a fast alternative to anisotropic diffusion for image enhancement. IEEE TPAMI 21(1), 42–48 (1999)
9. Gerig, G., Kubler, O., Kikinis, R., Jolesz, F.A.: Nonlinear anisotropic filtering of mri data. IEEE TMI 11(2), 221–232 (1992)
10. Hertzmann, A., Jacobs, C.E., Oliver, N., Curless, B., Salesin, D.H.: Image analogies. In: SIGGRAPH, pp. 327–340. ACM (2001)
11. Krissian, K., Aja-Fernández, S.: Noise-driven anisotropic diffusion filtering of mri. IEEE TIP 18(10), 2265–2274 (2009)
12. Mairal, J., Bach, F., Ponce, J., Sapiro, G., Zisserman, A.: Non-local sparse models for image restoration. In: CVPR, pp. 2272–2279. IEEE (2009)
13. Manjón, J.V., Coupé, P., Buades, A., Louis Collins, D., Robles, M.: New methods for mri denoising based on sparseness and self-similarity. Med. Image Anal. 16, 18–27 (2012)
14. Pizurica, A., Philips, W., Lemahieu, I., Acheroy, M.: A versatile wavelet domain noise filtration technique for medical imaging. IEEE TMI 22(3), 323–331 (2003)
15. Rousseau, F.: Brain hallucination. In: Forsyth, D., Torr, P., Zisserman, A. (eds.) ECCV 2008, Part I. LNCS, vol. 5302, pp. 497–508. Springer, Heidelberg (2008)
16. Roy, S., Carass, A., Prince, J.: A compressed sensing approach for mr tissue contrast synthesis. In: Székely, G., Hahn, H.K. (eds.) IPMI 2011. LNCS, vol. 6801, pp. 371–383. Springer, Heidelberg (2011)

# ToF Meets RGB: Novel Multi-Sensor Super-Resolution for Hybrid 3-D Endoscopy

Thomas Köhler[1,2], Sven Haase[1], Sebastian Bauer[1], Jakob Wasza[1],
Thomas Kilgus[3], Lena Maier-Hein[3], Hubertus Feußner[4],
and Joachim Hornegger[1,2]

[1] Pattern Recognition Lab, Friedrich-Alexander-Universität Erlangen-Nürnberg
[2] Erlangen Graduate School in Advanced Optical Technologies (SAOT)
{thomas.koehler,sven.haase}@fau.de
[3] Div. Medical and Biological Informatics Junior Group: Computer-Assisted
Interventions, German Cancer Research Center (DKFZ) Heidelberg
[4] Minimally Invasive Therapy and Intervention, Technical University of Munich

**Abstract.** 3-D endoscopy is an evolving field of research with the intention to improve safety and efficiency of minimally invasive surgeries. *Time-of-Flight* (ToF) imaging allows to acquire range data in real-time and has been engineered into a 3-D endoscope in combination with an RGB sensor ($640 \times 480$ px) as a hybrid imaging system, recently. However, the ToF sensor suffers from a low spatial resolution ($64 \times 48$ px) and a poor signal-to-noise ratio. In this paper, we propose a novel multi-frame super-resolution framework to improve range images in a ToF/RGB multi-sensor setup. Our approach exploits high-resolution RGB data to estimate subpixel motion used as a cue for range super-resolution. The underlying non-parametric motion model based on optical flow makes the method applicable to endoscopic scenes with arbitrary endoscope movements. The proposed method was evaluated on synthetic and real images. Our approach improves the peak-signal-to-noise ratio by 1.6 dB and structural similarity by 0.02 compared to single-sensor super-resolution.

## 1 Introduction

In minimally invasive procedures, reconstructing 3-D surfaces offers opportunities for new applications in addition to conventional 2-D endoscopes. This includes collision detection or augmented reality by registration with preoperative planning data [1]. In terms of hardware, during the past years, three technological directions for 3-D endoscopy emerged. (i) Stereoscopy [2] is a passive technique to acquire surface data. The drawback of stereo vision is the computationally demanding correspondence search and the unreliable results in texture-less regions. (ii) Structured light [3] is established as active acquisition technique. Therefore, the device requires the light source and a sensor for data acquisition placed at a certain distance to observe the situs from different perspectives, which is difficult to accomplish in one single endoscope. (iii) Recently, *Time-of-Flight* (ToF) technology was proposed for 3-D endoscopy to obtain range data in real-time (30 Hz) [4]. In a hybrid 3-D endoscope, the ToF sensor is augmented with an RGB camera to acquire range data fused with complementary color images [5].

K. Mori et al. (Eds.): MICCAI 2013, Part I, LNCS 8149, pp. 139–146, 2013.

Sensor fusion provides the surgeon a comprehensive view of a scene and is beneficial for image analysis [6]. However, today's ToF sensors suffer from a low spatial resolution and a poor signal-to-noise ratio (SNR) compared to color cameras. Thus, improvement of range data is essential to obtain reliable surface information.

Multi-frame super-resolution methods recover a high-resolution (HR) image from multiple low-resolution (LR) frames with known subpixel displacements [7]. Compared to single image upsampling, such techniques also increase the SNR and preserve edges essential for noisy range data. Recently, super-resolution were applied in 2-D endoscopy [8]. Approaches for color images were also adopted to ToF imaging [9]. An application independent challenge is accurate estimation of subpixel displacements having high impact to super-resolution quality [10]. In literature, several robust methods were proposed [11,12]. Here, super-resolution and motion estimation are formulated as joint optimization which is computationally demanding [12] or restricted to simplified motion models such as rigid motion [11] being an invalid assumption for the considered application.

In this paper, we propose a novel super-resolution framework for range data in a multi-sensor setup. Movements of the endoscope held by the surgeon are used as a cue for super-resolution. Our approach is based on sensor fusion of complementary RGB and range data, which is to the best of our knowledge not considered for multi-frame super-resolution yet. Motion is estimated by computing optical flow on RGB data to obtain accurate displacements for range images. This novelty of our method enables robust motion estimation without computationally demanding joint optimization whereas optical flow avoids restrictions of simplified models essential for realistic laparoscopic scenes. To the best of our knowledge, this is also the first application of super-resolution in 3-D endoscopy.

## 2 Methods

We address the problem of upsampling $K$ LR range images of resolution $M_1 \times M_2$ denoted as $\boldsymbol{Y}^{(1)} \ldots \boldsymbol{Y}^{(K)}$ and defined on domain $\Omega_r$. For convenience, we denote $\boldsymbol{Y}^{(k)}$ as vector $\boldsymbol{y}^{(k)} \in \mathbb{R}^M$ with $M = M_1 \cdot M_2$ by concatenating all pixels. For each $\boldsymbol{y}^{(k)}$ there exists a $L_1 \times L_2$ color image $\boldsymbol{C}^{(k)} \equiv \boldsymbol{c}^{(k)}$ defined on domain $\Omega_c$ captured simultaneously. Each $\boldsymbol{y}^{(k)}$ and $\boldsymbol{c}^{(k)}$ is related to a reference frame $\boldsymbol{y}^{(r)}$ and $\boldsymbol{c}^{(r)}$ by a geometric transformation modeling 3-D displacements.

Our aim is to determine an HR range image $\mathbf{x} \in \mathbb{R}^N$, $N = s^2 \cdot M$ from $K$ LR frames for the magnification factor $s \in \mathbb{R}$. First, we present sensor data fusion of range and RGB images as key idea in our framework. For super-resolution, an established maximum a-posteriori (MAP) estimation scheme is employed [7]. Finally, multi-sensor super-resolution is proposed based on the MAP approach and sensor data fusion for guidance in robust motion estimation.

### 2.1 Sensor Data Fusion

In hybrid ToF/RGB endoscopy, the incoming light is decomposed by a beam splitter in two components: near-infrared light for the ToF sensor and the residual for the RGB sensor (see Fig. 1). Fusion of both modalities can be tackled by

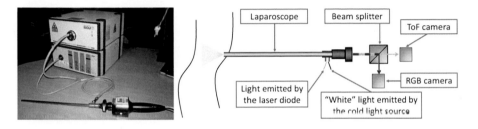

**Fig. 1.** 3-D endoscope to acquire range and RGB data simultaneously

stereo calibration [5] in general. In our work, we exploit the fact that a beam splitter is used and employ a homographic mapping. For a pair $(\tilde{\boldsymbol{u}}_r, \tilde{\boldsymbol{u}}_c)$ of corresponding range and RGB points in homogeneous coordinates, our mapping is given by $\tilde{\boldsymbol{u}}_c \cong \boldsymbol{H}_{cr}\tilde{\boldsymbol{u}}_r$. The homography $\boldsymbol{H}_{cr} \in \mathbb{R}^{3\times3}$ describes pixel-wise alignment and is estimated using a checkerboard calibration pattern with self-encoded markers and least-square estimation as proposed in [5]. Sensor fusion is performed by transforming each $\boldsymbol{c}^{(k)}$ into the coordinate system of $\boldsymbol{y}^{(k)}$.

### 2.2   Maximum A-posteriori Framework

The basic MAP framework [7] is based on a generative image model for mathematical modeling of image acquisition. Super-resolution is implemented by energy minimization based on this model to recover an HR image.

**Generative Image Model.** The generative image model states the relation between each LR frame $\boldsymbol{y}^{(k)}$ and the HR image $\boldsymbol{x}$ to be recovered according to:

$$\boldsymbol{y}^{(k)} = \gamma_m^{(k)}\boldsymbol{W}^{(k)}\boldsymbol{x} + \gamma_a^{(k)}\mathbf{1} + \boldsymbol{\epsilon}^{(k)}. \tag{1}$$

The system matrix $\boldsymbol{W}^{(k)}$ models geometric displacements between $\boldsymbol{x}$ and $\boldsymbol{y}^{(k)}$ as well as blur induced by the camera point spread function (PSF) and downsampling. To take out-of-plane movements and thus diverse range values in successive frames into account, we introduce $\gamma_m^{(k)}$ and $\gamma_a^{(k)}$, where $\mathbf{1} \in \mathbb{R}^M$ denotes the all-one vector. Spatially invariant noise is modeled by $\boldsymbol{\epsilon}^{(k)} \in \mathbb{R}^M$. For a space invariant Gaussian PSF of width $\sigma$, the matrix elements are obtained by:

$$W_{mn} = \exp\left(-||\boldsymbol{v}_n - \boldsymbol{u}'_m||_2^2 \,/\, 2\sigma^2\right), \tag{2}$$

where $\boldsymbol{v}_n \in \mathbb{R}^2$ are the coordinates of the $n^{th}$ pixel in $\boldsymbol{x}$ and $\boldsymbol{u}'_m \in \mathbb{R}^2$ are the coordinates of the $m^{th}$ pixel in $\boldsymbol{y}^{(k)}$ mapped to the HR grid [11]. For efficient memory management, we truncate $W_{mn}$ for $||\boldsymbol{v}_n - \boldsymbol{u}'_m||_2 > 3\sigma$. Please see our algorithm introduced in section 2.3 for details on the parametrization of this model for range super-resolution proposed in this paper.

**MAP Estimator.** The objective function to obtain an MAP estimate $\hat{\boldsymbol{x}}$ for the HR image $\boldsymbol{x}$ requires a data term and a regularizer weighted by $\lambda > 0$:

$$\hat{\boldsymbol{x}} = \arg\min_{\boldsymbol{x}} \left(\sum_{k=1}^{K} \left|\left|\boldsymbol{y}^{(k)} - \gamma_m^{(k)}\boldsymbol{W}^{(k)}\boldsymbol{x} - \gamma_a^{(k)}\mathbf{1}\right|\right|_2^2 + \lambda \sum_{n=1}^{N} h_\tau\left((\boldsymbol{D}\boldsymbol{x})_n\right)\right). \tag{3}$$

---

**Algorithm 1.** Multi-Sensor Super-Resolution (MSR)

---

**Input:** K range images $y^{(k)}$, RGB data $c^{(k)}$, reference frame $r = \lceil K/2 \rceil$
**Output:** Super-resolved range image $\hat{x}$
for $k = 1 \ldots K$ do
$\quad c^{(k)} := \text{Fuse}(y^{(k)}, c^{(k)})$                                    ▷ see Sect. 2.1
$\quad w_c(u_c) := \text{OpticalFlow}(c^{(t)}, c^{(r)})$
$\quad w_r(u_r) := \Delta((l_1 \cdot w_{c,1}(u_c) \; l_2 \cdot w_{c,2}(u_c))^\top)$      ▷ see Eq. (4)
$\quad W^{(k)} := \text{ComposeSystemMatrix}(w_r(u_r))$                      ▷ see Eq. (2)
$\quad \gamma_m^{(k)}, \gamma_a^{(k)} := \text{MSAC}(y^{(r)}, \text{Warp}(y^{(t)}, w_r(u_r)))$
$\hat{x}_0 := \text{BicubicUpsampling}(y^{(r)})$                            ▷ initial guess
$\hat{x} := \text{SCG}(\hat{x}_0, \{y^{(k)}\}, \{W^{(k)}\}, \{\gamma_m^{(k)}, \gamma_a^{(k)}\})$    ▷ see Eq. (3)

---

where $D$ is a high-pass filter and $h_\tau(z) = \tau^2(\sqrt{1 + (z/\tau)^2} - 1)$ is the pseudo Huber loss function used for regularization. For $D$ we choose a Laplacian to enforce smoothness for $x$, which guides the estimation to reliable solutions. However, since the regularizer based on the Huber function penalizes outlier less strictly than a Tikhonov regularization using the $L_2$ norm, edges are well preserved.

### 2.3   Multi-Sensor Super-Resolution

In our framework, each $c^{(k)}$ is aligned to $y^{(k)}$ after sensor fusion. Motion estimation is performed on RGB images employing optical flow and the displacement fields are projected to the range image domain to compose all system matrices $W^{(k)}$. The unknown $\gamma_m^{(k)}$ and $\gamma_a^{(k)}$ are determined using robust parameter estimation. We obtain $\hat{x}$ by minimizing (3) using Scaled Conjugate Gradients (SCG) optimization [13] with a bicubic upsampled version of reference frame $y^{(r)}$ coincident with $\hat{x}$ as initial guess. See Algorithm 1 for details of our method.

**Optical Flow Estimation.** For motion estimation, we determine displacement vector fields $w_c : \Omega_c \mapsto \mathbb{R}^2$, $w_c(u_c) = (w_{c,1}(u_c) \; w_{c,2}(u_c))^\top$ for RGB images between a reference frame $c^{(r)}$ and a template $c^{(t)}$ using optical flow. This transforms each point $u_c$ from $c^{(t)}$ to its position $u_c'$ in $c^{(r)}$ according to $u_c' = u_c + w_c(u_c)$. The central frame $c^{(r)}$ with $r = \lceil K/2 \rceil$ is chosen as reference to minimize the expected displacements between $c^{(r)}$ and $c^{(t)}$ for robust flow estimation. Optical flow is computed in a course-to-fine manner using the method proposed by Liu [14]. Once a displacement field $w_c$ is estimated, it is transformed yielding the range displacement field $w_r : \Omega_r \mapsto \mathbb{R}^2$:

$$w_r(u_r) = \Delta \left( l_1 \cdot w_{c,1}(u_c) \; l_2 \cdot w_{c,2}(u_c) \right)^\top, \tag{4}$$

for the resampling operator $\Delta : \mathbb{R}^2 \mapsto \mathbb{R}^2$. We implement $\Delta$ as the median of corresponding displacement vectors $w_c$ in both coordinate directions. To obtain $w_r$ in the dimension of range data, rescaling by $l_i$, $0 < l_i \leq 1$ is required, where

$l_i$ denotes the ratio of resolutions between $\boldsymbol{y}^{(k)}$ and $\boldsymbol{c}^{(k)}$. Then $\boldsymbol{w}_r$ is used to compose the system matrices for each frame according to Eq. 2.

**Range Diversity Correction.** If we allow general 3-D movements of the endoscope such as out-of-plane translation, this results in an offset for range values in successive frames. Neglecting this effect as implicitly done in related super-resolution approaches [9] leads to biased reconstructions. This problem can be mathematically compared to the fusion of intensity images differing photometrically. Therefore, we adopt a photometric registration scheme to range correction. First, two frames to be corrected are assumed to be geometrically aligned by warping them according to the precomputed optical flow displacement field. Let $y$ be a range value in reference frame $\boldsymbol{y}^{(r)}$. The corresponding range value $y'$ in template frame $\boldsymbol{y}^{(t)}$ is given according to the affine model $y' = \gamma_m \cdot y + \gamma_a$.

We utilize an M-estimator sample consensus (MSAC) for robust estimation of $\gamma_m$ and $\gamma_a$ as suggested by Capel [15] for photometric registration. These parameters are plugged into the generative image model (1) for $\gamma_m^{(k)}$ and $\gamma_a^{(k)}$. For the reference $\boldsymbol{y}^{(r)}$ we set $\gamma_m^{(r)} = 1$ and $\gamma_a^{(r)} = 0$ to obtain a super-resolved image having the same measurement range as the reference frame.

## 3 Experiments and Results

We compared multi-sensor super-resolution (MSR) to the conventional single-sensor approach (SSR) where optical flow is estimated on range data. The PSF width was set to $\sigma = 0.5$ and for regularization using Huber function we set $\lambda = 70$ and $\tau = 5 \cdot 10^{-3}$ determined empirically using a grid search. SCG was used with termination tolerance $10^{-3}$ for pixels of $\boldsymbol{x}$ and the objective function value. The maximum iteration number was set to 50. Super-resolution was applied with magnification $s = 4$ in a sliding window scheme over time using successive $K = 31$ frames (30 template and one reference frame) per window. This improves the robustness and our method is able to recover from failures caused e. g. by misregistration of single frames in highly dynamic scenes. Supplementary material for our experiments is available on our web page.[1]

**Synthetic Data.** For quantitative assessment, six synthetic data sets based on ground truth data were generated. We used a ToF/RGB simulator to obtain RGB and range data from a model of a laparoscopic scene designed in collaboration with a medical expert (see Fig 2). The resolutions for RGB (640×480 px) and range images (64×48 px) are equal to those of the hybrid 3-D endoscope used in experiments for real data. Each LR frame is a downsampled version of the ground truth and disturbed by a Gaussian PSF ($\sigma_b = 0.5$) as well as additive, zero-mean, Gaussian noise ($\sigma_n = 0.05$). Random motion of the camera was used to simulate movements of the endoscope held by a surgeon. Small displacements of endoscopic tools and organs simulated minimally invasive surgery. As quality metrics we employed the peak-signal-to-noise ratio (PSNR) and structural

---

[1] http://www5.cs.fau.de/research/data/

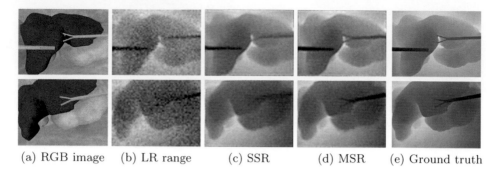

(a) RGB image     (b) LR range     (c) SSR     (d) MSR     (e) Ground truth

**Fig. 2.** Synthetic sequences S4 and S5: RGB data (a), LR range data (b), results for SSR (c) and the proposed MSR (d) compared to ground truth data (e)

**Table 1.** PSNR in dB (SSIM in brackets) for synthetic data. Each result is averaged over 10 sub-sequences per set. We compared bicubic upsampling (second column) to SSR (third column) and our MSR approach with the proposed range correction scheme (fourth column) and without range correction (last column).

| Sequence | Interpolation (bicubic) | Range corr. SSR | Range corr. MSR | No corr. MSR |
|----------|-------------------------|-----------------|-----------------|--------------|
| S1 | 24.28 (0.57) | 28.16 (0.87) | **29.85 (0.89)** | 29.83 (0.89) |
| S2 | 25.23 (0.59) | 30.78 (0.91) | **31.13 (0.92)** | 30.91 (0.91) |
| S3 | 25.83 (0.60) | 31.89 (0.92) | **32.72 (0.93)** | 31.93 (0.93) |
| S4 | 25.58 (0.59) | 29.06 (0.89) | **31.17 (0.91)** | 29.19 (0.91) |
| S5 | 26.58 (0.59) | 30.36 (0.91) | **32.77 (0.93)** | 31.35 (0.93) |
| S6 | 26.26 (0.57) | 28.43 (0.89) | **30.66 (0.92)** | 30.28 (0.92) |
| **Mean** | 25.63 (0.58) | 29.78 (0.90) | **31.38 (0.92)** | 30.58 (0.91) |

similarity (SSIM). For comparison, we also evaluated bicubic interpolation as a fast and simple upsampling technique. MSR was evaluated with and without range correction to justify our correction scheme. See Tab. 1 for PSNR and SSIM measures averaged over ten subsequent sequences in sliding window processing.

**Real Data.** For qualitative evaluation, we acquired real data using a hybrid 3-D endoscope prototype manufactured by Richard Wolf GmbH, Knittlingen, Germany. Therefore, a liver phantom and two surgical tools were measured with a frame rate of 30 fps. Range and RGB images were captured and the endoscope was slightly moved during acquisition. Raw data compared to super-resolved data is shown in Fig. 3. See Fig. 4 for a 3-D mesh created for one sequence.

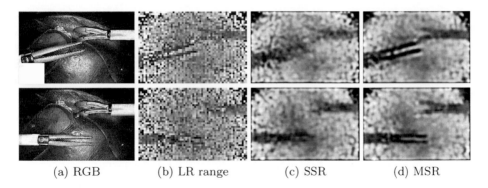

(a) RGB          (b) LR range          (c) SSR          (d) MSR

**Fig. 3.** Liver phantom acquired by a hybrid 3-D endoscope: RGB images (a), LR range data (b) and the results of SSR (c) as well as the proposed MSR (d)

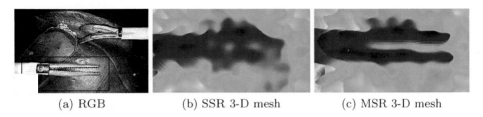

(a) RGB          (b) SSR 3-D mesh          (c) MSR 3-D mesh

**Fig. 4.** RGB image (a) and 3-D meshes for SSR (b) and the proposed MSR (c)

## 4    Discussion

For synthetic images, super-resolution yields more reliable 3-D surfaces compared to bicubic interpolation, especially due to denoising implicitly performed in MAP estimation (see Tab. 1). The proposed MSR approach clearly outperforms SSR indicated by increased mean PSNR (SSIM) of 1.6 dB (0.02). We could also verify improved reconstruction of depth discontinuities by visual inspection, e. g. for surgical tools (see Fig. 2). For sequences containing large out-of-plane movements (S4 and S5), we observed a particulary biased reconstruction if no range correction is applied indicated by decreased PSNR. For real data, the proposed MSR approach recovers the liver surface and endoscopic tools barley visible in raw data as well as in the result of SSR (see Fig. 3).

In our experiments, super-resolution was performed *off-line* to obtain one single HR image from multiple LR frames. Please note, that this limitation may be avoided by dynamic estimation schemes [10] to enable an *on-line* implementation, which is however beyond the scope of this paper.

## 5    Conclusions

In this paper, a multi-sensor framework for super-resolution in hybrid 3-D endoscopy has been introduced. Range super-resolution is guided by RGB images acquired simultaneously. Our method is a general-purpose technique to overcome low spatial resolutions and poor SNR of today's ToF sensors. For applications such as segmentation or classification, super-resolution holds great potential and may help to make the breakthrough of ToF imaging in minimally invasive surgery. Beyond ToF/RGB endoscopy, our method may also be applicable in related hybrid range imaging systems, which is part of our future work.

**Acknowledgments.** The authors gratefully acknowledge funding of the Erlangen Graduate School in Advanced Optical Technologies (SAOT) by the German National Science Foundation (DFG) in the framework of the excellence initiative and the support by the DFG under Grant No. HO 1791/7-1. This research was funded by the Graduate School of Information Science in Health (GSISH) and the TUM Graduate School. We thank the Metrilus GmbH for their support.

# References

1. Röhl, S., Bodenstedt, S., Suwelack, S., Kenngott, S., Mueller-Stich, P., Dillmann, R., Speidel, S.: Real-time surface reconstruction from stereo endoscopic images for intraoperative registration. In: Proc. SPIE, vol. 7964, p. 796414 (2011)
2. Field, M., Clarke, D., Strup, S., Seales, W.: Stereo endoscopy as a 3-d measurement tool. In: EMBC 2009, pp. 5748–5751 (2009)
3. Schmalz, C., Forster, F., Schick, A., Angelopoulou, E.: An endoscopic 3d scanner based on structured light. Med. Image Anal. 16(5), 1063–1072 (2012)
4. Penne, J., Höller, K., Stürmer, M., Schrauder, T., Schneider, A., Engelbrecht, R., Feußner, H., Schmauss, B., Hornegger, J.: Time-of-Flight 3-D Endoscopy. In: Yang, G.-Z., Hawkes, D., Rueckert, D., Noble, A., Taylor, C. (eds.) MICCAI 2009, Part I. LNCS, vol. 5761, pp. 467–474. Springer, Heidelberg (2009)
5. Haase, S., Forman, C., Kilgus, T., Bammer, R., Maier-Hein, L., Hornegger, J.: Tof/rgb sensor fusion for augmented 3d endoscopy using a fully automatic calibration scheme. In: Tolxdorff, T., Deserno, T.M., Handels, H., Meinzer, H.P. (eds.) Bildverarbeitung für die Medizin 2012, pp. 467–474. Springer, Heidelberg (2012)
6. Haase, S., Wasza, J., Kilgus, T., Hornegger, J.: Laparoscopic instrument localization using a 3-d time-of-flight/rgb endoscope. In: WACV 2013, pp. 449–454 (2013)
7. Park, S.C., Park, M.K., Kang, M.G.: Super-resolution image reconstruction: a technical overview. IEEE Signal Process Mag. 20(3), 21–36 (2003)
8. De Smet, V., Namboodiri, V., Van Gool, L.: Super-resolution techniques for minimally invasive surgery. In: Proceedings AE-CAI 2011, pp. 41–50 (2011)
9. Schuon, S., Theobalt, C., Davis, J., Thrun, S.: Lidarboost: Depth superresolution for tof 3d shape scanning. In: CVPR 2009, pp. 343–350 (2009)
10. Farsiu, S., Robinson, D., Elad, M., Milanfar, P.: Advances and challenges in super-resolution. Int. J. Imaging Syst. Technol. 14(2), 47–57 (2004)
11. Tipping, M.E., Bishop, C.M.: Bayesian image super-resolution. In: Adv. Neural Inf. Process. Syst., pp. 1303–1310. MIT Press (2003)
12. Fransens, R., Strecha, C., Van Gool, L.: Optical flow based super-resolution: A probabilistic approach. Comput. Vis. Image Underst. 106(1), 106–115 (2007)
13. Nabney, I.T.: NETLAB: Algorithms for Pattern Recognition, 1st edn. Advances in Pattern Recognition. Springer (2002)
14. Liu, C.: Beyond Pixels: Exploring New Representations and Applications for Motion Analysis. PhD thesis, Massachusetts Institute of Technology (2009)
15. Capel, D.: Image mosaicing and super-resolution. PhD thesis, Oxford (2004)

# Attenuation Correction Synthesis
# for Hybrid PET-MR Scanners

Ninon Burgos[1], Manuel Jorge Cardoso[1,2], Marc Modat[1,2], Stefano Pedemonte[1],
John Dickson[3], Anna Barnes[3], John S. Duncan[4], David Atkinson[5],
Simon R. Arridge[1], Brian F. Hutton[3,6], and Sebastien Ourselin[1,2]

[1] Centre for Medical Image Computing, University College London, London, UK
[2] Dementia Research Centre, University College London, London, UK
[3] Institute of Nuclear Medicine, University College London, London, UK
[4] Department of Clinical and Experimental Epilepsy, UCL IoN, London, UK
[5] Centre for Medical Imaging, University College London, London, UK
[6] Centre for Medical Radiation Physics, University of Wollongong, NSW, Australia

**Abstract.** The combination of functional and anatomical imaging technologies such as Positron Emission Tomography (PET) and Computed Tomography (CT) has shown its value in the preclinical and clinical fields. In PET/CT hybrid acquisition systems, CT-derived attenuation maps enable a more accurate PET reconstruction. However, CT provides only very limited soft-tissue contrast and exposes the patient to an additional radiation dose. In comparison, Magnetic Resonance Imaging (MRI) provides good soft-tissue contrast and the ability to study functional activation and tissue microstructures, but does not directly provide patient-specific electron density maps for PET reconstruction.

The aim of the proposed work is to improve PET/MR reconstruction by generating synthetic CTs and attenuation-maps. The synthetic images are generated through a multi-atlas information propagation scheme, locally matching the MRI-derived patient's morphology to a database of pre-acquired MRI/CT pairs. Results show improvements in CT synthesis and PET reconstruction accuracy when compared to a segmentation method using an Ultrashort-Echo-Time MRI sequence.

## 1 Introduction

Positron Emission Tomography/Magnetic Resonance Imaging (PET/MRI) scanners are expected to offer a new range of applications in neuro-oncology, neurodegenerative diseases, such as Alzheimer's disease, and epilepsy [1]. To accurately quantify the radionuclide uptake, PET data need to be corrected for photon attenuation. The attenuation information is usually obtained from a transmission scan in standalone PET or derived from a Computed Tomography (CT) image in combined PET/CT. As MRI intensities do not reflect the electron densities, alternative methods must be developed for PET/MRI acquisitions. These methods can be classified in three categories: segmentation, atlas, and emission-based approaches. In segmentation-based methods, uniform linear attenuation coefficients are assigned to tissue classes obtained by segmenting an MRI image.

K. Mori et al. (Eds.): MICCAI 2013, Part I, LNCS 8149, pp. 147–154, 2013.
© Springer-Verlag Berlin Heidelberg 2013

In atlas-based methods, an anatomical model or dataset is deformed to match the patient's anatomy in order to apply the attenuation map from the model to the patient data. The third class of methods exploits PET emission data from a time-of-flight PET system and anatomical information from MR images to compute the attenuation maps.

In the method from Martinez-Möller *et al.* [2], the body is segmented into four classes: background, lungs, fat and soft-tissues. While the results obtained in whole-body studies are satisfactory, the lack of bone information has a significant impact on the quantification of the radionuclide uptake in brain studies [3]. Keereman *et al.* [4] used Ultrashort-Echo-Time (UTE) sequences to distinguish cortical bone, air and soft tissue. Berker *et al.* [5] developed a 4-class tissue segmentation technique applied to brain studies. Cortical bone, air, fat and soft-tissues are segmented using a combined UTE/Dixon MRI sequence. Although the overall voxel classification accuracy reached is superior to the accuracy obtained without Dixon or UTE components, the bone segmentation is still inaccurate in complex regions such as nasal sinuses [5]. Johansson *et al.* [6] described a Gaussian mixture regression model that links the MRI intensity values to the CT Hounsfield units (HU). Schreibmann *et al.* [7] developed a multimodality optical flow deformable model that maps patient MRI images to a CT atlas. In the Hofmann *et al.* method [8], local information derived from a pattern recognition technique and global information obtained by an atlas registration are combined to predict a pseudo-CT image from a given MR image. All these methods assume a one-to-one correspondence between MRI and CT intensities. However, several materials such as cerebrospinal fluid, air and bone have similar intensities in a T1-weighted MRI image but distinct values in a CT image. Considering local information may enhance the results, but inaccuracies still remain at boundaries such as air and bone in the nasal sinuses.

The proposed method follows the principle of multi-atlas information propagation in order to synthesize an attenuation correction map from an MRI image. As an alternative to a one-to-one mapping from the observed MRI intensities to CT-like intensities, one can exploit the concept of morphological similarity between subjects. When used in the context of segmentation propagation [9], a set of segmented anatomical atlases from several subjects are mapped to a target subject and subsequently fused according to the morphological similarity between the mapped and the target anatomical images. This morphological similarity, normally interpreted as an image similarity measure, is used to enforce the fact that the most morphologically similar atlases should carry more weight during the fusion process [10]. This work will exploit the same idea in the context of intensity propagation and fusion. The developed algorithm makes use of a pre-acquired set of aligned MRI/CT image pairs from multiple subjects to propagate in a voxel wise fashion the CT intensities corresponding to similar MRIs. The proposed approach relies on the concept of morphological similarity rather than the assumption of one-to-one intensity mapping between the MRI and the CT. This enables the synthesization of a patient-specific pseudo CT image, from which the attenuation map is then generated.

## 2 Method

In PET/CT imaging, the main technique to correct for attenuation is to derive the attenuation coefficients from a CT image. In the case of a hybrid PET/MR scanner, the only anatomical and structural information available is an MR image. A diagram illustrating the proposed method in which a synthetic CT is obtained from a given MRI is shown in Figure 1.

### 2.1 MR-CT Database Preprocessing and Inter-subject Mapping

The database consists of pairs of T1-weighted MRI and CT brain images. For each subject, the MRI is affinely aligned to the CT using a symmetric approach based on Ourselin *et al.* [11]. Even though this is an intra-subject alignment, a full affine registration is used to compensate for possible gradient distortions in the MRI scans.

In order to synthesise the CT for a given MRI, one first needs to register all the MRIs in the atlas database to the target MRI. This inter-subject coordinate mapping is obtained using a symmetric global registration followed by a cubic B-spline parametrisation non-rigid registration, using normalised mutual information as a measure of similarity [12]. All the CTs in the atlas database are then mapped to the target subject using the transformation that maps the subject's corresponding MRI in the atlas database to the target MRI. Through this registration and resampling procedure, one obtains a series of MRI/CT pairs aligned to the MRI of the target subject.

### 2.2 CT Synthesis

The proposed framework uses a local image similarity measure between the target MRI and the set of registered MRIs as a metric of the underlying

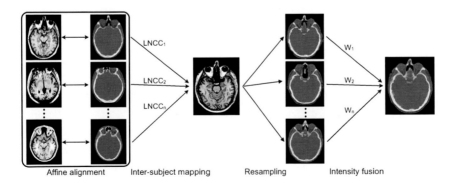

**Fig. 1.** CT synthesis diagram for a given MRI image. All the MRIs in the atlas set are registered to the target MRI. The CTs in the atlas set are then mapped using the same transformation to the target MRI. A similarity measure (LNCC) between the mapped and target MRIs is converted to weights (W) to reconstruct the target CT.

morphological similarity. Provided the local image similarity is a good approximation of the local morphological similarity between subjects, we assume that if two MRIs are similar at a certain spatial location, the two CTs will also be similar.

**Image/Morphological Similarity.** The morphological similarity between the target MRI and the registered MRIs from the atlas database is calculated locally using the normalised cross-correlation (LNCC) scheme proposed by Yushkevich *et al.* [13]. The LNCC similarity measure monitors the local quality of match between the MRI of the target subject and each of the warped MRIs from the atlas database. In this work, a convolution-based fast local normalised correlation coefficient proposed by Cachier *et al.* [14] is used. Let the target subject's MRI be denoted by $I^{MRI}$ and its corresponding unknown CT be denoted by $I^{CT}$. For each of the $N$ atlases in the database, let the mapped MRI and CT images of atlas $n$ be denoted by $J_n^{MRI}$ and $J_n^{CT}$ respectively. The LNCC between $I^{MRI}$ and $J_n^{MRI}$ at voxel $v$ is then given by:

$$\text{LNCC}_v = \frac{\langle I^{MRI}, J_n^{MRI} \rangle_v}{\sigma_v(I^{MRI})\sigma_v(J_n^{MRI})} \ . \tag{1}$$

As in [14], the means and standard deviations (std) at voxel $v$ are calculated using a Gaussian kernel $G$, with a kernel std equal to 5 voxels, using convolution:

$$\overline{I}_v = G * I(v) \qquad \sigma(I)_v = \sqrt{\overline{I^2}_v - \overline{I}_v^2} \qquad \langle I, J \rangle_v = \overline{I \cdot J}_v - \overline{I}_v \cdot \overline{J}_v \ ,$$

where $*$ denotes the convolution operator. High LNCC values indicate a better local match between the two MRI images.

As suggested by Yushkevich *et al.* [13], the range of LNCC can vary quite dramatically between subjects and locations. Thus, a ranking scheme similar to [13] is used. The LNCC at each voxel is ranked across all atlas images, with the rank being denoted by $R_{nv}$. The ranks $R_{nv}$ are then converted to weights by applying an exponential decay function:

$$W_{nv} = \begin{cases} e^{-\beta R_{nv}} & R_{nv} < \kappa, \\ 0 & \text{otherwise} \ . \end{cases} \tag{2}$$

with $W_{nv}$ being the weight associated with the $n^{th}$ subject image at voxel $v$ and $\kappa$ being a truncation parameter. The weight function is restricted to the highest $\kappa$ LNCCs, removing the influence of morphologically dissimilar subjects or mis-registration. Here, $N = 27$, $\kappa$ is set to 9 and $\beta$ to 0.5. Future work will involve an explicit optimisation of these values.

**Intensity Fusion.** Similarly to the label fusion framework suggested by Cardoso *et al.* [15], an estimate of the target subject's CT can be obtained by a spatially varying weighted averaging. The weights $W_{nv}$ are used to reconstruct the target CT image $I^{CT}$ at voxel $v$ as follows:

$$I_v^{CT} = \frac{\sum_{n=1}^N W_{nv} \cdot J_{nv}^{CT}}{\sum_{n=1}^N W_n} \ . \tag{3}$$

## 2.3   Attenuation Map

To obtain the attenuation map ($\mu$-map), the synthetic CT image is resampled to the PET resolution. The resampled CT image is then matched to the PET's point spread function (PSF) by filtering it with a 6mm full-width at half-maximum Gaussian filter. According to [16], the CT values expressed in HU are converted to PET attenuation coefficients in cm$^{-1}$ by a bilinear transformation:

$$\mu = \begin{cases} \mu_{\text{water}} \left(1 + \frac{I^{CT}}{1000}\right) & I^{CT} \leq 0 \text{ HU} \\ \mu_{\text{water}} \left(1 + \frac{I^{CT}}{1000} \frac{\rho_{\text{water}}(\mu_{\text{bone}} - \mu_{\text{water}})}{\mu_{\text{water}}(\rho_{\text{bone}} - \rho_{\text{water}})}\right) & I^{CT} > 0 \text{ HU} \end{cases} \tag{4}$$

where $\mu_{\text{water}}$ and $\mu_{\text{bone}}$ represent the attenuation coefficients at the PET 511 keV energy for water and bone respectively and $\rho_{\text{water}}$ and $\rho_{\text{bone}}$ represent the attenuation coefficients at the CT energy respectively. These values are set to $\mu_{\text{water}} = 0.096\,\text{cm}^{-1}$, $\mu_{\text{bone}} = 0.172\,\text{cm}^{-1}$, $\rho_{\text{water}} = 0.184\,\text{cm}^{-1}$ and $\rho_{\text{bone}} = 0.428\,\text{cm}^{-1}$

# 3   Validation and Results

**Data.** All the data used in this work were acquired with two scanners. The T1-weighted MRIs (3.0T; TR/TE, 1800ms/2.73ms; flip angle 9°; resolution 0.527 × 0.527 × 0.9 mm$^3$) and UTE attenuation maps (resolution 1.562 × 1.562 × 1.562 mm$^3$) were acquired on a Siemens Biograph mMR hybrid PET/MR scanner; the CTs (resolution 0.586 × 0.586 × 1.25 mm$^3$), and reconstructed PETs (radio-pharmaceutical: FDG; resolution 1.953 × 1.953 × 3.27 mm$^3$) on a GE Discovery ST PET/CT scanner.

**Validation Scheme.** The synthesization performance of the proposed algorithm is validated against ground truth data. The quantitative validation consists of three steps:

- The pseudo CT (pCT) is compared to the subject's ground truth CT image at the original resolution, validating the accuracy of the CT reconstruction.
- The pCT is resampled to the PET's resolution and convolved with the point spread function, validating how accurate the CT synthesis is at the resolution relevant for PET reconstruction.
- The PET image is reconstructed using the pCT-derived $\mu$-map and compared with the ground truth PET reconstructed using the CT-based $\mu$-map, validating the accuracy of the PET attenuation correction.

The dataset consists of T1-weighted MRI, CT and PET brain images from 28 subjects. In 17 cases, MRI data are truncated at the front and back of the head. As UTE $\mu$-map images are also available for 4 subjects, synthesization performance of the proposed algorithm is compared to the UTE-based synthesization method. All quantitative assessments are performed using a leave-one-out cross-validation scheme.

152    N. Burgos et al.

**Table 1.** Average (std) of the MAR between the ground truth (high-resolution CT, PET-resolution CT and CT-reconstructed PET) and the corresponding synthetic images, using both the proposed method (pCT) and UTE. The common datasets consist of 4 subjects with a non-truncated T1 and a known UTE $\mu$-map, the untruncated datasets consist of 7 subjects with a non-truncated T1 but no associated UTE $\mu$-map and the truncated datasets gather 17 subjects with a truncated T1 image. "No AC" corresponds to the residuals without attenuation correction. PETs are quantitatively normalised using the pons as the reference region.

| | High-res CT | | PET-res CT | | Reconstructed PET | | |
| | pCT | UTE | pCT | UTE | No AC | pCT | UTE |
|---|---|---|---|---|---|---|---|
| Common data (N=4) | 100 (3) | 190 (25) | 77 (4) | 194 (17) | 1.66 (0.15) | 0.23 (0.05) | 0.74 (0.09) |
| Untruncated data (N=7) | 102 (10) | - | 73 (15) | - | 0.85 (0.64) | 0.12 (0.09) | - |
| Truncated data (N=17) | 108 (10) | - | 84 (10) | - | 1.10 (0.51) | 0.18 (0.10) | - |

**Pseudo CT Reconstruction Accuracy.** Using only the MRI image of the subject, a pseudo CT image is generated using the proposed method. This generated CT is then compared to the ground truth CT. The metric used for validation is the mean absolute residual, defined as MAR $= \sum_v |GT_v^{CT} - I_v^{CT}|$. This metric is estimated between the ground truth CT ($GT^{CT}$) and the pseudo CT ($I^{CT}$) for every subject in the database. The same MAR metric is also used to assess the synthesis accuracy after resampling the pCT to the PET resolution and simulating the PET PSF. When available, the MAR is computed between the UTE $\mu$-map and the ground truth CT at both CT and PET resolutions. The average (std) MAR, measured in Hounsfield units, across all the subjects in the database and for both experiments is presented in Table 1. The error obtained with the pCT method is half that of the error obtained with the UTE method. The results also emphasize the robustness of the algorithm in the case of a truncated target MRI. Examples of ground truth CTs and $\mu$-maps, pseudo CTs and pseudo $\mu$-maps and UTE-based $\mu$-maps are presented in Figure 2.

**PET Reconstruction Accuracy.** Due to the unavailability of the raw PET data, we make use of the PET reconstruction provided by the PET/CT scan-

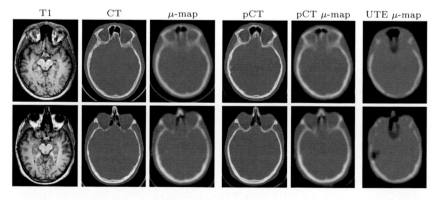

**Fig. 2.** Acquired T1-weighted MRI, CT and $\mu$-map, pseudo CT and $\mu$-map generated by the proposed method and UTE-based $\mu$-map for two subjects

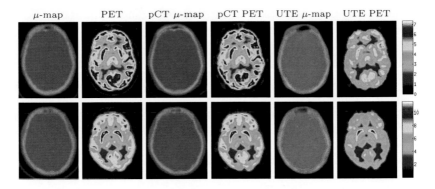

**Fig. 3.** (From left to right) The ground truth $\mu$-map and PET reconstruction followed by the equivalent images generated using the proposed method and UTE-based methods, for two subjects. All methods are normalised to the same scale.

ner. To reconstruct the PET with the pCT-based $\mu$-map, we follow a projection/reconstruction technique similar to Hofmann *et al.* [8]. The original PET, the original $\mu$-map and the pCT-based $\mu$-map are projected to obtain sinograms. The original attenuation correction is removed from the PET and the non-corrected PET is then corrected using the pCT $\mu$-map. Following the same pipeline, we also reconstruct PET images using the CT $\mu$-map (this PET is considered as the ground truth) and the UTE $\mu$-map. The iterative reconstruction is performed using a GPU accelerated rotation-based projection and backprojection algorithm developed by Pedemonte *et al.* [17]. Results of PET reconstructions using different attenuation maps are displayed in Figure 3. The MAR is computed between the ground truth PET and the non-corrected, pCT and UTE-PET. Results are shown in Table 1. The error obtained using the pCT $\mu$-map is three times smaller than the error obtained using the UTE $\mu$-map.

## 4    Conclusion

This paper presents a simple CT and attenuation map synthesis algorithm based on a multi-atlas information propagation scheme. While the sharpness of the synthetic CT images is lower than the ground-truth subject's CT at the original resolution, this problem is greatly reduced at the resolution and PSF of the PET image. Overall, the proposed algorithm provides an improvement in PET reconstruction accuracy when compared to the UTE-based correction.

**Acknowledgements.** This work was supported by an IMPACT studentship funded jointly by Siemens and the UCL FES, the EPSRC (EP/K005278/1 and EP/H046410/1) and the CBRC Strategic Investment Award (#168).

## References

1. Von Schulthess, G.K., Kuhn, F.P., Kaufmann, P., Veit-Haibach, P.: Clinical positron emission tomography/magnetic resonance imaging applications. Seminars in Nuclear Medicine 43(1), 3–10 (2013)

2. Martinez-Möller, A., Souvatzoglou, M., Delso, G., Bundschuh, R.A., Chefd'hotel, C., Ziegler, S.I., Navab, N., Schwaiger, M., Nekolla, S.G.: Tissue classification as a potential approach for attenuation correction in whole-body PET/MRI: evaluation with PET/CT data. Journal of Nuclear Medicine 50(4), 520–526 (2009)
3. Schleyer, P.J., Schaeffter, T., Marsden, P.K.: The effect of inaccurate bone attenuation coefficient and segmentation on reconstructed PET images. Nuclear Medicine Communications 31(8), 708–716 (2010)
4. Keereman, V., Fierens, Y., Broux, T., De Deene, Y., Lonneux, M., Vandenberghe, S.: MRI-based attenuation correction for PET/MRI using ultrashort echo time sequences. Journal of Nuclear Medicine 51(5), 812–818 (2010)
5. Berker, Y., Franke, J., Salomon, A., Palmowski, M., Donker, H.C.W., Temur, Y., Izquierdo-Garcia, D., Fayad, Z.A., Kiessling, F., Schulz, V.: MRI-based attenuation correction for hybrid PET/MRI systems: a 4-class tissue segmentation technique using a combined ultrashort-echo-time/Dixon MRI sequence. JNM 53(5) (2012)
6. Johansson, A., Karlsson, M., Nyholm, T.: CT substitute derived from MRI sequences with ultrashort echo time. Medical Physics 38(5), 2708 (2011)
7. Schreibmann, E., Nye, J.A., Schuster, D.M., Martin, D.R., Votaw, J., Fox, T.: MR-based attenuation correction for hybrid PET-MR brain imaging systems using deformable image registration. Medical Physics 37(5), 2101 (2010)
8. Hofmann, M., Steinke, F., Scheel, V., Charpiat, G., Farquhar, J., Aschoff, P., Brady, M., Schölkopf, B., Pichler, B.J.: MRI-based attenuation correction for PET/MRI: a novel approach combining pattern recognition and atlas registration. Journal of Nuclear Medicine 49(11), 1875–1883 (2008)
9. Heckemann, R.A., Hajnal, J.V., Aljabar, P., Rueckert, D., Hammers, A.: Automatic anatomical brain MRI segmentation combining label propagation and decision fusion. NeuroImage 33(1), 115–126 (2006)
10. Sabuncu, M.R., Van Leemput, K., Fischl, B., Golland, P.: A generative model for image segmentation based on label fusion. TMI 29(10) (2010)
11. Ourselin, S., Roche, A., Subsol, G.: Reconstructing a 3D structure from serial histological sections. Image and Vision Computing 19(2001), 25–31 (2000)
12. Modat, M., Ridgway, G.R., Taylor, Z.A., Lehmann, M., Barnes, J., Hawkes, D.J., Fox, N.C., Ourselin, S.: Fast free-form deformation using graphics processing units. Computer Methods and Programs in Biomedicine 98(3), 278–284 (2010)
13. Yushkevich, P.A., Wang, H., Pluta, J., Das, S.R., Craige, C., Avants, B.B., Weiner, M.W., Mueller, S.: Nearly automatic segmentation of hippocampal subfields in in vivo focal T2-weighted MRI. NeuroImage 53(4), 1208–1224 (2010)
14. Cachier, P., Bardinet, E., Dormont, D., Pennec, X., Ayache, N.: Iconic feature based nonrigid registration: the PASHA algorithm. CVIU 89(2-3) (2003)
15. Cardoso, M.J., Wolz, R., Modat, M., Fox, N.C., Rueckert, D., Ourselin, S.: Geodesic Information Flows. In: Ayache, N., Delingette, H., Golland, P., Mori, K. (eds.) MICCAI 2012, Part II. LNCS, vol. 7511, pp. 262–270. Springer, Heidelberg (2012)
16. Burger, C., Goerres, G., Schoenes, S., Buck, A., Lonn, A.H.R., Von Schulthess, G.K.: PET attenuation coefficients from CT images: experimental evaluation of the transformation of CT into PET 511-keV attenuation coefficients. European Journal of Nuclear Medicine and Molecular Imaging 29(7), 922–927 (2002)
17. Pedemonte, S., Bousse, A., Erlandsson, K., Modat, M., Arridge, S., Hutton, B.F., Ourselin, S.: GPU accelerated rotation-based emission tomography reconstruction. In: IEEE Nuclear Science Symposuim, pp. 2657–2661 (2010)

# Low-Rank Total Variation for Image Super-Resolution

Feng Shi[*], Jian Cheng[*], Li Wang, Pew-Thian Yap, and Dinggang Shen

Department of Radiology and BRIC, University of North Carolina at Chapel Hill, NC, USA
dgshen@med.unc.edu

**Abstract.** Most natural images can be approximated using their low rank components. This fact has been successfully exploited in recent advancements of matrix completion algorithms for image recovery. However, a major limitation of low-rank matrix completion algorithms is that they cannot recover the case where a whole row or column is missing. The missing row or column will be simply filled as an arbitrary combination of other rows or columns with known values. This precludes the application of matrix completion to problems such as super-resolution (SR) where missing values in many rows and columns need to be recovered in the process of up-sampling a low-resolution image. Moreover, low-rank regularization considers information globally from the whole image and does not take proper consideration of local spatial consistency. Accordingly, we propose in this paper a solution to the SR problem via simultaneous (global) low-rank and (local) total variation (TV) regularization. We solve the respective cost function using the alternating direction method of multipliers (ADMM). Experiments on MR images of adults and pediatric subjects demonstrate that the proposed method enhances the details of the recovered high-resolution images, and outperforms the nearest-neighbor interpolation, cubic interpolation, non-local means, and TV-based up-sampling.

## 1    Introduction

Matrix completion algorithms have been shown recently to be effective in estimating missing values in a matrix from a small sample of known entries [1]. For instance, it has been applied to the famous Netflix problem where one needs to infer user's preference for unrated movies based on only a small number of rated movies [2]. To address this ill-conditioned problem, matrix completion methods often assume that the recovered matrix is low-rank and then uses this as a constraint to minimize the difference between the given incomplete matrix and the estimated matrix. Candes *et al.* proved that, most low-rank matrices can be perfectly recovered from a small number of given entries [3].

Matrix completion is widely applied to image/video in-painting and decoding problems. However, matrix completion is limited when applied to matrices with a whole missing row or column (see white horizontal and vertical lines in Fig. 1). In this case, the missing row or column will be simply filled as an arbitrary combination of other

---

[*] F.S. and J.C. contributed equally to this work.

K. Mori et al. (Eds.): MICCAI 2013, Part I, LNCS 8149, pp. 155–162, 2013.

known rows or columns to keep the total rank small. This precludes the application of matrix completion to problems such as super-resolution (SR) where missing values for many rows and columns need to be recovered in the process of up-sampling a low-resolution image by a factor of 2 times or larger [4]. Note that the goal of SR is to recover the fine anatomical details from one or more low-resolution images to construct a high-resolution image. In MR applications, single-image based SR is widely used since it requires only a single input image. For example, non-local means (NLM) is broadly employed [5], sometimes with the help from other modalities [6]. In this work, we focus on recovering a high-resolution image from a single MR image.

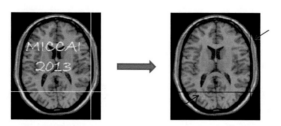

**Fig. 1.** Recovering missing values in a 2D image by using low-rank matrix completion [1]. The red arrows mark the horizontal and vertical lines that the algorithm fails to recover.

Another limitation of matrix completion algorithms is that they consider information globally from the whole image and does not exploit the local spatial consistency. Although local information may not be useful in applications such as the Netflix problem, where different rows (e.g., users) can be considered independently, it is valuable in image recovery. A solution to this problem is to integrate low-rank regularization with local regularization such as total variation [7]. By doing so, we can take advantage of both forms of regularization to harness remote information for effective image recovery and the local information to handle missing rows and columns.

Specifically, in this paper, we propose a novel low-rank total variation (LRTV) method for recovering a high-resolution image from a low-resolution image. Our method 1) explicitly models the effects of down-sampling and blurring on the low-resolution images, and 2) uses both low-rank and total variation regularizations to help solve the ill-conditioned inverse problem. Experiments on MR images of both adults and pediatric subjects demonstrate superior results of our method, compared to interpolation methods as well as NLM and TV-based up-sampling methods.

## 2     Method

For recovering the high-resolution image, our method 1) uses low-rank regularization to help retrieve useful information from remote regions; and 2) uses total variation regularization for keeping better local consistency.

## 2.1     Super-Resolution Problem

The physical model for the degradation effects involved in reducing a high-resolution (HR) image to a low-resolution (LR) image can be mathematically formulated as:

$$T = DSX + n \qquad (1)$$

where $T$ denotes the observed LR image, $D$ is a down-sampling operator, $S$ is a blurring operator, $X$ is the HR image that we want to recover, and $n$ represents the observation noise. The HR image can be estimated using this physical model by minimizing the below least-square cost function:

$$\min_{X} \|DSX - T\|^2 + \lambda \mathfrak{R}(X) \qquad (2)$$

where the first term is a data fidelity term used for penalizing the difference between the degraded HR image $X$ and the observed LR image $T$. The second term is a regularization term often defined based on prior knowledge. Weight $\lambda$ is introduced to balance the contributions of the fidelity term and regularization term.

## 2.2     Formulation of Low-Rank Total-Variation (LRTV) Method

The proposed LRTV method is formulated as follow:

$$\min_{X} \|DSX - T\|^2 + \lambda_{rank} \|X\|_* + \lambda_{tv} TV(X) \qquad (3)$$

where the second term is for low-rank regularization, and the third term is for total variation regularization. $\lambda_{rank}$ and $\lambda_{tv}$ are the respective weights.

**Low-Rank Regularization.** A $N$-dimensional image can be seen as a high order tensor, and its rank can be defined as the combination of trace norms of all matrices unfolded along each dimension [1]: $\|X\|_* = \sum_{i=1}^{N} \alpha_i \|X_{(i)}\|_{tr}$, where $N$ is the number of image dimensionality such as $N = 3$ for the 3D images. $\alpha_i$ are parameters satisfying $\alpha_i \geq 0$ and $\sum_{i=1}^{N} \alpha_i = 1$. $X_{(i)}$ is the unfolded $X$ along the $i$-th dimension: $unfold_i(X) = X_{(i)}$. For example, a 3D image with size of $U \times V \times W$ can be unfolded into three 2D matrices, with size of $U \times (V \times W)$, $V \times (W \times U)$, and $W \times (U \times V)$, respectively. $\|X_{(i)}\|_{tr}$ is the trace norm, which can be computed by summing the singular values of $X_{(i)}$. We employ the alternating direction method of multipliers (ADMM) [8] to solve this problem.

**Total-Variation Regularization.** The TV regularization term is defined as the integral of the absolute gradient of the image [9]: $TV(X) = \int |\nabla X| dx dy dz$. TV-regularization is formulated based on the observation that unreliable image signals usually have excessive and possibly spurious details, which lead to a high total variation. Thus, by minimizing the TV to remove such details, the estimated image will more likely match the original image. It has been proved quite effective in preserving edges. The TV-regularization problem can be solved by split Bregman method [10].

## 2.3    LRTV Optimization

We follow the alternating direction method of multipliers (ADMM) algorithm to solve the cost function in Eq. (3). ADMM is proven to be efficient for solving optimization problems with multiple non-smooth terms in the cost function [8]. We introduce redundant variables $\{M_i\}_{i=1}^N$ to obtain the following new cost function:

$$\min_{X,\{M_i\}_{i=1}^N} \|DSX - T\|^2 + \lambda_{rank} \sum_{i=1}^N \alpha_i \|M_{i(i)}\|_{tr} + \lambda_{tv} TV(X)$$

$$\text{subject to } X_{(i)} = M_{i(i)}, \ i = 1, \dots, N \tag{4}$$

Here, for each dimension $i$, we use $M_i$ to simulate $X$ by requiring that the unfolded $X$ along the $i$-th dimension $X_{(i)}$ should be equal to the unfolded $M_i$ along this dimension $M_{i(i)}$.

The cost function in Eq. (4) can be further rewritten as an unconstrained optimization problem by replacing the constraints between $X_{(i)}$ and $M_{i(i)}$ using a new term based on Augmented Lagrangian method of multiplier with multiplies $\{Y_i\}_{i=1}^N$ [8]:

$$\min_{X,\{M_i\}_{i=1}^N,\{Y_i\}_{i=1}^N} \|DSX - T\|^2 + \lambda_{rank} \sum_{i=1}^N \alpha_i \|M_{i(i)}\|_{tr} + \lambda_{tv} TV(X) +$$

$$\sum_{i=1}^N \frac{\rho}{2} (\|X - M_i + Y_i\|^2 - \|Y_i\|^2) \tag{5}$$

According to ADMM [8], we break Eq. (5) into three sub-problems below that need to be solved for iteratively updating the variables.

**Subproblem 1:** Update $X^{(k+1)}$ by minimizing:

$$\arg \min_X \|DSX - T\|^2 + \lambda_{tv} TV(X) + \sum_{i=1}^N \frac{\rho}{2} \|X - M_i^{(k)} + Y_i^{(k)}\|^2 \tag{6}$$

This subproblem can be solved by gradient descent with step size $dt$.

**Subproblem 2:** Update $\left\{M_i^{(k+1)}\right\}_{i=1}^N$ by minimizing:

$$\min_{\{M_i\}_{i=1}^N} \lambda_{rank} \sum_{i=1}^N \alpha_i \|M_{i(i)}\|_{tr} + \sum_{i=1}^N \frac{\rho}{2} \|X^{(k+1)} - M_i + Y_i^{(k)}\|^2 \tag{7}$$

which can be solved using a close-form solution according to [11]:

$$M_i = fold_i \left[ SVT_{\lambda_{rank}\alpha_i/\rho} \left( X_{(i)}^{(k+1)} + Y_{i(i)}^{(k)} \right) \right] \tag{8}$$

where $fold_i(\cdot)$ is the inverse operator of $unfold_i(\cdot)$, i.e., $fold_i(M_{i(i)}) = M_i$. $SVT(\cdot)$ is the Singular Value Thresholding operator [11] using $\lambda_{rank}\alpha_i/\rho$ as the shrinkage parameter.

**Subproblem 3:** Update $\left\{Y_i^{(k+1)}\right\}_{i=1}^N$ by:

$$Y_i^{(k+1)} = Y_i^{(k)} + \left( X^{(k+1)} - M_i^{(k+1)} \right) \tag{9}$$

Parameters are optimized based on a small set of datasets. In this work, we set $\alpha_1 = \alpha_2 = \alpha_3 = 1/3$, $\lambda_{rank} = 0.01$, $\lambda_{TV} = 0.01$, $dt = 0.1$, and the maximum iteration as

---

Algorithm 1. Low-Rank Total Variation (LRTV) for Image Super Resolution

---

Input:     Low-resolution image $T$;
Output:     Reconstructed high-resolution image $X$;
Initialize: $X = upsample(T)^*$, $M = 0$, $Y = 0$.
Repeat
1. Update $X$ based on Eq. (6);
2. Update $M$ based on Eq. (7);
3. Update $Y$ based on Eq. (9);
4. Until difference in the cost function (Eq. (5)) is less than $\varepsilon$;
End

---

\* The $upsample(\cdot)$ operator is implemented by nearest-neighbor interpolation.

200. The difference between iterations is measured by $\|X^k - X^{k-1}\|/\|T\|$, and the program is stopped when this difference is less than $\varepsilon = 1e - 5$.

## 3     Experiments

### 3.1     Low-Rank Representation

We first evaluated whether brain images can be sufficiently characterized using low-rank representations. We selected a representative 2D slice from an adult T1 MR image in Brainweb (http://www.bic.mni.mcgill.ca/brainweb/), which has a size of 181×181 and in-plane resolution of 1 mm (Fig. 2). We then performed singular value decomposition (SVD) on this image to obtain its 181 eigenvalues. As shown in Fig. 2, the eigenvalues decrease dramatically, with most values being close to zero. We reconstructed the image after removing the small eigenvalues, and compared it with the original image. Peak signal-to-noise ratio (PSNR) is used to evaluate the quality of reconstruction: $PSNR = 20 * log10(\|Truth\|/\|Truth - Recovered\|)$.

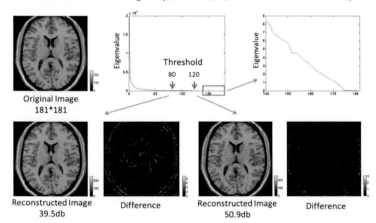

**Fig. 2.** Low-rank representation of brain images. Top row shows the original image, eigenvalue plot, and zoomed eigenvalue plot of indices from 140 to 181. Bottom row shows the two reconstructed images and their differences with the original image by using top 80 and 120 eigenvalues, respectively.

The result shows that, by using the top 80 eigenvalues, the reconstructed image has high PSNR (39.5db), although some edge information in the brain boundary is lost. However, when using the top 120 eigenvalues (out of 181), the resulting image does not show visual differences with respect to the original image. For the 3D Brainweb image with size of 181×217×181, its rank can actually be computed by the average rank of its 3 unfolded 2D images, which is thus less than its longest image size 217. This rank is very low, compared to its voxel number of $7.1×10^6$. Our analysis suggests that brain images can be represented using the low-rank approximations.

## 3.2    Experimental Setting

We applied our method to a set of down-sampled and blurred 3D brain images and evaluated whether our method can successfully recover the original high-resolution images (Fig. 3). Blurring was implemented using a Gaussian kernel with a standard deviation of 1 voxel. The blurred image was then down-sampled by averaging every 8 voxels (to simulate the partial volume effect), resulting in half of the original resolution. The quality of reconstruction of all methods was evaluated by comparing with the ground-truth images using PSNR.

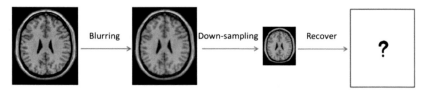

**Fig. 3.** Simulation of low-resolution image from high-resolution image

Our method was evaluated on two publicly available datasets. First, we randomly select 30 adult subjects from ADNI (http://www.loni.ucla.edu/ADNI), with 10 from Alzheimer's disease (AD), 10 from mild cognitive impairment (MCI), and 10 from normal controls. Their ages were 75±8 years at MRI scan. T1 MR images were acquired with 166 sagittal slices at the resolution of 0.95×0.95×1.2 $mm^3$. Second, we randomly select 20 pediatric subjects from NDAR (http://ndar.nih.gov/), with age of 11±3 years at MRI scan. T1 MR images were also acquired with 124 sagittal slices at the resolution of 0.94×0.94×1.3 $mm^3$.

## 3.3    Results

Fig. 4 shows the representative image SR results of an adult scan (upper panel) and a pediatric scan (lower panel). For the first row of each panel, from left to right show the input image, the results of nearest-neighbor interpolation, cubic interpolation, NLM based up-sampling [5], TV based up-sampling [10], proposed LRTV method, and ground truth. Of note, here we used the implementation of NLM released by authors (https://sites.google.com/site/pierrickcoupe/). We implemented TV through the proposed method by setting $\lambda_{rank} = 0$, $\rho = 0$, and solving only the subproblem 1.

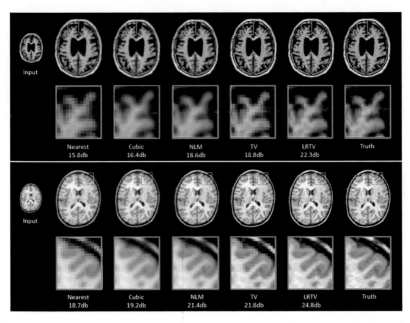

**Fig. 4.** Results for an adult scan (upper panel) and a pediatric scan (lower panel). In each panel, the first row is the input image and second row is the closeup view of selected regions.

Closeup views of selected regions are shown for better visualization. It can be observed that the results of both the nearest-neighbor and cubic interpolation methods show severe blurring artifacts. The contrast is enhanced in the results of NLM and TV up-sampling methods, while the proposed LRTV method preserves edges best and achieves the highest PSNR values.

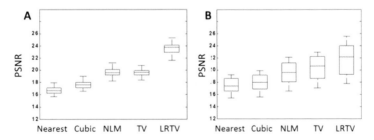

**Fig. 5.** Boxplot of PSNR results for (A) adult dataset and (B) pediatric dataset. The proposed LRTV method significantly outperforms all other comparison methods (p<0.01).

Quantitative results on the images of 30 adults and 20 pediatric subjects are shown in Fig. 5. Our proposed method significantly outperforms all other comparison methods (p<0.01). Results on adult subjects demonstrate less variance and higher accuracy than that of pediatric subjects, which may be because the image quality is higher in the matured brain and clearer gyri/sulci patterns appear in the adult images. No significant difference was found between the adult subjects of AD, MCI, and controls.

## 4    Conclusion and Future Work

We have presented a novel super-resolution method for recovering a high-resolution image from a single low-resolution image. For the first time, we show that estimation with a combined low-rank and total-variation regularization is a viable solution to the SR problem. This combination brings together global and local information for effective recovery of the high-dimensional image. Experimental results indicate that our method outperforms the nearest interpolation, cubic interpolation, NLM- and TV-based up-sampling. It is worth noting that the interpolation methods (nearest, cubic) do not estimate the image generation process, which is the intrinsic limitation of that kind of methods. While for TV and NLM, they used the same model as the proposed method, so the comparisons are fair. Meanwhile, although our method is developed for single-image SR, it can be easily generalized to multiple-image SR. Our future work will be dedicated to extend the proposed method to longitudinal scans, i.e., images acquired from the same subject at different time points.

## References

1. Liu, J., Musialski, P., Wonka, P., Ye, J.: Tensor Completion for Estimating Missing Values in Visual Data. IEEE Transactions on Pattern Analysis and Machine Intelligence 35, 208–220 (2013)
2. Netflix: Netflix prize webpage (2007), http://www.netflixprize.com/
3. Candès, E.J., Recht, B.: Exact matrix completion via convex optimization. Foundations of Computational Mathematics 9, 717–772 (2009)
4. Park, S.C., Park, M.K., Kang, M.G.: Super-resolution image reconstruction: a technical overview. IEEE Signal Processing Magazine 20, 21–36 (2003)
5. Manjón, J.V., Coupé, P., Buades, A., Fonov, V., Louis Collins, D., Robles, M.: Non-local MRI upsampling. Medical Image Analysis 14, 784–792 (2010)
6. Rousseau, F.: A non-local approach for image super-resolution using intermodality priors. Medical Image Analysis 14, 594 (2010)
7. Chambolle, A., Lions, P.-L.: Image recovery via total variation minimization and related problems. Numerische Mathematik 76, 167–188 (1997)
8. Boyd, S., Parikh, N., Chu, E., Peleato, B., Eckstein, J.: Distributed optimization and statistical learning via the alternating direction method of multipliers. Foundations and Trends in Machine Learning 3, 1–122 (2011)
9. Rudin, L.I., Osher, S., Fatemi, E.: Nonlinear total variation based noise removal algorithms. Physica D: Nonlinear Phenomena 60, 259–268 (1992)
10. Marquina, A., Osher, S.J.: Image super-resolution by TV-regularization and Bregman iteration. Journal of Scientific Computing 37, 367–382 (2008)
11. Cai, J.-F., Candès, E.J., Shen, Z.: A singular value thresholding algorithm for matrix completion. SIAM Journal on Optimization 20, 1956–1982 (2010)

# First Use of Mini Gamma Cameras for Intra-operative Robotic SPECT Reconstruction

Philipp Matthies[1], Kanishka Sharma[1], Aslı Okur[1,2], José Gardiazabal[1,2],
Jakob Vogel[1], Tobias Lasser[1,3], and Nassir Navab[1]

[1] Computer Aided Medical Procedures (CAMP),
Technische Universität München, Germany
[2] Department of Nuclear Medicine, Klinikum Rechts der Isar,
Technische Universität München, Germany
[3] Institute of Biomathematics and Biometry, Helmholtz Zentrum München, Germany

**Abstract.** Different types of nuclear imaging systems have been used in the past, starting with pre-operative gantry-based SPECT systems and gamma cameras for 2D imaging of radioactive distributions. The main applications are concentrated on diagnostic imaging, since traditional SPECT systems and gamma cameras are bulky and heavy. With the development of compact gamma cameras with good resolution and high sensitivity, it is now possible to use them without a fixed imaging gantry. Mounting the camera onto a robot arm solves the weight issue, while also providing a highly repeatable and reliable acquisition platform. In this work we introduce a novel robotic setup performing scans with a mini gamma camera, along with the required calibration steps, and show the first SPECT reconstructions. The results are extremely promising, both in terms of image quality as well as reproducibility. In our experiments, the novel setup outperformed a commercial fhSPECT system, reaching accuracies comparable to state-of-the-art SPECT systems.

## 1 Introduction

During the last years, evolving technology has enabled to move further towards intra-operative imaging. This is of tremendous interest, as pre-operative datasets can only be used to a limited extent during surgery. The reason are non-linear discrepancies between the older dataset and the actual situation, as caused for instance by a different patient position or organ deformations. Deformable registration methods exist, but their behavior is usually not sufficiently well-determined to be clinically applicable. Many intra-operative imaging modalities are now natural components of OR equipment, such as Ultrasound or X-ray C-Arm.

A rather recent example is freehand SPECT (fhSPECT) [1, 2] which aims at providing intra-operative nuclear imaging. In SPECT, a radioactive tracer will (ideally) concentrate within a certain targeted anatomical structure, and radioactivity counts acquired from known poses with intersecting perspectives can be used to tomographically reconstruct this distribution. Such information can, when provided in real time, be used for navigation purposes, or to check the

K. Mori et al. (Eds.): MICCAI 2013, Part I, LNCS 8149, pp. 163–170, 2013.

success of an ongoing procedure. Several groups report on the use of fhSPECT in different surgical procedures [3–5].

The fhSPECT system basically consists of a hand-held gamma probe (containing one detector, like a Geiger counter) yielding activity counts, and an optical tracking system for locating the former. The surgeon will move the probe over the surface of the region of interest and collect pose/activity pairs along the way. The major difference between a diagnostic SPECT system and fhSPECT is obviously the number and spatial distribution of measurements. While the gantry of a stationary scanner provides statistical significance and good coverage by design, the performance of fhSPECT depends strongly on the abilities of the human operator doing the scan. An inexperienced user will most likely collect biased input data, for instance by leaving out important probe poses or by aiming the probe towards an expected hotspot, thus leaving out important zero-measurements required to carve away regions of no activity. In order to improve the situation, several directions can be taken. One option is to replace the gamma probe, known to have problems in regions with higher background or overlapping activities, with a gamma camera [6], thus obtaining more readings and statistically more meaningful measurements at the same time. Providing measurements on a pixel grid, the device was very bulky while requiring very long acquisition times of $10[min]$ and more, and was therefore not suited for intra-operative use. Today, portable mini gamma cameras are available, which weigh less than $1[\mathrm{kg}]$, while offering good resolution and sensitivity.

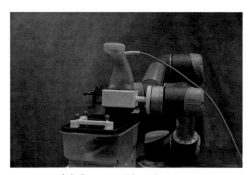
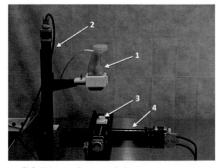

(a) Setup with robot arm          (b) Setup for model measurement

**Fig. 1.** (1a) Setup with gamma camera attached to robot arm. (1b) Positioning table with gamma camera (1) attached to acquire lookup tables. Custom made parts are used to align the mini gamma camera with the positioning table axes (2 and 4) and to guarantee alignment of radioactive source (3) in front of the detector.

Another important component is the use of a robot arm to guide the imaging sensor, making the scanning process and the image quality reproducible and reliable as it is still not practical to perform hand-held reconstructions on a regular basis. Several classical imaging modalities have recently been combined with robot technology such as C-arm X-ray [7] and laparoscopic ultrasound [8].

Bowsher et al. proposed a robotic multi-pinhole SPECT system [9], however only computer simulations were presented. Also for fhSPECT, first steps towards robotic guidance have been taken [10, 11]. For the gamma camera, due to its intrinsic weight and the need of holding it steadily to properly identify the origin of the gamma emission, a robot arm is a natural choice. This, plus the advantage of fast and precise mechanical tracking, provides a perfect match for the gamma camera setup Potential clinical applications of the robotic mini gamma camera include sentinel lymph node biopsies for breast or head and neck cancer as with fhSPECT, however with faster and more accurate reconstructions allowing to provide better images in more complicated cases such as cervix cancer.

## 2   Materials and Methods

### 2.1   Hardware Setup

The setup consists of a mini gamma camera (Crystal Imager, Crystal Photonics, Germany), mounted on a robot arm (UR5, Universal Robots, Denmark) using a custom-made holder, see Fig. 1a. An optical tracking system (Polaris Vicra, Northern Digital Inc., Canada) was used to track the phantom.

The mini gamma camera comprises of a $4 \times 4[cm^2]$ CdZnTe crystal which has $16 \times 16$ pixels. The collimator is made of lead and tungsten and measures $11.15[mm]$ in length. It has 256 square holes with sizes of $2.16 \times 2.16[mm^2]$ each.

To measure an approximate gamma camera model, the camera was mounted to a precision positioning system (OWIS, Germany), see Fig. 1b. This positioning system was preferred for its very low repeatability error ($< 15[\mu m]$).

For comparison, a fhSPECT system (declipseSPECT, SurgicEye, Germany) with a single pixel detector (HiSens, Crystal Photonics, Germany) was employed.

### 2.2   Gamma Camera Modeling

For SPECT reconstruction, a model of the gamma camera response is needed. We measure an approximation using a $^{57}$Co calibration source ($0.97[MBq]$ at time of acquisition) and a three axes precision positioning system. As illustrated in Fig. 1b, the mini gamma camera is mounted on a holder (1) that can move along the z-axis (2). The calibration source is mounted on a holder (3) that can be moved in x- and y-direction (4).

The source is scanned in a $150 \times 150 \times 150[mm^3]$ grid with step size $5[mm]$ over the centered source. A volume of $50 \times 50 \times 50[mm^3]$ directly centered in front of the camera is rastered with a finer step size of $1[mm]$. At each grid position, an image is acquired with $7[s]$ exposure time.

The resulting measurements were corrected by a homogeneity correction factor and an energy window of $\pm10\%$ was applied after energy calibration had been performed. For each detector pixel $k$ the measurements are then stored in a lookup table $\ell^k$ for later use in the reconstruction method. The area covered by the lookup table is illustrated in Fig. 2a. Fig. 2b shows a 3D rendering of the values of the lookup table for one example detector pixel.

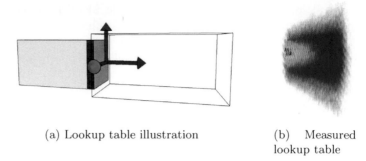

(a) Lookup table illustration          (b)    Measured
                                       lookup table

**Fig. 2.** (2a) Drawing of gamma camera with volume of lookup table in front of it illustrating the dimensions and orientations of the reference coordinate system. (2b) Graph showing an exemplary lookup table for an arbitrary pixel. The gamma camera is centered on the left face of the volume pointing to the right. Contributions of the different voxels in the volume in front of the camera to the specific pixel are shown. Red indicates a high contribution, blue a low one.

### 2.3    Coordinate Systems Calibration

Corresponding activity measurements and camera poses are the key to tomographic reconstruction. The optical tracking system provides pose information for a tracking target *cam* mounted to the camera, but in order to relate measurements via the lookup tables to the world system, the world locations of the detector pixels are required.

First, we define a *detector* coordinate system compatible to the lookup table (Fig. 2a), centered on the detector face, $x$- and $y$- axes aligned with the pixel grid and $z$ pointing away from the camera towards the measurement region. In order to obtain the respective transformation $^{cam}\mathbf{T}_{detector}$, we first compute the *detector* coordinate system in absolute terms and derive the relative transformation afterwards.

Consequently, we measure the four corner points of the detector face using a calibrated optical pointer (Fig. 3), yielding $\mathbf{c}_{\pm x, \pm y} \in \mathbb{R}^3$. From these four points, we compute the mean and obtain the center/base point $\mathbf{O}_{detector} = \mu(\mathbf{c}_{\pm x, \pm y})$ where $\mu$ denotes a function yielding the $n$-dimensional arithmetic mean. Using the averaged delta vectors $\mathbf{v}'_x = \mu(\mathbf{c}_{+x, \pm y} - \mathbf{c}_{-x, \pm y})$ and $\mathbf{v}'_y = \mu(\mathbf{c}_{\pm x, +y} - \mathbf{c}_{\pm x, -y})$, we then compute the $x$- and $y$-axes as $\mathbf{v}_x = \mathbf{v}'_x / \|\mathbf{v}'_x\|$ and $\mathbf{v}_y = \mathbf{v}'_y / \|\mathbf{v}'_y\|$. The $z$-axis is finally computed via the cross product as $\mathbf{v}_z = \mathbf{v}_x \times \mathbf{v}_y$. From the base point and the three axes we obtain the detector coordinate system, and compute the incremental transformation $^{cam}\mathbf{T}_{detector}$.

### 2.4    Reconstruction Method

Let $f : V \to \mathbb{R}$ denote the activity to be reconstructed in the volume of interest $V \subset \mathbb{R}^3$. Given a set of $n$ basis functions $b_i : V \to \mathbb{R}$, we discretize $f \approx \sum_{i=1}^{n} x_i b_i$

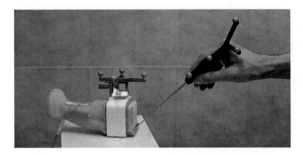

**Fig. 3.** An optical pointer was used to correlate the detector front face with the optical tracking target attached to the mini gamma camera

with a coefficient vector $\mathbf{x} = (x_i) \in \mathbb{R}^n$. In this work, the $b_i$ are voxel basis functions, chosen in a $56 \times 50 \times 22$ grid with voxel size $2.5 \times 2.5 \times 2.5 [mm^3]$.

The measured lookup tables $\ell^k$ at each gamma camera pixel $k$ are then used to map each voxel $b_i$ to a camera measurement $m_j^k$ at position $p_j$ via nearest neighbor interpolation, yielding a linear measurement model $\mathcal{M}_j^k(b_i)$. For each camera position $p_j$ and camera pixel $k$ we then have $\mathcal{M}_j^k(f) = m_j^k$ using the model $\mathcal{M}_j^k$, with $\mathbf{m} = (m_j^k) \in \mathbb{R}^l$ denoting the camera readouts. Together, this allows to formulate the discretized reconstruction problem as

$$m_j^k = \mathcal{M}_j^k(f) \approx \sum_{i=1}^{n} x_i \mathcal{M}_j^k(b_i).$$

Using the short notation $a_{ji}^k = \mathcal{M}_j^k(b_i)$ we define the system matrix $\mathbf{A} = (a_{ji}^k)$. Now the reconstruction problem can be formulated as solving an inconsistent system of linear equations $\mathbf{Ax} = \mathbf{m}$ [10]. After removal of columns and rows being entirely zero from $A$ to avoid singularities, we solve the least squares problem $\min_{\mathbf{x}} \|\mathbf{Ax} - \mathbf{m}\|^2$ using a standard maximum likelihood expectation maximization (MLEM) algorithm with 20 iterations. Finally, the computed approximation to $\mathbf{x}$ allows computation of the desired activity map $f$.

## 2.5   Experimental Procedure

A phantom was made mimicking a sentinel lymph node scenario. Three hollow spheres ($2 \times 0.2[ml]$ and $0.1ml$) were screwed into a plastic box and an optical tracking target was attached on the lid, as shown in Fig.4a. The spheres were filled with $^{99m}$Tc (650 [kBq] in sphere (1), 850 [kBq] in (2) and 500 [kBq] in (3), cf. Fig. 4b). Five robotic gamma camera scans were performed with an acquisition time of $60[s]$ for each scan from the directions shown in Fig. 4b. The robot was moving to 6 previously defined positions on 3 orthogonal planes and takes gamma camera acquisitions of $10[s]$. In each scan the angle, position and orientation of the gamma camera was slightly changed. For comparison we also scanned 5 times with the fhSPECT system with a duration of $60[s]$ and comparable scanning directions.

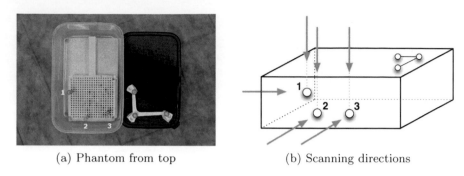

(a) Phantom from top                    (b) Scanning directions

**Fig. 4.** (4a) Phantom from top view with the three spheres filled with radioactive $^{99m}$Tc solution, the lid with the optical tracking target attached to it lies beneath the box to reveal the view inside. (4b) Scanning directions of the robot moving the mini gamma camera. All the spheres were scanned from one side and from the top. The freehand gamma probe scans covered the same three sides homogeneously.

## 3    Evaluation and Results

Five gamma camera scans were performed and compared to a CT image of the phantom as ground truth with the $^{99m}$Tc filled spheres clearly visible. The reconstructions yielded mean distances to their respective ground truth of $4.3[mm]$ ($\sigma = 0.3[mm]$, sphere 1), $4.0[mm](\sigma = 0.9[mm]$, sphere 2) and $5.6[mm]$ ($\sigma = 3.4[mm]$, sphere 3). In all five scans the three spheres could be reconstructed successfully, only in one reconstruction a larger artifact close to one sphere showed up, in two other scans one small artifact was visible close to the correctly reconstructed spheres and to the border of the volume. These artifacts result from the nature of the used model as the lookup tables contain the largest values close to the detector and when the volume of interest is very close to the detector positions, the border regions are intensified.

The fhSPECT reconstructions were then compared to the ground truth as well. Only in one case all three spheres could be reconstructed, although combined with additional artifacts (cp. arrows in Fig. 5b). In the remaining four scans 2 of the 3 hot spots could be detected without major artifacts in the images. The mean distance of the reconstructed spheres to their respective ground truth positions were $20.4[mm](\sigma = 3.1[mm])$, sphere 1) and $16.8[mm](\sigma = 2.2[mm])$, sphere 2). Sphere 3 could only be reconstructed in one scan with a distance of $27.2[mm]$ to its ground truth position. This resulted with the tradeoff of large artifacts in the image. However, total counts acquired with the mini gamma camera were more than 10 times higher and the fhSPECT scanning time is considered short compared to clinical practice.

Fig. 5a shows a reconstruction performed using a gamma camera mounted to a robot arm and scanning the phantom from 6 different positions for $10[s]$ each. Fig. 5b shows a reconstruction performed with fhSPECT device and a gamma probe after scanning the volume of interest for $60[s]$ from three orthogonal sides.

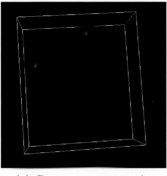

(a) Camera reconstruction

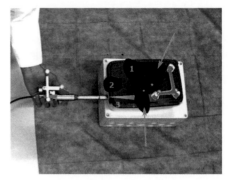

(b) Probe reconstruction

**Fig. 5.** Reconstruction performed using a gamma camera mounted to a robot arm (5a) and with fhSPECT device and a gamma probe (5b). Arrows indicate artifacts.

# 4   Discussion and Conclusion

The upgrade from a single gamma detector to a compact gamma camera for 3D freehand scans has a huge impact on the quality of the tomographic reconstructions achieved by comparable computation times ($< 1[min]$). The fact that camera data enables reconstructing hot-spots with lower activity, the novel system allows faster acquisitions and lower tracer doses, thus limiting the exposure, and therefore the risk associated with the procedure.

This is, of course, not without trade-offs, most importantly the weight of the camera. This can be solved by using a robot arm like it is proposed in this paper, or by a mechanical construction to support it.

The ability of reconstructing images with an accuracy close to a diagnostic SPECT machine, coupled with the low presence of artifacts and the increased precision of the hot-spot relocation are clear benefits for the medical workflow. However, the purpose of intra-operative SPECT is guidance and not diagnosis.

The use of a robot arm enables the use of optimized acquisition trajectories, or feedback loops, since it is also possible to use the current acquisitions to perform on-the-fly adaptive trajectories. This combination can lead to even shorter acquisition times, while keeping the quality constant. The robot used for the experiments is not a medical device, and it does not fulfill the minimum safety requirements for its use in the operation room [12]. However, it is possible to use for phantom studies and ex-vivo experiments.

Future applications could include radioembolization therapy [13] using $^{99m}$Tc-MAA in concordance with intra-operative CT images to better localize any suspicious foci of activity.

**Acknowledgements.** This work was partially funded by the DFG SFB 824 and the DFG cluster of excellence MAP.

# References

1. Wendler, T., Hartl, A., Lasser, T., Traub, J., Daghighian, F., Ziegler, S.I., Navab, N.: Towards Intra-operative 3D Nuclear Imaging: Reconstruction of 3D Radioactive Distributions Using Tracked Gamma Probes. In: Ayache, N., Ourselin, S., Maeder, A. (eds.) MICCAI 2007, Part II. LNCS, vol. 4792, pp. 909–917. Springer, Heidelberg (2007)
2. Wendler, T., Herrmann, K., Schnelzer, A., Lasser, T., Traub, J., Kutter, O., Ehlerding, A., Scheidhauer, K., Schuster, T., Kiechle, M., Schwaiger, M., Navab, N., Ziegler, S.I., Buck, A.K.: First demonstration of 3-D lymphatic mapping in breast cancer using freehand SPECT. Eur. J. Nucl. Med. 37(8), 1452–1461 (2010)
3. Schnelzer, A., Ehlerding, A., Blümel, C., Okur, A., Scheidhauer, K., Paepke, S., Kiechle, M.: Showcase of intraoperative 3D imaging of the sentinel lymph node in a breast cancer patient using the new freehand SPECT technology. Breast Care 7(6), 484–486 (2012)
4. Heuveling, D.A., Karagozoglu, K.H., van Schie, A., van Weert, S., van Lingen, A., de Bree, R.: Sentinel node biopsy using 3D lymphatic mapping by freehand SPECT in early stage oral cancer: a new technique. Clin. Otolaryngol. 37(1), 89–90 (2012)
5. Naji, S., Tadros, A., Traub, J., Healy, C.: Case report: Improving the speed and accuracy of melanoma sentinel node biopsy with 3D intra-operative imaging. J. Plast. Reconstr. Aes. 64(12), 1712–1715 (2011)
6. Weinberg, I., Zawarzin, V., Pani, R., De Vincentes, G.: Implementing reconstruction with hand-held gamma cameras. In: IEEE Nuclear Science Symposium Conference Record, vol. 104, pp. 21/101–21/104 (2000)
7. Ganguly, A., Fieselmann, A., Marks, M., Rosenberg, J., Boese, J., Deuerling-Zheng, Y., Straka, M., Zaharchuck, G., Bammer, R., Fahrig, R.: Cerebral CT Perfusion Using an Interventional C-Arm Imaging System: Cerebral Blood Flow Measurements. Am. J. Neuroradiol. 32, 1525–1531 (2011)
8. Schneider, C., Guerrero, J., Nguan, C., Rohling, R., Salcudean, S.: Intra-operative "Pick-Up" Ultrasound for Robot Assisted Surgery with Vessel Extraction and Registration: A Feasibility Study. In: Taylor, R.H., Yang, G.-Z. (eds.) IPCAI 2011. LNCS, vol. 6689, pp. 122–132. Springer, Heidelberg (2011)
9. Bowsher, J., Yan, S., Roper, J., Giles, W., Yin, F.: TU-A-BRA-01: a robotic multi-pinhole SPECT system for onboard and other region-of-interest imaging, vol. 39, pp. 3887–3888. AAPM (2012)
10. Vogel, J., Reichl, T., Gardiazabal, J., Navab, N., Lasser, T.: Optimization of acquisition geometry for intra-operative tomographic imaging. In: Ayache, N., Delingette, H., Golland, P., Mori, K. (eds.) MICCAI 2012, Part III. LNCS, vol. 7512, pp. 42–49. Springer, Heidelberg (2012)
11. Gardiazabal, J., Reichl, T., Okur, A., Lasser, T., Navab, N.: First flexible robotic intra-operative nuclear imaging for image-guided surgery. In: Barratt, D., Cotin, S., Fichtinger, G., Jannin, P., Navab, N. (eds.) IPCAI 2013. LNCS, vol. 7915, pp. 81–90. Springer, Heidelberg (2013)
12. Taylor, R., Paul, H., Kazanzides, P., Mittelstadt, B., Hanson, W., Zuhars, J., Williamson, B., Musits, B., Glassman, E., Bargar, W.: Taming the bull: safety in a precise surgical robot. In: Fifth International Conference on Advanced Robotics (ICAR), vol. 1, pp. 865–870 (1991)
13. Peynircioğlu, B., Çil, B., Bozkurt, F., Aydemir, E., Uğur, O., Balkancı, F.: Radioembolization for the treatment of unresectable liver cancer: initial experience at a single center. Diagn. Interv. Radiol. 16(1), 70–78 (2010)

# Robust Model-Based 3D/3D Fusion Using Sparse Matching for Minimally Invasive Surgery

Dominik Neumann[1,2], Sasa Grbic[2,3], Matthias John[4], Nassir Navab[3],
Joachim Hornegger[1], and Razvan Ionasec[2]

[1] Pattern Recognition Lab, University of Erlangen-Nuremberg, Germany
[2] Imaging and Computer Vision, Siemens Corporate Research, Princeton, USA
[3] Computer Aided Medical Procedures, Technical University Munich, Germany
[4] Siemens AG, Healthcare Sector, Forchheim, Germany

**Abstract.** Classical surgery is being disrupted by minimally invasive and transcatheter procedures. As there is no direct view or access to the affected anatomy, advanced imaging techniques such as 3D C-arm CT and C-arm fluoroscopy are routinely used for intra-operative guidance. However, intra-operative modalities have limited image quality of the soft tissue and a reliable assessment of the cardiac anatomy can only be made by injecting contrast agent, which is harmful to the patient and requires complex acquisition protocols. We propose a novel sparse matching approach for fusing high quality pre-operative CT and non-contrasted, non-gated intra-operative C-arm CT by utilizing robust machine learning and numerical optimization techniques. Thus, high-quality patient-specific models can be extracted from the pre-operative CT and mapped to the intra-operative imaging environment to guide minimally invasive procedures. Extensive quantitative experiments demonstrate that our model-based fusion approach has an average execution time of 2.9 s, while the accuracy lies within expert user confidence intervals.

## 1 Introduction

Fluoroscopy guided cardiac interventions such as endovascular stenting, atrial ablation, closure of atrial/ventricular septal defects and transcatheter valve repair or replacement are a rapidly growing market. Compared to conventional open-heart surgeries, these procedures are expected to be less invasive, reduce procedural morbidity, mortality, and intervention cost, while accelerating patient recovery. For inoperable or high-risk patients, minimally invasive surgery is the only treatment option [1]. However, without direct access to the affected anatomy, advanced imaging is required to secure a safe and effective execution.

Overlays of 3D anatomical structures based on pre-operative data [2] can potentially provide valuable information for interventional guidance when displayed on live fluoroscopy. High-quality pre-operative 3D data is routinely acquired for diagnostic and planning purposes by means of Computed Tomography, Magnetic Resonance Imaging or Echocardiography. However, direct 3D pre-operative to 2D fluoroscopy registration is difficult to solve, especially within the intra-operative setup that does not allow for user interaction or time-consuming processing.

K. Mori et al. (Eds.): MICCAI 2013, Part I, LNCS 8149, pp. 171–178, 2013.

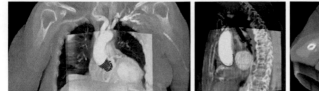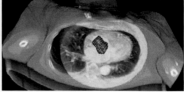

**Fig. 1.** Yellow: C-arm CT, gray: fused high-quality CT, blue: anatomical model

C-arm CT is emerging as a novel modality that can acquire 3D CT-like volumes directly in the OR in the same coordinate system as 2D fluoroscopy, which overcomes the need for 2D/3D registration. For most procedures, the patients are older and therefore, a safe execution of the procedure is the dominating factor [3]. Some methods work directly on the C-arm CT images [4] to extract patient-specific models for procedure guidance. However, acquiring high-quality, contrasted, and motion compensated C-arm CT images is challenging and clinicians would prefer a much simpler protocol without contrast or gating. Today, manual or semi-automatic tools are used to align the pre-operative CT and the intra-operative C-arm CT. Thus, C-arm CT serves as a bridge between 3D pre-operative data and 2D live fluoroscopy.

Multi-modal 3D/3D registration algorithms can be utilized to automate the process of aligning the pre-operative scan with the C-arm CT. [5] uses mutual information to cope with intensity inconsistencies between CT and MR and [6] presents an atlas-based approach to track the myocardium and ventricles from MR data. However, these methods are computationally expensive, and without appropriate guidance of a shape prior likely to converge into local minima.

We propose a method to fuse 3D pre-operative high-quality anatomical information with live 2D intra-operative imaging via non-contrasted 3D C-arm CT (Fig. 1). Robust learning-based methods are employed to automatically extract patient-specific models of target and anchor anatomies from CT. Anchor anatomies have correspondences in the pre- and intra-operative images, while target anatomies are not visible in the intra-operative image, but essential to the procedure. A novel sparse matching approach is employed to align the pre- and intra-operative anchor anatomies. Data and model uncertainties are learned and exploited during the matching process. Our method is able to cope with image artifacts, partially visible models, and does not require contrast agent.

## 2    Method

Our fully-automatic method (Fig. 2) fuses a pre-operative CT image $\mathcal{M}$ (moving) with an intra-operative C-arm CT image $\mathcal{F}$ (fixed), such that a target anatomy (aortic valve) is aligned. The process is based on an anchor anatomy $\mathcal{A}$ (pericardium) extracted from $\mathcal{M}$, and a probability map $\tilde{\mathcal{F}}$ derived from $\mathcal{F}$. Optimal transformation parameters $\hat{\boldsymbol{\theta}}$ are sought. $\boldsymbol{\theta} = (\boldsymbol{\phi_\theta}, \boldsymbol{t_\theta})$ represents a rigid transformation with Euler angles $\boldsymbol{\phi_\theta} = (\phi_x, \phi_y, \phi_z)$ and translation $\boldsymbol{t_\theta} = (t_x, t_y, t_z)$.

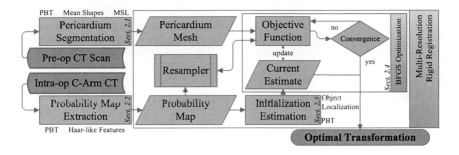

**Fig. 2.** Fusion workflow overview

## 2.1   Pericardium Segmentation

We use a recent method by Zheng et al. [7] to segment the patient-specific anchor anatomy $\mathcal{A}$ in $\mathcal{M}$ (Fig. 3(a)). Their technique consists of three main steps. First, the pose and scale of the heart is estimated using marginal space learning (MSL). Second, a mean shape based on manual annotations is aligned. In a third step, the parameters are refined using a boundary detector based on the probabilistic boosting tree (PBT) [8], followed by additional postprocessing.

## 2.2   Probability Map Extraction

A probability map $\tilde{\mathcal{F}}$ is created from $\mathcal{F}$ by evaluating a PBT classifier on each voxel (Fig. 3(b)). The classifier was trained to robustly delineate pericardium boundary regions in C-arm CT images utilizing Haar features to achieve robustness and computational efficiency. Medical experts created a database DB of pericardium annotations $\{\mathcal{P}\}$ on 393 interventional C-arm CT scans $\{\mathcal{V}\}$. For training, positive samples were generated with regard to the position of the voxels corresponding to points in the ground-truth mesh. The negative samples for each tuple in the database $(\mathcal{V}, \mathcal{P}) \in$ DB are based on randomly selected voxels $v \in \mathcal{V}$, where the distance of $v$ to all points in $\mathcal{P}$ exceeds a certain threshold.

## 2.3   Initialization Estimation

In order to find a reliable initialization $\theta^0 = (\phi_{\theta^0}, t_{\theta^0})$, our method recovers the offset $t_{\theta^0}$ between $\mathcal{M}$ and $\mathcal{F}$. We neglect the rotational error ($\phi_{\theta^0} = 0$), since it is rather small between the CT and the C-arm CT scan due to the acquisition protocols being similar as the patients adopt almost identical positions. Our solution is based on object localization, a concept from computer vision, which we formulate as a classification problem. We evaluate a PBT classifier trained using DB from Sect. 2.2 on each voxel and choose the one that is most likely to contain the pericardium center $c_{\mathcal{F}}$. Let $c_{\mathcal{A}}$ be the center of $\mathcal{A}$, then $\theta^0 = (\phi_{\theta^0}, -c_{\mathcal{A}} + c_{\mathcal{F}})$. Robust detections were achieved by utilizing $\tilde{\mathcal{F}}$ as the input for training and detection, since the probability maps look similar for both contrasted and non-contrasted images, because the classifier for $\tilde{\mathcal{F}}$ was trained on both types of volumes. Thus, the method can be used with or without contrast agent injected.

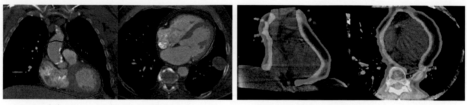

|  |  |
| --- | --- |
| (a) Pre-operative CT scan | (b) Intra-operative C-arm CT scan |

**Fig. 3.** Volume slices overlaid by (a) segmented pericardium, (b) probability map: red indicates high likelihood of pericardium occurrence, blue/transparent: low probability

### 2.4 Optimization Strategy

$\boldsymbol{\theta}$ is refined within a numerical quasi-Newton optimization framework utilizing the BFGS update rule. To compensate for potential initial coarse misalignment, the concept of multi-resolution optimization is exploited by optimizing in a coarse-to-fine manner on various granularity levels of $\tilde{\mathcal{F}}$ (4, 2 and 1 mm).

**Objective Function.** We aim to find the transformation $\hat{\boldsymbol{\theta}} = \operatorname{argmin}_{\boldsymbol{\theta}} f$ that yields the minimal objective function value. $f$ depends on $\mathcal{A}$ and $\tilde{\mathcal{F}}$:

$$f(\boldsymbol{\theta} \mid \mathcal{A}, \tilde{\mathcal{F}}) = \frac{\sum_{\boldsymbol{p} \in \mathcal{A}} \text{is\_inside}(\boldsymbol{\theta}(\boldsymbol{p}), \tilde{\mathcal{F}}) \cdot \psi(\boldsymbol{\theta}(\boldsymbol{p}), \tilde{\mathcal{F}})}{\sum_{\boldsymbol{p} \in \mathcal{A}} \text{is\_inside}(\boldsymbol{\theta}(\boldsymbol{p}), \tilde{\mathcal{F}})} \quad . \tag{1}$$

$\boldsymbol{p}$ denotes a point in $\mathcal{A}$ and $\boldsymbol{p}' = \boldsymbol{\theta}(\boldsymbol{p})$ is that point transformed w.r.t. $\boldsymbol{\theta}$. The indicator function is\_inside$(\boldsymbol{p}', \tilde{\mathcal{F}})$ evaluates to 1, if $\boldsymbol{p}'$ is inside the physical boundaries of the volume $\tilde{\mathcal{F}}$, otherwise 0. $\psi(\boldsymbol{p}', \tilde{\mathcal{F}})$ returns a value inversely proportional to the probabilistic prediction at the voxel $\in \tilde{\mathcal{F}}$ where $\boldsymbol{p}'$ is located. When the number of points within the boundaries of the volume is below a certain threshold, an alternative objective function prevents $\mathcal{A}$ and $\tilde{\mathcal{F}}$ from diverging.

**Gradient Computation.** The BFGS method relies on the gradient $\nabla$ in order to estimate an approximation of the inverse of the Hessian. Unfortunately, $f$ is highly complex and therefore does not allow for analytical derivations. Hence, we approximate $\tilde{\nabla} \approx \nabla f(\boldsymbol{\theta} \mid \mathcal{A}, \tilde{\mathcal{F}})$ component-wise with finite differences:

$$\tilde{\nabla}_i = f(\boldsymbol{\theta} + \boldsymbol{\delta}^i \mid \mathcal{A}, \tilde{\mathcal{F}}) - f(\boldsymbol{\theta} \mid \mathcal{A}, \tilde{\mathcal{F}}) \quad . \tag{2}$$

$\tilde{\nabla}_i$ denotes the $i^{\text{th}}$ component of $\tilde{\nabla}$ and $\boldsymbol{\delta}^i$ is a 6D offset vector where all components are zero, except for the $i^{\text{th}}$ component $\boldsymbol{\delta}_i^i$, which is set to a particular step size. Despite its asymmetric computation scheme, the gradient is sufficiently stable in this application. For the translational components, $\boldsymbol{\delta}_i^i$ equals the resolution of $\tilde{\mathcal{F}}$. This choice asserts that (2) does not evaluate to zero, since the majority of points in $\mathcal{A}$ transformed w.r.t. $\boldsymbol{\theta}$ will correspond to a different $\boldsymbol{v} \in \tilde{\mathcal{F}}$ than their corresponding points transformed w.r.t. $\boldsymbol{\theta} + \boldsymbol{\delta}^i$. Regarding the rotational components, we experimentally determined that a spacing proportional to the resolution of $\tilde{\mathcal{F}}$ (e.g. $\boldsymbol{\delta}_i^i = 1°$ when resolution is 1 mm) works properly.

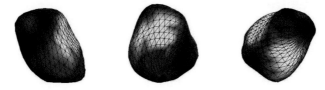

**Fig. 4.** Prior weights, dark colors: small weights, bright colors: high influence

While computing the translational gradient components is straightforward, rotation in 3D poses a major problem due to its inherent non-linearity and co-dependencies. We address these issues by utilizing a linearization of rotation matrices $\boldsymbol{R}$ using a first order approximation $\tilde{\boldsymbol{R}}$ as proposed by Mitra et al. [9]. Let $\boldsymbol{R_\theta}$ be the 3D rotation matrix defined by $\boldsymbol{\phi_\theta} = (\phi_x, \phi_y, \phi_z)$ with $\boldsymbol{R_\theta}^{-1} = \boldsymbol{R_\theta}^{\top}$ and $\det(\boldsymbol{R_\theta}) = 1$. Its first-order approximation is given by

$$\tilde{\boldsymbol{R}}_{\boldsymbol{\theta}} = \begin{pmatrix} 1 & -\phi_z & \phi_y \\ \phi_z & 1 & -\phi_x \\ -\phi_y & \phi_x & 1 \end{pmatrix} \approx \boldsymbol{R_\theta} \ . \tag{3}$$

It is important to mention that $\tilde{\boldsymbol{R}}_{\boldsymbol{\theta}} \approx \boldsymbol{R_\theta}$ only holds under small motion ($\|\boldsymbol{\phi}\|_2 \to 0$). Hence, we cannot use $\tilde{\boldsymbol{R}}_{\boldsymbol{\theta}}$ for large angles without introducing errors. Therefore, we compute the rotational components of $\tilde{\nabla}$ using a composite transformation. First, a point $\boldsymbol{p} \in \mathcal{A}$ is transformed w.r.t. the current $\boldsymbol{\theta}$ using the exact Euler-angle representation to generate an intermediate point $\boldsymbol{p}''$. Second, $\boldsymbol{p}''$ is rotated according to the minor rotation $\boldsymbol{\delta}^i$ to yield $\boldsymbol{p}'$ using $\tilde{\boldsymbol{R}}_{\boldsymbol{\theta}}$. Altogether, we get $\boldsymbol{p}' = \boldsymbol{\delta}^i(\boldsymbol{p}'') = \boldsymbol{\delta}^i(\boldsymbol{\theta}(\boldsymbol{p}))$. $\boldsymbol{p}'$ constitutes the first argument for is_inside and $\psi$ in (1) when computing the rotational components of $\tilde{\nabla}$ using (2).

**Prior Weights.** The classifier response (Sect. 2.2) is more reliable in some regions of the volumes compared to others. For instance see Fig. 3(b), where the areas close to the left ventricle and right atrium have high responses, while classification near the spine is noisy and the right ventricle region shows low confidence. Robustness and accuracy of our method could be improved significantly (cf. Sect. 3.1) by incorporating prior weights $\boldsymbol{w} = \{w_{\boldsymbol{p}} \mid \boldsymbol{p} \in \mathcal{A}\}$. Each point $\boldsymbol{p}$ in the pericardium model $\mathcal{A}$ is assigned a patient-independent weight $w_{\boldsymbol{p}}$. $\boldsymbol{w}$ increases the influence of those points that are likely to be located within a region of high confidence in $\tilde{\mathcal{F}}$, whereas a point that lies in a noisy or often falsely classified region gets penalized. Gradient magnitude, as well as the distance of a point to the upper and lower boundary of the pericardium were most useful for reliability predictions. Based on these observations and DB from Sect. 2.2, we computed values for $\boldsymbol{w}$ (Fig. 4). Incorporation of $\boldsymbol{w}$ into (1) yields

$$f(\boldsymbol{\theta} \mid \mathcal{A}, \tilde{\mathcal{F}}, \boldsymbol{w}) = \frac{\sum_{\boldsymbol{p} \in \mathcal{A}} \text{is\_inside}(\boldsymbol{\theta}(\boldsymbol{p}), \tilde{\mathcal{F}}) \cdot \psi(\boldsymbol{\theta}(\boldsymbol{p}), \tilde{\mathcal{F}}) \cdot w_{\boldsymbol{p}}}{\sum_{\boldsymbol{p} \in \mathcal{A}} \text{is\_inside}(\boldsymbol{\theta}(\boldsymbol{p}), \tilde{\mathcal{F}})} \ . \tag{4}$$

## 3   Experimental Results

We compiled a set of 88 corresponding clinical CT and C-arm CT volumes, each with an isotropic resolution of 1 mm. 18 image pairs are native, while 70 were acquired with contrast agent injected. Medical experts annotated the pericardium in each volume, 43 studies include annotations of the aortic valve (AV). The data is organized in a database $DB_{cl} = \{(\mathcal{V}_i, \check{\mathcal{V}}_i, \mathcal{P}_i, \check{\mathcal{P}}_i, \mathcal{R}_i, \check{\mathcal{R}}_i) \mid i = 1 \dots 88\}$. $\mathcal{V}_i$, $\mathcal{P}_i$ and $\mathcal{R}_i$ denote the $i^{\text{th}}$ CT volume, its pericardium and AV annotation. Analogously, $\check{\mathcal{V}}_i$, $\check{\mathcal{P}}_i$ and $\check{\mathcal{R}}_i$ denote these structures for the C-arm CT acquisition. The results are based on a symmetric mesh-to-mesh distance metric $\varepsilon$:

$$\varepsilon(\mathcal{X}, \mathcal{Y}) = \frac{1}{2} \left( \sum_{p \in \mathcal{X}} \min_{\triangle \in \mathcal{Y}} \varepsilon_{\text{p2t}}(p, \triangle) + \sum_{p \in \mathcal{Y}} \min_{\triangle \in \mathcal{X}} \varepsilon_{\text{p2t}}(p, \triangle) \right) , \tag{5}$$

where $\mathcal{X}$, $\mathcal{Y}$ are triangulated meshes and $\varepsilon_{\text{p2t}}(p, \triangle)$ denotes the point-to-triangle distance. Note that (5) might underestimate misalignment tangential to the surface. However, it is a fairly natural measure closely resembling visual assessment.

### 3.1   Quantitative Evaluation on Clinical Data

We evaluated our method on $DB_{cl}$ with both, prior weights (Sect. 2.4) enabled and disabled. In Table 1 (left), the left and right columns for each scenario show error statistics resulting from a comparison of the optimally transformed segmented pericardium $\hat{\theta}(\mathcal{A})$ and the ground-truth annotation in the C-arm CT volume $\check{\mathcal{P}}$, and results for a comparison of the transformed CT-based aortic valve $\hat{\theta}(\mathcal{R})$ and its C-arm based annotation $\check{\mathcal{R}}$, respectively. With prior weights incorporated, a registration accuracy of 5.60 ± 1.81 mm measured between the anchor anatomy (pericardium) is achieved. Furthermore, with an error of 4.63 ± 1.90 mm, the target anatomy (AV) is aligned very well. When the patient-independent weighting is ignored, the mean errors increase significantly by more than 35% regarding the pericardium and almost 55% for the AV. One reason is that more outliers are generated, having a strong influence on the overall errors. Hence, the prior information improves the fusion performance significantly.

### 3.2   Comparison to State-of-the-Art Fusion

We compared our model-to-image registration to an image-to-image fusion approach utilizing ITK, a state-of-the-art medical imaging library. Multi-resolution optimal parameters $\hat{\theta}_*$ were obtained by an optimizer for rigid versor transformations. We customized the maximum and minimum step lengths adaptively for each resolution, the maximum number of iterations was set to 200, and we initialized the procedure by aligning the center of both volumes. The similarity metric is based on mutual information. Quantitative results are presented in Table 1 (right). We excluded cases where the method failed ($\varepsilon > 20$ mm). Using this error-threshold rule, we disregarded almost half of all measurements. However, since this framework is not specifically designed to align the pericardium, the large number of fail cases is understandable. Many of the failures occurred for

**Table 1.** Errors [mm] with/without prior weights (left) and for state-of-the-art (right)

| Method | Prior | | No Prior | | State-of-the-Art | | Prior | |
|---|---|---|---|---|---|---|---|---|
| $\varepsilon(\cdot,\cdot)$ | $\hat{\theta}(\mathcal{A}),\check{\mathcal{P}}$ | $\hat{\theta}(\mathcal{R}),\check{\mathcal{R}}$ | $\hat{\theta}(\mathcal{A}),\check{\mathcal{P}}$ | $\hat{\theta}(\mathcal{R}),\check{\mathcal{R}}$ | $\hat{\theta}_*(\mathcal{P}),\check{\mathcal{P}}$ | $\hat{\theta}_*(\mathcal{R}),\check{\mathcal{R}}$ | $\hat{\theta}(\mathcal{P}),\check{\mathcal{P}}$ | $\hat{\theta}(\mathcal{R}),\check{\mathcal{R}}$ |
| #Studies | 88 | 43 | 88 | 43 | 47 | 21 | 47 | 21 |
| Mean | **5.60** | 4.63 | **7.57** | 7.17 | **7.19** | 6.33 | **5.03** | 4.45 |
| Std | 1.81 | 1.00 | 4.38 | 7.10 | 4.86 | 4.71 | 1.80 | 2.14 |
| Median | 5.29 | 4.64 | 6.91 | 5.52 | 4.96 | 4.56 | 5.02 | 4.32 |

images with significant differences in the size of the field of view between the CT and the C-arm CT scan. Still, a mean error of 7.19 mm is substantially larger than the error of our method, with a mean of 5.03 mm on the same dataset.

### 3.3   Inter-user Variability Study

Ascribing a rational meaning to quantitative results is challenging. In most cases, the true performance of a system would not only be measured in absolute terms but rather relative to the manual performance of experts. Thus, we compared our method to individual performances of a group of 10 experts on 10 datasets.

Let $\theta_{ji}$ be the $i^{th}$ expert's transform for the $j^{th}$ pair of volumes. We compare the fit of the $\theta_{ji}$-transformed CT pericardium to the ground-truth C-arm CT annotation, i.e. we evaluate $\varepsilon(\check{\mathcal{P}}_j, \theta_{ji}(\mathcal{P}_j))$. Our automated method exhibits lower errors than the median expert in 80% of all cases and shows high robustness with no outliers (see Fig. 5). There exists only one dataset, where the automatic fusion is inferior to more than 75% of the experts. Moreover, the experts' manual fusion time per data pair ranged from two to five minutes, while our method takes only $2.9 \pm 0.4$ s (in DB$_{cl}$) on average, which means a speedup of up to 99%.

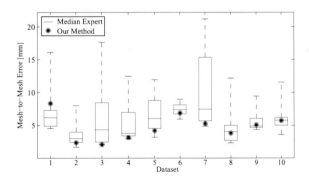

**Fig. 5.** Inter-user variability, box edges indicate $25^{th}$ and $75^{th}$ percentiles of user errors

## 4   Conclusion

We presented a method to fuse pre-operative CT and intra-operative 3D C-arm CT data. A novel sparse matching approach is employed to align the pre-operative anchor anatomy to the intra-operative setting. Data and model uncertainties are learned and exploited. Quantitative and qualitative evaluation demonstrate an accurate mapping of the target anatomy to the intra-operative modality. In direct comparison with a state-of-the-art registration framework, our method outperforms it significantly in robustness and accuracy. Furthermore, an inter-user variability study confirms that the accuracy of our fully-automatic method lies within the confidence interval of the expert group while reducing the duration of the alignment process from five minutes to three seconds. Thus, comprehensive patient-specific models can be estimated from high-contrast CT and fused into the imaging environment of operating rooms to facilitate guidance in cardiac interventions without tedious and time-consuming manual interactions.

# References

1. Leon, M.B., Smith, C.R., Mack, M., Miller, D.C., Moses, J.W., Svensson, L.G., Tuzcu, E.M., Webb, J.G., Fontana, G.P., Makkar, R.R., Brown, D.L., Block, P.C., Guyton, R.A., Pichard, A.D., Bavaria, J.E., Herrmann, H.C., Douglas, P.S., Petersen, J.L., Akin, J.J., Anderson, W.N., Wang, D., Pocock, S.: Transcatheter aortic-valve implantation for aortic stenosis in patients who cannot undergo surgery. N. Engl. J. Med. 363, 1597–1607 (2010)
2. Grbic, S., Ionasec, R., Vitanovski, D., Voigt, I., Wang, Y., Georgescu, B., Navab, N., Comaniciu, D.: Complete valvular heart apparatus model from 4D cardiac CT. Med. Image Anal. 16(5), 1003–1014 (2012)
3. Maddux, J.T., Wink, O., Messenger, J.C., Groves, B.M., Liao, R., Strzelczyk, J., Chen, S.Y., Carroll, J.D.: Randomized study of the safety and clinical utility of rotational angiography versus standard angiography in the diagnosis of coronary artery disease. Catheter. Cardiovasc. Interv. 62(2), 167–174 (2004)
4. Zheng, Y., John, M., Liao, R., Boese, J., Kirschstein, U., Georgescu, B., Zhou, S.K., Kempfert, J., Walther, T., Brockmann, G., Comaniciu, D.: Automatic aorta segmentation and valve landmark detection in C-arm CT: Application to aortic valve implantation. In: Jiang, T., Navab, N., Pluim, J.P.W., Viergever, M.A. (eds.) MICCAI 2010, Part I. LNCS, vol. 6361, pp. 476–483. Springer, Heidelberg (2010)
5. Wells, W., Viola, P., Nakajima, S., Kikinis, R.: Multi-modal volume registration by maximization of mutual information. Med. Image Anal. 1(1), 35–51 (1996)
6. Lorenzo-Valdés, M., Sanchez-Ortiz, G.I., Mohiaddin, R.H., Rueckert, D.: Atlas-based segmentation and tracking of 3D cardiac MR images using non-rigid registration. In: Dohi, T., Kikinis, R. (eds.) MICCAI 2002, Part I. LNCS, vol. 2488, pp. 642–650. Springer, Heidelberg (2002)
7. Zheng, Y., Vega-Higuera, F., Zhou, S.K., Comaniciu, D.: Fast and automatic heart isolation in 3D CT volumes: Optimal shape initialization. In: Wang, F., Yan, P., Suzuki, K., Shen, D. (eds.) MLMI 2010. LNCS, vol. 6357, pp. 84–91. Springer, Heidelberg (2010)
8. Tu, Z.: Probabilistic boosting-tree: Learning discriminative models for classification, recognition, and clustering. In: Tenth IEEE Int'l Conf. on Comp. Vision, vol. 2, pp. 1589–1596. IEEE (2005)
9. Mitra, N.J., Gelfand, N., Pottmann, H., Guibas, L.: Registration of point cloud data from a geometric optimization perspective. In: Proc. of the 2004 Eurographics/ACM SIGGRAPH Symp. on Geom. Proc., pp. 22–31. ACM, New York (2004)

# Iterative Closest Curve: A Framework for Curvilinear Structure Registration Application to 2D/3D Coronary Arteries Registration

Thomas Benseghir[1,2,*], Grégoire Malandain[2,**], and Régis Vaillant[1]

[1] GE-Healthcare, 78530 Buc, France
[2] INRIA, 06900 Sophia Antipolis, France

**Abstract.** Treatment coronary arteries endovascular involves catheter navigation through patient vasculature. The projective angiography guidance is limited in the case of chronic total occlusion where occluded vessel can not be seen. Integrating standard preoperative CT angiography information with live fluoroscopic images addresses this limitation but requires alignment of both modalities.

This article proposes a structure-based registration method that intrinsically preserves both the geometrical and topological coherencies of the vascular centrelines to be registered, by the means of a dedicated curve-to-curve distance pairs of closest curves are identified, while pairing their points. Preliminary experiments demonstrate that the proposed approach performs better than the standard Iterative Closest Point method giving a wider attraction basin and improved accuracy.

**Keywords:** registration, curvilinear structure, ICP, chronic total occlusion, CTO, coronary, X-ray, computed tomography angiography, CTA.

## 1 Introduction

Percutaneous Coronary Intervention (PCI) is a minimally invasive procedure where a catheter is navigated through the patient vasculature in order to gain access to the pathology location. X-ray projective angiographic images allow the interventional cardiologists to visualize the vessels and devices and guide the endovascular intervention. In the case of Chronic Total Occlusion (CTO) contrast agent could not go through the occluded vessel which remains invisible in the angiography. Moreover, projective images do not allow 3D perception of the vessels whose local orientation may not be estimated correctly from the projective images, especially when the vessel is curved along the direction of the X-ray beam. On the other hand, preoperative CT angiography (CTA) provides a static map of the entire vasculature, including occluded vessels and potential calcifications. Moreover, ambiguities due to the projective nature of angiography

---

*   Asclepios project-team, Inria Sophia Antipolis - Méditerranée.
**  Morpheme project-team, Inria Sophia Antipolis - Méditerranée, I3S, UMR 7271, iBV, UMR 7277.

are not present in CTA. CTA acquisition is now standard in clinical practice before starting a difficult CTO case, due to the obtained understanding of the anatomical and lesion geometry is of unique value [12].

Integrating information extracted from CTA into fluoroscopic 2D images may facilitate guidance but necessitate a preliminary step of registration. The registration of the pre-operative data shall reach an accuracy of few millimeters at maximum in order to bring improved guidance to the operator. We explore feature-based registration approaches for their potential to bring the level of accuracy that we look for and also because the considered images present salient features to be used. Indeed the vessels are curvilinear structures which can be conveniently segmented in both CTA and fluoroscopic images made during an injection of contrast agent.

Features are represented by centerlines, which correspond to the curves following the vessel center, sometimes with radius information or perpendicular vessel cross-section. Leveraging curvilinear structures for solving registration problems has been tested in multiple medical fields: coronary [8] or cerebral [13] angiograms, liver images [3], [6] or in other applications [11], for diagnosis, planning and guidance purposes.

Several methods can be used to match two sets of features. Besl and McKay developed the Iterative Closest Point (ICP) algorithm [2] that is applicable to large frameworks, considering features as set of points. The algorithm is formed of three consecutive steps which are iterated: (i) Pair each point of a data to its closest in the model; (ii) Compute the transformation minimizing the mean square error between the paired points; (iii) Apply the transformation to the data and go back to (i). The success of the algorithm depends a lot on pairing and therefore on initial pose estimation. Thus, many variants have been introduced to improve the pairing construction. In [5], ICP is embedded into an expectation maximization framework, which allows multiple correspondences. Several other variants are compared in [10], all aiming to better build the pairings in order to improve registration robustness and accuracy.

Another class of methods, such as [13], formulate this problem as a matching measure optimization process in the set of admissible transformations. However, the energy measure to be optimized may have multiple local minima. Hierarchical approaches (gradually increasing searched transformation complexity) or combination of different optimization methods [9] partially help dealing with this issue. These local minima of the matching metric mainly come from the underlying point-to-point distance, and are thus due to pairing done without respecting the structural coherency. To improve this, [8] propose a hybrid metric between augmented points, including local structural information such as local direction, involving Euclidean distance from point to point and similarity properties of the iconic features. This improves the similarity of matched points, but is still inefficient to ensure a global coherency between the structures to be matched.

Global coherency has been addressed in [3], [6] and [11] as a graph matching problem, where graph nodes (corresponding to vessel bifurcations or endpoints) are matched. However, such information may be unreliable in the aimed application because of the inherent characteristics of the 2D projective images (projection may induce error in bifurcation localization and introduces spurious ones by superposition of two vessels) and the potential segmentation errors.

We propose then to introduce a structure-based registration method, inspired by the ICP algorithm. It is dedicated to curvilinear structures, hence called Iterative Closest Curve, or ICC. Its main feature is that the built pairings conform with the vasculature structure of the images to be matched.

## 2    Iterative Closest Curve Method

The ICC-algorithm mimics the ICP algorithm introduced in [2], but with curves being considered instead of points. An intuitive notion of a curve allows one to understand the ICC framework and its capacity to preserve topological coherency during the registration process. Let the data $\mathcal{C}$ be a set of curves that can be registered to a model $\mathcal{X}$. The internal representation of $\mathcal{C}$ and $\mathcal{X}$ can be of any form but must allow one to extract curves from it.

The closest curve definition of an individual data curve $C \in \mathcal{C}$ in a model $\mathcal{X}$ is based upon a curve-to-curve distance $d$. We denote $X_C$ the closest curve of $C$ in $\mathcal{X}$ that satisfies

$$X_C = \operatorname*{argmin}_{X \in \mathcal{X}} d(C, X). \tag{1}$$

Contrary to standard closest point pairing, the resulting pairings insure topological and geometrical coherence since a curve is paired to another one.

Following the ICP framework we now define the best transformation $\hat{T}$ in a sense of least square curve registration:

$$\hat{T} = \operatorname*{argmin}_{T \in \Omega} \sum_{C \in \mathcal{C}} d^2 \left( T(C), X_C \right) \tag{2}$$

where $\Omega$ is the set of admissible transformations.

The ICC algorithm consists of the iteration of three steps:

1. Pair each curve $C$ in the set $\mathcal{C}$ to its closest curve $X_C$ in the set $\mathcal{X}$ (Eq. 1)
2. Compute the transformation $\hat{T}$ minimizing the mean square error between the paired curves (Eq. 2)
3. Apply the transformation $\hat{T}$ to the set $\mathcal{C}$ and go back to 1 until convergence.

Now we have provided a framework for general curvilinear structure registration, some steps must be described to implement the ICC algorithm.

**Data and Model.** The data $\mathcal{C}$ is defined as a set of $N_{\mathcal{C}}$ curves $(C_k)_{k=1..N_{\mathcal{C}}}$ of $\mathbb{R}^3$ representing the centerlines of a coronary vessel tree. These curves are traced from distal points to a common root point insuring a global coherence along an entire vessel during pairing. Concerning the model $\mathcal{X}$, curvilinear features are obtained from a 2D image by using a Hessian-based method [7] and then connected to obtain a non-directed graph structure. Therefore, $\mathcal{X}$ is composed of edges (centerline curves in $\mathbb{R}^2$) and nodes that are either extremities or bifurcations. Because of the projective nature of the image, detected bifurcations may be due to either a 3D bifurcation projection or a superimposition of two distinct vessels. No attempt to distinguish those cases has been attempted which may lead the graph to contain cycles.

**Curve-to-Curve Distance.** In the case of 3D/2D registration, the distance $d$ in Eq. 1 deals with curves in different spaces ($\mathbb{R}^3$ and $\mathbb{R}^2$). This problem can be overcome by applying a projective operator $P$ (given by system calibration) to the 3D curves when it is necessary. In practice, it is convenient to work with polygonal curves $C : [1, n] \rightarrow \mathbb{R}^3$ and $X_C : [1, m] \rightarrow \mathbb{R}^2$, constructed by linking $n$ points $\{C(p), p \in \{1...n\}\}$ (resp. $m$ and $\{X_C(p), p \in \{1...m\}\}$). A generic set-to-set distance based on these construction points, e.g. the Hausdorff distance, can be considered but does not take into account the curvilinear structure of the data. The Fréchet distance between continuous polygonal curves, which has been addressed in [1], intrinsically takes into account the topological structures of curves. This distance respects the ordering of points along curves but is computationally expensive. A faster discrete version presented in [4] called the "coupling distance" gives an upper bound of the Fréchet distance by minimizing the distance between coupled points for all possible couplings. A coupling is a sequence of $Q$ pairs of points $(C(\gamma(1)), X_C(\lambda(1))), \ldots, (C(\gamma(Q)), X_C(\lambda(Q)))$ where the dummy variable $Q$ is ranged between $\max(n, m)$ and $(n + m)$ and $\gamma$ (resp. $\lambda$) is a non-decreasing surjection from $1 \ldots Q$ to $1 \ldots n$ (resp. to $1 \ldots m$) called a reparameterization mapping.

We derive from the Fréchet distance [4] the distance $d$ defined as

$$d(C, X_C) = \sqrt{\min_{Q, \lambda, \gamma} \sum_{i=1...Q} ||P(C(\gamma(i))) - X_C(\lambda(i))||^2} \ . \qquad (3)$$

These surjective mappings ensure that the summation is done over the complete set of points, forming the discrete curves. We imposed them to be non-decreasing to take into account the order of points along curves and because the pairing strategy defined below gives a scan sense direction along the curves.

**Curves Pairing.** Eq. 1 requires to compute the Fréchet distance for all possible curves $X$ in the graph $\mathcal{X}$. A curve in $\mathcal{X}$ is defined as a path between two nodes, if it exists, without visiting twice the same edge. Yet, since the 2D graph may be noisy or complex the amount of possible curves can lead to a computationally explosive search. We propose to restrict the set of admissible curves by selecting candidates having their extremities in a neighborhood of the data curve extremities $C(1)$ and $C(n)$ projections. In practice, we identify edges (and nodes) in the vicinity of both $P(C(1))$ and $P(C(n))$ and construct the shortest path between them in the graph. If no 2D structure can be found close to the vessel distal part, a recursive shortening mechanism of the 3D curve is implemented to deal with topological differences between the data and the model. The shortest path is built upon distances along curves as edge weights.

**Transformation Computation.** Any optimization procedure can potentially be used to solve Eq. 2. Here we choose to take advantage of the underlying point-to-point pairing induced by the coupling realizing the Fréchet distance in

Eq. 3. Indeed, for each curve $C_k$ we have a couple of reparameterization function $\gamma_k$ and $\lambda_k$ and a dummy variable $Q_k$ constituting point pairings between $\mathcal{C}$ and $\mathcal{X}$ that can be grouped as a single notation $\gamma$, $\lambda$ and $Q$. Then Eq. 2 can be rewritten as

$$\hat{T} = \underset{T \in \Omega}{\operatorname{argmin}} \sum_{k=1}^{N_C} \min_{Q_k, \lambda_k, \gamma_k} \sum_{i=1}^{Q_k} ||P\left(T\left(C_k\left(\gamma_k(i)\right)\right)\right) - X_{C_k}(\lambda_k(i))||^2. \qquad (4)$$

We propose to solve this least square problem by alternatively optimizing the transformation $T$ and the coupling variables $\gamma$, $\lambda$ and $Q$. For a given transformation $T$ finding the best coupling variables is simply obtained by computing the Fréchet distance. Coupling variables allows one to construct point pairing between set $\mathcal{C}$ and $\mathcal{X}$. Finding the best transformation is then equivalent to a least square alignment between two point sets with a given correspondence between points. We compute iteratively: (a) point-pairing optimization by Fréchet distance (between paired curves, the curve pairing being unchanged in this transformation computation loop); (b) transformation optimization at a fixed point-pairing; (c) applying the transformation to paired curves. This transformation optimization in ICC is thus equivalent to an "ICP"-like algorithm where closest point pairing is replaced by the Fréchet pairing at a given curve-to-curve pairing.

**CTO Handling.** One major concern in registration is the topological difference between the data and the model. In the case of CTO, a part of a vessel or even the whole vessel is not visible in the 2D image, while it is present in the 3D CTA. This problem is solved in two different ways in the ICC algorithm. On the one hand, as mentioned in the curve pairing process, if no compatible curve can be found in the neighborhood of a vessel extremity we recursively shorten the 3D vessel. This approach can deal with missing parts of a vessel due to either CTO or lack of contrast leading to misdetection of 2D vessels. On the other hand, we implemented standard robust transformation estimators based on a loop of transformation optimization and pairing rejection based on a study of the residual error distribution. We introduce robust estimators in transformation computation at the ICC level (step 2.) by rejecting curve-pairings, but also inside the transformation computation when computing least square alignment (step b.) by rejecting point-pairings. The curve outlier rejection aims to deal with entire missing curves and point rejection with noisy detection.

## 3    Results

The goal of this result section is to give an example of applicability of the Iterative Closest Curve algorithm and prove its potential with respect to the standard Iterative Closest Point method. To this end we use four real data cases coming from three patients including one Chronic Total Occlusion (CTO) and one stenosis patient. One case is composed of a 3D segmentation of the left coronary tree (extracted via a commercial product), a fluoroscopic image and a manual pose estimation constituting the ground truth. Two cases were built from the CTO patient at different angulations. The sequences have been collected following standard clinical procedures and as such did not imply any additional procedural steps for the patient.

First, we want to highlight the structural coherency brought by the ICC methodology with respect to ICP in Fig. 1 and 2. For the same initial position (projected in blue) pairing are shown by segments linking data projection points and their paired corresponding points in the image. Fig. 1 presents the lack of coherence induced by closest point pairing along vessels. A single vessel in 3D presents different "jumps" in its pairing and is matched to multiple non-connected 2D detected curves. On the contrary, the ICC approach create a curve-to-curve pairing and the Fréchet distance imposes order coherence of the underlying point pairing along the two curves. As shown in Fig. 2, even if the pairing do not correspond to the expected one it seems more realistic. From the initial position presented in blue we run both ICC and ICP, leading to the results presented in Fig. 3. While the ICP algorithm gets stuck at a position where multiple vessels in 3D are transversally crossing 2D detected curves, the ICC algorithm converges to an acceptable 3D pose.

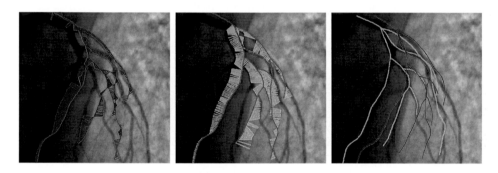

**Fig. 1.** Pairing obtained with the ICP algorithm  **Fig. 2.** Pairing obtained with the ICC algorithm  **Fig. 3.** ICC (green) and ICP (red) registration results

Secondly, to confirm the robustness of ICC with respect to rotations we evaluate the registration algorithms on 100 random perturbations of the ground truth pose (manually determined). The random 3D displacement has been applied to the coronary tree and a step of alignment between the 3D root node and its detection in the 2D image, i.e. a translation, has been applied. This later step is an initialization step that seems realistic either in a manual or automatic way, thus only rotation pertubations have been investigated. We conducted experiments on three ranges of angular perturbation: 5, 10 and 15 degrees.

We assessed the registration error by the means of the Mean Projective Error (MPE); that is the average residual distance between projected 3D points after registration with respect to their ground truth counterparts. Fig. 4 displays

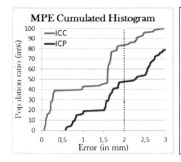

**Fig. 4.** Statistics on Mean Projected Error (MPE). **Left:** the cumulated MPE for case 1 obtained with 100 random rotations for $5°$ of rotation. **Right:** mean and 90th percentile of the MPE distribution for ICC and ICP algorithm.

| Case | MPE | $5°$ rotation | | $10°$ rotation | | $15°$ rotation | |
|---|---|---|---|---|---|---|---|
| | | ICC | ICP | ICC | ICP | ICC | ICP |
| 1 | mean | 1.4 | 2.1 | 3.2 | 5.0 | 6.9 | 9.3 |
| | 90% | 3.0 | 3.7 | 7.4 | 10.3 | 15.6 | 18.8 |
| 2 | mean | 1.3 | 2.3 | 2.0 | 3.9 | 4.2 | 8.3 |
| | 90% | 3.0 | 4.4 | 4.3 | 8.1 | 9.3 | 16.8 |
| 3 | mean | 1.7 | 3.4 | 4.0 | 6.9 | 7.1 | 10.6 |
| | 90% | 3.9 | 6.6 | 8.7 | 13.9 | 12.4 | 21.2 |
| 4 | mean | 1.3 | 1.8 | 2.6 | 4.3 | 7.5 | 8.7 |
| | 90% | 3.3 | 3.6 | 6.2 | 8.6 | 16.5 | 18.2 |

the cumulative MPE histogram for one patient and one angle (5 degrees). It demonstrates that the ICC (blue curve) performs better than the ICP (red curve). For example, a 2 mm MPE is reached in only 50% of tested positions for ICP and in more than 80% for ICC.

Fig. 4 (right) also shows a table capturing the behavior of ICC and ICP algorithms for the whole dataset by computing the average and ninetieth percentile of MPEs. ICC obtains lower values for both indicators, suggesting that ICC can be more accurate that ICP, and that point based methods can benefit from integration of global structural information.

Current implementation runs in around five seconds on an Intel CORE i5 cadenced at 1.5 GHz.

## 4    Conclusion

We proposed in this paper a general registration method for curvilinear structure taking into account geometrical and topological coherency of the data. We exemplified the ICC method with a 2D/3D registration implementation applied to coronary artery registration. By introducing curve-to-curve pairing and distance, we showed that ICC algorithm overpassed the standard ICP algorithm and significantly improved the resulting pairings. The improvement in the pairings has been visually evaluated in test experiments. We also estimated the improvement by comparing the mean projection error obtained with our approach to the reference ICP method.

For future work, the capacity of this algorithm to handle transformation scheme involving non-rigid deformations needs to be evaluated. Indeed, we observed in our test application that the rigid transformation is insufficient to describe the changes supported by the anatomy between the pre- and the peroperative imaging situation. Additional outlier rejection mechanisms shall also be added to extend further the attraction basin.

# References

1. Alt, H., Godau, M.: Measuring the resemblance of polygonal curves. In: Proceedings of the Eighth Annual Symposium on Computational Geometry, SCG 1992, pp. 102–109. ACM, New York (1992)
2. Besl, P.J., McKay, N.D.: A method for registration of 3-D shapes. IEEE Transactions on Pattern Analysis and Machine Intelligence 14(2), 239–256 (1992)
3. Charnoz, A., Agnus, V., Malandain, G., Forest, C., Tajine, M., Soler, L.: Liver registration for the follow-up of hepatic tumors. In: Duncan, J.S., Gerig, G. (eds.) MICCAI 2005. LNCS, vol. 3750, pp. 155–162. Springer, Heidelberg (2005)
4. Eiter, T., Mannila, H.: Computing discrete Fréchet distance. Technical Report CD-TR 94/64, Christian Doppler Laboratory for Expert Systems, TU Vienna, Austria (1994)
5. Granger, S., Pennec, X., Roche, A.: Rigid point-surface registration using an EM variant of ICP for computer guided oral implantology. In: Niessen, W.J., Viergever, M.A. (eds.) MICCAI 2001. LNCS, vol. 2208, pp. 752–761. Springer, Heidelberg (2001)
6. Groher, M., Zikic, D., Navab, N.: Deformable 2D-3D registration of vascular structures in a one view scenario. IEEE Transactions on Medical Imaging 28(6), 847–860 (2009)
7. Krissian, K., Malandain, G., Ayache, N., Vaillant, R., Trousset, Y.: Model-based detection of tubular structures in 3D images. Computer Vision and Image Understanding 80(2), 130–171 (2000)
8. Metz, C., Schaap, M., Klein, S., Baka, N., Neefjes, L., Schultz, C., Niessen, W., van Walsum, T.: Registration of 3D+t coronary CTA and monoplane 2D+t X-ray angiography. IEEE Transactions on Medical Imaging 32(5), 919–931 (2013)
9. Rivest-Henault, D., Sundar, H., Cheriet, M.: Nonrigid 2D/3D registration of coronary artery models with live fluoroscopy for guidance of cardiac interventions. IEEE Transactions on Medical Imaging 31(8), 1557–1572 (2012)
10. Rusinkiewicz, S., Levoy, M.: Efficient variants of the ICP algorithm. In: 3-D Digital Imaging and Modeling. IEEE (2001)
11. Serradell, E., Glowacki, P., Kybic, J., Moreno-Noguer, F., Fua, P.: Robust Non-Rigid Registration of 2D and 3D Graphs. In: Conference on Computer Vision and Pattern Recognition (2012)
12. Shah, P.B.: Management of coronary chronic total occlusion. Circulation 123(16), 1780–1784 (2011)
13. Sundar, H., Khamene, A., Xu, C., Sauer, F., Davatzikos, C.: A novel 2D-3D registration algorithm for aligning fluoro images with 3D pre-op CT/MR images. In: Medical Imaging, vol. 6141, p. 61412K. SPIE (2006)

# Towards Realtime Multimodal Fusion
# for Image-Guided Interventions Using
# Self-similarities

Mattias Paul Heinrich[1,2], Mark Jenkinson[2], Bartłomiej W. Papież[1],
Sir Michael Brady[3], and Julia A. Schnabel[1]

[1] Institute of Biomedical Engineering,
Department of Engineering, University of Oxford, UK
[2] Oxford University Centre for Functional MRI of the Brain, UK
[3] Department of Oncology, University of Oxford, UK
mattias.heinrich@eng.ox.ac.uk
http://users.ox.ac.uk/~shil3388

**Abstract.** Image-guided interventions often rely on deformable multi-modal registration to align pre-treatment and intra-operative scans. There are a number of requirements for automated image registration for this task, such as a robust similarity metric for scans of different modalities with different noise distributions and contrast, an efficient optimisation of the cost function to enable fast registration for this time-sensitive application, and an insensitive choice of registration parameters to avoid delays in practical clinical use. In this work, we build upon the concept of structural image representation for multi-modal similarity. Discriminative descriptors are densely extracted for the multi-modal scans based on the "self-similarity context". An efficient quantised representation is derived that enables very fast computation of point-wise distances between descriptors. A symmetric multi-scale discrete optimisation with diffusion regularisation is used to find smooth transformations. The method is evaluated for the registration of 3D ultrasound and MRI brain scans for neurosurgery and demonstrates a significantly reduced registration error (on average 2.1 mm) compared to commonly used similarity metrics and computation times of less than 30 seconds per 3D registration.

**Keywords:** multimodal similarity, discrete optimisation, neurosurgery.

## 1 Introduction

Deformable multi-modal registration plays an important role for image-guided interventions, where scans are often acquired using different modalities, e.g. to propagate segmentation information for image-guided radiotherapy [9]. The alignment of multi-modal scans is difficult, because there can be a large amount of motion between scans, the intra-operative scan is often of lower scan quality than diagnostic scans and no functional relationship between intensities across modalities exists. In this work, we address the registration of intra-operative 3D ultrasound (US) to pre-operative magnetic resonance imaging (MRI) for image-guided neurosurgery. The brain tissue exhibits non-rigid deformations after opening the skull (*brain shift* [11]), which needs to be compensate to relate

K. Mori et al. (Eds.): MICCAI 2013, Part I, LNCS 8149, pp. 187–194, 2013.

the intra-operative ultrasound to the MRI scan (which has a higher quality and can give a better guidance for tumour resection).

## 2    Previous Work

Mutual information (MI) has been frequently used in rigid multi-modal registration [10,17]. However, for deformable multi-modal registration, many disadvantages have been identified for MI-based similarity measures [13]. In particular, the locally varying noise distribution and speckle pattern of ultrasound make the estimation of a global intensity mapping difficult. The results in [14] suggest that using standard MI is insufficient for US-MRI registration. The authors propose the use a multi-feature $\alpha$-MI metric as presented in [16]. This, however, comes at a great computational cost, which is a disadvantage for this time sensitive application. Another possible approach is to use a simulated ultrasound-like image based on an MRI [1] or computed tomography (CT) scan [19] for registration. An accurate ultrasound simulation is, however, far from trivial, especially for interventional scans.

For these reasons, structural image representations have gained great interest for deformable multi-modal registration. The motivation is that, once the images are transformed into a representation independent of the underlying image acquisition, efficient monomodal optimisation techniques can be employed. In [18], a scalar structural representation based on local entropy has been successfully applied to the deformable registration of different MRI modalities and the rigid alignment of MRI and CT brain scans. De Nigris et al. [2] used gradient orientation to drive a rigid multi-modal registration of brain scans. In [4], we proposed a multi-dimensional "modality independent neighbourhood descriptor" (MIND) based on the concept of local self-similarities (LSS) [15] and applied it to the non-rigid registration of CT and MRI chest scans. Self-similarities were also employed in [14], however, not as a structural representation, but instead using the Earth Mover's Distance as self-similarity distance within the multi-dimensional feature-space of $\alpha$-MI. There are a number of limitations of these approaches. First, scalar representations [18] are often not sufficiently discriminative to drive a non-rigid registration with many degrees of freedom. Second, high-dimensional descriptors are often computationally too expensive for the use in interventional applications. Third, the inherent strong noise and imaging artefacts of US make a robust estimation of structural image representations challenging.

In this work, we address these challenges by introducing a novel contextual image descriptor: the "self-similarity context" (SSC). The motivation and derivation of SSC is presented in Sec. 3.1. A descriptor quantisation and an efficient point-wise distance metric are proposed. In Sec. 3.2 the employed discrete optimisation framework is described and a simple approach is presented, which ensures symmetric transformations. Quantitative experiments of a neurosurgical application are presented in Sec. 4 for an evaluation of our approach and a comparison to other similarity metrics and previously published methods on the same dataset, based on manual landmark correspondences.

## 3    Methods

SSC is estimated based on patch-based self-similarities in a similar way as e.g. LSS or MIND, but rather than extracting a representation of local shape or geometry, it aims to find the context around the voxel of interest. Therefore, the negative influence of noisy patches can be greatly reduced, making this approach very suitable for ultrasound registration. Spatial context has been successfully applied to object detection [7] and is the driving force of pictorial structures [3].

### 3.1    Self-similarity Context

Self-similarity can be described by a distance function between image patches within one image $I$ (sum of squared differences $SSD$ can be used within the same scan), a local or global noise estimate $\sigma^2$, and a certain neighbourhood layout $\mathcal{N}$ for which self-similarities are calculated. For a patch centred at $\mathbf{x}$, the self-similarity descriptor $\mathcal{S}(I, \mathbf{x}, \mathbf{y})$ is given by:

$$\mathcal{S}(I, \mathbf{x}, \mathbf{y}) = \exp\left(-\frac{SSD(\mathbf{x}, \mathbf{y})}{\sigma^2}\right) \quad \mathbf{x}, \mathbf{y} \in \mathcal{N} \tag{1}$$

where $\mathbf{y}$ defines the centre location of a patch within $\mathcal{N}$. In [4] and [15], the neighbourhood layout was defined to always include the patch centred around $\mathbf{x}$ for pairwise distance calculations. This has the disadvantage that image artefacts or noise within the central patch always have a direct adverse effect on the self-similarity descriptor. We therefore propose to completely avoid using the patch at $\mathbf{x}$ for the calculation of the descriptor for this location. Instead, all pairwise distances of patches within the six neighbourhood (with a Euclidean distance of $\sqrt{2}$ between them) are used. The spatial layout of this approach is visualised in Fig. 1 and compared to MIND (showing the central patch in red, patches in $\mathcal{N}$ in grey, and edges connecting pairs for which distances are calculated in blue). The aim of SSC is not to find a good structural representation of the underlying shape, but rather the context within its neighbourhood. The noise estimate $\sigma^2$ in Eq. 1 is defined to be the mean of all patch distances. Descriptors are normalised so that $\max(\mathcal{S}) = 1$.

**Pointwise Multimodal Similarity Using SSC:** Structural image representations are appealing, because they enable multi-modal registration using simple similarity metric across modalities. Once the descriptors are extracted for both images, yielding a vector for each voxel, the similarity metric between locations $\mathbf{x}_i$ and $\mathbf{x}_j$ in two images $I$ and $J$ can be defined as the sum of absolute differences (SAD) between their corresponding descriptors. The distance $D$ between two descriptors is therefore:

$$D(\mathbf{x}_i, \mathbf{x}_j) = \frac{1}{|\mathcal{N}|} \sum_{\mathbf{y} \in \mathcal{N}} |\mathcal{S}(I, \mathbf{x}_i, \mathbf{y}) - \mathcal{S}(J, \mathbf{x}_j, \mathbf{y})| \tag{2}$$

Equation 2 requires $|\mathcal{N}|$ computations to evaluate the similarity at one voxel. Discrete optimisation frameworks, as the one employed here, use many cost function evaluations per voxel. In order to speed up the computations, we propose to

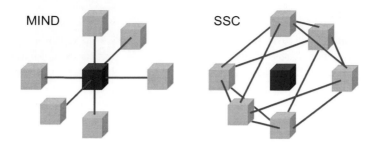

**Fig. 1.** Concept of self-similarity context (SSC) compared to MIND with six-neighbourhood (6-NH). The patch around the voxel of interest is shown in red, all patches within its immediate 6-NH are shown in grey. Left: All patch distances (shown with blue lines) used for MIND within the 6-NH take the centre patch into account. Right: Geometrical and structural context can be better described by SSC using all patch-to-patch distances, none of which is dependent on the central patch.

quantise the descriptor to a single integer value with 64 bits, without significant loss of accuracy. The exact similarity evaluation of Eq. 2 can then be obtained using the Hamming distance between two descriptors using only one operation per voxel. A descriptor using self-similarity context consists of 12 elements, for which we use 5 bits per element, which translates into 6 different possible values (note that we cannot use a quantisation of $2^5$ because the Hamming weight only counts the number of bits, which differ). Figure 2 illustrates the concept, which could also be employed for other multi-feature based registration techniques.

## 3.2   Discrete Optimisation

Discrete optimisation is used in this work, because it is computationally efficient, no derivative of the similarity cost is needed, local minima are avoided and large deformations can be covered by defining an appropriate range of displacements **u**. Here, we adopt our recent approach [5,6], which uses a block-wise parametric transformation model with belief propagation on a tree graph (BP-T) [3]. The regularisation term penalises squared differences of displacements for neighbouring control points and is weighted with a constant $\lambda$. Not all similarity terms within the influence region of each control point, but only a randomly chosen subset of them are taken into account. This concept, which has also been used in stochastic gradient descent optimisation [8] and in [2], greatly reduces the computation of the similarity term without loss of accuracy (as shown in [6]).

**Inverse Consistent Transformations:** We introduce a simple scheme to obtain inverse consistent mappings, given the forward and backward displacement fields $\mathbf{u}^n$ and $\mathbf{v}^n$ respectively (which are independently calculated), by iteratively updating the following equations:

$$\mathbf{u}^{n+1} = 0.5(\mathbf{u}^n - \mathbf{v}^n(\mathbf{x} + \mathbf{u}^n))$$
$$\mathbf{v}^{n+1} = 0.5(\mathbf{v}^n - \mathbf{u}^n(\mathbf{x} + \mathbf{v}^n))$$

$$(3)$$

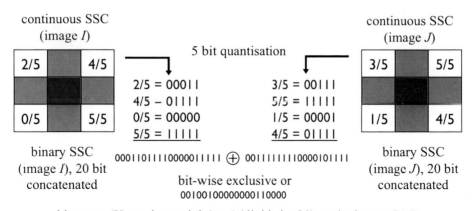

bit-count (Hamming weight) = 4 (divide by 20) equivalent to SAD

**Fig. 2.** Concept of using the Hamming distance to speed up similarity evaluations. Continuous valued descriptor entries (here: $|\mathcal{N}| = 4$) are quantised to a fixed number of bits and concatenated. The similarity of Eq. 2 can then be evaluated using only one bitwise XOR and bit-count operation.

## 4     Registration of US and MRI Scans for Neurosurgery

We applied the presented approach to a set of 13 pairs of pre-operative MRI and pre-resection 3D ultrasound (US) images of the Brain Images of Tumours for Evaluation (BITE) database [12] from the Montreal Neurological Institute[1]. The MRI scans have an isotropic resolution of 0.5 mm and the US are resampled to the same resolution (the MRI scans are then cropped to have the same dimensions and a similar field of view). Roughly 27 corresponding anatomical landmarks have been selected for each scan pair by a neurosurgeon and two experts. The same dataset was recently used by [14], and therefore enables a direct comparison. They apply multi-feature $\alpha$-MI [16] with a stochastic gradient descent optimisation [8], and extend this framework using a self-similarity weighting within the feature space, calling the new metric SeSaMI.

We use the following parameter settings for the discrete optimisation: three scales of control point spacings of $\{6, 5, 4\}$ mm, 50 similarity term samples per control point and a dense displacement search range of $\{12, 5, 2\}$ mm (with a spacing of $\{2, 1, 0.5\}$ mm). This corresponds to roughly $10^7$ degrees of freedom for the optimisation. We employ three different similarity metrics: blockwise MI, MIND [4] and SSC. For the self-similarity calculations a patch-size of $3 \times 3 \times 3$ voxels and a distance between neighbouring patches of 2 voxels was chosen. Blockwise MI is computed the same way as global MI [10], but a new joint histogram is estimated for each control point and each displacement using 100 samples within the cubic influence region of the control point. We empirically

---

[1] Publicly available at www.bic.mni.mcgill.ca/Services/ServicesBITE

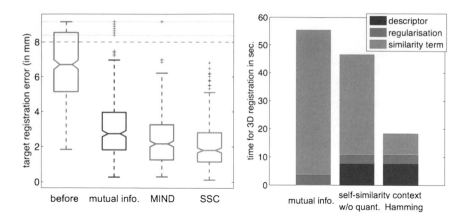

**Fig. 3.** Deformable registration of 13 cases of MRI-US brain scans, evaluated with ≈27 expert landmarks per case. The registration error of SSC (2.12±1.29 mm) is significantly lower than that of MIND (2.45±1.44 mm) and mutual information (3.07±1.74 mm) within the same discrete optimisation framework ($p = 7\times10^{-4}$ and $p < 10^{-6}$ respectively). The computation time per registration using SSC and the Hamming distance (≈20 sec per 3D pair) is more than twice as fast as MI and SSC without quantisation. The use of $\alpha$-MI with a continuous optimisation approach takes about 120 min. [14], which is too long for this time-concerning application.

found that 8 histogram bins give best results together with a Parzen window smoothing with $\sigma_P = 0.5$. An optimal regularisation parameter $\lambda = 0.5$ was found for MIND and SSC, and $\lambda = 0.25$ for MI. All resulting transformations are free from singularities (invertible) with an average complexity measured as standard deviation of the Jacobian of 0.08.

**Quantitative Results:** The average initial target registration error (TRE) in our experiments is $6.76 \pm 2.20$ mm (this value is only 4.12 mm in [14], because additional US-tracking information is used). SSC achieves the best overall registration accuracy of 2.12±1.29 mm (see Fig. 3), which is a significant improvement compared to MIND (2.45±1.44 mm) and mutual information (3.07±1.74 mm). The much more complex $\alpha$-MI metric and its SeSaMI variant used in [14] yield a higher TRE of 2.50 and 2.34 mm, respectively. The computation time of SSC (20 sec) is smaller than using MI (55 sec) within the same discrete optimisation framework and much smaller than using $\alpha$-MI (120 min). Additionally, when using SSC, the setting of the regularisation parameter $\lambda$ has a low sensitivity (less compared to MIND and MI) causing an increase of TRE of only 0.1 mm when choosing 4× larger or smaller values. Figure 4 shows an example of the registration problem and the resulting alignment using SSC.

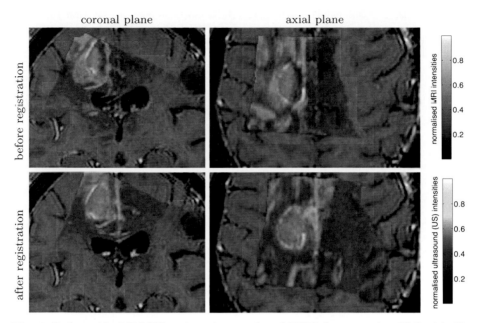

**Fig. 4.** Deformable MRI-US registration results of BITE dataset using SSC with discrete optimisation. The intra-operative ultrasound scan is shown as false colour overlay over the grayscale MRI intensities. A clearly improved alignment of the ventricles and the solid tumour is visible after registration (bottom row).

## 5    Conclusion

This paper addresses the challenging deformable registration of pre-operative MRI to intra-operative ultrasound for neurosurgery. A novel image descriptor the "self-similarity context" (SSC) is presented, with low sensitivity to image noise, and a quantisation scheme for fast distance evaluations using Hamming weights. When used in a discrete optimisation framework with a stochastic similarity term sampling, a computation time of less than half a minute is achieved on a standard CPU and state-of-the-art registration accuracy with an average error of 2.12 mm, which is a statistically significant improvement over previous self-similarity based metrics [4] and mutual information. In the future, we plan a GPU implementation (which could then lead to real-time performance) and further comparisons to other structural image representations (e.g. gradient orientation [2]) and the application of our approach to further applications of image-guided interventions.

**Acknowledgements.** We would like to thank EPSRC and Cancer Research UK for funding this work within the Oxford Cancer Imaging Centre.

## References

1. Arbel, T., Morandi, X., Comeau, R.M., Collins, D.L.: Automatic non-linear MRI-ultrasound registration for the correction of intra-operative brain deformations. In: Niessen, W.J., Viergever, M.A. (eds.) MICCAI 2001. LNCS, vol. 2208, pp. 913–922. Springer, Heidelberg (2001)

2. De Nigris, D., Collins, D., Arbel, T.: Multi-modal image registration based on gradient orientations of minimal uncertainty. IEEE Trans. Med. Imag. (2012)
3. Felzenszwalb, P.F., Huttenlocher, D.P.: Pictorial structures for object recognition. Int. J. Comp. Vis. 61, 55–79 (2005)
4. Heinrich, M.P., Jenkinson, M., Bhushan, M., Matin, T., Gleeson, F.V., Brady, S.M., Schnabel, J.A.: MIND: Modality independent neighbourhood descriptor for multi-modal deformable registration. Med. Imag. Anal. 16(7), 1423–1435 (2012)
5. Heinrich, M.P., Jenkinson, M., Brady, S.M., Schnabel, J.A.: Globally optimal deformable registration on a minimum spanning tree using dense displacement sampling. In: Ayache, N., Delingette, H., Golland, P., Mori, K. (eds.) MICCAI 2012, Part III. LNCS, vol. 7512, pp. 115–122. Springer, Heidelberg (2012)
6. Heinrich, M., Jenkinson, M., Brady, M., Schnabel, J.: MRF-based deformable registration and ventilation estimation of lung CT. IEEE Trans. Med. Imag. (2013)
7. Heitz, G., Koller, D.: Learning spatial context: Using stuff to find things. In: Forsyth, D., Torr, P., Zisserman, A. (eds.) ECCV 2008, Part I. LNCS, vol. 5302, pp. 30–43. Springer, Heidelberg (2008)
8. Klein, S., Staring, M., Pluim, J.: Evaluation of optimization methods for nonrigid medical image registration using mutual information and B-Splines. IEEE Trans. Image Proc. 16(12), 2879–2890 (2007)
9. Lu, C., Chelikani, S., Papademetris, X., Knisely, J.P., Milosevic, M.F., Chen, Z., Jaffray, D.A., Staib, L.H., Duncan, J.S.: An integrated approach to segmentation and nonrigid registration for application in image-guided pelvic radiotherapy. Med. Imag. Anal. 15(5), 772–785 (2011)
10. Maes, F., Collignon, A., Vandermeulen, D., Marchal, G., Suetens, P.: Multimodality image registration by maximization of mutual information. IEEE Trans. Med. Imag. 16(2), 187–198 (1997)
11. Maurer, C.R., Hill, D.L.G., Martin, A.J., Liu, H., McCue, M., Rueckert, D., Lloret, D., Hall, W.A., Maxwell, R.E., Hawkes, D.J., Truwit, C.L.: Investigation of intraoperative brain deformation using a 1.5 Tesla interventional MR system: Preliminary results. IEEE Trans. Med. Imaging 17(5), 817–825 (1998)
12. Mercier, L., Del Maestro, R., Petrecca, K., Araujo, D., Haegelen, C., Collins, D.: Online database of clinical MR and ultrasound images of brain tumors. Med. Phys. 39, 3253 (2012)
13. Pluim, J., Maintz, J., Viergever, M.: Image registration by maximization of combined mutual information and gradient information. IEEE Trans. Med. Imag. 19(8), 809–814 (2000)
14. Rivaz, H., Collins, D.L.: Self-similarity weighted mutual information: A new nonrigid image registration metric. In: Ayache, N., Delingette, H., Golland, P., Mori, K. (eds.) MICCAI 2012, Part III. LNCS, vol. 7512, pp. 91–98. Springer, Heidelberg (2012)
15. Shechtman, E., Irani, M.: Matching local self-similarities across images and videos. In: CVPR 2007, pp. 1–8. IEEE (2007)
16. Staring, M., van der Heide, U., Klein, S., Viergever, M., Pluim, J.: Registration of cervical MRI using multifeature mutual information. IEEE Trans. Med. Imag. 28(9), 1412–1421 (2009)
17. Viola, P., Wells III, W.: Alignment by maximization of mutual information. Int. J. Comput. Vision 24(2), 137–154 (1997)
18. Wachinger, C., Navab, N.: Entropy and laplacian images: Structural representations for multi-modal registration. Med. Imag. Anal. 16(1), 1–17 (2012)
19. Wein, W., Brunke, S., Khamene, A., Callstrom, M.R., Navab, N.: Automatic CT-ultrasound registration for diagnostic imaging and image-guided intervention. Med. Imag. Anal. 12(5), 577 (2008)

# Efficient Convex Optimization Approach to 3D Non-rigid MR-TRUS Registration

Yue Sun[1], Jing Yuan[1], Martin Rajchl[1], Wu Qiu[1], Cesare Romagnoli[2], and Aaron Fenster[1,2]

[1] Imaging Research Labs, Robarts Research Institute, Western University, Canada
[2] Department of Medical Imaging, Western University, Canada

**Abstract.** In this study, we propose an efficient non-rigid MR-TRUS deformable registration method to improve the accuracy of targeting suspicious locations during a 3D ultrasound (US) guided prostate biopsy. The proposed deformable registration approach employs the multi-channel modality independent neighbourhood descriptor (MIND) as the local similarity feature across the two modalities of MR and TRUS, and a novel and efficient duality-based convex optimization based algorithmic scheme is introduced to extract the deformations which align the two MIND descriptors. The registration accuracy was evaluated using 10 patient images by measuring the TRE of manually identified corresponding intrinsic fiducials in the whole gland and peripheral zone, and performance metrics (DSC, MAD and MAXD) for the apex, mid-gland and base of the prostate were also calculated by comparing two manually segmented prostate surfaces in the registered 3D MR and TRUS images. Experimental results show that the proposed method yielded an overall mean TRE of 1.74 mm, which is favorably comparable to a clinical requirement for an error of less than 2.5 mm.

**Keywords:** Non-rigid Image Registration, Convex Optimization, MR-TRUS prostate registration, MIND Similarity Measurement.

## 1 Introduction

Prostate cancer is the most common non-skin cancer in men of developed countries, with a large and increasing incidence in most countries, and the third leading cause of death due to cancer. It is estimated to affect 26,500 men in Canada in 2012 [1], 238,590 in United States in 2013 [2] and is the most common cancer in men in UK (40,975 new cases in 2010) [3]. To this end, transrectal ultrasound (TRUS) guided prostate biopsy is the standard approach for definitive diagnosis and guiding biopsy needles to suspicious regions in the prostate, due to its real-time and radiation-free imaging capability, low cost and operation simplicity [4]. However, its lack of image contrast to clearly visualize early-stage prostate cancer results in false-negative rates for systematic sextant biopsies ranging up to 30% [5] and thereby increasing the number of repeat biopsies.

Recent developments in Magnetic Resonance Imaging (MRI) have demonstrated a high sensitivity and specificity for the detection of early stage prostate

K. Mori et al. (Eds.): MICCAI 2013, Part I, LNCS 8149, pp. 195–202, 2013.
© Springer-Verlag Berlin Heidelberg 2013

cancer [6]. Reports have shown that MRI can achieve a high accuracy of diagnosing prostate cancer at approximately 72-76% [7]. Although MR prostate imaging is advancing, it cannot yet replace TRUS guided needle biopsy, especially when real-time guidance is required, due to the high cost and time consuming procedure associated with performing MR imaging and targeting. In this regard, MR-TRUS registration technique provides an effective way to use TRUS to target biopsy needles toward regions of the prostate containing MR identified suspicious lesions [8]. However, efficient and accurate 3D non-rigid MR-TRUS registration is a challenging task due to the totally different image appearances of these two image modalities, in spite of its great clinical interests in practice. Few works to date have contributed to this task. Hu *et al.* [9] used a patient-specific finite element-based statistical motion model trained by biomechanical simulations and registered the model to 3D TRUS images, which was done by maximizing the likelihood of a particular model shape given a voxel intensity-based feature that provided an estimate of surface normal vectors at the boundary of the gland. Mitra *et al.* [10] proposed a 2D thin-plate spline-based non-linear regularization approach to align the sampled points of the segmented prostate contours, which essentially match the Bhattacharyya distance of the applied statistical shape contexts; however, the proposed framework only worked in 2D, which limits its application in practice.

**Contributions:** In this work, we propose a novel duality-based approach to computing the challenging 3D MIND-based non-rigid MR-TRUS deformable registration. A coarse-to-fine scheme is applied to capture the large deformations, and at each resolution level, an efficient multiplier-based algorithm is employed to compute an updated incremental deformation field. We performed the proposed method to register 10 patient images. Our results demonstrate that the proposed method yields clinically sufficient accuracy with less user interactions, while the segmentation of prostate boundaries is not required. A mean TRE of 1.74 mm is obtained, which is favorably comparable to a clinical requirement for an error of less than 2.5 mm.

## 2   Method

The modality independent neighbourhood descriptor (MIND) introduced by Heinrich *et al.* [11] presents an image descriptor independent of the modality, contrast and noise of various image modalities, while sensitive to the inherent image features such as image corners or edges etc. It is actually based on the local image self-similarity feature, which was originally introduced by Buades *et al.* [12] for image denoising. In [11], Heinrich *et al.* demonstrated for image registration, especially with different image modalities, the point-wise MIND descriptor performs superior to the other proposed image information descriptors, such as the normalized mutual information (NMI) [13] or patch-based entropy descriptor [14] etc. In this work, we utilize MIND as the cross-modality measure to the introduced 3D non-rigid MR-TRUS deformable registration. Let $I^M(x)$ and $I^R(x)$ be the input 3D MR image and TRUS image respectively.

$\mathcal{M}(x) := (m_1(x), \ldots, m_k(x))^\mathsf{T}$ and $\mathcal{R}(x) := (r_1(x), \ldots, r_k(x))^\mathsf{T}$ be the computed $k$-channel MIND descriptor at $x$ associated with the MR image $I^M(x)$ and the TRUS image $I^R(x)$, where $k$ is the dimension of the applied MIND descriptor. We aim to minimize a difference measure between $\mathcal{M}(x)$ and the deformed $\mathcal{R}(x+u)$ over the deformation field $u(x) = (u_1(x), u_2(x), u_3(x))^\mathsf{T}$, which can be essentially formulated as

$$\min_u P(\mathcal{M}(x), \mathcal{R}(x+u)) := \sum_{i=1}^k \int p_i(m_i(x) - r_i(x+u)) \, dx, \qquad (1)$$

where the penalty function $p_i(v)$, $i = 1 \ldots k$, is often positive and convex. For example, when $p_i(v) = |v|^2/2$, $i = 1 \ldots k$, the above formulation defines the sum of squared difference measure (SSD). Clearly, the minimization of (1) is ill-posed, for which a smoothness regularization of the deformation field $u(x)$ is often added to (1) to restrict the solution space of $u(x)$. In this paper, we consider the convex regularization term $G(u) := \sum_{i=1}^3 \int |\nabla u_i|^2 \, dx$, which results in the following minimization problem

$$\min_u P(\mathcal{M}(x), \mathcal{R}(x+u)) + \alpha \, G(u) \qquad (2)$$

where $\alpha > 0$ is constant.

## 2.1  Linearization and Primal-Dual Optimization Approach

Note the function $\mathcal{R}(x+u)$ is often highly non-smooth, hence the energy function of (2). To efficiently address the challenging minimization problem of (2), we first linearize and approximate $\mathcal{R}(x+u) := (r_1(x+u), \ldots, r_k(x+u))$ by

$$r_i(x+u) \simeq (r_i + \nabla r_i \cdot u)(x), \quad i = 1 \ldots k. \qquad (3)$$

Therefore, we have the linearized approximation of (2) which amounts to

$$\min_u \sum_{i=1}^k \int p_i\Big(\big((m_i - r_i) - \nabla r_i \cdot u\big)(x)\Big) \, dx + \alpha \, G(u). \qquad (4)$$

Let $p_i^*(w)$, $i = 1 \ldots k$, be the conjugate of the convex function $p_i(v)$ such that

$$p_i(v_i(x)) = \max_{w_i(x)} v_i(x) \cdot w_i(x) - p_i^*(w_i(x)). \qquad (5)$$

However, we also have

$$\alpha \, G(u) = \max_q \sum_{j=1}^3 \langle \operatorname{div} q_j, u_j \rangle - \frac{1}{2\alpha} \sum_{j=1}^3 \int q_j^2(x) \, dx. \qquad (6)$$

In view of (3)-(6), through simple computation, we have the following *dual formulation* to the convex minimization problem (4):

$$\max_{w,q} E(w,q) := \sum_{i=1}^k \langle w_i, m_i - r_i \rangle - \sum_{i=1}^k \int p_i^*(w_i(x)) \, dx - \frac{1}{2\alpha} \sum_{j=1}^3 \int q_j^2(x) \, dx$$

$$(7)$$

subject to

$$F_j(x) := \sum_{i=1}^{k} w_i(x) \cdot \partial_j r_i(x) - \operatorname{div} q_j(x) = 0; \quad j \in \{1,2,3\}, \; \forall x \in \Omega. \quad (8)$$

By modern convex optimization theories, it is easy to prove that

**Proposition 1.** *The* convex minimization problem (4) *and the* dual optimization formulation (7) *are equivalent to each other, i.e.* (4) $\Longleftrightarrow$ (7).

In fact, each component of the deformation field $(u_1(x), u_2(x), u_3(x))^\top$ just works as the multiplier function to the respective linear equalities (8) under the perspective of primal and dual. Therefore, we can derive an efficient duality-based Lagrangian augmented algorithm, see [15,16] for details of the modern dual optimization theory and applications in image processing.

### 2.2 Coarse-to-Fine Incremental Scheme

To capture the large deformations, a coarse-to-fine scheme is applied. First, we construct a coarse-to-fine pyramid of each MIND descriptor function: let $\mathcal{M}^1(x)$ $\dots \mathcal{M}^L(x)$ be the $L$-level coarse-to-fine pyramid representation of $\mathcal{M}(x)$ from the coarsest resolution $\mathcal{M}_1(x)$ to the finest resolution $\mathcal{M}^L(x) = \mathcal{M}(x)$; and $\mathcal{R}^1(x)$ $\dots \mathcal{R}^L(x)$ the $L$-level coarse-to-fine pyramid representation of $\mathcal{R}(x)$.

At each $\ell$ level, $\ell = 1 \dots L$, we compute the deformation field $u^\ell(x)$ based on the two MIND functions $\mathcal{M}^\ell(x)$ and $\mathcal{R}^\ell(x + u^{\ell-1})$ at the same resolution level, where $\mathcal{R}^\ell(x + u^{\ell-1})$ is warped by the deformation field $u^{\ell-1}(x)$ computed at the previous level $\ell - 1$. For the coarsest level, i.e. $\ell = 1$, the so-called previous-level deformation is set to be 0.

## 3  Experiments and Evaluation

**Manual Initialization.** The MR image is first resampled to have the same dimensions and voxel size as the TRUS image. We initialize the registration using 3 manually placed approximately corresponding landmarks and the centroid of the three points as a default point on the 3D TRUS and MR images to generate a rigid transform as initial alignment. These manually selected landmarks are closely associated with geometric features that can be observed on both modalities. Fig. 1 shows an example of the landmarks on the prostate boundary on the axial MR and 3D TRUS slices, which correspond to the image with the largest view of the prostate.

**Materials.** In this study, T2-weighted MR images using a body coil and corresponding 3D TRUS images from 10 patients were acquired. The MR images were obtained at 3 Tesla using a GE Excite HD MRI system (Milwaukee, WI, USA) at an image size of $512 \times 512 \times 36$ voxels with a voxel size of $0.27 \times 0.27 \times 2.2$ mm$^3$. The 3D TRUS images were acquired using a 3D TRUS mechanical scanning system developed in our laboratory, using a Philips HDI-5000 US machine with a Philips C9-5 transducer. The 3D TRUS image size is $448 \times 448 \times 350$ voxels with a voxel size of $0.19 \times 0.19 \times 0.19$ mm$^3$.

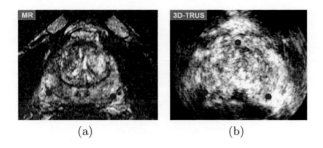

(a)                              (b)

**Fig. 1.** Red dots indicate corresponding anatomical landmarks on the MR (a) and TRUS images (b)

**Evaluation.** We measured the target registration error (TRE) as the overall misalignment of manually marked corresponding intrinsic fiducials in MR and 3D TRUS images. We selected 41 fiducial pairs, of which 17 were within the peripheral zone (PZ), in which up to 80% of the tumors can be located. The PZ is subject to the deformation caused by the US transducer during the biopsy, which must be corrected to allow accurate biopsy targeting. We also measured the fiducial localization error (FLE) [17] to allow determination whether fiducial identification dominates the TRE. We also compared the registered MR and corresponding 3D TRUS images by calculating the Dice similarity coefficient (DSC) [18], the mean absolute surface distance (MAD), and the maximum absolute surface distance (MAXD) [19]. All validation metrics were separately calculated for three prostate sub-regions: the apex, mid-gland and base, selected along the apex-base axis of the manual segmented TRUS prostates (0.3, 0.4, 0.3 of the length of the base-apex axis respectively) [20].

**Accuracy.** The frequency distributions of the TREs for the PZ, central gland (CG) and whole gland (WG) are plotted in Figure 3 and the mean TRE results are summarized in Table 1. The results of FLE are 0.21 mm for 3D TRUS and 0.18 mm for MR. Table 2 shows the mean DSC, MAD and MAXD for WG, apex, mid-gland, and base, respectively.

**Computation Time.** The proposed non-rigid MR-TRUS registration algorithm was implemented using parallel computing architecture (CUDA, NVIDIA Corp., Santa Clara, CA), and the user interface was developed in Matlab (Natick, MA). The experiments were conducted on a Windows desktop with an Intel i7-3770 CPU (3.4 GHz) and a GPU of NVIDIA Geforce 680GTX. The mean registration time of our method per patient was $90 \pm 5s$ in addition to $30 \pm 5s$ for initialization.

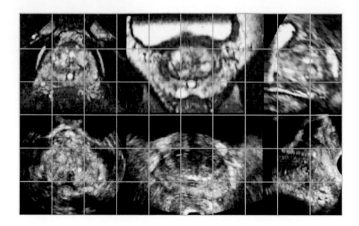

**Fig. 2.** Examples of axial (left column), coronal (middle column) and sagittal (right column) views through registered MR (top row) and 3D TRUS (bottom row) images

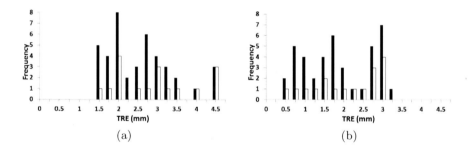

(a)                                    (b)

**Fig. 3.** WG (black) and PZ (white) frequency distributions of: (a) initial alignment TRE between all 41 fiducial pairs, and (b) non-rigid registration TRE

**Table 1.** Peripheral zone (PZ), central gland (CG) and whole gland (WG) mean TRE results for non rigid MR-TRUS registration

|          | PZ            | CG            | WG            |
|----------|---------------|---------------|---------------|
| TRE (mm) | $1.97 \pm 0.86$ | $1.58 \pm 0.82$ | $1.74 \pm 0.84$ |

**Table 2.** Results of DSC, MAD and MAXD for 10 patient images

|            | Apex           | Mid            | Base            | WG             |
|------------|----------------|----------------|-----------------|----------------|
| DSC (%)    | $83.0 \pm 5.6$ | $92.9 \pm 2.6$ | $80.1 \pm 4.7$  | $85.6 \pm 2.5$ |
| MAD (mm)   | $2.09 \pm 0.69$ | $1.36 \pm 0.44$ | $2.38 \pm 0.63$ | $1.79 \pm 0.36$ |
| MAXD (mm)  | $9.22 \pm 2.84$ | $4.81 \pm 0.76$ | $10.12 \pm 2.99$ | $7.86 \pm 2.99$ |

# 4    Discussion and Conclusion

In this work, we propose a convex optimization approach to non-rigid image-based MR-TRUS registration, which yielded PZ, CG and WG TRE values of 1.97 mm, 1.58 mm and 1.74 mm respectively (less than the clinically acceptable maximum TRE of 2.5 mm [21]). The higher value in PZ is due to the deformation caused by the US probe. Figure 3(b) shows that 80% of the TRE values for WG and 76% for PZ are below the desired values. The FLE was 0.21 mm for 3D TRUS images, and 0.18 mm for MR. Thus, the FLEs did not dominate the overall TRE. Table 2 shows that the proposed method generated a favorable DSC value of $92.9 \pm 2.6\%$ for the mid-gland, $83.0 \pm 5.6\%$ for the apex, and $80.1 \pm 4.7\%$ for the base. The lower DSC values for the apex and base compared to the mid-gland were caused by the low degree of structure recognition in these regions for MR and especially TRUS images. In addition, our method delivers similar consistent results of MAD and MAXD to the DSC. The mean TRE of $1.74 \pm 0.84$ mm is higher than the value of $1.60 \pm 1.17$ mm in Mitra *et al.* [10]. However, their method needed a segmented prostate surface for both MR and TRUS images, and also required the established MR-TRUS slice correspondence, which is difficult to achieve in practice. A median Root Mean Square (RMS) TRE of 2.4 mm was achieved in Hu *et al.* [9]; however, their biomechanical modeling required the additional segmentations of the MR prostate gland and lesion for the assistance (about 45 mins per patient).

In conclusion, to reduce the false negative rate for prostate biopsy, we developed an alternate approach using 3D TRUS images registered with MR images with targets identified to guide the biopsy. An efficient dual optimization approach is proposed to extracting the non-rigid MR-TRUS deformation field by registering the given two MIND descriptors, which does not require the segmentation of the prostate boundaries. Experimental results demonstrate that the proposed method yields clinically sufficient accuracy with less user interactions. In computation, once the deformation field is discretized, a dynamic prima-dual scheme [22] can also be adapted to extract the discrete-valued voxelwise correspondences.

**Acknowledgements.** The authors are grateful for the funding support from the Canadian Institutes of Health Research (CIHR), the Ontario Institute of Cancer Research (OICR), and the Canada Research Chairs (CRC) Program.

# References

1. Canadian Cancer Society (2012), http://www.cancer.ca
2. National Cancer Institute (2012), http://www.cancer.gov
3. Cancer Research UK (2013), http://www.cancerresearchuk.org
4. Rifkin, M.: Ultrasound of the prostate: imaging in the diagnosis and therapy of prostatic disease. Lippincott-Raven Publishers (1997)
5. Norberg, M., Egevad, L., Holmberg, L., Sparén, P., Norlén, B., Busch, C.: The sextant protocol for ultrasound-guided core biopsies of the prostate underestimates the presence of cancer. Urology 50(4), 562–566 (1997)

6. Zakian, K.L., Sircar, K., Hricak, H., Chen, H.N., Shukla-Dave, A., Eberhardt, S., Muruganandham, M., Ebora, L., Kattan, M.W., Reuter, V.E., Scardino, P.T., Koutcher, J.A.: Correlation of proton MR spectroscopic imaging with gleason score based on step-section pathologic analysis after radical prostatectomy. Radiology 234(3), 804–814 (2005)

7. Vilanova, J., Barceló-Vidal, C., Comet, J., Boada, M., Barceló, J., Ferrer, J., Albanell, J.: Usefulness of prebiopsy multifunctional and morphologic MRI combined with free-to-total prostate-specific antigen ratio in the detection of prostate cancer. American Journal of Roen 196, W715–W722 (2011)

8. Sonn, G.A., Natarajan, S., Margolis, D.J., MacAiran, M., Lieu, P., Huang, J., Dorey, F.J., Marks, L.S.: Targeted biopsy in the detection of prostate cancer using an office based magnetic resonance ultrasound fusion device. The Journal of Urology 189(1), 86–92 (2013)

9. Hu, Y., Ahmed, H.U., Taylor, Z., Allen, C., Emberton, M., Hawkes, D., Barratt, D.: MR to ultrasound registration for image-guided prostate interventions. Medical Image Analysis 16(3), 687–703 (2012)

10. Mitra, J., Kato, Z., Marti, R., Oliver, A., Llad, X., Sidib, D., Ghose, S., Vilanova, J.C., Comet, J., Meriaudeau, F.: A spline-based non-linear diffeomorphism for multimodal prostate registration. Medical Image Analysis 16(6), 1259–1279 (2012)

11. Heinrich, M.P., Jenkinson, M., Bhushan, M., Matin, T., Gleeson, F.V., Brady, S.M., Schnabel, J.A.: Mind: Modality independent neighbourhood descriptor for multi-modal deformable registration. MedIA 16(7), 1423–1435 (2012)

12. Buades, A., Coll, B., Morel, J.M.: A non-local algorithm for image denoising. In: CVPR, pp. 60–65 (2005)

13. Hermosillo, G., Chefd'Hotel, C., Faugeras, O.D.: Variational methods for multimodal image matching. International Journal of Computer Vision 50(3), 329–343 (2002)

14. Wachinger, C., Navab, N.: Entropy and laplacian images: Structural representations for multi-modal registration. Medical Image Analysis 16(1), 1–17 (2012)

15. Yuan, J., Bae, E., Tai, X.: A study on continuous max-flow and min-cut approaches. In: CVPR (2010)

16. Yuan, J., Bae, E., Tai, X.-C., Boykov, Y.: A continuous max-flow approach to potts model. In: Daniilidis, K., Maragos, P., Paragios, N. (eds.) ECCV 2010, Part VI. LNCS, vol. 6316, pp. 379–392. Springer, Heidelberg (2010)

17. Fitzpatrick, J., West, J., Maurer Jr., C.R.: Predicting error in rigid-body point-based registration. IEEE TMI 17(5), 694–702 (1998)

18. Zou, K., Warfield, S., Bharatha, A., Tempany, C., Kaus, M., Haker, S., Wells, W., Jolesz, F., Kikinis, R.: Statistical validation of image segmentation quality based on a spatial overlap index. Academic Radiology 11(2), 178–189 (2004)

19. Qiu, W., Yuan, J., Ukwatta, E., Tessier, D., Fenster, A.: Rotational-slice-based prostate segmentation using level set with shape constraint for 3D end-firing TRUS guided biopsy. In: Ayache, N., Delingette, H., Golland, P., Mori, K. (eds.) MICCAI 2012, Part I. LNCS, vol. 7510, pp. 537–544. Springer, Heidelberg (2012)

20. Mahdavi, S.S., Chng, N., Spadinger, I., Morris, W.J., Salcudean, S.E.: Semi-automatic segmentation for prostate interventions. Medical Image Analysis 15(2), 226–237 (2011)

21. Karnik, V., Fenster, A., Bax, J., Cool, D., Gardi, L., Gyacskov, I., Romagnoli, C., Ward, A.: Assessment of image registration accuracy in three-dimensional transrectal ultrasound guided prostate biopsy. Medical physics 37, 802 (2010)

22. Komodakis, N., Tziritas, G., Paragios, N.: Fast, approximately optimal solutions for single and dynamic MRFs. In: CVPR (2007)

# Left-Invariant Metrics for Diffeomorphic Image Registration with Spatially-Varying Regularisation

Tanya Schmah[1], Laurent Risser[2], and François-Xavier Vialard[3]

[1] Rotman Research Institute, Baycrest, Toronto, Canada
[2] CNRS, Institut de Mathématiques de Toulouse (UMR 5219), France*
[3] CEREMADE (UMR 7534), Université Paris Dauphine, France

**Abstract.** We present a new framework for diffeomorphic image registration which supports natural interpretations of spatially-varying metrics. This framework is based on *left-invariant diffeomorphic metrics* (LIDM) and is closely related to the now standard *large deformation diffeomorphic metric mapping* (LDDMM). We discuss the relationship between LIDM and LDDMM and introduce a computationally convenient class of spatially-varying metrics appropriate for both frameworks. Finally, we demonstrate the effectiveness of our method on a 2D toy example and on the 40 3D brain images of the LPBA40 dataset.

## 1 Introduction

Medical image registration often consists in estimating the transformation $\phi$ which "best" maps images $I$ and $J$. In diffeomorphic registration frameworks, $\phi$ is constrained to be a diffeomorphism, and in particular invertible. Successful diffeomorphic approaches include the Large Deformation Diffeomorphic Metric Matching framework (LDDMM) [13,3], and the closely-related Symmetric Normalisation (SyN) algorithm [2], as well as LogDemons [14]. In the LDDMM framework, we seek a path of diffeomorphisms $\phi(t)$, such that $\phi(0)$ is the identity and $\phi(1)$ is the final transformation of the image. The *spatial (Eulerian) velocity* of a path $\phi(t)$ is the time-varying vector field $v$ defined by

$$\partial_t \phi(t) = v(t) \circ \phi(t), \tag{1}$$

where the the symbol $\circ$ denotes composition. Given a Hilbert space $V$ of smooth vector fields with norm $\|.\|_V$, the matching problem is to find a time-varying vector field $v$ that minimises the functional

$$\mathcal{J}(v) = \frac{1}{2} \int_0^1 \|v(t)\|_V^2 \, dt + \frac{\lambda}{2} \|I \circ \phi(1)^{-1} - J\|_{L^2}^2, \tag{2}$$

under the constraint (1). The minimisation problem (2) is well-posed provided that the norm on $V$ is sufficiently strong in terms of smoothness. The first term

---

* The authors thank the AO1 grant from Université Paul Sabatier (Toulouse, France) and the ANR DEMOS project for funding.

K. Mori et al. (Eds.): MICCAI 2013, Part I, LNCS 8149, pp. 203–210, 2013.

of (2) is a "regularisation term" (or "energy term") that serves both to guarantee a well-posed problem and to force $\phi$ to stay "small". In practice, $V$ is defined by its reproducing kernel $K$ which is often chosen to be Gaussian.

Spatially-varying or non-isotropic regularisation is of great interest in medical applications, where it can represent variable deformability of tissue. For example, [7] models sliding conditions between the lungs and the ribs using piecewise-diffeomorphic transformations, *i.e.* transformations which are diffeomorphic in different regions only, and not in the whole image domain. Another recent example is the direction-dependent regularisation in [8], which computes displacement fields directly (and so large deformations may be non-invertible). Both of these papers use a fixed regularisation scheme based on prior anatomical knowledge. Neither paper uses fully diffeomorphic transformations.

Spatially-varying (or non-isotropic) regularisation within a diffeomorphic framework is clearly of interest, however it has not appeared in the literature until now. In LDDMM and SyN, we believe that this is because their standard interpretation in terms of moving source images does not support a natural interpretation of a spatially-varying regularisation kernel. Indeed in LDDMM, consider a deformation path $\phi(t)$ and a point $X$ in the source image. As $X$ moves along the path $\phi(t)(X)$, the contribution of its spatial velocity (defined by (1)) to the functional $\mathcal{J}(v)$ in (2) depends on the value of the regularisation kernel $K$ at the (moving) point $\phi(t)(X)$. Conversely the value of $K$ at a single point $x$ affects the regularisation along a whole curve of points in the source image. Thus there is no sense in which $K(x)$ at a single value of $x$ can be said to describe deformability at a single point of the source image.

With this motivation, we propose a new diffeomorphic registration framework that *does* support natural interpretations of spatially-varying metrics: Left-Invariant Diffeomorphic Matching (LIDM). This framework is analogous to LDDMM but based on a *left*-invariant metric, i.e. based on a norm in the body (Lagrangian) coordinates of the source image. This means that instead of the norm being applied to the spatial (Eulerian) velocity defined by (1), it is applied to the *convective velocity* defined by

$$\partial_t \phi(t) = d\phi(t) \cdot v(t)\,, \tag{3}$$

where $d\phi(t)$ is the spatial derivative of $\phi(t)$ and the symbol $\cdot$ denotes the multiplication of a matrix and a vector. The matching problem in LIDM is to minimise the same functional as in LDDMM (2) but under the "new" constraint (3). In this framework, the $v(t)$ in (2) is a convective velocity, which is expressed in body coordinates at all times $t$. At any given point $X$ in the source image, the contribution of $v(t)(X)$ to the energy term is controlled by $K(X)$ for all $t$. Hence $K(X)$ regularises the deformation at $X$, and in this sense describes *a priori* deformability of the source image at $X$. The parameters of $K$ can be learnt from data, a point to which we return in the Discussion.

In Section 2, we present the gradient calculation of the matching functional in the LIDM model. We then develop in Section 3 the correspondence between LIDM and LDDMM. Finally, the performance of the LIDM model is tested on synthetic and real data in Section 5.

## 2   A Gradient Descent Algorithm for LIDM

In this section, we apply a standard adjoint calculation in order to compute the gradient of the LIDM functional (2), which is the same as in LDDMM, subject to Eq. (3), and not Eq. (1). Our method is very similar to that in [11]. The first step is to write the constraint (3) in the following form:

$$\partial_t \phi_i(t) = \langle \nabla \phi_i, v(t) \rangle, \tag{4}$$

for $i = 1, \ldots, d$, where $d$ is the dimension of the ambient space, $\phi_i$ is the $i^{\text{th}}$ coordinate of $\phi$, and $\langle \cdot, \cdot \rangle$ the standard scalar product on $\mathbb{R}^d$. As usual, we introduce time dependent Lagrange multipliers denoted by $P_i(t) \in L^2(\mathbb{R}^d, \mathbb{R})$ in order to compute the adjoint equations, the augmented functional is then

$$\tilde{\mathcal{J}}(v, P) = \mathcal{J}(v) + \sum_{i=1}^{d} \int_0^1 \langle P_i, \partial_t \phi_i(t) - \langle \nabla \phi_i, v(t) \rangle_{\mathbb{R}^d} \rangle_{L^2(\mathbb{R}^d, \mathbb{R})} \, dt. \tag{5}$$

Note that the scalar product $\langle \cdot, \cdot \rangle_{L^2(\mathbb{R}^d, \mathbb{R})}$ is the usual pairing in $L^2(\mathbb{R}^d, \mathbb{R})$. The gradient of (5) can be computed by taking free variations of the augmented functional. Variations w.r.t. $v$ lead to

$$\nabla \tilde{\mathcal{J}}(v)(t) = v(t) - K \langle \nabla \phi(t), P(t) \rangle_{\mathbb{R}^d}, \tag{6}$$

where $K$ denotes the isomorphism from $V^*$ (the dual of $V$) to $V$ and $\langle \nabla \phi(t), P(t) \rangle_{\mathbb{R}^d} = \sum_{i=1}^{d} P_i \nabla \phi_i$. In addition, $P(t) = [P_i]_{i=1,\ldots,d}$ is equivalent to a vector field and solves $\dot{P}_i(t) = \nabla \cdot (P_i(t) v(t))$ where $\nabla \cdot$ stands for the divergence of a vector field. The previous equation is given by taking variations of functional (5) w.r.t. $\phi$. Note that variations w.r.t. $P_i$ lead to the reconstruction equation (3). Last, the boundary condition at time 1 for the case of the square of the $L^2$ norm that appears in (2) is:

$$P(1) = d\phi^{-T}(1)[|D\phi(1)|\Delta \circ \phi(1) \nabla I], \tag{7}$$

where $\Delta = \lambda(I \circ \phi^{-1}(1) - J)$ and $|D\phi(1)|$ denotes the Jacobian determinant of $\phi(1)$. The notation $d\phi^{-T}(1)$ denotes the inverse transpose of $d\phi(1)$. Combining equations (6) and (7), we obtain

$$\nabla \tilde{\mathcal{J}}(v)(t) = v(t) - K \, m(t), \tag{8}$$

where $m(t) = \nabla \hat{I}(t)|D\phi(t)| \left( \hat{I}(t) - J \circ \phi(t) \right)$ and $\hat{I}(t) := I \circ \left( \phi(1)^{-1} \circ \phi(t) \right)$.

Perhaps not unexpectedly, those equations are very close to the gradient of the standard LDDMM functional. In the next section, we detail the relations between the two models.

## 3   Relation to Standard LDDMM

The previous calculation guides us towards the strong relation between LIDM and LDDMM models. By comparing the LDDMM gradient (see [6,12] for instance) and the LIDM gradient, the reader may infer the following proposition.

**Proposition 1.** *The optimal LIDM path $\phi(t)$ is given by $\phi(t) = \psi_1 \circ \psi_{1-t}^{-1}$ for $\psi(t)$ the LDDMM optimal path. In particular, the final diffeomorphic mappings are the same in the two models, $\phi(1) = \psi(1)$.*

*Proof (Outline).* The minimization of the functional (2) can be written as:

$$\mathcal{J}(v) = \frac{1}{2} \int_0^1 \|v(t)\|_V^2 \, dt + \frac{\lambda}{2} \|I \circ \psi(1) - J\|_{L^2}^2 , \tag{9}$$

with $\partial_t \psi(t) = -v(t) \circ \psi(t)$. This is close to the standard LDDMM formulation but the two differences are (1) the use of $\psi^{-1}$ instead of $\psi$ and (2) the minus sign in the previous flow equation. Moreover, the first term of the functional is the square of the right-invariant distance $\mathsf{d}$ on the group of diffeomorphisms so that $\mathsf{d}(Id, \psi) = \mathsf{d}(\psi^{-1}, Id)$. Indeed, if $v_R(t)$ is a geodesic vector field for LDMMM between $Id$ and $\psi$, then $-v_R(1-t)$ is a geodesic between $Id$ and $\psi^{-1}$. We therefore have shown that to an optimal path $v(t)$ of functional (2) corresponds an optimal path $v_R(t)$ of the corresponding LDDMM functional such that $v(t) = v_R(1-t)$.

In summary, the final diffeomorphic mapping is the same in both approaches but the diffeomorphism paths do differ. There are two optimal paths from $Id$ to $\phi_1$: one left- and one right- geodesic. Fig. 1 illustrates the different optimal paths given by the two models in an exact matching problem of points (landmarks).

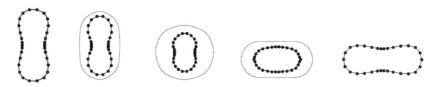

**Fig. 1.** Deformations from the left-most source image to the right-most target image. Green and blue curves show the optimal LDDMM and LIDM paths, respectively.

## 4    Spatially-Varying Metrics

The LIDM model opens up the opportunity to use spatially-varying and non-isotropic metrics, as explained in the Introduction. If some *a priori* information on the deformation intensity is known in body coordinates, then this can be modelled in the regularisation kernel. We now give a simple example of this.

As an idealised situation of interest, one can consider a partition of the template image domain $\Omega \subset \mathbb{R}^d$ into $n$ parts $(\Omega_i)_{i=1}^n$. To each part, one can associate a Gaussian kernel $k_{\sigma_i}$ with a given smoothing parameter $\sigma_i$ that incorporates some knowledge on the template. We also introduce a smooth partition of unity $\chi_i : \Omega \mapsto [0,1]$ satisfying $\sum_{i=1}^n \chi_i(x) = 1$ for $x \in \Omega$ and $\chi_i$ vanishing outside a compact containing $\Omega_i$. We can build the new kernel $K$:

$$K(x,y) = \sum_{i=1}^{n} \chi_i(x)k_{\sigma_i}(x,y)\chi_i(y) \text{ where } x, y \in \Omega \,.$$

In addition, this kernel has a variational interpretation (omitted here to save space) that justifies its form. This is the type of kernels we use for our experimental results on synthetic and real data in Section 5. Such a definition was motivated (1) by its simplicity to introduce different smoothing on the partition and (2) by computational considerations. Indeed, the computational cost of the kernel $K$ is $n$ times the cost of a single Gaussian kernel so that having two or three regions of interest is feasible in practical situations.

## 5    Results

### 5.1    Results on 2D Phantom Images

In this subsection, we register the phantom images shown in Fig. 2. We registered these images using: LIDM, Symmetric Normalization (SyN)[1] [2] and multi-kernel LDDMM[2] [6]. Note that SyN is closely-related to LDDMM, and its implementation in ANTS is considered to be state-of-the-art for neuroimaging [5]. Specifically, we used the following techniques: (**LIDM**) Considering the partition of unity shown in Fig. 2, we used Gaussian smoothing kernels with standard deviations 33 and 4 pixels in the white and black regions, respectively. These values were chosen because they are half of the width of the dark grey circle and the small black structures protruding from its inner surface, respectively. (**SyN**$_{\sigma_f,\sigma_d}$) We used the command "ANTS 2 -m MSQ[target,source,1,0] -i 100x100x1000 -r Gauss[$\sigma_f,\sigma_d$] -t SyN[0.4]". Gaussian kernels with various standard deviations to perform fluid-like ($\sigma_f$) and diffusion-like ($\sigma_d$) regularization were tested: After registering the images using a large kernel ($\sigma_f = 32$, $\sigma_d = 1$: SyN$_{init}$), we composed the deformation with those obtained using finer kernels ($\sigma_f = \{1, 2, 4, 8, 16\}$ and $\sigma_d = 0$, or $\sigma_f = 1$ and $\sigma_d = \{\frac{1}{8}, \frac{1}{4}, \frac{1}{2}, 1, 2, 4\}$). (**MK-LDDMM**) We used a kernel constructed as the sum of 7 Gaussian kernels having standard deviations linearly sampled between 1 and 50 and weights automatically tuned (option -M_Gauss_easier of uTIlzReg_LDDMM).

To evaluate the registration quality, we measured the sum of the square differences (SSD) between the registered images in the whole image domain $\Omega$ and in the ROI shown in Fig. 2, as well as the maximum determinant of the Jacobians (DetJ). SSDs were normalised by the corresponding SSD between the original images. Results are presented in Fig. 2 and Table 1. For SyN, we present a selection of results giving the best balance between SSD and DetJ.

The lowest SSDs, 0.14 for $\Omega$ and 0.21 in the ROI, were obtained by LIDM. A competitive strategy is (SyN) with fluid regularization ($\sigma_f > 0$), where SSD$_{\Omega} \in [0.20, 0.23]$ and SSD$_{\text{ROI}} \in [0.36, 0.38]$, for max DetJ $\in [3.59, 4.06]$. The matching is however higher using (LIDM) for a similar max DetJ.

---

[1] http://www.picsl.upenn.edu/ANTS/
[2] http://sourceforge.net/projects/utilzreg/

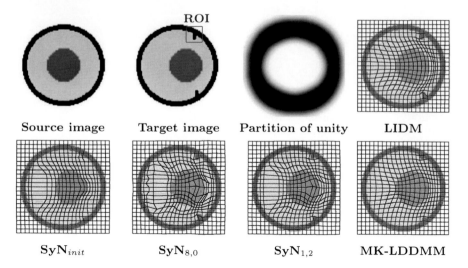

**Fig. 2.**   Results of image registration tests on a synthetic example

**Table 1.**   Quantitative results obtained on the synthetic images shown in Fig. 2. Subscripts after SyN indicate the degree of fluid- and diffusion-like regularisation $(\sigma_f, \sigma_d)$.

|  | LIDM | SyN$_{init}$ | SyN$_{2,0}$ | SyN$_{8,0}$ | SyN$_{1,0.25}$ | SyN$_{1,2}$ | MK-LDDMM |
|---|---|---|---|---|---|---|---|
| SSD$_\Omega$ | 0.14 | 0.46 | 0.21 | 0.23 | 0.19 | 0.28 | 0.29 |
| SSD$_{\mathrm{ROI}}$ | 0.21 | 0.73 | 0.36 | 0.37 | 0.37 | 0.63 | 0.68 |
| max DetJ | 3.70 | 2.06 | 4.06 | 3.59 | 3.67 | 2.35 | 2.6 |

## 5.2   Results on 3D Brain Images

We performed additional tests on the 40 subjects of the LONI Probabilistic Brain Atlas (LPBA40) [9], using the probabilistic tissue maps (white matter, grey matter and CSF). We first resampled all images to a resolution of 1 mm and aligned them to subject 09 using non-rigid registration with a very large smoothing kernel (SyN with the option -r Gauss[50,1]). We then constructed a partition of unity by dilating (structuring element of 2 mm) and smoothing (Gaussian kernel of 3 mm) the grey matter density map of subject 09. Finally, we registered subject 09 to all other ones using two strategies: **(LIDM)** We first used LIDM with the predefined partition of unity and Gaussian kernels having standard deviations of 7 mm around the grey matter and 33 mm elsewhere. The underlying idea here is that we allow more flexibility for the registration around the grey matter than in the rest of the image. **(SyN$_{\sigma_f,\sigma_d}$)** We also performed SyN registration with different regularisation parameters: -r Gauss[$\sigma_f,\sigma_d$], where $(\sigma_f, \sigma_d) = \{(7,2),(3,3),(10,4),(5,1),(2,2)\}$ as well as the parameters of Klein *et al* study [5]. We computed the SSD between each pair of registered images, the target overlaps between the segmented brain regions (see [5]), and the maximum DetJ of the deformations. SSDs were normalised by the SSD before registration.

As shown Table 2, SyN gives slightly better average results than LIDM here. However, normalised SSDs, overlaps and max DetJs are within the range of values produced by varying the SyN parameters. This shows the validity of LIDM for the analysis of 3D brain images and opens up interesting perspectives for further investigations with applications in medical imaging, as discussed in the next section.

**Table 2.** Average results obtained on the 40 3D brain images of the LPBA40 dataset

|          | LIDM  | $\text{SyN}_{7,2}$ | $\text{SyN}_{3,3}$ | $\text{SyN}_{10,4}$ | $\text{SyN}_{5,1}$ | $\text{SyN}_{2,2}$ | $\text{SyN}_{[5]}$ |
|----------|-------|--------|--------|---------|--------|--------|--------|
| SSD      | 0.28  | 0.21   | 0.23   | 0.30    | 0.17   | 0.21   | 0.21   |
| Overlap  | 0.723 | 0.717  | 0.716  | 0.713   | 0.715  | 0.708  | 0.728  |
| max DetJ | 5.02  | 4.55   | 3.20   | 2.81    | 6.38   | 4.85   | 5.36   |

## 6   Discussion

We have introduced a novel diffeomorphic matching framework, Left Invariant Diffeomorphic Matching (LIDM), in which spatially-varying and directionally-dependent regularisation kernels can encode local deformability properties of the source image. Through the relationship between LIDM and LDDMM described in Section 3, it also follows that spatially-varying and directionally-dependent kernels in LDDMM are interpretable in the same way, which has not been re-marked upon before.

We have demonstrated the value of spatially-varying kernels in registration, in experiments with both synthetic and real data (brain MRI). In both experiments, we applied LIDM with a fixed spatially-varying kernel, chosen on the basis of observed feature scales (for the synthetic example) and our experience with other algorithms (for the real data). We compared LIDM with two state-of-the-art algorithms: SyN (implemented in ANTS) and MK-LDDMM. For SyN, we explored a wide range of regularisation parameters. In the synthetic example, LIDM produced superior matches, as judged by sum of squared differences (SSD), while for the real data, LIDM produced results similar to SyN but not as good as the best SyN result. It is significant that in both cases, LIDM gave a good match with the first (and only) parameters that we chose, which suggests an important advantage in ease of use.

The main motivation driving our work is to automatically learn spatially-varying and directionally-dependent regularisation parameters, as has been done by Simpson et al. [10] for global regularisation parameters. Our contribution justifies this project in the diffeomorphic context, in LIDM and LDDMM and also, by extension, in SyN. Various methods could be used to optimise the parameters for a population of targets, including Bayesian methods related to those in [1,4].

# References

1. Allassonnière, S., Amit, Y., Trouvé, A.: Towards a coherent statistical framework for dense deformable template estimation. J. R. Statist. Soc. B 69(1), 3–29 (2007)
2. Avants, B.B., Epstein, C.L., Grossman, M., Gee, J.C.: Symmetric diffeomorphic image registration with cross-correlation: Evaluating automated labeling of elderly and neurodegenerative brain. Medical Image Analysis 12, 26–41 (2008)
3. Beg, M.F., Miller, M.I., Trouvé, A., Younes, L.: Computing large deformation metric mappings via geodesic flows of diffeomorphisms. Int. J. Comput. Vision 61(2), 139–157 (2005)
4. Cotter, C.J., Cotter, S.L., Vialard, F.X.: Bayesian data assimilation in shape registration. ArXiv e-prints (December 2012)
5. Klein, A., Ghosh, S.S., Avants, B.B., Yeo, B.T.T., Fischl, B., Ardekani, B.A., Gee, J.C., Mann, J.J., Parsey, R.V.: Evaluation of volume-based and surface-based brain image registration methods. NeuroImage 51(1), 214–220 (2010)
6. Risser, L., Vialard, F.X., Wolz, R., Murgasova, M., Holm, D.D., Rueckert, D.: Simultaneous Multi-scale Registration Using Large Deformation Diffeomorphic Metric Mapping. IEEE Transactions on Medical Imaging 30(10), 1746–1759 (2011)
7. Risser, L., Vialard, F.X., Baluwala, H.Y., Schnabel, J.A.: Piecewise-diffeomorphic image registration: Application to the motion estimation between 3D CT lung images with sliding conditions. Medical Image Analysis 17, 182–193 (2012)
8. Schmidt-Richberg, A., Werner, R., Handels, H., Ehrhardt, J.: Estimation of slipping organ motion by registration with direction-dependent regularization. Medical Image Analysis 16, 150–159 (2012)
9. Shattuck, D.W., Mirza, M., Adisetiyo, V., Hojatkashani, C., Salamon, G., Narr, K.L., Poldrack, R.A., Bilder, R.M., Toga, A.W.: Construction of a 3D probabilistic atlas of human cortical structures. NeuroImage 39, 1064–1080 (2008)
10. Simpson, I.J.A., Schnabel, J.A., Groves, A.R., Andersson, J.L.R., Woolrich, M.W.: Probabilistic inference of regularisation in non-rigid registration. NeuroImage 59(3), 2438–2451 (2012)
11. Singh, N.P., Hinkle, J., Joshi, S., Fletcher, P.T.: A vector momenta formulation of diffeomorphisms for improved geodesic regression and atlas construction. In: IEEE Proceedings of ISBI 2013 (2013)
12. Sommer, S., Nielsen, M., Lauze, F., Pennec, X.: A multi-scale kernel bundle for LDDMM: Towards sparse deformation description across space and scales. In: Székely, G., Hahn, H.K. (eds.) IPMI 2011. LNCS, vol. 6801, pp. 624–635. Springer, Heidelberg (2011)
13. Trouvé, A.: Diffeomorphic groups and pattern matching in image analysis. Int. J. Comput. Vision 28, 213–221 (1998)
14. Vercauteren, T., Pennec, X., Perchant, A., Ayache, N.: Symmetric log-domain diffeomorphic registration: A demons-based approach. In: Metaxas, D., Axel, L., Fichtinger, G., Székely, G. (eds.) MICCAI 2008, Part I. LNCS, vol. 5241, pp. 754–761. Springer, Heidelberg (2008)

# A Generalised Spatio-Temporal Registration Framework for Dynamic PET Data: Application to Neuroreceptor Imaging

Jieqing Jiao[1,2,*], Julia A. Schnabel[1], and Roger N. Gunn[1,2,3]

[1] Institute of Biomedical Engineering, Department of Engineering Science,
University of Oxford, UK
[2] Imanova Limited, Hammersmith Hospital, London, UK
[3] Department of Medicine, Imperial College, London, UK

**Abstract.** This work presents a novel pharmacokinetic model based registration algorithm for the motion correction of dynamic positron emission tomography (PET) images. The algorithm employs a generalised model that derives the input function from the tomographic data itself to model the PET tracer kinetics and thus eliminates the need of arterial blood sampling. Both the temporal constraint from the tracer kinetic behaviour and spatial constraint from the image similarity are integrated in a joint probabilistic model, in which the subject motion and tracer kinetic parameters are iteratively optimised, leading to a groupwise registration framework of motion corrupted dynamic PET data. The algorithm is evaluated with simulated and measured human dopamine D3 receptor imaging data using $[^{11}C]$-(+)-PHNO. The simulation-based validation demonstrates that the new algorithm has a subvoxel registration accuracy on average for noisy data with simulated motion artefacts. The algorithm also shows reductions in motion on initial experiments with measured clinical $[^{11}C]$-(+)-PHNO brain data.

**Keywords:** Groupwise spatio-temporal registration, dynamic PET, motion correction, basis pursuit denoising.

## 1 Introduction

Positron emission tomography (PET) is a powerful non-invasive imaging tool that can provide valuable biological measurements of physiology, biochemistry and pharmacology. These measurements readily enable the investigation of normo-patho-physiology and aid in drug development by providing important information on whether a drug reaches and engages with its target. A modern PET scanner has a spatial resolution of $4mm$, and subject motion inevitably alters the voxel-to-tissue mapping during a dynamic scan of between 30 minutes to 2 hours. The corrupted tissue activity curves measured cause inaccuracies

---

* This work is supported by Chinese Ministry of Education - University of Oxford Scholarships and Clinical Imaging Centre, GlaxoSmithKline.

K. Mori et al. (Eds.): MICCAI 2013, Part I, LNCS 8149, pp. 211–218, 2013.

in quantifying the relevant biological/physiological processes. Thus, motion correction for quantitative dynamic PET is critical. For image-based registration methods, this is technically challenging since the similarities of morphological features or temporally consistent information is more limited in PET frames compared with magnetic resonance imaging (MRI) or computed tomography (CT) [1]. To address such image registration problems in dynamic imaging, kinetic models have been introduced to account for temporal changes in MRI data [2]. For dynamic PET data, we previously presented an approach [3] that incorporates a tracer pharmacokinetic model into the registration framework to correct for subject motion. This data-driven pharmacokinetic model required a blood input function to describe different tracer behaviour across the images. This means that the method is limited to data sets that have associated measurements of the arterial input function, which represent only a small fraction of dynamic PET studies. The goal of this work is to develop a method which generalises to dynamic PET studies that do not have such measurements.

In this paper we develop a novel registration framework for dynamic PET images using a generalised pharmacokinetic model. A reference region is selected in the imaged volume with no (or lowest) specific binding. The input function is derived from the reference region and therefore eliminates the blood-dependence. The unknown compartmental system is solved with a set of kinetic basis functions and basis pursuit denoising. The basis pursuit denoising approach depends on the estimation of a relaxation parameter which determines the parsimony of the kinetic model. We propose an efficient approach for its estimation. To the best of our knowledge, this work presents the first algorithm in literature to correct for subject motion by incorporating a generalised pharmacokinetic model into the registration of dynamic PET data.

## 2    Method

### 2.1    Joint Probabilistic Model of Tracer Kinetics and Subject Motion

Whist the process of radioactive decay gives rise to a Poisson distribution, in reconstructed PET image data, the distribution resembles a Gaussian due to the aggregation of a number of noise sources [4]. For each image volume, the tracer kinetics of the injected tracer determines the intensity of photon emission. However, any subject motion will affect the voxel-to-tissue mapping. Therefore, given the measured PET data $\mathbf{Y}$, the probability of tracer kinetics $\mathbf{\Phi}$ and subject motion $\mathbf{T}$ can be formulated as:

$$p(\mathbf{\Phi}, \mathbf{T}|\mathbf{Y}) = \prod_{j=1}^{M} \prod_{k=1}^{F} \frac{1}{\sqrt{2\pi\sigma^2(t_k)}} exp\left(-\frac{(\mathbf{Y}(\mathbf{T}_k^{-1}(\mathbf{x}_j), t_k) - \mathbf{Y}_{\mathbf{\Phi}}(\mathbf{x}_j, t_k))^2}{2\sigma^2(t_k)}\right),$$

(1)

where $Y_{\mathbf{\Phi}}$ is the tracer activity in the image volume determined by $\mathbf{\Phi}$, $\mathbf{x}_j$ are the coordinates of voxel $j$, $t_k$ is the mid-frame time for the $k-$th frame, and $M$ and $F$ are the numbers of voxels and time frames, respectively. $\sigma^2(t_k) = c \times \mathbf{Y}(t_k)$ is the noise variance where $c$ is a noise level constant.

## 2.2    Basis Pursuit Reference Tissue Model

The tracer activity, $\mathbf{Y_\Phi}$, can be described by a generalised reference tissue model [5]. Let $C_T(t)$ and $C_R(t)$ be tracer concentration time courses in a target and reference tissue, respectively. Then, the general equation for a reference tissue input compartmental model is $C_T(t) = \phi_0 C_R(t) + \sum_{i=1}^{m+n-1} \phi_i e^{-\theta_i t} \otimes C_R(t)$, where $m$ and $n$ are the total numbers of tissue compartments in the target and reference tissues, and $\otimes$ denotes convolution [5].

This can be expressed as an expansion on a basis, $C_T(t) = \sum_{i=1}^{N} \phi_i \psi_i = \mathbf{\Phi\Psi}$, with $\psi_i = e^{-\theta_i t} \otimes C_R(t)$. A discrete set of $N = m + n - 1$ values for $\theta_i$ can be chosen from a physiologically plausible range spaced in a logarithmic manner to elicit a suitable coverage of the kinetic spectrum.

The tissue observation $\mathbf{y} = Y(x_j)$, corresponds to $C_T(t)$ as $\mathbf{y} = [y_1 \cdots y_F]^T$, $y_k = \frac{1}{t_k^e - t_k^s} \int_{t_k^s}^{t_k^e} C_T dt$, where $t_k^s$ and $t_k^e$ are the start and end frame times ($k = 1 \ldots F$). Accordingly, the basis function $\psi_i$ can be written as $\psi_i = [\psi_{i1} \ldots \psi_{iF}]^T$, $\psi_{ik} = \frac{1}{t_k^e - t_k^s} \int_{t_k^s}^{t_k^e} e^{-\theta_i t} \otimes C_R dt$ and $\mathbf{\Psi} = [\psi_1 \ldots \psi_N]$. Using the measured PET data $\mathbf{Y}$ and pre-calculated $\mathbf{\Psi}$, the unknown $\mathbf{\Phi}$ can be determined by $\mathbf{Y} \cong \mathbf{\Psi\Phi}$. To account for the temporally varying statistical uncertainty of the measurements, the weighted least squares problem $\mathbf{W}^{\frac{1}{2}}\mathbf{Y} \cong \mathbf{W}^{\frac{1}{2}}\mathbf{\Psi\Phi}$ can be considered, where $\mathbf{W}$ is the inverse of the covariance matrix.

To solve for $\mathbf{\Phi}$, standard least squares techniques are not usually applicable because an overcomplete basis ($N > F - 1$) leads to an under-determined set of equations. In [5], the problem is transformed by applying the method of basis pursuit denoising [6] by introducing a regularising term on sparsity, to $\min_{\mathbf{\Phi}} ||\mathbf{W}^{\frac{1}{2}}(\mathbf{Y} - \mathbf{\Psi\Phi})||_2^2 + \mu||\mathbf{\Phi}||_p$. The regularisation parameter $\mu > 0$ balances the approximation error and sparseness of $\mathbf{\Phi}$ to impose a unique solution. This is based on prior knowledge that the observed data can be accurately described by a few compartments. For computational purposes, this corresponds to $p = 1$ being chosen for the $L_p$ norm and the problem is solved by basis pursuit denoising as $\min \frac{1}{2}\mathbf{x}^T \mathbf{H}\mathbf{x} + \mathbf{c}^T \mathbf{x}$ $s.t.$ $x_i \geq 0$ where $\mathbf{H} = \begin{bmatrix} \mathbf{\Psi}^T \mathbf{W}\mathbf{\Psi} & -\mathbf{\Psi}^T \mathbf{W}\mathbf{\Psi} \\ -\mathbf{\Psi}^T \mathbf{W}\mathbf{\Psi} & \mathbf{\Psi}^T \mathbf{W}\mathbf{\Psi} \end{bmatrix}$, $\mathbf{c} = \mu \mathbf{1} - \begin{bmatrix} \mathbf{\Psi}^T \mathbf{W}\mathbf{\Psi} \\ -\mathbf{\Psi}^T \mathbf{W}\mathbf{\Psi} \end{bmatrix}$ and $\mathbf{x} = \begin{bmatrix} \mathbf{\Phi}^+ \\ \mathbf{\Phi}^- \end{bmatrix}$. $\mathbf{\Phi}$ is given by $\mathbf{\Phi} = \mathbf{\Phi}^+ - \mathbf{\Phi}^-$ finally yielding $\mathbf{Y_\Phi} = \mathbf{\Psi\Phi}$.

## 2.3    Determination of Regularisation Parameter $\mu$

$\mu$ regularises the number of compartmental components and should be determined by the tracer-target interaction. In [5], $\mu$ is selected by leave-one-out cross-validation (LOOCV) using measured $\mathbf{Y}$. For the motion correction task, if determined by LOOCV using data with motion artefacts, $\mu$ can be too small, which leads to overfitting of unwanted motion artefacts. Therefore, we optimise $\mu$ using a different approach:

Firstly a numerical phantom is needed for the given tracer to provide reconstructed noiseless motion-free 4D PET data $\mathbf{Y_0}$ as the ground truth. In the volume, we can sample $\mathbf{y}_0$ from $\mathbf{Y}_0$ for each voxel, and add Gaussian noise at a random level to simulate the measured $\mathbf{y}$. Then a set $\mathbb{T} = \{z_1 \dots z_n\}, z_i = (\mathbf{y}, \mathbf{y}_0)$ can be obtained. For $\mathbf{y}$, the basis pursuit denoising regularised by $\mu$ can predict a fitted $f_\mu(\mathbf{y})$. For $\mathbb{T}$, the average squared error of $f_\mu$ is $L_\mu = \mathbb{E}(f_\mu(\mathbf{Y}) - \mathbf{Y}_0)$. Then we choose the $\mu$ that minimises $L$.

### 2.4 Iterative Optimisation of $\mathbf{\Phi}$ and T: A Spatio-Temporal Registration

The joint probability distribution $p(\mathbf{\Phi}, \mathbf{T}|\mathbf{Y})$ is optimised with the Iterated Conditional Modes (ICM) optimisation algorithm [7], consisting of iterating the optimisation of two subsets of the unknowns: $\mathbf{\Phi}$ and $\mathbf{T}$. The iterative optimisations of $p(\mathbf{\Phi}|\mathbf{T}, \mathbf{Y})$ and $p(\mathbf{T}|\mathbf{\Phi}, \mathbf{Y})$ are equivalent to performing basis pursuit denoising to update $\mathbf{\Phi}$, and a spatial similarity minimisation to update $\mathbf{T}$.

---

**Algorithm.** Spatio-temporal pharmacokinetic model based registration of 4D PET data

---

**Input**: Motion-corrupted PET data $\mathbf{Y}(\mathbf{x}, t)$
**Output**: Motion-corrected PET data $\mathbf{Y}(\mathbf{T}^{-1}(\mathbf{x}), t)$. The estimated
         motion $\mathbf{T}$ and tracer pharmacokinetic parameter $\mathbf{\Phi}$.
Initialization $\mathbf{T} = \mathbf{Id}$, $\mathbf{Y}(\mathbf{T}^{-1}(\mathbf{x}), t) = \mathbf{Y}(\mathbf{x}, t)$;
**while** *not converged* **do**
    | - Derive reference input $C_R(t)$ from $\mathbf{Y}(\mathbf{T}^{-1}(\mathbf{x}), t)$ and calculate basis
    |   function $\Psi$ as in Sec 2.2;
    | - Do basis pursuit denoising using $\mathbf{Y}(\mathbf{T}^{-1}(\mathbf{x}), t)$ and $\Psi$, calculating the
    |   kinetic parameter $\mathbf{\Phi}$ and the model-predicted PET data $\mathbf{Y_\Phi} = \Psi\mathbf{\Phi}$ as
    |   in Sec 2.2;
    | - Selectively scale $\mathbf{Y}$ and $\mathbf{Y_\Phi}$ using the noise variance term $\sigma$ as in
    |   Sec 2.1, ruling out the voxels containing mainly noise;
    | - Do image registration on scaled $\mathbf{Y}$ and $\mathbf{Y_\Phi}$ using SSD as the cost
    |   function to obtain motion $\mathbf{T}$ and the motion-corrected PET data
    |   $\mathbf{Y}(\mathbf{T}^{-1}(\mathbf{x}), t)$;
**end**

---

## 3 Experiments and Results

We applied the proposed method on data from human dopamine D3 receptor imaging studies with $[^{11}\text{C}]$-(+)-PHNO. Dopamine D3 receptors are involved in the pathophysiology of a number of neuropsychiatric conditions such as addiction, schizophrenia, and Parkinson's disease (PD). $[^{11}\text{C}]$-(+)-PHNO is a D3 preferring PET tracer which has recently opened the possibility of imaging D3 receptors in the human brain *in vivo* [8] in various brain structures, such as the substantia nigra (SN), globus pallidus (GP), ventral striatum (VST), dorsal putamen (PU), dorsal caudate (CD) and thalamus (THA). The cerebellum is used as the reference region as it has a low level of specific binding and has been determined to be an appropriate reference tissue for $[^{11}\text{C}]$-(+)-PHNO previously [8].

We used a software phantom to determine the regularisation parameter $\mu$ and quantify the motion correction accuracy. The Zubal brain phantom is widely applied in simulating PET neurological images [1,9] but lacks the delineation of SN and VST, which are ROIs in this study. We thus derived the motion free phantom by fitting the tracer kinetic model to measured [$^{11}$C]-(+)-PHNO 4D data from a healthy subject with visually negligible motion. The PET image voxel size is $2 \times 2 \times 2mm^3$ and the phantom comprises 26 temporal frames (durations: $8 \times 15$ s, $3 \times 1$ min, $5 \times 2$ min, $5 \times 5$ min, $5 \times 10$ min). Accuracy of registration was quantified as the target registration error (TRE) [10], averaged over all voxels and time frames.

## 3.1   Regularisation Parameter $\mu$

A set $\mathbb{T}$, $n(\mathbb{T}) = 3000$, was generated using the phantom described above. A mask was applied to discard background voxels with noise only. 50 values for $\mu$ were logarithmically spaced in $[10^{-2}, 10^2]$. The average squared error $L_\mu$ was calculated and is shown in Fig. 1. It is consistent with a histogram of $\mu$ that minimises the fitting error for each data point in $\mathbb{T}$. A value of $\mu = 8.6850$ was chosen to be optimal.

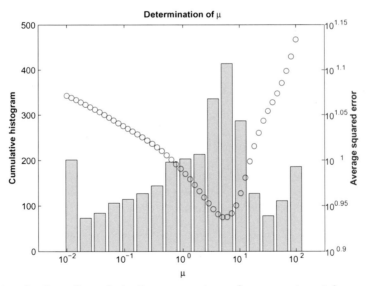

**Fig. 1.** Determination of regularisation parameter $\mu$ for compartmental sparsity for basis pursuit denoising in the registration framework. For 50 $\mu$ values logarithmically spaced in $[10^{-2}, 10^2]$, the average squared error $L_\mu$ (in blue) is consistent with the histogram of $\mu$ minimising the fitting error for each data point in $\mathbb{T}$ (in yellow) for an optimal value of $\mu = 8.6850$.

An intuitive way of determining $\mu$ is to update its value using $\mathbf{Y}(\mathbf{T}^{-1}(\mathbf{x}), t)$ by LOOCV in each iteration. We compared the TRE of updating $\mu$ to that of the fixed $\mu = 8.6850$, and the results show that the fixed $\mu$ has similar registration accuracy and is computationally more efficient. Therefore, we used the fixed $\mu$ approach for the following experiments.

## 3.2    Simulation-Based Validation

Simulated data sets were generated by introducing random rigid head translations and rotations to each temporal frame of the phantom. Ten simulations were conducted for a large motion level ($\sim 10mm$) and a small motion level ($\sim 5mm$) respectively, noise was added at a normal level in clinical data and a higher level. 5 simulations were carried out at each noise level to each motion-corrupted data set, generating 220 data sets. We performed motion correction using three methods: a frame-by-frame registration of each PET frame to the one with highest uptake based on normalised mutual information (FBF), the groupwise registration of all frames with spectral analysis that requires the blood input (GIR_SA) *red* previously proposed by us in [3], and the reference tissue groupwise registration of all frames using basis pursuit (GIR_BP) that avoids blood measurement proposed in this paper. The TREs are shown in Fig. 2.

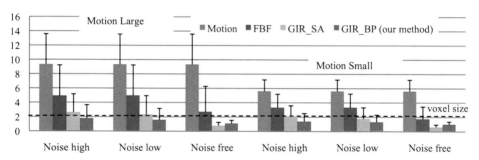

**Fig. 2.** Registration accuracy, quantified as target registration error (TRE, in $mm$) of the spatio-temporal groupwise image registration with basis pursuit (proposed GIR_BP), with spectral analysis (GIR_SA, required blood input) and frame-by-frame registration based on normalised mutual information (FBF) on simulated data sets. The dashed line indicates the voxel size. For each simulation, the TREs were averaged over all time frames. The mean TREs at each motion level and noise level before and after correction are shown, along with the standard deviations as error bars. The proposed GIR_BP achieves on average subvoxel ($< 2mm$) accuracy and has smaller errors for noisy data compared to GIR_SA, which requires arterial blood sampling.

## 3.3    Clinical Data

We applied the GIR_BP method to measured clinical data from a healthy subject with visually obvious motion shown in Fig. 3. [11C]-(+)-PHNO was injected as an intravenous bolus over approximately 30 seconds at the start of a 90 minute 3D-mode dynamic PET acquisition using a Siemens Biograph 6 PET-CT with Truepoint gantry. PET data were reconstructed using 2D filtered back projection with corrections for attenuation (based on a low-dose CT acquisition) and scatter. Dynamic data were binned in the same way as phantom data.

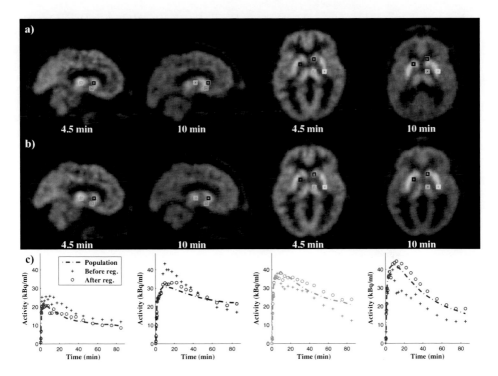

**Fig. 3.** Selected temporal frames (times are mid-frame times) from sagittal and axial slices from dynamic PET [$^{11}$C]-(+)-PHNO data of a healthy subject: a) before motion correction, b) after registration using the proposed GIR_BP method. Voxels from various ROIs are depicted in colours which are spatially fixed to demonstrate the displacement. c) PET data from these voxels before and after registration. Mean population PET data (from a larger group of healthy subjects scanned with [$^{11}$C]-(+)-PHNO) for the ROIs scaled to this subject to account for differences in dose and subject weight is shown by dashed lines. Colours correspond to ROIs as: ■ SN, ▨ VST, ■ CD, ■ PU, ■ GP and ▨ TH. The subject exhibited obvious rotation of $\sim 10°$ which was corrected considerably by the proposed method, and the tracer kinetics in these ROIs determined by the target densities showed consistency with population data after correction.

## 4    Discussion and Conclusion

We have introduced a generic registration framework to correct for subject motion in dynamic PET data that incorporates a reference tissue pharmacokinetic model into the groupwise registration process. This represents a significant increase in scope over the previous groupwise PET registration method [3] which required arterial blood data and as a consequence would only be applicable to a small number of dynamic PET studies. The new approach incorporates a generic reference tissue model which is implemented in a basis function framework and solved by the method of basis pursuit denoising. We have proposed an efficient approach to determine the relaxation factor that regularises the sparsity of kinetic components in the registration framework. We tested the proposed method on human dopamine D3 receptor PET data with [$^{11}$C]-(+)-PHNO with the cerebellum as the reference region. Results on realistic simulated data show subvoxel ($< 2mm$) registration accuracy. Initial evaluation on clinical data from a healthy subject with obvious motion provides evidence that motion can be reduced substantially in line with expectations from the simulated data. The proposed method is in principle applicable to all dynamic PET studies data given the selection of an appropriate reference tissue, as the method is based on an adaptive kinetic model derived from the general properties of compartmental tracer kinetics. Future evaluation over a range of different tracers, and extensions to differing applications requiring higher-order transformations and additional constraints will determine the full utility of the method. In addition, by describing the measured PET data using tracer kinetics and subject motion, the proposed registration framework could be integrated into the reconstruction of sinogram or list-mode data.

# References

1. Costes, N., Dagher, A., Larcher, K., Evans, A.C., Collins, D.L., Reilhac, A.: Motion correction of multi-frame PET data in neuroreceptor mapping: simulation based validation. Neuroimage 47(4), 1496–1505 (2009)
2. Buonaccorsi, G.A., Roberts, C., Cheung, S., Watson, Y., Davies, K., Jackson, A., Jayson, G.C., Parker, G.J.M.: Tracer kinetic model-driven registration for dynamic contrast enhanced MRI time series. Med. Image Comput. Comput. Assist. Interv. 8(pt. 1), 91–98 (2005)
3. Jiao, J., Searle, G.E., Tziortzi, A.C., Salinas, C.A., Gunn, R.N., Schnabel, J.A.: Spatial-temporal Pharmacokinetic Model Based Registration of 4D Brain PET Data. In: Durrleman, S., Fletcher, T., Gerig, G., Niethammer, M. (eds.) STIA 2012. LNCS, vol. 7570, pp. 100–112. Springer, Heidelberg (2012)
4. Oikonen, V.: Noise model for PET time-radioactivity curves. Turku PET Centre Modelling report TPCMOD0008 (2003)
5. Gunn, R.N., Gunn, S.R., Turkheimer, F.E., Aston, J.A.D., Cunningham, V.J.: Positron emission tomography compartmental models: a basis pursuit strategy for kinetic modeling. J. Cereb. Blood Flow Metab. 22(12), 1425–1439 (2002)
6. Chen, S.S., Donoho, D.L., Michael, S.A.: Atomic decomposition by basis pursuit. SIAM Journal on Scientific Computing 20, 33–61 (1998)
7. Besag, J.: On the statistical analysis of dirty pictures. Journal of the Royal Statistical Society, Series B (Methodological) 48(3), 259–302 (1986)
8. Searle, G.E., Beaver, J.D., Tziortzi, A., Comley, R.A., Bani, M., Ghibellini, G., Merlo-Pich, E., Rabiner, E.A., Laruelle, M., Gunn, R.N.: Mathematical modelling of [(11)C]-(+)-PHNO human competition studies. Neuroimage 68, 119–132 (2013)
9. Zubal, I.G., Harrell, C.R., Smith, E.O., Rattner, Z., Gindi, G., Hoffer, P.B.: Computerized three-dimensional segmented human anatomy. Med. Phys. 21(2), 299–302 (1994)
10. Fitzpatrick, J., West, J., Maurer Jr., C.R.: Predicting error in rigid-body point-based registration. IEEE Trans. Med. Imaging 17(5), 694–702 (1998)

# Constructing an Un-biased Whole Body Atlas from Clinical Imaging Data by Fragment Bundling

Matthias Dorfer[1,*], René Donner[1], and Georg Langs[1,2]

[1] CIR Lab, Department of Radiology, Medical University of Vienna, Austria
[2] CSAIL, Massachusetts Institute of Technology, Cambridge, MA, USA
{matthias.dorfer,rene.donner,georg.langs}@meduniwien.ac.at

**Abstract.** Atlases have a tremendous impact on the study of anatomy and function, such as in neuroimaging, or cardiac analysis. They provide a means to compare corresponding measurements across populations, or model the variability in a population. Current approaches to construct atlases rely on examples that show the same anatomical structure (e.g., the brain). If we study large heterogeneous clinical populations to capture subtle characteristics of diseases, we cannot assume consistent image acquisition any more. Instead we have to build atlases from imaging data that show only parts of the overall anatomical structure. In this paper we propose a method for the automatic contruction of an un-biased whole body atlas from so-called *fragments*. Experimental results indicate that the fragment based atlas improves the representation accuracy of the atlas over an initial whole body template initialization.

**Keywords:** Anatomical atlas construction, Medical imaging fragments, Average shape and intensity model, Landmark transformation accuracy.

## 1   Introduction

Models that represent common characteristics of a specific anatomical structure, or *atlases* are at the center of medical imaging analysis in the context of quantitative morphometric population analysis, or as a reference frame to summarize functional data across large cohorts. In computational anatomy anatomical atlases have been constructed for single organs such as the brain [3], or for entire body regions such as the abdomen [6]. Anatomical atlases help to automatically distinguish between healthy and pathological subjects [4] or to segment or annotate anatomical structures contained in the imaging data [8]. Existing approaches commonly rely on the presence of the same anatomical structure of interest in all examples that form the training data for the atlas, and the target data the atlas is applied to. This is feasible for organ specific studies, such as in

* This work has received funding from the Austrian Sciences Fund (P 22578-B19, PULMARCH), EU (FP7/2007-2013) under grant agreements 318068 (VISCERAL), 257528 (KHRESMOI).

K. Mori et al. (Eds.): MICCAI 2013, Part I, LNCS 8149, pp. 219–226, 2013.

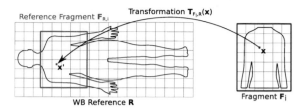

**Fig. 1.** Overview of fragment to WB reference space registration. The goal is to find a transformation $\mathbf{T}_{F_i,R}$ which registers a fragment $\mathbf{F}_i$ with the WB reference template $\mathbf{R}$.

neuroimaging, where the brain is the focus of analysis [1]. It is not feasible for building a representative model of the entire human body. In clinical practice, only those parts of the anatomy relevant for diagnosis are imaged [2]. We call these imaging data *fragments*. To use this data for population studies, to represent anatomical variability, or to identify characteristics of pathologies we need methodology to build an atlas from fragment data.

The contribution of this work is an atlas construction framework to construct an un-biased template from clinical medical imaging fragment data. Fragments acquired during clinical routine cover the human body in overlapping regions. The proposed atlas construction allows for the dense sampling of a wide range of anatomical regions in a clinical population. It goes beyond building and stitching individual atlases that represent individual anatomical regions. Furthermore, the atlas adds structure to arbitrary clinical imaging data examples, that constitute its training population. The framework provides functionality to localize the region of a fragment in relation to a Whole Body (WB) reference template and to register the fragment within the WB reference space. Based on the fragments the average shape and intensity template is updated. The method is closely related to Guimond et. al. [3] but extends it to image fragments. This fragment based model enables the bundling of imaging fragments within a single common WB reference space.

The results indicate that our approach is feasible, and is able to construct an atlas in situations where a large fraction of the data shows only part of the structure of interest. After an initial fit to a WB template the fragment registrations, and the template are updated and refined in an iterative process that further reduces bias.

## 2   Methods

Given a set of fragments $\mathbf{F}_1, ..., \mathbf{F}_N$, where $\mathbf{F}_i \in \mathbb{R}^{m_i \times n_i \times h_i}$, we seek to find a reference template $\mathbf{R} \in \mathbb{R}^{m \times n \times h}$ and corresponding transformations $\mathbf{T}_{F_i,R}$ so that $\mathbf{T}_{F_i,R}$ maps each position between the reference template and the individual fragment. To initialize the group-wise registration, all fragments are registered to a WB volume, that can either be a single individual, or the result of group-wise registration of multiple WB volumes. For each fragment the corresponding region (reference space fragment) $\mathbf{F}_{R,i}$ in $\mathbf{R}$ is determined. Then, the fragments $\mathbf{F}_i$ are

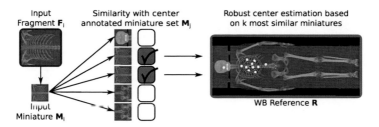

**Fig. 2.** Overview of miniature similarity based robust center estimation

registered to their corresponding region $\mathbf{F}_{R,i}$. After initialization the template is updated to represent both shape and appearance variation in the fragment population, and the fragments are registered to the updated template iteratively. This leads to an increasinlgy un-biased template $\mathbf{R}_F$ representing the population of fragments [3]. Fig. 1 illustrates all components contributing to the registration problem addressed. The main computation steps of the algorithm are: (1) For each fragment $\mathbf{F}_i$ estimate the center $\mathbf{c}_i$ in $\mathbf{R}$. (2) Estimate the corresponding reference fragment $\mathbf{F}_{R,i}$. (3) Non-rigidly register $\mathbf{F}_i$ to $\mathbf{F}_{R,i}$. (4) Compute updated fragment based shape and intensity population model $\mathbf{R}_F$ based on the registered fragments. In the following we describe the steps in detail.

## 2.1 Fragment Center Estimation

The first step to register $\mathbf{F}_i$ to $\mathbf{R}$ is to estimate its center position $\mathbf{c}_i$ in $\mathbf{R}$. This is based on calculating the appearance similarity of the fragment $\mathbf{F}_i$ and a set of fragments $\mathbf{F}_j^c$ with known center points $\mathbf{c}_j^c$, following an approach proposed in [2]. Fig. 2 provides an overview of the center estimation algorithm. For each $\mathbf{F}_j^c$ we construct a miniature $\mathbf{M}_j$ by resizing it to dimensions of $32 \times 32 \times 32$ voxels. $\mathbf{F}_i$ is downscaled analogously. We compute the Normalized Cross Correlation (NCC) and select those $k$ miniatures for whom this similarity is highest.

Given the centers $\mathbf{c}_1^c, ..., \mathbf{c}_k^c$ of of the $k$ top ranked miniatures, we calculate the median position, and keep the 50 percent of estimates closest to the median. The region containing these estimates is denoted as Region of Trimmed Estimates (RTE). From this set we calculate the center estimate by $\mathbf{c}_i = \frac{1}{k/2} \sum_{\mathbf{c}_j^c \in RTE} \mathbf{c}_j^c$ for $\mathbf{F}_i$. This estimate is used to initialize the transformation and the fragment region in the WB template.

## 2.2 Fragment Region Estimation

Based on $\mathbf{c}_i$ we estimate the region in $\mathbf{R}$ corresponding to the fragment. We refine the fragment center estimate $\mathbf{c}_i$ as well as the region $\mathbf{I}_{F_{R,i}}$ (voxel coordinates) of the reference fragment $\mathbf{F}_{R,i}$ (intensity volume) with respect to $\mathbf{R}$ iteratively. The initial region $\mathbf{I}_{F_{R,i}}$ corresponding to the fragment is spanned by the bounding box, with same dimensions as the fragment, centered around $\mathbf{c}_i$, defined by coordinates of two opposite corners $\mathbf{x}_{cor1,i}$ and $\mathbf{x}_{cor2,i}$. The input fragment $\mathbf{F}_i$ is affinely registered to the corresponding reference fragment $\mathbf{F}_{R,i} = \mathbf{R}(\mathbf{I}_{F_{R,i}})$ resulting in an affine transformation $\mathbf{T}_{F_i,R}^a$. Based on $\mathbf{T}_{F_i,R}^a$, we update $\mathbf{I}_{F_{R,i}}$. For the region update the two homogeneous corner coordinates $\mathbf{x}_{cor1,i}$ and $\mathbf{x}_{cor2,i}$ are transformed by the inverse of $\mathbf{T}_{F_i,R}^a$. i.e., $\mathbf{x}_{cor\,l,i}^1 = \mathbf{T}_{F_i,R}^{a,-1}(\mathbf{x}_{cor\,l,i})$ with $l = 1, 2$. The updated corresponding region $\mathbf{I}_{F_{R,i}}^1$ of the fragment is now spanned by the transformed corner points $\mathbf{x}_{cor1,i}^1$ and $\mathbf{x}_{cor2,i}^1$ leading to an updated reference space fragment $\mathbf{F}_{R,i}^1$ and a rigid component $\mathbf{T}_{F_i,R}^r$ of the transformation $\mathbf{T}_{F_i,R}$. The updated center position $\mathbf{c}_i^1$ is computed as the arithmetic mean of the transformed corner points.

The localization procedure is iterated with the updated reference fragment until the region estimate $\mathbf{I}_{F_{R,i}}^k$ converges. We keep the affine transformation $\mathbf{T}_{F_i,R}^a$ of the final iteration $k$ as initialization for the non-rigid registration.

## 2.3   Non-rigid Registration of the Fragment to the WB Template

The previous computation step estimates the corresponding reference space fragment $\mathbf{F}_{R,i}$ and region $\mathbf{I}_{F_{R,i}}$ of the input fragment $\mathbf{F}_i$ in the WB template $\mathbf{R}$. The final step of fragment to WB registration is the non-rigid registration of the query fragment $\mathbf{F}_i$ with the reference space fragment $\mathbf{F}_{R,i}$ yielding the non-rigid transformation $\mathbf{T}_{F_i,R}^{nr}$. For registration B-spline based Free Form Deformation (FFD) is used [7],[5]. The final result is an embedding of the non-rigidly registered fragment $\mathbf{F}_i'$ in the WB reference template $\mathbf{R}$ as well as the corresponding transformation $\mathbf{T}_{F_i,R} = \mathbf{T}_{F_i,R}^{nr} \circ \mathbf{T}_{F_i,R}^a \circ \mathbf{T}_{F_i,R}^r$.

## 2.4   Fragment Based Un-biased WB Reference Template Update

With the algorithm described in the previous subsections, we register fragments $\mathbf{F}_i$ with $i = 1, ..., N$ to a common reference template $\mathbf{R} \in \mathbb{R}^{m \times n \times h}$. In the first stage fragments are registered to an initial template $\mathbf{R}^0$. After the first iteration, this template is updated based on the fragment appearance, and deformation information, to obtain an un-biased template. For each fragment $\mathbf{F}_i$ we have the corresponding region $\mathbf{I}_{F_{R,i}}$ in $\mathbf{R}$, the reference fragment $\mathbf{F}_{R,i}$, the transformation $\mathbf{T}_{F_i,R}$, and the transformed fragment $\mathbf{F}_i' = \mathbf{F}_i(\mathbf{T}_{F_i,R}^{-1}(\mathbf{x}))$.

Based on these components the shape and intensity averaging, proposed by Guimond et. al. [3] is enhanced to a fragment based model. For a region constrained shape and intensity averaging we calculate for every voxel $\mathbf{x}$ in $\mathbf{R}$, the set of fragments $\mathcal{I}(\mathbf{x}) = \{i | \mathbf{T}_{F_i,R}^{-1}(\mathbf{x}) \in \mathbf{F}_i\}$ that contribute to it as well as the corresponding number of contributors $\mathbf{N}(\mathbf{x}) = |\mathcal{I}(\mathbf{x})|$. Based on $\mathbf{N}(\mathbf{x})$ the average fragment registration $\overline{\mathbf{F}}' \in \mathbb{R}^{m \times n \times h}$ is formalized as $\overline{\mathbf{F}}'(\mathbf{x}) = \frac{1}{\mathbf{N}(\mathbf{x})} \sum_{i \in \mathcal{I}(\mathbf{x})} \mathbf{F}_i(\mathbf{T}_{F_i,R}^{-1}(\mathbf{x}))$. The transformations of the fragments towards $\mathbf{R}$ are averaged in each voxel $\mathbf{x}$, i.e., $\overline{\mathbf{T}}_F = \mathcal{M}(\mathbf{T}_{F_i,R}^{nr})$ where $i \in \mathcal{I}(\mathbf{x})$. In practice we follow Guimond et. al [3] and estimate the mean by averaging the vector fields of the non-rigid transformations. We exclude rigid and affine transformations from un-biasing, since they mainly capture variability in image acquisition (e.g., body

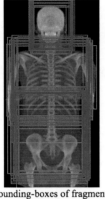 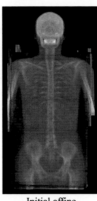 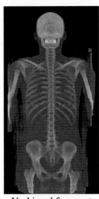

| Bounding-boxes of fragments contributing to $\mathbf{R}_F$ | Initial affine bundling of fragments | Un-biased fragment based model $\mathbf{R}_F$ |

**Fig. 3.** Construction results of the fragment based WB shape and intensity model $\mathbf{R}_F$ on 60 head, thorax, and abdomen fragments

region imaged, resolution), and assume that the population variability is encoded in the non-rigid component of the transformations. The fragment based average shape and intensity model $\mathbf{R}_F^1$ of iteration one is computed by applying the region dependent inverse average deformation $\overline{\mathbf{T}}_F^{-1}$ to the region dependent average intensity registration image $\overline{\mathbf{F}}'$. This results in $\mathbf{R}_F^1(\mathbf{x}) = \overline{\mathbf{F}}'(\overline{\mathbf{T}}_F^{-1}(\mathbf{x}))$ and draws the shape of the average intensity registration $\overline{\mathbf{F}}'$ towards the geometric population center of the training fragments [3]. The result is an un-biased fragment based model $\mathbf{R}_F^1$ representing the underlying fragment population $\mathbf{F}_1, ..., \mathbf{F}_N$. We proceed by again registering the fragments to this template, and updating the template $\mathbf{R}_F^k$ iteratively, until convergence.

## 3   Experimental Results

We evaluate the fragment based WBA construction on data that includes a single initial WB Computed Tomography (CT) volume $\mathbf{R}$ and 60 CT fragments $\mathbf{F}_i$ encompassing parts of the body including head, thorax, or abdomen. All volumes are isotropic and have a voxel dimension of 2 mm. In each fragment expert annotated bone landmarks are placed for evaluation, if present. They are used as reference for validation of registration accuracy, and the representational power of the atlas. The aim of the experiment is to show, (1) that the proposed method is capable to register medical imaging fragments containing locally limited anatomical regions to a common WB reference template $\mathbf{R}$ and (2) that the fragment based model $\mathbf{R}_F$ improves the representation of the imaging data in comparison to the initialization $\mathbf{R}$.

### 3.1   Experimental Setup

All 60 fragments $\mathbf{F}_i$ are registered with the WB template $\mathbf{R}$ resulting in the registered fragments $\mathbf{F}_i'$ and the corresponding transformations $\mathbf{T}_{F_i,R}$ (see sub section 2.2 and Subsection 2.3). Fragment center estimation was based on 1200 annotated fragments. The registrations are used to compute the average fragment model $\mathbf{R}_F$ as described in sub section 2.4. Fig. 3 summarizes the results and shows the resulting fragment based model $\mathbf{R}_F$. Additionally the contribution of each training fragment $\mathbf{F}_i$ to the respective region of $\mathbf{R}_F$ is highlighted. In Fig. 3(c) blue rectangles indicate the bounding boxes of the fragments in the reference space.

After model computation all fragments are registered to the updated, unbiased fragment based template $\mathbf{R}_F$. The registration transformations $\mathbf{T}_{F_i,R}$ and $\mathbf{T}_{F_i,R_F}$ are applied to the coordinates of the landmarks annotated in the respective fragments. This yields landmark distributions containing the position estimates for each of the landmark positions in the two reference spaces $\mathbf{R}$ and $\mathbf{R}_F$. As evaluation measure the centroid of these landmark distributions as well as the mean distance of all landmarks in a distribution to their centroid are computed. If the method proposed is valid, the average distance to the centroids is expected to decrease for the fragment based model $\mathbf{R}_F$.

### 3.2  Evaluation of Landmark Transformation Accuracy

Fig. 4 shows the initial WB template $\mathbf{R}$ in comparison to the fragment based model $\mathbf{R}_F$. In addition to the maximum intensity projections the one, two, and three standard deviation areas of the transformed landmark distributions are visualized as ellipses. The numbers identify individual landmarks, annotated in the fragments. For both cases we registered the individual fragments to the template. We interpret a lower spread of the mapped positions as an indicator that the template is a better representative of the population. The fragment based model provides an improved representation of the fragment data, in particular in the abdominal region (landmark 32, 47-52). The bar plot in Fig. 5a presents the mean distances of the landmarks in a distribution to their centroid. The original WB template $\mathbf{R}$ is shown in blue; the fragment based model $\mathbf{R}_F$ in red.

In the abdominal region the transformation error decreases for the fragment based model in each of the seven landmarks (32, 47-52). The average distance over all seven landmarks decreases from 8.7 mm to 7.1 mm (-1.6 mm). Landmark 52 shows a maximum decrease of -2.58 mm. For the thorax region, the average distance shows a decrease for the first four landmarks (29, 30, 31, 33) and an increase for the remaining four of the eight landmarks (34, 47, 48, 49). The accuracy improvement over all thorax landmarks is summarized by an average transformation error decrease from 6.23 mm to 6.08 mm (-0.15 mm). The average distance to the center of the landmark distribution in the head fragments decreases for landmark 35, 36, 37, 41 and 42. The average distance of landmark 40 and 50 is not effected by the model. Landmark 38 and 39 show an increased distance. The accuracy improvement over all head landmarks is summarized by an average transformation error decrease from 3.96 mm to 3.82 mm (-0.14 mm).

Fig. 5b summarizes the average landmark transformation improvement achieved by the fragment based model for each landmark. Values below zero indicate that the model performs correct in the region of the respective landmark.

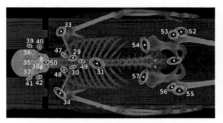
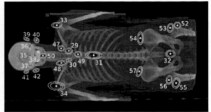

(a) Initial WB template **R**.          (b) Fragment based WB model **R**$_F$.

**Fig. 4.** Landmark distributions before and after fragment based un-biased WB template computation. The ellipses indicate the distribution of landmarks mapped from all fragments the template. Ideally they should coincide. The fragment based model improves the agreement.

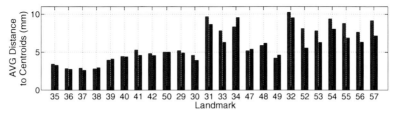

(a) Average distance of landmark distributions to their centroids.

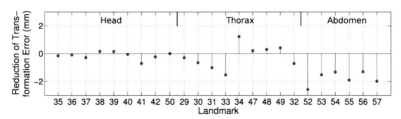

(b) Average improvement of landmark transformation accuracy.

**Fig. 5.** Landmark transformation accuracy of abdominal fragments before and after fragment based WB template update. (blue: initial WB reference **R**, red: fragment based WB template **R**$_F$).

The landmark transformation accuracy is increased for 16 landmarks, remains the same for landmark 40 and 50, and decreases for 6 of the 24 landmarks. The best results are achieved in the abdominal region.

This increased landmark transformation accuracy indicates that it is feasible to construct a whole body template from fragments. All fragment positions were located reliably during the initial center estimate. The decreased registration error of the landmarks shows that the fragment based WB model improves the representation of the underlying fragment population. Note that we did not explicitly evaluate the effect of pathologies present in the fragments at this point.

# 4    Conclusion

We propose methodology for constructing a WBA from fragments. The fragment based atlas is motivated by the fact, that typically individual medical imaging data recorded in hospitals do not cover the entire body region, while their inclusion into atlas building is necessary if we aim for a representative model of a large population [2,3]. This is relevant to represent the natural variability for model learning [3], disease characterization [4], or epidemiological research [9]. Existing approaches take only examples that cover identical anatomical structures into account (e.g., the brain [4]). The present work overcomes this limitation. The method estimates the position as well as the precise mapping between coordinates of a fragment and the WB reference fully automatically. In an iterative procedure the fragments are registered to a WB template, and this template is updated to reduce bias. The results show that our approach is feasible if the majority of the data consists of fragments, and reduces bias compared to an initial WB template.

# References

1. Dale, A.M., Fischl, B., Sereno, M.I.: Cortical surface-based analysis – i. segmentation and surface reconstruction. Neuroimage 9, 179–194 (1999)
2. Donner, R., Haas, S., Burner, A., Holzer, M., Bischof, H., Langs, G.: Evaluation of fast 2d and 3d medical image retrieval approaches based on image miniatures. In: Müller, H., Greenspan, H., Syeda-Mahmood, T. (eds.) MCBR-CDS 2011. LNCS, vol. 7075, pp. 128–138. Springer, Heidelberg (2012)
3. Guimond, A., Meunier, J., Thirion, J.P.: Average brain models: A convergence study. Computer Vision and Image Understanding 77(2), 192–210 (2000)
4. Joshi, S., Davis, B., Jomier, B.M., Gerig, G.: Unbiased diffeomorphic atlas construction for computational anatomy. Neuroimage 23 (suppl. 1), 151–160 (2004)
5. Modat, M., Ridgway, G.R., Taylor, Z.A., Lehmann, M., Barnes, J., Hawkes, D.J., Fox, N.C., Ourselin, S.: Fast free-form deformation using graphics processing units. Comput. Methods Prog. Biomed. 98(3), 278–284 (2010)
6. Park, H., Bland, P.H., Meyer, C.R.: Construction of an abdominal probabilistic atlas and its application in segmentation. IEEE TMI 22(4), 483–492 (2003)
7. Rueckert, D., Sonoda, L.I., Hayes, C., Hill, D.L.G., Leach, M.O., Hawkes, D.J.: Nonrigid registration using free-form deformations: application to breast MR images. IEEE TMI 18(8), 712–721 (1999)
8. Sabuncu, M.R., Yeo, B.T.T., Van Leemput, K., Fischl, B., Golland, P.: A Generative Model for Image Segmentation Based on Label Fusion. IEEE TMI 29(10), 1714–1729 (2010)
9. Sabuncu, M.R., Balci, S.K., Shenton, M.E., Golland, P.: Image-driven population analysis through mixture modeling. IEEE TMI 28(9), 1473–1487 (2009)

# Learning a Structured Graphical Model with Boosted Top-Down Features for Ultrasound Image Segmentation

Zhihui Hao[1], Qiang Wang[1], Xiaotao Wang[1], Jung Bae Kim[2],
Youngkyoo Hwang[2], Baek Hwan Cho[3], Ping Guo[1], and Won Ki Lee[1]

[1] Medical Imaging Group, China Lab
[2] Medical System Lab
[3] Data Analytics Group, Samsung Advanced Institute of Technology

**Abstract.** A key problem for many medical image segmentation tasks is the combination of different-level knowledge. We propose a novel scheme of embedding detected regions into a superpixel based graphical model, by which we achieve a full leverage on various image cues for ultrasound lesion segmentation. Region features are mapped into a higher-dimensional space via a boosted model to become well controlled. Parameters for regions, superpixels and a new affinity term are learned simultaneously within the framework of structured learning. Experiments on a breast ultrasound image data set confirm the effectiveness of the proposed approach as well as our two novel modules.

## 1 Introduction

Pathological structure segmentation is one of the core tasks for medical image processing. In recent years, studies on image segmentation are often categorized as one of the two paradigms: top-down or bottom-up ones [1]. The former involves a detection of object bounding-box and a follow-up refining of object contour. A high-precision detector becomes the key to rank the huge amount of sliding windows. The latter is committed to a classification of all image atoms, *i.e.* pixels or superpixels, and a holistic grouping based on their affinities.

The two paradigms suffer their own troubles, however, especially when dealing with medical images. Take breast sonograms for example, the various shapes of lesion make them hardly be handled by box-fashioned detector and the insufficiency of uniform structural features increases the difficulty of detection model training. On the other side, classifying and grouping image atoms often fails without a wide range of inspection, since many pixels in lesion and subcutaneous fat lobules barely have any difference. As discussed in [2], ultrasound image segmentation relies on an organic integration of low- and high-level image knowledge to remedy these problems.

In fact, many efforts have been made towards a combination of top-down and bottom-up segmentation [1,3,4]. We will compare them with ours in Sec. 2. The main contribution of this work is a novel scheme of embedding detection windows into a superpixel based graphical model, which enables an automatic

K. Mori et al. (Eds.): MICCAI 2013, Part I, LNCS 8149, pp. 227–234, 2013.

process of lesion detection and segmentation. Properties of these windows are not simply used for a ranking [5] or heuristically treated as superpixel features [2]. Their impacts to superpixels are well controlled independently after boosted into higher-dimensional space. Furthermore, all parameters for detection window properties, superpixel features and a new superpixel affinity term are trained in the framework of structured learning [6], thereby ensuring a full leverage of them. The simplicity and generality of these features allows a potentially fast execution of our approach, as well as an immediate application of the model to other segmentation problems.

## 2    Related Works

Conditional random field (CRF) models have been used for solving segmentation problems in both medical images [7,2] and natural images [8,9,3,10]. Structured support vector machine (SSVM) is firstly introduced to CRF by Szummer *et al.* [8] to learn the weights that balance all data terms. As in [9,7], the unary term in [8] is defined based on the posterior probability of graph node. Lucchi *et al.* [10] moves a step forward by co-training the interior coefficients with a linearization of the energy function. Our work belongs to this strand. But different from both, our work is committed to integrating region information into CRF. We put our attention on the design of region model and a corresponding pairwise term.

Many studies have made efforts to combine top-down and bottom-up image cues for object segmentation. Levin and Weiss [1] define a location bias term in CRF, which calculates the cost of aligning pixel-wise segmentation mask with object-part regions. The regions are selected from a large pool and used directly without a discussion of their validities. Ladický *et al.* [3] introduce detection windows into CRF in the form of a higher order potential. The windows could be accepted or rejected based on the harmony with other-level potentials. The work most related to ours is [2], where the authors treat a set of features extracted from detection hypotheses as auxiliary features of superpixel. Our work differs from them in two main aspects: *first*, image regions and atoms have independent features and they interact with, instead of filtering each other; *second*, parameters in the model are freed from individual assignments, but are packaged up and optimized within the structured learning framework.

The necessity of learning a specific pairwise term has also been observed by [11,7]. The novelty of our work is, instead of training an affinity function, we optimize the parametric pairwise term together with the unary term, thus obtain a model with potentially better compatibility.

## 3    The Problem and Energy Function

Our work is based on the bottom-up strategy. The task of lesion segmentation is treated as that of labeling variables in a conditional random field. Let $X = \{\mathbf{x}_i\}_i$ be the set of random variables that correspond to image atoms (superpixels here) and $Y = \{y_i\}_i$ be one of many possible labelings. The CRF model finds the optimal $Y^*$ by minimizing an energy function, which consists of a unary term $D(y_i, \mathbf{x}_i; \mathbf{w}^A)$ for all node variables and a pairwise term $V(y_i, y_j, \mathbf{x}_i, \mathbf{x}_j; \mathbf{w}^V)$ for all neighboring pairs $(i, j)$. Let us abbreviate the two terms by $D_i^A(\mathbf{w}^A)$ and $V_{ij}(\mathbf{w}^V)$. In this paper, we will learn a graphical model with the energy function of

$$\mathcal{E}(Y, X, R; \mathbf{w}) = \sum_i \left( D_i^A(\mathbf{w}^A) + D_i^R(y_i; \mathbf{w}^R, \mathbf{x}^R) \right) + \sum_{(i,j)} V_{ij}(\mathbf{w}^V). \qquad (1)$$

This equation reveals the problem to be addressed. The energy function contains a new unary term (with a superscript of $R$), which is introduced by image regions in contrast to the one by image atoms (with superscript $A$). The regions are generated from some top-down object locating paradigm, *e.g.* from sliding-window detector [12] in this paper. We preserve about 20 detection hypotheses for each image. The impact of this new term $D^R$ is controlled by an unknown parameter $\mathbf{w}^R$ as well as the state of the regions, $\mathbf{x}^R$.

The main goal of this work is to efficiently define the data terms and simultaneously learn their parameters, thereby building a graphical model with structured outputs for image atoms and regions. We simply call it a structured graphical model (SGM) in the paper. With such a model, we can combine different-level image cues and leverage them effectively for the final cut of CRF.

The image regions acceptable to the energy function in Eq. (1) are not limited to detection windows. In medical images with strong ambiguity, different-scale fragments can provide different perspectives on the object of interest, for example, superpixels and maximally stable extremal regions (MSER) [13]. The proposed model allows an alternation of the region finding method and since the energy function is additive, it also allows the overlapping of multiple sets of regions. These regions are possibly from several different methods, or even from different imaging modalities.

## 4   Learning a Structured Graphic Model

### 4.1   The Unary Terms for Image Atoms and Regions

The unary term of $D_i^A$ measures the cost of assigning label $y_i$ to the feature vector $\mathbf{x}_i$. As in [10], we define it as a sum of inner products of $\mathbf{x}_i$ with class-dependent parameters:

$$D_i^A(\mathbf{w}^A) = \delta(y_i = 1)D_i^{A+} + \delta(y_i = -1)D_i^{A-} = \delta^+ \langle \mathbf{w}^{A+}, \mathbf{x}_i \rangle + \delta^- \langle \mathbf{w}^{A-}, \mathbf{x}_i \rangle, \quad (2)$$

where $\mathbf{w}^A = [(\mathbf{w}^{A+})^T, (\mathbf{w}^{A-})^T]^T$. Although expressed with binary symbols for clarity, it can be extended to multi-class cases without much effort. Next we use similar notations to define the region term $D_i^R$.

Suppose there is a detection window $R$ that covers superpixel $i$ with a confidence of $x^R$. We define the data term from $R$ to $i$ as a non-linear step function: $D_i^{R+}(w^R, x^R) = w^{R+}\delta(x^R \gtrless \tau)$, where $\gtrless$ takes one from *greater-than* and *less-than* signs. By adjusting the gain $w^{R+}$ and the threshold $\tau$, we can easily control

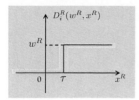 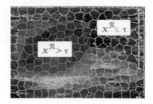 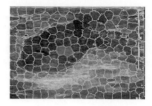

**Fig. 1.** The *left* and *middle* figures illustrate the simplified region model and an application example, where the detection windows will release energies of $w^R$ and 0 respectively to superpixels they cover. The *right* figure shows a positive (red) and a negative (green) pair of superpixels for training the pairwise term.

and discriminate the impacts of different region instances that come from a same paradigm. The $D_i^{R-}$ is defined in the same way, with the parameter of $w^{R-}$. The region model is shown in Fig. 1.

Moreover, the regions could have multiple properties. For example, the *objectness* measures in [5] describe the saliency of the region, the color contrast with the surrounding, and *etc*. We can then derive a more complex version of the region term:

$$D_i^{R+}(\mathbf{w}^{R+}, \mathbf{x}^R) = \sum_{(k)} w_{(k)}^{R+} \delta(x_{i(k)}^R \gtrless \tau_{(k)}) \triangleq \langle \mathbf{w}^{R+}, \phi(\mathbf{x}_i^R) \rangle. \tag{3}$$

Note that the region states could behave very different when projected on different image atoms, for example, on those they cover and miss, thereby represented by $\mathbf{x}_i^R$ in practical calculating. As indicated by Eq. (3), the set of the step functions can be regarded as a mapping function, which transforms the state $\mathbf{x}^R$ into a potentially higher dimensional feature vector $\phi(\mathbf{x}^R)$. Therefore, the whole term can be expressed as an inner product as in Eq. (2). The mapping function can be trained with $(\mathbf{x}_i^R, y_i)_i$ by off-the-shelf boosting learning algorithm [14], which returns an ensemble model composed of organized decision stumps and their associated weights. We preserve the first $K$ decision stumps as our step functions. The weight parameters $\mathbf{w}^R$ will be re-trained as a part of our structured model.

From another perspective, the unary term equals to a weighted sum of image atom features and boosted region features, rather than with raw region features. This is the foundation that our method can outperform previous ones. We will show the related comparisons in the experiment section.

## 4.2    The Parametric Pairwise Term

The pairwise term measures the affinity of any superpixel pair in the graph. A general-purpose pairwise term in CRF involves a product of several image factors (such as the color similarity between superpixels and their shared boundary length [9]) with a single, scalar parameter. In our case, however, the intervention of region hypotheses creates many artificial edges in the probability map along the region boundaries, which brings much trouble for tuning the pairwise term.

**Table 1.** Features extracted for the data terms in our structured graphical model

| Unary Terms | | Parametric Pairwise Term |
|---|---|---|
| From Image Atoms (Superpixels) | Intensity histogram; Centroid Location (x,y). | Intensity contrast; Length of shared boundary (LSB); |
| From Regions* (Detection Windows [12]) | Detection confidence; Objectness measures [5]; Localized version† of above; | Edge strength; Edge strength averaged by LSB; Localized version† of above features. |

*For any atom covered by multiple regions, take their maximum features as the atom features.
†A feature in image $I$ is localized by $\tilde{x} = (x - \mu)/\sigma$, where the mean $\mu$ and standard deviation $\sigma$ are estimated from the feature instances in $I$.

We need a new definition with higher degrees of freedom to accommodate our new unary term.

Again, we enforce the non-linear mapping function in Eq. (3) to boost the raw pair-features. Our pairwise term is defined as follows:

$$V_{ij}(\mathbf{w}^V) = \delta(y_i = y_j) f(\mathbf{x}^{ij}, \mathbf{w}^V) = \delta(y_i = y_j) \sum_k w_k^V \delta(x_k^{ij} \gtrless \tau_k). \quad (4)$$

Training samples are collected around the groundtruth of lesion to learn the mapping function. As shown in Fig. 1(c), pairs that cross the lesion boundary are regarded as positive samples with edge labels of 1 and pairs inside the lesion are negatives. The other cases are ignored.

The feature $\mathbf{x}^{ij}$ characterizing a neighboring atom pair is extracted from different aspects of image cues. We summarize the feature types in Tab. 1. The edge strength in the table is an accumulation of Canny edge within a narrow band along the shared boundary. Note that we also introduce a set of localized version of these features by calculating their standard scores. The localized features can focus the mapping function on local contrast especially during training to highlight ambiguous lesion boundaries. Besides those in Tab. 1, we believe that a concatenation of the individual features $\mathbf{x}_i$ and $\mathbf{x}_j$ [7] could be a valid supplement.

### 4.3 Learning the Parameters

The parameter $\mathbf{w}$ consists of $\mathbf{w}^A$, $\mathbf{w}^R$ and $\mathbf{w}^V$. After simple transformations, we can see that the energy in Eq. (1) becomes linearly expressible in $\mathbf{w}$. In order to recover the segmentation by minimizing this $\mathcal{E}_{\mathbf{w}}$, the following inequality should hold for any image $X$ with a groundtruth labeling $G$.

$$\mathcal{E}(Y) - \mathcal{E}(G) = \mathbf{w}^T \Psi(Y) - \mathbf{w}^T \Psi(G) \geq 0, \ \forall Y \neq G. \quad (5)$$

The optimal $\mathbf{w}$ can be learned in the framework of structured support vector machine [6]. Given a set of training images and their groundtruth labelings, the SSVM optimizes the parameter by enlarging the margins between $\mathcal{E}(G)$ and any other $\mathcal{E}(Y)$:

$$\min_{\xi, \mathbf{w}} \sum_{n=1}^{N} \xi^{(n)}, \text{ s.t. } \xi \succeq 0, \ \mathbf{w} \succeq 0, \ \|\mathbf{w}\|_1 = 1, \tag{6}$$

$$\mathbf{w}^T \Psi(Y) - \mathbf{w}^T \Psi(G^{(n)}) \geq \Delta(Y, G^{(n)}) - \xi^{(n)}, \ \forall Y \neq G^{(n)}, \ \forall n$$

We constrain the 1-norm of $\mathbf{w}$ to encourage its sparsity. The term of $\Delta(Y, G^{(n)})$ applies re-scaled margins [6] to different cases of $Y$. Instead of using the hamming loss, it has a slightly different definition in our work:

$$\Delta(Y, \ G^{(n)}) = \sum_n \delta(y_i = 0, \ g_i^{(n)} = 1), \tag{7}$$

which means that we only punish the cases where lesion superpixels are falsely classified into backgrounds. This is very important to our problem considering in most cases breast lesion possesses only a small percentage of area. The biased penalty prevents them from being overshadowed by redundant negatives in the model learning phase.

The number of possible constraints could be nearly infinite. The SSVM solves this problem by employing the column-generation technique. At each iteration, only the most violated constraint for each training sample is added into the working set. The corresponding labeling can be found using the standard graph cut method [15] as in inference. We refer the reader to [6,10] for similar details. We stop the learning when $\mathbf{w}$ converges. With a tolerance of $1e - 5$ on $\|\mathbf{w}^t - \mathbf{w}^{t-1}\|_2$, the learning process usually takes about 30 iterations in our experiments.

## 5    Experiments

We evaluate the proposed approach on a 2D breast ultrasound image data set, which contains 469 B-mode ultrasound images with about 52% benign cases and 48% malignant cases. The image size is about $780 \times 540$ with a spatial resolution of 0.23mm/pixel. The malignant cases have been confirmed with biopsy, and the benign cases have been followed up for at least 3 years. Lesion boundaries are delineated manually by experienced radiologists. We have provided them a special assisting software for gently refining the contours.

The dimension of boosted features in our graphical model, i.e. the number of step functions, is set to 100 for both the unary term and the pairwise term. About 200 SLIC superpixels [16] are generated in each image (also, for competitors in the following experiments). We randomly select 75% images for model training and the other 25% images for testing. Fig. 2 has shown some results of lesion segmentation. In the 4-th column, detection windows with $D^{R+} > D^{R-}$ are drawn. Note that our approach can handle the cases that contain multiple lesions, whereas detection windows with highest confidence (shown as valid rectangles) often miss one of the targets and lead to incomplete results.

Next, we compare the proposed approach with some baselines to highlight the contribution of each module. Considering the primary purpose of this work, we mainly focus on these three aspects: 1) Boosted Features (BF) vs. Raw Features (RF) provided by regions; 2) Parametric Pairwise-term (PP) vs. Ordinary

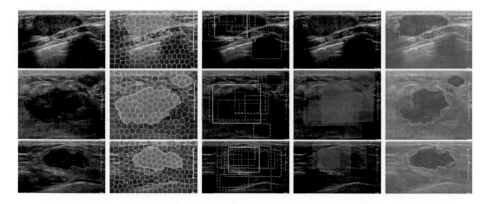

**Fig. 2.** Experiment results of lesion segmentation in breast ultrasound images. Each column shows 1) the input images, 2) superpixels with outlined groundtruth, 3) top-10 detection windows, 4) windows selected by our region model that have positive impacts to superpixels, and 5) the final segmentations.

**Table 2.** Experiment results of 5-time random subsampling cross-validations

| Approaches | Average Jaccard | Hausdorff Distance | Average Distance |
|---|---|---|---|
| SGM(BF+PP) | $0.693 \pm 0.012$ | $38.7 \pm 3.1$ | $15.6 \pm 1.3$ |
| SGM(BF+OP) | $0.681 \pm 0.025$ | $50.1 \pm 3.8$ | $17.8 \pm 1.8$ |
| SGM(RF+OP) | $0.669 \pm 0.028$ | $52.9 \pm 5.4$ | $20.8 \pm 2.0$ |
| Hao12 [2] | $0.654 \pm 0.028$ | $53.0 \pm 4.8$ | $25.4 \pm 5.1$ |
| Fulkerson09 [9] | $0.580 \pm 0.052$ | $69.5 \pm 6.7$ | $36.3 \pm 7.2$ |

Pairwise-term (OP); 3) the proposed vs. other segmentation approaches. Specifically, the following methods are compared:

- SGM(BF+PP), where all modules proposed in this paper are included;
- SGM(BF+OP), where the pairwise term is defined as in [9];
- SGM(RF+OP), where raw region features are treated as atom features;
- Hao12 [2], similar to SGM(RF+OP) but with more powerful features and without structured learning;
- Fulkerson09 [9], a typical CRF based segmentation approach without regions involved.

The comparison tests are repeated 5 times with a 3:1 random train/test split. A quantitative result is reported in Tab. 2. The measurements are the average overlapping ratio (*i.e.* the *Jaccard*), the maximum (*i.e.* the *hausdorff*) and the average contour-to-contour distances. Details of the latter two measurements can be found in [17]. The mean and standard derivation of 5 tests are reported. We can see that the proposed method with boosted features and parametric pairwise term outperforms the variants, and also obtains a better result than the previous methods.

## 6  Conclusion

We have proposed a structured graphical model to efficiently combine the region-level features and superpixel-level features. Relationships between regions and superpixels can also be captured by defining new energy terms. Also, a structured labeling and segmentation for multi-class objects (if there are) could be studied based on our method. These are some directions of our future work.

# References

1. Levin, A., Weiss, Y.: Learning to combine bottom-up and top-down segmentation. In: Leonardis, A., Bischof, H., Pinz, A. (eds.) ECCV 2006. LNCS, vol. 3954, pp. 581–594. Springer, Heidelberg (2006)
2. Hao, Z., Wang, Q., Seong, Y.K., Lee, J.-H., Ren, H., Kim, J.: Combining crf and multi-hypothesis detection for accurate lesion segmentation in breast sonograms. In: Ayache, N., Delingette, H., Golland, P., Mori, K. (eds.) MICCAI 2012, Part I. LNCS, vol. 7510, pp. 504–511. Springer, Heidelberg (2012)
3. Ladický, Ľ., Sturgess, P., Alahari, K., Russell, C., Torr, P.H.S.: What, where and how many? combining object detectors and crfs. In: Daniilidis, K., Maragos, P., Paragios, N. (eds.) ECCV 2010, Part IV. LNCS, vol. 6314, pp. 424–437. Springer, Heidelberg (2010)
4. Kuettel, D., Ferrari, V.: Figure-ground segmentation by transferring window masks. In: CVPR, pp. 558–565. IEEE (2012)
5. Alexe, B., Deselaers, T., Ferrari, V.: What is an object? In: CVPR, pp. 73–80. IEEE (2010)
6. Tsochantaridis, I., Hofmann, T., Joachims, T., Altun, Y.: Support vector machine learning for interdependent and structured output spaces. In: ICML, p. 104. ACM (2004)
7. Lucchi, A., Smith, K., Achanta, R., Lepetit, V., Fua, P.: A fully automated approach to segmentation of irregularly shaped cellular structures in em images. In: Jiang, T., Navab, N., Pluim, J.P.W., Viergever, M.A. (eds.) MICCAI 2010, Part II. LNCS, vol. 6362, pp. 463–471. Springer, Heidelberg (2010)
8. Szummer, M., Kohli, P., Hoiem, D.: Learning crfs using graph cuts. In: Forsyth, D., Torr, P., Zisserman, A. (eds.) ECCV 2008, Part II. LNCS, vol. 5303, pp. 582–595. Springer, Heidelberg (2008)
9. Fulkerson, B., Vedaldi, A., Soatto, S.: Class segmentation and object localization with superpixel neighborhoods. In: CVPR, pp. 670–677. IEEE (2009)
10. Lucchi, A., Li, Y., Smith, K., Fua, P.: Structured image segmentation using kernelized features. In: Fitzgibbon, A., Lazebnik, S., Perona, P., Sato, Y., Schmid, C. (eds.) ECCV 2012, Part II. LNCS, vol. 7573, pp. 400–413. Springer, Heidelberg (2012)
11. Batra, D., Sukthankar, R., Chen, T.: Learning class-specific affinities for image labelling. In: CVPR, pp. 1–8. IEEE (2008)
12. Felzenszwalb, P., Girshick, R., McAllester, D., Ramanan, D.: Object detection with discriminatively trained part-based models. PAMI 1627–1645 (2009)
13. Feng, X., Shen, X., Wang, Q., Kim, J., et al.: Learning based ensemble segmentation of anatomical structures in liver ultrasound image. In: SPIE Medical Imaging, Citeseer (2013)
14. Freund, Y., Schapire, R.: A decision-theoretic generalization of on-line learning and an application to boosting. J. Comput. Syst. Sci. 55(1), 119–139 (1997)
15. Boykov, Y., Veksler, O., Zabih, R.: Fast approximate energy minimization via graph cuts. PAMI 23(11), 1222–1239 (2001)
16. Achanta, R., Shaji, A., Smith, K., Lucchi, A., Fua, P., Susstrunk, S.: Slic superpixels compared to state-of-the-art superpixel methods. PAMI 34(11), 2274–2282 (2012)
17. Madabhushi, A., Metaxas, D.: Combining low-, high-level and empirical domain knowledge for automated segmentation of ultrasonic breast lesions. IEEE Trans. Med. Imaging 22(2), 155–169 (2003)

# Utilizing Disease-Specific Organ Shape Components for Disease Discrimination: Application to Discrimination of Chronic Liver Disease from CT Data

Dipti Prasad Mukherjee[1,2], Keisuke Higashiura[3], Toshiyuki Okada[2], Masatoshi Hori[2], Yen-Wei Chen[3], Noriyuki Tomiyama[2], and Yoshinobu Sato[2]

[1] Indian Statistical Institute, Kolkata, West Bengal, India
[2] Department of Radiology, Graduate School of Medicine, Osaka University, Japan
[3] Graduate School of Information Science and Engineering, Ritsumeikan University, Japan

**Abstract.** We describe a method to capture disease-specific components in organ shapes. A statistical shape model, constructed by the principal component analysis (PCA) of organ shapes, is used to define the subspace representing inter-subject shape variability. The first PCA is applied to the datasets of healthy organ shapes to define the subspace of normal variability. Then, the datasets of diseased shapes are projected onto the orthogonal complement (OC) of the subspace of normal variability, and the second PCA is applied to the projected datasets to derive the subspace representing the disease-specific variability. To calculate the OC of an n-dimensional subspace, a novel closed-form formulation is developed. Experiments were performed to show that the support vector machine classification in the OC subspace better discriminated healthy and diseased liver shapes using 99 CT data. The effects of the number of training data and the difference in segmentation methods on the classification accuracy were evaluated to clarify the characteristics of the proposed method.

**Keywords:** Statistical shape model, orthogonal complement, support vector machine, liver fibrosis, computer-aided diagnosis.

## 1 Introduction

Discriminating diseased organs from healthy ones based on the variations of organ shapes is one of the important goals of computational anatomy. The early structural change in cortical grey matter caused by Alzheimer's disease is a well-studied problem [1]. This work studied the shape variations based on the local geometric measurement from an average representation of the shape. However, global deformation patterns may be more important for studying some pathological anatomies such as chronic liver disease (CLD). To our knowledge, the development of computational tools for modeling disease-specific global deformation patterns is still insufficient.

To study the variability of normal anatomy or pathological structures caused by the disease, the statistical shape model (SSM), which is constructed by the principal component analysis (PCA) of organ shapes, is one of the basic representation schemes [2].

K. Mori et al. (Eds.): MICCAI 2013, Part I, LNCS 8149, pp. 235–242, 2013.

However, it would be ideal if it was possible to eliminate the normal variability of organ shapes from the variability of diseased organs to effectively study disease-specific behavior.

We propose to use the disease-specific shape component SSM that objectively eliminates the variability of healthy shapes. We generate an SSM with a given set of healthy organ shapes and then design a subspace that is the orthogonal complement (OC) of the healthy shape SSM. The projection of a new healthy shape sample into the OC subspace is ideally expected to result in sufficiently small components. Subsequently, the projections of diseased shapes into this OC subspace are expected to mostly consist of the disease-specific components after eliminating the normal variability. In our literature survey, the OC subspace was utilized for content-based image retrieval [3]. However, it has not been applied to discriminate subtle variations in anatomical shapes caused by the disease, such as those addressed by Golland et al. [4]. Here, we do not assume that the components of shape changes caused by the disease are in the OC subspace, but assume and demonstrate that using the disease-specific components in the OC subspace is useful for disease discrimination.

In this study, we address the problems of shape-based discrimination of CLD. With respect to computer-assisted diagnosis (CAD) of CLD, the local shape has been studied [5]. However, its usefulness is limited to the discrimination of serious stages, where bumpy contours of the liver surface are clearly observed. Although the radiologists' observations of the global changes of CLD are typically used in clinical diagnosis, the modeling of global liver shape changes in CAD has been insufficient. Because these shape change patterns are often subtle, their detection may be a difficult task even for experienced radiologists. The purpose of this work is to objectify and quantify these shape changes by statistical shape analysis, and in particular, the shape components specific to CLD using the OC subspace. We eventually aim to develop a CT-based imaging biomarker for staging liver fibrosis.

The main contributions of this study are as follows: (1) We have shown that the anatomical difference of shape is clarified in the OC space, which improves the support vector machine (SVM) classification accuracy. (2) We combine the OC-based SVM classifier with automated CT segmentation of the liver to evaluate its performance and limitations in clinical use. (3) In addition, a complete closed-form solution of estimation of n-dimensional OC space is provided from the methodological point of view.

## 2     Methodology

SSM provides a family of shape vectors, $\mathbf{x} \in \mathbb{R}^n$, $\mathbf{x} = \bar{\mathbf{x}} + \mathbf{P}b$, where $\bar{\mathbf{x}}$ represents the mean shape and $\mathbf{P}$ represents the eigenvector of some shape space samples, $\chi$. The SSM parameter $b$ is varied within $\pm \kappa \sigma$, $\sigma = \sqrt{\lambda}$, where $\lambda$ represents the eigenvalue of the SSM space $\chi$. In general, the $\kappa$ value of 2 or 3 is chosen and the probability of the parameter $b$ is assumed to follow a Gaussian distribution. Given the sample shape S, which is not included in $\chi$, the estimation of $b$ could be a multidimensional optimization of the distance $\|\mathbf{S} - \mathbf{x}(b)\|$. This distance could be either

Euclidean or Mahalanobis distance between the point clouds S and $x$ for a given $b$. However, in case the new shape $\mathbf{S} \notin \chi$ is already registered with the family $\chi$, then $b = \mathbf{P}^T(\mathbf{S} - \bar{\mathbf{x}})$, where $^T$ represents the transpose. If $\chi$ represents a healthy or disease class of organs, the SSM parameter $b$ can be estimated using $b_N = \mathbf{P}_N^T(\mathbf{x}_N - \bar{\mathbf{x}}_N)$, where subscript N represents a healthy organ class. Assuming that a global deformation of the organ shape caused by a specific disease is represented by the eigenvectors $\mathbf{P}_D$, the disease shape $\mathbf{x}_D$ is represented as

$$\mathbf{x}_D = \bar{\mathbf{x}}_N + \mathbf{P}_N b_N + \mathbf{P}_D c_D, \tag{1}$$

where $c_D$ is the SSM parameter. Let $\mathbf{P}_{OCN}$ be the sub-components of $\mathbf{P}_D$ projected onto the OC of the healthy SSM. Thus, we can modify Eq. (1) as,

$$\mathbf{x}_D = \bar{\mathbf{x}}_N + \mathbf{P}_N b'_N + \mathbf{P}_{OCN} c_{OCN}. \tag{2}$$

$\mathbf{P}_{OCN}$ is calculated as the principal component (PC) of the OC-transformed disease samples $\mathbf{x}_D$ that is projected onto the OC of the healthy SSM. Therefore, to create the OC-transformed disease-specific SSM, we obtain $c_{OCN}$ by $c_{OCN} = \mathbf{P}_{OCN}^T(\mathbf{x}_D - \bar{\mathbf{x}}_N - \mathbf{P}_N b'_N)$. Next, we present a complete closed-form solution for the estimation of $n$-dimensional OC space.

## 2.1    Orthogonal Complement of Principal Components

The OC of a subspace $M \subset \mathbb{R}^n$ is given by $M^\perp = \{w \in \mathbb{R}^n : w^T v = 0, \forall v \in M\}$. $M^\perp$ represents a subspace and $\mathbb{R}^n = M \oplus M^\perp$. If dim $M = q$, then dim $M^\perp = n - q$. We are interested in finding the OC of a subset of PCs of a covariance matrix. The OC of a correlation matrix is used for tracking principal and/or minor subspaces for applications in signal processing involving time series data [6]. In that case, the OCs weigh the correlation matrix in each iteration of tracking. In our case, the orthogonal complement of a few leading PCs defining healthy organ shape will be used to project the disease specific shape.

Assuming that $n$-D shape space is split into the $r$ and $p$-D subspaces, such that the first $p$ PCs of the shape space are chosen to calculate the OC and $\boldsymbol{\phi}$ is $(r + p) \times p$ eigenvectors of a covariance matrix $\mathbf{Z}$ ($(r + p) \times (r + p)$ dimension), we can decompose $\boldsymbol{\phi}$ into two matrices as,

$$\boldsymbol{\phi}^T = [\boldsymbol{\alpha}^T \boldsymbol{\beta}^T] \tag{3}$$

where, $\boldsymbol{\alpha}$ represents the $(r \times p)$ matrix containing the *first r rows* of $\boldsymbol{\phi}$ and $\boldsymbol{\beta}$ represents the $(p \times p)$ matrix *containing p last* rows of $\boldsymbol{\phi}$. To find out the OC of the p-dimensional dominant subspace, we need to do orthogonal decomposition of $\boldsymbol{\beta}$. Three promising orthogonal decompositions are the QR decomposition, SVD decomposition, and polar decomposition. The most stable and suitable way is to use polar decomposition, where factors are unique and coordinate-independent [7]. Using polar decomposition, $\boldsymbol{\beta} = \boldsymbol{\theta} \mathbf{U}$, where $\mathbf{U}$ represents the positive definite and $\boldsymbol{\theta}$ represents the orthogonal matrix. The orthogonal factor $\boldsymbol{\theta}$ represents the closest possible orthogonal matrix to $\boldsymbol{\beta}$ [7]. The physical interpretation of polar decomposition is that the orthogonal factor $\boldsymbol{\theta}$ provides a rotation and the positive definite *factor U provides* a stretch along the basis vectors *defined in U*.

Therefore, $(r \times p)$ upper sub-matrix $\boldsymbol{\alpha}$ of $\boldsymbol{\phi}$ has to be rotated along the orthogonal part of the remaining lower $(p \times p)$ sub-matrix $\boldsymbol{\beta}$ of $\boldsymbol{\phi}$. Therefore, we define $\mathbf{f}_1 = \boldsymbol{\alpha}\boldsymbol{\theta}^T$ and $\mathbf{f}_2 = \mathbf{f}_1(\mathbf{I} + \mathbf{U})^{-1}$. Note that $(\mathbf{I} + \mathbf{U})$ is always positive definite. Then, the OC of $p$ dimensional subspace of $\boldsymbol{\phi}$ is given by,

$$\mathbf{O} = \begin{bmatrix} \mathbf{I}_r - \mathbf{f}_1\mathbf{f}_2^T \\ -\mathbf{f}_1^T \end{bmatrix}. \tag{4}$$

The matrices $\mathbf{f}_1$ and $\mathbf{f}_2$ are of dimensions $(r \times p)$, so $\mathbf{O}$ is $(r + p) \times r$ dimensional orthonormal matrix. In Eq. (4) the lower $(p \times r)$ part of $\mathbf{O}$ represents the orthogonal rotation of the upper $(r \times p)$ part of $\boldsymbol{\phi}$ in the direction orthonormal to the lower $(p \times p)$ part of $\boldsymbol{\phi}$. The $[(\mathbf{I} + \mathbf{U})^{-1}][(\boldsymbol{\alpha}\boldsymbol{\theta}^T)^T]$ part of the right hand side of the upper $(r \times p)$ part of $\mathbf{O}$ represents the pseudo-inverse of $[\boldsymbol{\alpha}\boldsymbol{\theta}^T]$ and acts as OC projector from the theory of least square. It can be easily shown that $\mathbf{O}^T\mathbf{O} = \mathbf{I}$. Therefore, $\mathbf{O}$ represents the OC of the $p$ dimensional subspace defined *by the p PCs* of the covariance matrix $\mathbf{Z}$. Then, because $\boldsymbol{\phi}$ is also an orthogonal matrix, $\mathbf{O}^T\boldsymbol{\phi} = \mathbf{0}$.

Therefore, by taking the *first p eigenvectors* of the healthy organ subspace $\mathbf{P}_N$, Eq. (4) yields the OC of the healthy organ subspace. Next, we define the diseased organ subspace in the OC of the healthy shape.

## 2.2    Diseased Organ Subspace

The generation of healthy shape subspace is straightforward and provides the basis vectors $f_1$, $f_2$, ..., $f_k$, of normal variations of the $k$ dimensional healthy subspace. For an $n$ dimensional shape sample $\mathbf{x}_N$, we define the $(n-k)$ dimensional subspace as the OC of the healthy subspace. The OC is calculated using Eq. (4). Let the basis vectors of the OC be $o_1$, $o_2$, ..., $o_{n-k}$. We project each of the $n$ dimensional vectors $(\mathbf{x}_D - \bar{\mathbf{x}}_N)$ of the disease datasets to the $(n - k)$ dimensional OC subspace. The projected vectors are given by

$$\mathbf{x}_D' = \sum_{i=1}^{(n-k)} \langle (\mathbf{x}_D - \bar{\mathbf{x}}_N), o_i \rangle o_i. \tag{5}$$

Then, PCA is performed on the projected $(n - k)$ vectors $\mathbf{x}_D'$. The *first l basis* vectors of this projected disease data set provides the disease specific subspace, $g_1'$, $g_2'$, $g_3'$, ..., $g_l'$. Note that $g_i = \sum_{j=1}^{(n-k)} \langle g'_j, e_j \rangle o_j$, where $e_j$ denotes a $(n - k)$ dimensional unit vector *whose j-th element* is one and others are zero. Therefore, we obtain the disease subspace $g_1$, $g_2$, $g_3$, ..., $g_l$, where all the basis vectors are orthogonal to each other and to the healthy subspace.

# 3    Experimental Results

## 3.1    Dataset and Experimental Methods

We evaluated the conventional and proposed methods using 99 (53 healthy and 46 diseased) liver shape data. All the shape data represented as polygon models are registered to have the same topology of polygon models. The method for correspondence among the shape data was as follows. One reference data was initially selected, to which all other data were non-rigidly registered [8] to obtain the average shape. All the data were then registered to the average shape to obtain the final correspondence. The liver shape and size was normalized using the standard space defined by an approximation of the abdominal cavity according to a previous report [9]. The conventional method used SSM constructed from the mixed datasets of healthy and diseased liver shapes [4], whereas the proposed method used the OC-transformed disease-specific SSM described in Section 2. The SSM parameters were used for SVM classification of healthy and disease. SVM classification using the conventional method is basically the same as the method described by Golland et al. [4].

The diseased liver shapes were segmented from contrast-enhanced CT data taken from 46 CLD patients. Among them, the livers of 29 patients were histologically diagnosed (through biopsy or tissue resection) to be fibrotic, i.e., stage F1 or higher according to the established criteria [10], and 17 patients underwent minimally invasive liver therapy. The healthy liver shapes were derived from the CT data of 53 potential liver donors. All the data were retrospective. Figure 1 shows typical healthy and diseased liver shapes.

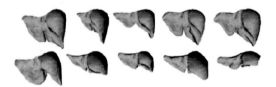

**Fig. 1.** Examples of liver shapes. Top (blue): Healthy livers. Bottom (red): Diseased livers.

We used two types of CT segmentation methods: manual tracing and fully automated. The average accuracy of automated segmentation in the Jaccard index was 0.897 for healthy and 0.867 for diseased livers. We evaluated the results under three segmentation conditions: (1) both training and test data were manually traced ("Both-manual"); (2) the training data were manually traced but the test data were automated ("Training-manual & test-automated"); and (3) both were automated ("Both-automated"). The first condition is unrealistic in a clinical setting because manual segmentation for each patient is a large burden for the clinical staff. The second condition will be clinically feasible because each patient data is automatically processed once the classifier has been trained. The third condition is also clinically feasible and has an advantage that automated addition of the training data is possible in the clinical routine.

We performed $k$-fold cross validation. Only within the training data, we further performed another (leave-one-out) cross validation to select the optimal parameter values involved in the classifier so that the highest classification accuracy was attained. Note that the test data were totally separated from the classifier training as well as the parameter optimization. In the parameter optimization, the number of PCs was optimized. In the disease-specific SSM, the number of PCs in the healthy SSM, whose OC was used, was also optimized. We used a linear SVM and no parameter was involved in it. A Gaussian-RBF SVM was not used because its lower performance in our problem was confirmed via a preliminary cross-validation study. The above $k$-fold cross validation was performed for 30 different $k$ partitions of the data, which were randomly generated, and the results were averaged.

## 3.2    Results

We plotted the ROC curves by shifting the discrimination hyper-plane of SVM along its normal for the proposed and conventional methods [4]. We also evaluated the classification accuracy that is defined as the ratio of the numbers of correctly classified shapes to all the shapes when the SVM hyper-plane is not shifted.

Figure 2 shows the ROC curves and classification accuracy under the three segmentation conditions, when $k = 15$, i.e., 15-fold cross-validation was performed. The number of PCs was approximately 37 in the conventional method, whereas it was 8 for the healthy SSM and 20 for the OC-transformed disease-specific SSM in the proposed method. The proposed method showed higher performance on ROC and classification accuracy under the conditions "Both-manual" and "Both-automated" than the conventional method. Under "Training-manual & testing-automated," the classification accuracy was the worst. The reduction of the accuracy from "Both-manual" to "Both-automated" was larger in the proposed method than in the conventional method, although the accuracy was still better in "Both-automated." Overall, the proposed method shows better performance, even though a larger accuracy reduction was observed when the automated segmentation was used.

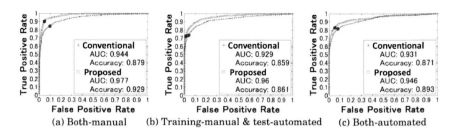

(a) Both-manual        (b) Training-manual & test-automated        (c) Both-automated

**Fig. 2.** ROC curves. Conventional: Blue, Proposed: Red. The knots on the curves denote the classification results when the discrimination plane was not shifted, i.e., they represent original SVM classification results. AUC represents the area under the curve.

Figure 3 shows the effects of the number of training data on the classification accuracy using different $k$ values in $k$-fold cross-validation. The number of training data was 50, 66, and 92 for $k = 2$, 3, and 15, respectively. The accuracy improvement was large in the proposed method for increased number of training data compared with the conventional method.

Figure 4 visualizes the shape deformation patterns corresponding to the normal of the SVM hyper-plane (See captions of Fig. 4 for the details). As in Fig. 4(b), the proposed method showed more subtle shape deformation for the discrimination than the conventional method.

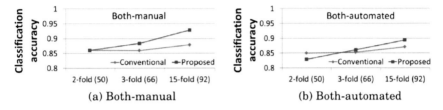

(a) Both-manual                    (b) Both-automated

**Fig. 3.** Effects of number of training data on classification accuracy (Conventional: Blue, Proposed: Red). The number of training data is shown in parenthesis along the horizontal axis.

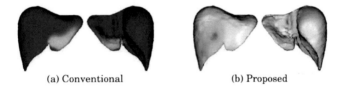

(a) Conventional                    (b) Proposed

**Fig. 4.** Deformation patterns corresponding to the normal vector of the discrimination hyperplane of SVM. The liver shape is the projection of the average shape onto the discrimination plane. The normal vector originates from the discrimination plane and heads to the disease side. Blue and cyan represent large and slight atrophy (shrinkage), respectively, and yellow represents slight hypertrophy (dilation).

## 4    Discussion and Conclusions

The proposed method showed better accuracy than the conventional method when the same segmentation method was used in training and testing. However, the accuracy difference became small in automated segmentation (Fig. 2), suggesting that the proposed method is more sensitive to segmentation error. As shown in Fig. 4, the proposed method appears to capture more subtle disease-specific shape deformations, which are considered to be easily affected by the segmentation error. However, among the existing methods, the segmentation method used in this study may not be the most accurate. Further, the liver segmentation accuracy may improve with future research.

The accuracy improvement by increasing the training data was larger in the proposed method than in the conventional method. One potential reason is because the healthy subspace covered a more accurate variability due to the increasing training data; thus, the disease subspace was less contaminated by the normal variability. When the automated segmentation is used for training, increasing the training data will be easy in the clinical routine; thus, this feature is advantageous for the proposed method.

In our dataset, the patients of the dataset belonged to the same race. Healthy livers have large inter-subject variability, but it may be smaller within the same race. To clinically accept these results, further validations, including multi-race and prospective studies, are essential. Furthermore, the fibrosis diagnosis is clinically important. In our dataset, 63% of the disease data were histologically diagnosed to be fibrotic. We tested the classifier for the dataset consisting of healthy and fibrotic livers, and obtained similar classification accuracy (0.924 for "Both-manual" and 0.889 for "Both-automated"). Thus, the proposed method will also be promising for diagnosis of fibrosis.

We have shown that the OC subspace projection pronounces the diseased components of an organ shape and more clearly clusters the healthy and diseased organs. In addition, the results showed the necessity of more accurate segmentation. Future work will include the application of the proposed method to different diagnostic problems.

**Acknowledgments.** This work is partly supported by KAKENHI No. 21103003.

# References

1. Thompson, P., Mega, M., Woods, R., Zoumalan, C., Lindshield, C., Blanton, R., Moussai, J., Holmes, C., Cummings, J., Toga, A.: Cortical Change in Alzheimer's Disease Detected with a Disease-specific Population-based Brain Atlas. Cerebral Cortex 11(1), 1–16 (2001)
2. Heimann, T., Meinzer, H.: Statistical Shape Models for 3D Medical Image Segmentation: A review. Med. Image Anal. 13(4), 543–563 (2009)
3. Dacheng, T., Xiaoou, T.: Orthogonal Complement Component Analysis for Positive Samples in SVM Based Relevance Feedback Image Retrieval. Computer Vision and Pattern Recognition 2, 586–591 (2004)
4. Golland, P., Grimson, E., Shenton, M., Kikinis, R.: Detection and analysis of statistical differences in anatomical shape. Med. Image Anal. 9(1), 69–86 (2005)
5. Goshima, S., Kanematsu, M., Koayashi, T., Furukawa, T., Zhang, X., Fujita, H., Watanabe, H., Kondo, H., Moriyama, N., Bae, K.: Staging Hepatic Fibrosis: Computer-Aided Analysis of Hepatic Contours on Gadolinium Ethoxybenzyl Diethylenetriaminepentaacetic Acid-Enhanced Hepatocyte-Phase Magnetic Resonance Imaging. Hepatology 55(1), 328–329 (2012)
6. Badeau, R., Richard, G., Bertrand, D.: Fast and stable YAST algorithm for principal and minor subspace tracking. IEEE Trans. Signal Process. 56(8), 3437–3446 (2008)
7. Higham, N.: Computing the polar decompositions-with applications. SIAM Journal on Scientific and Statistical Computing 7(4), 1160–1174 (1986)
8. Rueckert, D., Sonoda, L.I., Hayes, C., Hill, D.L.G., Leach, M.O., Hawkes, D.J.: Non-rigid registration using free-form deformations: Application to breast MR images. IEEE Trans. Med. Imaging 18(8), 712–721 (1999)
9. Okada, T., Shimada, R., Hori, M., Nakamoto, M., Chen, Y.W., Nakamura, H., Sato, Y.: Automated segmentation of the liver from 3D CT images using probabilistic atlas and multi-level statistical shape model. Acad. Radiol. 15(11), 1390–1403 (2008)
10. Ichida, F., Tsuji, T., Omata, M., Ichida, T., Inoue, K., Kamimura, T., Yamada, G., Hino, K., Yokosuka, O., Suzuki, H.: New Inuyama classification; new criteria for histological assessment of chronic hepatitis. International Hepatology Communications 6(2), 112–119 (1996)

# Visual Phrase Learning and Its Application in Computed Tomographic Colonography

Shijun Wang, Matthew McKenna, Zhuoshi Wei, Jiamin Liu, Peter Liu,
and Ronald M. Summers

Imaging Biomarkers and Computer-Aided Diagnosis Laboratory,
Radiology and Imaging Sciences, Clinical Center, National Institutes of Health,
Bldg 10, Room 1C224, Bethesda, MD 20892-1182, U.S.
rms@nih.gov

**Abstract.** In this work, we propose a visual phrase learning scheme to learn an optimal visual composite of anatomical components/parts from CT colonography images for computer-aided detection. The key idea is to utilize the anatomical parts of human body from medical images and associate them with biological targets of interest (organs, cancers, lesions, etc.) for joint detection and recognition. These anatomical parts of the human body are not necessarily near each other regarding their physical locations, and they serve more like a human body navigation system for detection and recognition. To show the effectiveness of the proposed learning scheme, we applied it to two sub-problems in computed tomographic colonography: teniae detection and classification of colorectal polyp candidates. Experimental results showed its efficacy.

## 1 Introduction

To help radiologists read images and identify lesions, various computer-aided detection (CADe) and computer-aided diagnosis (CADx) systems have been developed [1, 2]. In the majority of CAD systems developed for radiology, anatomical knowledge is highly embedded into the algorithm design. In other words, interaction with radiologists during algorithm development, and integration of expert human knowledge into the algorithm, is crucial to the success of these CAD systems. However, instead of relying on a radiologist to define the anatomical knowledge used in a CAD system, we believe that a computer could learn what parts of the human anatomy are useful in performing the detection task. Particularly, this work focuses on how to automatically build an anatomical model of human body using only statistical information from CT images.

In recent years, significant progress has been made in the field of computerized object detection and recognition due to the application of statistical learning on large-scale data. Some cutting edge methods include bag of words (BoW) [3], deformable templates [4], and part-based models [5]. BoW methods are built from codebooks, or collections, of visual patches extracted from images. BoW methods usually employ affine invariant descriptors to characterize image patches. Furthermore, the efficient

K. Mori et al. (Eds.): MICCAI 2013, Part I, LNCS 8149, pp. 243–250, 2013.
© Springer-Verlag Berlin Heidelberg 2013

creation of useful codebooks for visual object recognition is a critical step in BoW methods [5]. In the deformable templates technique, the key idea is to fit a model to an image by minimizing the error between the input image and the closest model instance. Finally, with part-based models, the target object is modeled by mixtures of multi-scale deformable part models [5]. In the work of [6] on part-based models, they proposed an explicit way to utilize auxiliary/accompanied objects to detect and recognize a main target object. They called their approach visual phrase recognition [6], where a visual phrase is a complex visual composite containing several objects (i.e. "a person riding a horse").

In this work, we propose a visual phrase learning scheme to learn visual composites in medical images. The key motivation is to develop an automatic way to learn visual phrases, instead of the manual way in the original work [6]. We utilize the anatomical parts of human body from medical images by composing them with a target of interest (e.g. organs, cancers, lesions) for joint detection and recognition. Unlike the work of [6], the relevant anatomical parts of human body are not necessarily near each other, and they serve more as a human body navigation system for detection and recognition. To show the efficacy of our new visual phrase, we applied our learning scheme to two problems encountered in CTC: the identification of the teniae coli and the classification of polyp candidates in a CAD system (Fig.1).

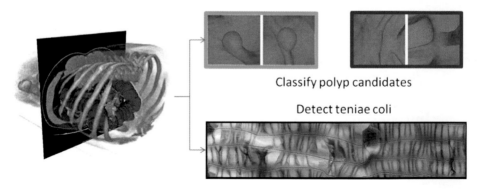

Classify polyp candidates

Detect teniae coli

**Fig. 1.** Overview of CTC and two applications: colonic polyp classification (green square shows a true polyp and blue square shows a false positive) and teniae coli detection

## 2    Visual Phrase Learning

We show a diagram of our proposed system in Fig. 2. In the work of Sadeghi and Farhadi [6], the visual phrases were determined by prior knowledge using bounding boxes. All components belonging to a visual phrase were in close spatial proximity, making the system a top-down approach in which a visual phrase is determined beforehand and then applied to test images. What happens if we do not know the visual parts of the phrase a priori, or if we have a large pool of visual parts (codebook) and do not know which combination will be helpful for the detection of the target object? Also, how can visual phrases be developed for visual parts that are distributed in different spatial locations? In the following subsections, we address these problems

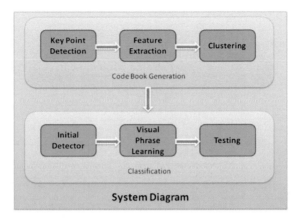

**Fig. 2.** System diagram of the proposed visual phrase learning algorithm

by proposing a bottom-up method to learn the optimal visual phrase for joint object detection and recognition from a codebook of visual parts.

## 2.1    Problem Formulation

For a two-class classification problem, given training samples $\{(X_1,y_1),\ldots,(X_n,y_n)\}$, $y_i \in \{-1,+1\}$, where each training sample $X$ is a composition of detection $x$ and auxiliary data (visual patches coming from a codebook with $m$ items) associated with each detection $\{x_1^c,\ldots,x_m^c\}$, the visual phrase learning problem is formulated as follows:

$$\min_{w_c} \min_{w_1,b,\xi} \frac{1}{2}\|w_1\|^2 + C_1 \sum_{i=1}^{n} \xi_i , \tag{1}$$

$$\text{s.t. } y_i\left(w_1^T X_i w_c + b\right) \geq 1 - \xi_i, \xi_i \geq 0, \forall_{i=1}^n, w_c \geq 0, \sum_{i=0}^{m} w_{ci} = 1,$$

where $w_1$ is a linear classifier in feature space; $b$ is the bias item of the classifier; $w_c \geq 0$ is a parameter vector to learn visual phrase from a codebook; and $C_1$ is a trade-off parameter to control the classifier complexity and slack variables $\xi_i$, $i = 1,2,\ldots,n$; Please note that each training sample, $X_i$, is a $d \times (m+1)$ matrix in which each column represents a detection/instance, each row corresponds to a feature and $d$ is the feature's dimension. The first column is the detection we wish to classify. The next $m$ columns represent $m$ parts from a code book. The column-wise order of detection and code book items is fixed to maintain consistency across all training and test samples. The purpose of the above learning problem is to learn the visual phrase (specified by $w_c$) which has the best performance regarding classification, given a codebook from the image data. Our hypothesis is that a visual phrase (composed of detection and its surrounding structures) has better discriminating power than a single detection object. Eq. (1) is a new formulation which contains the key idea on visual phrase learning proposed in this paper. Please note that $X_i$ in Eq. (1) is a 2D matrix which differentiates the proposed formulation from traditional support vector machines formulation.

## 2.2    Linear SDP Solution

To solve the above optimization problem, we propose the following theorem:

**Theorem 1.** The above visual phrase learning problem can be formulated as the following semi-definite programming (SDP) problem:

$$\min_{w_c,\ v,\delta,\lambda} t \quad \text{s.t.} \quad \begin{bmatrix} K & \dfrac{(e+v-\delta+\lambda y)}{\sqrt{2}} \\ \dfrac{(e+v-\delta+\lambda y)^T}{\sqrt{2}} & \left(t-C_1\delta^T e\right) \end{bmatrix} \geq 0, \tag{2}$$

$$W_c = W_c^T,\ e^T W_c e = 1,\ v \geq 0, \delta \geq 0,$$

where $K_{ij} = y_i y_j trace\left(X_i^T X_j \times W_c^T\right); v \geq 0, \delta \geq 0$ and $\lambda$ are dual variables introduced in the dual problem; $e$ is a vector filled with all ones. Our SDP solution provides a closed-form solution to the optimization problem in (1), which is guaranteed to be global optimal. The proof is omitted due to page limit.

It is interesting to note that the solution we show in Theorem 1 has connections with multi-kernel learning [7] and sequence kernel learning [8]. Multi-kernel learning can be viewed as special cases of our visual phrase learning framework.

## 2.3    Kernelization

In the previous subsection we showed the linear solution for the visual phrase learning problem in the original feature space. Now let's consider its nonlinear solution. First let us define a mapping function $\Phi$ which maps the data in the original Euclidean space to a new reproducing kernel Hilbert space (RKHS): $\mathbb{R}^d \rightarrow H$. More specifically, the mapping function $\Phi$ maps each column of the input sample (detection plus codebook items) to the same RKHS. $H$ may be infinite dimensional. Utilizing a different mapping function and RKHS for detection and codebook is also feasible but beyond the scope of this paper. The visual phrase learning problem in the new Hilbert space can be formulated as follows:

$$\min_{w_c} \min_{w_1,b,\xi} \frac{1}{2}\|w_1\|^2 + C_1 \sum_{i=1}^{n} \xi_i, \tag{3}$$

$$\text{s.t. } y_i\left(w_1^T\Phi(X_i)w_c + b\right) \geq 1-\xi_i,\ \xi_i \geq 0,\ \forall_{i=1}^{n}, w_c \geq 0, \sum_{i=0}^{m} w_{ci} = 1.$$

$\Phi(X_i)$ is the mapping of detection $x_i$ and its corresponding codebook items. Each column of $\Phi(X_i)$ corresponds to one vector in the new RKHS. We define a symmetric kernel function for the input samples (detection plus codebook items) as follows: $K_f\left(X_i, X_j\right) = trace\left(\Phi(X_i)^T \Phi(X_j) \times W_c^T\right)$. Let us define the corresponding symmetric kernel function for the mapping function $\Phi$ as follows: $K_c\left(X_{im}, X_{jn}\right) = \Phi(X_{im})^T \Phi(X_{jn})$

where subscripts $m$ and $n$ correspond to $m$'th and $n$'th columns of sample $X_i$ and $X_j$. Then we have the following Theorem:

**Theorem 2.** The symmetric kernel function $K_f\left(X_i, X_j\right) = trace\left(\Phi(X_i)^T \Phi(X_j) \times W_c^T\right)$ fulfills the Mercer's condition for any kernel function $K_c\left(X_{im}, X_{jn}\right) = \Phi(X_{im})^T \Phi(X_{jn})$ fulfilling the Mercer's condition when $w_c \geq 0$ (element-wise).

**Proof:** For any square integrable functions g(x),

$$\iint K_f\left(X_i, X_j\right) g(X_i) g\left(X_j\right) dX_i dX_j = \iint trace\left(\Phi(X_i)^T \Phi(X_j) \times W_c^T\right) g(X_i) g\left(X_j\right) dX_i dX_j$$

$$= \sum_{u=0}^{m} \sum_{v=0}^{m} w_{cu} w_{cv} \iint \Phi(X_{iu})^T \Phi(X_{jv}) g(X_i) g\left(X_j\right) dX_i dX_j \geq 0 \qquad \square$$

By using the Lagrange multiplier optimization method, we obtain the theorem:

**Theorem 3.** The nonlinear visual phrase learning problem can be formulated as the following semi-definite programming (SDP) problem:

$$\min_{w_c, \, v, \delta, \lambda} t \quad \text{s.t.} \quad \begin{bmatrix} K & \dfrac{(e+v-\delta+\lambda y)}{\sqrt{2}} \\ \dfrac{(e+v-\delta+\lambda y)^T}{\sqrt{2}} & (t-C_1\delta^T e) \end{bmatrix} \geq 0, \qquad (4)$$

$W_c = W_c^T$ and $e^T W_c e = 1$, $v \geq 0, \delta \geq 0$, where

$K_{ij} = y_i y_j trace\left(\Phi(X_i)^T \Phi(X_j) \times W_c^T\right)$. Proof is omitted due to the page limit.

## 3    Experiments: Teniae Coli

Teniae coli are three longitudinal smooth muscle bands in the colon surface. They are parallel, equally distributed, and form a triple helix structure from the appendix to the sigmoid colon. Fig.1 illustrates a human colon and the configuration of the teniae coli. Teniae are anatomically meaningful landmarks and can be used to estimate the circumferential positions of potential lesions in CT colonography.

To detect teniae coli, colon segmentation was first performed on the original CTC slice. The segmented colon surface was reconstructed and unfolded into a 2D flattened colon using a reversible projection. The unfolded images then were converted into 2D height maps. The height maps are 2D intensity images that record the elevation of the colon surface relative to the unfolding plane, where haustral folds correspond to high elevation points and teniae to low elevation points.

We used CTC data from 20 patients, dividing patients into separate training (17) and testing (3) sets. The separation of training/test sets was determined empirically. We cropped each image to only include the middle segment of each image as the teniae were very difficult to define at either end of the colon.

To generate the codebook used in our approach, we utilized a multiscale Harris operator to detect points of interest on our images [9]. The detector located corners and edges at various scales. We extracted a small patch around each detected point. Fig. 3(a) shows some typical keypoints detected by the Harris operator. Note that these visual words are not adjacent to each other. We utilized a range of features to describe each keypoint, including HOG, shape context, and SIFT. We also included the location of each detection and a histogram of intensity values as additional features. A k-means clustering scheme (k=5) was used to learn the elements in our codebook. The number of visual words was empirically determined based on performance of the system on the training set. For kernel computation and classification, we used a radial basis function (RBF) kernel with a kernel width parameter set as the 90th percentile of pairwise distances between all training samples. We applied the same kernel to the following colonic polyp detection data. The RBF kernel was chosen because its efficacy on many real applications.

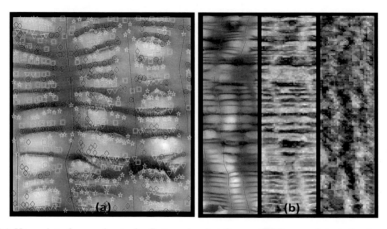

**Fig. 3.** (a) Keypoints from subset of a flattened colon from a CTC scan, detected using a Harris detection scheme. Different markers denote different clusters. Note the regular pattern around the folds. (b) Detection results of teniae coli. From left to right: original height map of a colon with ground truth (red lines); detection results of using detection features only; detection results using the proposed visual phrase approach. The brighter the detection block, the higher the probability it is a tenia coli.

In Fig. 3(b) we show comparisons between the proposed method and an SVM that used detection features only. As is evident in the above figure, the visual phrase classifier is able to learn the pattern of the teniae falling between and orthogonal to folds. All the non-teniae structures, like folds and colon walls, were suppressed by the visual phrase. The SVM, which is blind to surrounding structures, mistakes areas between folds (running horizontally, orthogonal to the teniae) as teniae.

## 4    Experiments: Colonic Polyp Detection in CTC

In the polyp detection problem, we used CTC data from 50 patients, dividing patients into separate training (25) and testing (25) sets. We extracted the colon from each scan and performed a curvature-based analysis to generate an initial list of lesions of interest. After initial filtering, we identified 880 polyp candidates (detections) which include 62 true polyps.

For each polyp candidate, our system generated 5 intraluminal, volume-rendered images focusing on the detection from various viewpoints (Fig. 1 shows two viewpoints as illustration). Averaged prediction scores of the 5 images were used as the final prediction score for the polyp candidate. We used 2D HOG features to describe the images (the first column of sample X in Section 2.1). To generate a codebook of auxiliary data, traditional 3D curvature based features were extracted from original CT slices. These 3D features are widely used in traditional CTC CAD to capture the anatomical shapes of the polyp candidate and its surrounding structures.

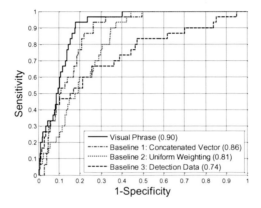

**Fig. 4.** ROC comparison of the proposed visual phrase method and baseline methods. The difference between the visual phrase method and the highest-performing baseline method (concatenated vector) is significant ($p<0.05$).

We produced receiver operating curves (ROC) to analyze the performance of the visual phrase. We compared the visual phrase with 3 baseline methods. For the first method, we concatenated the detection data and all codebook items into a single vector that was fed to the classifier. For the second method, we set the Wc matrix to equally weight the detection data and each codebook item. We also compared the visual phrase classifier to a system that only used the detection features. In Fig. 5 the ROC's of the four methods are compared. Use of visual phrases improved the classification performance compared with the baseline methods. The AUC's of each method were 0.90 ($\pm 0.04$), 0.86 ($\pm 0.04$), 0.81 ($\pm 0.05$), and 0.74 ($\pm 0.05$) respectively. The difference between the visual phrase method and the highest-performing baseline method (concatenated vector) was significant (p<0.05).

## 5     Conclusion and Discussion

In this work, we proposed a visual phrase learning scheme to learn a visual composite of anatomical parts from medical images for medical computer-aided detection.

In theory, components of a visual phrase are not necessarily "meaningful" anatomical parts. In the proposed method, useful visual words were identified by the learning process with the guidance of training labels. Any visual words which were useful for the classification were highly weighted and selected. For example, visual words on the colon folds and colon wall near the folds were highly weighted and therefore anatomically "meaningful". Experimental results on two CTC applications showed improved performance with the proposed method.

Our proposed method has several advantages. First, we do not need manual identification of the visual phrase. In Sadeghi and Farhadi's work on recognition using visual phrase [6], the appearance models for each category were learned using deformable part models which required manually labeled bounding boxes for training patches. Second, our method has more flexibility. We allow the learned visual parts to be distributed across the whole image, not limited to local patches.

**Acknowledgements.** This work was supported by the Intramural Research Programs of the NIH Clinical Center and by a Cooperative Research and Development Agreement with iCAD. This study utilized the high-performance computational capabilities of the Biowulf Linux cluster at the National Institutes of Health.

# References

1. Doi, K.: Computer-aided diagnosis in medical imaging: Historical review, current status and future potential. Computerized Medical Imaging and Graphics 31, 198–211 (2007)
2. Wang, S.J., Summers, R.M.: Machine learning and radiology. Medical Image Analysis 16, 933–951 (2012)
3. Csurka, G., Dance, C.R., Fan, L., Willamowski, J., Bray, C.: Visual Categorization with Bags of Keypoints. In: ECCV Workshop on Statistical Learning in Computer Vision (2004)
4. Cootes, T.F., Edwards, G.J., Taylor, C.J.: Active appearance models. IEEE Transactions on Pattern Analysis and Machine Intelligence 23, 681–685 (2001)
5. Felzenszwalb, P.F., Girshick, R.B., McAllester, D., Ramanan, D.: Object Detection with Discriminatively Trained Part-Based Models. IEEE Transactions on Pattern Analysis and Machine Intelligence 32, 1627–1645 (2010)
6. Sadeghi, M.A., Farhadi, A.: Recognition Using Visual Phrases. In: Proceedings of the IEEE Conference on Computer Vision and Pattern Recognition (2011)
7. Lanckriet, G.R.G., Cristianini, N., Bartlett, P., El Ghaoui, L., Jordan, M.I.: Learning the kernel matrix with semidefinite programming. Journal of Machine Learning Research 5, 27–72 (2004)
8. Cortes, C., Mohri, M., Rostamizadeh, A.: Learning sequence kernels. In: IEEE Workshop on Machine Learning for Signal Processing, pp. 2–8 (2008)
9. Mikolajczyk, K., Schmid, C.: Indexing based on scale invariant interest points. In: Proceedings of the Eighth IEEE International Conference on Computer Vision, ICCV 2001, vol. 521, pp. 525–531 (2001)

# Fusing Correspondenceless 3D Point Distribution Models

Marco Pereañez[1], Karim Lekadir[1], Constantine Butakoff[2],
Corné Hoogendoorn[1], and Alejandro Frangi[3]

[1] CISTIB, Universitat Pompeu Fabra and CIBER-BBN, Barcelona, Spain
[2] PhySense, Universitat Pompeu Fabra, Barcelona, Spain
[3] CISTIB, University of Sheffield, Sheffield, UK

**Abstract.** This paper presents a framework for the fusion of multiple point distribution models (PDMs) with unknown point correspondences. With this work, models built from distinct patient groups and imaging modalities can be merged, with the aim to obtain a PDM that encodes a wider range of anatomical variability. To achieve this, two technical challenges are addressed in this work. Firstly, the model fusion must be carried out directly on the corresponding means and eigenvectors as the original data is not always available and cannot be freely exchanged across centers for various legal and practical reasons. Secondly, the PDMs need to be normalized before fusion as the point correspondence is unknown. The proposed framework is validated by integrating statistical models of the left and right ventricles of the heart constructed from different imaging modalities (MRI and CT) and with different landmark representations of the data. The results show that the integration is statistically and anatomically meaningful and that the quality of the resulting model is significantly improved.

## 1 Introduction

Despite their widespread use in medical imaging, point distribution models (PDMs) [2] often suffer from over-fitting, or lack of sufficient generalization ability. This is due to the fact that typically too few training examples are available compared to the dimensionality of the shapes themselves. Extensive work has been dedicated to improving the generalization ability of statistical shape models. These works can be roughly categorized into: a) methods that *add artificial variation to a model*, b) methods that *combine statistical and physical models*, and c) methods that *model object ensembles, and/or object hierarchies*. However, little attention has been placed on methods that aggregate preexisting statistical models into a single more robust model. Yet, this would allow to unify PDMs from different research centers, patient groups and imaging modalities, without the need for the original data, which is not always available and cannot be freely exchanged across centers for various legal and practical reasons.

In the recent years, a few techniques have been published to fuse means and eigenvectors [4,11,1]. However, they require point correspondence between models, a constraint which is rarely valid in practice as the PDMs are derived from

K. Mori et al. (Eds.): MICCAI 2013, Part I, LNCS 8149, pp. 251–258, 2013.

datasets delineated at different clinical centers, using distinct delineation protocols and observers. Unlike for shapes [6], the problem of establishing point correspondence between eigenspaces has not been yet investigated.

In this paper we present a method for the normalization and fusion of statistical models of anatomical shape. To achieve this, an inter-model barycentric mapping is estimated by combining rigid and nonrigid registrations of the means, with the aim to transform the PDMs into a common landmark representation. Subsequently, a model fusion technique is applied which, unlike existing methods [5], takes into account the weights of each model in the final result, thus obtaining a model that is statistically and anatomically meaningful. The proposed framework is validated by integrating anatomical models of various geometrical and statistical complexity, based on left and right ventricular MRI and CT datasets.

## 2   Normalization Algorithm

The goal of the proposed algorithm is the creation of a single fused model from a set of models built from shapes that do not share point correspondence and hence, have different eigenspace representations, and different dimensionality. Since we do not have the original datasets, we need to solve the point correspondence problem among the different model means, and find a transformation that re-parametrizes all eigenvectors into a common space.

For the remainder of the paper, let $\Omega_i = (\bar{\mathbf{x}}_i, \boldsymbol{\Phi}_i, \boldsymbol{\Lambda}_i, K_i, V_i)$, be the $i$-th model in the set $\{\Omega_i : i = 1, \ldots, N\}$ of pre-built models of the same object with different landmark placement strategy. Here $\bar{\mathbf{x}}_i$ is a vector of concatenated vertex coordinates representing the mean shape, $\boldsymbol{\Phi}_i$ and $\boldsymbol{\Lambda}_i$ are the eigenvector and eigenvalue matrices, respectively, and $K_i$ and $V_i$ are the number of observations used to build the model, and their triangulation. Now, let $\mathcal{M}_i = (\bar{\mathbf{x}}_i, V_i)$ be the model mean surfaces defined by the vertices $\bar{\mathbf{x}}_i$ and triangulations $V_i$.

### 2.1   Computing Surface Correspondence

Selecting a reference surface mesh is the first step in computing surface correspondence across all models. Here, we choose the highest resolution mesh (*i.e.* CT) as reference, to retain as much shape information – high frequency detail – as possible from the different models. The aim is to establish surface correspondence between each of the models' mean surfaces $\mathcal{M}_i$, and the chosen reference mean surface $\mathcal{M}_{ref}$. This should produce a mapping that linearly transforms the shape representation of each PDM to match that of the reference PDM. To achieve this, we first perform an initial rigid registration using the iterative closest point (ICP) algorithm in order to resolve pose differences between the means. Subsequently we apply the currents-based diffeomorphic registration method [3] to obtain a more accurate surface correspondence. In other words, we estimate a combined transformation $\varphi_i : \mathcal{M}_i \to \mathcal{M}_{ref}$ such that $\varphi_i(\mathcal{M}_i)$ is as close as possible to $\mathcal{M}_{ref}$. Note that neither ICP nor the currents approach rely on point correspondences, thus making them fit for this purpose.

## 2.2   Computing Inter-model Landmark Mapping

Once surface correspondence has been obtained, we proceed to find a suitable transformation that re-parametrizes all meshes to match the parametrization found on the reference mesh.

Specifically, we seek a transformation matrix $\mathbf{T}_i$ that expresses every point on $\mathcal{M}_{ref} = (\bar{\mathbf{x}}_{ref}, V_{ref})$ as a linear combination of the vertices on the previously registered mean meshes $\mathcal{M}_i = (\varphi_i(\bar{\mathbf{x}}_i), V_i)$.

Let $\varphi_i(\bar{\mathbf{x}}_i)$, for $i = 1, \ldots, N$, be the points of the $i$-th mean shape on the reference surface $\mathcal{M}_{ref}$. Without any loss of generality we can use the same triangulation that is already present in the surface $\mathcal{M}_{ref}$. Let $\mathbf{T}_i$ be a linear transformation matrix such that $\bar{\mathbf{x}}_{ref} \approx \mathbf{T}_i \varphi_i(\bar{\mathbf{x}}_i)$. It follows naturally that this is achieved when $\mathbf{T}_i$ contains the barycentric coordinates of the points $\bar{\mathbf{x}}_{ref}$ expressed in terms of points $\varphi_i(\bar{\mathbf{x}}_i)$ and triangulation $V_i$. $\mathbf{T}_i \bar{\mathbf{x}}_i$ will change the triangulation of the surface $\mathcal{M}_i$ to match that of $\mathcal{M}_{ref}$ and therefore it can be represented by the pair $\mathcal{M}'_i = (\mathbf{T}_i \bar{\mathbf{x}}_i, V_{ref})$.

For every point in the reference shape we compute the normal to its mesh surface, and the point of intersection with a plane described by a triangle on the target mesh. We then compute barycentric coefficients $c_{i,1}$, $c_{i,2}$, $c_{i,3}$ for each point in the triangle, and construct a point transformation matrix $\mathbf{P}_i$ as

$$\mathbf{P}_i = \begin{bmatrix} & 0 \; c_{i,1} \; 0 & 0 \; 0 & & 0 \; c_{i,2} \; 0 & 0 \; 0 & & 0 \; c_{i,3} \; 0 & 0 \; 0 & \\ \cdots & 0 \; 0 \; c_{i,1} & 0 \; 0 \cdots & 0 \; 0 \; c_{i,2} & 0 \; 0 \cdots & 0 \; 0 \; c_{i,3} & 0 \; 0 \cdots \\ & 0 \; 0 \; 0 & c_{i,1} \; 0 & & 0 \; 0 \; 0 & c_{i,2} \; 0 & & 0 \; 0 \; 0 & c_{i,3} \; 0 & \end{bmatrix}_{3 \times 3m},$$

where the column-wise position of every $3 \times 3$ diagonal matrix $\mathbf{C_i}$ encodes the indexing of a simplex on the target mesh, thus preserving point correspondence between the reference and target meshes. $m$ is the number of points in the target mesh. Finally the complete transformation matrix $\mathbf{T}_i$ is a row-wise concatenation of point transformation matrices $\mathbf{P}_i$,

$$\mathbf{T}_i = \left[ \mathbf{P}_i^{(1)} \cdots \mathbf{P}_i^{(n)} \right]^T_{3n \times 3m}$$

where $n$ is the number of points in the reference mesh. Due to the linearity of $\mathbf{T}_i$, any shape $\mathbf{x}_i \approx \bar{\mathbf{x}}_i + \mathbf{\Phi}_i \mathbf{b}_i$ can also be re-parametrized as $\mathbf{T}_i \mathbf{x}_i \approx \mathbf{T}_i \bar{\mathbf{x}}_i + \mathbf{T}_i \mathbf{\Phi}_i \mathbf{b}_i$. Thus, the models to be fused are $\Omega'_i = (\mathbf{T}_i \bar{\mathbf{x}}_i, \mathbf{T}_i \mathbf{\Phi}_i, \mathbf{\Lambda}_i, K_i, V_{ref})$.

## 3   Fusion Algorithm

Once all eigenspaces have been transformed to having a common triangulation, the models $\Omega'_i = (\mathbf{T}_i \bar{\mathbf{x}}_i, \mathbf{T}_i \mathbf{\Phi}_i, \mathbf{\Lambda}_i, K_i, V_{ref}), i = 1, \ldots, N$ are fused. To simplify notation, we denote the newly transformed mean shapes and eigenvector matrices as $\bar{\mathbf{x}}'_i = \mathbf{T}_i \bar{\mathbf{x}}_i$ and $\mathbf{\Phi}'_i = \mathbf{T}_i \mathbf{\Phi}_i$, respectively.

The goal of fusion is to compute an eigenspace $\Omega = (\bar{\mathbf{x}}, \mathbf{\Phi}, \mathbf{\Lambda}, K)$, using only information from $\Omega'_i = (\bar{\mathbf{x}}'_i, \mathbf{\Phi}'_i, \mathbf{\Lambda}_i, K_i)$, for $i = 1, \ldots, N$ as described in the previous section. The resulting model should be equivalent to one built from the full set of original observations.

### 3.1   Global Alignment

Since every PDM has a different mean shape and a different pose, the first step is to align the means $\bar{\mathbf{x}}_i'$ of all PDMs using Procrustes Analysis [8]. Then the aligned means $\bar{\mathbf{x}}_i'$ are used to estimate the fused mean $\bar{\mathbf{x}}$.

During alignment of the means, shapes are centered and rescaled to unit size and a $d \times d$ matrix accounting for rotation is estimated, where $d$ is the dimensionality of landmarks (*i.e.*, $d = 3$). Let $\mathbf{S}_i$ be the $d \times d$ rotation matrix from the transformation that aligns the shape $\bar{\mathbf{x}}_i'$ to the mean $\bar{\mathbf{x}}$. Let $\mathbf{\Xi}_i$ be a $dn \times dn$ block-diagonal matrix with repeating $\mathbf{S}_i$ along its diagonal. We use transformations $\mathbf{\Xi}_i$ to reorient eigenvectors $\mathbf{\Xi}_i\mathbf{\Phi}_i$, such that we work with eigenspaces $\Omega_i'' = (\mathbf{\Xi}_i\bar{\mathbf{x}}_i', \mathbf{\Xi}_i\mathbf{\Phi}_i', \mathbf{\Lambda}_i, K_i)$, assuming the mean shapes are already translation and scale-independent.

### 3.2   Determining the Basis of the Fused Space

The fused model eigenvalues and eigenvectors should satisfy $\mathbf{D} = \mathbf{\Phi}\mathbf{\Lambda}\mathbf{\Phi}^T$, where $\mathbf{D}$ is a combined covariance matrix that can be obtained solely from information in models $\Omega_i'$, and where each covariance matrix $\mathbf{D}_i = \mathbf{\Phi}_i\mathbf{\Lambda}_i\mathbf{\Phi}_i^T$ is weighted according to the number of contributed shapes of each of the models. For the complete mathematical derivation of $\mathbf{D}$ we refer to [1].

The fused space is obtained as follows:

1. *Find an eigenspace that spans all models' eigenspaces:* Construct an orthonormal basis set $\mathbf{\Gamma}$, that spans all the eigenspaces $\mathbf{\Xi}_i\mathbf{\Phi}_i$ of the input models. This is done by orthonormalization of the matrix $\mathbf{H}$, defined as $\mathbf{H} = [\mathbf{\Xi}_1\mathbf{\Phi}_1', \ldots, \mathbf{\Xi}_N\mathbf{\Phi}_N', \delta_{1,2}, \ldots, \delta_{1,N}, \ldots, \delta_{N-1,N}]$, where $\delta_{i,j} = (\mathbf{\Xi}_i\bar{\mathbf{x}}_i' - \mathbf{\Xi}_j\bar{\mathbf{x}}_j')$, for $i, j = 1, \ldots, N$, and $j > i$.
2. *Determine an intermediate eigenproblem:* Use $\mathbf{\Gamma}$ to derive an intermediate eigenproblem: $\mathbf{\Gamma}\mathbf{D}\mathbf{\Gamma}^T = \mathbf{R}\mathbf{\Lambda}\mathbf{R}^T$, whose solution provides the fused model eigenvalues $\mathbf{\Lambda}$ and eigenvectors $\mathbf{R}$ needed to correctly orient basis $\mathbf{\Gamma}$.
3. *Compute the fused eigenvector matrix:* Finally, the eigenvectors $\mathbf{\Phi}$ of the fused model are obtained from $\mathbf{\Phi} = \mathbf{\Gamma}\mathbf{R}$.

## 4   Results

### 4.1   Quantitative Evaluation

Numerical assessment of the proposed fusion is carried out using a set of 42 cardiac MRI datasets acquired using a GE Signa CVi-HDx 1.5T scanner (General Electric, Milwaukee, USA). The images were manually delineated by an expert clinician using 880 landmarks for the LV and 1200 landmarks for the RV. The following experiment was then carried out:

1. For each $\mathbf{x}_i = \mathbf{x}_{\text{test}}$, define a ground truth PDM $\Omega_{OM}$ (Original Model) constructed from $S_{OM} = S_{\text{all}} \setminus \mathbf{x}_{\text{test}}$ (leave-one-out).

2. Partition $S_{OM}$ into randomly selected subsets $S_A$, $S_B$, $S_C$ such that $S_A \cap S_B \cap S_C = \emptyset$, $S_A \cup S_B \cup S_C = S_{OM}$ (repeated 100 times).
3. Without loss of generality, choose subsets $S_B$ and $S_C$ and resample all shapes to obtain $S'_B$ and $S'_C$ such that point correspondence between sets $S_A$, $S_B$ and $S_C$ is lost.
4. Construct the models $\Omega_{S_A}$, $\Omega_{S'_B}$, and $\Omega_{S'_C}$ from $S_A$, $S'_B$, and $S'_C$, respectively.
5. Apply the normalization and fusion algorithm to PDMs $\Omega_{S_A}$, $\Omega_{S'_B}$, and $\Omega_{S'_C}$ to obtain the fused model $\Omega_{NF}$.
6. Compare the accuracy of shape reconstruction achieved by the $\Omega_{OM}$, and $\Omega_{NF}$ PDMs by computing the mean point-to-surface distance between $\tilde{\mathbf{x}}_{\text{test},OM}$ and $\tilde{\mathbf{x}}_{\text{test},NF}$, the reconstructions obtained $\Omega_{OM}$ and $\Omega_{NF}$, respectively.

Note that all models were built preserving 98% of total variance, and allowing $\pm 3$ standard deviations from the mean. Resampling of $S_B$ and $S_C$ in step 3 was done through two iterations of Loop-subdivision [9] of the original meshes, followed by a centroidal Voronoi diagram algorithm [10] to remove the correspondence.

We performed the experiments on both the LV and the RV shapes. Table 1 summarizes the results as Hausdorff distances, where it can seen that a low reconstruction error is found, which shows that the unified model is similar to the one obtained directly from the original data. The small reconstruction errors are due to the change in surface parameterization in step 3 which inevitably leads to a loss of geometrical information. However, this is kept under 0.5 mm and with a low maximum error for both the LV and RV. This also shows that the proposed fusion can handle models corresponding to different geometrical complexities and anatomical variabilities (*e.g.*, LV and RV).

In order to demonstrate the capability of the technique to fuse multiple models (more than two), Figs. 1(a) and 1(c) illustrate the first mode of variation of three models obtained through random partition of the original dataset (columns 1-3), their fusion (col. 4), and the original shapes model (col. 5). It can be seen visually that the modes obtained for the $\Omega_{OM}$ and $\Omega_{NF}$ models are almost identical. Also, Figs. 1(b) and 1(d) show the eigenvalues for both the $\Omega_{OM}$ and $\Omega_{NF}$ of the same models (Figs. 1(a) and 1(c)), organized by descending variance. It can be seen from the eigenvalue curves that our method is able to accurately merge the statistical qualities of the models, regardless of shape parametrization, and in absence of the original data.

**Table 1.** Point-to-surface distance statistics between reconstructions ($\Omega_{OM}$ and $\Omega_{NF}$)

| Structure | Mean ± Stdev (mm) | Max (mm) |
|---|---|---|
| Left Ventricle | 0.319 ± 0.107 | 0.674 |
| Right Ventricle | 0.497 ± 0.157 | 0.723 |

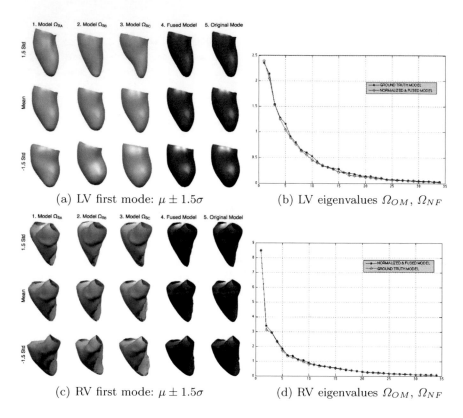

(a) LV first mode: $\mu \pm 1.5\sigma$     (b) LV eigenvalues $\Omega_{OM}$, $\Omega_{NF}$

(c) RV first mode: $\mu \pm 1.5\sigma$     (d) RV eigenvalues $\Omega_{OM}$, $\Omega_{NF}$

**Fig. 1.** First modes of variation of three models $\Omega_{S_A}$, $\Omega_{S_B'}$ and $\Omega_{S_C'}$ (cols. 1, 2 and 3), the fused model $\Omega_{NF}$ (col. 4) and original model $\Omega_{OM}$ (col. 5); for (a) the LV and (c) the RV. Also shown are the eigenvalues of $\Omega_{OM}$ and $\Omega_{NF}$ for (b) LV and (d) RV.

## 4.2   Fusion of MR and CT Models

In this section we evaluate the applicability of the technique by fusing the MR model as described in the previous section with an online PDM constructed from a population of 134 CT datasets[1]. The LV and RV shapes were segmented using an atlas-based approach [7], and described by 1347 and 1748 landmarks, respectively. The original CT datasets are not publicly available and therefore only the obtained means and eigenvectors are used in this validation. The first mode of variation of the MR and CT models are shown in Fig. 2(a) for the LV, and 2(b) for the RV (cols. 1, and 3), respectively. It can be seen that the variability captured by the MR and CT models differ, as can be expected, since they were constructed from different populations. In particular, more localized variation is encoded by the CT statistical model for both the LV and the RV.

We then apply the normalization algorithm to the MR model in order to establish point correspondence, and as observed from comparing Fig. 2 (cols. 1

---

[1] http://www.cistib.upf.edu/cistib/index.php/
   downloads/Statistical_Cardiac_Atl

and 2), the shape variability is well preserved. This suggests that no significant loss of geometrical and statistical information results from the proposed eigenvector transformation despite the complex geometries involved. We then apply the fusion stage to merge the MR and CT PDMs and the result is displayed in Fig. 2 (col. 4). Visually, it is evident that features of variation found in both the MR and CT models are incorporated into the unified model. In particular, for both the LV and RV, the first mode of variation for the fused model incorporates a pattern describing a transition from the high resolution CT model to the smoother representation found in MRI. In other words, the unified model integrates detailed, as well as smoother surface representations. Inter-modality differences in resolution are encoded as patterns of shape variability into the fused model. In the case of the RV, the regional variation at the valvular level is mostly related to the MR model, while the CT model contributes with the global variation in morphology.

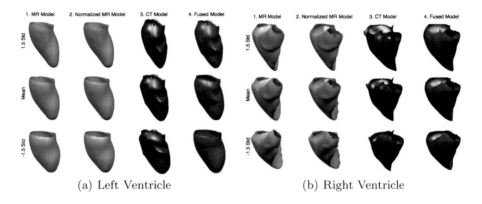

(a) Left Ventricle                    (b) Right Ventricle

**Fig. 2.** First modes of variation of two models constructed from imaging modalities MR (col. 1) and CT (col. 3). Also shown are the fused model (col. 4) and the normalized (pre-fusion) MR model (col. 2).

In order to show quantitatively how well the fusion improves shape representation over the individual models, we performed reconstruction of the MR datasets following a leave-one-out scheme based on the MR model alone and then on the fused MR-CT model. The results of the reconstruction are summarized in Table 2. The mean error obtained with the MR-only model for the LV was of 0.953 mm, whereas with the $\Omega_{NF}$ it was reduced to 0.465 mm. This is a significant improvement of 51% over the MR model. Also, for the RV, the mean error with the MR-only model is equal to 1.315 mm, while the fusion reduced the reconstruction error to 0.805 mm, which represents a 38% improvement over the MR model. On average the total improvement is 44.5%. These results demonstrate the benefit of the proposed approach to obtain models that generalize better to new instances without the need for any additional datasets but merely by taking advantage of pre-existing PDMs.

**Table 2.** Reconstruction statistics for the MR dataset (LV, RV), comparing the performance of $\Omega_{MR}$, and a $\Omega_{MR-CT}$

| Structure | Model | Mean ± Stdev (mm) | Max (mm) |
|---|---|---|---|
| Left Ventricle | MR model | 0.953 ± 0.259 | 1.800 |
| | MR+CT model | 0.465 ± 0.153 | 0.006 |
| Right Ventricle | MR model | 1.315 ± 0.310 | 2.225 |
| | MR+CT model | 0.805 ± 0.197 | 1.246 |

## 5   Conclusion

We present a framework to construct unified multi-modal statistical shape models by normalizing and merging pre-existing PDMs, without the need for the original or any additional datasets. The fused model can be obtained despite differences in the clinical population, delineation protocols and imaging modalities. With the proposed technique, a unique statistical shape model with good specificity and generalization ability is obtained for improved interpretation of medical images.

## References

1. Butakoff, C., Frangi, A.F.: A framework for weighted fusion of multiple statistical models of shape and appearance. IEEE Trans. Pattern Anal. Machine Intell. 28(11), 1847–1857 (2006)
2. Cootes, T.F., Taylor, C.J., Cooper, D.H., Graham, J.: Active shape models—their training and application. Comput. Vis. Image Understand. 61(1), 38–59 (1995)
3. Durrleman, S., Pennec, X., Trouvé, A., Ayache, N.: Statistical models of sets of curves and surfaces based on currents. Med. Image Anal. 13(5), 793–808 (2009)
4. Franco, A., Lumini, A., Maio, D.: Eigenspace merging for model updating. In: Proc. Int. Conf. Pattern Recognition (ICPR), vol. 2, pp. 156–159 (2002)
5. Hall, P., Marshall, D., Martin, R.: Merging and splitting eigenspace models. IEEE Trans. Pattern Anal. Machine Intell. 22(9), 1042–1049 (2000)
6. Heimann, T., Meinzer, H.P.: Statistical shape models for 3D medical image segmentation: A review. Med. Image Anal. 13(4), 543–563 (2009)
7. Hoogendoorn, C., Duchateau, N., Sánchez-Quintana, D., Whitmarsh, T., De Craene, M., Sukno, F.M., Lekadir, K., Frangi, A.F.: A high-resolution atlas and statistical model of the human heart from multislice CT. IEEE Trans. Med. Imaging 32(1), 28–44 (2013)
8. Horn, B.K.P.: Closed-form solution of absolute orientation using unit quaternions. J. Opt. Soc. Am. A Optic. Image Sci. Vis. 4(4), 629–642 (1987)
9. Loop, C.: Smooth subdivision surfaces based on triangles. Master's thesis, Department of mathematics, University of Utah, Utah, USA (1987)
10. Valette, S., Chassery, J.M.: Approximated centroidal Voronoi diagrams for uniform polygonal mesh coarsening. Comput. Graph. Forum 24(3), 381–389 (2004)
11. Zhou, X.S., Gupta, A., Comaniciu, D.: An information fusion framework for robust shape tracking. IEEE Trans. Pattern Anal. Machine Intell. 27(1), 115–129 (2005)

# Robust Multimodal Dictionary Learning

Tian Cao[1], Vladimir Jojic[1], Shannon Modla[3], Debbie Powell[3],
Kirk Czymmek[4], and Marc Niethammer[1,2]

[1] University of North Carolina at Chapel Hill, NC
[2] Biomedical Research Imaging Center, UNC Chapel Hill, NC
[3] University of Delaware, DE
[4] Carl Zeiss Microscopy, LLC
tiancao@cs.unc.edu

**Abstract.** We propose a robust multimodal dictionary learning method
for multimodal images. Joint dictionary learning for both modalities may
be impaired by lack of correspondence between image modalities in training data, for example due to areas of low quality in one of the modalities. Dictionaries learned with such non-corresponding data will induce
uncertainty about image representation. In this paper, we propose a
probabilistic model that accounts for image areas that are poorly corresponding between the image modalities. We cast the problem of learning
a dictionary in presence of problematic image patches as a likelihood
maximization problem and solve it with a variant of the EM algorithm.
Our algorithm iterates identification of poorly corresponding patches and
refinements of the dictionary. We tested our method on synthetic and real
data. We show improvements in image prediction quality and alignment
accuracy when using the method for multimodal image registration.

## 1   Introduction

Sparse representation model represents a signal with sparse combinations of
items in a dictionary and shows its power in numerous low-level image processing applications such as denoising and inpainting [4] as well as discriminative
tasks such as face and object recognition [10]. Dictionary learning plays a key
role in applications using sparse models. Hence, many dictionary learning methods have been introduced [1,11,6,7]. In [1], a dictionary is learned for image
denoising, while in [6], supervised learning is performed for classification and
recognition tasks. In [7], a multimodal dictionary is learned from audio-visual
data. Mutltimodal dictionaries can be applied to super-resolution [11], multi-
modal image registration [3] and tissue synthesis [9].

However, multimodal dictionary learning is challenging: it may fail or provide
inferior dictionary quality without sufficient correspondences between modalities in the training data. This problem has so far not been addressed in the
literature. For example, a low quality image deteriorated by noise in one modality can hardly match a high quality image in another modality. Furthermore,
training images are pre-registered. Resulting registration error may harm image

K. Mori et al. (Eds.): MICCAI 2013, Part I, LNCS 8149, pp. 259–266, 2013.

correspondence and hence dictionary learning. Such noise- and correspondence-corrupted dictionaries will consequentially produce inferior results for image reconstruction or prediction. Fig. 1 shows an example of multimodal dictionary learning for both perfect and imperfect corresponding image pairs.

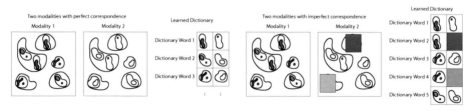

**Fig. 1.** An illustration of perfect (left) and imperfect (right) correspondence between multimodal images and their learned dictionaries. The imperfect correspondence (gray part in right images) could result in learning an imperfect dictionary (gray dictionary words) which is not desirable. Our goal is to *robustly* recover a compact dictionary of *corresponding* elements.

In this paper, instead of directly learning a multimodal dictionary from training data [3], we distinguish between image regions with and without good correspondence in the learning process. Our main contributions are as follows

- *We propose a probabilistic model for dictionary learning which discriminates between corresponding and non-corresponding patches.* This model is generally applicable to multimodal dictionary learning.
- *We provide a method robust to noise and mis-correspondences.* We demonstrate this using real and synthetic data and obtain "cleaner" dictionaries.
- *We demonstrate consistency of performance for a wide range of parameter settings.* This indicates the practicality of our approach.

The paper is organized as follows: Sec. 2 describes the multimodal dictionary learning method and its probabilistic model. Sec. 3 provides an interpretation of the proposed model. We apply the model to synthetic and real data in Sec 4. The paper concludes with a summary of results and an outlook on future work.

## 2     Dictionary Learning Method

Let $I_1$ and $I_2$ be two different training images acquired from different modalities for the same area or object. Assume the two images have been registered already.

### 2.1     Sparse Multimodal Dictionary Learning

To learn a multimodal dictionary $\tilde{D}$ using a sparse representation, one solves

$$\{\hat{\tilde{D}}, \hat{\alpha}\} = \arg\min_{\tilde{D},\alpha} \sum_{i=1}^{N} \frac{1}{2}\|\tilde{x}_i - \tilde{D}\alpha_i\|_2^2 + \lambda\|\alpha_i\|_1, \tag{1}$$

where $\|.\|_1$ is the $\ell_1$ norm of a vector and the $\ell_1$ regularization induces sparsity in $\alpha$, $N$ is the number of training samples, $\tilde{D} = [D_1, D_2]^T$ is the corresponding multimodal dictionary (dictionaries are stacked for the two modalities) and $\tilde{x}_i = R_i[I_1, I_2]^T$ ($R_i$ is an operator to select the $i$th image patch). Note that there is only one set of coefficients $\alpha_i$ per patch, which relates the two dictionaries.

## 2.2   Confidence Measure for Image Patch

The confidence can be defined as a conditional probability $p(h|x_i)$. Given image patches $\{x_i\}_{i-1}^N$ we want to reconstruct them with our learned multimodal dictionary. Here, $h$ is the hypothesis of whether the reconstruction of $x_i$ uses some 'noise' dictionary items (i.e. non-corresponding dictionary items); $h = 1$ indicates that the reconstruction $x_i$ uses 'noise' dictionary elements.

Applying Bayes Rule [8,2], $p(h = 1|x_i)$ can be represented as,

$$p(h = 1|x_i) = \frac{p(x_i|h = 1)p(h = 1)}{p(x_i|h = 1)p(h = 1) + p(x_i|h = 0)p(h = 0)}. \tag{2}$$

Assuming the independence of each image patch $x_i$ and that the pixels in each patch follow a Gaussian distribution, for $p(x_i|h)$ we assume

$$p(x_i|h = 1, \theta_1) = \mathcal{N}(x_i; \mu_1, \sigma_1^2), \; p(x_i|h = 0, \theta_0; D, \alpha_i) = \mathcal{N}(x_i - D\alpha_i; 0, \sigma_0^2). \tag{3}$$

The parameters we need to estimate are $\theta_1 = \{\mu_1, \sigma_1\}$ and $\theta_0 = \sigma_0$, as well as the prior probability $p(h)$, where $p(h = 1) = \pi$ and $p(h = 0) = 1 - \pi$.

Based on the assumption of conditional independence of the random variable $x_i$ given $h$ and $\theta$ [8], we can use either maximum likelihood (ML) or maximum a posteriori (MAP) estimation for these parameters [8].

## 2.3   Robust Multimodal Dictionary Learning Based on EM

For robust multimodal dictionary learning, we want to estimate $\theta = \{\tilde{D}, \alpha\}$ considering the latent variable $h$. Based on the probabilistic framework of dictionary learning [1], we have $p(\tilde{x}|\theta) = \sum_h p(\tilde{x}, h|\theta)$. The ML estimation for $\theta$ is as follows

$$\hat{\theta} = \arg\max_\theta p(\tilde{x}|\theta) = \arg\max_\theta \log \sum_h p(\tilde{x}, h|\theta) = \arg\max_\theta \ell(\theta). \tag{4}$$

Instead of directly maximizing $\ell(\theta)$, we maximize the lower bound $Q(\theta) = \sum_h p(h|\tilde{x}, \theta) \log p(\tilde{x}, h|\theta)$ [8]. $p(h|\tilde{x}, \theta)$ is the confidence in section 2.2. We can apply the following EM algorithm to maximize $Q(\theta)$,

$$\mathbf{E\text{-step}} : Q(\theta|\theta^{(t)}) = E[\log p(\tilde{x}, h|\theta^{(t)})]; \; \mathbf{M\text{-step}} : \theta^{(t+1)} = \arg\max_\theta E[\log p(\tilde{x}, h|\theta)].$$

In the E-step we compute $p(h_i|\tilde{x}, \theta)$, $h_i \in \{1, 0\}$, which provides a confidence level for each training patch given $\tilde{D}$ and $\alpha$. In the M-step $p(h_i|\tilde{x}, \theta)$ is a weight for each image patch for updating $\theta$. We use a variant of the EM algorithm for multimodal dictionary learning. We replace $p(h_i|\tilde{x}, \theta)$ by $\delta_p(p(h_i|\tilde{x}, \theta))$. Here, $\delta_p(p)$ is an indicator function and $\delta_p(p) = 1$, if $p \geq 0.5$, $\delta_p(p) = 0$, otherwise. Thus in each iteration we rule out the image patches which have high confidence that they are noise patches. We then refine the multimodal dictionary using the corresponding training samples. The detailed algorithm is shown in Alg. 1.

---

**Algorithm 1.** EM algorithm for Multimodal Dictionary Learning

---

**Input:**     Training multimodal image patches: $\{\tilde{x}_i\}$, $i \in 1, ..., N$;
                Initialize multimodal dictionary $\tilde{D} = \tilde{D}_0$, $\tilde{D}_0$ is trained on all of the $\tilde{x}_i$;

**Output:**   Refined dictionary $\hat{\tilde{D}}$

1: (**E-step**) compute $\delta_p(p(h = 0|\tilde{x}_i, \theta))$, where

$$\delta_p(p) = \begin{cases} 1, & \text{if } p \geq 0.5, \\ 0, & \text{otherwise.} \end{cases} \tag{5}$$

$$p(h = 0|\tilde{x}_i, \theta) = \frac{p(\tilde{x}_i|h = 0, \theta)p(h = 0)}{p(\tilde{x}_i|h = 1, \theta)p(h = 1) + p(\tilde{x}_i|h = 0, \theta)p(h = 0)}. \tag{6}$$

update $\theta_1$ and $\theta_0$ in (3) based on $\delta_p(p(h = 0|\tilde{x}_i, \theta))$.

2: (**M-step**) update $\tilde{D}$ and $\alpha$ as follows[1],

$$\tilde{D}^{(t)} = \arg\min_{\tilde{D}} \sum_{i=1}^{N} \delta_p(p(h = 0|\tilde{x}_i, \theta))(\frac{1}{2}\|\tilde{x}_i - \tilde{D}\alpha_i\|_2^2 + \lambda\|\alpha_i\|_1),$$

$$\text{s.t. } \|\tilde{D}_j\|_2^2 \leq 1, \ j = 1, 2, ..., k. \tag{7}$$

$$\alpha_i^{(t)} = \arg\min_{\alpha_i} \delta_p(p(h = 0|\tilde{x}_i, \theta))(\frac{1}{2}\|\tilde{x}_i - \tilde{D}^{(t)}\alpha_i\|_2^2 + \lambda\|\alpha_i\|_1).$$

3: Iterate E and M steps until convergence reached.

---

## 3     Interpreting the Model

If there is no prior information about $p(h)$, we assume $p(h = 1) = p(h = 0) = 0.5$. If $p(h = 0|\tilde{x}_i, \theta) > 0.5$, based on (3), (5), (6), we have

$$\|\tilde{x}_i - \tilde{D}\alpha\|_2^2 \leq \sigma_0^2/\sigma_1^2\|\tilde{x}_i - \mu_i\mathbf{1}\|_2^2 = c\|\tilde{x}_i - \mu_i\mathbf{1}\|_2^2. \tag{8}$$

Here $\|\tilde{x}_i - \tilde{D}\alpha\|_2^2$ is the sum of squares of reconstruction residuals of image patch $\tilde{x}_i$, and $\|\tilde{x}_i - \mu_i\mathbf{1}\|_2^2$ is the sum of squares of centered intensity values (with mean $\mu_i\mathbf{1}$ removed) in $\tilde{x}_i$.

Thus equation (8) defines the criterion for corresponding multimodal image patches as those patches which can be explained by the multimodal dictionary $\tilde{D}$ better than the patch's mean intensity, i.e. the sum of squared residuals should be smaller than a threshold $T$, and $T$ is dependent on the variance of $\tilde{x}_i$, $\sigma_1^2$, and the variance of the reconstruction residual, $\sigma_0^2$.

---

[1] We use SPAMS (http://spams-devel.gforge.inria.fr) for dictionary learning and sparse coding[5].

Intuitively, a small $\sigma_1$ favors more corresponding image patches and a large $\sigma_1$ considers more image patches as non-corresponding.

# 4    Experimental Validation

We consider the image prediction problem (for a known dictionary $\tilde{D}$) solving

$$\{\hat{\alpha}_i\} = \arg\min_{\alpha_i} \sum_i^N \|\tilde{x}_i' - \tilde{D}\alpha_i\|_2^2 + \lambda\|\alpha_i\|_1. \tag{9}$$

Unlike for eq. 1, where $\tilde{x}_i = R_i[I_1, I_2]^T$, here $\tilde{x}_i' = R_i[I_1, u_2]^T$ where $u_2$ is the prediction of $I_2$. Since $I_2$ is not measured, we can effectively set $R_i u_2 = D_2\alpha_i$ or equivalently remove it from the optimization. Given $\{\hat{\alpha}_i\}$ we can then compute the predicted image. Most applications using multimodal dictionary are concerned about the prediction residuals, such as super-resolution and multimodal registration [11,3]. We therefore first validate our algorithm based on the resulting sum of squares of prediction residuals (SSR).

We test our proposed multimodal dictionary learning method on synthetic and real data. For the synthetic data, we generate non-corresponding multimodal image patches using the following generative model. We choose $p(h = 1)$ which defines the noise level in the training set, i.e. the percentage of non-corresponding multimodal image patches in the training set. For each non-corresponding patch $x_i^1$, we generate $\mu_i \mathbf{1}$ as the mean of all training patches and add Gaussian noise $\epsilon_\mu$. We generate a noise patch by adding Gaussian noise $\epsilon_{x_i^1}$ to the mean $\mu_i \mathbf{1}$.

## 4.1    Synthetic Experiment on Textures

We create multimodal textures by smoothing a given texture with a Gaussian kernel and inverting the intensity of the smoothed image. Fig. 2 shows an example of our generated multimodal textures. We generate both training and testing multimodal textures from Fig. 2, i.e. use half of the multimodal textures for training (add noise as non-correspondence regions) and the other half of the multimodal textures for testing. We extract $10 \times 10$ image patches in both training images, and add 'noise' with non-corresponding image patches to replace corresponding patches. The $\sigma$ for the Gaussian noise is set to 0.2.

We test how $\sigma_1$ influences our dictionary learning method at a fixed noise level $p(h = 1) = 0.5$. Fig. 2 shows the result. In practice, we can either learn $\sigma_1$ with an EM algorithm or manually choose it. When $\sigma_1$ is close to 0.2 (the $\sigma$ for the noise), to be specific, $\sigma_1 \in (0.15, 0.4)$, we get consistently lower SSRs. This indicates that our algorithm is robust for a wide range of $\sigma_1$ values and noise. For $\sigma_1 < 0.15$, all the patches are considered as corresponding patches while for $\sigma_1 > 0.4$, all the patches are classified as non-corresponding patches. Our method has the same performance as the standard method in [3] in these two cases. The learned multimodal dictionaries are illustrated in Fig. 2 showing that our algorithm successfully removes non-corresponding patches.

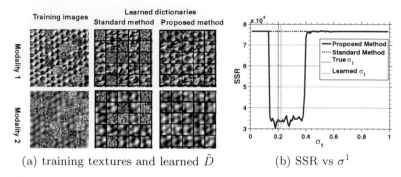

(a) training textures and learned $\tilde{D}$          (b) SSR vs $\sigma^1$

**Fig. 2.** $\tilde{D}$ is learned from training images with Gaussian noise (left). Standard method cannot distinguish corresponding patches and non-corresponding patches while our proposed method can remove non-corresponding patches in the dictionary learning process. The curve (right) shows the robustness with respect to $\sigma_1$. The vertical green dashed line indicates the learned $\sigma_1$.

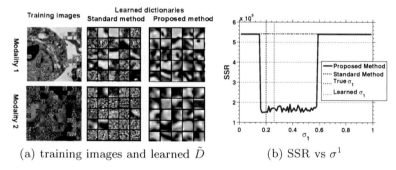

(a) training images and learned $\tilde{D}$          (b) SSR vs $\sigma^1$

**Fig. 3.** $\tilde{D}$ is learned from training SEM/confocal images with Gaussian noise (left). The curve (right) shows the robustness with respect to $\sigma_1$. The vertical green dashed line indicates the learned $\sigma_1$.

## 4.2  Synthetic Experiment on Multimodal Microscope Images

We also test the proposed algorithm on correlative microscope images. We have 8 pairs of Scanning Electron Microscopy (SEM) and confocal images. Image pairs have been aligned with fiducials. Fig. 3 (a) illustrates an example of SEM/confocal images. We add non-corresponding patches using the same method as in sec. 4.1. Fig 3 (a) shows the results. The dictionary learned with our method shows better structure and less noise compared with the standard dictionary learning method. Fig. 3 (b) shows the interaction between $\sigma_1$ and SSR with fixed $p(h = 1) = 0.5$. For $\sigma_1 < 0.16$, all the image patches are categorized as corresponding patches while for $\sigma_1 > 0.6$, all the patches are classified as non-corresponding patches. Our method has the same performance as the standard method under these conditions. We observe a large range of $\sigma_1$ values resulting in improved reconstruction results indicating robustness.

## 4.3   Multimodal Registration on Correlative Microscopy

We use the proposed multimodal dictionary learning algorithm for multimodal registration [3]. The multimodal image registration problem simplifies to a monomodal one using the multimodal dictionary in a sparse representation framework. The test data is Transmission Electron Microscopy (TEM) and confocal microscopy. We have six pairs of TEM/confocal images. We train the multimodal dictionary using leave-one-out cross-validation. Fig. 4 shows an example of our test data. We first registered the training images with manually chosen landmarks (no ground truth available), then learned the multimodal dictionary and applied it to predict the corresponding image for a given source image. We resampled the predicted images with up to $\pm 2.07 \mu m$ (30 pixels) in translation in the x and y directions (at steps of 10 pixels) and $\pm 20°$ in rotation (at steps of 10 degrees). Then we registered the resampled predicted image to the corresponding target using a rigid transformation model. $\sigma_1$ is chosen as 0.15 based on cross-validation for the prediction errors in this experiment. Tab. 1 shows a comparison of our method with the method in [3]. The result shows about 15% improvement in prediction error and a statistically significant improvement in registration errors.

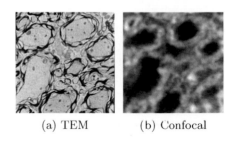

(a) TEM          (b) Confocal

**Fig. 4.** TEM/Confocal images

**Table 1.** Prediction and registration results. Prediction is based on the method in [3], and we use SSR to evaluate the prediction results. Here, MD denotes our proposed multimodal dictionary learning method and ST denotes the dictionary learning method in [3]. The registrations use Sum of Squared Differences (SSD) and mutual information (MI) similarity measures. We report the results of mean and standard deviation of the absolute error of corresponding landmarks in micron (0.069 micron = 1 pixel). The p-value is computed using a paired t-test.

|            | Metric | Method | mean | std | p-value |
|------------|--------|--------|------|-----|---------|
| Prediction | SSR    | MD     | $\mathbf{6.28 \times 10^4}$ | $3.61 \times 10^3$ | |
|            |        | ST     | $7.43 \times 10^4$ | $4.72 \times 10^3$ | |
| Registration | SSD  | MD     | **0.760** | 0.124 | 0.0004 |
|            |        | ST     | 0.801 | 0.139 | |
|            | MI     | MD     | **0.754** | 0.127 | 0.0005 |
|            |        | ST     | 0.795 | 0.140 | |

## 5   Conclusion

In this paper, we proposed a robust multimodal dictionary learning method based on a probabilistic formulation. We directly model corresponding and non-corresponding multimodal training patches. Our method is based on a variant of the EM algorithm which classifies the non-corresponding image patches and updates the multimodal dictionary iteratively. We validated our method using synthetic and real data. Our algorithm demonstrated its robustness to noise (non-corresponding image patches). We also applied our method to multimodal registration showing an improvement in alignment accuracy compared with the traditional dictionary learning method. The proposed method is expected to be of general use for multimodal dictionary learning. While our method is based on a Gaussian noise model, it can easily be adapted to other noise model such as Poisson noise. Future work will address multimodal dictionary learning in the context of deformable image registration.

**Acknowledgments.** This work was supported by NSF (EECS-1148870, EECS-0925875), NIH (5P41EB002025-28, 5R01GM097587-03, 2P41EB002025-26A1), Delaware INBRE program (NIH NIGMS 8P20GM103446-13) and Lineberger Comprehensive Cancer Center startup funds.

# References

1. Aharon, M., Elad, M., Bruckstein, A.: K-svd: An algorithm for designing overcomplete dictionaries for sparse representation. IEEE Transactions on Signal Processing 54(11), 4311–4322 (2006)
2. Besag, J.: On the statistical analysis of dirty pictures. Journal of the Royal Statistical Society. Series B (Methodological), 259–302 (1986)
3. Cao, T., Zach, C., Modla, S., Powell, D., Czymmek, K., Niethammer, M.: Registration for correlative microscopy using image analogies. Biomedical Image Registration, 296–306 (2012)
4. Elad, M., Aharon, M.: Image denoising via sparse and redundant representations over learned dictionaries. IEEE Transactions on Image Processing 15(12), 3736–3745 (2006)
5. Mairal, J., Bach, F., Ponce, J., Sapiro, G.: Online dictionary learning for sparse coding. In: Proceedings of the 26th Annual International Conference on Machine Learning, pp. 689–696. ACM (2009)
6. Mairal, J., Bach, F., Ponce, J., Sapiro, G., Zisserman, A.: Supervised dictionary learning. In: NIPS, pp. 1033–1040 (2008)
7. Monaci, G., Jost, P., Vandergheynst, P., Mailhe, B., Lesage, S., Gribonval, R.: Learning multimodal dictionaries. IEEE Transactions on Image Processing 16(9), 2272–2283 (2007)
8. Neal, R., Hinton, G.: A view of the em algorithm that justifies incremental, sparse, and other variants. NATO ASI Series D Behavioural and Social Sciences 89, 355–370 (1998)
9. Roy, S., Carass, A., Prince, J.: A compressed sensing approach for mr tissue contrast synthesis. In: Székely, G., Hahn, H.K. (eds.) IPMI 2011. LNCS, vol. 6801, pp. 371–383. Springer, Heidelberg (2011)
10. Wright, J., Yang, A., Ganesh, A., Sastry, S., Ma, Y.: Robust face recognition via sparse representation. IEEE Transactions on Pattern Analysis and Machine Intelligence 31(2), 210–227 (2009)
11. Yang, J., Wright, J., Huang, T., Ma, Y.: Image super-resolution via sparse representation. IEEE Transactions on Image Processing 19(11), 2861–2873 (2010)

# Bayesian Atlas Estimation for the Variability Analysis of Shape Complexes

Pietro Gori[1,2], Olivier Colliot[1,2], Yulia Worbe[2], Linda Marrakchi-Kacem[1,2,3],
Sophie Lecomte[1,2,3], Cyril Poupon[3], Andreas Hartmann[2], Nicholas Ayache[4],
and Stanley Durrleman[1,2]

[1] Aramis Project-Team, Inria Paris-Rocquencourt, Paris, France
[2] CNRS UMR 7225, Inserm UMR-S975, UPMC, CRICM, Paris, France
[3] Neurospin, CEA, Gif-Sur-Yvette, France
[4] Asclepios Project-Team, Inria Sophia Antipolis, Sophia Antipolis, France

**Abstract.** In this paper we propose a Bayesian framework for multi-object atlas estimation based on the metric of currents which permits to deal with both curves and surfaces without relying on point correspondence. This approach aims to study brain morphometry as a whole and not as a set of different components, focusing mainly on the shape and relative position of different anatomical structures which is fundamental in neuro-anatomical studies. We propose a generic algorithm to estimate templates of sets of curves (fiber bundles) and closed surfaces (sub-cortical structures) which have the same "form" (topology) of the shapes present in the population. This atlas construction method is based on a Bayesian framework which brings to two main improvements with respect to previous shape based methods. First, it allows to estimate from the data set a parameter specific to each object which was previously fixed by the user: the trade-off between data-term and regularity of deformations. In a multi-object analysis these parameters balance the contributions of the different objects and the need for an automatic estimation is even more crucial. Second, the covariance matrix of the deformation parameters is estimated during the atlas construction in a way which is less sensitive to the outliers of the population.

## 1 Introduction

In the last years statistical analysis of shapes has acquired a central role in medical imaging. One of the main applications is to find morphological differences between a population of controls and one of patients or to highlight the effects of a treatment (i.e. drug) on a group of patients. Most studies focus their attention on a single anatomical structure [6, 8–10, 12]. Others propose multi-object analysis considering only a particular kind of shape, either only surfaces (sub-cortical structures) [2, 11, 13] or only curves (fiber-bundles) [5]. However, brain anatomy consists of an intricate network of white matter fiber bundles and sub-cortical structures which need to be studied together in many neuro-anatomical studies. One example is the study of the neural circuits whose morphological changes are often correlated with neurodevelopmental disorders, such as in Gilles de la

K. Mori et al. (Eds.): MICCAI 2013, Part I, LNCS 8149, pp. 267–274, 2013.
© Springer-Verlag Berlin Heidelberg 2013

Tourette syndrome (GTS) [3]. To this end, we propose here a new atlas construction method based on the framework of currents which permits to deal simultaneously with curves and surfaces. Given a set of shape complexes, each one is seen as a deformation of a common template complex. Both the template complex and the deformations, together called "atlas", need to be estimated and they characterize the anatomical invariants and the variability of the population. Every deformation is based on one single diffeomorphism of the whole 3D space which preserves the spatial organization of the objects and prevents shape components to intersect, fold or shear during deformation. In the case of neuro-anatomical studies, this makes possible a more realistic analysis since one can study the brain as a whole and not as a series of independent components. Moreover the metric between shape complexes is derived from the metric on deformations that consistently integrates the variations of each component of the complex. The use of currents allows to estimate such deformations without relying on point or fiber correspondence.

We extend to shape complexes (curves and surfaces) the methodology of [2] proposed only for surfaces and we enrich it. The aspects borrowed from [2] aim not to increase the dimensionality of the deformation parametrization between a single and a multi-object analysis and to make the results more useful for neuro-anatomical studies. The first one is achieved by separating the parametrization of the deformations from the one of the template complex and therefore making it not dependent on the size and number of objects. A second aspect is to construct templates with the same form (topology) of the shapes. This was not the case in previous works based on currents like in [5] where the template was a set of disconnected Dirac delta currents or in [6] where it was the superimposition of warped surfaces. Now templates of closed surfaces have a mesh structure defined by the user while templates of fiber bundles have the form of sets of curves connecting cortical to sub-cortical structures. This makes easier the interpretation of the results since the template complex can be compared with the shapes of the population and it is also possible to study the relations between objects of the template complex which is crucial in neuro-anatomical studies like in [3].

In this paper, the atlas is estimated using the same generative model as in [1, 2]. We propose to estimate the atlas of shape complexes using similar Bayesian priors as in [1] for images. This enables to automatically estimate the trade-off between the data term and the regularity of the deformations instead of being fixed by the user as in [2]. This parameter is important in the context of statistical analysis since a value too small might weight too much the data term leading to a situation of over-fitting. On the contrary, a value too large might penalize the deformations making less accurate the analysis of the variability of the population. Moreover, the situation is even more complicated in multi-object analysis where each object is characterized by its own parameter which weights the contribution of the object in the criterion to be optimized. Objects characterized by a bigger norm than the others should be weighted lesser in order to balance all the contributions for the atlas estimation. The automatic estimation of the different parameters takes into account also this aspect in only one simulation.

Previously [2] it was necessary more than one simulation in order to understand the "best" trade-off and the choice was very subjective.

A second improvement is the estimate of the covariance matrix of the deformation parameters during the atlas construction in a more statistically robust way. This should lead to a PCA less influenced by the outliers in contrast to an analysis based on a covariance matrix computed at the end of the procedure.

## 2    Bayesian Framework for Atlas Estimation

In the first paragraph we recall how to build diffeomorphic deformations with the new control point scheme defined in [2]. Afterwards, we explain the novelty of our new Bayesian formulation, highlighting the methodological differences with respect to [2] linked to the use of priors. Eventually we introduce an innovative solution to initialize templates of shape complexes (curves and surfaces).

*Diffeomorphism.* Assume that we have $M$ different structures segmented from structural and diffusion images for $N$ subjects. All structures belonging to subject $i$ can be seen as a shape complex $\boldsymbol{S}_i = \{S_{ij}\}_{j=1\ldots M}$ which is modeled as the deformation of a common template complex $\phi^i(\boldsymbol{T})$ plus a residual $\epsilon_i$ where $\boldsymbol{T} = \{T_j\}_{j=1\ldots M}$ and $\epsilon_i = \{\epsilon_{ij}\}_{j=1\ldots M}$. Shape complexes, deformed template complex and residuals are modelled as currents. The deformation $\phi^i$ depends only on subject $i$. The whole 3D space is deformed by a single diffeomorphism using the control point formulation presented in [2]. Diffeomorphic deformations are built by integrating a time-varying vector field $v_t(x)$ over the interval $[0, 1]$. Calling $\phi_t(x)$ the position of a point $x$ at time $t$, its evolution is given by: $\dot{\phi}_t(x) = v_t(\phi_t(x))$ and under some smoothness constraints of $v_t$ satisfied here [7] the set of deformations $\{\phi_t\}_{t \in [0,1]}$ is a flow of diffeomorphisms. The speed vector field $v_t$ is defined by a dynamical system of $C_p$ control points $c=\{c_k\}$, shared among the whole population and a set of momenta $\boldsymbol{\alpha}^i=\{\alpha_k^i\}$ linked to each control point and specific to each subject: $\dot{x}(t) = v_t(x(t)) = \sum_{p=1}^{C_p} K(x(t), c_p(t))\alpha_p^i(t)$, where $K$ is an interpolating kernel (i.e. gaussian). This equation defines the motion of all the points in the 3D space: both template and control points. The momenta $\boldsymbol{\alpha}^i$ parametrize the deformation of the template complex towards the shapes of subject $i$. If we assume that there are no external forces in the system, the total energy is conserved and it is equal to the Hamiltonian $\sum_{k=1}^{C_p} \sum_{p=1}^{C_p} \alpha_k^i(t)^T K(c_k(t), c_p(t))\alpha_p^i(t)$. Control points and momenta satisfy therefore the Hamiltonian system:

$$\begin{cases} \dot{c}_k(t) = v_t(c_k(t)) = \sum_{p=1}^{C_p} K(c_k(t), c_p(t))\alpha_p^i(t) \\ \dot{\alpha}_k^i(t) = - \sum_{p=1}^{C_p} \alpha_k^i(t)^T \alpha_p^i(t) \nabla_1 K(c_k(t), c_p(t)) \end{cases} \quad (1)$$

Integrating Eq.1 and $\dot{\boldsymbol{T}}(t) = v_t(\boldsymbol{T}(t))$ with $\boldsymbol{T}(0) = \boldsymbol{T}$ from $t=0$ to $t=1$, one obtains the deformed template complex $\boldsymbol{T}(1)=\phi^i(\boldsymbol{T})$. The last diffeomorphism $\phi^i$ at time $t=1$ is completely parametrized by the initial conditions of the system. Since the control points are shared among the population, the only subject-specific deformation parameters are the $C_p$ initial momenta $\{\alpha_k^i(0)\}=\boldsymbol{\alpha}_0^i$.

*Currents.* The aim of our atlas construction is to estimate simultaneously the $C_p$ control points $c$, the $N$ sets of initial momenta $\{\alpha_0^i\}$ and the template complex $T$ optimizing at the same time the residuals $\{\epsilon_i\}$ in a Bayesian framework sense. More formally this can be achieved by maximizing the joint posterior distribution of $c$, $\{\alpha_0^i\}$ and $T$ given $\{S_i\}$. The space of currents is of infinite dimension and therefore *pdf* are not defined. In order to overcome this problem we fix M finite dimensional spaces $W_{\Lambda j}^*$, one for each object $j$, constituted by grids on which shapes and templates are projected ($\Pi$) and where *pdf* are defined. As demonstrated in [7], the norm in this space is: $\Pi(S_{ij} - \phi^i(T_j))^T K_W^j \Pi(S_{ij} - \phi^i(T_j))$ which is precisely the numerical scheme used in [7] to compute the continuous norm on currents. $K_W^j$ is the currents kernel sampled at the grid points of $W_{\Lambda j}^*$ and it is defined as a block matrix whose blocks are 3D gaussian kernels characterized by the same standard deviation. In this way, both the $\alpha_0^i$ and the residuals $\epsilon_{ij}$ can be modelled with Gaussian distributions. Assuming independence of observations, their likelihoods are: $p(\alpha_0^i|\Gamma_\alpha) \propto \frac{1}{|\Gamma_\alpha|^{1/2}} \exp\left[-\frac{1}{2}(\alpha_0^i)^T \Gamma_\alpha^{-1} \alpha_0^i\right]$ and $p(\epsilon_{ij}|\sigma_{\epsilon j}^2) \propto \frac{1}{|\sigma_{\epsilon j}^2|^{\Lambda_j/2}} \exp\left[-\frac{1}{2\sigma_{\epsilon j}^2}\|(S_{ij} - \phi^i(T_j))\|_{W_{\Lambda j}^*}^2\right]$, where $\Lambda_j$ is the number of points of the $j$-th grid. $\Gamma_\alpha$ and $\sigma_{\epsilon j}^2(K_W^j)^{-1}$ are two covariance matrices. The scalar $\sigma_{\epsilon j}^2$ depends on the object $j$ and it is the variance of $\epsilon_j = \{\epsilon_{ji}\}_{i=1...N}$.

*Bayesian Framework.* As in [1] for images, it is possible to estimate both $\Gamma_\alpha$ and $\sigma_{\epsilon j}^2$ in a Bayesian framework using the standard conjugate prior of the Gaussian distribution, the Inverse Wishart: $\Gamma_\alpha \sim W^{-1}(P_\alpha, \frac{w_\alpha}{N})$ and $\sigma_{\epsilon j}^2 \sim W^{-1}(P_{\epsilon j}, \frac{w_{\epsilon j}}{N})$ where the matrix $P_\alpha$ and the scalars $w_\alpha, \{P_{\epsilon j}\}, \{w_{\epsilon j}\}$ are new hyper-parameters fixed by the user. Using an uniform prior distribution for the template complex $T$ and for the control points $c_0$ and assuming all random variables independent, it is possible to write explicitly the posterior distribution $F$ of $T$, $\{\alpha_0^i\}, c_0, \Gamma_\alpha, \{\sigma_{\epsilon j}^2\}$ given the shapes $\{S_i\}$. Maximizing $F$ is equivalent to minimize $E = -\log(F) =$

$$\frac{M}{2}\sum_{i=1}^{N}(\alpha_0^i)^T \Gamma_\alpha^{-1} \alpha_0^i + \sum_{j=1}^{M}\sum_{i=1}^{N}\frac{1}{2\sigma_{\epsilon j}^2}\left(\|(S_{ij} - \phi^i(T_j))\|_{W_{\Lambda j}^*}^2 + \frac{P_{\epsilon j}w_{\epsilon j}}{N}\right) +$$
$$\frac{M}{2}(w_\alpha + N)\log(|\Gamma_\alpha|) + \frac{M}{2}w_\alpha tr(\Gamma_\alpha^{-1}P_\alpha) + \sum_{j=1}^{M}\frac{1}{2}(w_{\epsilon j} + \Lambda_j N)\log(\sigma_{\epsilon j}^2) \tag{2}$$

where the first two terms were present also in [2]. The use of two conjugate priors makes possible to compute the optimal values for $\Gamma_\alpha$ and $\sigma_{\epsilon j}^2$ in a closed form:

$$\hat{\Gamma}_\alpha = \frac{\sum_{i=1}^{N}\left[(\alpha_0^i)(\alpha_0^i)^T\right] + w_\alpha P_\alpha^T}{(w_\alpha + N)} \qquad \hat{\sigma}_{\epsilon j}^2 = \frac{\sum_{i=1}^{N}\|(S_{ij} - \phi^i(T_j))\|_{W_{\Lambda j}^*}^2 + w_{\epsilon j}P_{\epsilon j}}{(w_{\epsilon j} + N\Lambda_j)}$$

$\hat{\Gamma}_\alpha$ is equal to a weighted sum between the sample covariance matrix and the prior. A good choice for the prior seems to be: $P_\alpha = K_V^{-1}$, where $K_V$ is a block matrix whose blocks are 3D gaussian kernels between two different control points. If all $\alpha_0^i$ are equal to zero, $\hat{\Gamma}_\alpha \sim K_V^{-1}$ and this means that the "deformation regularity" part in Eq.2 becomes $\sum_{i=1}^{N}(\boldsymbol{\alpha}_0^i)^T K_V \boldsymbol{\alpha}_0^i$, which is the sum of the geodesic distances from the template complex to all the shapes as in [2].

The second parameter $\hat{\sigma}_{\epsilon j}^2$ is equal to a weighted sum between the data-term of the $j$-th object and the prior and it was previously fixed by the user. The results were highly dependent on its value as shown in the next section. Now it is automatically estimated in a way which balances the contributions of the different objects in order that objects characterized by bigger norms do not stand above the smaller ones. With this new technique the sample covariance matrix penalizes the deformations of the template complex towards "outliers" at each iteration. Thus adjusting also the residual variance $\boldsymbol{\sigma}_\epsilon^2 = \{\sigma_{\epsilon j}^2\}_{j=1...M}$, contrary to [2] where both $\Gamma_\alpha'$ and $\boldsymbol{\sigma}_\epsilon^2$ were fixed during optimization.

*Gradient Descent.* For the other parameters $\boldsymbol{T}, \{\boldsymbol{\alpha}_0^i\}, \boldsymbol{c}_0$ there is not a closed form and they are computed using a gradient descent algorithm. Their gradients are: $\nabla_{T_k} E = \sum_{i=1}^{N} \nabla_{T_k}\left[\frac{1}{2\sigma_{\epsilon k}^2} D_{ik}\right]$, $\nabla_{\boldsymbol{\alpha}_0^s} E = \sum_{j=1}^{M} \nabla_{\boldsymbol{\alpha}_0^s}\left[\frac{1}{2\sigma_{\epsilon j}^2} D_{sj}\right] + M\Gamma_\alpha^{-1}\boldsymbol{\alpha}_0^s$ and $\nabla_{\boldsymbol{c}_0} E = \sum_{i=1}^{N}\sum_{j=1}^{M} \nabla_{\boldsymbol{c}_0}\left[\frac{1}{2\sigma_{\epsilon j}^2} D_{ij}\right]$. The differentiation of the data term $D_{ij} = ||(S_{ij} - \phi^i(T_j))||_{W_{\Lambda j}^*}^2$ is exactly the same as in [2]. The gradient of the prior $P_\alpha$ with respect to $\boldsymbol{c}_0$ is not taken into account since its norm is negligible. The use of a gradient descent method implies the choice of an initial template. Its "form" (topology) is preserved during the minimization process. We propose to initialize templates of 3D closed surfaces as centred and scaled ellipsoids. Templates of fiber bundles are initialized in two steps. First, it is selected randomly 10% of the fibers of each subject bundle from its most dense part. After, all the fibers are grouped and it is used a greedy approximation method based on the framework of currents to select the $H$ most representative fibers, where $H$ is the average number of fibers in the subject bundles.

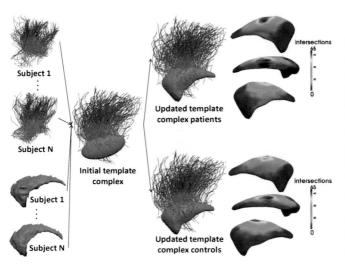

**Fig. 1.** <u>Left</u>: template update process for left caudate (LC) and left caudate bundle (LCB) in patients and controls. <u>Center</u>: updated template complexes starting from the same initial template complex but using only the population of patients or controls. <u>Right</u>: number of intersections between fibers and surface.

## 3  Experiments and Discussion

In the following experiments the data set is composed of left caudate (LC) and left caudate bundle (LCB) of 10 controls and 10 patients with GTS. The segmentation of the shapes was performed from T1-weighted MRI and DWI respectively [3, 4]. We use the non-oriented currents metric, also called varifold metric [14], which allows not to orient shapes in a consistent way across population.

The initial template process ends with two updated template complexes for the population of controls and patients respectively (Fig.1). These two template complexes reveal the common anatomical features of their populations. In Fig.1-right are highlighted the number of fibers intersecting the surface. Fibers seem to be more spread on the template surface of patients with respect to controls.

In Fig.2 we show the updated template complexes deformed according to the first mode of PCA for both groups using the estimated covariance matrix. In the set of controls there is mainly a variability in the distribution of fibers along the upper part of the surface. For patients there is especially a spread/concentration of the fibers on the surface towards the sides of the nucleus. There is also an elongation/shortening of the surface but it is common to both populations.

Eventually we evaluate the robustness of our method w.r.t. the hyper-parameter values and we compare its performance with the same optimization scheme using $\Gamma_\alpha = K_V^{-1}$ and different fixed values for $\sigma_\epsilon^2$, leading to the same results as with the method in [2]. In Fig.3 we show the norm of the difference between the updated template complex and a reference template complex which we choose arbitrarily equal to the one with a fixed $\sigma_\epsilon^2$ equal to 0.01 for all the

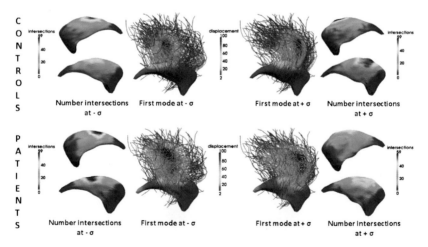

**Fig. 2.** PCA based on the covariance matrix of the deformation parameters. The central panels show the deformed updated template complexes at $\pm\,\sigma$ along the first principal direction. The colors refer to the magnitude of the displacement of the points from the template complex. The lateral panels show the number of intersections between the bundle and the surface at $\pm\,\sigma$.

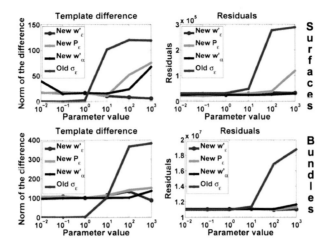

**Fig. 3.** Comparison of the robustness of the results w.r.t. hyper-parameters values ("New") and previously manually set trade-off ("Old"). Each result for the "New" method comes from an atlas estimation where it has been changed only one of the hyper-parameters fixing the others equal to 1. Both $w_\epsilon$ and $w_\alpha$ have been normalised ($w_\epsilon = w'_\epsilon N\Lambda$, $w_\alpha = w'_\alpha N$) so that the results can be compared using the same range of values for both the hyper-parameters and the trade-off.

objects. We show also the residuals $\epsilon$ obtained at the end of the atlas procedure. In both cases we show results using different normalised hyper-parameter values or different fixed values for $\sigma_\epsilon^2$. It is possible to conclude that the results with a fixed $\sigma_\epsilon^2$ (as in [2]) lead to results more variable than with the hyper-parameters which can therefore have a "universal" value, for example equal to 1. We obtained similar results for different sets of parameters using only surfaces, only bundles or both.

## 4   Conclusions

We have presented here a new multi-object atlas construction method based on a Bayesian framework and we have compared its performance with the one of a previous technique described in [2]. We have shown that this new formulation permits to have results less sensitive to the parameters fixed by the user. Moreover the covariance matrix of the deformation parameters is estimated throughout the atlas construction penalizing the contributions of the outliers. This new method can be applied simultaneously to fiber bundles (curves) and sub-cortical structures (closed surfaces) for which we propose also a generic template initialization procedure. Initial templates show the same "form" of the shapes which is also preserved during the atlas estimation. Moreover this technique allows to preserve the underlying organization of the structures under examination. This permits to study the relative positions of different objects in the template complex and how they interact. In this way it is possible, for example, to highlight precisely the anatomical differences between a population of controls and patients. Our preliminary results in a GTS study show differences in neuronal connexions which still need to be discussed in regards to the hypothesis put forth in [3]. The use of currents, which minimizes the need of user intervention, gives the possibility to apply full brain morphometry to large data sets.

# References

1. Allassonnière, S., Amit, Y., Trouvé, A.: Toward a Coherent Statistical Framework for Dense Deformable Template Estimation. J. R. Statist. Soc. B 69(1), 3–29 (2007)
2. Durrleman, S., Prastawa, M., Korenberg, J.R., Joshi, S.C., Trouvé, A., Gerig, G.: Topology Preserving Atlas Construction from Shape Data without Correspondence using Sparse Parameters. In: Proc. Med. Image Comput. Comput. Assist. Interv. (2012)
3. Worbe, Y., Gerardin, E., Hartmann, A., Valabrègue, R., Chupin, M., Tremblay, L., Vidailhet, M., Colliot, O., Lehéricy, S.: Distinct structural changes underpin clinical phenotypes in patients with Gilles de la Tourette syndrome. Brain 133, 3649–3660 (2010)
4. Marrakchi-Kacem, L., Delmaire, C., Guevara, P., Poupon, F., Lecomte, S., Tucholka, A., Roca, P., Yelnik, J., Durr, A., Mangin, J., Lehéricy, S., Poupon, C.: Mapping Cortico-Striatal Connectivity onto the Cortical Surface: A New Tractography-Based Approach to Study Huntington Disease. PLoS One 8(2), e53135 (2013)
5. Durrleman, S., Fillard, P., Pennec, X., Trouvé, A., Ayache, N.: Registration, Atlas Estimation and Variability Analysis of White Matter Fiber Bundles Modeled as Currents. NeuroImage 55(3), 1073–1090 (2011)
6. Glaunès, J., Joshi, S.C.: Template estimation from unlabeled point set data and surfaces for Computational Anatomy. In: Proc. International Workshop on the Mathematical Foundations of Computational Anatomy (2006)
7. Durrleman, S.: Statistical models of currents for measuring the variability of anatomical curves, surfaces and their evolution. PhD thesis, University of Nice (2010)
8. Hufnagel, H., Pennec, X., Ehrhardt, J., Ayache, N., Handels, H.: Computation of a Probabilistic Statistical Shape Model in a Maximum-a-posteriori Framework. Methods Inf. Med. 48(4), 314–319 (2009)
9. Kurtek, S., Klassen, E., Ding, Z., Avison, M.J., Srivastava, A.: Parameterization-invariant shape statistics and probabilistic classification of anatomical surfaces. Inf. Process. Med. Imaging 22, 147–158 (2011)
10. Joshi, S.H., Klassen, E., Srivastava, A., Jermyn, I.: A Novel Representation for Riemannian Analysis of Elastic Curves in Rn. In: IEEE Comput. Soc. Conf. Comput. Vis. Pattern Recognit., pp. 1–7 (2007)
11. Chen, T., Rangarajan, A., Eisenschenk, S.J., Vemuri, B.C.: Construction of a neuroanatomical shape complex atlas from 3D MRI brain structures. NeuroImage 60(3), 1778–1787 (2012)
12. Davies, R.H., Twining, C.J., Cootes, T.F., Taylor, C.J.: Building 3-D Statistical Shape Models by Direct Optimization. IEEE Trans. Med. Imag. 29(4), 961–981 (2010)
13. Gorczowski, K., Styner, M., Jeong, J.Y., Marron, J.S., Piven, J., Hazlett, H.C., Pizer, S.M., Gerig, G.: Multi-object analysis of volume, pose, and shape using statistical discrimination. IEEE Trans. Pattern. Anal. Mach. Intell. 32(4), 652–661 (2010)
14. Charon, N., Trouvé, A.: Functional currents: a new mathematical tool to model and analyse functional shapes. CoRR abs/1206.3564 (2012)

# Manifold Regularized Multi-Task Feature Selection for Multi-Modality Classification in Alzheimer's Disease

Biao Jie[1,2], Daoqiang Zhang[1,*], Bo Cheng[1], and Dinggang Shen[2,*]

[1] Dept. of Computer Science and Engineering,
Nanjing University of Aeronautics and Astronautics, Nanjing 210016, China
[2] Dept. of Radiology and BRIC, University of North Carolina at Chapel Hill, NC 27599
dqzhang@nuaa.edu.cn, dgshen@med.unc.edu

**Abstract.** Accurate diagnosis of Alzheimer's disease (AD), as well as its pro-dromal stage (i.e., mild cognitive impairment, MCI), is very important for poss-ible delay and early treatment of the disease. Recently, multi-modality methods have been used for fusing information from multiple different and complemen-tary imaging and non-imaging modalities. Although there are a number of exist-ing multi-modality methods, few of them have addressed the problem of joint identification of disease-related brain regions from multi-modality data for clas-sification. In this paper, we proposed a manifold regularized multi-task learning framework to jointly select features from multi-modality data. Specifically, we formulate the multi-modality classification as a multi-task learning framework, where each task focuses on the classification based on each modality. In order to capture the intrinsic relatedness among multiple tasks (i.e., modalities), we adopted a group sparsity regularizer, which ensures only a small number of fea-tures to be selected jointly. In addition, we introduced a new manifold based Laplacian regularization term to preserve the geometric distribution of original data from each task, which can lead to the selection of more discriminative fea-tures. Furthermore, we extend our method to the semi-supervised setting, which is very important since the acquisition of a large set of labeled data (i.e., diag-nosis of disease) is usually expensive and time-consuming, while the collection of unlabeled data is relatively much easier. To validate our method, we have performed extensive evaluations on the baseline Magnetic resonance imaging (MRI) and fluorodeoxyglucose positron emission tomography (FDG-PET) data of Alzheimer's Disease Neuroimaging Initiative (ADNI) database. Our experi-mental results demonstrate the effectiveness of the proposed method.

## 1    Introduction

Alzheimer's disease (AD) is the most common type of dementia, accounting for 60-80 percent of age-related dementia cases. It is predicted that the number of affected people will double in the next 20 years, and 1 in 85 people will be affected by 2050 [1]. Since the AD-specific brain changes begin years before the patient becomes symptomatic, early clinical diagnosis becomes a challenging task. Therefore, many

---

[*] Corresponding authors.

K. Mori et al. (Eds.): MICCAI 2013, Part I, LNCS 8149, pp. 275–283, 2013.
© Springer-Verlag Berlin Heidelberg 2013

studies have focused on possible identification of such changes at the early stage, i.e., mild cognitive impairment (MCI), by leveraging neuroimaging data [2-4].

Recently, machine learning and pattern classifications methods have been widely used in neuroimaging analysis of AD and MCI, including both group comparison (i.e., between clinically different groups) and individual classification. Early researches mainly focus on extracting features (e.g., regions of interest (ROIs) based or voxel-based) from single imaging modality such as structural magnetic resonance imaging (MRI) or fluorodeoxyglucose positron emission tomography (FDG-PET), etc. More recently, researchers have begun to integrate multiple imaging modalities to further improve the accuracy of disease diagnosis.

Different imaging modalities provide different views of brain function or structure. For example, structural MRI provides information about the tissue type of the brain, while FDG-PET measures the cerebral metabolic rate for glucose. Intuitively, integration of multiple modalities may uncover the previously hidden information that cannot be found by using single modality. A number of studies have exploited the fusion of multiple modalities to improve the AD or MCI classification performance [2, 3, 5]. For example, Zhang et al. [2] combined three modalities, i.e., MRI, FDG-PET, and cerebrospinal fluid (CSF), to discriminate AD/MCI and normal controls. Existing studies have indicated that different imaging modalities can provide essential complementary information that can improve accuracy in disease diagnosis.

For imaging modalities, even after feature extraction (i.e., from brain regions), there may still exist the irrelevant features. So, feature selection is commonly used to remove the irrelevant features. However, due to the complexity of brain and the disease, it is challenging to detect all relevant disease-related regions from a single modality alone, especially in early stage of the disease. Different imaging modalities may provide essential complementary information that can help identify these dysfunctional regions implicated by the same underlying pathology. In addition, recent studies also show that there is overlap between the disease-related brain regions detected by MRI and FDG-PET, such as regions in the hippocampus and the mesia temporal lobe [3]. Some feature selection techniques (e.g., t-test) have been used for identifying the disease-related regions from multi-modality data, while an obvious disadvantage of these techniques is that they don't consider the intrinsic relatedness between features across different modalities. To the best of our knowledge, only a few works have exploited to jointly select features from multi-modality neuroimaging data for AD/MCI classification. For example, Huang et al. [3] proposed to jointly identify disease-related brain features from multi-modality data by using sparse composite linear discrimination analysis (SCLDA) method. Zhang et al. [5] proposed a multimodal multi-task learning for joint feature selection for AD classification, and achieved the state-of-the-art performance in AD classification.

In this paper, as motivated by the work in [5], we proposed a new multi-task-based joint feature selection model that considers both the intrinsic relatedness among multi-modality data and the geometric distribution of each modality data. To this end, we formulate the classification of multi-modality data as a multi-task learning (MTL) problem, where each task focuses on the classification of each modality. The aim of MTL is to improve the generalization performance by jointly learning a set of related tasks [6]. Specifically, two regularization items are included in the proposed model. The first item is group Lasso regularizer [7], which ensure only a small number of features to be jointly selected across different tasks (i.e., modalities). The second item is Laplacian regularization term, which can preserve the geometric distribution information of the whole data from each task. This information may help to capture more discriminative features. Furthermore, we extend our method to the semi-supervised setting (i.e., learning from both labeled and unlabeled data), which is of great importance in practice since the acquisition of labeled data (i.e., diagnosis of disease) is generally expensive and time-consuming, while the collection of unlabeled data is relatively much easier.

## 2     Manifold Regularized Multi-Task Feature Selection

In this section, we first briefly introduce the existing multi-task feature selection method [5]. Then, we derive our proposed manifold regularized multi-task feature selection models as well as the corresponding optimization algorithm.

### 2.1     Multi-Task Feature Selection (MTFS)

Assume that there are $M$ supervised learning tasks (i.e., the number of modalities), Denote $X^m = [x_1^m, x_2^m, ..., x_N^m]^T \in R^{N \times d}$ as the training data matrix on $m$-th task (i.e., $m$-th modality) from $N$ training subjects, and $Y = [y_1, y_2, ..., y_N]^T \in R^N$ as the response vector from these training subjects, where $x_i^m$ represents feature vector of the $i$-th subject, and $y_i$ is the corresponding class label (i.e., patient or normal control). Let $w^m \in R^d$ parameterizes a linear discriminant function for task $m$. Then the multi-task feature selection (MTFS) model is to solve the following objective function:

$$\min_W \frac{1}{2} \sum_{m=1}^{M} \|Y - X^m w^m\|_2^2 + \lambda_1 \|W\|_{2,1} \tag{1}$$

where $W = [w^1, w^2, ..., w^M] \in R^{d \times M}$ is the weight matrix whose row $w_j$ is the vector of coefficients associated with the $j$-th feature across different tasks. Here, $\|W\|_{2,1} = \sum_{j=1}^{d} \|w_j\|_2$ is the sum of the $\ell_2$-norms of the rows of matrix $W$, as was used in the Group Lasso [7]. The use of $\ell_{2,1}$-norm encourages matrix with many zero rows. In other words, this $\ell_{2,1}$-norm combines multiple tasks and ensures that a small number of common features will be selected across different tasks. The parameter $\lambda_1$ is a regularization parameter which balances the relative contributions of the two terms.

### 2.2     Manifold Regularized Multi-Task Feature Selection (M2TFS)

In the MTFS model, a linear mapping function (i.e., $f(x) = x^T w = w^T x$) was adopted to transform the data from the original high-dimensional space to one-dimensional space. In this model, for each task we only consider the relationship between data and class label, while the mutual dependence among data is ignored, which may result in large deviations even for very similar data after mapping.

To address this problem, we introduced a new regularization term which preserves the geometric distribution information of the whole data:

$$\min_{W} \sum_{m=1}^{M} \sum_{i,j}^{N} \|f(x_i^m) - f(x_j^m)\|_2^2 S_{ij}^m = 2 \sum_{m=1}^{M} (w^m)^T (X^m)^T L^m X^m w^m \quad (2)$$

where $S^m = [s_{ij}^m]$ denotes a similarity matrix that defines the similarity on task $m$ across different subjects. $L^m = D^m - S^m$ represents combinatorial Laplacian matrix for task $m$, where $D^m$ is the diagonal matrix defined as $D_{ii}^m = \sum_{j=1}^{N} s_{ij}^m$. Here, the similarity matrix can be defined as:

$$s_{ij}^m = \begin{cases} 1, \text{if } x_i^m \text{ and } x_j^m \text{ are from the same class.} \\ 0, \text{otherwise.} \end{cases} \quad (3)$$

This penalized item can be explained as follows. The more similar between $x_i^m$ and $x_j^m$ (i.e., $x_i^m$ and $x_j^m$ come from the same class), the distance between $f(x_i^m)$ and $f(x_j^m)$ shoud be smaller, and *vice versa*. It is easy to see that Eq. (2) aims to preserve the local neighboring structure of *same-class* data during the mapping. With the regularizer in Eq. (2), the proposed manifold regularized multi-task feature selection model (M2TFS) has the following objective function:

$$\min_{W} \frac{1}{2} \sum_{m=1}^{M} \|Y - X^m w^m\|_2^2 + \lambda_1 \|W\|_{2,1} + \lambda_2 \sum_{m=1}^{M} (w^m)^T (X^m)^T L^m X^m w^m \quad (4)$$

where $\lambda_1$ and $\lambda_2$ are the two positive constants. Their values can be determined via inner cross-validation on training data.

## 2.3     Semi-supervised M2TFS (Semi-M2TFS)

Generally, semi-supervised learning methods attempt to exploit the intrinsic data distribution disclosed by the unlabeled data and thus help to construct a better learning model [8]. It is easy to find that, in the proposed M2TFS model, only the first item and the similarity matrix $S^m$ in Eq. (2) involve the supervised information (i.e., the class labels of subjects), so we can easily extend our model to semi-supervised version as follows.

We first define a diagonal matrix $P \in R^{N \times N}$ to indicate labeled data, i.e., $P_{ii} = 0$ if the class label of subject $i$ is unknown, and $P_{ii} = 1$ otherwise. Then, according to [9], we redefine the similarity matrix $S^m$ with the following Gaussian function

$$s_{ij}^m = \exp\left(\frac{-\|x_i^m - x_j^m\|}{2\sigma^2}\right) \quad (5)$$

Finally, based on the formulation in Eq. (4), the objective function of our semi-supervised M2TFS model (denoted as Semi-M2TFS) can be written as follows:

$$\min_{W} \frac{1}{2} \sum_{m=1}^{M} \|P(Y - X^m w^m)\|_2^2 + \lambda_1 \|W\|_{2,1} + \lambda_2 \sum_{m=1}^{M} (w^m)^T (X^m)^T L^m X^m w^m \quad (6)$$

where $L^m$ is the corresponding Laplacian matrix based on the new defined similarity matrix $S^m$ in Eq. (5). It is worth noting that Eq. (4) is a special case of Eq. (6) except the definition of similarity matrix. Below, we will develop a new method for optimizing the objective function in Eq. (6).

## 2.4   Optimization Algorithm

To optimize the problem in Eq. (6), we resort to the widely applied Accelerated Proximal Gradient (APG) method [10]. In this paper, we have implemented an APG optimization procedure similar to that of [11]. Specifically, we first separate the objective function in Eq. (6) to the smooth part:

$$f(W) = \frac{1}{2} \sum_{m=1}^{M} (\|P(Y - X^m w^m)\|_2^2 + 2\lambda_2 (w^m)^T (X^m)^T L^m X^m w^m) \qquad (7)$$

and non-smooth part:

$$g(W) = \lambda_1 \|W\|_{2,1} \qquad (8)$$

Then, the following function is constructed for approximating the composite function $f(W) + g(W)$:

$$\Omega_l(W, W_k) = f(W_k) + \langle W - W_k, \nabla f(W_k) \rangle + \frac{l}{2} \|W - W_k\| + g(w) \qquad (9)$$

where $\nabla f(W_k)$ denotes the gradient of $f(W)$ at point $W_k$ of the $k$-th iteration, and $l$ is the step size.

Finally, the update step of AGP algorithm is defined as:

$$W_{k+1} = arg \min_W \frac{1}{2} \|W - V_k\|_2^2 + \frac{1}{l} g(W) \qquad (10)$$

where $l$ can be determined by line search, and $V_k = W_k - \frac{1}{l} \nabla f(W_k)$

The key of AGP algorithm is how to solve the update step efficiently. The study in [11] shows that this problem can be decomposed into $d$ separate subproblems, and the analytical solutions of these subproblems can be easily obtained.

In addition, according to technique used in [10], instead of performing gradient descent based on $W_k$, we can compute the following formulation as:

$$Q_k = W_k + \alpha_k (W_k - W_{k-1}) \qquad (11)$$

where $\alpha_k = \frac{(1-\beta_{k-1})\beta_k}{\beta_{k-1}}$ and $\beta_k = \frac{2}{k+3}$.

The algorithm for Eq. (6) can achieve a convergence rate of $O(1/K^2)$, where $K$ is the maximum iteration.

## 3   Classification

Following in [2], we adopted the multi-kernel based support vector machine (SVM) method for classification. Specifically, for each modality of training subjects, a linear kernel was first calculated based on features selected by the above-proposed method. Then, the multi-kernel SVM used in [2] was adopted to combine the multi-modality data for classification.

## 4     Experiments

To evaluate the effectiveness of our proposed method, we perform a series of experiments on the multi-modality data from the Alzheimer's Disease Neuroimaging Initiative (ADNI) database (www.loni.ucla.edu/ADNI). We used a total of 202 subjects with corresponding baseline MRI and PET data, which includes 51 AD patients, 99 MCI patients (including 43 MCI converters and 56 MCI non-converters), and 52 normal controls (NC).

Image pre-processing is performed for all MRI and FDG-PET images. Specifically, we use the specific application tool for image pre-processing as similarly used in [2], i.e., spatial distortion, skull-stripping, and removal of cerebellum. Then, for structural MR images, we use the FSL package [12] to segment each image into three different tissues: gray matter (GM), white matter (WM), and CSF. With atlas warping, each subject was registered to a template with 93 manually labeled regions-of-interest (ROIs) [13]. For each ROI, the volume of GM tissue in that ROI was computed as a feature. For FDG-PET image, we use a rigid transformation to align it onto its respective MR image of the same subject, and then compute the average intensity of each ROI in the FDG-PET image as a feature. Overall, for each subject, we can acquire 93 features from MRI image and another 93 features from PET image.

To evaluate the performance of proposed method, we adopt the classification accuracy, area under receiver operating characteristic (ROC) curve (AUC), sensitivity (i.e., the proportion of patients that are correctly predicted), and specificity (i.e., the proportion of normal controls that are correctly predicted), as performance measures. Two sets of experiments, i.e., supervised classification and semi-supervise classification, were performed on 202 ADNI baseline MRI and PET data, respectively. In both sets of experiments, multiple binary classifiers, i.e., AD vs. NC, MCI vs. NC, and MCI converters (MCI-C) vs. MCI non-converters (MCI-NC), are built, respectively.

### 4.1     Supervised Classification

In this experiment, 10-fold cross-validation strategy was adopted to evaluate the classification performance. This process is repeated for 10 times independently to avoid any bias introduced by randomly partitioning dataset in the cross-validation. In current studies, we compared our proposed method with the state-of-the-art multi-modality-based methods, including multi-modality method proposed in [2] (denoted as MM and MML, corresponding to 'without feature selection' and 'lasso as feature selection', respectively) and multi-task feature selection method [5] (denoted as MTFS). In addition, for more comparisons, we also concatenate all features from MRI and FDG-PET into a long feature vector, and then perform two different feature selection methods, i.e., t-test, Lasso and sequential floating forward selection (SFFS) [14]. Finally, the standard SVM with linear kernel was used for classification. The detailed experimental results are summarized in Table 1.

As we can see from Table 1, our proposed M2TFS method consistently outperforms the other methods on three classification groups. Specifically, our proposed M2TFS method achieves the classification accuracy of 95.03%, 79.27% and 68.94% for AD vs. NC, MCI vs. NC, and MCI-C vs. MCI-NC, respectively, while the best classification accuracy of other methods are 92.25%, 74.34% and 61.67%, respectively. Also, M2TFS is consistently superior to other methods in sensitivity measure as well as AUC value.

Besides, we performed the significance test between accuracy of our proposed and those of compared methods, using the standard paired t-test. The results show that our proposed method is significantly better than the comparison methods (i.e., all the corresponding p-value are less than 0.01). All these results show that our proposed M2TFS method can take advantage of geometric distribution of data to seek out the most discriminative subset of features.

**Table 1.** Classification performance of different methods

| Methods | AD vs. NC (%) | | | | MCI vs. NC (%) | | | | MCI-C vs. MCI-NC (%) | | | |
| | ACC | SEN | SPE | AUC | ACC | SEN | SPE | AUC | ACC | SEN | SPE | AUC |
|---|---|---|---|---|---|---|---|---|---|---|---|---|
| CON-L | 91.02 | 90.39 | 91.35 | 0.95 | 73.44 | 76.46 | 67.12 | 0.78 | 58.44 | 52.33 | 63.04 | 0.60 |
| CON-T | 90.94 | 91.57 | 90.00 | 0.97 | 73.02 | 78.08 | 63.08 | 0.77 | 59.11 | 53.49 | 63.57 | 0.64 |
| SFFS | 86.78 | 87.06 | 86.15 | 0.93 | 69.21 | 82.12 | 45.38 | 0.73 | 56.28 | 44.42 | 64.82 | 0.55 |
| MM | 91.65 | 92.94 | 90.19 | 0.96 | 74.34 | 85.35 | 53.46 | 0.78 | 59.67 | 46.28 | 69.64 | 0.60 |
| MML | 92.25 | 92.16 | 92.12 | 0.96 | 73.84 | 77.27 | 66.92 | 0.77 | 61.67 | 54.19 | 66.96 | 0.61 |
| MTFS | 92.07 | 91.76 | 92.12 | 0.95 | 74.17 | 81.31 | 60.19 | 0.77 | 61.61 | 57.21 | 65.36 | 0.62 |
| M2TFS | 95.03 | 94.90 | 95.00 | 0.97 | 79.27 | 85.86 | 66.54 | 0.82 | 68.94 | 64.65 | 71.79 | 0.70 |

## 4.2    Semi-supervised Classification

In the experiment, we validated the classification performance of our proposed method under semi-supervised setting. Specifically, we first fixed a ratio $r_1 = 50\%$ of positive and negative subjects as labeled data. At the following procedure, we used a fraction $r_2 \in \{10\%, 20\%, 40\%, 60\%, 80\%\}$ of the rest of subjects as unlabeled data. We evaluated our methods with selected labeled data and unlabeled data by using 10-fold cross validation. This process is also repeated 10 times independently. For any chosen fraction $r_2$ of unlabeled data, we also repeated 10 times to avoid any bias introduced by randomly choosing unlabeled data. The experiment was also repeated 10 times to avoid any bias introduced by randomly choosing labeled data. Fig. 1 shows the classification accuracy of our proposed method with respect to the use of different number of unlabeled samples.

As we can see from Fig. 1, the classification accuracy can be consistently improved with the increase of unlabeled samples on three classification groups, which show that the proposed method can lead to the selection of more discriminative features by using geometric distribution of data, and as a result the classification performance was significantly improved with increase of number of unlabeled data. These results also demonstrate the significant gain obtained by adding the distribution information of data.

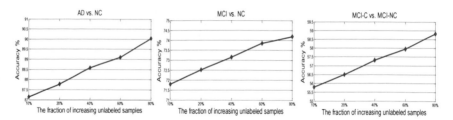

**Fig. 1.** Classification accuracy with different number of unlabeled samples

# 5    Conclusion

In summary, this paper addresses the problem of exploiting the geometric distribution of data to build the multi-task feature selection method for jointly selecting features from multi-modalities data. By introducing the manifold regularization item into the multi-task learning framework, we used the accelerated proximal gradient algorithm to seek the optimal solution for seeking out the most informative features subset. We have developed the manifold regularized multi-task feature selection method for both supervised and semi-supervised cases, and the corresponding algorithms are denoted as M2TFS and Semi-M2TFS, respectively. Experimental results on ADNI dataset validate the efficacy of our proposed method. Different from the existing multi-task feature selection method, our method utilizes the geometric distribution knowledge of data for early diagnosis of AD with better results.

**Acknowledgments.** This work was supported in part by NIH grants EB006733, EB008374, EB009634, and AG041721, SRFDP grant (No. 20123218110009), NUAAFRF grant (No. NE2013105), and also UNSFA grant (No. KJ2013Z095).

# References

1. Brookmeyer, R., Johnson, E., Ziegler-Graham, K., Arrighi, H.M.: Forecasting the global burden of Alzheimer's disease. Alzheimers & Dementia 3, 186–191 (2007)
2. Zhang, D., Wang, Y., Zhou, L., Yuan, H., Shen, D.: Multimodal classification of Alzheimer's disease and mild cognitive impairment. Neuroimage 55, 856–867 (2011)
3. Huang, S., Li, J., Ye, J., Chen, K., Wu, T.: Identifying Alzheimer's Disease-Related Brain Regions from Multi-Modality Neuroimaging Data using Sparse Composite Linear Discrimination Analysis. In: Proceedings of Neural Information Processing Systems Conference (2011)
4. Cheng, B., Zhang, D., Shen, D.: Domain Transfer Learning for MCI Conversion Prediction. In: Ayache, N., Delingette, H., Golland, P., Mori, K. (eds.) MICCAI 2012, Part I. LNCS, vol. 7510, pp. 82–90. Springer, Heidelberg (2012)
5. Zhang, D., Shen, D.: Multi-modal multi-task learning for joint prediction of multiple regression and classification variables in Alzheimer's disease. Neuroimage 59, 895–907 (2012)
6. Argyriou, A., Evgeniou, T., Pontil, M.: Multi-task Feature Learning. In: NIPS (2006)

 7. Yuan, M., Lin, Y.: Model selection and estimation in regression with grouped variables. J. Roy. Stat. Soc. B 68, 49–67 (2006)
 8. Zhu, X., Goldberg, A.B.: Introduction to semi-supervised learning. Morgan & Claypool, San Rafael (2009)
 9. Belkin, M., Niyogi, P., Sindhwani, V.: Manifold regularization: A geometric framework for learning from labeled and unlabeled examples. J. Mach. Learn. Res. 7, 2399–2434 (2006)
10. Chen, X., Pan, W., Kwok, J.T., Carbonell, J.G.: Accelerated gradient method for multi-task sparse learning problem. In: ICDM (2009)
11. Liu, J., Ye, J.: Efficient L1/Lq Norm Regularization. Technical report, Arizona State University (2009)
12. Zhang, Y., Brady, M., Smith, S.: Segmentation of brain MR images through a hidden Markov random field model and the expectation maximization algorithm. IEEE Transactions on Medical Imaging 20, 45–57 (2001)
13. Shen, D., Davatzikos, C.: HAMMER: Hierarchical attribute matching mechanism for elastic registration. IEEE Transactions on Medical Imaging 21, 1421–1439 (2002)
14. Pudil, P., Novovičová, J., Kittler, J.: Floating search methods in feature selection. Pattern Recognition Letters 15, 1119–1125 (1994)

# Similarity Guided Feature Labeling
# for Lesion Detection

Yang Song[1], Weidong Cai[1], Heng Huang[2], Xiaogang Wang[3], Stefan Eberl[4],
Michael Fulham[4,5], and Dagan Feng[1]

[1]BMIT Research Group, School of IT, University of Sydney, Australia
[2]Computer Science and Engineering, University of Texas at Arlington, USA
[3]Department of Electronic Engineering, Chinese University of Hong Kong, China
[4]Department of PET and Nuclear Medicine, Royal Prince Alfred Hospital, Australia
[5]Sydney Medical School, University of Sydney, Australia

**Abstract.** The performance of automatic lesion detection is often affected by the intra- and inter-subject feature variations of lesions and normal anatomical structures. In this work, we propose a similarity-guided sparse representation method for image patch labeling, with three aspects of similarity information modeling, to reduce the chance that the best reconstruction of a feature vector does not provide the correct classification. Based on this classification model, we then design a new approach for detecting lesions in positron emission tomography – computed tomography (PET-CT) images. The approach works well with simple image features, and the proposed sparse representation model is effectively applied for both detection of all lesions and characterization of lung tumors and abnormal lymph nodes. The experiments show promising performance improvement over the state-of-the-art.

## 1 Introduction

Automatic lesion detection is highly desirable for computed aided diagnosis. The detection system can be used in early screening or to provide second opinions for decision making. While it is conceptually simple that lesions are just regions with features distinctive from the normal anatomical structures, the detection performance is often hindered by large intra- and inter-subject variations of visual patterns. Such variations are common for both normal anatomical structures and lesions within the same subject or across different subjects.

Lesion detection is usually based on customized feature extraction and classification [6,8]. These classifiers are mainly based on parametric models and work well if there is good feature separation between lesions and normal structures. Complex and domain-specific feature design might be necessary, but could become ineffective for unseen data. Non-parametric classifications, such as multi-atlas and sparse representation methods, have also been recently proposed [4,5,11,3]. The basic principle of both types of approaches can be considered as weighted combination of reference images. While the weights for multi-atlas are normally computed using predetermined formula, the weights in sparse representation are derived by minimizing the reconstruction error.

K. Mori et al. (Eds.): MICCAI 2013, Part I, LNCS 8149, pp. 284–291, 2013.

A potential issue with sparse representation is that, since it is aimed at minimizing the reconstruction errors, it does not necessarily lead to good classification. Various improvements have thus been proposed to incorporate extra constraints into the formulation, such as discriminative labeling [2], group and locality information [10,12], and similarity relationships between references [1]. To better address problem of lesion detection, we design a new similarity-guided sparse representation method for image patch classification. Based on the basic sparse representation, we model the between-reference similarity, similarities between the testing patch and references, and similarities between the testing patch and its neighborhood. The design is motivated by the propositions that 1) to achieve labeling-consistent reconstruction, similar references should get similar weights, and references that are more similar to the testing patch should have higher weights; and 2) neighboring patches should get similar labels if they exhibit similar visual features.

The proposed classification model is common to different application domains. As a case study, in this work, we design a new three-stage approach based on the proposed similarity-guided sparse representation method for lesion detection on FDG PET-CT images of the thorax. The objectives are: 1) to detect different types of lesions; and 2) to characterize a lesion that is detected as a lung tumor or an abnormal lymph node. Compared to the lesion detection method [8], the proposed approach relies on much simpler feature design and uses a single classification model for detection and characterization.

## 2 Similarity-Guided Sparse Representation

Suppose an image $I$ contains $N_I$ non-overlapping patches, and given that some patches exhibiting typical anatomical features are already labeled (Section 3.1), the objective is to label the remaining patches. Denote the feature vector of an image patch $p_i$ as $f_i$, with $f_i \in \mathbb{R}^{H \times 1}$. A reference dictionary $D_l$ of class $l$ can be constructed by concatenating the feature vectors of $Q_l$ labeled patches of class $l$ into a matrix: $D_l \in \mathbb{R}^{H \times Q_l}$. To determine the labeling of a testing patch $p$ with feature $f$, a sparse representation approach can be used, by first deriving the reconstructed feature vectors $\{f_l'\}$ for all classes:

$$x_l = \underset{x_l}{\operatorname{argmin}} \|f - D_l x_l\|_2^2 \ s.t. \|x_l\|_0 \leq C; \quad f_l' = D_l x_l \tag{1}$$

where $x_l \in \mathbb{R}^{Q_l \times 1}$ is a weight vector. Then the patch $p$ is labeled as the class with the lowest reconstruction difference: $L(p) = \operatorname{argmin}_l \|f - f_l'\|_2$. The classification performance, however, is often found unsatisfactory, since the linear combination is actually optimized for reconstruction but not classification. To improve the classification performance using sparse representation, we propose a similarity-guided design, which is detailed below.

## 2.1   Pairwise Reference Similarity

It is natural to expect that visually similar references in a dictionary would preferably contribute similarly to the reconstruction. We thus design a modified sparse reconstruction to obtain similar weights in $x_l$ for similar references:

$$x_l = \text{argmin}_{x_l} \|f - D_l x_l\|_2^2 + \Theta(x_l) \quad s.t. \ \|x_l\|_0 \leq C$$
$$\Theta(x_l) = \sum_{(a,b),a<b} s(q_a, q_b)|x_l(a) - x_l(b)| \tag{2}$$

where $q_a$ and $q_b$ denote the feature vectors of two reference patches $a$ and $b$, $s(q_a, q_b)$ measures the similarity between $a$ and $b$, and $x_l(a)$ and $x_l(b)$ denote the corresponding weight elements in the vector $x_l$. The addition of the $\Theta(x_l)$ term helps to encourage similar weights $x_l(a)$ and $x_l(b)$ if $q_a$ and $q_b$ are similar.

To represent the similarity between references, a pairwise distance $d(q_a, q_b)$ between a pair of references is computed: $d(q_a, q_b) = \|q_a - q_b\|_2$. Then based on the normalized distance $\bar{d}(q_a, q_b) \in [0, 1]$, a degree of similarity is derived: $s(q_a, q_b) = \exp\{-\bar{d}(q_a, q_b)\}$ Next, to make Eq. (2) easier to solve, we construct a similarity matrix $U_l \in \mathbb{R}^{0.5Q_l(Q_l-1) \times Q_l}$, with each element defined as [1]:

$$U_l((a,b), k) = \begin{cases} s(q_a, q_b) & \text{if } k = a \\ -s(q_a, q_b) & \text{if } k = b \\ 0 & \text{otherwise} \end{cases} \tag{3}$$

where $(a, b)$ and $k$ are the row and column indexes of $U_l$. Each row of $U_l$ corresponds to a pair of references $a$ and $b$. Then the $\Theta(x_l)$ term can be rewritten as: $\Theta(x_l) = \|U_l x_l\|_1$. We relax it with L2 norm $\|U_l x_l\|_2^2$ so that Eq. (2) would be easily solvable using orthogonal matching pursuit (OMP) [9].

## 2.2   Patch Reference Similarity

It is also expected that references that are more similar to the testing patch should be assigned with higher weights, so that it becomes more likely to obtain a good reconstruction only for the correct dictionary. To incorporate the similarity preference between the testing patch and the references, the sparse reconstruction is further modified as:

$$x_l = \text{argmin}_{x_l} \|f - D_l x_l\|_2^2 + \|U_l x_l\|_2^2 + \Phi(x_l) \quad s.t. \ \|x_l\|_0 \leq C$$
$$\Phi(x_l) = \sum_c \bar{d}(f, q_c)x_l(c) \tag{4}$$

where $c$ indexes the reference patches and $q_c$ denotes its feature vector, $x_l(c)$ is the corresponding weight element in the vector $x_l$, and $\bar{d}(f, q_c)$ measures the normalized distance between patch $p$ and the reference $c$. Here minimization of the $\Phi(x_l)$ term would lead to a smaller weight $x_l(c)$ if $\bar{d}(f, q_c)$ is larger.

Similarly, by defining a distance vector $V_l \in \mathbb{R}^{1 \times Q_l}$ with each element of $\bar{d}(f, q_c)$, and relaxing with L2 norm, $\Phi(x_l)$ can be rewritten as: $\Phi(x_l) = \|V_l x_l\|_2^2$.

And the overall sparse reconstruction is thus now defined as:

$$
\begin{aligned}
x_l &= \operatorname{argmin}_{x_l} \|f - D_l x_l\|_2^2 + \|U_l x_l\|_2^2 + \|V_l x_l\|_2^2 \\
&= \left\| \begin{pmatrix} f \\ 0^{0.5 Q_l (Q_l - 1) \times 1} \\ 0 \end{pmatrix} - \begin{pmatrix} D_l \\ U_l \\ V_l \end{pmatrix} x_l \right\|_2^2 = \|\mathbf{f} - \Omega_l x_l\|_2^2 \quad s.t. \ \|x_l\|_0 \le C
\end{aligned}
\tag{5}
$$

The OMP algorithm is applied to solve $x_l$ efficiently, and the reconstructed vector is thus: $\mathbf{f}'_l = \Omega_l x_l$, and the labeling is $L(p) = \operatorname{argmin}_l \|\mathbf{f} - \mathbf{f}'_l\|_2$.

## 2.3   Neighborhood Similarity

Considering that label of a testing patch would be similar to its neighboring patches (if they are visually similar), the collective information of the neighborhood is thus also important. To refine the label based on the neighborhood information surrounding $p$, a different labeling scheme is designed:

$$
L(p) = \operatorname*{argmin}_l \|\mathbf{f} - \mathbf{f}'_l\|_2 + \sum_j s(f, g) \gamma(j, l) \tag{6}
$$

where $j$ indexes a neighboring patch of $p$ and $g$ denotes its feature vector, $s(f, g)$ measures the degree of similarity between $p$ and $j$, and $\gamma(j, l)$ is the cost of $j$ labeled as class $l$:

$$
\gamma(j, l) = \left\{ \begin{array}{ll} 0 & \text{if } L(j) = l \\ \|\mathbf{f} - \mathbf{f}'_l\|_2 & \text{if } L(j) \ne l \\ \|\mathbf{g} - \mathbf{g}'_l\|_2 & \text{if } L(j) \text{ unknown} \end{array} \right\} \tag{7}
$$

If the label $L(j)$ of the neighboring patch $j$ is already known after the initial labeling (Section 3.1), $\gamma(j, l)$ is then determined based on the reconstruction difference of $p$. Otherwise, $\gamma(j, l)$ is equal to its own reconstruction difference. In this way, spatial smoothness is encouraged, and the contribution from $j$ is higher if it is more similar to $p$.

## 3   Lesion Detection

### 3.1   Initial Tissue Labeling

In PET-CT images, the lung field normally exhibits low CT densities. Lesions are usually prominent on PET because they display increased FDG uptake. However, some lesions can exhibit relatively low uptake, and non-lesion high uptake regions can also occur in the mediastinum. Such cases might cause incorrect classification between lesions and mediastinal regions. Therefore, in the first step, we would like to label areas that are obviously representative of the lung field (LF), mediastinum (MS) or lesion (LS). The MS and LS areas then serve as references to further classify the unlabeled (UN) areas (Section 3.2).

To do this, we first divide the image into non-overlapping $5 \times 5$ voxel patches. An image patch $p_i$ can be confidently categorized as LF if its average CT density is less than a domain-knowledge based value (e.g. 800). Then for non-LF patches, labeling is derived based on its average FDG uptake $v$: $L(p_i)$ =MS if $v < \alpha(Z)$, or $L(p_i)$ =LS if $v > 2\alpha(Z)$, with $\alpha(Z)$ an image set specific threshold [7]. The remaining patches with $v \in [\alpha(Z), 2\alpha(Z)]$ are thus the UN ones (Fig. 1a).

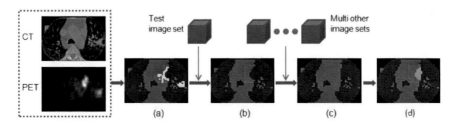

**Fig. 1.** Method illustration. (a) The initial tissue labeling output, with LF depicted as dark gray, MS as light gray, LS as red and UN patches as yellow. (b) The lesion detection output, derived based on reference dictionaries constructed from the test image set. (c) The labeling output for LF and MS patches, derived based on reference dictionaries constructed from multiple other image sets. (d) The lesion characterization output, with tumor shown as purple and abnormal lymph nodes as blue.

### 3.2   Intra-image Lesion Detection

In the second step, we further classify the UN patches as LS or MS, so that all true lesions would be detected (Fig. 1b). To do this, first, for each $p_i$, a 4-dimensional feature vector is computed: its mean and standard deviation of the CT densities, and mean and standard deviation of the FDG uptake. Next, two reference dictionaries $D_{LS}(Z)$ and $D_{MS}(Z)$ are constructed, by concatenating the feature vectors of the labeled LS or MS patches. Note that instead of using the entire database, such patches are gathered from the 3D image set containing $p_i$ only, to avoid inter-image variations. Then, for a UN patch $p_i$, its labeling $L(p_i) \in \{LS,MS\}$ is determined using the similarity-guided sparse representation Eq. (6). The logic here is that, if $p_i$ is more similar to the LS patches, it is more likely that $p_i$ is also LS; and similarly for the MS case.

### 3.3   Inter-image Lesion Characterization

In the last step, the detected lesion is characterized as a tumor or an abnormal lymph node (Fig. 1d). Similar to [8], we estimate what normal anatomical structure (LF or MS) could be present at the lesion location if the subject had been healthy. Then, if this anatomical region is originally LF (or MS), the lesion would be a tumor (or abnormal lymph node). Different from [8], here we use the proposed similarity-guide sparse representation method.

The objective is to relabel each LS patch $p_i$ as LF or MS (Fig. 1c). We consider that at similar spatial locations, collective information from multiple image sets would estimate well the original anatomical structure of $p_i$. Therefore, two reference dictionaries $D_{LF}(p_i)$ and $D_{MS}(p_i)$ are constructed for $p_i$, using labeled LF and MS patches at similar locations as $p_i$ but from images excluding the test subject. A patch is considered spatially similar to $p_i$ if the distance between them is less than 10% of the thorax size. In order to reduce the dictionary size for computational efficiency, only 1/5 of the database is used for dictionary construction. Then, with the two reference dictionaries, $L(p_i)$ is derived as LF or MS, using Eq. (6). Note that the $x$ and $y$ coordinates of the patch center are also included in the feature vector for location-based estimation. The patch-wise labels are finally combined by majority voting to classify a lesion object as tumor or abnormal lymph node.

Based on this approach, a small number of detected lymph nodes, however, would actually be tumors (those affecting mostly the mediastinum rather than lung fields) or myocardium (large bright area in the mediastinum). Therefore, for the detected abnormal lymph nodes that are very large, those in the upper left area of the medastinum are filtered as myocardium, and others are marked as tumors. The size criteria are determined based on two-fold cross validation.

## 4   Experimental Results

Our dataset comprises 50 sets of 3D thoracic FDG PET-CT images from subjects with non-small cell lung cancer, provided by the Royal Prince Alfred Hospital, Sydney. An expert reader of the images annotated 54 lung tumors and 35 abnormal lymph nodes. During preprocessing, the background and soft tissue areas outside of the lung and mediastinum are removed automatically with Otsu thresholding and connected component analysis. The 3D image sets are also aligned in the $z$-direction based on the location of the carina in the central part of the thorax, to obtain the spatially-similar reference patches (Section 3.3).

**Table 1.** Patch-level labeling performance. (a) Initial tissue labeling. (b) Lesion detection. (c) LF/MS labeling for detected lesions.

| Ground truth | Labeling | | | Ground truth | Labeling | | Ground truth | Labeling | |
|---|---|---|---|---|---|---|---|---|---|
| | MS | LS | UN | | MS | LS | | LF | MS |
| MS | 0.962 | 0 | 0.038 | MS | 0.991 | 0.009 | LF | 0.927 | 0.073 |
| LS | 0.024 | 0.405 | 0.571 | LS | 0.011 | 0.989 | MS | 0.249 | 0.751 |
| (a) | | | | (b) | | | (c) | | |

As shown in Table 1a, after initial tissue labeling, most of the patches that are labeled as MS or LS are indeed MS or LS types. Then, with the intra-image lesion detection, the UN patches are further categorized, and most of the MS and LS patches are now correctly labeled (Table 1b). Mislabeled patches are mainly in areas with relatively high uptake in the mediastinum or where there is lower uptake than is expected for tumors. Finally, with the inter-image lesion characterization, the detected lesions are categorized as tumors or abnormal lymph nodes. The performance of labeling LS patches as LF or MS is listed in Table 1c. In cases with lymph nodes adjacent to the lung fields, about 1/4 of patches are labeled as LF rather than the expected MS. However, this is usually not a problem for characterizing abnormal lymph nodes, since the majority of patches are correctly labeled. The performance comparison using different constructs of the sparse representation is shown in Fig. 2.

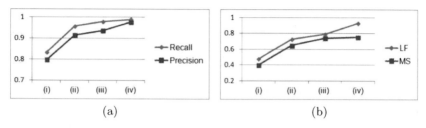

(a)                                    (b)

**Fig. 2.** (a) Patch labeling performance for LS (Section 3.2). (b) True positive rates of labeling LF and MS (Section 3.3). Comparing (iv) proposed similarity-guided sparse representation with: (i) basic sparse representation, (ii) basic plus pairwise reference similarity, and (iii) basic plus pairwise reference and patch reference similarities.

The performance of object-level detection is listed in Table 2. A lesion object is counted as true positive if at least 60% of its volume is labeled correctly. Some false positive lesions are detected in the mediastinum where there is elevated uptake, and are thus mostly characterized as lymph nodes. This affects the precision of detecting abnormal lymph nodes. The lymph nodes, especially those at the hilum, are sometimes difficult to differentiate from lung tumors and this then affects the recall of lymph nodes and precision of detecting tumors. Our results are overall better than the state-of-the-art [8]. On a standard PC with a Matlab implementation, the detection method takes on average 50s per 3D PET-CT image. Compared to [8], this method is more efficient without requiring additional structure delineation.

**Table 2.** The object-level detection performance for tumors and abnormal lymph nodes, compared with state-of-the-art [8].

|  | Tumor | Node | Tumor [8] | Node [8] |
|---|---|---|---|---|
| Recall (%) | 96.3 | 91.4 | 90.7 | 88.6 |
| Precision (%) | 92.9 | 86.5 | 89.1 | 88.6 |

# 5    Conclusion

In this work, we present a new similarity-guided sparse representation model for patch-wise feature classification, incorporating the pairwise reference similarity, patch reference similarity and neighborhood similarity. Based on this model, we then design a new three-stage approach to detect lung tumors and abnormal lymph nodes from thoracic FDG PET-CT images. Our method tackles the challenges caused by intra- and inter-subject variations effectively, and achieves promising performance improvement. In future work, we will investigate if more comprehensive feature design helps to improve the detection performance.

# References

1. Han, Y., Wu, F., Shao, J., Tian, Q., Zhuang, Y.: Graph-guided sparse reconstruction for region tagging. In: CVPR, pp. 2981–2988 (2012)
2. Jiang, Z., Lin, Z., Davis, L.S.: Learning a discriminative dictionary for sparse coding via label consistent K-SVD. In: CVPR, pp. 1697–1704 (2011)
3. Liao, S., Gao, Y., Shen, D.: Sparse patch based prostate segmentation in CT images. In: Ayache, N., Delingette, H., Golland, P., Mori, K. (eds.) MICCAI 2012, Part III. LNCS, vol. 7512, pp. 385–392. Springer, Heidelberg (2012)
4. Liu, M., Lu, L., Ye, X., Yu, S., Salganicoff, M.: Sparse classification for computer aided diagnosis using learned dictionaries. In: Fichtinger, G., Martel, A., Peters, T. (eds.) MICCAI 2011, Part III. LNCS, vol. 6893, pp. 41–48. Springer, Heidelberg (2011)
5. Parisot, S., Duffau, H., Chemouny, S., Paragios, N.: Graph-based detection, segmentation & characterization of brain tumors. In: CVPR, pp. 988–995 (2012)
6. van Ravesteijin, V.F., van Wijk, C., Vos, F.M., Truyen, R., Peters, J.F., Stoker, J., van Vliet, L.J.: Computer-aided detection of polyps in CT colonography using logistic regression. IEEE Trans. Med. Imag. 29(1), 120–131 (2010)
7. Song, Y., Cai, W., Eberl, S., Fulham, M.J., Feng, D.: Automatic detection of lung tumor and abnormal regional lymph nodes in PET-CT images. J. Nucl. Med. 52(supp. 1), 211 (2011)
8. Song, Y., Cai, W., Zhou, Y., Feng, D.: Thoracic abnormality detection with data adaptive structure estimation. In: Ayache, N., Delingette, H., Golland, P., Mori, K. (eds.) MICCAI 2012, Part I. LNCS, vol. 7510, pp. 74–81. Springer, Heidelberg (2012)
9. Tropp, J.: Greed is good: algorithmic results for sparse approximation. IEEE Trans. Inf. Theory 50, 2231–2242 (2004)
10. Wang, J., Yang, J., Yu, K., Lv, F., Huang, T., Gong, Y.: Locality-constrained linear coding for image classification. In: CVPR, pp. 3360–3367 (2010)
11. Wolz, R., Chu, C., Misawa, K., Mori, K., Rueckert, D.: Multi-organ abdominal CT segmentation using hierarchically weighted subject-specific atlases. In: Ayache, N., Delingette, H., Golland, P., Mori, K. (eds.) MICCAI 2012, Part I. LNCS, vol. 7510, pp. 10–17. Springer, Heidelberg (2012)
12. Xu, D., Huang, Y., Zeng, Z., Xu, X.: Human gait recognition using patch distribution feature and locality-constrained group sparse representation. IEEE Trans. Image Process. 21(1), 316–326 (2012)

# Large Deformation Image Classification
# Using Generalized Locality-Constrained Linear Coding*

Pei Zhang[1], Chong-Yaw Wee[1], Marc Niethammer[2], Dinggang Shen[1],
and Pew-Thian Yap[1,**]

[1] Department of Radiology,
[2] Department of Computer Science,
Biomedical Research Imaging Center (BRIC),
The University of North Carolina at Chapel Hill, USA
peizhang@email.unc.edu, mn@cs.unc.edu,
{chongyaw_wee,ptyap,dgshen}@med.unc.edu

**Abstract.** Magnetic resonance (MR) imaging has been demonstrated to be very useful for clinical diagnosis of Alzheimer's disease (AD). A common approach to using MR images for AD detection is to spatially normalize the images by non-rigid image registration, and then perform statistical analysis on the resulting deformation fields. Due to the high nonlinearity of the deformation field, recent studies suggest to use initial momentum instead as it lies in a linear space and fully encodes the deformation field. In this paper we explore the use of initial momentum for image classification by focusing on the problem of AD detection. Experiments on the public ADNI dataset show that the initial momentum, together with a simple sparse coding technique—locality-constrained linear coding (LLC)—can achieve a classification accuracy that is comparable to or even better than the state of the art. We also show that the performance of LLC can be greatly improved by introducing proper weights to the codebook.

## 1 Introduction

Alzheimer's disease (AD) is a brain disorder that causes progressive memory loss and intellectual disabilities. Treatment can be most efficacious if AD can be detected as early as possible. While clinical diagnostic criteria are still routine practice for AD detection, many recent studies have shown that brain imaging, e.g., magnetic resonance imaging (MRI), can greatly facilitate clinical diagnosis.

---

* Data used in the preparation of this article were obtained from the Alzheimer's Disease Neuroimaging Initiative (ADNI) database (adni.loni.ucla.edu). As such, the investigators within the ADNI contributed to the design and implementation of ADNI and/or provided data but did not participate in analysis or writing of this report. A complete listing of ADNI investigators can be found at http://adni.loni.ucla.edu/wp-content/uploads/how_to_apply/ADNI_Acknowledgement_List.pdf

** Corresponding author. This work was supported in part by a UNC start-up fund, NSF grants (EECS-1148870 and EECS-0925875) and NIH grants (EB006733, EB008374, EB009634, MH088520, AG041721, MH100217, and MH091645).

K. Mori et al. (Eds.): MICCAI 2013, Part I, LNCS 8149, pp. 292–299, 2013.
© Springer-Verlag Berlin Heidelberg 2013

To use MR images for AD detection, a common approach is to spatially align all the images to a common template and perform statistical analysis on the resulting deformation fields. Examples are statistical deformation models [2] and deformation-based morphometry [7]. However, the deformation field often lies in a highly nonlinear space, which is harder to work with compared with linear space. As such, recent advances in large deformation diffeomorphic metric mapping (LDDMM) methods [5,11,14] suggest to use initial momentum since it lies in a linear space. Moreover, when convolved with an appropriate kernel, the initial momentum generates a series of velocity fields that can be used to obtain the deformation field. As such, the initial momentum uniquely encodes and parameterizes the deformation field.

In this paper we explore the use of initial momentum for image classification, particularly for distinguishing AD or mild cognitive impairment (MCI) patients from healthy controls (HCs). Our work is closely related to [11] and [14]. In [11] principal component analysis (PCA) is applied to a set of initial momenta, and the resulting eigenvalues are used to train a logistic regression model to detect hippocampal shape abnormality in AD. Instead of PCA, Yang et al. [14] used locally linear embedding (LLE) [6] together with initial momenta to represent hippocampal shape in a low-dimensional space.

Our work differs from the above two methods mainly in two aspects. First, we use a recent sparse coding (SC) technique, locality-constrained linear coding (LLC) [10], for classification. Second, our goal is different. We explore the use of initial momentum for image classification, while the above works use it for shape classification [11] and low-dimensional shape embedding [14].

Our main contributions include (1) we propose a generalized LLC that uses a weighted codebook, leading to improved performance; (2) we describe how to use initial momentum to approximate geodesic distance to speed up image coding in the generalized LLC framework.

## 2   Methodology

Suppose we have a group of training images from multiple classes, a test image and a predefined template image. The problem is to tell which class the test image belongs to. We first align the template to the test image and each training image to obtain a set of initial momenta. This is achieved by the LDDMM algorithm [16], which will be briefly reviewed in Sect. 2.1. Then, for the test image and each training image, their geodesic distance can be approximated using the associated initial momenta as described in Sect. 2.2. Based on the geodesic distance, a subset of training images can be selected as the basis vectors (or codebook). By feeding the codebook to the generalized LLC introduced in Sect. 2.3, we can then classify the test image. Details are given below.

### 2.1   The LDDMM Algorithm

Let $I_0$ be the source image and $I_1$ be the target image. We would like to minimize

$$E(v_t) = \frac{1}{2}\int_0^1 ||v_t||_V^2 \, dt + \frac{1}{\sigma^2} ||I_0 \circ \phi_{1,0} - I_1||_{\ell^2}^2 ,$$

$$\text{s.t. } \dot{\phi}_{t,0} + (D\phi_{t,0})v_t = 0, \quad \phi_{0,0} = \texttt{id},$$

(1)

where $v_t$ is a time-dependent velocity field to be solved, $\sigma > 0$ is a regularization constant, $\phi_{s,t}$ is a map induced by $v_t$, mapping a voxel from its position at time $s$ to its position at time $t$, and id is an identity map. $||v_t||_V^2 = \langle L^\dagger L v_t, v_t \rangle_{\ell^2}$, where $L$ is a proper differential operator. Usually a smoothing kernel $K = (L^\dagger L)^{-1}$ is defined instead of $L$. $\dot{\phi}_{t,0} = \partial \phi_{t,0}/\partial t$ and $D\cdot$ is the Jacobian operator.

To minimize (1) we use the method of Lagrange multipliers to convert (1) to an unconstrained energy functional, compute the functional variation w.r.t $v_t$, $\phi_{t,0}$ as well as the Lagrange multipliers, and obtain a set of optimality conditions by setting the variation to zero (see [16] for details). Based on the optimality conditions and conservation of momentum (see [5] for details), we can prove that the gradient of (1) w.r.t $v_t$ is equivalent to the gradient w.r.t the initial momentum $\lambda_0$

$$\nabla_{\lambda_0} E = \lambda_0 - |D\phi_{0,1}|\lambda_1 \circ \phi_{0,1}, \tag{2}$$

where $\lambda_1$ is the final adjoint. The proof is beyond the scope of this paper and is thus omitted.

Equation (2) implies that the gradient descent can be directly performed on $\lambda_0$ by pulling $\lambda_1$ back to $t = 0$. The pullback can be achieved by computing a forward map (from $t = 0$ to $t = 1$) on the fly during a backward integration. Specifically, we compute the momentum at time $t$ by $\lambda_t = |D\phi_{t,0}|\lambda_0 \circ \phi_{t,0}$, and then the velocity field at time $t$ by convolving $\lambda_t$ with the kernel $K$ (i.e. $v_t = K\lambda_t$). In this way we can obtain a series of velocity fields $\{v_{t_0}, v_{t_1}, \ldots, v_{t_{N-1}}\}$ at time $\{t_0, t_1, \ldots, t_{N-1}\}$ (suppose we have $N$ uniformly spaced time points). According to [1], the forward map $\phi_{0,1}$ and backward map $\phi_{1,0}$ can be then computed by concatenating a set of small deformation fields, i.e.

$$\phi_{0,1} = (\text{id} + \frac{1}{N}v_{t_{N-1}}) \circ (\text{id} + \frac{1}{N}v_{t_{N-2}}) \circ \cdots \circ (\text{id} + \frac{1}{N}v_{t_0}),$$
$$\phi_{1,0} = (\text{id} - \frac{1}{N}v_{t_0}) \circ (\text{id} - \frac{1}{N}v_{t_1}) \circ \cdots \circ (\text{id} - \frac{1}{N}v_{t_{N-1}}). \tag{3}$$

Then we can pull $\lambda_1$ back to $t = 0$ by $|D\phi_{0,1}|\lambda_1 \circ \phi_{0,1}$ to update the gradient. In this work we use line search for gradient descent. Note that our formulation avoids the computational complexity of a full adjoint compared with [9].

The above process also reveals that $\lambda_0$ parameterizes the map by $\lambda_t = |D\phi_{t,0}|\lambda_0 \circ \phi_{t,0}$, from which a set of velocity fields can be obtained at each time point. Integrating all the velocity fields over the whole time interval leads to the final map $\phi_{1,0}$. The length $\rho$ of the optimal trajectory from $\phi_{0,0}$ to $\phi_{1,0}$ can be computed as $\rho = \langle \lambda_0, K\lambda_0 \rangle_{\ell^2}$, and represents the geodesic distance between $I_0$ and $I_1$ [5].

## 2.2   Approximate Geodesic Distance

The LLC emphasizes the use of a small set of training images that are most similar to the test image for coding (see Sect. 2.3). This requires us to compute the similarity (or distance) between the test image and each training image, leading to the complexity of $O(M)$, where $M$ is the number of training images. Obviously, this will be very time-consuming if $M$ is large. Below we describe an approximation to the geodesic distance $\rho$, which will reduce the complexity to $O(1)$.

Let $I_T$ be a template image. We register it to two images $I_i$ and $I_j$. Ideally, we have $I_T = I_i \circ \phi_{0,1}^i = I_j \circ \phi_{0,1}^j$. Hence, $I_j$ can be represented by $I_i$ using $I_j = I_i \circ \phi_{0,1}^i \circ \phi_{1,0}^j$. By replacing $\phi_{0,1}^i$ and $\phi_{1,0}^j$ with a set of small deformation fields using (3) we have

$$I_j = I_i \circ (\mathrm{id} + \frac{1}{N}\boldsymbol{v}_{t_{N-1}}^i) \circ \cdots \circ (\mathrm{id} + \frac{1}{N}\boldsymbol{v}_{t_0}^i) \circ (\mathrm{id} - \frac{1}{N}\boldsymbol{v}_{t_0}^j) \circ \cdots \circ (\mathrm{id} - \frac{1}{N}\boldsymbol{v}_{t_{N-1}}^j).$$

By expanding the above equation and discarding the higher order terms, we can obtain a first-order approximation to the true map between $I_i$ and $I_j$ by

$$I_j \approx I_i \circ \left( \mathrm{id} + \frac{1}{N}(\boldsymbol{v}_{t_0}^i - \boldsymbol{v}_{t_0}^j) + \frac{1}{N}(\boldsymbol{v}_{t_1}^i - \boldsymbol{v}_{t_1}^j) + \cdots + \frac{1}{N}(\boldsymbol{v}_{t_{N-1}}^i - \boldsymbol{v}_{t_{N-1}}^j) \right).$$

This indicates that we can approximate the geodesic distance between $I_i$ and $I_j$ by

$$\rho \approx \left\langle \boldsymbol{\lambda}_0^i - \boldsymbol{\lambda}_0^j, K(\boldsymbol{\lambda}_0^i - \boldsymbol{\lambda}_0^j) \right\rangle_{\ell^2}. \tag{4}$$

Although a similar result can be found in [14], here we derive from a different perspective. To estimate the distance between the test image and each training image, we only need to register the template image to the test image once and use (4) for approximation (given that we have already registered the template to all the training images).

## 2.3 Generalized Locality-Constrained Linear Coding

The LLC [10] is a kind of sparse coding (SC) techniques [4,13], where a codebook and a set of weights are used to represent a given data. The weights are sparse in the sense that most are zeros. Compared with other SC approaches, the LLC emphasizes locality, that is, a small set of basis vectors close to the given data instead of the whole codebook should be used for coding. It has been shown that this locality constraint can give better reconstruction and can help avoid similar data to be encoded by different basis vectors.

Let $a \in \mathbb{R}^n$ be the data point to be encoded. Given a set of training data points, the first step of the LLC is to compute the distance between $a$ and each training data point, and choose the $k$ nearest neighbors of $a$ based on the distance in the training set as the codebook. We use $B = \{b_1, b_2, \ldots, b_k\} \in \mathbb{R}^{n \times k}$ to represent the selected codebook. In this work the data point is simply the intensity values across the whole image and the set of initial momenta is used to compute distance as described in Sect. 2.2.

Once we have $B$, we can then code $a$ by solving the following equation

$$\arg\min_{c} ||a - Bc||^2 + \alpha ||d \odot c||^2, \quad \text{s.t. } \mathbf{1}^{\mathrm{T}}c = 1, \tag{5}$$

where $c \in \mathbb{R}^k$ is the weight vector, $\odot$ stands for element-wise multiplication and $d \in \mathbb{R}^k$ represents the distance between $a$ and each basis vector in $B$. Equation (5) essentially estimates a set of weights such that they can be used to best reconstruct $a$ together with the codebook under the locality constraint. However, there are a large number of confounding elements that will adversely affect coding precision. To penalize those confounding elements, we instead use the following equation for coding

$$\arg\min_{c} ||\tilde{a} - \tilde{B}c||^2 + \alpha ||d \odot c||^2, \quad \text{s.t. } \mathbf{1}^{\mathrm{T}}c = 1, \tag{6}$$

where $\tilde{a} = z \odot a$ and $\tilde{B} = \{w_1 \odot b_1, w_2 \odot b_2, \ldots, w_k \odot b_k\}$. $z$ and $\{w_k\}$ are weighting vectors for penalization. The analytical solution to (6) is given by

$$\tilde{c} = (C + \alpha \mathrm{diag}^2(d))\backslash 1, \tag{7}$$

$$c = \tilde{c}/1^{\mathrm{T}}c, \tag{8}$$

where $C = (\tilde{B}^{\mathrm{T}} - 1\tilde{a}^{\mathrm{T}})(\tilde{B}^{\mathrm{T}} - 1\tilde{a}^{\mathrm{T}})^{\mathrm{T}}$. In this work $z$ and $\{w_k\}$ are pre-computed using all the data points for efficiency (see Sect. 3 for details).

Once we have the weights $c$, we use the method described in [12] for classification, i.e. $\arg\min_i \|\tilde{a} - \tilde{B}\hat{c}_i\|_{\ell^2}$, where $\hat{c}_i \in \mathbb{R}^k$ is a vector whose nonzero elements are the elements in $c$ associated with class $i$. As each element of $c$ is associated with a basis $b_k$, which is, in turn, associated with a class, $\hat{c}_i$ can be obtained by identifying the class of $b_k$.

## 3    Experiments

We demonstrate the efficacy of our method using the ADNI database by comparing with one of the state-of-the-art approaches [15]. We used the same dataset as [15] to test our method. The dataset contains 51 AD patients, 99 MCI patients and 52 HCs (see [15] for detailed subject information and the list of subject IDs). We only used the MR images associated with those subjects for our experiment.

We preprocessed the dataset using the FreeSurfer [3]. The procedure includes non-uniform intensity normalization, Talairach transform computation, intensity normalization and skull stripping.

For each image in the dataset we aligned it to a template image using affine registration. Here we used the AAL atlas [8] as the template. Then we registered the template to each of the aligned images using the LDDMM algorithm described in Sect. 2.1. The template image and an example of the initial momentum are shown in Fig. 1a-b. We then used the resulting deformation fields to further warp each affinely aligned image (Fig. 1c) onto the template. Examples of the resulting images are shown in Fig. 1d.

To evaluate the performance of our algorithm we grouped the warped images from the AD patients and the HCs, and randomly split the image pool into 10 even subsets. Note that one subset contains more images than the others since the numbers of images of the AD patients and the HCs are unequal. We evaluated our algorithm using 10-fold cross-validation, which was repeated 10 times with 10 random splits. Similar to [15], we computed the mean of classification accuracy, sensitivity and specificity as performance indicators. We repeated the above process by using the set of warped images grouped from the MCI patients and the HCs.

We first compared the original LLC [10] with the generalized LLC introduced in Sect. 2.3. In all the experiments throughout this paper we set $k = 10$ and $\alpha = 0.001$. We find that smaller $k$ and larger $\alpha$ failed to give satisfactory results. For the generalized LLC, we pre-computed $z$ and $\{w_k\}$ using all the warped images from the two classes (e.g., AD and HC or MCI and HC). This was achieved by performing Welch's (two-tailed) $t$-test between voxels at corresponding positions in the images. We used hard assignment, that is, all voxels with $p$-value below a threshold (0.05) are ones, otherwise zeros. The resulting image was converted into a column vector and used as $w_k$.

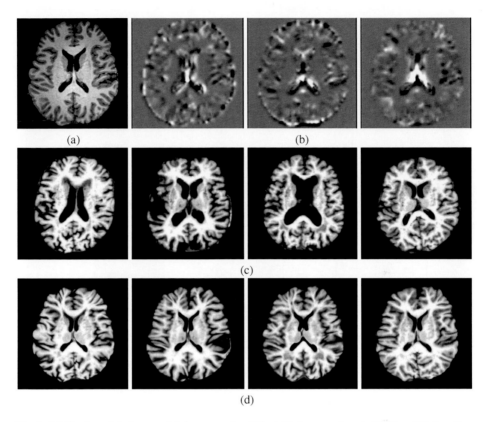

**Fig. 1.** (a) The template image. (b) An example of the initial momentum in X, Y and Z directions (from left to right). (c) Examples of affinely registered images. (d) Examples of the registered images using the LDDMM algorithm. Note that the initial momentum has been normalized for a better view.

In this work we used the same $w_k$ to weight each basis vector in the selected codebook and set $z = w_k$. Hence, the test images were also weighted using $w_k$. Although more sophisticated methods can be used to compute $z$ and $\{w_k\}$, below we show that this simple technique is good enough to lead to promising results. A similar $t$-test was also performed on the set of initial momenta in each direction. The resulting vector image was used to weight each initial momentum, and the geodesic distance was estimated as described in Sect. 2.2 using the weighted momenta, which are found to give a better estimate of distance than the original momenta. We ran our algorithm using the two kinds of LLC respectively. The results shown in Fig. 2 clearly indicate that the generalized LLC significantly outperforms the original one.

We further compared our approach with [15], where linear support vector machines are applied to multi-modal data for classification. We summarize the comparison in Fig. 3. We can see that our method significantly outperforms [15] when only MR images are used. Compared with the results obtained by [15] on multi-modal data, our algorithm yields comparable classification accuracy when distinguishing AD patients from HCs, and significantly better result when distinguishing MCI patients from HCs.

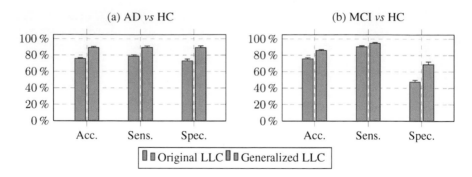

**Fig. 2.** Comparison of the original LLC and the generalized LLC

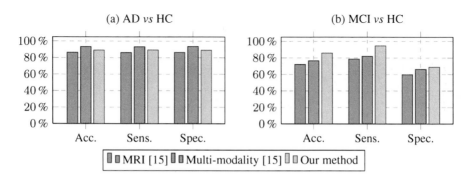

**Fig. 3.** Comparison of our method and the work in [15]

## 4    Discussion and Conclusions

We have described an image classification method by virtue of the initial momentum. This is achieved by using a generalized LLC algorithm together with an approximate geodesic distance between images. Experimental results show that the generalized LLC algorithm significantly outperforms the original one [10]. This demonstrates that the performance can be greatly improved by focusing on the discriminative voxels during coding. We also show that our algorithm can achieve comparable or even better classification accuracy rate when compared with one of the state-of-the-art methods.

We implemented the system in C++ using the Insight Segmentation and Registration Toolkit[1] (ITK). The typical running time of our LDDMM algorithm is 8~10 minutes. The timing is based on an iMac with an Intel® Core™ i5 processor (3.1 GHz).

In the future we will explore how to extract and select various features from the initial momentum to further improve classification accuracy. We also plan to investigate more sophisticated methods to learn the weighting matrix for the generalized LLC algorithm.

---

[1] http://www.itk.org/

# References

1. Ashburner, J., Friston, K.J.: Diffeomorphic registration using geodesic shooting and Gauss-Newton optimisation. NeuroImage 55(3), 954–967 (2011)
2. Caban, J., Rheingans, P.: Relational statistical deformation models for morphological image analysis and classification. In: Proceedings of International Symposium on Biomedical Imaging, pp. 1333–1336 (2010)
3. Fischl, B.: Freesurfer. NeuroImage 62(2), 774–781 (2012)
4. Lee, H., Battle, A., Raina, R., Ng, A.: Efficient sparse coding algorithms. In: Proceedings of Advances in Neural Information Processing Systems, pp. 801–808 (2007)
5. Miller, M.I., Trouvé, A., Younes, L.: Geodesic shooting for computational anatomy. Journal of Mathematical Imaging and Vision 24(2), 209–228 (2006)
6. Roweis, S.T., Saul, L.K.: Nonlinear dimensionality reduction by locally linear embedding. Science 290(5500), 2323–2326 (2000)
7. Teipel, S.J., Born, C., Ewers, M., Bokde, A.L., Reiser, M.F., Mller, H.J., Hampel, H.: Multivariate deformation-based analysis of brain atrophy to predict Alzheimer's disease in mild cognitive impairment. NeuroImage 38(1), 13–24 (2007)
8. Tzourio-Mazoyer, N., Landeau, B., Papathanassiou, D., Crivello, F., Etard, O., Delcroix, N., Mazoyer, B., Joliot, M.: Automated anatomical labeling of activations in SPM using a macroscopic anatomical parcellation of the MNI MRI single-subject brain. NeuroImage 15(1), 273–289 (2002)
9. Vialard, F.X., Risser, L., Rueckert, D., Cotter, C.: Diffeomorphic 3D image registration via geodesic shooting using an efficient adjoint calculation. International Journal of Computer Vision 97(2), 229–241 (2012)
10. Wang, J., Yang, J., Yu, K., Lv, F., Huang, T., Gong, Y.: Locality-constrained linear coding for image classification. In: Proceedings of IEEE Conference on Computer Vision and Pattern Recognition, pp. 3360–3367 (2010)
11. Wang, L., Beg, F., Ratnanather, T., Ceritoglu, C., Younes, L., Morris, J.C., Csernansky, J.G., Miller, M.I.: Large deformation diffeomorphism and momentum based hippocampal shape discrimination in dementia of the Alzheimer type. IEEE Transactions on Medical Imaging 26(4), 462–470 (2007)
12. Wright, J., Yang, A.Y., Ganesh, A., Sastry, S.S., Ma, Y.: Robust face recognition via sparse representation. IEEE Transactions on Pattern Analysis and Machine Intelligence 31(2), 210–227 (2009)
13. Yang, J., Yu, K., Gong, Y., Huang, T.: Linear spatial pyramid matching using sparse coding for image classification. In: Proceedings of IEEE Conference on Computer Vision and Pattern Recognition, pp. 1794–1801 (2009)
14. Yang, X., Goh, A., Qiu, A.: Locally linear diffeomorphic metric embedding (LLDME) for surface-based anatomical shape modeling. NeuroImage 56(1), 149–161 (2011)
15. Zhang, D., Wang, Y., Zhou, L., Yuan, H., Shen, D.: Multimodal classification of Alzheimer's disease and mild cognitive impairment. NeuroImage 55(3), 856–867 (2011)
16. Zhang, P., Niethammer, M., Shen, D., Yap, P.-T.: Large deformation diffeomorphic registration of diffusion-weighted images with explicit orientation optimization. In: Mori, K., Sakuma, I., Sato, Y., Barillot, C., Navab, N. (eds.) MICCAI 2013, Part II. LNCS, vol. 8150, pp. 27–34. Springer, Heidelberg (2013)

# Persistent Homological Sparse Network Approach to Detecting White Matter Abnormality in Maltreated Children: MRI and DTI Multimodal Study

Moo K. Chung[1], Jamie L. Hanson[1], Hyekyoung Lee[2], Nagesh Adluru[1], Andrew L. Alexander[1], Richard J. Davidson[1], and Seth D. Pollak[1]

[1] University of Wisconsin-Madison, USA
[2] Seoul National University, Korea
mkchung@wisc.edu

**Abstract.** We present a novel persistent homological sparse network analysis framework for characterizing white matter abnormalities in tensor-based morphometry (TBM) in magnetic resonance imaging (MRI). Traditionally TBM is used in quantifying tissue volume change in each voxel in a massive univariate fashion. However, this obvious approach cannot be used in testing, for instance, if the change in one voxel is related to other voxels. To address this limitation of univariate-TBM, we propose a new persistent homological approach to testing more complex relational hypotheses across brain regions. The proposed methods are applied to characterize abnormal white matter in maltreated children. The results are further validated using fractional anisotropy (FA) values in diffusion tensor imaging (DTI).

## 1 Introduction

Traditionally tensor-based morphometry (TBM) in magnetic resonance imaging (MRI) has been massively univariate in that response variables are fitted using a linear model at each voxel producing massive number of test statistics (Figure 1). However, univariate approaches are ill-suited for testing more complex hypotheses about multiple anatomical regions. For example, the univariate-TBM cannot answer how the volume increases in one voxel is related to other voxels. To address this type of more complex relational hypothesis across different brain regions, we propose a new persistent homological approach.

The Jacobian determinant is the most often used volumetric mesurement in TBM. We propose to correlate the Jacobian determinant across different voxels and quantify how the volume change in one voxel is correlated to the volume changes in other voxels. However, existing multivariate statistical methods exhibit serious defects in applying to the whole brain regions due to the *small-n large-p problem* [2]. Specifically, the number of voxels $p$ are substantially larger than the number of subjects $n$ so the often used maximum likelihood estimation (MLE) of the covariance matrix shows the rank deficiency and it is no longer

K. Mori et al. (Eds.): MICCAI 2013, Part I, LNCS 8149, pp. 300–307, 2013.

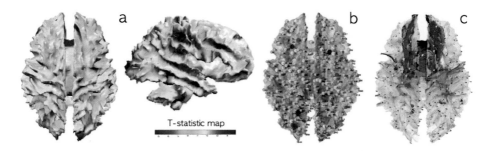

**Fig. 1.** (a) $T$-statistic map of group differences (PI-controls) on Jacobian determinants. (b) 548 uniformly sampled nodes in MRI where the persistent homology is applied. The nodes are sparsely sampled in the template to guarantee there is no spurious high correlation due to proximity between nodes. (c) The same nodes are taken in DTI to check the consistency against the MRI results.

positive definite. In turn, the estimated correlation matrix is not considered as a good approximation to the true correlation matrix. The small-$n$ large-$p$ problem can be addressed by regularizing the ill-conditioned correlation or covariance matrices by sparse regularization terms.

Sparse model $\mathcal{A}$ is usually parameterized by a tuning parameter $\lambda$ that controls the sparsity of the representation. Increasing the sparse parameter makes the representation more sparse. Instead of performing statistical inference at one fixed $\lambda$ that may not be optimal, we propose to quantify how the topology of sparse solution changes over the increasing $\lambda$ using the persistent homology. Then it is possible to obtain additional characterization of a population that cannot be obtained in the univariate-TBM.

The proposed framework is applied in characterizing abnormal white matter alterations in children who experienced maltreatment while living in post-institutional (PI) settings before being adopted by families in the US. The main contributions of the paper are (i) the introduction of a novel persistent homological approach to characterizing white matter abnormality and (ii) its application to MRI and DTI showing consistent results between the modalities.

## 2   Motivation

Let $\mathbf{J}_{n \times p} = (J_{ij})$ be the matrix of Jacobian determinant for subject $i$ at voxel position $j$. The subscripts denote the dimension of matrix. There are $p$ voxels of interest and $n$ subjects. The Jacobian determinants of all subjects at the $j$-th voxel is denoted as $\mathbf{x}_j = (J_{1j}, \cdots, J_{nj})'$. The Jacobian determinants of all voxels for the $i$-th subject is denoted as $\mathbf{y}_i = (J_{i1}, \cdots, J_{ip})'$. $\mathbf{x}_j$ is the $j$-th column and $\mathbf{y}_i$ is the $i$-th row of the data matrix $\mathbf{J}$. The covariance matrix of $\mathbf{y}_i$ is given by $\mathrm{Cov}\,(\mathbf{y}_i) = \mathbf{\Sigma}_{p \times p} = (\sigma_{kl})$ and estimated using the sample covariance matrix $S$ *via* MLE. To remedy this small-$n$ and large-$p$ problem, the likelihood is regularized with $L_1$-penalty:

$$L(\mathbf{\Sigma}^{-1}) = \log \det \mathbf{\Sigma}^{-1} - \operatorname{tr}\left(\mathbf{\Sigma}^{-1}S\right) - \lambda \|\mathbf{\Sigma}^{-1}\|_1, \tag{1}$$

where $\|\cdot\|_1$ is the sum of the absolute values of the elements. $L$ is maximized over all possible symmetric positive definite matrices. (1) is a convex problem and it is usually solved using the graphical-lasso (GLASSO) algorithm [4,6].

Since the different choice of parameter $\lambda$ will produce different solutions, we propose to use the collection of $\mathbf{\Sigma}^{-1}(\lambda)$ for every possible value of $\lambda$ for the subsequent statistical inference. This avoids the problem of identifying the optimal sparse parameter that may not be optimal in practice. The question is then how to use the collection of $\mathbf{\Sigma}^{-1}(\lambda)$ in a coherent mathematical fashion.

Consider a sparse model $\mathcal{A}(\lambda)$, which gets more sparse as $\lambda$ increases. Then under some condition, it is possible to have $\mathcal{A}(\lambda_1) \supset \mathcal{A}(\lambda_2) \supset \mathcal{A}(\lambda_3) \supset \cdots$ for $\lambda_1 \leq \lambda_2 \leq \cdots$. Within the persistent homological framework [5], $\mathcal{A}(\lambda)$ is said to be *persistent* if it has this type of nested subset structure. The collection of the nested subsets is called *filtration*.

## 3 Persistent Structures for Sparse Network Models

**Sparse Correlations.** We assume the measurement vector $\mathbf{x}_j$ at the $j$-th node is centered with zero mean and unit variance. These condition is achieved by centering and normalizing data. Let $\mathbf{\Gamma} = (\gamma_{jk})$ be the correlation matrix, where $\gamma_{jk}$ is the correlation between the nodes $j$ and $k$. *Sparse correlation* $\mathbf{\Gamma}$ is then estimated as

$$\widehat{\mathbf{\Gamma}} = \arg \min_{\beta} \frac{1}{2} \sum_{j=1}^{p} \sum_{k \neq j} \| \mathbf{x}_j - \beta_{jk}\mathbf{x}_k \|_2^2 + \lambda \|\beta\|_1, \tag{2}$$

where $\beta = (\beta_{jk})$. When $\lambda = 0$, the sparse correlation is simply given by the sample correlation, i.e. $\widehat{\gamma}_{jk} = \mathbf{x}_j'\mathbf{x}_k$. As $\lambda$ increases, the correlation becomes more sparse. Using the sparse solution (2), we will explicitly construct a persistent structure on $\widehat{\mathbf{\Gamma}}(\lambda)$ over changing $\lambda$.

Let $A = (a_{jk})$ be the adjacency matrix defined using the sparse correlation:

$$a_{jk}(\lambda) = \begin{cases} 1 & \text{if } \widehat{\gamma}_{jk} \neq 0; \\ 0 & \text{otherwise.} \end{cases}$$

Let $\mathcal{G}(\lambda)$ be the graph induced from the adjacency matrix $A$. It can be algebraically shown that the induced graph is persistent and from a filtration:

$$\mathcal{G}(\lambda_1) \supset \mathcal{G}(\lambda_2) \supset \mathcal{G}(\lambda_3) \supset \cdots \tag{3}$$

for $\lambda_1 \leq \lambda_2 \leq \lambda_3$. The proof follows by simplifying the adjacency matrix $A$ into a simpler but equivalent adjacency matrix $B = (b_{jk})$:

$$b_{jk}(\lambda) = \begin{cases} 1 & \text{if } |\mathbf{x}_j'\mathbf{x}_k| > \lambda; \\ 0 & \text{otherwise.} \end{cases} \tag{4}$$

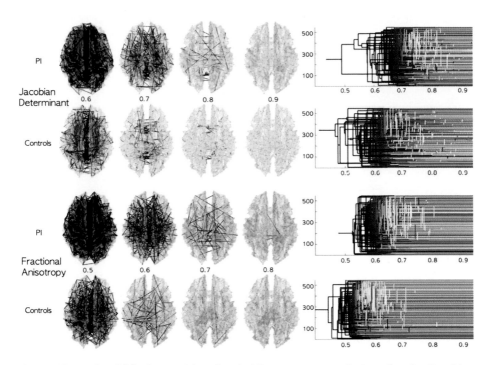

**Fig. 2.** Networks $\mathcal{G}(\lambda)$ obtained by thresholding sparse correlations for the Jacobian determinant from MRI and fractional anisotropy from DTI at different $\lambda$ values. The collection of the thresholded graphs forms a filtration. PI shows more dense network at a given $\lambda$ value. Since PI is more homogenous, in the white matter region, there are more dense high correlations between nodes. The filtration is visualized using the equivalent dendrogram [5], which also shows more dense linkages for PI at high correlations.

Then it is not difficult to see the graph induced from the adjacency matrix $B$ should be persistent. Hence, *the filtration on $\mathcal{G}(\lambda)$ can be constructed by simply thresholding the sample correlation $\mathbf{x}'_j \mathbf{x}_k$ for each $\lambda$ without solving the optimization problem (2)*. Figure 2 shows filtrations obtained from sparse correlations between Jacobian determinants on preselected 548 nodes in the two groups showing group difference. It is not necessary to perform filtrations for infinitely many possible filtration values. For an $n$-node network, it can be algebraically shown that at most $n-1$ increments are sufficient to obtain a unique filtration.

**Sparse Likelihood.** The identification of a persistent homological structure out of the inverse covariance $\widehat{\mathbf{\Sigma}}^{-1}(\lambda)$ in (1) is similar. However, it is more involved than the sparse correlation case. Let $A = (a_{ij})$ be the adjacency matrix

$$a_{ij}(\lambda) = \begin{cases} 1 & \text{if } \widehat{\sigma^{ij}} \neq 0; \\ 0 & \text{otherwise.} \end{cases} \tag{5}$$

The adjacency matrix $A$ induces a graph $\mathcal{G}(\lambda)$ consisting of $\kappa(\lambda)$ number of partitioned subgraphs

$$\mathcal{G}(\lambda) = \bigcup_{l=1}^{\kappa(\lambda)} G_l(\lambda) \text{ with } G_l = \{V_l(\lambda), E_l(\lambda)\},$$

where $V_l$ and $E_l$ are vertex and edge sets of the subgraph $G_l$ respectively. Unlike the sparse correlation case, we do not have full persistency on the induced graph $\mathcal{G}$. The partitioned graphs can be proven to be partially nested in a sense that only the partitioned node sets are persistent [4,6], i.e.

$$V_l(\lambda_1) \supset V_l(\lambda_2) \supset V_l(\lambda_3) \supset \cdots \tag{6}$$

for $\lambda_1 \leq \lambda_2 \leq \lambda_3$ and all $l$. Subsequently the collection of partitioned vertex set $\mathcal{V}(\lambda) = \bigcup_{l=1}^{\kappa(\lambda)} V_l(\lambda)$ is also persistent. On the other hand, the edge sets $E_l$ may not be persistent. The identification of the vertex filtration can be fairly time consuming since it requires solving the convex optimization problem (1) for multiple $\lambda$ values. However, it can be easily obtained by identifying a simpler adjacency matrix $B$ that gives the identical vertex sets $V_l$ (Figure 3).

Let $B(\lambda) = (b_{ij})$ be another adjacency matrix given by

$$b_{ij}(\lambda) = \begin{cases} 1 & \text{if } |\widehat{s}_{ij}| > \lambda; \\ 0 & \text{otherwise.} \end{cases} \tag{7}$$

where $\widehat{s}_{ij}$ is the sample covariance matrix. The adjacency matrix $B$ similarly induces the graph $\mathcal{H}$ with $\tau(\lambda)$ disjoint subgraphs:

$$\mathcal{H}(\lambda) = \bigcup_{l=1}^{\tau(\lambda)} H_l(\lambda)$$

with $H_l = \{W_l(\lambda), F_l(\lambda)\}$. $W_l$ and $F_l$ are vertex and edge sets of the subgraph $H_l$ respectively. Then trivially the node set $W_l$ forms a filtration over the sparse parameter:

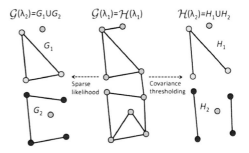

**Fig. 3.** Schematic of graph filtrations obtained by sparse-likelihood (5) and sample covariance thresholding (7). The vertex set of $\mathcal{G}(\lambda_1) = \mathcal{H}(\lambda_1)$ consists of gray nodes. For the next filtration value $\lambda_2$, $\mathcal{G}(\lambda_1) \neq \mathcal{H}(\lambda_1)$. However, the partitioned vertex sets (yellow and red) of $\mathcal{G}(\lambda_1)$ and $\mathcal{H}(\lambda_1)$ match.

$$W_l(\lambda_1) \supset W_l(\lambda_2) \supset W_l(\lambda_3) \supset \cdots \tag{8}$$

It can be further shown that $\kappa(\lambda) = \tau(\lambda)$ and $V_l(\lambda) = W_l(\lambda)$ for all $\lambda > 0$ [6]. Hence, *the filtration on the vertex set $V_l(\lambda)$ is constructed by simply thresholding the sample covariance $\widehat{s}_{ij}(\lambda)$ for each $\lambda$ without solving the time consuming optimization problem (2).* Figure 3 shows the schematic of constructing the filtration on sparse likelihood by the covariance thresholding.

# 4    Application to Maltreated Children Study

**MRI Data and Univariate-TBM.** T1-weighted MRI were collected using a 3T GE SIGNA scanner for 23 children who experienced maltreatment while living in post-institutional (PI) settings before being adopted by families in the US, and age-matched 31 normal control subjects. The average age for PI is 11.26 ⊥ 1.71 years while that of controls is $11.58 \pm 1.61$ years. A study specific template was constructed using the diffeomorphic shape and intensity averaging technique through Advanced Normalization Tools (ANTS) [1]. Image normalization of each individual image to the template was done using symmetric normalization with cross-correlation as the similarity metric. The 1mm deformation fields are then smoothed out with Guassian kernel with bandwidth $\sigma = 4$mm.

The computed Jacobian maps were fed into univariate-GLM at each voxel for testing the group effect while accounting for age and gender difference. Figure 1 shows the significant group difference between PI and controls. Any region above the $T$-statistic value of 4.86 or below -4.86 is considered significant at 0.05 (corrected). However, what the univariate-TBM can not determine is the dependency of Jacobian determinants at two different positions. It is possible that structural abnormality at one region of the brain might be related to the other regions due to interregional dependency. For this type of more complex hypothesis, we need the proposed persistent homological approach.

**Inference on Barcodes.** Since Jacobian determinants at neighboring voxels are highly correlated, we uniformly subsampled $p = 548$ number of nodes along the white matter template mesh vertices in order not to have spurious high correlation between two adjacent nodes (Figure 1). The proposed method is very robust under the change of node sizes. For the node sizes between 548 and 1856, the choice of node sizes did not affect the subsequent analysis. Following the proposed method, we constructed the filtrations on sparse correlations and inverse covariance without solving the optimizations (1) and (2). The filtrations are quantified using the barcode representation, which plots the change of Betti numbers over filtration values [5] (Figure 4). The first Betti number $\beta_0(\lambda)$ counts the number of connected components of the graph $\mathcal{G}(\lambda)$ at the filtration value $\lambda$.

Given the barcode $\beta_0^i(\lambda)$ for group $i$, we tested if the barcodes were different between the groups, i.e. $\beta_0^1(\lambda) \neq \beta_0^2(\lambda)$ for some $\lambda \in [0,1]$. A Kolmogorov-Smirnov (KS) like test statistic $T = \sup_{\lambda \in [0,1]} \left| \beta_0^1(\lambda) - \beta_0^2(\lambda) \right|$ is used. Since each group produces one barcode, we used the Jackknife resampling technique for inference. For a group with $n$ subjects, one subject is removed and the remaining $n-1$ subjects are used in constructing the barcode. This process is repeated for each subject to produce $n$ barcodes (Figure 4). The Jackknife resampling produces 23 and 31 barcodes respectively for PI and controls. In order for the permutation test to converge for our data set, it requires tens of thousands permutations and it is really time consuming. So we used a much simpler Jackknife resampling. Then the test statistic $T$ is constructed between $23 \times 31$ pairs of barcodes. Under the null, $T$ is expected to be zero. One-sample T-test on the collection of $T$ is then subsequently performed to show huge group discrimination for sparse

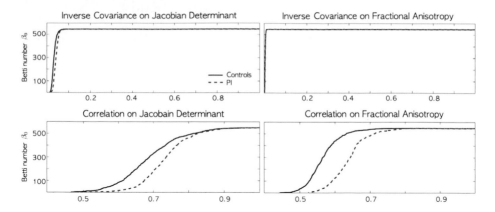

**Fig. 4.** The barcodes on the sparse inverse covariance (top) and correlation (bottom) for Jacobian determinant (left) and FA (right). Unlike the inverse sparse covariance, the sparse correlation shows huge group separation between normal controls and post-institutionalized (PI) children ($p$-value < 0.001).

correlations in Figure 4 ($p$-value < 0.001). The barcodes for normal controls show much higher Betti numbers at the given threshold. This suggests higher non-uniformity in Jacobian determinants across the brain that causes increased disconnections in correlations. The inverse covariance was not able to discriminate the groups. The MATLAB codes for constructing barcodes and statical inference is given in http://brainimaging.waisman.wisc.edu/~chung/barcodes.

**Validation Against DTI.** For children who suffered early neglect and abuse, white matter microstructures are more diffusely organized [3]. So we expect less white matter variability not only in the Jacobian determinants but also in the fractional anisotropy (FA) values in DTI as well. The MRI data in this study has the corresponding DTI. The DTI acquisition are done in the same 3T GE SIGNA scanner and the acquisition parameters can be found in [3]. We applied the proposed persistent homological method in obtaining the filtrations for sparse correlations and inverse covariances in the same 548 nodes (Figure 1). The resulting filtration patterns also show similar pattern of rapid increase in disconnected components (Figure 2 and 4) for sparse correlations. The Jackknife-based one-sample T-test also shows significant group difference for correlations ($p$-value < 0.001). This results are due to consistent abnormality observed in both MRI and DTI modalities. PI exhibited stronger white matter homogeneity and less spatial variability compared to normal controls in both MRI and DTI measurements. The inverse covariance was not able to discriminate the groups.

## 5   Conclusions and Discussions

Using the persistent homological framework, we have shown that PI group shows less anatomic variation in MRI compared to the normal controls. This result is consistent with DTI, which shows similar patterns. The reason we did not detect the group difference in the inverse covariances might be that, as shown in Figure 4, the changes in the first Betti number are occurring in a really narrow window and losing the discrimination power. On the other hand the sparse correlations exhibit more slow changes in the Betti number over the wide window making it easier to discriminate the groups. The proposed method is general enough to run on any type of volumetric imaging data that is spatially normalized.

**Acknowledgements.** This work was supported by NIH Research Grants MH61285 and MH68858 to S.D.P., NIMH Grant MH84051 to R.J.D. and US National Institute of Drug Abuse (Fellowship DA028087) to J.L.H. The authors like to thank Matthew Arnold of University of Bristol for the discussion on the KS-test procedure and pointing out the reference [6].

# References

1. Avants, B.B., Epstein, C.L., Grossman, M., Gee, J.C.: Symmetric diffeomorphic image registration with cross-correlation: Evaluating automated labeling of elderly and neurodegenerative brain. Medical Image Analysis 12, 26–41 (2008)
2. Friston, K.J., Holmes, A.P., Worsley, K.J., Poline, J.-P., Frith, C.D., Frackowiak, R.S.J.: Statistical parametric maps in functional imaging: a general linear approach. Human Brain Mapping 2, 189–210 (1995)
3. Hanson, J.L., Adluru, N., Chung, M.K., Alexander, A.L., Davidson, R.J., Pollak, S.D.: Early neglect is associated with alterations in white matter integrity and cognitive functioning. In: Child Development (in press, 2013)
4. Huang, S., Li, J., Sun, L., Ye, J., Fleisher, A., Wu, T., Chen, K., Reiman, E.: Learning brain connectivity of Alzheimer's disease by sparse inverse covariance estimation. NeuroImage 50, 935–949 (2010)
5. Lee, H., Chung, M.K., Kang, H., Kim, B.-N., Lee, D.S.: Computing the shape of brain networks using graph filtration and Gromov-Hausdorff metric. In: Fichtinger, G., Martel, A., Peters, T. (eds.) MICCAI 2011, Part II. LNCS, vol. 6892, pp. 302–309. Springer, Heidelberg (2011)
6. Mazumder, R., Hastie, T.: Exact covariance thresholding into connected components for large-scale graphical lasso. The Journal of Machine Learning Research 13, 781–794 (2012)

# Inter-modality Relationship Constrained Multi-Task Feature Selection for AD/MCI Classification

Feng Liu[1,2], Chong-Yaw Wee[2], Huafu Chen[1], and Dinggang Shen[2]

[1] Key Laboratory for NeuroInformation of Ministry of Education, School of Life Science and Technology, University of Electronic Science and Technology of China, Sichuan, China
[2] Department of Radiology and Biomedical Research Imaging Center (BRIC), University of North Carolina at Chapel Hill, NC, USA
dgshen@med.unc.edu

**Abstract.** In conventional multi-modality based classification framework, feature selection is typically performed separately for each individual modality, ignoring potential strong inter-modality relationship of the same subject. To extract this inter-modality relationship, $L_{2,1}$ norm-based multi-task learning approach can be used to jointly select common features from different modalities. Unfortunately, this approach overlooks different yet complementary information conveyed by different modalities. To address this issue, we propose a novel multi-task feature selection method to effectively preserve the complementary information between different modalities, improving brain disease classification accuracy. Specifically, a new constraint is introduced to preserve the inter-modality relationship by treating the feature selection procedure of each modality as a task. This constraint preserves distance between feature vectors from different modalities after projection to low dimensional feature space. We evaluated our method on the Alzheimer's Disease Neuroimaging Initiative (ADNI) dataset and obtained significant improvement on Alzheimer's Disease (AD) and Mild Cognitive Impairment (MCI) classification compared to state-of-the-art methods.

**Keywords:** Alzheimer's Disease, Multi-task learning, Sparse representation, Multi-modality, Multi-kernel support vector machine.

## 1    Introduction

Alzheimer's Disease (AD) that is highly related to the central nervous system is a genetically complex and irreversible neurodegenerative disorder. AD is the most common form of dementia diagnosed in people over 65 years of age, and is characterized by a decline in cognitive and memory functions [1]. Efforts have been made for the past few decades to understand the pathophysiological underpinnings of AD and its intermediate stage, i.e., Mild Cognitive Impairment (MCI) [2]. Previous study suggest that individuals with MCI tend to progress to AD at a rate of approximately 10% to 15% per year, compared to Normal Controls (NC) who tend to develop dementia at a rate of 1% to 2% per year [3]. Due to high progression rate, it is crucial to accurately identify AD in its early stage for possible treatment and intervention.

K. Mori et al. (Eds.): MICCAI 2013, Part I, LNCS 8149, pp. 308–315, 2013.
© Springer-Verlag Berlin Heidelberg 2013

There is ample evidence showing individuals with AD are significantly affected in their brain functions and structures. For example, Greicius *et al.* found that disrupted connectivity between posterior cingulate and hippocampus accounted for the posterior cingulate hypometabolism [4]. In addition, Guo *et al.* reported that patients with AD exhibited significant decrease of gray matter volume in the hippocampus, parahippo-campal gyrus, insula and superior temporal gyrus, suggesting the potential of using these regions as an imaging marker for AD [5]. However, these findings are solely based on univariate or group-level statistical methods, and thus are of limited utility for individual-level disease diagnosis. In fact, disease diagnosis at individual level is important for clinical usage that can be accomplished through pattern classification technique. This technique is sensitive to the fine-grained spatial discriminative patterns and is effective in providing predictive value to diseases. To date, pattern classification method has been widely used on neuroimaging data to identify AD and MCI from NC [6, 7].

Recent studies demonstrate that complementary information from different neuroimaging modalities can be used jointly to improve AD/MCI diagnosis [8, 9]. However, feature selection procedure in these studies is typically performed separately for each individual modality, ignoring strong within-subject inter-modality relationship. Recently, $L_{2,1}$ norm-based multi-task learning has been proposed to simultaneously select features from different tasks based on intrinsic relationship between different tasks [10]. Learning multiple related tasks simultaneously has shown to often perform better than learning each task separately [11]. This learning approach, although enables the joint selection of common features from different modalities, unfortunately may overlook different yet complementary information conveyed by different modalities.

To address this issue, a novel multi-task learning based feature selection method is proposed to better preserve the complementary information conveyed by different modalities. In the proposed feature selection method, a new constraint is imposed to preserve the inter-modality relationship after feature projection while enforcing the sparseness of the selected features. A multi-kernel Support Vector Machine (SVM) is then adopted to combine these selected features. The proposed method has been evaluated on ADNI dataset and obtained promising results.

## 2      Materials and Methods

### 2.1      Data Acquisition and Preprocessing

Data used in this study are obtained from the ADNI dataset (http://www.loni.ucla.edu/ADNI). In total, we use 202 subjects from ADNI dataset: 51 patients with AD, 99 patients with MCI, and 52 NC. Image preprocessing is carried out separately for magnetic resonance imaging (MRI) and Fluorodeoxyglucose (FDG) Positron-Emission Tomography (PET) data. The preprocessing steps of MRI data include skull-stripping [12], dura removal, intensity inhomogeneity correction, cerebellum removal, spatial segmentation and registration. We then parcellate the preprocessed images into 93 regions according to the template in [13]. Only gray matter volume of these 93 regions-of-interest is used in the study. For the preprocessing of PET images, we align the PET image of each subject to its corresponding MRI image using a rigid transformation and the average intensity of each regions-of-interest is calculated as a feature. Therefore, we have two 93-dimensional feature vectors for each subject.

## 2.2    Multi-Task Feature Selection

Feature selection is treated as a multi-task regression problem that incorporates the relationship between different modalities. Let $X^j = \left[x_1^j, \ldots, x_i^j, \ldots, x_n^j\right]^T$ be a $n \times d$ matrix that represents $d$ features of $n$ training samples for modality $j$, $j = 1, \ldots, m$, where $m$ is the total number of modalities. Let $y^j = \left[y_1^j, \ldots, y_i^j, \ldots, y_n^j\right]^T$ be a $n$ dimensional corresponding target vector (with classification labels as values of $+1$ or $-1$ in this study) for modality $j$. In our application, we have two modalities (MRI and PET) and the same target vectors, i.e., $m = 2$ and $y^1 = y^2$. According to [14], the linear model used for prediction is defined as follows:

$$\hat{y}^j = X^j w^j \tag{1}$$

where $w^j \in R^{d \times 1}$ and $\hat{y}^j$ are the regression coefficient vector and the predicted label vector of the $j$-th modality, respectively. One of the popular approaches to estimate $W = [w^1, \ldots, w^j, \ldots, w^m]$ is by minimizing the following objective function:

$$\min_W \sum_{j=1}^m \left\|X^j w^j - y^j\right\|_F^2 + \lambda_1 \|W\|_1 \tag{2}$$

where $\lambda_1 > 0$ is a regularization parameter, and $\|W\|_1$ is the $L_1$ norm of $W$ defined as $\sum_{i=1}^d \sum_{j=1}^m |w_{i,j}|$. The first term of Eq. (2) measures the empirical error on the training data while the second term controls the sparseness. This regression model is known as Least Absolute Shrinkage and Selection Operator (LASSO) [15].

The limitation of this regression model is that all tasks are assumed to be independent. Although we can use group sparsity (i.e., $L_{2,1}$ norm) to guide the selection of features for same regions from different modalities, the complementary information conveyed by different modalities might be eliminated after this group constraint. To address this problem, one effective way is to preserve the relative distance between feature vectors of different modalities of the same subject (also called as inter-modality relationship) after feature projection via the following constraint:

$$D = \sum_{i=1}^n \sum_{j=1}^m \sum_{k=1, k \neq j}^m \frac{\left\|x_i^j w^j - x_i^k w^k\right\|_F^2}{\left\|x_i^j - x_i^k\right\|_F^2} \tag{3}$$

where $x_i^j$ and $x_i^k$ denote the feature vectors of the $j$-th and $k$-th modalities in the $i$-th subject, respectively. $\left\| x_i^j - x_i^k \right\|_F^2$ measures the relative distance between the feature vectors $x_i^j$ and $x_i^k$ before feature projection, and $\left\| x_i^j w^j - x_i^k w^k \right\|_F^2$ measures the respective distance after feature projection (or the distance between the corresponding predictions). Basically, for two initial vectors with small distance, they are constrained to have small distance after projection. While for the two initial vectors with very large distance, we will put less constraint on their mapping since the inverse of their initial distance is almost zero. This constraint preserves the inter-modality relationship after projection of feature vectors from different modalities onto the low-dimensional feature space.

By incorporating this constraint into Eq. (2), we can obtain a new objective function:

$$\min_w \sum_{j=1}^m \left\| X^j w^j - y^j \right\|_F^2 + \lambda_1 \|W\|_1 + \lambda_2 D \qquad (4)$$

where $\lambda_2 > 0$ is the regularization parameter that controls the degree of preserving the inter-modality relationship. Of note, features from different modalities are normalized to have zero mean and unit standard deviation to enable direct combination of different types of features. In this study, we use Accelerated Proximal Gradient method [16] to optimize the objective function in Eq. (4). After feature selection, only those features with non-zero regression coefficients are used for final classification.

## 2.3    Multi-kernel SVM Classification

A multi-kernel SVM method is applied to integrate features from different modalities (i.e., PET and MRI) for classification via a weighted linear combination [8]. In brief, for each modality, we calculate the corresponding kernel on the basis of the features selected by the aforementioned feature selection method. Subsequently, multi-kernel SVM is used to construct a mixed kernel matrix by linearly combining kernels from different modalities. It is worth noting that the optimal parameters used for combining different kernels are determined by using grid search approach. SVM classifier with linear kernel is implemented via the LIBSVM toolbox [17].

A nested ten-fold cross-validation strategy is used to evaluate classification performance. Specifically, the inner cross-validation loop is used to determine the parameters, i.e., the regularization parameters $\lambda_1$, $\lambda_2$ and the above-mentioned kernel combination parameter from training set. The outer loop is then used to evaluate the generalizability of the SVM model by using an independent testing set. SVM model that perform the best during the inner cross-validation stage is considered as the optimal model and is used to classify unseen test samples. This process is repeated 10 times to avoid the bias introduced by randomly partitioning dataset in the cross-validation. Accuracy, sensitivity, and specificity are calculated to quantify the performance of all compared methods.

An overview of the proposed AD/MCI classification pipeline is illustrated in **Fig.1**.

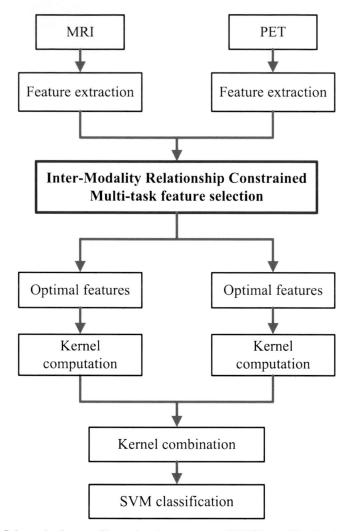

**Fig. 1.** Schematic diagram illustrating the proposed AD/MCI classification framework

## 3    Experimental Results

The performance of our method is compared with the 1) Single-Task feature selection (i.e., LASSO) integrated with the Multi-modality Multi-kernel (STMM) SVM, 2) Single-Task feature selection integrated with the Single-modality Single-kernel (STSS) SVM, and 3) Joint feature Selection (i.e., $L_{2,1}$ norm) integrated with Multi-modality Multi-kernel (JSMM) SVM. It is worth noting that we use the same training and testing data across the experiments for all the methods for fair comparison. For each comparison, the performance of each comparison method is evaluated through the classification of AD vs. NC and MCI vs. NC, respectively.

As shown in **Table 1** and **Fig. 2**, the proposed method outperforms all comparison methods in AD/MCI classification. Specifically, for distinguishing AD from NC, our method achieves accuracy of 94.37%, with a sensitivity of 94.71%, a specificity of 94.04%, and the Area Under the receiver operating characteristic Curve (AUC) of 0.9724. On the other hand, for distinguishing MCI from NC, our method achieves a classification accuracy of 78.8%, with a sensitivity of 84.85%, a specificity of 67.06%, and the AUC of 0.8284. We also perform paired $t$-tests on the accuracies of all comparison methods with our method and obtain $p$ values smaller than 0.05 for all comparisons, indicating significant improvement by our method on AD/MCI classification. These results demonstrate that preserving inter-modality relationship improves the classification performance. The numbers of support vectors used in our method are 29~40 and 57~69 for AD and MCI classifications, respectively. The numbers of selected features used for final classification are 8~14 and 41~64 for AD and MCI classifications, respectively. The whole classification pipeline requires 10 and 30 minutes for AD and MCI classifications, respectively.

**Table 1.** Classification performance of all comparison methods. ACC, SEN, SPE stand for the accuracy, sensitivity, and specificity, respectively.

| Method | AD vs. NC | | | | MCI vs. NC | | | |
|---|---|---|---|---|---|---|---|---|
| | ACC (%) | SEN (%) | SPE (%) | AUC | ACC (%) | SEN (%) | SPE (%) | AUC |
| STMM | 91.02 | 89.02 | 92.88 | 0.9655 | 72.08 | 75.56 | 65.38 | 0.7826 |
| STSS | 88.25 | 84.91 | 91.54 | 0.9004 | 71.41 | 77.78 | 59.23 | 0.7575 |
| JSMM | 91.10 | 91.57 | 90.58 | 0.9584 | 73.54 | 81.01 | 59.23 | 0.7706 |
| **Proposed** | **94.37** | **94.71** | **94.04** | **0.9724** | **78.80** | **84.85** | **67.06** | **0.8284** |

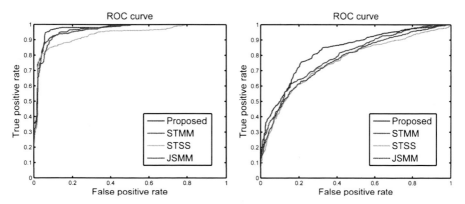

**Fig. 2.** Receiver Operating Characteristic (ROC) curves of different methods (with feature selection) for AD (left) and MCI (right) classifications

In order to validate the effectiveness of the proposed feature selection method, we compare the AD/MCI classification performance with and without the proposed feature selection step. The same multi-kernel SVM framework is applied for both the comparison methods. As seen in **Table 2**, the proposed feature selection method out-performs the approach without feature selection. For further comparison, we summar-ize the results of recent multi-modal classification studies. Hinrichs *et al.* used 48 AD patients and 66 NC for classification, and obtained an accuracy of 87.6% by using two modalities (PET + MRI), and an accuracy of 92.4% by using five types of fea-tures (MRI + PET + cerebrospinal fluid (CSF) + Apolipoprotein E (APOE) + cogni-tive scores) [8]. Gray *et al.* used 37 AD patients, 75 MCI patients and 35 NC, report-ing an accuracy of 89% for AD classification and an accuracy of 74.6% for MCI clas-sification by using four types of features (CSF + MRI + PET + Genetic features) [9]. As seen in **Table 3**, our method performs better than the two aforementioned studies, even though they used more modalities. Although direct comparison with these stu-dies is not appropriate due to possible use of different subjects (although from the same ADNI dataset), the obtained results validate the promising performance of our method for AD classification to some extent.

**Table 2.** Classification performance with and without feature selection step

| Method | Subjects | Modalities | AD vs. NC (%) | MCI vs. NC (%) |
|--------|----------|------------|---------------|----------------|
| Without | 51AD+99MCI+52NC | PET+MRI | 89.90 | 70.89 |
| **With** | **51AD+99MCI+52NC** | **PET+MRI** | **94.37** | **78.80** |

**Table 3.** Comparison of classification accuracies reported in the literature

| Method | Subjects | Modalities | AD vs. NC (%) | MCI vs. NC (%) |
|--------|----------|------------|---------------|----------------|
| Hinrichs *et al.* [8] | 48AD+66NC | PET+MRI | 87.60 | - |
| Hinrichs *et al.* [8] | 48AD+66NC | MRI+PET+CSF+APOE +cognitive scores | 92.40 | - |
| Gray *et al.* [9] | 37AD+75MCI+35NC | PET+MRI+CSF+Genetic | 89.00 | 74.60 |
| **Proposed** | **51AD+99MCI+52NC** | **PET+MRI** | **94.37** | **78.80** |

# 4     Conclusion

We propose a novel multi-task learning based feature selection method to effectively integrate the complementary information from multiple modalities neuroimaging data to improve AD/MCI identification. Specifically, we treat the selection of features from each modality as a task and preserve the inter-modality relationship after projec-tion of feature vectors from different modalities onto the low-dimensional feature space. Experimental results on ADNI dataset demonstrate that our proposed multi-task feature selection technique, integrated with the multi-kernel SVM, outperforms all comparison methods. In the future, we will extend our work to include more modalities (such as CSF or genetic features) to improve AD/MCI classification performance.

# References

1. Delbeuck, X., Van der Linden, M., Collette, F.: Alzheimer's disease as a Disconnection Syndrome? Neuropsychology Review 13, 79–92 (2003)
2. Petersen, R.C., Smith, G.E., Waring, S.C., Ivnik, R.J., Kokmen, E., Tangelos, E.G.: Aging, memory, and mild cognitive impairment. Int. Psychogeriatr. 9(suppl. 1), 65–69 (1997)
3. Bischkopf, J., Busse, A., Angermeyer, M.C.: Mild cognitive impairment–a review of prevalence, incidence and outcome according to current approaches. Acta Psychiatr. Scand. 106, 403–414 (2002)
4. Greicius, M.D., Srivastava, G., Reiss, A.L., Menon, V.: Default-mode network activity distinguishes Alzheimer's disease from healthy aging: evidence from functional MRI. Proc. Natl. Acad. Sci. U. S. A. 101, 4637–4642 (2004)
5. Guo, X., Wang, Z., Li, K., Li, Z., Qi, Z., Jin, Z., Yao, L., Chen, K.: Voxel-based assessment of gray and white matter volumes in Alzheimer's disease. Neurosci. Lett. 468, 146–150 (2010)
6. Fan, Y., Rao, H., Hurt, H., Giannetta, J., Korczykowski, M., Shera, D., Avants, B.B., Gee, J.C., Wang, J., Shen, D.: Multivariate examination of brain abnormality using both structural and functional MRI. Neuroimage 36, 1189–1199 (2007)
7. Zhang, D., Shen, D.: Multi-modal multi-task learning for joint prediction of multiple regression and classification variables in Alzheimer's disease. Neuroimage 59, 895–907 (2012)
8. Hinrichs, C., Singh, V., Xu, G., Johnson, S.C.: Predictive markers for AD in a multi-modality framework: an analysis of MCI progression in the ADNI population. Neuroimage 55, 574–589 (2011)
9. Gray, K.R., Aljabar, P., Heckemann, R.A., Hammers, A., Rueckert, D.: Random forest-based similarity measures for multi-modal classification of Alzheimer's disease. Neuroimage 65, 167–175 (2013)
10. Liu, J., Ji, S., Ye, J.: Multi-task feature learning via efficient l 2, 1-norm minimization. In: Proceedings of the Twenty-Fifth Conference on Uncertainty in Artificial Intelligence, pp. 339–348. AUAI Press (2009)
11. Evgeniou, A.A.T., Pontil, M.: Multi-task feature learning. In: Advances in Neural Information Processing Systems 19: Proceedings of the 2006 Conference, p. 41. MIT Press (2007)
12. Wang, Y., Nie, J., Yap, P.T., Shi, F., Guo, L., Shen, D.: Robust deformable-surface-based skull-stripping for large-scale studies. Med. Image Comput. Comput. Assist. Interv. 14, 635–642 (2011)
13. Kabani, N.J.: 3D anatomical atlas of the human brain. Neuroimage 7, S717 (1998)
14. Zhou, J., Yuan, L., Liu, J., Ye, J.: A multi-task learning formulation for predicting disease progression. In: Proceedings of the 17th ACM SIGKDD International Conference on Knowledge Discovery and Data Mining, pp. 814–822. ACM (2011)
15. Tibshirani, R.: Regression shrinkage and selection via the lasso. Journal of the Royal Statistical Society. Series B (Methodological), 267–288 (1996)
16. Nesterov, Y.: Introductory lectures on convex optimization: A basic course. Springer (2003)
17. Chang, C.-C., Lin, C.-J.: LIBSVM: a library for support vector machines. ACM Transactions on Intelligent Systems and Technology (TIST) 2, 27 (2011)

# The Impact of Heterogeneity and Uncertainty on Prediction of Response to Therapy Using Dynamic MRI Data

Manav Bhushan[1,2], Julia A. Schnabel[1], Michael Chappell[1], Fergus Gleeson[3], Mark Anderson[3], Jamie Franklin[3], Sir Michael Brady[4], and Mark Jenkinson[2]

[1] Institute of Biomedical Engineering (Department of Engineering Science), University of Oxford, UK[*]
[2] The Oxford Centre for Functional MRI of the Brain, Nuffield Department of Clinical Neurosciences, University of Oxford, UK
[3] Department of Radiology, Churchill Hospital, Oxford, UK
[4] Department of Oncology, University of Oxford, UK

**Abstract.** A comprehensive framework for predicting response to therapy on the basis of heterogeneity in dceMRI parameter maps is presented. A motion-correction method for dceMRI sequences is extended to incorporate uncertainties in the pharmacokinetic parameter maps using a variational Bayes framework. Simple measures of heterogeneity (with and without uncertainty) in parameter maps for colorectal cancer tumours imaged before therapy are computed, and tested for their ability to distinguish between responders and non-responders to therapy. The statistical analysis demonstrates the importance of using the spatial distribution of parameters, and their uncertainties, when computing heterogeneity measures and using them to predict response on the basis of the pre-therapy scan. The results also demonstrate the benefits of using the ratio of $K^{trans}$ with the bolus arrival time as a biomarker.

## 1 Introduction

In the past decade, dynamic contrast-enhanced magnetic resonance imaging (dceMRI) has become a widespread and very effective tool for diagnosis and treatment planning in cancer patients [1]. In the case of certain cancers such as breast [2], and cervical cancer [3], the predictive and diagnostic value of dceMRI has already been proven to a large extent. Even though colorectal cancer is the second-biggest cause of cancer-related deaths in Europe, a reliable imaging biomarker is yet to emerge. It is notoriously difficult to constrain motion during dceMRI scans of colorectal tumours, and the importance of motion-correction in estimating pharmacokinetic (PK) modelling has been shown previously in [4], [5]. There are various studies that predict response to treatment by comparing PK parameters before and during treatment, but it is more desirable to predict

---

[*] Acknowledgements: This work was funded by the CRUK/EPSRC Oxford Cancer Imaging Centre.

response only based on the pre-therapy scan. It is widely acknowledged that intra-tumoural heterogeneity is crucial in this regard [6], [7].

In the analysis of spatial distributions of PK parameters, two principal questions arise: (1) which parameter(s) to consider; (2) what kind of spatial features to look for. The parameters that have been examined most often in the case of dceMRI data, are the transfer coefficients $k_{ep}$ and $K^{trans}$ (in min$^{-1}$), that are indicators of vessel permeability (leakiness) and perfusion. Recent literature shows that the bolus arrival time ($t_0$) is clinically important since it is an indicator of necrosis [8]. In this study, the prognostic value of spatial heterogeneity in $k_{ep}$, $K^{trans}$, and a derived biomarker, $r_{kt} = K^{trans}/t_0$ with units min$^{-2}$, is investigated. Physiologically, $r_{kt}$ can be likened to a measure of the acceleration experienced by the bolus when it comes into contact with the vasculature. It signifies the ability of the vasculature to respond to the force exerted by the bolus, per unit mass.

In this study, we correct for motion, estimate PK parameters, and then compare some simple measures of heterogeneity. Another crucial aspect of dceMRI data analysis that has been investigated in this paper is the effect of uncertainty in the PK parameter estimates on prediction of response to therapy. The different sources of error and uncertainty in dceMRI data analysis have been analyzed in [9], but the uncertainty has not been integrated into the calculation of heterogeneity in tumours earlier. The model is also parametrized differently in [9], and patient motion is not explicitly taken into account. This study presents a comparison between the predictive values of different measures of heterogeneity calculated with and without taking uncertainty into account.

## 2   Methods

### 2.1   Pharmacokinetic Modelling

In a dceMRI scan, the patient is injected with a low molecular-weight contrast agent (CA), and MRI volumes are acquired at regular intervals after injection. The basic assumption of PK modelling is that the concentration of CA at each voxel in the image space is a function of some matrix physiological parameters ($\theta$) of the tissue. The changing concetration of CA leads to changes in the MRI signal, which depend on the physiological parameters $\theta$, the MRI acquisition parameters ($\alpha$), the motion applied during the scan (parametrized by the matrix $T$), and a noise process ($\epsilon$). Thus, the observed data $Y$ is given by:

$$Y = f(T, \theta, \alpha) + \epsilon \tag{1}$$

This generic formulation allows any PK model, $f$, and any noise model, $\epsilon$, to be used. In this study, we have used the Tofts one-compartment PK model [10], and assumed $\epsilon$ to be a Gaussian noise process with mean 0 and precision $\phi$, i.e. $\epsilon \sim N\left(0, \phi^{-1}\right)$. According to the Tofts model, for a given Arterial Input Function (AIF), the concentration of CA at time $t$, $C(t)$, can be written as:

$$C(t) = AIF(t - t_0) \otimes k_{ep} v_e e^{-k_{ep}(t-t_0)} \quad (for \; t > t_0) \tag{2}$$

Here $\otimes$ denotes a convolution, $t_0$ denotes the time at which the CA reaches the voxel under consideration, $k_{ep}$ denotes the rate of transfer of CA from the extra-cellular extra-vascular space (EES) to the blood plasma, $v_e$ denotes the proportion of space in that voxel occupied by the EES and $K^{trans} = k_{ep} \cdot v_e$. In order to restrict the number of variables, and to make the analysis more tractable, we have elected to use the Orton (population-averaged) AIF in this study (Model 2 from [11]). We are now interested in extracting the 'true' PK parameter matrix ($\theta = [K^{trans}, v_e, t_0]$), which best explain the data $Y$, and the uncertainties associated with these parameters.

## 2.2   The Variational Bayes Framework

In order to accomplish this task, a variational Bayes (VB) framework has been employed for the dceMRI analysis [12]. The objective is to maximize the probability of the PK parameters given the data. Thus, using Bayes' rule, we seek to maximize the posterior probability of the parameters given the data:

$$P(\theta \mid Y, T, \alpha) \propto P(Y \mid \theta, T, \alpha) \cdot P(\theta) \tag{3}$$

Here, $P(\theta)$ represents the prior probability of the PK parameters, which in this study is assumed to be a multi-variate normal (MVN) distribution, i.e:

$$P(\theta) = MVN(m_o, \Sigma_0) \tag{4}$$

Where the matrix $m_0 = [m_{k_{ep}}, m_{v_e}, m_{t_0}]$ represents the prior means of the PK parameters and $\Sigma_0$ represents their prior covariance matrix. The VB algorithm takes the mean-field approximation of the posterior distribution, in this case using a MVN for the distribution over the PK parameters. By choosing this conjugate distribution, an iterative update procedure can be derived to find the mean and precision of the distribution. Since the MRI acquisition parameters $\alpha$ remain fixed throughout, and since the VB updates for the PK parameters ($\theta$) are independent of the motion parameters $T$, we can express $f(T, \theta, \alpha)$ as $f(\theta)$. Now, using Eq (1), due to the assumption of Gaussian noise, we can re-write the likelihood term (for $N$ voxels) from Eq (3) as:

$$P(Y \mid \theta, T, \alpha) = \qquad P(\epsilon = f(\theta) - Y)$$
$$= \left(\frac{\phi}{2\pi}\right)^{N/2} \exp\left(-\frac{1}{2}\left((f(\theta) - Y) \cdot \phi \cdot (f(\theta) - Y)^T\right)\right) \tag{5}$$

Now, combining the likelihood term and the prior distributions, we can write the negative log-posterior ($L = -\log P(\theta \mid Y, T, \alpha)$) as:

$$L = \frac{1}{2}\left((f(\theta) - Y) \cdot \phi \cdot (f(\theta) - Y)^T\right) - \frac{N}{2}\log\phi$$
$$+ \frac{1}{2}(\theta - m)\Sigma(\theta - m)^T \qquad + \quad const \tag{6}$$

In order to minimize $L$, the function $f(\theta)$ is approximated by a first-order Taylor-series expansion about the mean of the posterior (MVN) distribution to give: $f(\theta) = f(m) + J(\theta - m)$, where $J$ denotes the Jacobian (row vector of partial

derivatives), calculated at the current estimate of the mean, i.e. $J_i = \left. \frac{\partial f(\theta)}{\partial \theta_i} \right|_{\theta=m}$.
Using this Taylor-series approximation, and following the procedure described in [12], the updates to the mean and covariance matrix for the PK parameters can be computed as:

$$\Sigma_{new} = aJ^T J + \Sigma_0 \tag{7}$$

$$m_{new}\Sigma_{new} = aJ^T (k + m_{old}J) + m_0\Sigma_0 \tag{8}$$

Here, $k = |f(\theta) - Y|$, and $a$ is a scalar function of the noise precision updated at each iteration. In addition, after each iteration of the VB algorithm, we register the raw data to the best-fit model-prediction available at that iteration using a non-linear logDemons deformation framework [13], and obtain a new estimate of the motion parameters $T$, and thereby a new estimate of the data $Y$.

The final covariance matrix $\Sigma$ can be used to estimate the uncertainties in different derived parameters. In order to estimate the uncertainties for derived parameters $(P)$, such as $K^{trans} = k_{ep} \cdot v_e$ and $r_{kt} = k_{ep} \cdot v_e/t_0$, we use the Taylor series expansion of $P = g(\theta) = g(k_{ep}, v_e, t_0)$, that is: $g(\theta+\partial\theta) = g(\theta)+\nabla g.(\partial\theta)^T$, to approximate the variance of $P$ as:

$$
\begin{aligned}
var(P) = & E\left\{(P - P_{mean})^2\right\} & \approx E\left\{(\nabla g \cdot (\partial\theta)^T)^2\right\} \\
= & (\nabla g) \cdot E\left\{(\partial\theta)^T \cdot (\partial\theta)\right\} \cdot (\nabla g)^T = & (\nabla g) \cdot \Sigma \cdot (\nabla g)^T
\end{aligned}
\tag{9}
$$

Here $\Sigma$ denotes the covariance matrix of the PK parameters obtained as part of the VB estimation. In this manner, the variance of $K^{trans}$ can be calculated as:

$$var(K^{trans}) = [v_e, k_{ep}] \cdot cov(k_{ep}, v_e) \cdot [v_e, k_{ep}]^T \tag{10}$$

Similarly, the variance of $r_{kt} = k_{ep} \cdot v_e/t_0$ can be calculated as:

$$var(r_{kt}) = \left[\frac{v_e}{t_0}, \frac{k_{ep}}{t_0}, \frac{-k_{ep} \cdot v_e}{t_0^2}\right] \cdot cov(k_{ep}, v_e, t_0) \cdot \left[\frac{v_e}{t_0}, \frac{k_{ep}}{t_0}, \frac{-k_{ep} \cdot v_e}{t_0^2}\right]^T \tag{11}$$

## 2.3   Heterogeneity Metrics

In this study, we use some standard measures of spatial heterogeneity [6], [7] and compare them with two newly formulated ones. An examination of the dceMRI data available to us showed that most of the tumours had a clearly defined enhancing rim and intra-tumoural vascular structures. It was evident that the enhancing rim and intra-tumoural vascular structures appeared brighter and enhanced sooner than the neighbouring areas. Thus, apart from looking at only the $K^{trans}$ and $k_{ep}$ maps, we also examined the map of the ratio $r_{kt=}K^{trans}/t_0$ (Fig 1) after additively scaling the values of $t_0$ so that the minimum was set to 1. Physiologically, $r_{kt}$ (having units $min^{-2}$) can be likened to the acceleration experienced by the bolus when it comes in contact with the tissue.

Due to the irregular enhancing vascular structures present in the tumours, we chose to examine the following measures for each parameter map $P$:

1. A measure of the fractal nature of the parameter map was estimated by calculating $S_T = \frac{1}{2}\sum_{x \in T}\left[\sum_{y \in \Omega_x}|P(x) - P(y)|\right]/N_T$. Here $T$ represents the tumour region, $N_T$ is the number of voxels in the tumour region, and $\Omega_x$ represents the six neighbours of the voxel $x$ in 3D.

2. In order to characterize the rim and other intra-tumoural vascular structures that are visible as sharp, high-value edges in the PK parameter maps, we define the product of $P$ with the gradient map of $P$ as a measure of 'sharpness'$= \frac{1}{2}\sum_{x \in T}P(x)\left[\sum_{y \in \Omega_x}(|P(x) - P(y)|)\right]/N_T$.

3. The eigenvalues ($[e_1, e_2, e_3]$, where $e_1 > e_2 > e_3$) of the structure tensor of $P$ can also be used to characterize the linearity or 'planarity' of the parameter map at every position. Since we expect strongly planar parts of the parameter map to be characterized by one dominant eigenvalue, we chose to examine the 'planarity'$= \sum_{x \in T}P(x)\frac{(e_1(x) - (e_2(x) + e_3(x)))}{e_1(x) + e_2(x) + e_3(x)}/N_T$.

We calculate each of these three measures for all chosen parameters ($r_{kt}$, $K^{trans}$ and $k_{ep}$), as well as versions that are weighted by uncertainties associated with them (Fig 2), as calculated from the VB algorithm. In order to compute each parameter map *with* uncertainty, the parameter map was divided point-wise by its corresponding variance (normalized by the average variance across all voxels).

# 3  Experiments and Results

Sixteen patients with locally advanced rectal adenocarcinomas underwent dceMRI scans before treatment with long-course CRT. All the data were acquired on a 1.5T GE scanner using a T1-weighted, gradient-echo, fat-suppressed sequence (LAVA) with TR=4.5ms, TE=2.2ms and flip angle of 12 degrees. Four image acquired before the dynamic series, and at different flip angles (3, 9, 12 and 15 degrees), were used to calculate the $T_{10}$ map. The contrast agent (MultiHance) was injected via a peripheral vein and MRI volumes with resolution $1 \times 1 \times 2\,mm^3$ were acquired every 12 seconds for the next 5 minutes.

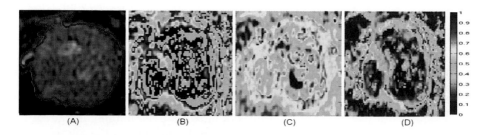

**Fig. 1.** The anatomical image showling the outline of the tumour (A), the $k_{ep}$ map in $min^{-1}$ (B), the $K^{trans}$ map in $min^{-1}$ (C) and the $r_{kt}$ map in $min^{-2}$ (D) for a rectal adenocarcinoma.

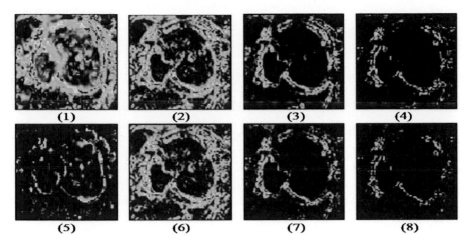

**Fig. 2.** The $r_{kt}$ map for a tumour (1), the map showing $S_T$ (2), sharpness (3) and planarity (4). The normalized variance map of $r_{kt}$ (5) is then used to weight each of the other three maps: $S_T$ (6), sharpness (7) and planarity (8). The display ranges are scaled between the minimum and the maximum values for each parameter map.

An expert radiologist segmented the tumour on high-resolution T2-weighted volumes acquired before the dynamic sequence. This volume was rigidly registered to the first volume of the dynamic scan, and the motion-correction and VB parameter estimation algorithm was applied to a rectangular ROI containing the tumour delineated by the radiologist. In order to compare the predictive values of all the measures of heterogeneity (computed within the segmented tumour), they were compared with the modified Tumour Regression Grade (mTRG) for each patient, calculated after resection at eight weeks [14]. According to the mTRG, eight of the sixteen patients were found to be partial responders (mTRG= 2), while the other eight were found to be non-responders (mTRG= 3).

The ability of each heterogeneity measure to predict response was statistically evaluated in two ways: (1) By computing the $p$-value between the quantities measured for the responder and non-responder groups; (2) Leave-one-out validation (LOOV) – each sample was classified (by fitting a multivariate normal density to each group) using all other samples as the training data, and the average proportion of samples that were mis-classified was recorded (Table 1).

The heterogeneity measures were also compared with the mean and standard deviations of each parameter (across all voxels), in order to evaluate the importance of using spatial distributions as opposed to summary values. The parameter, $r_{kt}$ was found to be the best predictor of response, showing a significant ($p < 0.05$) difference between responders and non-responders for the mean, $S_T$, sharpness and planarity measures (Fig 3). Furthermore, all the measures of spatial heterogeneity showed consistently better results than the corresponding mean and standard deviation, and would remain significant even after correcting for multiple comparisons. It is also clear from Table 1, that the inclusion of

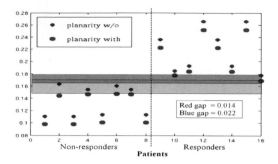

**Fig. 3.** Plots for the measured 'planarity' in the $r_{kt}$ map across all 16 patients. The red dots indicate the values obtained *without* incorporating uncertainty, and the red gap is the minimum difference between responders and non-responders for the same. The blue dots indicate the values obtained *with* uncertainty, and the blue gap is the minimum difference between responders and non-responders for the same.

**Table 1.** Statistical measures for the difference between the responder ($n = 8$) and non-responder ($n = 8$) groups for five measures using three PK parameters. Each measure is calculated on each parameter map with and without taking uncertainty into account. LOOV represents the proportion of samples mis-classified during leave-one-out validation. The minimum value in each row is indicated in bold.

| | | Mean | | St-Dev | | $S_T$ | | Sharpness | | Planarity | |
|---|---|---|---|---|---|---|---|---|---|---|---|
| **Uncertainty →** | | w/o | with | w/o | with | w/o | with | w/o | with | w/o | with |
| $k_{ep}$ | $p$-value | 0.10 | 0.09 | 0.21 | 0.16 | 0.13 | 0.10 | 0.09 | ***0.08*** | 0.12 | 0.10 |
| | LOOV | 0.52 | ***0.43*** | 0.61 | 0.53 | 0.51 | 0.48 | 0.46 | 0.43 | 0.50 | 0.46 |
| $K^{trans}$ | $p$-value | 0.07 | 0.05 | 0.13 | 0.11 | 0.04 | 0.03 | 0.04 | ***0.02*** | 0.09 | 0.07 |
| | LOOV | 0.42 | 0.38 | 0.48 | 0.41 | 0.24 | 0.21 | 0.25 | ***0.19*** | 0.38 | 0.33 |
| $r_{kt}$ | $p$-value | 0.04 | 0.03 | 0.08 | 0.07 | 0.03 | 0.02 | 0.01 | 0.01 | 0.004 | ***0.002*** |
| | LOOV | 0.28 | 0.25 | 0.41 | 0.38 | 0.25 | 0.20 | 0.14 | 0.10 | 0.10 | ***0.08*** |

uncertainty in the calculations of different measures consistently improves the ability of each measure to distinguish between responders and non-responders.

## 4   Conclusion

The results indicate that spatial heterogeneity of PK parameters in general, and the new biomarker $r_{kt} = K^{trans}/t_o$ in particular, show very promising potential for predicting response to therapy on the basis of only the pre-therapy dceMRI scan. The results also show that the inclusion of uncertainty in the calculation of heterogeneity measures causes a marked improvement in their ability to distinguish between responders and non-responders to CRT. In future, this model will also be tested with $v_p$ as part of the PK model.

# References

1. Zahra, M.A., Hollingsworth, K.G., Sala, E., Lomas, D.J., Tan, L.T.: Dynamic contrast-enhanced MRI as a predictor of tumour response to radiotherapy. The Lancet Oncology 8(1), 63–74 (2007)
2. He, D., Ma, D., Jin, E.: Dynamic MRI-derived parameters for hot and cold spots: correlation with breast cancer histopathology. Journal of the Balkan Union of Oncology 17(1), 57–64
3. Loncaster, J.A., Carrington, B.M., Sykes, J.R., Jones, A.P., Todd, S.M., Cooper, R., Buckley, D.L., Davidson, S.E., Logue, J.P., Hunter, R.D., West, C.M.: Prediction of radiotherapy outcome using dynamic contrast enhanced MRI of carcinoma of the cervix. Int. J. Radiat. Oncol. Biol. Phys. 54(3), 759–767 (2002)
4. Bhushan, M., Schnabel, J.A., Risser, L., Heinrich, M.P., Brady, J.M., Jenkinson, M.: Motion correction and parameter estimation in dceMRI sequences: application to colorectal cancer. In: Fichtinger, G., Martel, A., Peters, T. (eds.) MICCAI 2011, Part I. LNCS, vol. 6891, pp. 476–483. Springer, Heidelberg (2011)
5. Buonaccorsi, G.A., Roberts, C., Cheung, S., Watson, Y., Davies, K., Jackson, A., Jayson, G.C., Parker, G.J.M.: Tracer kinetic model-driven registration for dynamic contrast enhanced {MRI} time series. In: Duncan, J.S., Gerig, G. (eds.) MICCAI 2005. LNCS, vol. 3749, pp. 91–98. Springer, Heidelberg (2005)
6. Yang, X., Knopp, M.V.: Quantifying tumor vascular heterogeneity with dynamic contrast-enhanced magnetic resonance imaging: a review. Journal of Biomed. and Biotech., 732–848 (2011)
7. O'Connor, J.P.B., Rose, C.J., Jackson, A., Watson, Y., Cheung, S., Maders, F., Whitcher, B.J., Roberts, C., Buonaccorsi, G.A., Thompson, G., Clamp, A.R., Jayson, G.C., Parker, G.J.M.: DCE-MRI biomarkers of tumour heterogeneity predict CRC liver metastasis shrinkage following Bevacizumab and FOLFOX-6. Br. J. Cancer 105, 139–145 (2011)
8. McPhee, K.C.: Delayed Bolus Arrival Time with High Molecular Weight Contrast Agent, an Indicator of Necrosis. Proc. Intl. Soc. Mag. Reson. Med. 20 (2012)
9. Garpebring, A., Brynolfsson, P., Yu, J., Wirestam, R., Johansson, A., Asklund, T., Karlsson, M.: Uncertainty estimation in dynamic contrast-enhanced MRI. Magn. Reson. in Med. 2, 1–11 (2012)
10. Tofts, P.S., Brix, G., Buckley, D.L., Evelhoch, J.L., Henderson, E., Knopp, M.V., Larsson, H.B., Lee, T.Y., Mayr, N.A., Parker, G.J., Port, R.E., Taylor, J., Weisskoff, R.M.: Estimating kinetic parameters from dynamic contrast-enhanced T(1)-weighted MRI of a diffusable tracer: standardized quantities and symbols. J. Magn. Reson. Imaging. 10(3), 223–232 (1999)
11. Orton, M.R., D'Arcy, J.A., Walker-Samuel, S., Hawkes, D.J., Atkinson, D., Collins, D.J., Leach, M.O.: Computationally efficient vascular input function models for quantitative kinetic modelling using DCE-MRI. Physics in Medicine and Biology 53, 1225–1239 (2008)
12. Chappell, M., Groves, A., Whitcher, B., Woolrich, M.: Variational Bayesian Inference for a Nonlinear Forward Model. IEEE Transactions on Signal Processing 57, 223–236 (2009)
13. Vercauteren, T., Pennec, X., Perchant, A., Ayache, N.: Symmetric log-domain diffeomorphic registration: A demons-based approach. In: Metaxas, D., Axel, L., Fichtinger, G., Székely, G. (eds.) MICCAI 2008, Part I. LNCS, vol. 5241, pp. 754–761. Springer, Heidelberg (2008)
14. Bateman, A.C., Jaynes, E., Bateman, A.: Rectal cancer staging post neoadjuvant therapy–how should the changes be assessed? Histopathology 54, 713–721 (2009)

# Contrast-Independent Liver-Fat Quantification from Spectral CT Exams

Paulo R.S. Mendonça[1], Peter Lamb[1], Andras Kriston[2],
Kosuke Sasaki[3], Masayuki Kudo[3], and Dushyant V. Sahani[4]

[1] GE Global Research, One Research Circle, Niskayuna, NY 12309, USA
[2] GE Healthcare, Szikra u.2, Szeged, 6725, Hungary
[3] GE Healthcare Japan, 4-7-127, Asahigaoka, Hino-shi, Tokyo, Japan
[4] Massachusetts General Hospital, 55 Fruit St., Boston, MA 02114, USA
{mendonca,peter.lamb,a.kriston,kosuke.sasaki,
masayuki.kudo}@ge.com, dsahani@partners.org

**Abstract.** The diagnosis and treatment of fatty liver disease requires accurate quantification of the amount of fat in the liver. Image-based methods for quantification of liver fat are of increasing interest due to the high sampling error and invasiveness associated with liver biopsy, which despite these difficulties remains the gold standard. Current computed tomography (CT) methods for liver-fat quantification are only semi-quantitative and infer the concentration of liver fat heuristically. Furthermore, these techniques are only applicable to images acquired without the use of contrast agent, even though contrast-enhanced CT imaging is more prevalent in clinical practice. In this paper, we introduce a method that allows for direct quantification of liver fat for both contrast-free and contrast-enhanced CT images. Phantom and patient data are used for validation, and we conclude that our algorithm allows for highly accurate and repeatable quantification of liver fat for spectral CT.

## 1 Introduction

Accurate quantification of liver fat is of utmost importance for the diagnosis, characterization, and treatment of fatty liver disease [2]. This need is highlighted since early diagnosis can prevent the onset of more serious liver diseases and associated health risks [12], and even reverse forms of fatty liver disease [1]. Furthermore, concentration of liver fat is an important clinical consideration in liver resection [6].

Although liver biopsy is still accepted as the gold standard for liver-fat quantification, results are often disputed due to sampling error. Non-invasive imaging with magnetic resonance (MR), ultrasound (US), and computed tomography (CT), therefore, is of increasing interest [11]. Of these three modalities, MR is most often cited as the superior choice for liver-fat quantification [6,9]. However, alternatives to MR are desired since it is a costly and time-consuming exam [9]. The use of US in liver-fat quantification is disputed due to prevalent concerns about inexact quantification methods and inter-observer and inter-equipment reproducibility of results [2,13].

Three techniques currently exist for the quantification of liver fat with CT, and all rely on the assumption of an approximate inverse relationship between liver-fat content and liver attenuation [13]. The first method is the direct measurement of liver attenuation

K. Mori et al. (Eds.): MICCAI 2013, Part I, LNCS 8149, pp. 324–331, 2013.

in Hounsfield units (HU). The second and third techniques compute the average HU value of the liver and of the spleen, and then compute differences (liver minus spleen) or ratios (typically, spleen to liver). The use of the spleen, however, has not necessarily proven to be a better metric than direct measurement of liver attenuation [6].

The key limitation of these three methods is that they are impractical for contrast-enhanced CT acquisitions [6], where the presence of contrast agent greatly skews HU values. Spectral CT has offered a solution to the contrast-enhanced limitation via material decomposition, a technique that allows for the virtual removal of contrast from contrast-enhanced images, or *virtual un-enhancement* (VUE) [5,7]. However, liver-fat quantification via VUE ultimately relies on heuristic rules mapping HU values and fat content, and thus remains semi-quantitative in nature [12].

We propose a method for direct and accurate quantification of liver fat using spectral CT. Results on phantom data were compared to the MR IDEAL IQ technique [10], an MR-based method for liver-fat quantification. Results verify repeatability for both contrast-free and contrast-enhanced scans, thereby increasing the clinical usefulness of CT for the treatment of patients with fatty liver disease.

## 2  Material Decomposition via Spectral CT

Spectral CT explores the dependence of linear attenuation coefficient on x-ray energy to generate CT images decomposed into a *material basis*, typically including a water and an iodine component. Key to many material decomposition methods is the assumption that the mix of materials in the human body behaves as an *ideal solution* which, among many equivalent definitions, can be described as a mixture for which a volume-preservation law applies. Under such a model, it can be shown that the linear attenuation coefficient $\mu_L(E)$ at energy $E$ of a mixture of $N$ materials, each with linear attenuation coefficient $\mu_{L,i}(E)$, is given by $\mu_L(E) = \sum_{i=1}^{N} \alpha_i \mu_{L,i}(E)$, where $\alpha_i$ is the volume fraction of the $i$-th material in the mix, such that $\sum_{i=1}^{N} \alpha_i = 1$ and $\alpha_i \geq 0$ [8].

Spectral CT data consists of a pair of water and iodine density images, denoted $\rho_{H_2O}$ and $\rho_I$. This image pair is converted into images in units of linear attenuation at two pre-specified photon energies $E_i$, $i = 1,2$, according to the expression $\mu_L(E_i) = \rho_{H_2O}\mu_{M,H_2O}(E_i) + \rho_I\mu_{M,I}(E_i)$, where $\mu_{M,*}(E_i)$ is the (density-independent) *mass attenuation coefficient* of material "$*$" at energy $E_i$, readily obtained from standardized tables [4]. For a fixed pair of photon energies $E_j$, $j = 1,2$, we define $\mu_{L,*} = (\mu_{L,*}(E_1), \mu_{L,*}(E_2))$ for an arbitrary material "$*$". For a mix with materials $i = 1,2,3$, we have

$$\begin{bmatrix} \mu_{L,1} & \mu_{L,2} & \mu_{L,3} \\ 1 & 1 & 1 \end{bmatrix} \begin{bmatrix} \alpha_1 \\ \alpha_2 \\ \alpha_3 \end{bmatrix} = \begin{bmatrix} \mu_L \\ 1 \end{bmatrix} \quad \text{subject to } 0 \leq \alpha_i \leq 1, i = 1,2,3. \tag{1}$$

The complex compositional makeup of organs and tissues in the human body imposes great difficulties for material decomposition methods that can cope with only two or three materials in the material basis. This is particularly relevant for CT-based liver-fat quantification, in which fat, blood, liver tissue, and contrast agent are present. To address this problem, we propose an algorithm consisting of a sequence of two independent material decompositions of spectral CT data.

# 3   Algorithms and Methods

The input for the proposed liver-fat quantification algorithm can be either contrast-free or contrast-enhanced spectral CT data. In the contrast-enhanced case, *virtual un-enhancement* [5,7] is applied to produce images from which the effect of contrast enhancement has been digitally removed. In the contrast-free case, the VUE step is skipped and fat quantification can be directly performed.

## 3.1   Virtual Un-Enhancement of the Liver

To achieve consistency between contrast-free and contrast-enhanced results, we apply an algorithm for *virtual un-enhancement* (VUE) [5,7] to contrast-enhanced data. VUE produces images from which the effect of contrast enhancement has been removed. This is achieved by applying (1) using fat, blood, and contrast agent as the material triplet. General VUE methods make use of a non-negativity constraint over the parameters $\alpha_i$ in (1) as an indicator to select, among a large number of material triplets, which one is most adequate to represent the input data at a given voxel. For an appropriate selection, the condition $0 \leq \alpha_i \leq 1$, $i = 1, 2, 3$ should be immediately satisfied. Since the focus of our application is on liver-fat quantification, we are not concerned about representing materials such as bone or calcifications, which are typical confounding factors for general VUE methods. Moreover, we may also disregard the constraint $\alpha_i \geq 0$ introduced in [8]. In the specific context of liver-fat quantification, and assuming a fat ($i = 1$), blood ($i = 2$), and contrast agent ($i = 3$) material triplet, the violation of this constraint may in fact be expected. Healthy liver tissue, for example, has a higher attenuation than that of blood, in which case the equations $\sum_{i=1}^{3} \alpha_i \mu_{L,i}(E_j) = \mu_L(E_j)$ and $\sum_{i=1}^{3} \alpha_i = 1$, for photon energies $E_1$ and $E_2$, can only be satisfied if $\alpha_1$ is negative. Furthermore, the presence of noise may result in the above equations yielding a slightly negative value for $\alpha_3$ in the case of contrast-free exams.

Once the decomposition in (1) is completed and the coefficients $\alpha_i$, $i = 1, 2, 3$ are obtained, we proceed as in [7] and *replace* the contrast agent component of a voxel by its equivalent volume in blood, thereby producing a final VUE image with linear attenuation coefficients $\mu_L'(E_j)$ given by $\mu_L'(E_j) = \alpha_1 \mu_{L,1}(E_j) + (\alpha_2 + \alpha_3)\mu_{L,2}(E_j)$, for photon energies $E_j$, $j = 1, 2$. Graphically, this corresponds to the projection operation indicated by the arrow mapping "Input data" to "VUE" depicted in Fig. 1.

## 3.2   Fat Quantification of the Liver

For contrast-free spectral CT data, or for contrast-enhanced spectral CT data after the application of VUE, fat quantification is performed through dual-material decomposition using fat and healthy liver tissue as the material pair. The energy-dependent linear attenuation coefficient of healthy liver tissue is not directly available from standardized tables, and we therefore obtained it experimentally. Note that this is an off-line process, executed only once prior to algorithm implementation, and the resulting attenuation coefficient is valid for any input clinical data. To obtain the coefficient of healthy liver tissue, we first observed that the contrast-free (or VUE) attenuation of healthy liver tissue is accurately represented as a point along the line connecting the linear attenuations of fat and blood, as shown in Fig. 2. We then manually selected several regions of interest (ROIs) of healthy livers from images in our patient dataset. The linear attenuation coefficients at energies $E_j$, $j = 1, 2$ for the data of the selected ROIs was extracted, resulting in a set $\{\mu_{\text{L,liver}}^k, k = 1, \ldots, K\}$, where $K$ is the total number of voxels within the ROIs. Finally, we solve the simple convex optimization problem

$$\mu_{\text{L,liver}} = \arg\min_{\mu_{\text{L}}} \sum_{k=1}^{K} \|\mu_{\text{L}} - \mu_{\text{L,liver}}^k\|^2 \tag{2a}$$

$$\text{subj.} \quad \begin{vmatrix} \mu_{\text{L,fat}} & \mu_{\text{L,blood}} & \mu_{\text{L}} \\ 1 & 1 & 1 \end{vmatrix} = 0 \tag{2b}$$

yielding $\mu_{\text{L,liver}}$ (which corresponds to the large green point shown in Fig. 2). The basic cost function in (2a) favors estimates of $\mu_{\text{L,liver}}$ that are good approximations for the training data, and the constraint on the determinant of the $3 \times 3$ matrix in (2b) enforces that the points corresponding to the linear attenuations of fat, blood, and liver at energies $E_j$, $j = 1, 2$ are indeed aligned.

By imposing the constraint expressed in (2b), we can perform fat quantification on contrast-free (or VUE) data through dual-material decomposition, and the liver-fat quantification problem is now formulated as

$$\begin{bmatrix} \mu_{\text{L},1} & \mu_{\text{L,liver}} \\ 1 & 1 \end{bmatrix} \begin{bmatrix} \alpha_1 \\ \alpha_{\text{liver}} \end{bmatrix} = \begin{bmatrix} \mu_{\text{L}} \\ 1 \end{bmatrix} \tag{3}$$

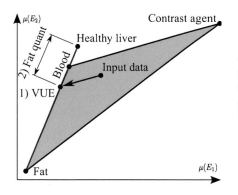

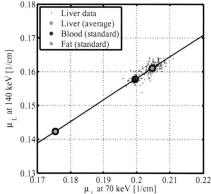

**Fig. 1. Steps of liver-fat quantification algorithm.** For contrast-enhanced spectral CT data, we first apply VUE to digitally remove the effect of contrast enhancement. After VUE, or for contrast-free spectral CT data, fat quantification is performed through dual-material decomposition using fat and healthy liver as the material pair.

**Fig. 2. Linear attenuation coefficient of healthy liver tissue.** Whereas the linear attenuation coefficients of fat (large gold point) and blood (large red point) can be obtained from standardized tables, the linear attenuation coefficient of healthy liver tissue (large green point) had to be derived experimentally.

**Table 1. Fat quantification results on phantom data.** The table shows mean ($\mu$) and standard deviation ($\sigma$) of the results of fat quantification for phantom data. Results of the proposed CT algorithm are quantitatively accurate, performing comparably to the MR IDEAL IQ technique.

| Ground truth | 0% | 10% | 20% | 30% | 50% | 100% |
|---|---|---|---|---|---|---|
| CT % fat ($\mu \pm \sigma$) | $1.1 \pm 1.5$ | $8.8 \pm 2.6$ | $16.8 \pm 2.8$ | $27.0 \pm 2.6$ | $46.5 \pm 3.0$ | $97.2 \pm 1.9$ |
| MR % fat ($\mu \pm \sigma$) | $1.8 \pm 1.7$ | $13.1 \pm 1.7$ | $23.9 \pm 1.6$ | $34.2 \pm 1.1$ | $53.0 \pm 1.2$ | $99.6 \pm 0.9$ |

subject to $0 \leq \alpha_i \leq 1, i = 1$, liver. Note that now we do impose the inequality constraints over the volume fractions $\alpha$, so as to avoid (due to noise) a volume fraction that is either negative or greater than 100%. For VUE data, (3) could be exactly satisfied if it were not for the inequality constraints. For contrast-free data (which does not undergo VUE), the inequality constraints can be violated (and may never be satisfied) since (3) is a linear system of three equations in two variables. Therefore, for both VUE and contrast-free data the final fat quantification result $\alpha = (\alpha_{\text{fat}}, \alpha_{\text{liver}})$ is obtained through the solution of a convex constrained least-squares problem, given by

$$\alpha(x) = \arg\min_{\alpha^*} \left\| \begin{bmatrix} \mu_{\text{L,fat}} & \mu_{\text{L,liver}} \\ 1 & 1 \end{bmatrix} \alpha^* - \begin{bmatrix} \mu_{\text{L}}(x) \\ 1 \end{bmatrix} \right\|^2$$
$$\text{subj.} \sum_{i=1}^{2} \alpha_i^* = 1, \alpha_i^* \geq 0, i = 1, 2. \tag{4}$$

Typically, material concentrations are reported as mass fractions, which we denote by $\beta$. An elementary calculation then yields $\beta_{\text{fat}} = \alpha_{\text{fat}}\rho_{\text{fat}}/(\alpha_{\text{fat}}\rho_{\text{fat}} + \alpha_{\text{liver}}\rho_{\text{liver}})$. The dependency of $\alpha$ on $x$ has been introduced in (4) to highlight that the input data $\mu_{\text{L}}$ (or $\mu_{\text{L}}(x)$) is the pair of linear attenuation coefficients at energies $E_1$ and $E_2$ *at the voxel* $x$, and that the complete algorithm is executed for every voxel within the liver, naturally lending itself towards a parallel implementation. Furthermore, only two inputs in $\mu_{\text{L}}(x)$ are required for each voxel, allowing further speed improvements through the use of lookup tables. Our implementation can process over $1.5 \times 10^7$ voxels (the size of a typical abdominal CT exam) per second on a 3.2 GHz quad-core Intel Xenon system.

## 4    Experiments and Results with Phantoms

Clinical ground truth for liver-fat content is difficult; even biopsy may be misleading, due to sampling errors. Therefore we used a physical phantom with carefully measured fat content as our ground truth for evaluating accuracy. Pig liver (in food) and titrated fat (lard) were mixed homogeneously to simulate fatty liver with concentrations of 0%, 10%, 20%, 30%, 50%, and 100% fat (by mass) and scanned using a GE Discovery CT750 HD scanner. For comparison, two MR scans were also performed using a GE Discovery MR750W and the commercially available IDEAL IQ technique [10], which provides a quantitative assessment of triglyceride fat content in the liver.

Fat quantification results for the phantom data using our algorithm are shown in Table 1. MR results using the IDEAL IQ technique are also presented for comparison.

While the MR results have a slightly smaller variance, our CT results have a smaller bias. Note that MR-based fat quantification methods, such as IDEAL IQ, face a number of confounding factors such as $T_1$ bias, $T_2^*$ decay, multiple fat peaks, noise bias, and eddy currents [3]. Furthermore, these techniques actually measure proton density fat fraction, which is correlated, but not equivalent, to true mass fat fraction. With this in mind, our results indicate that the proposed algorithm can match the performance of MR-based fat quantification methods, thereby increasing the clinical utility of CT.

## 5   Experiments and Results with Clinical Data

Study protocol was reviewed and approved by an institutional review board in Kinki University Hospital (Osaka-sayama City, Osaka, Japan) and informed consent was obtained from all participants. Spectral CT imaging was performed using a GE Discovery CT750 HD scanner on fifty patients with various stages of fatty liver disease. Multiphase scans consisting of contrast-free and contrast-enhanced (at the arterial, portal venous, and delayed) phases were acquired. Note that all patients underwent contrast-free scanning, but not all contrast-enhanced phases of scanning (13 patients underwent arterial phase scanning, 50 patients underwent portal venous phase scanning, and 40 patients underwent delayed phase scanning). The proposed algorithm was run on all

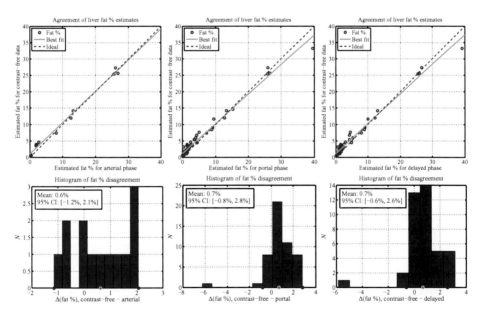

**Fig. 3. Repeatability of clinical liver-fat quantification results.** Top row: Scatterplots of liver-fat quantification results. Each red circle is the average liver-fat % reported by our algorithm for the contrast-free phase plotted against a particular contrast-enhanced phase. The dotted blue line is the region of perfect agreement. The solid green line is a fit to our results. Bottom row: Histograms of differences between the contrast-free and contrast-enhanced fat quantification results, with mean (green circle) and 95% confidence intervals (red circles) reported.

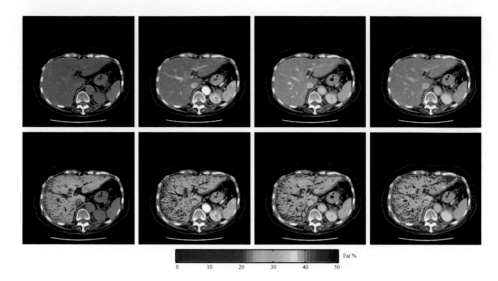

**Fig. 4. Overlay of fat quantification results.** Top row: From left to right, registered CT images of non-contrast, arterial, portal venous, and delayed phases of a liver exam. Bottom row: Overlay of fat % maps obtained from the proposed algorithm, showing consistent fat quantification results across all phases of imaging. Images are roughly aligned, but not fully registered.

multi-phase images, and liver-fat quantification results were aggregated on a 3D-basis for the voxels of the liver. Patient data is courtesy of Prof. Takamichi Murakami (Kinki University: Osaka-sayama City, Osaka, Japan).

Naturally, the concentration of hepatic fat of a given patient does not change with the injection of contrast agent. As shown in Fig. 3, all but one of the estimated fat concentrations for the contrast-enhanced scans are within $\pm 3$ %, in absolute terms, of the estimated fat concentration for the contrast-free scans. (The single exception comes from an exam severely corrupted by metal artifacts.) This demonstrates a key benefit of the present work: The consistent ability to estimate fat concentration regardless of the presence of contrast agent or the phase of imaging. As shown in Fig. 4, our algorithm produces consistent results across all phases of imaging. This naturally allows clinicians to incorporate our algorithm into any stage of their liver imaging workflow. Furthermore, fat % maps such as the ones displayed in Fig. 4 allow for easy visualization of the spatial distribution of fat content in the liver, which can greatly aid in procedures such as biopsy and surgery planning.

## 6   Conclusion

In this paper, we have presented a novel method for the accurate and repeatable quantification of liver fat using spectral CT. The innovation of this work lies in a sequential approach for material decomposition, which allows for liver-fat quantification for both contrast-free and contrast-enhanced images. We validate our algorithm with phantom data, which demonstrates absolute quantitative accuracy, and clinical data, which demonstrates the repeatability of the algorithm across multi-phase imaging. Results indicate that our algorithm has the potential to improve the utility of CT — and perhaps even obviate the need for biopsy — for the diagnosis, characterization, and treatment of fatty liver disease. Future work will extend the capabilities of the algorithm to allow for the detection and characterization of iron deposition, thus providing a more comprehensive tool for the analysis of patients with fatty liver disease.

# References

1. Asano, K., Bayram, E., Yu, H., Reeder, S.B.: Quantitative fat imaging for evaluating diffuse liver diseases. In: SignaPULSE, pp. 75–78. GE Healthcare (2011)
2. Duman, D., Celikel, C., Tüney, D., Imeryüz, N., Avsar, E., Tözün, N.: Computed tomography in nonalcoholic fatty liver disease. Digestive Diseases and Sciences 51(2), 346–351 (2006)
3. Hu, H.H., Börnert, P., Hernando, D., Kellman, P., Ma, J., Reeder, S., Sirlin, C.: ISMRM workshop on fat-water separation: Insights, applications and progress in MRI. Magnetic Resonance in Medicine 68(2), 378–388 (2012)
4. Hubbell, J.H., Seltzer, S.M.: Tables of X-ray mass attenuation ceofficients and mass energy-absorption coefficients. Technical Report NISTIR 5632, National Institute of Standards and Technology, Gaithersburg, MD, USA (May 1995)
5. Johnson, T.R.C., Krauß, B., Sedlmair, M., Grasruck, M., Bruder, H., Morhard, D., Fink, C., Weckbach, S., Lenhard, M., Schmidt, B., Flohr, T., Reiser, M.F., Becker, C.R.: Material differentiation by dual energy CT: Initial experience. European Radiology 17(6), 1510–1517 (2007)
6. Kodama, Y., Ng, C.S., Wu, T.T., Ayers, G.D., Curley, S.A., Abdalla, E.K., Vauthey, J.N., Charnsangavej, C.: Comparison of CT methods for determining the fat content of the liver. Am. J. Roentgenol. 188(5), 1307–1312 (2007)
7. Maddah, M., Mendonça, P.R.S., Bhotika, R.: Physically meaningful virtual unenhanced image reconstruction from dual-energy CT. In: IEEE Int. Symposium on Biomedical Imaging: From Nano to Macro, Rotterdam, The Netherlands (April 2010)
8. Mendonça, P.R.S., Bhotika, R., Thomsen, B.W., Licato, P.E., Joshi, M.C.: Multi-material decomposition of spectral CT images. In: SPIE Medical Imaging, San Diego, CA, USA, vol. 7622, pp. 76221W–76221W-9 (February 2010)
9. Patel, K.D., Abeysekera, K.W.M., Marlais, M., McPhail, M.J.W., Thomas, H.C., Fitzpatrick, J.A., Lim, A.K.P., Taylor-Robinson, S.D., Thomas, E.L.: Recent advances in imaging hepatic fibrosis and steatosis. Eur. J. Gastr. Hepat. 5(1), 91–104 (2011)
10. Reeder, S.B., Robson, P.M., Yu, H., Shimakawa, A., Hines, C.D.G., McKenzie, C.A., Brittain, J.H.: Quantification of hepatic steatosis with MRI: The effects of accurate fat spectral modeling. J. Magn. Reson. Imaging. 29(6), 1332–1339 (2009)
11. Sanai, F.M., Keeffe, E.B.: Liver biopsy for histological assessment: The case against. Saudi J. Gastroenterol. 16(2), 124–132 (2010)
12. Sanyal, A.J.: American Gastroenterological Association. AGA technical review on nonalcoholic fatty liver disease. Gastroenterology 123(5), 1705–1725 (2002)
13. Schwenzer, N.F., Springer, F., Schraml, C., Stefan, N., Machann, J., Schick, F.: Non-invasive assessment and quantification of liver steatosis by ultrasound, computed tomography and magnetic resonance. J. Hepatology 51(3), 433–445 (2009)

# Semi-automated Virtual Unfolded View Generation Method of Stomach from CT Volumes

Masahiro Oda[1], Tomoaki Suito[1], Yuichiro Hayashi[2], Takayuki Kitasaka[3],
Kazuhiro Furukawa[4], Ryoji Miyahara[4], Yoshiki Hirooka[5], Hidemi Goto[4],
Gen Iinuma[6], Kazunari Misawa[7], Shigeru Nawano[8], and Kensaku Mori[2,1]

[1] Graduate School of Information Science, Nagoya University
[2] Information and Communications Headquarters, Nagoya University
[3] School of Information Science, Aichi Institute of Technology
[4] Graduate School of Medicine, Nagoya University
[5] Department of Endoscopy, Nagoya University Hospital
[6] National Cancer Center
[7] Aichi Cancer Center
[8] International University of Health and Welfare Mita Hospital

**Abstract.** CT image-based diagnosis of the stomach is developed as a new way of diagnostic method. A virtual unfolded (VU) view is suitable for displaying its wall. In this paper, we propose a semi-automated method for generating VU views of the stomach. Our method requires minimum manual operations. The determination of the unfolding forces and the termination of the unfolding process are automated. The unfolded shape of the stomach is estimated based on its radius. The unfolding forces are determined so that the stomach wall is deformed to the expected shape. The iterative deformation process is terminated if the difference of the shapes between the deformed shape and expected shape is small. Our experiments using 67 CT volumes showed that our proposed method can generate good VU views for 76.1% cases.

**Keywords:** Stomach, virtual unfolding, CT image.

## 1 Introduction

In Japan, the mortality rate of stomach cancer is the second highest among cancer-related mortality [1]. Treatment of stomach cancer in the early stages is crucial. Gastric roentgenography and gastrofiberscopy are currently performed as the diagnostic methods of stomach cancer. But these methods are physically and mentally painful for patients. In recent years, a CT image-based diagnostic method of the stomach has been developed as an alternative choice [2] that utilizes virtual gastroscopic views generated from CT images. Although CT image-based stomach diagnosis systems greatly reduce the inspection time for patients, physicians need to manually change the viewpoints and the viewing directions of the virtual gastroscopic views many times during diagnosis. To reduce this load

K. Mori et al. (Eds.): MICCAI 2013, Part I, LNCS 8149, pp. 332–339, 2013.

of physicians, a virtual unfolded (VU) view of the stomach is suitable for displaying the stomach wall. This view enables physicians to observe the stomach wall at a glance.

Much research has been reported on the VU view generation of hollow organs. Most generate VU views of the colon [3,4]. Because these methods generate views in real-time, their unfolding processes do not follow the physical properties of organ deformation. VU view generation methods of the stomach have been proposed based on surface model [5] and volumetric model [6]. Although these methods simulate realistic deformations, they require the following complicated manual operations: (1) incision line determination, (2) unfolding force determination, and (3) the termination of unfolding processes. Truong et al. [7] automated (2) the unfolding force determination process. However, the results of their method heavily depend on the results of incision line determination. Their method requires many trial-and-error corrections in incision line determination. Suito et al. [8] presented an automated method of (1) the incision line determination process. These researches only automate one of the manual processes. Therefore, these VU view generation methods of the stomach still require complicated manual operations. They are time-consuming and the quality of their generated VU views heavily depends on the skill of the user.

In this paper, we propose a semi-automated method for generating VU views of the stomach from CT volumes. The contribution of this paper is first presentation of semi-automated method that can drastically reduce manual operations in generation of VU views of the stomach. Manual operation required in our method is just specifying two positions on CT images: the cardia and the pylorus. All other processes are automated in our method. We determine the incision line using a previous method [8]. Then a stomach wall model is generated from a stomach wall region extracted from a CT volume. Unfolding forces are added to the model. We newly introduce a method that automatically calculates the direction of the unfolding forces for this. The expected unfolded shape is estimated based on its diameter. Unfolding force is determined so that the stomach wall is deformed to the expected shape. Newmark-$\beta$ [9] method is introduced to simulate elastic deformation of the model. Because the unfolding process is performed iteratively, it must be terminated after appropriate iterations. For the termination of the unfolding process, we define a criterion that evaluates the progress of the unfolding process based on the differences of the shapes between the deformed stomach shape and the expected unfolded shape of the stomach.

## 2    Method

### 2.1    Preprocessing

In the preprocessing step, we extract an air region in the stomach, a stomach wall region, and the centerline of the stomach region from abdominal CT volumes [8]. Then the incision lines are determined using the methods shown in [8]. Since the incision line determination process [8] requires the positions of the cardia and the pylorus, these points are manually specified on CT volumes by mouse-click.

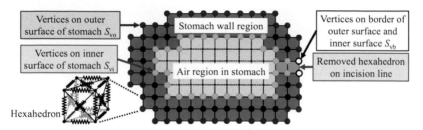

**Fig. 1.** Sets of vertices of hexahedra $S_{\text{vo}}$, $S_{\text{vi}}$, and $S_{\text{vb}}$ on stomach wall model

## 2.2   Definition of Stomach Wall Model

We utilize a previously proposed stomach wall model [7] to simulate the deformation. The model consists of a set of hexahedra covering the stomach wall region. The center of each hexahedron is a voxel in the stomach wall region. The length of each hexahedron edge in the $x, y$, and $z$ directions are $d, d$, and $\hat{d}$ voxels, respectively. Here, $\hat{d} = d \cdot (\text{pixel spacing})/(\text{slice spacing})$. The hexahedra on the incision line are removed from the stomach wall model. Each hexahedron is converted into elastic model by placing mass-points, springs, and dampers on vertices, edges, and diagonal lines [7].

We define three sets of the hexahedra vertices in the stomach wall model: $S_{\text{vo}}$, $S_{\text{vi}}$, and $S_{\text{vb}}$. A set of vertices on the outer and inner surfaces of the stomach wall model is represented as $S_{\text{vo}}$ and $S_{\text{vi}}$, respectively. The inner surface of the stomach wall model is a set of the faces of hexahedra in contact with the air region in the stomach and the incision line. A set of vertices near the incision line, which is included in both $S_{\text{vo}}$ and $S_{\text{vi}}$, are defined as $S_{\text{vb}}$ (Fig. 1).

## 2.3   Determination of Unfolding Force

The unfolding forces are added to the vertices of hexahedra on the incision line, which is unfolded to a planar shape by the forces. We first define an *unfolded plane* on which the stomach wall model is stretched. Then we obtain the *destination points* on the plane, where the vertices on the incision line must reach after unfolding.

**Determination of Unfolded Plane.** Unfolded plane $\Omega$ is uniquely defined by its normal vector $\mathbf{n}_\Omega$ and point $\mathbf{b}_\Omega$ on it as

$$\mathbf{n}_\Omega = (\mathbf{u}_{J/2} - \mathbf{x})/\parallel \mathbf{u}_{J/2} - \mathbf{x} \parallel, \tag{1}$$

$$\mathbf{b}_\Omega = \mathbf{r}_m^{(0)}, \quad m = \text{argmax}_{V_i \in S_{\text{vi}}} \left( \mathbf{r}_i^{(0)} \cdot \mathbf{n}_\Omega \right), \tag{2}$$

where $\mathbf{u}_j \ (j = 1, \ldots, J)$ is a point sequence forming the incision line. $\mathbf{x}$ is a point on a line segment, which connects $\mathbf{u}_1$ and $\mathbf{u}_J$, and satisfies $(\mathbf{x} - \mathbf{u}_1) \cdot (\mathbf{u}_{J/2} - \mathbf{x}) = 0$. $V_i \ (i = 1, \ldots, I)$ is the $i$-th vertex in the stomach wall model. $\mathbf{r}_i^{(\alpha)}$ is the position of $V_i$ after $\alpha$ iterations of the unfolding process. The positions of $\mathbf{n}_\Omega$ and $\mathbf{b}_\Omega$ are shown in Fig. 2(a) and (b).

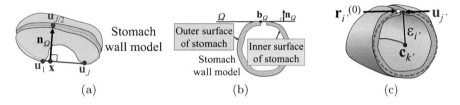

**Fig. 2.** (a) Normal vector $\mathbf{n}_\Omega$, (b) point $\mathbf{b}_\Omega$ on $\Omega$, and (c) radius of stomach $\epsilon_{i'}$ at $V_{i'}$

**Determination of Destination Point.** This process consists of three steps: (Step 1) Calculation of stomach radius, (Step 2) Calculation of base line, and (Step 3) Determination of destination point. The thick and thin parts of the stomach wall must be unfolded widely and narrowly. We compute the width of the unfolded view based on the radius of the stomach at each point on the incision line. Step 1 calculates the radius of the stomach. Step 2 computes the base line around which the stomach is unfolded. Step 3 determines the points where each vertex of the incision line is forced to be moved.

**(Step 1) Calculation of Stomach Radius:** We obtain the radius of the stomach for each vertex existing on the incision line. The point sequence on the centerline of the stomach is described as $\mathbf{c}_k$ $(k = 1, \dots, K)$. $\mathbf{c}_k$ that is closest to $\mathbf{u}_j$ is obtained as $\mathbf{c}_{k'}$ whose index is calculated by

$$k' = \operatorname{argmin}_{1 \le k \le K} \| \mathbf{c}_k - \mathbf{u}_j \| . \tag{3}$$

$V_{i'} \in S_{\mathrm{vb}}$ $(i' = 1, \dots, I')$ is the $i'$-th vertex existing on the incision line on the stomach wall model. The index of $\mathbf{u}_j$, which is closest to $\mathbf{r}_{i'}^{(0)}$ is obtained by

$$j' = \operatorname{argmin}_{1 \le j \le J} \| \mathbf{r}_{i'}^{(0)} - \mathbf{u}_j \| . \tag{4}$$

The radius of the stomach (Fig. 2(c)) at $V_{i'}$ is calculated by

$$\epsilon_{i'} = \| \mathbf{c}_{k'} - \mathbf{u}_{j'} \| . \tag{5}$$

**(Step 2) Calculation of Base Line:** The base line is a long axis of the point set on the incision line projected on the unfolded plane. Each point $\mathbf{u}_j$ is projected onto the closest point $\mathbf{u}'_j$ on the unfolded plane. We apply principal component analysis to $\mathbf{u}'_j$ to obtain the first and second eigenvectors of $\mathbf{u}'_j$. The first and second eigenvectors are $\mathbf{v}'_1$ and $\mathbf{v}'_2$. The direction of the base line is given by

$$\mathbf{v}_1 = \begin{cases} \mathbf{v}'_1 / \| \mathbf{v}'_1 \|, & if \ \mathbf{v}'_1 \cdot (\mathbf{u}'_J - \mathbf{u}'_1) < 0, \\ -\mathbf{v}'_1 / \| \mathbf{v}'_1 \|, & otherwise. \end{cases} \tag{6}$$

The base line is represented as a set of points and defined by

$$\mathbf{p}_j = \begin{cases} \mathbf{u}'_{J/2} - \mathbf{v}_1 \sum_{z=j}^{J/2-1} \| \mathbf{u}'_{z+1} - \mathbf{u}'_z \|, & if \ j = 1, \dots, J/2 - 1, \\ \mathbf{u}'_{J/2}, & if \ j = J/2, \\ \mathbf{u}'_{J/2} + \mathbf{v}_1 \sum_{z=J/2}^{j-1} \| \mathbf{u}'_{z+1} - \mathbf{u}'_z \|, & if \ j = J/2 + 1, \dots, J. \end{cases} \tag{7}$$

The position of $\mathbf{p}_j$ is shown in Fig. 3(a).

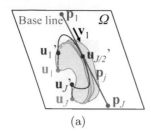
(a)

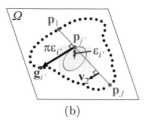
(b)

**Fig. 3.** (a) Base line $\mathbf{p}_j$ calculated from projected incision line $\mathbf{u}'_j$. (b) Destination point $\mathbf{g}_{i'}$ corresponds to $V_{i'}$.

**(Step 3) Determination of Destination Point**: Destination points $\mathbf{g}_{i'}$ are determined based on the base line and the radius of the stomach. $\mathbf{g}_{i'}$ is positioned $\pi\epsilon_{i'}$[mm] away from the base line on the unfolded plane (Fig. 3(b)):

$$\mathbf{g}_{i'} = \begin{cases} \mathbf{p}_{j'} + \pi\epsilon_{i'}\mathbf{v}_2, & if\ \{(\mathbf{u}_{j'} - \mathbf{c}_{k'}) \times (\mathbf{r}_{i'}^{(0)} - \mathbf{c}_{k'})\} \cdot (\mathbf{u}_{j'} - \mathbf{u}_{j'-1}) \geq 0, \\ \mathbf{p}_{j'} - \pi\epsilon_{i'}\mathbf{v}_2, & otherwise, \end{cases} \quad (8)$$

$\mathbf{v}_2$ is unit vector perpendicular to the base line obtained by

$$\mathbf{v}_2 = \begin{cases} \mathbf{v}'_2/ \parallel \mathbf{v}'_2 \parallel, & if\ (\mathbf{v}'_2 \times \mathbf{v}_1) \cdot \mathbf{n}_\Omega < 0, \\ -\mathbf{v}'_2/ \parallel \mathbf{v}'_2 \parallel, & otherwise. \end{cases} \quad (9)$$

**Unfolding Force Determination.** The direction of the unfolding force for $V_{i'}$ calculated as

$$\mathbf{e}_{i'}^{(\alpha)} = \mathbf{g}_{i'} - \mathbf{r}_{i'}^{(\alpha)}, \quad (10)$$

where $\alpha$ is the number of iterations in the iterative unfolding process. $\mathbf{e}_{i'}^{(\alpha)}$ is updated at each iteration step in the unfolding process.

## 2.4    Unfolding Process Based on Elastic Deformation

We deform the stomach wall model by Newmark-$\beta$ method [9] with the forces computed above. The shell-like volumetric model between the inner and outer surfaces shown in Fig. 1 is deformed here. We employ the elastic deformation procedure shown in [7]. This method [7] manually terminated the iterative unfolding process. We propose a criterion to evaluate progress of the unfolding process in order to determine termination of deformation.

We introduce new metric that measures the average distance between $\mathbf{r}_{i'}^{(\alpha)}$ and its destination point. The metric is described as

$$D^{(\alpha)} = \frac{1}{N} \sum_{V_{i'} \in S_{\mathrm{vb}}} \parallel \mathbf{r}_{i'}^{(\alpha)} - \mathbf{g}_{i'} \parallel, \quad (11)$$

where $N$ is the number of vertices included in $S_{\mathrm{vb}}$. If the change of the average distance is small in the iteration of the unfolding process, the stomach is adequately stretched. The iterative unfolding process is terminated if condition

$$\| D^{(\alpha-1)} - D^{(\alpha)} \| \leq \kappa \tag{12}$$

is satisfied.

## 2.5   Unfolded View Generation

After the stomach wall model deformation, we generate an unfolded volume by using relationship between the stomach wall models of pre- and post-deformations. The unfolded view is generated by volume-rendering of the unfolded volume.

## 3   Experiments and Results

We evaluated the proposed method by using 67 CT volumes that were taken from the distended state of the stomach using a foaming agent at two hospitals. The followings are the acquisition parameters of the CT volumes: image size: 512×512 pixels, number of slices: 371-644, pixel spacing: 0.625-0.774 mm, slice

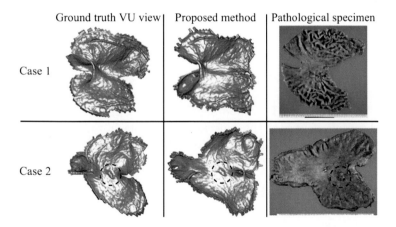

**Fig. 4.** Ground truth VU views, VU views generated by proposed method, and flattened pathological specimens of two cases. Circles indicate positions of a cancer.

**Table 1.** Numbers of good results and numbers of cases that caused overlapping, bending, and broken parts of stomach wall on generated VU views for various $\kappa$

| $\kappa$ | 0.1 | 0.2 | 0.3 | 0.4 | 0.5 | 0.6 | 0.7 | 0.8 | 0.9 | 1.0 |
|---|---|---|---|---|---|---|---|---|---|---|
| Good | 7 | 10 | 10 | 10 | 10 | 9 | 8 | 7 | 7 | 7 |
| Overlapping | 5 | 4 | 2 | 2 | 2 | 2 | 1 | 0 | 0 | 0 |
| Bending | 10 | 7 | 8 | 7 | 6 | 7 | 7 | 7 | 7 | 7 |
| Broken | 1 | 1 | 2 | 2 | 2 | 2 | 3 | 4 | 4 | 4 |

spacing: 0.4-1.0 mm, slice thickness: 0.5-1.0 mm. Parameter values $d = 8$ voxels and $\kappa = 0.5$ were experimentally chosen. The quality of the VU views was visually evaluated by surgeons and engineering researchers by giving *excellent* (All region on VU view is visible from a view point), *good* (One small failure part (overlapping, bending, or broken) exists on VU view), *fair*, and *bad* (Area of VU view where there are not visible from a view point by influence of failure parts is over 30% and 50%, respectively) classifications. The generated VU views were compared with the flattened pathological specimens of the resected stomachs from the patients. We prepared ground truth VU views with manual input of the incision lines and the unfolding forces. The generated VU views are shown in Fig. 4. The numbers of cases rated as top one (*excellent*) and two (*excellent* or *good*) classifications were 26 (38.8%) and 51 (76.1%) cases.

Since the quality of the VU views depends on the value of $\kappa$, we generated VU views by changing $\kappa$ values for 19 cases. Table 1 shows the numbers of good results and cases that caused overlapping, bending, and broken parts of the stomach wall in the VU views.

We compared the computation time in VU view generation of the proposed and a previous [6] methods (Computer: two Intel Xeon 3.33GHz processors, 4GB RAM). It took about 19 seconds for the manual input and 458 seconds for the automated process. In the previous method [6], manual processes including the incision line determination, the unfolding force determination, and the termination of the unfolding processes took about 900 seconds.

## 4    Discussion

From Fig. 4, the VU views generated by our proposed method clearly represent the shapes of a cancer and the stomach wall. Although the shapes of the views generated by the proposed method slightly differ from the ground truth VU views, such surface shapes as the cancer on the stomach wall were well observed. The surface shape is important for finding lesions. These results are applicable to other data judged as "Good". Therefore, the VU views generated using our proposed method are applicable for diagnosis.

From Table 1, the numbers of broken parts in the VU views become larger when large values of $\kappa$ are used. When $\kappa$ is large, the iteration of the unfolding process is terminated even if the stomach wall model is still largely being deformed. In such cases, several parts of the stomach wall model are greatly stretched. Largely stretched parts of the stomach wall model may cause broken parts in the VU views. The numbers of the overlapping parts on the VU view becomes larger for smaller $\kappa$. In this case, the iteration number of the unfolding process becomes large because the iteration continues until the incision lines of the model reach the destination points. In the unfolding process [7], forces are added to the vertices on the outer and inner surfaces of the stomach wall models. The magnitude of these forces increase as iteration progresses. This cause overlapping of the VU views. To minimize broken or overlapping parts, $\kappa = 0.5$ was selected as an optimal value for testing 67 cases.

This paper presented a semi-automated VU view generation method of the stomach. The automation of VU view generation also achieves qualitative stable VU views. Quality of VU views of the previous method heavily depends on experience levels of users. Our method generates VU views with minimal influence of user experience level. It also has potential to explore new diagnostic method of the stomach like as screening examinations of early gastric cancers or planning of gastric cancer surgery.

## 5    Conclusion

This paper presented a semi-automated VU view generation method. The determination of the unfolding forces and the termination of the unfolding were automated in our method. Experiments using 67 CT volumes showed that our proposed method can generate VU views with same quality as manually generated ones. Future work includes the automation of cardia and pylorus detection, unfolding of twisted stomachs, and evaluation using more samples.

**Acknowledgments.** Parts of this research were supported by the MEXT, the JSPS KAKENHI Grant Numbers 21103006, 25242047, and the Kayamori Foundation of Informational Science Advancement.

## References

1. Isobe, Y., Nashimoto, A., Akazawa, K., Oda, I., Hayashi, K., Miyashiro, I., Katai, H., Tsujitani, S., Kodera, Y., Seto, Y., Kaminishi, M.: Gastric cancer treatment in Japan: 2008 annual report of the JGCA nationwide registry. Gastric Cancer 14(4), 301–316 (2011)
2. Furukawa, K., Miyahara, R., Itoh, A., Ohmiya, N., Hirooka, Y., Mori, K., Goto, H.: Diagnosis of the invasion depth of gastric cancer using MDCT with virtual gastroscopy: comparison with staging with endoscopic ultrasound. Am. J. Roentgenology 197(4), 867–875 (2011)
3. Wang, G., McFarland, E.G., Brown, B.P., Vannier, M.W.: GI tract unraveling with curved cross sections. IEEE Trans. Med. Imag. 17(2), 318–322 (1998)
4. Bartroli, A.V., Wegenkittl, R., Konig, A., Groller, E.: Virtual colon unfolding. In: IEEE Visualization (2001)
5. Mori, K., Hoshino, Y., Suenaga, Y., Toriwaki, J., Hasegawa, J., Katada, K.: An improved method for generating virtual stretched view of stomach based on shape deformation. In: Proc. CARS 2001, pp. 425–430 (2001)
6. Mori, K., Oka, H., Kitasaka, T., Suenaga, Y.: A method for generating unfolded views of the stomach based on volumetric image deformation. In: Proc. SPIE Medical Imaging, vol. 5746, pp. 340–351 (2005)
7. Truong, T.D., Kitasaka, T., Mori, K., Suenaga, Y.: A physically-based method for unfolding the stomach from 3D CT images. In: Proc. IASTED Int. Conf. Computer Graphics and Imaging, pp. 231–236 (2008)
8. Suito, T., Oda, M., Kitasaka, T., Iinuma, G., Misawa, K., Nawano, S., Mori, K.: Automated incision line determination for virtual unfolded view generation of the stomach from 3D abdominal CT images. In: Proc. SPIE Medical Imaging, vol. 8315, pp. 83151M-1–7 (2012)
9. Newmark, N.M.: A method of computation for structural dynamics. Journal of Engineering Mechanics, Proc. ASCE 85(EM3), 67–94 (1959)

# Manifold Diffusion for Exophytic Kidney Lesion Detection on Non-contrast CT Images

Jianfei Liu[1], Shijun Wang[1], Jianhua Yao[1], Marius George Linguraru[2], and Ronald M. Summers[1]

[1] Imaging Biomarkers and Computer-Aided Diagnosis Laboratory, Radiology and Imaging Science, National Institutes of Health Clinical Center, Bethesda, MD 20892
[2] Sheikh Zayed Institute for Pediatric Surgical Innovation, Childrens National Medical Center, Washington, DC 20010

**Abstract.** Kidney lesions are important extracolonic findings at computed tomographic colonography (CTC). However, kidney lesion detection on non-contrast CTC images poses significant challenges due to low image contrast with surrounding tissues. In this paper, we treat the kidney surface as manifolds in Riemannian space and present an intrinsic manifold diffusion approach to identify lesion-caused protrusion while simultaneously removing geometrical noise on the manifolds. Exophytic lesions (those that deform the kidney surface) are detected by searching for surface points with local maximum diffusion response and using the normalized cut algorithm to extract them. Moreover, multi-scale diffusion response is a discriminative feature descriptor for the subsequent classification to reduce false positives. We validated the proposed method and compared it with a baseline method using shape index on CTC datasets from 49 patients. Free-response receiver operating characteristic analysis showed that at 7 false positives, the proposed method achieved 87% sensitivity while the baseline method achieved only 22% sensitivity. The proposed method showed far fewer false positives compared with the baseline method which makes it feasible for clinical practice.

**Keywords:** Kidney lesion detection, computed tomographic colonography, manifold diffusion, extracolonic finding, Riemannian manifold.

## 1 Introduction

Extracolonic findings on CT colonography (CTC) increase the chance of early detection of high-risk lesions with economic benefits[11]. Kidney lesions are one important extracolonic finding, belonging to C-RADS E2-E4 types[17]. Existing kidney lesion detection methods[8] take advantage of contrast in the intensity values of lesions on contrast-enhanced CT images. For CTC, however, intravenous contrast material is not given since it is not necessary for colonic polyp detection. On non-contrast CTC images, the intensity values of kidneys, lesions, and adjacent organs are similar as shown in Fig. 1a. Lack of texture cues makes the detection task substantially challenging in the image domain.

K. Mori et al. (Eds.): MICCAI 2013, Part I, LNCS 8149, pp. 340–347, 2013.

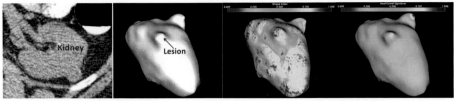

(a) CTC image      (b) Kidney surface      (c) Shape index      (d) Manifold diffusion

**Fig. 1.** Kidney lesion detection on the non-contrast CT. (a) An exophytic lesion is located in the left kidney. (b) The lesion presents as a protuberance on the kidney surface. (c) Shape index fails to identify the lesion because it is noisily distributed on the kidney surface. Blue to red represents small to large values. (d) Manifold diffusion accurately identifies shape changes at the lesion location.

Exophytic kidney lesions are located at kidney edges, and they appear as protuberances on the kidney surface in Fig. 1b. We thus resort to shape analysis approaches to identify lesion-caused protuberances. Shape index[6] is a single-value measurement of local surface topology and widely applied to tumor detection in colon[16] and breast[5]. Fig. 1c shows the distribution of shape index over kidney surface of Fig. 1b. Although shape index values are large at lesion regions and small at flat or concave areas, almost all protrusion surfaces are in red in Fig. 1c, partly due to noise, which introduces many false positives. Geometric noises can be smoothed based on local curvatures[4]. However, over-smoothing easily causes lesion protuberances to vanish. To compensate for this issue, the heat kernel diffusion[13] is often used to extract global shape spectrums by treating models as manifolds in Riemanian space. Semantic geometry features are preserved by choosing small spectrums. Due to this beneficial property, Lai et al.[7] applied this approach to extract geometric features to perform supine and prone colon registration. Unfortunately, high complexity of heat kernel smoothing makes it difficult to create simple feature descriptors for kidney lesion detection.

In this paper, we present a manifold diffusion method to create a compact, multi-scale heat kernel feature for detection and classification of exophytic kidney lesions. Fig. 1d illustrates our manifold diffusion response among the kidney surface. Note that the kidney lesion is located at the region with local maximum response (yellow) in comparison to its neighborhoods (green). In addition, diffusion response varies smoothly over the kidney surface, which is a desirable property to reduce false positives. Our kidney lesion detection framework is built on this diffusion process. Lesion candidates are extracted by the normalized cut algorithm on the vertex-weighted graph with the diffusion response as the weight. The multi-scale diffusion response is also discriminative to classify kidney lesions and reduce false positives. We validated our detection algorithm on CTC datasets from 49 patients and free response receiver operating characteristic analysis showed that the proposed method significantly outperformed shape index approach with high detection accuracy and low false positive rate.

## 2   Methodology

Kidneys are segmented from CTC image using our earlier work[9]. The marching cubes algorithm[10] is then applied to extract the kidney surface, which usually contains 35000-45000 vertices.

### 2.1   Manifold Diffusion

The kidney surface can be treated as a three-dimensional complete Riemannian sub-manifold $M$ of $\mathbb{R}^3$. A diffusion process on $M$ is governed by the heat equation,

$$\left( \frac{\partial}{\partial t} + \Delta_M \right) u(x,t) = 0 \tag{1}$$

where $\Delta_M$ is the Laplace-Beltrami operator[15]. If $M$ has boundaries and $f(0,x) = \delta_x : M \to \mathbb{R}$ denotes an initial heat distribution on $M$, the solution $u(x,t)$ is called the heat distribution at a point $x$ at time $t$ and $\lim_{t \to 0} u(x,t) = f$. Here, $\delta_x$ is the Dirac delta function. For any $M$, there exists a function $k_t(x,y) : \mathbb{R}^+ \times \mathbb{R}^3 \times \mathbb{R}^3 \to \mathbb{R}$, which leads to

$$u(x,t) = \int_M k_t(x,y)f(y)dy \tag{2}$$

$k_t(x,y)$ is called the heat kernel and measures the amounts of the heat transferred from $x$ to $y$ at time $t$. According to graph spectral theory[3], $k_t(x,y)$ can be decomposed as

$$k_t(x,y) = \sum_{i \geq 0} e^{-\lambda_i t} \phi_i(x) \phi_i(y) \tag{3}$$

Here, $\lambda_i$ and $\phi_i$ are, respectively, the $i^{th}$ eigenvalue and the $i^{th}$ eigenfunction of the Laplace-Beltrami operator. The parameter $t$ takes the scale role in the shape analysis as adjusting it can produce a family of $k_t(x,y)$. However, local geometrical descriptor using $k_t(x,y)$ is very complex because it involves both spatial and temporal variables. Instead, we set $x = y$ and create a compact manifold diffusion process by collecting a set of auto-diffusivity functions $\{k_t(x,x)\}_{t>0}$, where $k_t(x,x)$ means the remaining heat at a point $x$ after time $t$. Fig. 2 illustrates manifold diffusion response at different temporal scales. Fine scale response is maximized at the location of a small lesion protrusion (A) in Fig. 2a. The kidney surface with local maximum scale response is gradually shifted to large protrusions at lesions (B) and (C) in Fig. 2a, and eventually stops at two kidney tips in Fig. 2d because they are the most stable protrusions. Therefore, our manifold diffusion process at small temporal scales is a good fit for kidney lesion detection.

Manifold diffusion response is also useful to create semantic shape descriptors for kidney lesion classification. First, the Laplace-Beltrami operator is intrinsically defined on $M$, and the feature descriptor established on this operator is invariant under isometric transformation. In other words, our feature descriptor is insensitive to the variability among kidney lesions. Second, it is a compact

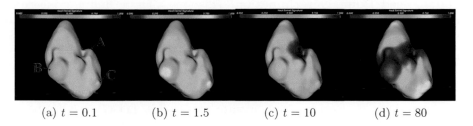

(a) $t = 0.1$       (b) $t = 1.5$       (c) $t = 10$       (d) $t = 80$

**Fig. 2.** Manifold diffusion response at different temporal scales. Here, three kidney lesions marked as A, B, and C are used to illustrate multi-scale diffusion response on their detection.

shape descriptor that can densely measure shape variance on the kidney surface. Third, the feature descriptor is informative, as it keeps all information about the intrinsic geometry of the manifold[15]. Lastly, in contrast to conventional surface smoothing algorithms[4] that cause lesions to fade, the feature descriptor from manifold diffusion is built on the kidney surfaces with original resolutions.

## 2.2 Kidney Lesion Detection and Classification

After manifold diffusion is established, we exploit scale response to assign the vertex weight of the kidney surface graph. Because kidney lesions are highlighted at small temporal scales in Fig. 2, we choose a sequence of fine scale responses to allow for our framework to identify lesions with different sizes. In our implementation, we choose $t \in \{0.1, 0.3, 0.5, 0.8, 1.0, 1.2, 1.5\}$ in Eq. 3. The kidney graph is then partitioned to search for sub-graphs with local maximum scale response, as kidney lesions typically stay in these regions. Fig. 3 summarizes the process of our kidney lesion detection, which consists of four main steps.

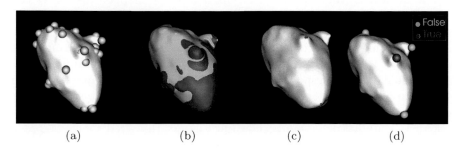

(a)       (b)       (c)       (d)

**Fig. 3.** Process of kidney lesion detection contains four main steps. (a) Seed point determination, (b) graph partition, (c) kidney lesion candidate selection, and (d) lesion detection and classification.

**Step 1: Seed Point Determination.** This step aims to find a sequence of vertices with local maximum diffusion response at each temporal scale level to facilitate graph partitioning. A seed point $v_s$ is determined if it fulfills $k_t(v_s, v_s) = \arg\max_{v \in ring(3)}(k_t(v, v))$, where $ring$ means the neighbors of $v$ on the graph[4]. The detected seed points are illustrated as green points in Fig. 3a.

**Step 2: Graph Partitioning.** Because kidney surface is represented as a graph, the normalized cut algorithm[14] is used to partition it. Let $G = (E, V)$ be the graph with the edge set $E$ and the vertex set $V$. The edge weight is assigned with the sum of scale response difference across a sequence of temporal scales.

$$d(v_1, v_2) = \left( \int_{0.1}^{1.5} (k_t(v_1, v_1) - k_t(v_2, v_2))^2 \right)^{1/2}, (v_1, v_2) \in E \qquad (4)$$

A cut is to find a set of edges $cut(A, B) = \sum_{v_1 \in A, v_2 \in B} d(v_1, v_2)$ to separate $G$ into two disjoint sets A and B with similar scale response values. Normalized cut is computed as

$$Ncut = \frac{cut(A, B)}{assoc(A, V)} + \frac{cut(A, B)}{assoc(B, V)} \qquad (5)$$

where $assoc(A, V) = \sum_{v_1 \in A, v_2 \in V} d(v_1, v_2)$ and $assoc(B, V)$ is similarly defined. Normalized cut is iteratively performed until no graph partitions contain two seed points. Fig. 3b shows the partition results where each sub-graph is represented as a color band.

**Step 3: Candidate Selection.** A partition is regarded as a lesion candidate if its scale response is the local maximum and its area is less than a experimentally determined threshold, $\alpha = 400mm^2$, because the partition includes parts of the lesion surface and the size of a lesion is limited. Fig. 3c illustrates the lesion candidates in red regions.

**Step 4: Lesion Detection and Classification.** We mapped the center point of the lesion candidates to the original CT image. A $10 \times 10 \times 10$ sub-image centered at the mapped point is constructed for computing appearance features. Mean and standard deviation of intensity values as well as speeded up robust feature (SURF) descriptor[1] are used to describe the lesion appearance. Multi-scale manifold diffusion response is used to characterize lesion shape. We combine appearance and shape information to formulate the final feature vector and train the support vector machine classifier[2] using Gaussian radial basis function as the kernel. The final detection is shown in Fig. 3d. Here, red spheres represent true detections and green ones false positives.

## 2.3   Validation Datasets and Methods

The framework for kidney lesion detection was validated on non-contrast CTC images from 49 patients. The slice thickness was 1mm. 25 patients have at least one kidney lesion, and the total number of lesions is 50. 46 of them are situated on the kidney surface. All lesions are marked by an experienced radiologist as the groundtruth. 19 lesions are located in the left kidney, and the remaining 31 are in the right kidney. Their size range is 3.2-40.5mm. Retrospective analyses of CTC images were approved by Office of Human Subjects Research. To better understand our approach, shape index is chosen as the baseline method for its popularity in tumor detection[5,16]. We follow the same strategy described above to find lesion candidates at graph regions with shape index value larger than 0.9.

# 3   Experimental Results

Our training dataset contains 15 patients and the test set 34 patients. There were 14 true kidney lesions in the training set and 36 true lesions in the test set. For our method, there were 18 true detections (TP) (from 13 unique kidney lesions) and 128 false positives (FP) in the training set; 33 TP (31 unique) and 277 FP in the test set. For the baseline method, there were 16 TP (7 unique) and 354 FP in the training set; 76 TP (18 unique) and 1080 FP in the test set. Our method generated 8 false positives per patient while shape index apporach 32 false positives per patient. Shape index also missed many lesions because the areas of their graph partitions are large than $\alpha$ at step 3 in the section 2.2.

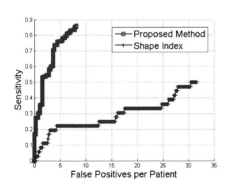

**Fig. 4.** Comparison of FROC curves of the proposed method and the baseline detection method based on shape index

In Fig. 4, we show the free-response receiver operating characteristic (FROC) curves on the test set with and without anatomical guidance. Fig. 4 shows that at 7 FPs, the sensitivity of the proposed method is 86.1% and the baseline method based on shape index is only 22%. These promising results demonstrated that our algorithm can accurately detect kidney lesions from non-contrast CTC images. Note that there were five true kidney lesions missed by the proposed method due to their locations (inside the kidney, not on the surface).

Fig. 5 illustrates kidney lesion detection on images of four patients with kidney lesions. In Fig. 5a, a kidney lesion was located in the left kidney. Our detection strategy identified it with two FPs. FP (B) stayed at the tip of kidney, similar to the lesion (F) in Fig. 5c. FP (C) was close to the renal vein, which was one of the main sources of false positives. Fig. 5b shows a challenging case as the left kidney was improperly segmented. However, our algorithm can still find lesion (D) with only two FPs. FP (E) was caused by the incorrect kidney segmentation. The patient in Fig. 5c has four lesions. Three of them were located in the left kidney, and the remaining one in the right kidney. Our detection algorithm accurately found all of them. There were two lesions in Fig. 5d.

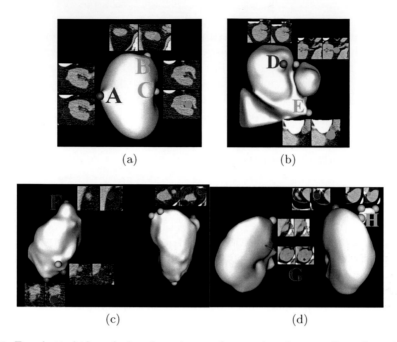

**Fig. 5.** Exophytic kidney lesion detection on four patient images. True detections are labeled in red and false detections in green. Sub-images are also extracted from the original CT to illustrate the detection. In Fig. 5b, inaccurate kidney segmentation contains part of liver (triangular object), and the inferior vena cava (round blob).

Our algorithm detected the one on the right kidney surface, while missed the Lesion (G) indicated by the red arrow internal to the left kidney because of no shape variance on the kidney surface. There were several FPs caused by the renal vein, such as (H). Nevertheless, experimental results demonstrated that our detection algorithm can accurately identify exophytic kidney lesions with a few FPs due to the renal vein, inaccurate kidney segmentation, and kidney tips.

## 4 Conclusion and Future Work

In this work, we developed a novel manifold diffusion method and showed its application to detect exophytic kidney lesions. It treated kidney surfaces as manifolds in the Riemannian space and generated a heat diffusion process on the manifolds by only considering temporal scale changes. Therefore, our manifold diffusion was a compact process, which can assist in kidney lesion detection and classification. The experiments demonstrated that our algorithm outperformed shape index with high detection accuracy and low false positive rate.

In the future, we will be investigating the renal vein atlas to reduce false positives as well as identifying texture and shape characteristics of internal kidney lesions. We are also developing an automatic scale selection metric for manifold diffusion instead of fixing a set of scales. Moreover, we are comparing our method with other shape descriptors, such as shape-DNA[12] and heat kernel smoothing[13].

**Acknowledgement.** This work was supported by the Intramural Research Program of the National Institutes of Health, Clinical Center.

# References

1. Bay, H., Ess, A., Tuytelaars, T., Gool, L.: Surf: Speeded up robust features. computer vision and image understanding. CVIU 110(3), 346–359 (2008)
2. Chang, C., Lin, C.: Libsvm: a library for support vector machines. ACM Trans. Intell Sys. Tech. 2(27), 1–27 (2011)
3. Chung, F.: Spectral Graph Theory (CBMS Regional Conference Series in Mathematics, No. 92). American Mathematical Society (1996)
4. Desbrun, M., Meyer, M., Schrder, P., Barr, A.H.: Implicit fairing of irregular meshes using diffusion and curvature flow (1999)
5. Irishina, N., Moscoso, M., Dorn, O.: Microwave imaging for early breast cancer detection using a shape-based strategy. IEEE Trans. Biomed. Eng. 56(4), 1143–1153 (2009)
6. Koenderink, J., Doorn, A.: Surface shape and curvature scales. Image and Vision Computing 10(8), 557–564 (1992)
7. Lai, Z., Hu, J., Liu, C., Taimouri, V., Pai, D., Zhu, J., Xu, J., Hua, J.: Intra-patient supine-prone colon registration in ct colonography using shape spectrum. In: Jiang, T., Navab, N., Pluim, J.P.W., Viergever, M.A. (eds.) MICCAI 2010, Part I. LNCS, vol. 6361, pp. 332–339. Springer, Heidelberg (2010)
8. Linguraru, M., Wang, S., Shah, F.: et al: Automated noninvasive classification of renal cancer on multi-phase ct. Med. Phys. 38, 5738–5746 (2011)
9. Liu, J., Linguraru, M.G., Wang, S., Summers, R.M.: Automatic segmentation of kidneys from non-contrast ct images using efficient belief propagation. In: SPIE Medical Imaging (2013)
10. Lorensen, W., Cline, H.: Marching cubes: A high resolution 3d surface construction algorithm. In: Computer Graphics, vol. 21, pp. 163–169 (1987)
11. Pickhardt, P., Hanson, M., Vanness, D.: et al: Unsuspected extracolonic findings at screening ct colonography: clinical and economic impact. Radiology 249, 151–159 (2008)
12. Reuter, M., Wolter, F.E., Peinecke, N.: Laplace-beltrami spectra as "shape-dna" of surfaces and solids. Computer-Aided Design 38(4), 342–366 (2006)
13. Seo, S., Chung, M.K., Vorperian, H.K.: Heat kernel smoothing using laplace-beltrami eigenfunctions. In: Jiang, T., Navab, N., Pluim, J.P.W., Viergever, M.A. (eds.) MICCAI 2010, Part III. LNCS, vol. 6363, pp. 505–512. Springer, Heidelberg (2010)
14. Shi, J., Malik, J.: Normalized cuts and image segmentation. IEEE Trans. PAMI 22(8), 888–905 (2000)
15. Sun, J., Ovsjanikov, M., Guibas, L.: A concise and provably informative multi-scale signature-based on heat diffusion. Comp. Graph. Forum 28, 1383–1392 (2008)
16. Yoshida, H., Nappi, J., MacEneaney, P.: et al: Computer-aided diagnosis scheme for detection of polyps at ct colonography. Radio Graphics 22, 963–979 (2002)
17. Zalis, M.E.: et al: Ct colonography reporting and data system: A consensus proposal. Radiology 236, 3–9 (2005)

# Errors in Device Localization in MRI Using Z-Frames

Jeremy Cepek[1,2], Blaine A. Chronik[1,3], and Aaron Fenster[1,2]

[1] Robarts Research Institute, The University of Western Ontario, London, Canada
{jcepek,afenster}@robarts.ca, bchronik@uwo.ca
[2] Biomedical Engineering, The University of Western Ontario, London, Canada
[3] Department of Physics and Astronomy, The University of Western Ontario, London, Canada

**Abstract.** The use of a passive MRI-visible tracking frame is a common method of localizing devices in MRI space for MRI-guided procedures. One of the most common tracking frame designs found in the literature is the z-frame, as it allows six degree-of-freedom pose estimation using only a single image slice. Despite the popularity of this design, it is susceptible to errors in pose estimation due to various image distortion mechanisms in MRI. In this paper, the absolute error in using a z-frame to localize a tool in MRI is quantified over various positions of the z-frame relative to the MRI isocenter, and for various levels of static magnetic field inhomogeneity. It was found that the error increases rapidly with distance from the isocenter in both the horizontal and vertical directions, but the error is much less sensitive to position when multiple contiguous slices are used with slice-select gradient nonlinearity correction enabled, as opposed to the more common approach of only using a single image slice. In addition, the error is found to increase rapidly with an increasing level of static field inhomogeneity, even with the z-frame placed within 10 cm of the isocenter.

**Keywords:** MRI-guided, stereotactic, z-frame, passive tracking.

## 1 Introduction

### 1.1 Background

The use of MRI for guiding interventional or diagnostic tools into human tissues is becoming increasingly prevalent. The choice of MRI as the guiding imaging modality is often due to its ability to produce high-resolution, high contrast images of soft tissues, and its intrinsic 3D acquisition capability: *i.e.* the ability to acquire single or contiguous image slices or image volumes in any arbitrary orientation. MRI allows multiple different tissue contrast mechanisms, the combination of which can provide unique information to radiologists for disease detection and grading. If a mechanical or robotic device is to be used for an MRI-guided procedure, a method of mapping coordinates between MRI space and device space is required. This mapping is generally performed by finding a rigid transformation that relates the two coordinate systems.

A common method of estimating the transform between device and MRI space in MRI-guided procedures is with the use of passive MRI-visible tracking frames. Passive tracking frames employ MRI-visible markers arranged in a known geometric

K. Mori et al. (Eds.): MICCAI 2013, Part I, LNCS 8149, pp. 348–355, 2013.
© Springer-Verlag Berlin Heidelberg 2013

configuration. Once imaged, a relationship between the device and MRI coordinate systems can be established, allowing any point in MRI space to be targeted by the interventional device. One of the tracking frames most commonly used for device localization in MRI is any one of the variations of designs based on the Brown-Roberts-Wells (BRW) frame, initially developed for CT-guided neurosurgical interventions.[1] This frame will hereafter be referred to simply as the 'z-frame'. This frame is attractive for many applications, because a full six degree-of-freedom estimate of a device's pose in MRI coordinates can be obtained using a single image slice of the frame (in principle). However, the nature of geometric distortion in MRI is much different from that in CT, and it is therefore necessary to consider the sources of error in localizing this frame in MRI. Geometric distortion in MRI is highly dependent on the level of magnetic field inhomogeneity (which can be both substantial and unpredictable in the region surrounding a patient's body and near devices containing magnetic materials), as well as the frame's location relative to the scanner's isocenter, which may be unfavorable due to patient positioning.

There are currently several devices in the literature employing the use of a z-frame for registering MRI-guided devices, and several authors have attempted to quantify its performance.[2-6] In [2], DiMaio et al. quantified the tracking accuracy of a z-frame with images acquired at varying slice positions and angles. However, their errors were defined relative to the orientation of the z-frame determined in a baseline image, and therefore give no indication of absolute error in localizing the frame in MRI. They also did not measure localization accuracy at an appreciable distance from the isocenter, which is important for devices with tracking frames positioned external to the patient's body. In [6], Tokuda et al. used a z-frame to register a needle template for MRI-guided transperineal prostate biopsy, and performed tests to quantify the error in z-frame registration; however, they did not consider positioning of the z-frame at a distance from the isocenter along the z-axis (in the LPS patient coordinate system, with the patient positioned head-first supine). Such a configuration is important to consider for applications such as handheld device tracking, as demonstrated by DiMaio et al. [2]. It has also been suggested by Cepek et al. [7] that some clinical MRI scanners may not be able to accurately model the motion of the scanner table, indicating the need to quantify errors in off-isocenter frame localization independently of scanner table motion errors. Tokuda et al. [6] also presented tooltip localization error for a needle lying 100 mm from the center of the z-frame, but this error would not be sensitive to rotational error in the z-axis. Finally, as was the case in [2], the errors reported in [6] were computed relative to the pose estimate of the z-frame in a baseline MRI scan, and therefore do not quantify absolute error. In [8], Tokuda et al. reported absolute error in localizing targets in a phantom using a z-frame, and found an RMS error of 3.7 mm for outer targets and 1.8 mm for inner targets (representative of targets within the prostate capsule). However, their results are only valid for one configuration of the z-frame relative to one specific type of anatomy (prostate). The authors in [4] presented results of needle placement accuracy in MRI using a device employing a z-frame, but these results include other sources of error and cannot be used to predict the error in z-frame registration alone.

In this work, the absolute error in using a z-frame to localize a tooltip in MRI is quantified for: a) varied position of the z-frame relative to the MRI isocenter, and b) various levels of static field inhomogeneity. In addition, the effect of slice-select error due to gradient field nonlinearity is quantified by imaging the z-frame with either a single image slice or multiple contiguous slices with slice-select gradient nonlinearity correction enabled (hereafter referred to as 3D distortion correction). This is achieved by fixing an MRI-visible spherical marker to a holder of known geometry, onto which a z-frame is mounted. The holder allows the spherical marker to be placed at the MRI isocenter for accurate imaging, and for the position of z-frame to be varied relative to the marker in an accurate manner. The estimated position of the spherical marker, as calculated using the z-frame registration, is compared to its true position, which is measured in tri-planar, high-resolution spin echo images.

## 2     Methods

### 2.1     Z-Frame Registration

The z-frame consists of an arrangement of seven MRI-visible cylinders. A single image slice will show seven ellipses, the centroids of which are used for localizing the frame. The frame is shown in Figure 1.

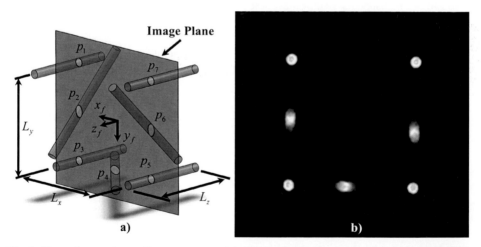

**Fig. 1.** The z-frame: a) coordinate system and image intersection points, b) MR image showing the seven ellipses

The three corresponding points in the frame coordinate system can be found as

$$P_{2_f} = \left[ -\frac{L_x}{2}, L_y \left( \frac{1}{2} - \frac{d_{23}}{d_{13}} \right), L_z \left( -\frac{1}{2} + \frac{d_{23}}{d_{13}} \right) \right], \tag{1}$$

$$P_{4_f} = \left[ L_x \left( \frac{1}{2} - \frac{d_{45}}{d_{35}} \right), \frac{L_y}{2}, L_z \left( -\frac{1}{2} + \frac{d_{45}}{d_{35}} \right) \right], \text{ and} \tag{2}$$

$$P_{6_f} = \left[ \frac{L_x}{2}, L_y \left( -\frac{1}{2} + \frac{d_{67}}{d_{57}} \right), L_z \left( -\frac{1}{2} + \frac{d_{67}}{d_{57}} \right) \right], \tag{3}$$

where $d_{ij}$ is the Euclidean distance between two points $p_i$ and $p_j$, which are the centroids of ellipses identified in the MR images. The transformation between these three points and those in MRI coordinates can be used to locate any point known in frame coordinates in MRI coordinates, or *vice versa*. Due to geometric distortion in the images of the frame, an exact rigid transformation between these points will not generally exist. Thus, a rigid transformation that minimizes the sum of squared distances between corresponding points is sought. Once this rigid transformation is found, any point known in the frame coordinate system can be found in the MRI coordinate system as:

$$P_{mr} = R_f P_f + T_f, \tag{4}$$

where $P_{mr}$ and $P_f$ are the coordinates of a point in the MR and frame coordinate systems, respectively, $R_f$ is a rotation matrix, and $T_f$ is a translation vector.

## 2.2    Experimental Apparatus

A holder was constructed that allows the spherical marker and z-frame to be fixed at precisely-known, discrete distances from each other. Varying the position of the z-frame is possible in both the y and z directions over a 3 x 3 grid of positions. The holder is designed so that, in any configuration, the spherical marker can be positioned at the MRI isocenter for accurate localization, and the z-frame can be imaged at a distance from the isocenter. Note that bed movement was not permitted during imaging, so that errors in z-frame localization due to offsets in the z direction could be quantified. The holder and z-frame were constructed from acetyl homopolymer, and the z-frame and spherical marker were filled with a 1% solution (by volume) of Gd-DTPA (Magnevist, Bayer Healthcare, Berlin, Germany) in distilled water. Localization error is defined as the Euclidean distance between the predicted marker location, computed from the z-frame registration, and its true position as measured in the high-resolution spin echo images. Accordingly, this measure is representative of the error in estimating the location of a tooltip or needle fixed to an interventional device at various distances from the localization frame. The z-frame has a size of Lx = Ly = Lz = 50.8 mm, as defined in Figure 1. The holder is shown in Figure 2.

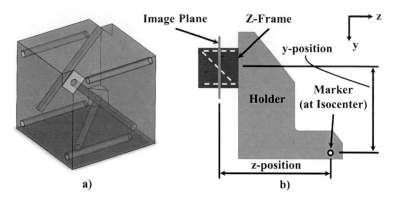

**Fig. 2.** The z-frame testing apparatus: a) CAD model of the z-frame used for the tests, b) setup of the z-frame and spherical marker on the holder. The spherical marker was positioned within 2 cm of the isocenter, and the position of the z-frame was varied in the y and z directions (in the LPS coordinate system for a patient positioned head-first supine).

## 2.3    MRI Acquisitions

The MRI sequence parameters for imaging of the spherical marker were selected to provide high-resolution images of the marker for accurate localization at the isocenter. Those for the z-frame images were chosen to be typical of the types of scans found in the literature for imaging this type of frame, which are usually tuned for fast image acquisition. The effect of uniform static field inhomogeneity was simulated by varying the scanner's center frequency. All images were acquired in a 3T MRI scanner (MR750, GE Healthcare, Milwaukee, WI). The parameters are shown in Table 1.

**Table 1.** MRI parameters used for accuracy test

| Parameter | Spherical Marker | Z-Frame | Units |
|---|---|---|---|
| Sequence Type | Spin echo | Fast gradient recalled echo | - |
| Repetition Time | 350 | 150 | ms |
| Echo Time | 12 | 4 | ms |
| Flip Angle | 90 | 60 | ° |
| Bandwidth | 230 | 244 | Hz/pixel |
| Slice Thickness | 1.5 | 3 | mm |
| Field-of-view | 60 x 60 | 100 x 100 | mm |
| Acquisition Matrix | 128 x 128 | 128 x 128 | - |
| # of Averages | 1 | 1 | - |
| rf coil | Whole body | Whole body | - |

Centroiding of objects in each image was performed following the method described in [7]. For each z-frame position, four image sets were acquired: single slices with frequency-encoding in both the x and y directions, and sets of multiple contiguous slices with 3D distortion correction enabled and frequency-encoding in both the x and y directions. Measurements of centroids were only made in the phase-encoded direction of each image. Using this method, which has been described in [7], two images are acquired at the same location, each with the direction of frequency encoding switched. Then, by combining the components of centroids from each image that were taken in the phase-encoded direction, a final in-plane measurement that is insensitive to in-plane distortion due to field inhomogeneity is obtained. The term "distortion correction" refers to a technique whereby a model of the profile of the magnetic field gradients is used to correct distortion in MR images due to gradient field nonlinearity.[9] Most clinical MR scanners feature a factory implementation of such an algorithm. The 2D version of distortion correction only corrects in-plane distortion, and can therefore be applied to single-slice acquisitions. Correction of out-of-plane distortion can be achieved using a 3D algorithm, but this requires either a 3D acquisition, or an acquisition of multiple contiguous slices. It is important to understand, however, that this method can only correct out-of-plane distortion (slice-select error) caused by gradient nonlinearity; slice-select error due to static field inhomogeneity will still be present. For all images acquired in this work, the factory 2D algorithm was enabled, and the effect of the factory 3D algorithm on localization error was tested.

## 3    Results

Figure 3 shows the error in localizing the spherical marker at different distances along the y- and z-axis of the z-frame from the isocenter. Errors are shown for images acquired with 3D distortion correction on (using multiple contiguous slices) and 3D distortion correction off (single slice). These measurements are representative of the error in localizing an interventional tool located at the MRI isocenter using a z-frame. Variation in localization error due to image noise was quantified by repeating the experiment five times with the z-frame at its furthest position from the isocenter. At this position, the sensitivity of the localization error to measurement errors is maximized. The standard deviation of error over these five acquisitions was 0.21 mm.

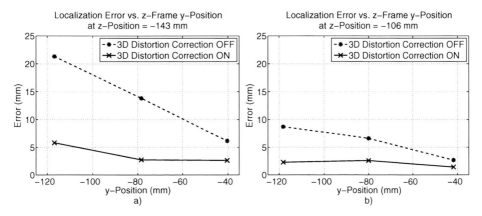

**Fig. 3.** Tooltip localization error vs. z-frame y-coordinate (relative to isocenter) at three distances from the isocenter along the z-axis. The use of a multi-slice acquisition with 3D distortion correction greatly reduced the error and its sensitivity to the position of the frame relative to the isocenter.

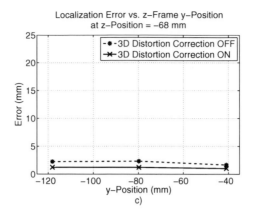

Fig. 3. (*continued*)

Figure 4 shows the variation in tooltip localization error with increasing static field inhomogeneity with the z-frame at its closest position to the isocenter.

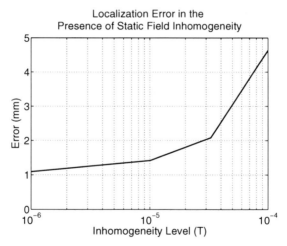

**Fig. 4.** Tooltip localization error vs. magnitude of static field inhomogeneity with the z-frame located at x = 0, y = -40 mm, z = -70 mm and the spherical marker at the isocenter

## 4    Summary

This work investigated the error in using a z-frame to localize the tooltip of an MRI-guided device. It was found that, when using a single image slice, the error increased rapidly with z-frame displacement from the isocenter. However, the use of multiple contiguous slices with 3D distortion correction enabled greatly reduced the dependence of the error on distance from the isocenter, reducing the error to less than 3 mm in most cases. It was also found that there is a strong dependence of error on static field inhomogeneity, even with the z-frame within 10 cm of the isocenter. This is likely due to the fact that the z-frame pose estimate is sensitive to slice-select error – a major downfall of this frame's design. It is important to note that variation of the z-frame's position strictly along the x-axis is expected to have the same effect as that along the y-axis, due to the expected symmetry of gradient hardware and the static field. However, the effect of a combined translation in the x-y plane cannot be extracted from this work. The results of this work will assist anyone developing MRI-guided devices to understand the effects of z-frame location, static field inhomogeneity, and 3D distortion correction on device localization accuracy.

# References

1. Brown, R.A.: A stereotactic head frame for use with CT body scanners. Invest. Radiol. 14, 300 (1979)
2. DiMaio, S., Samset, E., Fischer, G., Iordachita, I., Fichtinger, G., Jolesz, F., Tempany, C.: Dynamic MRI scan plane control for passive tracking of instruments and devices. In: Ayache, N., Ourselin, S., Maeder, A. (eds.) MICCAI 2007, Part II. LNCS, vol. 4792, pp. 50–58. Springer, Heidelberg (2007)
3. Fischer, G.S., DiMaio, S.P., Iordachita, I.I., Fichtinger, G.: Robotic assistant for transperineal prostate interventions in 3T closed MRI. In: Ayache, N., Ourselin, S., Maeder, A. (eds.) MICCAI 2007, Part I. LNCS, vol. 4791, pp. 425–433. Springer, Heidelberg (2007)
4. Song, S., Tokuda, J., Tuncali, K., Tempany, C., Zhang, E., Hata, N.: Development and Preliminary Evaluation of a Motorized Needle Guide Template for MRI-guided Targeted Prostate Biopsy. IEEE Trans. Biomed. Eng. (2013)
5. Su, H., Cardona, D.C., Shang, W., Camilo, A., Cole, G.A., Rucker, D.C., Webster, R., Fischer, G.S.: A MRI-guided concentric tube continuum robot with piezoelectric actuation: A feasibility study. In: IEEE International Conference on Robotics and Automation (ICRA), pp. 1939–1945 (2012)
6. Tokuda, J., Tuncali, K., Iordachita, I., Song, S.-E., Fedorov, A., Oguro, S., Lasso, A., Fennessy, F.M., Tempany, C.M., Hata, N.: In-bore setup and software for 3T MRI-guided transperineal prostate biopsy. Phys. Med. Biol. 57, 5823 (2012)
7. Cepek, J., Chronik, B., Lindner, U., Trachtenberg, J., Davidson, S., Bax, J., Fenster, A.: A system for MRI-guided transperineal delivery of needles to the prostate for focal therapy. Med. Phys. 40, 012304 (2013)
8. Tokuda, J., Fischer, G.S., DiMaio, S.P., Gobbi, D.G., Csoma, C., Mewes, P.W., Fichtinger, G., Tempany, C.M., Hata, N.: Integrated navigation and control software system for MRI-guided robotic prostate interventions. Computerized Medical Imaging and Graphics: the Official Journal of the Computerized Medical Imaging Society (2009)
9. Wang, D., Strugnell, W., Cowin, G., Doddrell, D.M., Slaughter, R.: Geometric distortion in clinical MRI systems: Part I: evaluation using a 3D phantom. Magn. Reson. Imaging 22, 1211–1221 (2004)

# 3-D Operation Situs Reconstruction with Time-of-Flight Satellite Cameras Using Photogeometric Data Fusion

Sven Haase[1], Sebastian Bauer[1], Jakob Wasza[1],
Thomas Kilgus[3], Lena Maier-Hein[3], Armin Schneider[4],
Michael Kranzfelder[4], Hubertus Feußner[4], and Joachim Hornegger[1,2]

[1] Pattern Recognition Lab, Friedrich-Alexander-Universität Erlangen-Nürnberg
sven.haase@fau.de
[2] Erlangen Graduate School in Advanced Optical Technologies (SAOT)
[3] Div. Medical and Biological Informatics Junior Group: Computer-assisted
Interventions, German Cancer Research Center (DKFZ) Heidelberg
[4] Minimally Invasive Therapy and Intervention, Technical University of Munich

**Abstract.** Minimally invasive procedures are of growing importance in modern surgery. Navigation and orientation are major issues during these interventions as conventional endoscopes only cover a limited field of view. We propose the application of a Time-of-Flight (ToF) satellite camera at the zenith of the pneumoperitoneum to survey the operation situs. Due to its limited field of view we propose a fusion of different 3-D views to reconstruct the situs using photometric and geometric information provided by the ToF sensor. We were able to reconstruct the entire abdomen with a mean absolute mesh-to-mesh error of less than 5 mm compared to CT ground truth data, at a frame rate of 3 Hz. The framework was evaluated on real data from a miniature ToF camera in an open surgery pig study and for quantitative evaluation with a realistic human phantom. With the proposed approach to operation situs reconstruction we improve the surgeons' orientation and navigation and therefore increase safety and speed up surgical interventions.

## 1 Introduction

Minimally invasive procedures gained a lot of attention, recently. In comparison to conventional surgery, endoscopic interventions aim at reducing pain, scars, recovery time and thereby hospital stay. Therefore, minimally invasive procedures hold benefits for both the patients and the hospital. Navigation and orientation are of particular relevance for the surgeon in minimally invasive surgery due to the limited field of view with conventional endoscopes. To improve both, different concepts to insert additional cameras have been proposed [1,2]. For instance, Cadeddu et al. describe a video camera that is positioned on the posterior abdominal wall and guided by an anterior magnetic device. Instead, we propose the concept of *3-D satellite cameras* as illustrated in Fig. 1(a). These cameras are inserted into the abdomen via a trocar and positioned at the top

K. Mori et al. (Eds.): MICCAI 2013, Part I, LNCS 8149, pp. 356–363, 2013.

of the pneumoperitoneum. Here, the imaging device can survey the operation field. Nevertheless, due to size limitations in endoscopic procedures, satellite cameras have shortcomings related to the hardware and optical systems. One of these is a narrow field of view. To expand the limited field of view the camera will reconstruct the entire situs initially by rotating and acquiring images from different areas for data fusion and then focus on the operation field. With no further repositioning of the patient the assumption of rigidity is acceptable for navigation assistance. Opposed to related work, our satellite camera delivers Time-of-Flight (ToF) 3-D surface and photometric information instead of pure 2-D video data. This enables a broad field of medical applications, e.g. collision detection, automatic navigation or registration with preoperative data.

Different approaches for data fusion with real-time capability have been proposed recently [3,4,5]. Warren et al. proposed a simultaneous localization and mapping based approach for natural orifice transluminal endoscopic surgery [3]. For stereo endoscopy, Röhl et al. presented a novel hybrid recursive matching algorithm that performs matching on the disparity map and the two input images [5]. Areas with little textural diversity are challenging scenarios for those color-based approaches regarding 3-D reconstruction. Instead of using conventional endoscopes we propose to navigate a 3-D satellite camera for reconstruction of the whole situs to enable a better orientation within the pneumoperitoneum. A ToF sensor acquires photogeometric data, i.e. both range data and intensity images encoding the amplitudes of the measured signal. By exploiting both complementary information we are able to reconstruct surfaces in areas with low textural diversity as well as areas with low topological diversity. In-vivo experiments on real data from a miniature ToF camera indicate the feasibility of using 3-D satellite cameras for situs reconstruction during minimally invasive surgery.

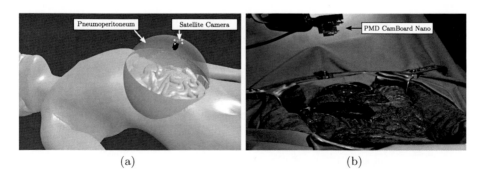

(a)                                            (b)

**Fig. 1.** (a) Illustration of the 3-D Time-of-Flight satellite camera hovering above the situs at the zenith of the pneumoperitoneum. (b) Experimental setup for acquiring in-vivo data in a pig study. Note the physical dimension of the miniature ToF camera.

## 2    Methods

We use a truncated signed distance function (TSDF) [6] to reconstruct the interior abdominal space. The advantage of this approach is threefold. First, by incorporating successive frames, details are refined. Second, the TSDF allows incorporating additional information for regions that were seen from different perspectives. This allows implicit denoising of data with lower quality. Third, the TSDF representation is computational efficient with both constant run time and memory. Inspired by the work of Whelan et al. [7], we enhanced the traditional TSDF from 3-D to 4-D to incorporate the amplitude domain. In this context, a major contribution is the incorporation of confidence weights derived from ToF characteristics into the TSDF reconstruction. To cope with real-time requirements in medical environments we apply a GPU-based photogeometric registration approach [8]. Below we detail the initial preprocessing for ToF data.

### 2.1    Time-of-Flight Data Processing

As ToF devices exhibit a low signal-to-noise ratio [9], preprocessing range data is an essential step. We apply a real-time capable framework that combines three processes. First, we interpolate invalid pixels based on a normalized convolution [10]. Second, we decrease temporal noise by averaging successive frames, allowed by the high acquisition speed of our sensor (see Sect. 3). Third, we perform bilateral filtering for edge-preserving denoising. The amplitude data depend not only on the material but also on the distance to the light source. Therefore, normalizing this data is necessary for incorporating the photometric domain into the registration process. We normalize amplitude data according to a simplified physical model $\tilde{a}(\boldsymbol{x}) = a(\boldsymbol{x})r^2(\boldsymbol{x})$ [11]. Here, $a$ denotes the amplitude value at the pixel coordinate $\boldsymbol{x}$ and $r$ denotes the measured radial distance. Furthermore, we also apply edge-preserving denoising in the amplitude domain. Nevertheless, photometric registration would still be affected by glare lights. To cope with this, we detect glare lights by basic thresholding and label them as invalid pixels.

### 2.2    Photogeometric Data Fusion into a Volumetric TSDF Model

The preprocessed data deliver photogeometric information of the situs from different points of view. For estimating the rotation matrix $\boldsymbol{R}_k$ and the translation vector $\boldsymbol{t}_k$ between the camera coordinate system of frame $k$ and the global world coordinate system we align two successive frames by applying an approximate iterative closest point (ICP) implementation [8]. The approach extends the traditional 3-D nearest neighbor search within ICP to higher dimensions, thus enabling the incorporation of additional complementary information, e.g. photometric data. It is based on the random ball cover acceleration structure for efficient nearest neighbor search on the GPU [12]. For 4-D data considered in this paper, the photogeometric distance metric $d$ is defined as:

$$d(\boldsymbol{m}, \mathcal{F}) = \min_{\boldsymbol{f} \in \mathcal{F}} \left( (1 - \chi) \|\boldsymbol{f}_g - \boldsymbol{m}_g\|_2^2 + \chi \|f_p - m_p\|_2^2 \right) , \tag{1}$$

where $\chi \in [0, 1]$ is a non-negative constant weighting the influence of the photometric data. $\boldsymbol{f}_g$ and $\boldsymbol{m}_g$ denote the position of an individual 3-D point in the fixed point set $\mathcal{F}$ and the moving point set $\mathcal{M}$, respectively. $f_p$ and $m_p$ denote the photometric scalar value given by the normalized amplitude data $\tilde{a}$.

Our reconstruction is based on a volumetric model defined by a TSDF along the lines of [6]. The TSDF is based on an implicit surface representation given by the zero level set of an approximated signed distance function of the acquired surface. For each position $\boldsymbol{p} \in \mathbb{R}^3$, the TSDF $\mathcal{T}_S$ holds the distance to the closest point on the current range image surface w.r.t. the associated inherent projective camera geometry:

$$\mathcal{T}_S (\boldsymbol{p}) = \eta \left( \| S \left( \boldsymbol{P}_s \left( \boldsymbol{p}_k \right) \right) \|_2 - \| \boldsymbol{p}_k \|_2 \right) C \left( \boldsymbol{P}_s \left( \boldsymbol{p}_k \right) \right), \tag{2}$$

where $\boldsymbol{p}_k = \boldsymbol{R}_k \boldsymbol{p} + \boldsymbol{t}_k$ denotes the transformation of $\boldsymbol{p}$ from world space into the moving local camera space. $\boldsymbol{P}_s : \mathbb{R}^3 \mapsto \mathbb{R}^2$ performs the projection of each 3-D point $\boldsymbol{p}_k$ into the image plane. $S$ reconstructs the 3-D surface point to a given range value in the sensor domain and $\eta$ is a truncation operator that controls the support region, i.e. outside this region the distance function is cut off. $C$ is a confidence weight that is introduced below.

For improved reconstruction, e.g. in terms of loop closures, we fuse our data in a frame-to-model manner [6], i.e. the current frame is not registered to the previous frame directly but to a raycasted image of the reconstructed model seen from the camera of the previous frame. Due to our high acquisition frame rate the rigid assumption for frame-to-model transformation estimation is tolerable.

To enable photogeometric reconstruction in a frame-to-model manner, our approach stores and fuses amplitude information. The amplitude value $\mathcal{T}_A$ is described by:

$$\mathcal{T}_A (\boldsymbol{p}) = \tilde{a} \left( \boldsymbol{P}_s \left( \boldsymbol{p}_k \right) \right) C \left( \boldsymbol{P}_s \left( \boldsymbol{p}_k \right) \right). \tag{3}$$

For robust data fusion we assign a confidence weight to each TSDF value to describe the reliability of the new measurement. In particular, we introduce the confidence function $C$ as:

$$C(\boldsymbol{x}) = e^{-\frac{\alpha}{\tilde{a}(\boldsymbol{x})}} e^{-\frac{\| \boldsymbol{x} - \boldsymbol{c} \|}{\beta}} v(\boldsymbol{x}), \tag{4}$$

with $\alpha$ and $\beta$ controlling the influence of the first terms and $\boldsymbol{c}$ denoting the pixel position of the center in the range image. Here, we exploit three characteristics of ToF cameras. With higher distances to the center or lower amplitude values the confidence decreases. The binary validity information $v(\boldsymbol{x})$ is provided by the ToF sensor and combined with the result of our glare light detection.

To provide temporal denoising we benefit from different frames that acquired the same spots by:

$$\tilde{\mathcal{T}}^t = \gamma \mathcal{T}^t + (1 - \gamma) \mathcal{T}^{t-1}, \tag{5}$$

where $\tilde{\mathcal{T}}^t$ denotes the temporal denoised result and $\mathcal{T}^t$ denotes the current result of Eq. 2 and Eq. 3. The weight $\gamma$ describes the influence of the previously reconstructed result $\mathcal{T}^{t-1}$.

## 3   Experiments

The experiments are split into two parts. For qualitative evaluation we acquired real in-vivo data in a pig study. For quantitative evaluation we acquired real data of a human abdomen phantom and compared it to CT ground truth data. In both experiments the satellite camera was moved across the situs at a typical measuring distance of 20 cm, while reconstructing the 3-D geometry of the operation field. For both experiments we applied the same preprocessing pipeline and used 25 frames for data fusion. In particular, we acquired a scene of 250 frames and fused every 10th frame to obtain a sufficient frame-to-frame movement. We averaged data over 3 successive frames to reduce temporal noise for the registration process. The parameters for the bilateral filter and the normalized convolution were set empirically. The temporal denoising parameter was set to $\gamma = 0.95$. The weightings of the confidence terms were set to $\alpha = 2000$ and $\beta = 100$. The photometric weighting was set to $\chi = 0.00025$. Regarding the scale of the parameter the maximum amplitude value of 40000 has to be taken into account. In the considered scenario, the texture is rather homogeneous. Hence, we set $\chi$ comparably low. Nonetheless, it guides the registration in flat regions. Our framework was implemented in CUDA and evaluated on an off-the-shelf laptop with an NVIDIA Quadro FX 1800M GPU and an i7-940XM CPU. For our experiments we used a CamBoard Nano miniature ToF camera from PMD Technologies GmbH, Siegen, Germany. It acquires ToF data at 60 Hz with a resolution of $160 \times 120$ px. The data is available online [1].

Even though being a compact device the CamBoard Nano ($37 \times 30 \times 25 mm^3$) exceeds the physical dimension needed for minimally invasive surgery. Hence, we performed our experiments in an open surgery scenario. For qualitative evaluation a pig was examined under artificial respiration, see Fig. 1(b). We compare the frame-to-frame data fusion to our frame-to-model approach and point out the benefits of our contributions - incorporating photometric data into the registration process and adding confidence weights to the TSDF. Furthermore, we reconstructed the whole operation situs from a ToF sequence of 25 frames.

Quantitative evaluation is performed by scanning an ELITE phantom [13] with CT and then acquiring data with the CamBoard Nano, while reconstructing the abdomen with our proposed framework. To compare the ToF reconstruction with the ground truth surface data, anatomical landmarks on both meshes were detected manually and registered. Then, we calculated the Hausdorff distance for a volume of interest to compare both surfaces in a mesh-to-mesh manner.

## 4   Results and Discussion

To investigate the performance on in-vivo data we reconstructed the abdomen of a pig, see Fig. 2. In addition, Fig. 3 illustrates the weakness of the frame-to-frame reconstruction compared to our frame-to-model result. Note that the blood vessel labeled in Fig. 3(c) is visible when reconstructing the scene using the proposed

---

[1] http://www5.cs.fau.de/research/data/

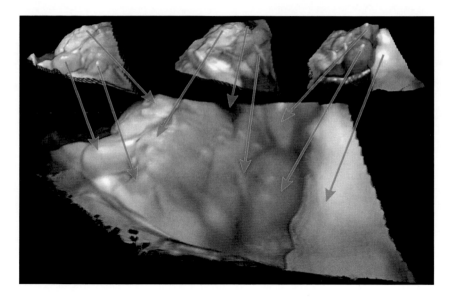

**Fig. 2.** The first row depicts 3 single frames of a 25-frames ToF sequence, acquired in an experimental in-vivo pig study. Below, the reconstructed operation situs is illustrated. Note that salient structures of individual frames are clearly visible in the reconstruction.

confidence weighting scheme and 4-D data, while it is blurred when considering the geometric data alone in the registration process, see Fig. 3(d). Compared to the frame-to-frame data fusion and the frame-to-model approach without confidence weights we achieve a smoother result while preserving the shape. In experiments with CT ground truth data we achieved a mean absolute mesh-to-mesh distance of 4.73 mm. The color-coded Hausdorff distance of the considered volume of interest is illustrated in Fig. 4(b). Note that substantial distance errors occur at the boundaries were only few data were available. The reconstruction accuracy in the central region was substantially better, see Fig. 4(c).

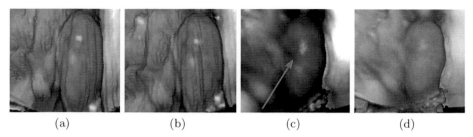

(a)                  (b)                  (c)                  (d)

**Fig. 3.** Closeup of the reconstructed operation situs at the position of the upper right image in Fig. 2. Reconstruction results for (a) 4-D frame-to-frame data fusion, (b) 4-D frame-to-model fusion without confidence weights, (c) 4-D frame-to-model approach with confidence weights, (d) frame-to-model approach using geometric information only. Note that the blood vessel marked with the blue arrow is best visible in (c).

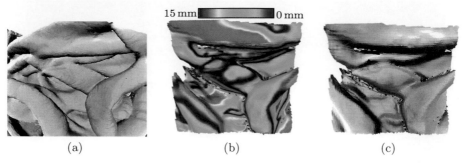

**Fig. 4.** (a) Ground truth data of the ELITE phantom. (b) Time-of-Flight surface with color coded Hausdorff distances. (c) Time-of-Flight reconstruction.

The experiments on real data illustrate that our framework is capable to provide reliable reconstructions even in the presence of severe noise ($\sigma_{ToF} \sim 5\,\mathrm{mm}$). Nevertheless, the distance map in Fig. 4(b) indicates that systematic errors in the ToF data and insufficient data at boundaries lead to locally imperfect reconstructions with higher mesh-to-mesh errors. The results on in-vivo data stress the benefits of our contributions. With our proposed 4-D frame-to-model data fusion we achieved more robust results compared to the 3-D approach. The introduced confidence weights for the TSDF produced a smoother reconstruction.

## 5   Conclusions

In this paper we proposed the use of a miniature ToF device as a 3-D satellite camera for minimally invasive surgery to reconstruct the operation situs. To extend the camera's field of view, we introduced a fusion framework that allows to reconstruct the operation situs for better orientation and navigation using both geometric and photometric information. Our proof-of-concept GPU implementation runs at 3 Hz on an off-the-shelf laptop. Experiments on real data showed that we benefit from our proposed confidence weights and resulted in a mean absolute mesh-to-mesh distance of less than 5 mm compared to ground truth CT data. Future work will investigate the upcoming generation of miniaturized ToF cameras that are expected to feature a geometry that fits through a trocar.

**Acknowledgments.** We gratefully acknowledge the support by the Deutsche Forschungsgemeinschaft (DFG) under Grant No. HO 1791/7-1. This research was supported by the Graduate School of Information Science in Health (GSISH) and the TUM Graduate School. The authors acknowledge funding of the Erlangen Graduate School in Advanced Optical Technologies (SAOT) by the DFG in the framework of the German excellence initiative. We also thank the Dr. Pfleger Stiftung for their partial support. This work was supported in the context of the R&D program IuK Bayern under Grant No. IUK338/001.

# References

1. Oleynikov, D., Rentschler, M., Hadzialic, A., Dumpert, J., Platt, S.R., Farritor, S.: Miniature robots can assist in laparoscopic cholecystectomy. Surgical Endoscopy 19(4), 473–476 (2005)
2. Cadeddu, J., Fernandez, R., Desai, M., Bergs, R., Tracy, C., Tang, S.J., Rao, P., Desai, M., Scott, D.: Novel magnetically guided intra-abdominal camera to facilitate laparoendoscopic single-site surgery: initial human experience. Surgical Endoscopy 23, 1894–1899 (2009)
3. Warren, A., Mountney, P., Noonan, D., Yang, G.Z.: Horizon Stabilized—Dynamic View Expansion for Robotic Assisted Surgery (HS-DVE). International Journal of Computer Assisted Radiology and Surgery 7(2), 281–288 (2012)
4. Mountney, P., Yang, G.Z.: Dynamic view expansion for minimally invasive surgery using simultaneous localization and mapping. IEEE Engineering in Medicine and Biology Society 1, 1184–1187 (2009)
5. Röhl, S., Bodenstedt, S., Suwelack, S., Kenngott, H., Mueller-Stich, B., Dillmann, R., Speidel, S.: Dense gpu-enhanced surface reconstruction from stereo endoscopic images for intraoperative registration. Medical Physics 39(3), 1632–1645 (2012)
6. Newcombe, R.A., Davison, A.J., Izadi, S., Kohli, P., Hilliges, O., Shotton, J., Molyneaux, D., Hodges, S., Kim, D., Fitzgibbon, A.: KinectFusion: Real-time dense surface mapping and tracking. In: 10th IEEE International Symposium on Mixed and Augmented Reality, pp. 127–136 (2011)
7. Whelan, T., Johannsson, H., Kaess, M., Leonard, J., McDonald, J.: Robust real-time visual odometry for dense RGB-D mapping. In: IEEE Robotics and Automation (2013)
8. Bauer, S., Wasza, J., Lugauer, F., Neumann, D., Hornegger, J.: Real-Time RGB-D Mapping and 3-D Modeling on the GPU Using the Random Ball Cover. In: Fossati, A., Gall, J., Grabner, H., Ren, X., Konolige, K. (eds.) Consumer Depth Cameras for Computer Vision - Research Topics and Applications, pp. 27–48 (2013)
9. Kolb, A., Barth, E., Koch, R., Larsen, R.: Time-of-flight cameras in computer graphics. Computer Graphics Forum 29(1), 141–159 (2010)
10. Knutsson, H., Westin, C.F.: Normalized and Differential Convolution: Methods for Interpolation and Filtering of Incomplete and Uncertain Data. In: IEEE Computer Vision and Pattern Recognition, pp. 515–523 (1993)
11. Oprisescu, S., Falie, D., Ciuc, M., Buzuloiu, V.: Measurements with ToF Cameras and Their Necessary Corrections. In: International Symposium on Signals, Circuits and Systems, vol. 1, pp. 1–4 (2007)
12. Cayton, L.: Accelerating nearest neighbor search on manycore systems. CoRR abs/1103.2635 (2011)
13. Gillen, S., Gröne, J., Knödgen, F., Wolf, P., Meyer, M., Friess, H., Buhr, H.J., Ritz, J.P., Feussner, H., Lehmann, K.: Educational and training aspects of new surgical techniques: experience with the endoscopic–laparoscopic interdisciplinary training entity (elite) model in training for a natural orifice translumenal endoscopic surgery (notes) approach to appendectomy. Surgical Endoscopy 26, 2376–2382 (2012)

# Multi-section Continuum Robot for Endoscopic Surgical Clipping of Intracranial Aneurysms

Takahisa Kato[1,3,*], Ichiro Okumura[2], Sang-Eun Song[3], and Nobuhiko Hata[3]

[1] Healthcare Optics Research Laboratory, Canon U.S.A., Inc., MA, USA
[2] Advanced Systems R&D Center, Canon Inc., Japan
[3] National Center for Image Guided Therapy, Brigham and Women's Hospital and Harvard Medical School, MA, USA

**Abstract.** We propose the development and assessment of a multi-section continuum robot for endoscopic surgical clipping of intracranial aneurysms. The robot has two sections for bending actuated by tendon wires. By actuating the two sections independently, the robot can generate a variety of posture combinations by these sections while maintaining the tip angle. This feature offers more flexibility in positioning of the tip than a conventional endoscope for large viewing angles of up to 180 degrees. To estimate the flexible positioning of the tip, we developed kinematic mapping with friction in tendon wires. In a kinematic-mapping simulation, the two-section robot at the target scale (i.e., an outer diameter of 1.7 mm and a length of 60 mm) had a variety of tip positions within 50-mm ranges at the 180°-angled view. In the experimental validation, the 1:10 scale prototype performed the three salient postures with different tip positions at the 180°-angled view.

**Keywords:** Continuum robot, Tendon drive, Robotic surgery, Aneurysm clipping, Endoscope-assisted microsurgery, Endoscopy.

## 1    Introduction

Intracranial aneurysms occur at the branching point of the major arteries in the anterior circulation near the base of the brain [1]. Intracranial aneurysms cause subarachnoid hemorrhage with a frequency of six to eight per 100,000 in western populations [2]. Such hemorrhages cause the death of 12% of patients before treatment and death for as many as 40% of patients even after treatment [1].

The treatment for intracranial aneurysms is to isolate the aneurysmal sac from circulation and prevent the thin wall of the blood vessel from rupturing. This treatment can be performed either surgically or endoluminally. In the surgical approach, a clip is placed at the neck of the aneurysmal sac to achieve thrombosis. In the endoluminal approach, a soft, metallic coil is placed within the lumen of the aneurysm. While the indications for the choice of surgical clipping or endoluminal coiling are still yet to be fixed [3, 4], surgical clipping remains the treatment of choice for intracranial

---

* Corresponding author.

K. Mori et al. (Eds.): MICCAI 2013, Part I, LNCS 8149, pp. 364–371, 2013.
© Springer-Verlag Berlin Heidelberg 2013

aneurysms [5, 12]. The interdisciplinary approach remains a safe and useful strategy when the configuration of aneurysms is difficult for endoluminal coiling [12].

For the surgical clipping procedure, the quality of clipping affects the outcome of the procedure. Thus, endoscopic visualization is necessary to attain the following three clinical goals, i.e., 1) inspection before clipping, 2) clipping under endoscopic view, and 3) postclipping evaluation. For inspection before clipping, the endoscope provides topographic information of the relationship of the aneurysm to the parent, branching, and perforating vessels, and to adjacent structures. For postclipping evaluation, the endoscope is utilized to assess clip position, to confirm the completeness of aneurysm obliteration, and to preclude the occlusion or constriction of parent, branching, or perforating vessels.

The literature suggests that one of the limitations of endoscopic clipping surgery at the present time is the inability to use the endoscope to inspect around or behind aneurysms without displacing neurovascular structures, which is a prerequisite for safe and efficient surgeries. As Fischer et al. indicate in [5], there are cases in which the visual inspection of the surrounding critical structure is vitally important ensure the safety of the procedure and to evaluate the positioning of the clips to minimize the risk of future rupturing. Some aneurysms are not amenable to direct clipping because of their location and the lack of a method for complete inspection. A flexible endoscope cannot be used for clipping surgery because the minimal space that is available in the basal cisterns precludes the safe use of a flexible endoscope for the required viewing angles of 30 to 70 degrees, or even higher [6].

The objective of this study is to develop an alternative to the use of conventional, rigid and flexible endoscopes so that wide-angled visualization and flexible positioning of the tip are possible. We propose the development and assessment of a novel, multi-section, continuum robot that can use a tendon wire. The approach we propose is unique since the robot will take into account the salient features of friction in a tendon wire when we control the curvature of the robot using tension as an input. We created and validated kinematic mapping with friction in a tendon wire between the input tension and the posture of the robot to estimate the position of the tip for a large viewing angle of the robot. To the best of our knowledge, such an approach considering the salient features of tendon friction in kinematic mapping by a continuum robot is original and has not been reported.

## 2    Materials and Methods

### 2.1    Mechanical Design

Figure 1 shows the structure of the robot, which is composed of a monolithic backbone, tendon wire, and wire guides. The robot has an outer diameter (O.D.) of 1.7 mm, a length of 60 mm and consists of the two sections, each with one degree of freedom. The robot has a 0.7 mm-diameter tool channel for imaging fibers. Three antagonistic pairs of tendon wires run through the wire guides. The two pairs end at the robot's midpoint, and the other pair ends at the distal end. The pair of tendon wires was spread apart from 0.65 mm from the centroid of the robot. Through differential variation of the tensions in the tendon wires, the tensions are transduced into torque at the wire guides. The torque bends the backbone at the distal section or the proximal section.

The backbone is an elastic tube, with flexible and rigid portions periodically spaced along its length. The wire guides align with the rigid portions so that the torques are applied only at the rigid portions. The flexible portion between two rigid portions and the guides is regarded as a constant-curvature element within one section under bending (hereafter referred to as a "cell"). Each cell has a length of 1 mm, with a bending stiffness of $2.0 \times 10^{-2}$ Nm/rad with imaging fiber stiffness for endoscopy. As we discuss below, the cells make kinematic modeling of both uneven curvatures and frictions simple. A material of the backbone and the tendon wires is superelastic nickel-titanium (NiTi) alloy. The wire guides are made of stainless steel. The wire guides have eyelets for holding tendon wires of 0.2 mm diameter. The tendon wires are 0.16 mm diameter wire ropes. The tension limitation is 5 N for one tendon wire due to the distortion tolerance for a linear elastic region (0.5 %). The structure was designed in CAD software, SolidWorks. The bending stiffness of the backbone was calculated by a finite-element analysis software, ANSYS.

Using two sections offers the advantages of active curvature compensation. By actuating two sections independently, the robot can generate a variety of posture combinations with curvatures at the distal and the proximal section while holding the tip angle.

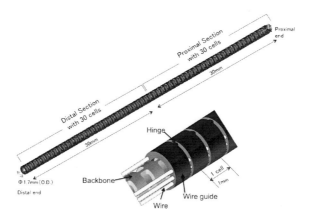

**Fig. 1.** Two-sections continuum robot design

## 2.2    Kinematic Mapping with Friction in Tendon Wire

We formulated the forward kinematic mapping (FKM) of the robot from the input tension in a tendon wire to the posture of the robot. For the FKM, we introduced arc parameters, which are curvature, length of arc and an angle of a bending plane containing the arc, as configuration parameters of the continuum robot. We mapped the tension to the arc parameters followed by mapping from the arc parameters to the posture of the robot to complete the FKM.

For accurate mapping between the tension and the arc parameters, we introduced a friction model that is a ratio of the tension variation in a tendon wire due to frictional forces between the tendon wire and eyelets in the wire guides. To express this tension variation, we created a concept of "cell." A cell is a unit of a linear elastic system consisting of a rotational spring, torque arms, and constant tensions within one cell. By concatenating cells, both tension variation and the corresponding curvature variation within one section can be handled in the FKM. Figure 2 shows this decomposition of a single section consisting of three cells.

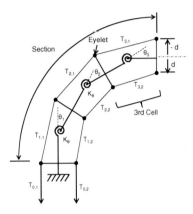

**Fig. 2.** Section consisting of a linear elastic system of cells

We assumed that system remains in quasistatic equilibrium. Frictional forces are equal to maximum static frictional forces proportional to the normal forces with friction coefficient $\mu$ at eyelets. By considering geometrical layout of the tendons and cells, we defined $\alpha_{i,j}$, which is the ratio of the tension variation in a tendon $i$ between cell $j$ and cell $(j+1)$, as:

$$\alpha_{i,j} = \frac{T_{j+1,i}}{T_{j,i}} \approx \left( \frac{1-\mu \cdot \sin\frac{\theta_j}{2}}{1+\mu \cdot \sin\frac{\theta_j}{2}} \right)^{Sgn(d_i) \cdot Sgn(\Sigma_i d_i \cdot T_{j,i})} \tag{1}$$

where Sgn(x) is Sign function, $T_{j,i}$ represents the tension in tendon $i$ in cell $j$, $\theta_j$ is the angular displacement of the distal end in the cell $j$. The magnitude of $d_i$ is the distance of tendon $i$ from the centroid of cell $j$ and the sign of $d_i$ represents the direction of the tendon $i$ from the centroid of cell $j$.

The rotational spring $K_\theta$ of cell $j$ maps the tension in a tendon wire to the arc parameters as:

$$\theta_j = \kappa_j \cdot s_j \approx \frac{\Sigma_i(d_i \cdot T_{j,i})}{K_\theta} \tag{2}$$

where $\kappa_j$ is the curvature of the cell $j$ and $s_j$ is the arc length of the cell $j$. Since $K_\theta$, $s_j$ and $d_i$ are known parameters, equations (1) and (2) allow us to map the tension in a tendon wire into the curvature by sequential calculation from the cell at the proximal end to the one at the distal end.

For the mapping from the arc parameters to the posture of the robot, we utilized a homogeneous transformation matrix parameterized by the arc parameters in [8] and applied the matrix for the cells. Our approach is completely different from the approach outlined in [8] because the matrix is applied to cells, not sections. The decomposition into cells allows us to calculate the posture of the robot with uneven curvatures by a simple calculation. Moreover, our mechanical design provides good consistency between this kinematic model and physical structure of cells.

## 2.3    Experimental Design

We conducted two sets of studies to validate the advantages of a two-section robot over a conventional one-section endoscope for an angled-view task. The first set assessed the flexibility of the tip position at a 180°-angled view task attained by a 1:1 scale robot by using FKM. The second set validated the postures when positioning the tip flexible at a 180°-angled view by developing a 1:10 scale prototype of the two-section robot.

**Performance Analysis**

We analyzed the flexibility of the tip position at a 180°-angled view as advantageous performance of the two-section robot. The analysis was conducted using FKM with a friction coefficient that we measured experimentally. The averaged measurement value was 0.31 for friction between test pieces of eyelets and wires. All data presented in this section were obtained using this friction coefficient.

To assess the flexibility of the tip position, we defined the tip position along a longitudinal direction of the robot (tip height) as a performance metric. We tabulated maximum, median and minimum values of this metric. The details of the procedure for this analysis are as follows:

First, a 1:1-scale robot with two-sections was analyzed. As the input of the FKM, we generated possible combinations of the tensions in the tendon wires ($T_{proxL}$, $T_{distR}$) or ($T_{proxR}$, $T_{distL}$) at intervals of 0.1 N. There was a minimum pre-tension value in the tendon wires to avoid slack. By inputting these combinations of the tensions in tendon wires to the FKM, we computed a corresponding group of postures for the robot. From this group we selected postures with a tip angle of 180 degrees. From all of these postures, we tabulated maximum, median and minimum values of the tip height.

Second, a one-section endoscope with the same mechanical specifications as the two-section robot was analyzed. We generated the possible tension in a tendon wire $T_{distR}$ at intervals of 0.1 N as the input for the FKM. Unlike the two-section robot, the one-section endoscope has only one tension as the input. The rest of the procedure to tabulate the tip height was the same as for the two-section robot.

Finally, we compared the tip height at a tip angle of 180 degrees between the two-section robot and one-section endoscope.

**Posture Validation**

To prove the concept of achieving flexibility with an angled view utilizing a two-section robot, we developed a 1:10 scale prototype of the two-section robot manually actuated by the tendon wires (Figure 3). The prototype has an outer diameter of 14.6 mm, a length of 208 mm and consists of the two sections actuated by tendon wires. The prototype had a similar mechanical structure to the 1:1 scale robot.

We set 180 degrees as a target angled view. For the input for these views, we converted the tensions in the tendon wires into the pull amount for the tendon wires. After placing the prototype on the surface of a stage, we pulled the tendon wires at these pull amounts and observed the postures of the prototype.

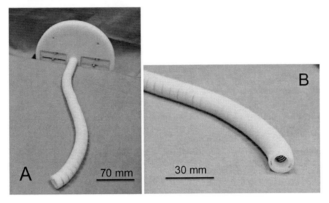

**Fig. 3.** 1:10 scale prototype. A: perspective view. B: enlarged view of the tip

# 3     Results

## 3.1     Performance Analysis

The results of the tip height test at a 180°-angled view are shown in Table 1. The two-section robot had a variety of tip heights from -36.3 mm to 12.5 mm; more than that of the one-section endoscope, which had only one solution at -14.5 mm. The postures of these tip heights are shown in Figure 4 A. The two-section robot varied the posture while retaining the tip angle through changes in the tensions of the tendon wires. Figure 4 B shows the angular displacement per cell of the two-section robot. From the maximum tip height to the minimum, a cell number with a larger angular displacement shifted from the distal section to the proximal section.

**Table 1.** Comparison of tip-height results between two sections and one section

| Tip height | One section (mm) | Two sections (mm) |
|---|---|---|
| Maximum | - | 12.5 |
| Median | -14.5 | -14.1 |
| Minimum | - | -36.3 |

370    T. Kato et al.

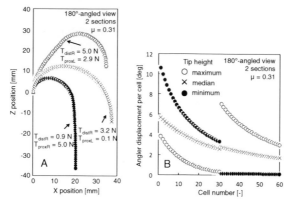

**Fig. 4.** Result of performance analysis of a two-section robot at 180°-angled view.  A, Postures of robot grounded at (0,0) mechanically. B, Angular displacement per cell.

## 3.2    Posture Validation

We validated the posture of the two-section prototype at a 180°-angled view (Figure 5 A-D). The prototype performed with a variety of tip heights while maintaining a tip angle at 180 degrees by changing the curvature distribution between the two sections. Figure 5 shows three salient postures of maximum (Figure 5 B), median (Figure 5 C) and minimum (Figure 5 D) values of the tip height at a 180°-angled view.

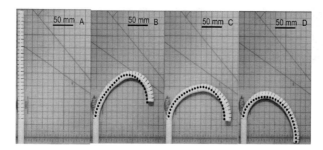

**Fig. 5.** Postures of 1:10 scale prototype at 180°-angled view with prediction by FKM (dots). A: initial straight posture. B: maximum tip height. C: median tip height. D: minimum tip height.

## 4    Discussion

In this study, we proposed the development and assessment of a multi-section continuum robot to enable a wide-angled visualization and flexible positioning of the tip of an endoscope. In the performance analysis done through forward kinematic mapping (FKM), the two-section robot had a larger variety of tip heights than the one-section endoscope, which had only one height.

The FKM in our study incorporates the piecewise constant-curvature approximation presented in prior art [7, 8]. Likewise, this approximation has been applied to many multi-section continuum robots in the medical field [9-11], because the constant curvature can facilitate analytical frame transformations [8]. In our study, to manage friction in tendon wires for more realistic estimation of the tip position, we introduced cells with good consistency in their physical structures. Because friction is eminent at a large tip angle, our FKM is useful for the analysis of a large-angled-view task.

In summary, we have shown that a two-section continuum robot has an advantage of flexible positioning of the tip at angled-view tasks over one-section endoscopes. This feature can expand the use of the endoscope to inspect around or behind aneurysms without displacing neurovascular structures.

**Acknowledgments.** Research reported in this publication was supported by Canon USA Inc. and the National Institutes of Health under Award Number P41EB015898, P01CA067165, R01CA138586, R01CA111288, R01CA124377 and R42CA137886. The content is solely the responsibility of the authors and does not necessarily represent the official views of the National Institutes of Health.

# References

1. Schievink, W.I.: Intracranial aneurysms. The New England Journal of Medicine 336(28), 1267 (1997)
2. de Rooij, N.K., et al.: Incidence of subarachnoid haemorrhage: a systematic review with emphasis on region, age, gender and time trends. Journal of Neurology, Neurosurgery, and Psychiatry 78, 1365 (2007)
3. Molyneux, A.J., et al.: International subarachnoid aneurysm trial (ISAT) of neurosurgical clipping versus endovascular coiling in 2143 patients with ruptured intracranial aneurysms: a randomised comparison of effects on survival, dependency, seizures, rebleeding, subgroups, and aneurysm occlusion. Lancet 366, 809 (2005)
4. Molyneux, A., et al.: International Subarachnoid Aneurysm Trial (ISAT) of neurosurgical clipping versus endovascular coiling in 2143 patients with ruptured intracranial aneurysms: a randomised trial. Lancet 360, 1267 (2002)
5. Fischer, G., et al.: Endoscopy in aneurysm surgery. Neurosurgery 70, 184 (2012)
6. Taniguchi, M., et al.: Microsurgical Maneuvers under Side-Viewing Endoscope in the Treatment of Skull Base Lesions. Skull Base-an Interdisciplinary 21, 115 (2011)
7. Jones, B.A., et al.: Kinematics for multisection continuum robots. IEEE Transactions on Robotics 22(1), 43–55 (2006)
8. Webster III, R.J., et al.: Design and Kinematic Modeling of Constant Curvature Continuum Robots: A Review. International Journal of Robotics Research 29(13), 1661–1683 (2010)
9. Camarillo, D.B., et al.: Configuration Tracking for Continuum Manipulators With Coupled Tendon Drive. IEEE Transactions on Robotics 25 (2009)
10. Webster III, R.J., et al.: Mechanics of Precurved-Tube Continuum Robots. IEEE Transactions on Robotics 25, 67–78 (2009)
11. Xu, K., et al.: An investigation of the intrinsic force sensing capabilities of continuum robots. IEEE Transactions on Robotics 24 (2008)
12. Proust, F., et al.: Quality of life and brain damage after microsurgical clip occlusion or endovascular coil embolization for ruptured anterior communicating artery aneurysms: neuropsychological assessment. Journal of Neurosurgery 110, 19 (2009)

# Inter-operative Trajectory Registration for Endoluminal Video Synchronization: Application to Biopsy Site Re-localization

Anant Suraj Vemuri[1,3], Stephane A. Nicolau[2], Nicholas Ayache[3],
Jacques Marescaux[2], and Luc Soler[2]

[1] IHU, Strasbourg, France
[2] IRCAD, Virtual-Surg, Strasbourg, France
[3] INRIA, Sophia Antipolis, France
anant.vemuri@inria.fr

**Abstract.** The screening of oesophageal adenocarcinoma involves obtaining biopsies at different regions along the oesophagus. The localization and tracking of these biopsy sites inter-operatively poses a significant challenge for providing targeted treatments. This paper presents a novel framework for providing a guided navigation to the gastro-intestinal specialist for accurate re-positioning of the endoscope at previously targeted sites. Firstly, we explain our approach for the application of electromagnetic tracking in acheiving this objective. Then, we show on three *in-vivo* porcine interventions that our system can provide accurate guidance information, which was qualitatively evaluated by five experts.

## 1 Introduction

Oesophageal adenocarcinoma (OAC) is rapidly increasing in frequency in the United States and other western countries. Gastroesophageal reflux disease, a benign complication caused by the stomach acid coming into the esophagus, as a chronic condition, leads to Barrett's esophagus (BE). It refers to the metaplasia in the cells of the lower esophagus and in most cases is a precursor to OAC. The evolution of BE to an adenocarcinoma is observed to progress from low-grade to a high-grade dysplasia. The guidelines [1] prescribe different levels of surveillance intervals depending on the degree of dysplasia with a minimum of two biopsies per year. A typical surveillance procedure involves taking four quadrant biopsies every 2cms towards the distal end of the esophagus and in suspicious regions. The biopsied tissue is sent to the pathology for evaluation. With the introduction of devices such as the probe-based confocal laser endomicroscopy real-time visualization and diagnosis of suspected regions can be performed intera-operatively. High resolution narrow band imaging has also been used for diagnosis and surveillance by visual inspection of the mucosa and the subepithelium. In each of these cases, during a follow-up inspection, the gastro-intestinal (GI) specialist is required to locate the previously biopsied or surveyed location. This problem in the literature has been termed as the re-localization

K. Mori et al. (Eds.): MICCAI 2013, Part I, LNCS 8149, pp. 372–379, 2013.

issue. Typically, the GI specialist uses the markings on the endoscope, which can be highly unreliable and which limit his or her ability to accurately re-position the endoscope and the optical biopsy probe and hence to effectively track the disease. Due to the lack of deterministic tools for providing such re-localization inter-operatively, the GI specialist has to survey or biopsy the entire affected oesophagus region, which prevents targeted treatments.

## 2   Related Works

To our knowledge, there is no previous work which tackles this issue of re-localization of the flexible endoscope inter-operatively. However, several approaches to track the biopsy points intraoperatively exist [2,3,4]; each of them relying on the recovery of the 3D structure of the anatomy, to map and track the biopsy sites as they move in and out of the field-of-view of the endoscope frame. Allain et al. [2,4] employ epipolar geometry, Mountney et al. [3] propose a simultaneous localization and mapping (SLAM) based method. Atasoy et al. [5], propose a probabilistic region matching approach in narrow-band images by using feature matches obtained from affine invariant anisotropic feature detector.

More recently Atasoy et al. [6] propose to formulate the re-localization as image-manifold learning process. By projecting endoscopic images on low dimensional space they propose to classify and cluster the images collected during multiple interventions into manageable segments, which they claim would aid in re-localization of the biopsy sites. However, they do not provide any spatial relations of the extracted segments inter-operatively, and so have not sufficiently clarified the application of their result in a clinical context for re-localization. We believe that, relying only on image based information for information extraction, that has to be mapped across multiple interventions can be highly unreliable; especially, due to temporal changes in tissue texture over multiple procedures, coupled with a highly deformable endoscopic scene, where repeatability of feature extraction, matching and tracking poses a significant challenge.

This paper proposes to solve the above problem, by introducing an Electromagnetic tracking system (EMTS) into the loop and providing a framework for utilizing it for re-localization inter-operatively. Firstly, we define the re-localization problem using a two-step approach; a) *Gross localization*: referring to an approximate positioning of the endoscope close to a reference point (typically a biopsy site) in a previously conducted procedure; and b) *Fine positioning*: referring to a mapping of the biopsy points taken during a previous procedure onto the images in the current intervention. Here, we address the gross localization issue. By attaching an electromagnetic (EM) sensor to the tip of a flexible endoscope, its movement within the body can be tracked with respect to a fixed external reference frame. By computing the correspondence between the EM sensor positions in two successive interventions, we propose to provide a guided-view to the GI specialist. This guided-view consists of a matching image extracted from the previously recorded intervention that best matches the live view (Fig. 3). This can, as will be shown, provide more information during the intervention to the GI specialist. The rest of the paper is organized as follows: Sec. 3 presents the system set-up and the work-flow of our approach. Sec. 4 describes the evaluation strategy and results.

## 3    System Setup and Methodology

The system setup consists of an EM field generator with a working volume of $50 \times 50 \times 50 \text{cm}^3$, which is placed roughly above the chest of the patient and fixed in position using a titanium arm, as shown in Fig. 1. A 6-*dof* EM sensor is inserted into the working channel of the endoscope and fixed at the tip of the endoscope (Fig. 1b). The EMTS and the endoscope are connected to a laptop, that synchronously records the data. A recording of an intervention consists of a list of EM sensor poses (trajectory of the endoscope tip), with the corresponding image frames captured from the endoscope. During a live procedure, given the recording of a previously conducted intervention, we find a corresponding image in the recording, that spatially matches the endoscope's current location in the oesophagus. Fig. 2 provides an overview of the work-flow of our method. The process is divided into three parts *a*) *Acquisition phase*: in which the recorded data is tagged and stored for further processing; *b*) *Registration phase*: to perform registration of EMTS reference frames of the live procedure and a previously recorded intervention chosen for providing a guided view.; and *c*) *Synchronization phase*: to perform spatial synchronization between the trajectories of the live intervention and the recording that was previously registered.

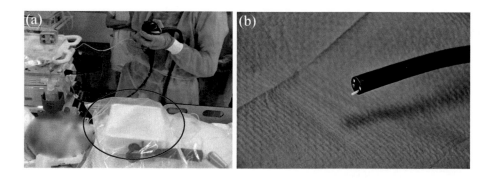

**Fig. 1.** (a) The apparatus setup in the operating room; (b) Placement of the sensor in the endoscope working channel

### 3.1    Acquisition Phase

During this phase, the GI specialist performs the recording of an intervention and tagging of relevant images. The flexible endoscope is slowly guided through the oesophagus, while the EM sensor pose and the corresponding image acquired from the endoscope are recorded to the database. The recording contains many uninformative frames; with bubbles, motion-blur, specular highlights, and out-of-focus images. Firstly, these uninformative frames are detected and left out from further processing using the method described in [7]. The GI specialist tags the images containing the sphincter as it is used as a landmark in the registration phase (Sec. 3.2). We use the sphincter as the anatomical landmark because it is stable and can be reached with good repeatable accuracy (∼3mm). The endoscopic frames that contain the biopsy procedure are tagged and in an offline step, the expert reviews the tagged biopsy images and selects those most relevant for the procedure. At this stage the expert can choose to add supplementary information to the images of the recordings, which will be available during the sychronization phase.

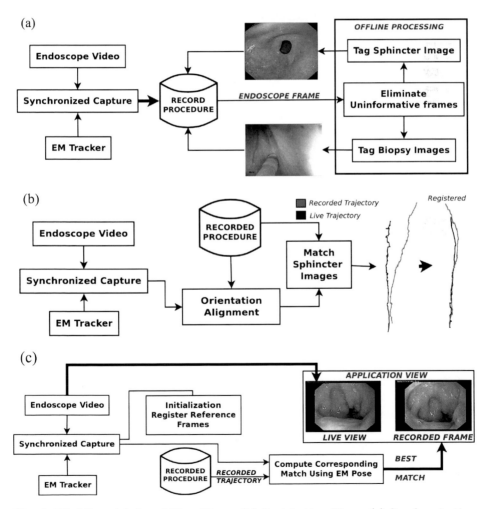

**Fig. 2.** Workflow, (a) Acquisition Phase; (b) Registration Phase; (c) Synchronization Phase

## 3.2    Registration Phase

Since the set-up of the EMTS would always change inter-operatively; registration must be performed between the EMTS reference frames of the live and a recording of a previous intervention chosen for providing a guided-view. We propose an on-line registration, without introducing additional constraints in the operating room. To achieve this, firstly, the EM sensor position is recorded while the GI specialist introduces the endoscope into the oesophagus and guides it until the sphincter. We use the contextual knowledge that the oesophagus is fairly linear and exhibits very minimal lateral movement. Hence, the largest principal components of the live trajectory and the trajectory of the previous intervention can be used to obtain 3D orientation alignment $(R)$ along $\hat{z} = [0\ 0\ 1]^T$ for each trajectory. The tagged sphincter positions can then used to obtain translation $t$, which along with $R$ provides an intialization for the iterative closest point (ICP) for further registration refinement.

## 3.3    Synchronization Phase

Once the reference frames have been aligned, a spatial correspondence between the sensor position from the current intervention and the previously recorded intervention is computed. By partitioning the trajectory of the previous intervention as a binary tree, a search for the closest neighbour (in euclidean sense) to the current sensor position is made. Due to localized deformations of the oesophagus during navigation, the trajectories are not smooth and exhibit deviations (Fig. 3a) from the central oesophagus line (connecting the throat to the sphincter, along $\hat{z}$), which can lead to a false match with marked depth difference. Since the trajectories have been aligned along $\hat{z}$, the search space is constrained to lie within $\Delta z$ ($\approx$ 2mm). The closest neighbour gives the corresponding best matching image of the region in the oesophagus taken during the previous procedure. In particular, the matched images that were tagged to contain locations of biopsy sites, provide the GI specialist a more localized region for review. Fig. 3 presents the result of the the synchronization phase. ICP finds the transform up to a rotation along $\hat{z}$, however, since the search space is constrained along this direction, the determination of the closet neighbour is unaffected by it.

## 4    Results

For the purposes of the experiments we used a NDI ©Aurora EMTS (accuracy of 0.5mm in a working volume of $30 \times 30 \times 30cm^3$). The proposed approach was tested on three sets of *in-vivo* sequences on different porcines, with each set consisting of four recordings. Prior marking were made on the oesophagus using a dual knife at every 2cm to simulate biopsy locations. To replicate realistic surgical procedures conducted at different times, the EM field emitter was randomly repositioned before each recording. The steps as explained in Sec. 3

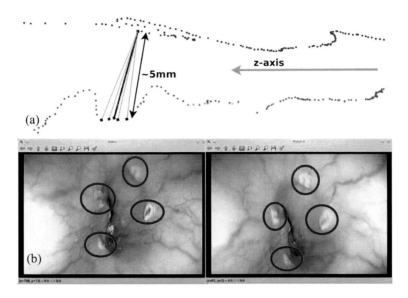

**Fig. 3.** View of the application window. (a) The magnified view of the live and previously recorded trajectories and the corresponding matches; (b) The image from the live view (left) and best matched image (right) from previously recorded intervention. The encircled regions indicate markings made using the dual knife.

were performed, with the first recording as the reference and three other recordings to mimic a follow-up procedure. A qualitative evaluation of the approach was performed by presenting the output of the synchronization phase to five experts. As shown in Fig. 3(b) two images were presented, one displaying frames to emulate the live stream from an intervention and the second, displaying the corresponding matching frame from a previously recorded intervention. Using the markings made by the dual knife and other visible landmarks as reference, the expert assessed the relevance and quality of the matched image presented

**Table 1.** Each question is rated on a scale of 1 (definitely not) to 5 (definitely yes). Five experts were asked to evaluate the results. All showed strong agreement for usefulness of the approach.

| Question | E1 | E2 | E3 | E4 | E5 | Mean | Stdv |
|---|---|---|---|---|---|---|---|
| Does the proposed image contain the information that you expected? | 4 | 4 | 5 | 4 | 5 | 4.4 | 0.55 |
| Would the information be helpful for your procedure? | 5 | 5 | 4 | 4 | 4 | 4.4 | 0.55 |
| Would this information change the way you would explore the oesophagus? | 3 | 4 | 4 | 3 | 3 | 3.4 | 0.55 |
| Do you think the approach would reduce the duration of exploration? | 4 | 4 | 3 | 3 | 4 | 3.4 | 0.55 |
| Are you likely to be interested in using such an application in the future? | 5 | 5 | 5 | 5 | 5 | 5 | 0 |
| Would you recommend it to a fellow colleague? | 4 | 5 | 5 | 5 | 5 | 4.8 | 0.45 |
| Rate the quality of information? | 5 | 5 | 5 | 4 | 5 | 4.8 | 0.45 |

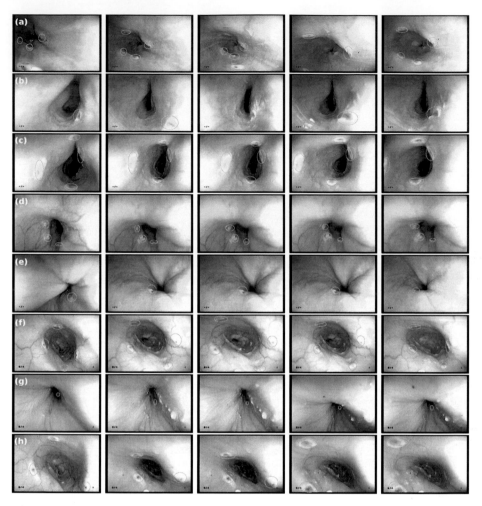

**Fig. 4.** The 1st column shows the frames from the live video, the 2nd column shows the closest match. Columns 3,4 and 5 present frames randomly selected from the 20 best matches obtained from the synchronization phase.

using our approach. We quantified the feedback of their experience using a questionnaire presented in Table. 1. The evaluation experiment clearly shows that the experts found the current system very useful for re-localizing the simulated biopsy sites. However, it was suggested that the matched image did not necessarily provide the ideal viewpoint (Fig 4a,b and e). Upon added investigation we observed that by considering ($\sim$) 20 best neighbours, the selection of best image can be refined to accommodate the best viewpoint. Fig. 4 shows a sample of these frames. While our current approach already provides the GI specialist with a more advanced guidance, we can further improve the frame selection by performing image analysis on these best neighbours.

# 5    Conclusion

This paper introduces a novel framework for combining images with instrument tracking information for inter-operative biopsy site re-localization. An application of this approach using EMTS for Barrett's oesophagus has been presented. To our knowledge, this is the first time such a system has been proposed in the literature. The system set-up is quite straightforward, it works in real-time (trajectory matching $\sim$ 100Hz), can be used with minimal change to the operating room protocol and most of the offline steps can easily be automated. Moreover, because the system is scalable in time, the recordings can be shared between GI specialists without loss of information. Finally, since our method does not rely on the quality of images, it is robust to typical endoscopic image artefacts for inter-operative comparison. In future, we will tackle the issue of best viewpoint selection and the mapping of recorded regions of interest to the live view. Currently the accuracy of the approach relies on the repeatability of accurately localizing the sphincter inter-operatively by the GI specialist, we would also address this issue in the future.

**Acknowledgement.** This work is part of the "ARFlex" project supported by IHU, Strasbourg. We would like to extend our thanks to Dr. Hyunsoo Chung, Dr. Jérôme Huppertz, Prof. Gérard Gay and Prof. Michel Delvaux for their invaluable support.

# References

1. Wang, K.K., Sampliner, R.E.: Updated guidelines 2008 for the diagnosis, surveillance and therapy of Barrett's esophagus. The American Journal of Gastroenterology 103(3), 788–797 (2008)
2. Allain, B., Hu, M., Lovat, L.B., Cook, R., Ourselin, S., Hawkes, D.: Biopsy site re-localisation based on the computation of epipolar lines from two previous endoscopic images. In: Yang, G.-Z., Hawkes, D., Rueckert, D., Noble, A., Taylor, C. (eds.) MICCAI 2009, Part I. LNCS, vol. 5761, pp. 491–498. Springer, Heidelberg (2009)
3. Mountney, P., Giannarou, S., Elson, D., Yang, G.-Z.: Optical biopsy mapping for minimally invasive cancer screening. In: Yang, G.-Z., Hawkes, D., Rueckert, D., Noble, A., Taylor, C. (eds.) MICCAI 2009, Part I. LNCS, vol. 5761, pp. 483–490. Springer, Heidelberg (2009)
4. Allain, B., Hu, M., Lovat, L.B., Cook, R.J., Vercauteren, T., Ourselin, S., Hawkes, D.J.: A system for biopsy site re-targeting with uncertainty in gastroenterology and oropharyngeal examinations. In: Jiang, T., Navab, N., Pluim, J.P.W., Viergever, M.A. (eds.) MICCAI 2010, Part II. LNCS, vol. 6362, pp. 514–521. Springer, Heidelberg (2010)
5. Atasoy, S., Glocker, B., Giannarou, S., Mateus, D., Meining, A., Yang, G.-Z., Navab, N.: Probabilistic region matching in narrow-band endoscopy for targeted optical biopsy. In: Yang, G.-Z., Hawkes, D., Rueckert, D., Noble, A., Taylor, C. (eds.) MICCAI 2009, Part I. LNCS, vol. 5761, pp. 499–506. Springer, Heidelberg (2009)
6. Atasoy, S., et al.: Endoscopic video manifolds for targeted optical biopsy. IEEE Transactions on Medical Imaging 31(3), 637–653 (2012)
7. Bashar, M.K., et al.: et al. Automatic detection of informative frames from wireless capsule endoscopy images. Medical Image Analysis 14(3), 449–470 (2010)

# System and Method for 3-D/3-D Registration between Non-contrast-enhanced CBCT and Contrast-Enhanced CT for Abdominal Aortic Aneurysm Stenting

Shun Miao[1], Rui Liao[1], Marcus Pfister[2], Li Zhang[1], and Vincent Ordy[1]

[1] Siemens Corporation, Corporate Technology, Princeton, NJ, USA
[2] Siemens Healthcare, Erlangen, Germany

**Abstract.** In this paper, we present an image guidance system for abdominal aortic aneurysm stenting, which brings pre-operative 3-D computed tomography (CT) into the operating room by registering it against intra-operative non-contrast-enhanced cone-beam CT (CBCT). Registration between CT and CBCT volumes is a challenging task due to two factors: the relatively low signal-to-noise ratio of the abdominal aorta in CBCT without contrast enhancement, and the drastically different field of view between the two image modalities. The proposed automatic registration method handles the first issue through a fast quasi-global search utilizing surrogate 2-D images, and solves the second problem by relying on neighboring dominant structures of the abdominal aorta (i.e. the spine) for initial coarse alignment, and using a confined and image-processed volume of interest around the abdominal aorta for fine registration. The proposed method is validated offline using 17 clinical datasets, and achieves 1.48 mm target registration error and 100% success rate in 2.83 s. The prototype system has been installed in hospitals for clinical trial and applied in around 30 clinical cases, with 100% success rate reported qualitatively.

**Keywords:** 3-D/3-D registration, cone-beam computed tomography, abdominal aortic aneurysm, global optimization.

## 1   Introduction

Abdominal aortic aneurysm (AAA) causes 15,000 death yearly in the U.S. [1]. As an alternative to the well-established open surgery, minimally invasive AAA stenting is a rapidly emerging technology that is especially suitable for high-risk surgical candidates. Contrast-enhanced computed tomography (CT) provides detailed anatomical assessment of the abdominal aorta and therefore is routinely performed in pre-operative planning. Overlay of pre-operative CT and intra-operative fluoroscopy is also used during the procedure, especially for complicated aneurysms, to guide the catheterization of the side branches and positioning of the stents. However, the current clinical practice is hindered by the cumbersome workflow, including (semi-)manual registration.

K. Mori et al. (Eds.): MICCAI 2013, Part I, LNCS 8149, pp. 380–387, 2013.

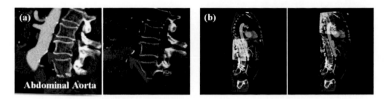

**Fig. 1.** (a) Sagittal slices of CT (white) and CBCT (yellow). Abdominal aorta (pointed out by red arrows) has high contrast in contrast-enhanced CT, but is barely visible in non-contrast-enhanced CBCT. (b) Overlay of CT (white) and CBCT (yellow) before and after registration, showing the large difference in FOVs and the need for a global optimization scheme.

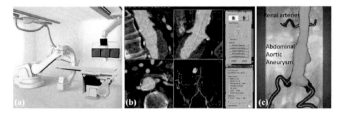

**Fig. 2.** (a) Angiographic C-Arm system to acquire interventional 3-D CBCT volumes in an operating room. (b) 3-D/3-D registration system for AAA stenting. (c) Overlay of the 3-D model on a real-time 2-D fluoroscopy.

This paper describes a 3-D/3-D registration system that brings the pre-operative contrast-enhanced CT into the operating room by registering it against the intra-operative non-contrast-enhanced cone-beam CT (CBCT). Because renal insufficiency is highly prevalent in patients undergoing AAA stenting, extensive use of iodine contrast may cause renal failure and needs to be avoided. Therefore, we use non-contrast CBCT for registration purpose, which is a challenging problem due to the relatively poor image quality of the non-contrast-enhanced CBCT, where the abdominal aorta has a very low image contrast (Fig. 1a). Another challenge is that abdominal CT typically has a much larger field of view (FOV) than CBCT (Fig. 1b), leading to many local optima in the registration space.

To the best of our knowledge, there is no literature reporting on automatic registration of abdominal aorta between contrast-enhanced CT and non-contrast-enhanced CBCT due to the aforementioned difficulties. Normalized Mutual Information (NMI) has been widely applied for general multi-modality image registration [2]. However NMI is driven mainly by large structures with high contrast and therefore is not directly applicable to our application, where the target object to be registered is relatively small and homogeneous compared to other neighboring structures. Multi-resolution strategy has been used with local optimizers for an increased capture range in registration [3], which, however, does not work adequately when the FOVs vary in a great extent like in our case. Global search has been mainly limited to 2-D image registration tasks due to its high computational complexity. Some heuristic semi-global optimization schemes, e.g. simulated annealing [4] and genetic algorithm [5], are proposed for the trade off between capture range and efficiency. However, their computational cost for 3-D/3-D registration is still prohibitively high for interventional use.

## 2    System Overview

Our 3-D/3-D registration system has been prototypically integrated into an angiographic C-arm system (Siemens Artis zee/zeego, Fig. 2a). Fig. 2b shows the prototype system with an example registration. Mesh models are used for representing the abdominal aorta segmented from CT, which is then overlaid onto intra-operative 2-D X-ray images for the purpose of real-time navigation and guidance during AAA stenting procedures (Fig. 2c).

To facilitate visual check of registration accuracy by physicians, CT and CBCT volumes are displayed and blended in both volume rendering and multi-planar reformatting (MPR). Multiple options are provided for the blending effect for an intuitive check, such as summation, subtraction, side by side, and embedded MPR of CT into CBCT volume. Cutting planes of the MPRs are automatically determined based on the abdominal aorta segmented from CT and the detected landmarks including renal artery ostia and illiac artery bifurcations, so that physicians can verify the registration result at the target area without any manual operation.

## 3    Registration Method

### 3.1    Quasi-global Search

A good pose initialization is important for intensity-based registration methods, especially for our application where the FOVs of CT and CBCT volumes are dramatically different. However, a complete global search in 3-D space is not computationally practical. To achieve a reliable and efficient initialization, we follow the concept of using 2-D anatomy targeted projections to surrogate the original volume [6]. A similarity measure is then defined on the lower-dimensional (2-D) surrogate images, instead of the 3-D volume, which significantly reduces the computation cost of similarity evaluation, thereby making quasi-global search in the registration space computationally feasible.

To compute the surrogate image, the Maximum Intensity Projections (MIPs) are computed along three directions $(x, y, z)$, as shown in Fig. 3. For example, given the CT volume $I_{CT}$, the surrogate image of CT along $x$ direction is defined as:

$$MCT_x = \max_x I_{CT}(x, y, z) \tag{1}$$

Surrogate images along $x, y, z$ directions are denoted as $MCT_x$, $MCT_y$, $MCT_z$ for CT and $MCB_x$, $MCB_y$, $MCB_z$ for CBCT, respectively. The similarity between CT and CBCT volumes for the purpose of pose initialization is then defined as the summation of the NMIs of all three pairs of surrogate images:

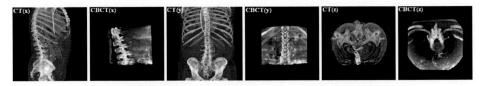

Fig. 3. Surrogate images for CT and CBCT

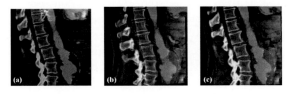

Fig. 4. (a) Initial position before registration. (b) Registration using the whole volume. (c) Registration using the spine segmentation.

$$S(I_{CT}, I_{CB}) = \sum_{i=x,y,z} NMI(MCT_i, MCB_i) \tag{2}$$

For AAA intervention, typically both CT and CBCT volumes are acquired with the patient lying in the supine position. Therefore the two volumes have similar initial orientations and the main objective of pose initialization is to estimate 3-D translation. If the transformation $T$ is translation-only, the similarity can be computed as:

$$S(T(I_{CT}), I_{CB}) = \sum_{i=x,y,z} NMI(T_i^{2D}(MCT_i), MCB_i) \tag{3}$$

where $T_i^{2D}, i = x, y, z$ are the corresponding 2-D translations of the three surrogate images using the 3-D translation parameters from $T$. Note that 2-D translation of the surrogate images as a result of 3-D translation of the original volume can be computed efficiently without re-computation of the MIPs.

Several hundred positions in the registration space are sampled, and translation only local optimization in multi-resolution pyramid is performed starting from each selected position based on the similarity measure defined in Eqn. 3. In addition, the spatial location of the structure of interest in image domain and the likely location of local optima in parameter domain are used to best choose the starting points globally in the registration space. For example, denser and more points are sampled in the head-foot direction because it is known that the largest variance between the FOVs of CT and CBCT volumes lies in this direction, and local optima happen more likely along this direction due to the repetition pattern of the spine in thoracic-abdominal CT/CBCT. Pose initialization is then obtained as the global optimal position with the highest similarity measure among all the registration results.

## 3.2   Spine Registration

After coarse alignment of CT and CBCT volumes through pose initialization, a structure-targeted rigid-body registration is performed to align the spine, which is a dominant structure in both image modalities and as a result can be much more reliably registered in this step compared to the abdominal aorta. In addition, registration of the spine brings the abdominal aorta close to the correct position because these two structures are anatomically adjacent to each other.

To focus the registration on the spine, we first coarsely segment the spine from both CT ($P_{CT}$) and CBCT ($P_{CB}$) volumes via thresholding using the known range of Hounsfield Unit (HU) for bony structures. This simple and coarse segmentation is sufficient for registration purpose because the most dominant features of the spine, such as the bright edge of the vertebrae, can always be reliably segmented. In addition, those large organs that potentially interfere with spine registration, such as the liver, can be reliably excluded. The spine segmentation results from both CT and CBCT volumes are combined as:

$$P = P_{CT} \cap P_{CB} \tag{4}$$

And the NMI similarity measure is defined on the spine as

$$NMI_s(I_{CT}, I_{CB}) = \frac{H(I_{CT}(P)) + H(I_{CB}(P))}{H(I_{CT}(P), I_{CB}(P))} \tag{5}$$

where $H(I_1)$ and $H(I_2)$ are entropy of $I_1$ and $I_2$, respectively, and $H(I_1, I_2)$ is the joint entropy. By defining the NMI similarity measure on the spine only, the registration is targeted and as a result most accurate on the spine, as shown in Fig. 4. In addition, to ensure the smoothness of the joint histogram and thus reduce the number of local optima in the registration space, we estimate the joint histogram on the basis of Parzen windows made of Gaussian density function [7].

## 3.3   Aorta Registration

Registration of the abdominal aorta is difficult due to the very low signal-to-noise ratio of the vessel structures in CBCT without contrast medium. In addition, for AAA stenting, the main stent graft needs to be deployed very close to the renal artery ostia with a sufficient supporting zone but without occluding them. Registration thus needs to be highly accurate in the area around renal artery ostia, which is a relatively small object compared to other neighboring structures, such as the spine, the liver, and etc. To handle this problem, we use a confined and image-processed VOI around the abdominal aorta and the renal ostia, to eliminate irrelevant interfering structures and enforce the registration algorithm focusing on the target organ for aorta registration.

To calculate the confined VOI, we first automatically segment vessel structures from CT using a graph-cut based method [8]. This segmentation is straightforward because vessel structures are contrast-enhanced in the CT volume. The VOI in CT is then defined as a bounding box that contains the segmented renal

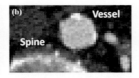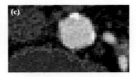

**Fig. 5.** (a) Abdominal aorta segmentation (red), centerline (green) and VOI automatically calculated based on the segmentation (yellow). Five target points that are used for computing TRE are shown as blue dots. (b) Spine is included in the VOI because it is very close to the abdominal aorta. (c) Spine is eliminated from the VOI by the proposed spine removal process.

arteries, the renal ostia and the upper part of the abdominal aorta, as shown in Fig. 5a. Since the abdominal aorta in CBCT is already relatively close to that in CT after spine registration, the VOI in CBCT is a dilated version of the VOI in CT, eliminating the need for explicit segmentation on CBCT which is a much more difficult task without contrast enhancement.

The spine can still possibly be included in the confined VOI due to its close proximity to the abdominal aorta (Fig. 5b). To eliminate the impact of the spine, image processing is applied on the CT to remove the spine. Once the spine is removed from the CT, the spine in the CBCT has no matching structure and therefore has little influence during registration process. The spine mask is generated by thresholding CT intensities within the VOI by a heuristic HU value corresponding to the bone and excluding the voxels in the vessel segmentation. The intensity mean and variance of the VOI excluding the spine and the vessel are computed and denoted as $\mu$ and $\sigma$, respectively. The spine is then removed by filling those spine voxel with intensities from a Gaussian distribution $N(\mu, \sigma)$, as shown in Fig. 5c.

In the confined and image-processed VOI, the abdominal aorta and the renal arteries become the only dominant structures, and therefore can be reliably registered using standard intensity-based registration methods, starting from the position obtained by spine registration. We again use NMI as the similarity measure and Hill Climbing (HC) as the optimizer. Two examples of aorta registration are shown in Fig. 6.

## 4   Algorithm Implementation

Our system is based on a highly optimized implementation: 1. Multi-resolution strategy is used in all steps. 2. Recursive Gaussian filtering is used in Parzen window joint histogram estimation for computational efficiency [9]. Furthermore, the implementation of the filtering is optimized to ensure coalesce memory access. 3. A relatively small joint histogram (128 × 128 bins) is used to reduce the cost of evaluating NMI, and the upper and lower bound of the histogram are carefully chosen to ensure sufficient intensity resolution of the target object. 4. OpenMP is used to take advantage of multi-core CPU.

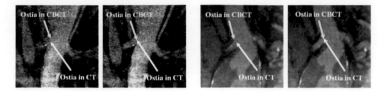

**Fig. 6.** Two examples of CT and CBCT overlay before (left) and after (right) aorta registration. Renal ostia (annotated by arrows) are about 7 mm off originally, and are perfectly aligned after aorta registration.

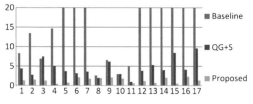

**Fig. 7.** TRE for 17 datasets

**Table 1.** Summary of Results

|  | μTRE (mm) | maxTRE (mm) | Success rate |
|---|---|---|---|
| Baseline | 43.15 | 176.15 | 5.89% |
| QG+S | 4.59 | 9.56 | 23.53% |
| Proposed | 1.48 | 2.39 | 100% |

## 5   Experiments and Results

We conducted experiments using 17 AAA clinical datasets to validate the proposed method. Registration accuracy is measured by 3-D target registration error (TRE), which is defined as the average 3-D Euclidean distance between the transformed landmarks and the corresponding ground truth (manually annotated and confirmed by domain experts) for 5 landmarks: 2 renal ostia and 3 points along the centerline of the abdominal aorta. We calculated the average TRE ($\mu$TRE) and the maximum TRE (maxTRE) for all datasets. Success rate is evaluated based on the criterion that TRE<2.5 mm is clinically useful (according to our collaborating physicians) and thus a successful registration.

Experimental results are summarized in Table 1 and Fig. 7. In Fig. 7, the errors by baseline registration for some datasets far exceeding the range are not fully plotted. We first evaluated the baseline intensity-based 3-D/3-D registration, which uses NMI as the similarity measure and HC as the optimizer. The initial position before registration is provided by overlaying the center of mass of the two volumes. This method has a small capture range, leading to a low success rate (5.89%) and a large $\mu$TRE (43.15 mm). We also evaluated the performance of applying only the first two steps (quasi-global search and spine registration, denoted as QG+S) of the proposed method. This method achieved maxTRE of 9.56 mm, demonstrating that it successfully brings the target object close to the correct position for all the test cases. However, the $\mu$TRE (4.59 mm) and the low success rate (23.53%) indicates that the registration accuracy in the target area after these two steps is insufficient for clinical use. By performing the last step of aorta registration, the proposed method achieved $\mu$TRE of 1.48 mm and 100% success rate.

Due to the high efficiency of the proposed algorithm for quasi-global search as well as our highly optimized implementation, our method achieved 2.83 s computation time on average (Intel Xeon E5-5620, volume size $512\times512\times781$), which is critical for the system to be well accepted clinically. This is about one order of magnitude faster compared to other existing methods. For example, DIRECT (Dividing Rectangles) deterministic global optimization algorithm takes 36 s to complete 3D3D registration using 8 CPUs [10].

Besides offline experiments, our system is currently under clinical trial and has been used during 30 clinical cases. So far we have received 100% success rate from qualitative clinical feedbacks. This system meets the clinical requirements of AAA stenting procedures in terms of accuracy, robustness and speed.

## 6   Discussions and Conclusions

In this paper, we presented an image guidance system that brings pre-operative CT into the operating room to support interventional AAA stenting. The proposed 3-D/3-D registration method is fully automatic and highly efficient, and the system (including visualization) is seamlessly integrated into AAA stenting workflow. The presented work focus on the initial alignment of CT volumes and the support on the deployment of AAA main stent graft. Our future works include: 1. 2-D/3-D registration to compensate for patient movement during the procedure. 2. local deformable registration of iliac arteries to support the deployment of the branch stent graft during AAA.

## References

1. Creager, M.A., et al.: Aneurysmal disease of the aorta and its branches. In: Vascular Medicine: A Textbook of Vascular Biology and Disease, pp. 901–925 (1996)
2. Pluim, J.P.W., et al.: Mutual-information-based registration of medical images: a survey. TMI 22(8), 986–1004 (2003)
3. Thévenaz, P., et al.: Optimization of mutual information for multiresolution image registration. TMI 9(12), 2083–2099 (2000)
4. Matsopoulos, G.K., et al.: Automatic retinal image registration scheme using global optimization techniques. TITB 3(1), 47–60 (1999)
5. Rouet, J.M., et al.: Genetic algorithms for a robust 3-d mr-ct registration. TITB 4(2), 126–136 (2000)
6. Zhang, L., et al.: A knowledge-driven quasi-global registration of thoracic-abdominal ct and cbct for image-guided interventions. In: SPIE (2013)
7. Wells, W.M., et al.: Multi-modal volume registration by maximization of mutual information. Medical Image Analysis 1(1), 35–51 (1996)
8. Lombaert, H., et al.: A multilevel banded graph cuts method for fast image segmentation. In: ICCV, vol. 1, pp. 259–265. IEEE (2005)
9. Gunnar, F., et al.: Improving deriche-style recursive gaussian filters. JMIV 26(3), 293–299 (2006)
10. Dru, F., et al.: An itk framework for deterministic global optimization for medical image registration. In: Medical Imaging, p. 61442. International Society for Optics and Photonics (2006)

# Beyond Current Guided Bronchoscopy: A Robust and Real-Time Bronchoscopic Ultrasound Navigation System

Xiongbiao Luo and Kensaku Mori

Information and Communications Headquarters, Nagoya University
xiongbiao.luo@gmail.com, kensaku@is.nagoya-u.ac.jp

**Abstract.** This paper develops a new bronchoscopic ultrasound navigation system that fuses multimodal sensory information including preoperative images, bronchoscopic video sequences, ultrasound images, and external position sensor measurements. To construct such a system, we must align these information coordinate systems. We use hand-eye calibration to align the video camera and its attached external sensor and introduce a phantom-free method to calibrate the ultrasonic probe and its fixed external sensor. More importantly, we propose a marker-free registration method that uses the bronchoscope and the bronchial tree center information to register the sensor and the pre-operative coordinate systems. We constructed a bronchial phantom to validate our system, whose navigation accuracy was about 2.6 mm. Furthermore, compared to the current navigated bronchoscopy, the main advantage of our system is that it navigates the bronchoscope and the ultrasonic mini probe simultaneously and provides bronchial structures inside and outside the bronchial walls, particularly lymph node structures in ultrasonic images.

## 1 Introduction

Guided bronchoscopy fuses different modal sensory information to assist physicians to perform endoscopic interventions, e.g., transbronchial lung biopsy (TBLB) for lung cancer staging. Numerous papers have discussed guided bronchoscopy in the literature. Image registration (IR) methods are widely used in guided bronchoscopy [1,2], although they still suffer from problematic video images, e.g., surface mucus. Electromagnetic tracking (ET) systems are increasingly employed in bronchoscopic navigation [3,4,5]. Both IR- and ET-based techniques navigate the bronchoscope well to the target regions. After reaching the suspicious regions, fluoroscopy must be performed to guide the tissue biopsies since biopsy needles cannot be observed in the suspicious regions beyond the bronchial walls from the CT and video images [3]. The ultrasound mini probe is a promising device to observe needles and structures beyond bronchial walls in ultrasound images [6]. However, it cannot navigate itself to targets during interventions.

Beyond current guided bronchoscopy that performs biopsies with fluoroscopy, we construct a real-time bronchoscopic ultrasound guidance system that can navigate a bronchoscope and a ultrasound mini probe simultaneously and observe

K. Mori et al. (Eds.): MICCAI 2013, Part I, LNCS 8149, pp. 388–395, 2013.

biopsy needles and pulmonary structures beyond the bronchial walls. Our system combines bronchoscopic video, an ultrasound probe, an ET system, and CT slices to navigate the bronchoscope and the probe and guide the bronchoscopic accessory tools. To establish different alignments in our system, we propose phantom-free and marker-free registration methods after hand-eye calibration.

The contribution of this work is threefold. To the best of our knowledge, no guided bronchoscopy systems have been reported that resemble our system. Our system can track not only the bronchoscope and the ultrasound probe synchronously but it can also observe endoscopic accessory tools and pulmonary structure without fluoroscopy. We propose an improved marker-free registration approach to align an external tracking sensor and pre-operative images. Our method, which uses both bronchoscope and bronchial tree center information, was demonstrated to be more accurate than the others. Additionally, we introduce phantom-free calibration to align the ET and ultrasound systems.

## 2    Navigation System Design

### 2.1    Hardware

Our system includes the following hardware: (1) an ET system and two electromagnetic sensors (ES), (2) an ultrasound (US) miniature radial probe, (3) a bronchoscopic camera (BC) integrated into a bronchoscope in an endoscopy system, and (4) a host computer with an user interface display. We use an ET system with two sensors fixed to collect bronchoscope and US miniature probe movements. Additionally, we need to acquire the CT images of the anatomy. In general, our system involves five coordinate spaces: ET, ES, BS, US, and CT (Fig. 2).

### 2.2    Software

We designed our system interface with five displays: (1) unmodified and real-time bronchoscopic video, (2) axial view of reformatted CT slices, synchronized with video and US images, (3) unchanged and real-time US images, (4) real-time virtual rendering images that correspond to video and US sequences, and (5) segmented three-dimensional lung structures that include airway trees and lymph nodes and real-time US images that are transformed in the CT space.

## 3    Approaches in Navigation

To realize our navigation system, we determine four transformations, $^{ES_1}\mathbf{T}_{BC}$, $^{ES_2}\mathbf{T}_{US}$, $^{CT}\mathbf{T}_{ET}$, and $^{CT}\mathbf{T}_{US}$, among five coordinate systems: ET, ES, BS, US, and CT. Two sensor outputs, $^{ET}\mathbf{T}_{ES_1}$ (to record the bronchoscope motion) and $^{ET}\mathbf{T}_{ES_2}$ (to measure the US probe motion), indicate the transformation between the ET and ES coordinate systems. We must determine these transformations of $^{ES_1}\mathbf{T}_{BC}$, $^{ES_2}\mathbf{T}_{US}$, $^{CT}\mathbf{T}_{ET}$, and $^{CT}\mathbf{T}_{US} = {}^{CT}\mathbf{T}_{ET}{}^{ET}\mathbf{T}_{ES_2}{}^{ES_2}\mathbf{T}_{US}$ to navigate the bronchoscope and the US probe in our system. We propose phantom-free and marker-free methods for obtaining $^{ES_2}\mathbf{T}_{US}$ and $^{CT}\mathbf{T}_{ET}$.

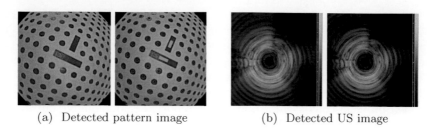

(a)  Detected pattern image          (b)  Detected US image

**Fig. 1.** Images for BC-ES spatial alignment and phantom-free US-ES calibration

## 3.1  BC-ES Spatial Alignment

To compute $^{ES_1}\mathbf{T}_{BC}$, we perform a hand-eye calibration, which establishes the hand (e.g., a robot gripper) and eye (e.g., a camera) relationship that can be calculated using a number of acquired camera and gripper motions. In our case, *"hand"* corresponds to the ET sensor, and *"eye"* relates to the bronchoscope camera. Using pattern images (Fig. 1 (a)), $^{ES_1}\mathbf{T}_{BC}$ can be solved by [7]:

$$\begin{cases} \Delta^{ES_1}\mathbf{T}_{ij} \cdot {}^{ES_1}\mathbf{T}_{BC} = {}^{ES_1}\mathbf{T}_{BC} \cdot \Delta^{BC}\mathbf{T}_{ij} \\ \Delta^{ES_1}\mathbf{T}_{ij} = {}^{ES_1}\mathbf{T}_{ET}^i \cdot {}^{ET}\mathbf{T}_{ES_1}^j \\ \Delta^{BC}\mathbf{T}_{ij} = {}^{BC}\mathbf{T}_{P}^i \cdot {}^{P}\mathbf{T}_{BC}^j \end{cases}, \tag{1}$$

where $\Delta^{ES_1}\mathbf{T}_{ij}$ is the relative sensor motion measured by the EM system and $\Delta^{BC}\mathbf{T}_{ij}$ is the camera movement relative to the calibration pattern frame for the bronchoscope moving from the $i$-th pose to the $j$-th pose. Bronchoscopic camera pose $^{BC}\mathbf{T}_P^i$ is computed by the camera calibration [7].

## 3.2  Phantom-Free US-ES Calibration

We here propose a phantom-free method to calculate $^{ES_2}\mathbf{T}_{US}$. Since we attach an ET sensor to the US probe, the sensor shape can be observed in the US images (Fig. 1(b)). We segment such a shape and get its center point $\mathbf{a}_k^{us}$ that is represented by homogeneous coordinates: $\mathbf{a}_k^{us} = (a_k^x, a_k^y, 0, 1)^T$ ($k$ indicates the US frame number). We perform the following minimization to compute $^{ES_2}\mathbf{T}_{US}$:

$$^{ES_2}\tilde{\mathbf{T}}_{US} = \arg \min_{^{ES_2}\mathbf{T}_{US}} \left\| \mathbf{p}_k - {}^{ET}\mathbf{T}_{ES_2} \cdot {}^{ES_2}\mathbf{T}_{US} \cdot \mathbf{a}_k^{us} \right\|, \tag{2}$$

where position $\mathbf{p}_k = (p_k^x, p_k^y, p_k^z, 1)^T$ is from the sensor attached at the US probe.

## 3.3  Real-Time Marker-Free ET-CT Registration

Since the accuracy of our system is heavily influenced by the ET-CT registration error, we modify the marker-free method to compute $^{CT}\mathbf{T}_{ET}$ more accurately. To synchronize the ET and CT coordinate systems, we could use either the marker-based or marker-free methods [3,5]. Although the marker-based method

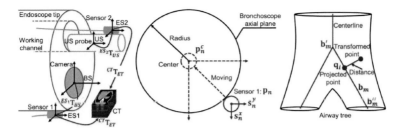

**Fig. 2.** Coordinate systems involved in our navigation system (*left*), moving original sensor position $\mathbf{p}_n$ to bronchoscope center $\mathbf{p}_n^c$ (*middle*), and assigning bronchus centerline $\mathbf{b}_m$ to modified sensor position $\mathbf{p}_n^c$ (*right*)

works well [3], it is somewhat difficult to perform it operating rooms. Without additional setups (e.g., anatomical marker selection), the marker-free method assumes that the bronchoscope is operated along the bronchial centerlines in the bronchoscopy; such an assumption is easily violated in practice.

To address the above assumption, we move the sensor measurements much closer to the bronchial centerlines. We believe that the center of the bronchoscope axial plane is closer to the bronchial centerlines than the position of the sensor attached to the bronchoscope surface. Therefore, we can move the sensor measurement to the center of the bronchoscope axial plane (Fig. 2). Changing the sensor position to the bronchoscope center (close to the bronchial centerlines) will prove very effective in our experiments.

Suppose $(\mathbf{p}_n, \mathbf{s}_n^x, \mathbf{s}_n^y, \mathbf{s}_n^z)$ (i.e., $^{ET}\mathbf{T}_{ES_1}$) is the measurement with position $\mathbf{p}_n$ and the orientation $(\mathbf{s}_n^x, \mathbf{s}_n^y, \mathbf{s}_n^z)$ of the $x$-, $y$-, and $z$-directions from the sensor is attached to the bronchoscope surface ($n$ is the measurement number). Based on sensor output directions $\mathbf{s}_n^x$ and $\mathbf{s}_n^y$, bronchoscope center $\mathbf{p}_n^c$ is calculated by:

$$\mathbf{p}_n^c = \mathbf{p}_n - r_b \cdot (\mathbf{s}_n^x + \mathbf{s}_n^y), \tag{3}$$

where $r_b$ is the bronchoscope radius. Fig. 2 shows the relation of $\mathbf{p}_n^c$ and $\mathbf{p}_n$. After we segment the CT images to get bronchial centerline $\mathbf{b}_m = (\mathbf{b}_m', \mathbf{b}_m'')$ ($m$ is the bronchus number, $\mathbf{b}_m'$ and $\mathbf{b}_m''$ are the start and end points of $\mathbf{b}_m$), we assign closest centerline $\hat{\mathbf{b}}_m$ to $\mathbf{p}_n^c$ by minimizing distance $E(^{CT}\mathbf{T}_{ET} \cdot \mathbf{p}_n^c, \mathbf{b}_m)$:

$$\hat{\mathbf{b}}_m = \arg\min_{\mathbf{b}_m} E(^{CT}\mathbf{T}_{ET} \cdot \mathbf{p}_n^c, \mathbf{b}_m), \tag{4}$$

where $^{CT}\mathbf{T}_{ET} \cdot \mathbf{p}_n^c$ is the transformed point and $E(^{CT}\mathbf{T}_{ET} \cdot \mathbf{p}_n^c, \mathbf{b}_m)$ is defined as (Fig. 2)

$$\mathbf{E}(^{CT}\mathbf{T}_{ET} \cdot \mathbf{p}_n^c, \mathbf{b}_m) = \begin{cases} ||^{CT}\mathbf{T}_{ET} \cdot \mathbf{p}_n^c - \mathbf{b}_m'|| & \lambda < 0 \\ ||^{CT}\mathbf{T}_{ET} \cdot \mathbf{p}_n^c - \mathbf{b}_m''|| & \lambda > ||\mathbf{b}_m'' - \mathbf{b}_m'|| \, , \\ \sqrt{||^{CT}\mathbf{T}_{ET} \cdot \mathbf{p}_n^c - \mathbf{b}_m'||^2 - \lambda^2} & otherwise \end{cases} \tag{5}$$

where $\lambda = (^{CT}\mathbf{T}_{ET} \cdot \mathbf{p}_n^c - \mathbf{b}_m') \cdot (\mathbf{b}_m'' - \mathbf{b}_m') \cdot ||\mathbf{b}_m'' - \mathbf{b}_m'||^{-1}$. Since we might obtain several centerlines $\{\hat{\mathbf{b}}_m\}$, we choose optimal centerline $\mathbf{b}_{m*}$ by computing the difference between vector $(\hat{\mathbf{b}}_m'' - \hat{\mathbf{b}}_m') \cdot ||\hat{\mathbf{b}}_m'' - \hat{\mathbf{b}}_m'||^{-1}$ and sensor $z$-direction $\mathbf{s}_n^z$:

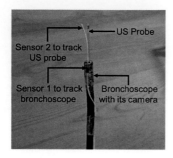 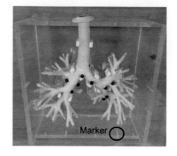

**Fig. 3.** Sensor, bronchoscope, US probe, and phantom used in experiments

$$\mathbf{b}_{m*} = \arg \min_{\{\hat{\mathbf{b}}_m\}} \arccos < \frac{\hat{\mathbf{b}}''_m - \hat{\mathbf{b}}'_m}{||\hat{\mathbf{b}}''_m - \hat{\mathbf{b}}'_m||}, \frac{^{CT}\mathbf{T}_{ET} \cdot \mathbf{s}^z_n}{||^{CT}\mathbf{T}_{ET} \cdot \mathbf{s}^z_n||} >, \tag{6}$$

where $<, >$ represents the dot product. We project transformed point $^{CT}\mathbf{T}_{ET} \cdot \mathbf{p}^c_n$ on optimal centerline $\mathbf{b}_{m*}$ and obtain projected point $\mathbf{q}_n$ (Fig. 2):

$$\mathbf{q}_n = \mathbf{b}'_{m*} + \frac{(^{CT}\mathbf{T}_{ET} \cdot \mathbf{p}^c_n - \mathbf{b}'_{m*}) \cdot (\mathbf{b}''_{m*} - \mathbf{b}'_{m*})}{||\tilde{\mathbf{B}}''_i - \tilde{\mathbf{B}}'_i||} \cdot \frac{(\mathbf{b}''_{m*} - \mathbf{b}'_{m*})}{||\mathbf{b}''_{m*} - \mathbf{b}'_{m*}||}. \tag{7}$$

Finally, we obtain bronchoscope center points $\mathcal{M} = \{(\mathbf{p}^c_n, \mathbf{s}^x_n, \mathbf{s}^y_n, \mathbf{s}^z_n)\}^N_{n=1}$ and projected points $\mathcal{P} = \{\mathbf{q}_n\}^N_{n=1}$ (total sensor measurement number $N$) and determine optimal $^{CT}\tilde{\mathbf{T}}_{ET}$ by ($r_{m*}$ is the radius of $\mathbf{b}_{m*}$):

$$^{CT}\tilde{\mathbf{T}}_{ET} = \arg \min_{\mathbf{p}^c_n \in \mathcal{M}, \mathbf{q}_n \in \mathcal{P}} \sum_n \frac{||^{CT}\mathbf{T}_{ET} \cdot \mathbf{p}^c_n - \mathbf{q}_n||}{r_{m*}}. \tag{8}$$

## 4   Navigation Accuracy Analysis

**Experimental Settings** In our experiments, we used a 3-D Guidance med-SAFE tracker (Ascension Technology Corporation, USA) as our ET system. Two electromagnetic sensors (1.5 mm, 6DoF) were attached to a bronchoscope (BF Type 200, Olympus, Tokyo) and US probe (UM-S20-17S, Olympus, Tokyo) for tracking their movements (Fig. 3). The tip diameter of the bronchoscope and the probe was 4.0 and 1.7 mm. We constructed a bronchial phantom to evaluate our methods. Its CT space parameters were $512 \times 512 \times 611$ voxels and $0.892 \times 0.692 \times 0.5$ mm$^3$. We placed twenty markers on the phantom (Fig. 3) and used them to evaluate the registration error of $^{CT}\mathbf{T}_{ET}$ by: $Err = \sum^{20}_{o=1} ||\mathbf{q}^{CT}_o - {}^{CT}\mathbf{T}_{ET} \cdot \mathbf{p}^{ET}_o||/20$.

**Accuracy Analysis.** Our constructed system interface with five displays (Fig. 4) provides physicians with different visualization information. We used twelve pattern images with twelve sensor measurements to perform the hand-eye calibration. The calibration error was about 0.5 mm. We also used ten frames of US

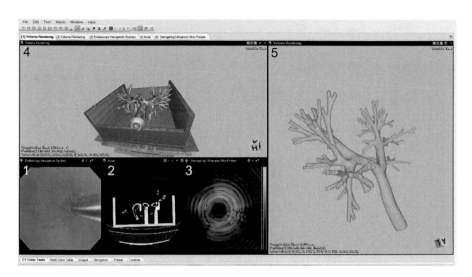

**Fig. 4.** Our system interface with five displays: 1, 2, 3, 4, and 5

**Table 1.** Quantitative comparison of average registration error and average distance (Eq. 5) between sensor measurements and bronchial centerlines

| Methods<br>Experiments | Deguchi et al. [5] | | Our method | |
|:---:|:---:|:---:|:---:|:---:|
| | Accuracy | Distance | Accuracy | Distance |
| 1 | 6.9 mm | 5.2 mm | 3.2 mm | 4.2 mm |
| 2 | 4.0 mm | 5.1 mm | 2.6 mm | 4.1 mm |
| 3 | 3.9 mm | 4.8 mm | 1.4 mm | 3.9 mm |
| 4 | 4.8 mm | 5.2 mm | 2.9 mm | 4.2 mm |
| 5 | 4.9 mm | 6.1 mm | 3.1 mm | 3.1 mm |
| **Average** | **4.9 mm** | **5.3 mm** | **2.6 mm** | **3.9 mm** |

images to align the US and sensor coordinate systems. The current alignment error was around 0.8 mm. Table 1 quantifies the average ET-CT registration error and the average distance (computed by Eq. 5) between the sensor measurements and the bronchial centerlines in the five experiments. The distance to the bronchial centerlines of the methods of Deguchi et al. [5] and ours was around 5.3 and 3.9 mm. The average registration error was reduced from 4.9 to 2.6 mm. Fig. 5 shows the registration accuracy, the distance, and the sensor measurement points distributed inside the bronchial trees of Experiment 5. Fig. 6 compares the registration results of the two methods. Since the virtual images generated from the registered results of our method more closely resemble the video images than Deguchi et al. [5], our method outperforms it [5].

Compared with current guided bronchoscopy, we believe that our system is promising since it provides different visualization information, e.g., the current bronchoscope and US probe positions in the CT coordinate system and the pulmonary structures and the biopsy needle locations inside and outside the bronchial walls, to assist physicians to perform bronchoscopic interventions. We

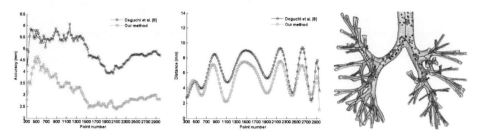

**Fig. 5.** Plotted registration accuracy (*left*) and distance to bronchial centerlines (*middle*). *Right*: *Green* points based on our method were closer to *blue* bronchial centerlines than *red* points generated from Deguchi et al. [5]

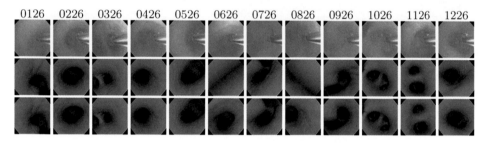

**Fig. 6.** Visual comparison of ET-CT registration results. Top row shows uniformly selected frame numbers, and second row shows their corresponding video images. Third and fourth rows display virtual images registered by Deguchi et al. [5] and our method. Our method shows better performance.

also improved the registration accuracy of the marker-free method. We attribute such an improvement to moving the original sensor position to the bronchoscope center to reduce the distance between the sensor positions and the bronchial centerlines (Fig. 5). Our experimental results demonstrated that our idea can significantly diminish the assumption of moving the bronchoscope along the bronchial centerlines. However, our system navigation error still originated mainly from the ET-CT registration step due to static and dynamic errors of our ET system. The inherent static error is 1.4 mm. The dynamic error, which is difficult to correct without optical trackers, is caused by the dynamic magnetic field distortion that results from metals in the working volume of our ET system. Note that, in our current validation, we did not consider the respiratory motion problem, which also challenges our system's navigation accuracy. It is possible to track the breathing motion by attaching several sensors to the thorax to compensate the accuracy. We will evaluate our method on patient datasets or a dynamic phantom that can simulate breathing motion in the future.

# 5    Conclusions

This paper proposed a new bronchoscopic ultrasound navigation system that combines pre-operative images, bronchoscopic video sequences, ultrasound images, and external position sensor measurements. The most advantageous point of our system enables physicians to navigate the bronchoscope and the ultrasonic mini probe simultaneously, locating bronchial structures inside and outside the bronchial walls in the video and US images, particularly pulmonary lymph nodes where biopsies may be performed. We also modified a marker-free method to perform CT-to-physical registration on the basis of moving sensor positions to the bronchoscope axial centers. The current registration accuracy can be improved from 4.9 to 2.6 mm, which approximates the clinical requirement of 2.0 mm. Future work includes further improvement of our system navigation accuracy under respiratory motion and validating our system on patient datasets.

**Acknowledgment.** This work was partly supported by the center of excellence project "Development of high-precision bedside devices for early metastatic cancer diagnosis and surgery" (01-D-D0806) funded by the Aichi Prefecture, the JSPS Kakenhi "Modality-seamless navigation for endoscopic diagnosis and surgery assistance based on multi-modality image fusion" (25242047), and the project "Computational anatomy for computer-aided diagnosis and therapy: frontiers of medical image sciences" (21103006) funded by a Grant-in-Aid for Scientific Research on Innovative Areas, MEXT, Japan.

# References

1. Deligianni, F., Chung, A.J., Yang, G.Z.: Nonrigid 2-D/3-D registration for patient specific bronchoscopy simulation with statistical shape modeling: Phantom validation. IEEE TMI 25(11), 1462–1471 (2006)
2. Luo, X., Feuerstein, M., Deguchi, D., Kitasaka, T., Takabatake, H., Mori, K.: Development and comparison of new hybrid motion tracking for bronchoscopic navigation. MedIA 16(3), 577–596 (2012)
3. Schwarz, Y., Greif, J., Becker, H.D., Ernst, A., Mehta, A.: Real-time electromagnetic navigation bronchoscopy to peripheral lung lesions using overlaid CT images: The first human study. Chest 129(4), 988–994 (2006)
4. Luo, X., Kitasaka, T., Mori, K.: Bronchoscopy navigation beyond electromagnetic tracking systems: a novel bronchoscope tracking prototype. In: Fichtinger, G., Martel, A., Peters, T. (eds.) MICCAI 2011, Part I. LNCS, vol. 6891, pp. 194–202. Springer, Heidelberg (2011)
5. Deguchi, D., Feuerstein, M., Kitasaka, T., Suenaga, Y., Ide, I., Murase, H., Imaizumi, K., Hasegawa, Y., Mori, K.: Real-time marker-free patient registration for electromagnetic navigated bronchoscopy: a phantom study. IJCARS 7(3), 359–369 (2012)
6. Herth, F.J.F., Schuler, H., Gompelmann, D., Kahn, N., Gasparini, S., Ernst, A., Schuhmann, M., Eberhardt, R.: Endobronchial ultrasound-guided lymph node biopsy with transbronchial needle forceps: a pilot study. Eur. Respir. J. 39, 373–377 (2012)
7. Wengert, C., Reeff, M., Cattin, P.C., Szekely, G.: Fully automatic endoscope calibration for intraoperative use. In: BFDM 2006, pp. 419–423. Springer (2006)

# A Stochastic Model for Automatic Extraction of 3D Neuronal Morphology

Sreetama Basu[1], Maria Kulikova[2], Elena Zhizhina[3],
Wei Tsang Ooi[1], and Daniel Racoceanu[2,4]

[1] National University of Singapore, Singapore
[2] University Pierre and Marie Curie, Paris, France
[3] Institute of Information Transmission Problems, Russia
[4] CNRS, France

**Abstract.** Tubular structures are frequently encountered in bio-medical images. The center-lines of these tubules provide an accurate representation of the topology of the structures. We introduce a stochastic Marked Point Process framework for fully automatic extraction of tubular structures requiring no user interaction or seed points for initialization. Our Marked Point Process model enables unsupervised network extraction by fitting a configuration of objects with globally optimal associated energy to the centreline of the arbors. For this purpose we propose special configurations of marked objects and an energy function well adapted for detection of 3D tubular branches. The optimization of the energy function is achieved by a stochastic, discrete-time multiple birth and death dynamics. Our method finds the centreline, local width and orientation of neuronal arbors and identifies critical nodes like bifurcations and terminals. The proposed model is tested on 3D light microscopy images from the DIADEM data set with promising results.

## 1 Introduction

Advances in imaging technologies generate huge volume of microscopy data. Manual analysis of such data is prohibitively expensive in terms of the expert man-hours required. At present, high resolution, high content 3D data is becoming more and more prevalent. Thus, a fully automatic, stochastic rather than deterministic data exploration strategy, combining both local and global image evidence, is desired [1].

Neurite tracing methods connect paths of maximum neuriteness voxels locally between sets of seed points to extract the global neurite structure. A common drawback of existing methods is their dependence on seed points [2]. Often, manual intervention is required to select the optimal seed points. Unavailability of seed points can even lead to entire branches going undetected. Not only for neurons, seed points are a relevant concern for all kinds of tubular structure extraction scenarios [3]. Commonly, multiscale Eigen-analysis [4], in combination with gradient information [5] or intensity ridge traversal [6] are used to detect seeds on tubule centrelines. These filters find voxels maximizing a vesselness measure by collecting responses over a range of filter scales. They are computationally intensive as multiple scales and orientations of the filters are convolved with the image data at every voxel. With increasing volume of data and considering 3D orientations of neurites, deterministic filter response maximization

K. Mori et al. (Eds.): MICCAI 2013, Part I, LNCS 8149, pp. 396–403, 2013.

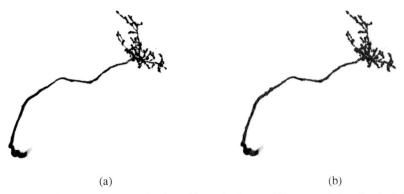

(a)            (b)

**Fig. 1.** (a) Minimum intensity projection of intensity inverted (for ease of visualisation) Olfactory Projection Fibers (OPF) data obtained by confocal microscopy. (b) The extracted network with the proposed model visualised on a projection of the OPF data. We restrict overlap of object to have a sparse density on the branches and yet get a sense of the continuity of the neurites.

is an infeasible option, considering the huge solution space that is required to be explored. The results will be sensitive to initialization, necessitating human intervention. Machine learning techniques like SVMs for automatic seed selection have been proposed in the literature [7]. But their dependence on availability and quality of learning data, however, make them an unattractive choice.

We develop an efficient Marked Point Process (MPP) framework for extraction of neuronal structures from 3D data without greatly increasing the computational complexity of sampling and estimation, in contrast to existing MPP based 2D methods [8],[9]. Firstly, spheres are chosen as MPP objects, in particular because it gives one dimensional object space but allows to simultaneously extract center line, size and local orientation of branches. Secondly, to find the Maximum A Posteriori (MAP) estimate of the optimal configuration, we sample from the object configuration space using a Multiple Birth and Death (MBAD) dynamics embedded in a Simulated Annealing scheme [10]. The MBAD dynamics reduces computational cost over traditional Reversible Jump Monte Carlo Markov Chain samplers by avoiding proposal kernel computations and leads to faster convergence.

## 2 3D Marked Point Process Model

The *Point Process* models were first introduced in [11] to exploit random fields whose realizations are configurations of random points describing a spatial distribution of data.

### 2.1 From Point to Parametric Marked Point Process

We consider a point process $\mathcal{X}$ existing in $K = [0, X_{max}] \times [0, Y_{max}] \times [0, Z_{max}]$, where $K$ is a bounded, connected subset of $\mathbb{V}^3$, the image domain. In the Marked Point Processes, each point $x_i$ is associated with additional parameters (marks) $m_i$ to define an object $\omega_i = (x_i, m_i)$. Here, $x_i \in K$ and $m_i \in M$ and the Marked Point Process $\mathcal{Y}$ is defined on $K \times M$. The *configuration space* of the objects is given by $\Omega = \cup_{n=0}^{\infty} \Omega_n$, where $\Omega_0$ is the empty set, each $\Omega_n, n \in \mathbb{N}$ is the set of unordered sets (configurations) containing $n$ objects and $\gamma_n \in \Omega_n, \gamma_n = \{\omega_1, \ldots, \omega_n\}$. Note that $n$ can be arbitrary, and in the following sections of the paper the elements of configuration $\gamma \in \Omega$ (with an arbitrary number of elements) will be denoted as $\omega_i$, where $i = 1 \ldots n$.

## 2.2    Gibb's Distribution and Energy of Configuration

The Marked Point Processes are defined by their probability density w.r.t. the reference Poisson process. Given a real, bounded below function $U(\gamma)$ in $\Omega$, the Gibbs distribution $\mu_\beta$ in terms of the density $p(\gamma) = \frac{d\mu_\beta}{d\lambda}(\gamma)$ w.r.t. Lebesgue-Poisson measure $\lambda$ on $\Omega$ is defined as:

$$p(\gamma) = \frac{z^{|\gamma|}}{Z_\beta} \exp[-\beta U(\gamma)]. \tag{1}$$

Here, parameters $z, \beta > 0$ and $Z_\beta$ is a normalizing factor. In the Gibbs energy model, the optimum object configuration $\hat{\gamma}$ corresponds to the minimum global energy, where $\gamma$ represents the configuration of objects:

$$\hat{\gamma} = \arg \max_\gamma p(\gamma) = \arg \min_\gamma U(\gamma). \tag{2}$$

$$U(\gamma) = \sum_{\omega_i \in \gamma} U_d(\omega_i) + \sum_{\substack{\omega_i, \omega_j \in \gamma; \\ \omega_i \sim \omega_j}} U_i(\omega_i, \omega_j) + \sum_{\omega_i \in \gamma} U_c(\omega_i), \tag{3}$$

where the operation $\sim$ is defined as a neighborhood relation: $\omega_i \sim \omega_j = |\omega_i, \omega_j \in \gamma :$ $|x_i - x_j| < tD|$ and $D$ is distance between centres of objects $\omega_i$ and $\omega_j$, and $t \in \mathbb{N}$. $U_d$ represents the data energy, $U_i$ is the interaction prior energy and $U_c$ is the connection prior energy. We seek to minimize the global energy $U(\gamma)$. To find the minimizer $\hat{\gamma}$ means to find the number $n$ of objects in the required configuration and to find positions of all $n$ objects in the configuration $\hat{\gamma}$.

# 3    Energy Modeling for 3D Neuronal Network Extraction

Our aim is to extract the neuronal branches by generating a configuration of objects fitted to the points of maximum medialness measure on the image volume. For this purpose, we adopt spheres as objects $\omega_i = (x_i, r_i)$, $x_i \in \mathbb{V}^3$, $r_i \in [r_{min}, r_{max}]$ and $\omega_i(x_i, r_i) = (y_i : |x_i - y_i| \le r_i)$ where $y_i$ are voxels in the image domain $\mathbb{V}^3$. The stochastic optimization and random sampling strategy of the object configuration space, which also defines our filter space, extracts an optimal configuration of objects whose radii correspond to the scales of the filters maximizing the responses at their centre voxels in the image data. In the following section we describe each of the energy components in detail.

## 3.1    Data Energy

Our data energy response is based on the tubularity filter proposed in [12] and the interested reader may refer it for complete details. The Hessian is a second order partial derivative of image data containing local structural information. Its principal components determine the tangent direction and normal plane of the local neurite structures.

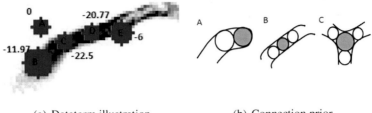

(a) Dataterm illustration              (b) Connection prior

**Fig. 2.** (a) High negative energies indicate "good" objects (eg. objects B,C,D) i.e. objects situated on the branch centreline and the same size as the local branch width. "Bad" objects, for example, on the background (object A) or not centred correctly on the branch (object E) have low probabilities of survival in the configuration during the energy minimization scheme. (b) Each sub configuration is identified by its characteristic connection energy - evaluated w.r.t. the number of neighbors with direct data connection with the current object (shaded in the image). A: Terminal. B: Anchor points along the length of a branch. C: Bifurcation junction.

The scale of the Hessian $\sigma_H$ is uniformly sampled from the radius range $[r_{min}, r_{max}]$. The medialness measure $M(\omega_i)$ is obtained by taking an integral of the image gradient at scale $\sigma_G$ along the circumference of the cut of the spherical object on the normal plane defined by $V1$ and $V2$ -

$$M(\omega_i) = |\frac{\pi}{2} \int_{\theta=0}^{2\pi} \nabla I^{(\sigma_G)}(x_i + r_i V_\theta) d\theta|. \tag{4}$$

Here, $V_\theta = cos(\theta)V_1 + sin(\theta)V_2$ is a rotating phasor in the normal plane sampling gradient information at radial distance $r$ from the center $x_i = [x, y, z]^T, x_i \in \mathbb{V}^3$ of the object. The medialness measure varies greatly for thin or weakly contrasted neurite branches, a common occurrence in case of microscopy images due to injection of noise and non-homogeneous staining of the neurons. Thus, a user defined optimal global threshold to reject structured noise and background artifacts is difficult to obtain. So, to discriminate between "good" and "bad" objects an adaptive thresholding of the medialness response is performed based on the gradient response at the tube's center $M_c(\omega_i) = |\nabla I^{(\sigma_H)}(x_i)|$. The data energy term is then defined as follows:

$$U_d(\omega_i) = \begin{cases} -(M(\omega_i) - M_c(\omega_i)), & \text{if } M(\omega_i) > M_c(\omega_i) \\ 0, & \text{otherwise.} \end{cases} \tag{5}$$

### 3.2 Pair-Wise Interaction Prior Energy

This term is a pair-wise interaction potential for objects in each other's zone of influence. It avoids crowding together of spheres along the neuronal processes and favors continuity of network by merging of close lying disconnected fragments, a common occurrence in microscopy data due to inhomogeneity in branch intensity and poor contrast with background. Around every object exists an immediate zone of repulsion followed by a concentric zone of attraction. Two energy potentials are defined: $U_+$ is repulsive in nature to penalize objects lying too close to each other, and $U_-$ is attractive in nature to favor objects in reasonable distances of each other.

$$U_i(\omega_i, \omega_j) = \begin{cases} U_+, & \text{if } d < d_r \\ U_-, & \text{if } d_r \leq d \leq d_a \\ 0, & \text{if } d > d_a. \end{cases} \quad (6)$$

Here, $d$ is the Euclidean distance between the centres of the spheres; $d_r$ and $d_a$ ($d_r < d_a$) are respectively the repulsive and attractive distances, $d_r, d_a$ are multiples of $r_i + r_j$. By varying $d_r$ and $d_a$, density of spheres along the neuronal branches can be controlled.

### 3.3 Connection Prior Energy

The second prior is a multi-object interaction potential, incorporating constraints on the connection among objects. Depending on the number of objects $k(\omega_i) = |\omega_j \in \gamma : d_r < d(\omega_i, \omega_j) < d_a|$, in the neighborhood, the prior term can also be used to determine branching points and termination points along neuronal processes, see Fig. 2(b).

$$U_c(\omega_i) = \begin{cases} E_1, & \text{if } k(\omega_i) = 0 \\ -E_1, & \text{if } k(\omega_i) = 1 \\ -E_2, & \text{if } k(\omega_i) = 2, 3 \\ -E_2, & \text{if } k(\omega_i) = 4 \\ E_1, & \text{if } k(\omega_i) > 4. \end{cases} \quad (7)$$

This association of favorable energy potentials $E_1$ and $E_2$ with particular local subconfigurations encourage accurate detection of critical nodes. At the same time, it discourages isolated objects in the configuration, which are likely to correspond to cell nuclei or other such background structures.

### 3.4 Optimization

The complexity of optimization of the global energy depends directly on the size of the sampling space of the objects, which we limit by the adoption of spherical objects, with a 1-dimensional parameter space. The optimum global energy is defined over the space of union of all possible configurations, considering an unknown a-priori number of objects. To obtain the optimal configuration of the objects on the image data, we use MAP estimation (Eq.2). We sample from the probability distribution $\mu_\beta$ using a Markov chain of the discrete-time Multiple Birth and Death dynamics defined on $\Omega$ and apply a Simulated Annealing scheme. At every iteration, a transition is considered from current configuration $\gamma$ to $\gamma' \cup \gamma''$ where $\gamma' \subset \gamma$ and $\gamma''$ is any new configuration. The corresponding transition probability is given by:

$$P(\gamma \to \gamma' \cup \gamma'') \sim (z\delta)^{|\gamma''|} \prod_{\omega_i \in \gamma \setminus \gamma'} \frac{\alpha_\beta(\omega_i, \gamma)\delta}{1 + \alpha_\beta(\omega_i, \gamma)\delta} \prod_{\omega_i \in \gamma'} \frac{1}{1 + \alpha_\beta(\omega_i, \gamma)\delta}, \quad (8)$$

where $\alpha_\beta(\omega_i, \gamma) = \exp(-\beta(U(\gamma \setminus \omega_i) - U(\gamma)))$. The convergence properties of the Markov Chain to the global minimum under a decreasing scheme of parameters $\delta$ and $\frac{1}{\beta}$ are proved in [10]. The probability of death of an object depends on both the

---

**Algorithm 1.** Multiple Birth and Death

---

**Initialize**

Discrete time-step $\delta = \delta_0$ and inverse temperature $\beta = \beta_0$.

Now, alternate between birth and death step until stop condition is met:

**Birth**

(a) Generate a configuration of spheres $\gamma \in \Omega$, from the Lebesgue-Poisson distribution with intensity $z = \delta z_0$ for centers, with independent radii uniformly distributed on $[r_{min}, r_{max}]$. A hard core repulsion $\delta_\epsilon$ is added with $\epsilon$ equal to one pixel.

(b) $\gamma' \cup \gamma''$: Add the new set of objects $\gamma''$ to the "surviving" ones $\gamma' \subset \gamma$ to get the current configuration $\gamma$.

**Death**

(a) Sort the objects of the current configuration according to their data energy $U_d(\omega_i)$, for the purpose of accelerating computation;

(b) Each object $\omega_i$ in the configuration $\gamma$, is removed with probability $p(\omega_i, \gamma) = \frac{\delta \alpha_\beta(\omega_i, \gamma)}{1 + \delta \alpha_\beta(\omega_i, \gamma)}$;

**Termination**

Terminate if all and only objects added in the birth step of current iteration are removed. Else, update $\gamma$, decrease $\delta$, $\frac{1}{\beta}$ according to a geometric annealing schedule and go to the birth step.

---

temperature and its relative energy in the sub-configuration; whereas, birth of object is independent of both energy and temperature and is spatially homogenous. In this way, the iterative process finds a configuration $\hat{\gamma}$ minimizing the global energy Eq. 3.

## 4    Experiments and Results

We test the performance of our proposed model on 3D light microscopy image stacks from the DIADEM Challenge database [13]. See Fig.3 and Fig.1. Although our method is not sensitive to the initialization of the configuration, to speed up convergence to the optimum configuration, the birth of the objects are restricted to a region of interest defined by the dilation of the maximum intensity projection of the original data stack for OPF and NL1 datasets. On the CCF data, obtained by Brightfield Microscopy, the configuration space is limited to a layered depth map obtained by a maximum intensity projection of the data. Our unoptimized Matlab implementation takes 57 mins, 3 hrs 29 mins, 1hr 33 mins to converge on NL1, OPF and CCF respectively, on a PC running Intel Core i7 processor, 3.4 GHz with 8GB RAM.

The *parameters of the priors* are set to - $U_+ = 10$, $U_- = -2$, $E_1 = 1.5$ and $E_2 = 2.0$, as described in the literature [14]. The *sampling parameters* are learnt from experiments and set as $\beta_0 = 1$ and $\delta_0$ to approximately three to five times the number of objects expected in the final configuration. The objects are sampled uniformly from the radius ranges $[1, 10]$, $[1, 3]$ and $[1, 25]$ for OPF, NL1 and CCF datasets respectively. The deviation of the extracted points set (P) using our proposed model from gold standard manually delineated centrelines (G) is compared in Table 1 in the following way:

$$max(P, G) = max(\min_{p \in P, g \in G}(f(p, g))) \tag{9}$$

$$avg(P, G) = avg(\min_{p \in P, g \in G}(f(p, g))) \tag{10}$$

$$err_r(P, G) = avg(|r_p - r_g| : \min_{p \in P, g \in G}(f(p, g))) \tag{11}$$

where $f(p,g)$ represents Euclidean distance of the concerned points and $r_p$ and $r_g$ are radius at point $p$ and $g$ respectively. Thus, our method produces an automatic and reliable extraction of neuronal morphology. It is robust to small branch discontinuities, intensity variations due to inhomogeneous labeling, noise and background interference.

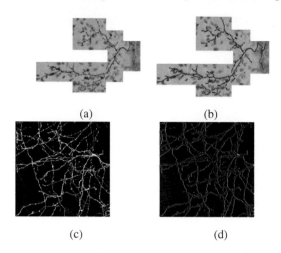

(a)                                (b)

(c)                                (d)

**Fig. 3.** (a) Minimum intensity projection of Cerebellar Climbing Fibers (CCF) obtained by Transmitted Light Brightfield microscopy. (b) The neuronal network extraction with the proposed model visualised on a slice CCF data. (c) Maximum intensity projection of Neocortical Layer 1 Axons (NL1) obtained by 2-photon Laser Scanning microscopy. (d) The neuronal network extraction with the proposed model on the projection of the NL1 data. These results are obtained with a high density of objects, allowing overlap to fully reconstruct the fuzzy and blurred segments of the neurites.

**Table 1.** Evaluation of our proposed method against Gold Standard manual extraction. The units of reporting error are anisotropic image voxels. The errors are higher along the z-axis due to the differential resolution of original data. *: ground truth radius not available.

| Dataset | Resolution | Centreline deviation | | | Radius |
|---------|------------|----------|----------|-----------------------------|-----------|
| | | $avg(P,G)$ | $max(P,G)$ | Points under 1 voxel error | $err_r(P,G)$ |
| OP1 | 512x512x60 | 1.231 | 3.9 | 80.14% | 0.5243 |
| OP2 | 512x512x88 | 1.065 | 2.5319 | 78.72% | * |
| OP4 | 512x512x67 | 1.4064 | 2.7154 | 83.71% | 0.5786 |
| CCF1 | 6120x4343x34 | 2.67 | 6.5869 | 66.23% | 1.7656 |
| NC01 | 512x512x60 | 1.1398 | 2.0119 | 79.12% | * |

## 5    Conclusion

To conclude, we present a MPP model for unsupervised network extraction that is fully automatic and requires neither seed points nor manual intervention. The proposed method significantly improves network detection by reconstructing blurred and fuzzy segments of networks due to connectivity priors of the energy function. Our work can also be viewed as a stochastic optimization of scale-orientation space for matched filters, developing a connected network of maximum vesselness points on tubular structures. The stochastic optimization to the global minimum and the random nature of data exploration makes it preferable for large, high content microscopy data-sets. The obtained results demonstrate its reliability and robustness for fully automated analysis of neuronal morphology.

So far, we only extract the neuronal structures by a configuration of uniformly spaced MPP objects. A future extension of our work might be neuronal reconstruction, where the extracted centreline, local width and orientation information along with detected critical nodes will aid in a connected, tree hierarchical representation of the neuronal arbors. Additionally, studies of the sensitivity and robustness of our model w.r.t. the model parameters and automatic estimation of the critical parameters are important, as that would increase the applicability of the family of Marked Point Process based methods.

# References

1. Meijering, E.: Neuron tracing in perspective. Cytometry Part A 77(7), 693–704 (2010)
2. Türetken, E., Blum, C., González, G., Fua, P.: Reconstructing geometrically consistent tree structures from noisy images. In: Jiang, T., Navab, N., Pluim, J.P.W., Viergever, M.A. (eds.) MICCAI 2010, Part I. LNCS, vol. 6361, pp. 291–299. Springer, Heidelberg (2010)
3. Kirbas, C., Quek, F.: A review of vessel extraction techniques and algorithms. ACM Computing Surveys 36(2), 81–121 (2004)
4. Frangi, A.F., Niessen, W.J., Vincken, K.L., Viergever, M.A.: Muliscale vessel enhancement filtering. In: Wells, W.M., Colchester, A.C.F., Delp, S.L. (eds.) MICCAI 1998. LNCS, vol. 1496, pp. 130–137. Springer, Heidelberg (1998)
5. Krissian, K., Malandain, G., Ayache, N., Vaillant, R., Trousset, Y.: Model-based multiscale detection of 3d vessels. In: CVPR, pp. 722–727 (1998)
6. Aylward, S.R., Bullitt, E.: Initialization, noise, singularities and scale in height ridge traversal for tubular object centerline extraction. IEEE Trans. Med. Imaging 21(2), 61–75 (2002)
7. González, G., Fleuret, F., Fua, P.: Learning rotational features for filament detection. In: CVPR, pp. 1582–1589 (2009)
8. Lacoste, C., Finet, G., Magnin, I.E.: Coronary tree extraction from x-ray angiograms using marked point processes. In: ISBI, pp. 157–160 (2006)
9. Sun, K., Sang, N., Zhang, T.: Marked point process for vascular tree extraction on angiogram. In: Yuille, A.L., Zhu, S.-C., Cremers, D., Wang, Y. (eds.) EMMCVPR 2007. LNCS, vol. 4679, pp. 467–478. Springer, Heidelberg (2007)
10. Descombes, X., Minlos, R., Zhizhina, E.: Object extraction using a stochastic birth-and-death dynamics in continuum. Journal of Math. Imaging and Vision 33(3), 347–359 (2009)
11. Baddeley, A., Van Lieshout, M.: Stochastic geometry models in high-level vision. Journal of Applied Statistics 20(5-6), 231–256 (1993)
12. Pock, T., Janko, C., Beichel, R., Bischof, H.: Multiscale medialness for robust segmentation of 3d tubular structures. In: Proceedings of the Computer Vision Winter Workshop, pp. 93–102 (2005)
13. Brown, K., Barrionuevo, G., Canty, A., De Paola, V., Hirsch, J., Jefferis, G., Lu, J., Snippe, M., Sugihara, I., Ascoli, G.: The diadem data sets: Representative light microscopy images of neuronal morphology to advance automation of digital reconstructions. Neuroinformatics, 1–15 (2011)
14. Cariou, P., Descombes, X., Zhizhina, E.: A point process for fully automatic road network detection in satellite and aerial images. Problems of Information Transmission 10(3), 247–256 (2010)

# A Viterbi Approach to Topology Inference for Large Scale Endomicroscopy Video Mosaicing

Jessie Mahé[1], Tom Vercauteren[1], Benoît Rosa[2], and Julien Dauguet[1]

[1] Mauna Kea Technologies, Paris, France
julien.dauguet@maunakeatech.com
[2] ISIR, UPMC-CNRS UMR7222, Paris, France

**Abstract.** Endomicroscopy allows in vivo and in situ imaging with cellular resolution. One limitation of endomicroscopy is the small field of view which can however be extended using mosaicing techniques. In this paper, we describe a methodological framework aiming to reconstruct a mosaic of endomicroscopic images acquired following a noisy robotized spiral trajectory. First, we infer the topology of the frames, that is the map of neighbors for every frame in the spiral. For this, we use a Viterbi algorithm considering every new acquired frame in the current branch of the spiral as an observation and the index of the best neighboring frame from the previous branch as the underlying state. Second, the estimated transformation between each spatial pair previously found is assessed. Mosaicing is performed based only on the pairs of frames for which the registration is considered successful. We tested our method on 3 spiral endomicroscopy videos each including more than 200 frames: a printed grid, an ex vivo tissue sample and an in vivo animal trial. Results were statistically significantly improved compared to reconstruction where only registration between successive frames was used.

## 1 Endomicroscopy during Surgical Intervention

Probe-based Confocal Laser Endomicroscopy (pCLE) is an imaging technique that provides in vivo video sequences of soft tissues at cellular level [8]. The work presented in this paper is part of a gastrointestinal surgery project where we aim to perform an *optical biopsy* during the procedure using pCLE. Like most microscopy imaging techniques, pCLE offers high resolution images at the expense of the field of view. Mosaicing techniques can be used to extend the field of view by stitching series of overlapping images and create a large field of view image. Mosaicing algorithms can be separated in two classes. In the first category are methods with no a priori on the acquisition trajectory (e.g. handheld microscopes) based on topology inference [6] where the configuration of the frames has to be entirely recovered from registration [1,4,7]. These methods are powerful but by definition do not take advantage of any topology information which tends to make them less robust and more computationally demanding on long videos. In the second category are methods adapted for known - usually robotized - acquisition trajectories (e.g. microscope with motorized platform) where the a

K. Mori et al. (Eds.): MICCAI 2013, Part I, LNCS 8149, pp. 404–411, 2013.

priori knowledge directly provides the topology [3]. For our project, a dedicated device was designed to allow video mosaic acquisitions wherein a robot holds the probe and follows a pre-defined spiral trajectory [2]. The theoretical trajectory given as a command to the robot can be actually very disturbed due to tissue friction and mechanical distortions (see Fig. 5, right). In a similar context, the mechanical perturbations were considered so dramatic that the estimation of the transformation between successive frames actually served as a velocity sensor to control the robot [5]. For mosaic reconstruction of videos acquired with our setup, theoretically we fall into the category of known trajectory. However, surgical conditions imply that we can not entirely rely on the trajectory information to infer the acquisition topology. Moreover, the actual neighbors might offer very little overlap preventing from performing reliable registration. The contribution of this paper is to propose a strategy to tackle the problem of mosaic reconstruction with weak a priori on the trajectory. We propose a three step method: first we infer the frames topology using Viterbi algorithm, second we estimate for each neighboring frames previously found the quality of the registration, and finally we rely on the best associations only to perform the final mosaic reconstruction.

## 2   Material and Method

### 2.1   Material

We used three film sequences acquired following the same spiral trajectory. The first sequence is a test sequence; it was acquired on a sheet of white paper with a printed image of a regular black grid using an industrial robot. The second sequence was acquired ex vivo on chicken breast using the same industrial robot. The last sequence was acquired in vivo on pig liver using the surgical actuator. Trajectories were three loop Archimedean spirals of polar equation $r = a\theta$ with $a = d_0/2\pi$ where $d_0 = 150\mu m$ is the theoretical inter-branch distance. The field of view of the mini-probe is approximately circular with a size of $200\mu m$, which implies a maximum theoretical overlap of $50\mu m$ between two frames from successive branches belonging to the same radius (see Fig. 1).

### 2.2   Method

The baseline information most video mosaicing algorithms rely on is the temporal registration between successive frames. Although fallible, this registration is considered sufficiently reliable since successive frames usually offer good overlapping provided that the speed of the probe is low enough. The goal of the topology inference is to add some extra associations between frames that are not temporal neighbors to constrain the global reconstruction and to prevent error propagation. We will refer to these extra associations as spatial neighbors. In this work, we will consider that the transformation between frames can be modeled by a translation estimated by maximization of the absolute value of correlation coefficient: we will refer to the estimated transformation as the *best* translation in the following.

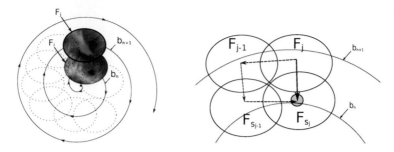

**Fig. 1.** The configuration of the spiral trajectory acquisition (left). The principle of checking the current spatial transformation by checking the registration consistency with previous frames (right).

**Viterbi Algorithm.** The first part of the method consists of estimating the spatial neighbor frames. Let us consider a hidden Markov model where at a given time index $j$, the observation is the current frame $F_j$ and the hidden state $s_j$ is the index of the frame in the previous branch that has the largest overlap with $F_j$ (see Fig. 1). The frame $F_{s_j}$ corresponding to the hidden state $s_j$ will also be referred to as the *best match* for $F_j$. Following the Viterbi algorithm, we aim at recovering the most probable sequence of hidden states, $s^{0 \to j} = \{s_0, s_1, \cdots, s_j\}$, given the sequence of observed frames, $F^{0 \to j} = \{F_0, F_1, \cdots, F_j\}$:

$$\hat{s}^{0 \to j} = \arg \max_{s^{0 \to j}} P(s^{0 \to j} | F^{0 \to j}). \qquad (1)$$

Let $\delta_j(i) = \max_{s^{0 \to j-1}} P(s^{0 \to j-1}, s_j = i, F^{0 \to j})$ be the probability of the best sequence of states ending at state $s_j = i$. Similarly to the standard Viterbi algorithm but keeping the complete set of observations in the emission probability we find that:

$$\delta_j(i) = P(F_j | s_j = i, F^{0 \to j-1}) \cdot \max_{i'} [P(s_j = i | s_{j-1} = i') \cdot \delta_{j-1}(i')]. \qquad (2)$$

Thanks to (2), the dynamic programing approach of the Viterbi algorithm allows us to solve for (1) by keeping back-pointers to the antecedent of each possible last hidden state. In this work, the transition probability $P_j^T$ is taken such that, if $F_j$ has $F_i$ as *best match*, i.e. $s_j = i$, the most likely a priori *best match* for $F_{j+1}$ will be $F_{i+1}$, i.e. $s_{j+1} = i + 1$:

$$P_j^T(i, i') = P(s_{j+1} = i' | s_j = i) = \mathcal{N}(i'; i + 1, \sigma_T), \qquad (3)$$

where $\mathcal{N}(i'; i + 1, \sigma_T)$ is the Gaussian probability function of mean $i + 1$ and standard deviation $\sigma_T$, with $\sigma_T$ controlling the strength of the a priori on the temporal smoothness of the sequence of states. The emission probability $P_j^E$ is chosen such that a frame $F_j$ is likely to have $F_i$ as *best match* if the registration between $F_j$ and $F_i$ leads to a good similarity criterion and to a transformation that is close to the expected one:

$$P_j^E(i, F_j) = P(F_j | s_j = i, F^{0 \to j-1}) = \mathcal{N}(d_{ij}; d_0, \sigma_D) \cdot Corr(F_i, F_j), \qquad (4)$$

where $d_{ij}$ is the euclidean distance between frames $F_i$ and $F_j$, $d_0$ is the expected distance between successive branches, $\sigma_D$ reflects the expected precision of the robot and $Corr(F_i, F_j)$ is the best absolute value of the correlation coefficient when registering frames $F_i$ and $F_j$ with translation transformations.

**Filtering of Associations.** We deduct from the Viterbi path the global topology providing spatial associations between frames of the video sequence. However, some of these associations might be erroneous and even correct associations might not offer sufficient overlap and features for successful registration. To only keep pairs of frames that are both actual neighbors and successfully registered, we operate a filtering of the pairs. For a given pair of frames $F_i$ of branch $b_n$ and $F_j$ of branch $b_{n+1}$ supposedly spatial neighbors, we compute the following transformation consistency criterion $TC$: $TC_{ij} = \|T_{ji} - T_{(i-1)i} \circ T_{(j-1)(i-1)} \circ T_{j(j-1)}\|$ where $T_{ji}$ is the best estimated translation between $F_i$ and $F_j$ (see Fig. 1). We then evaluate the reliability of the association between frames $F_i$ and $F_j$ based on three criteria: the transformation consistency $TC_{ij}$, the absolute value of the correlation coefficient $CC_{ij}$ and the distance consistency $DC_{ij} = | d_0 - d_{ij} |$. We only keep spatial pairs respecting one of the following conditions:

- $TC_{ij} < TC_{strict}$ and $CC_{ij} > CC_{loose}$ and $DC_{ij} < DC_{loose}$
- $TC_{ij} < TC_{loose}$ and $CC_{ij} > CC_{strict}$ and $DC_{ij} < DC_{loose}$
- $TC_{ij} < TC_{loose}$ and $CC_{ij} > CC_{loose}$ and $DC_{ij} < DC_{strict}$
- $TC_{ij} < TC_{mid}$ and $CC_{ij} > CC_{mid}$ and $DC_{ij} < DC_{mid}$

where subscript tags $\{strict, mid, loose\}$ refer to $10^{th}, 20^{th}, 30^{th}$ percentiles of the set of values $TC$, $DC$ and $90^{th}, 80^{th}, 70^{th}$ percentiles of the set of values $CC$ estimated for all the pairs of frames derived from the Viterbi path and ranked in increasing order.

**Mosaic Reconstruction.** For the final mosaic reconstruction, we modified the mosaicing algorithm described in [7] so as to be able to inject the spatial pairs previously obtained to impose the topology. The rest of the algorithm remains unchanged: the best transformation is estimated between successive frames (temporal neighbors) as well as between given spatial pairs. A robust Fréchet mean of all the transformations - temporal and spatial - is then computed leading to the estimation of one unique transformation to the common reference per frame. Each point of each frame is then transformed to populate the final common reference. A smooth scattered data approximation is finally performed to construct the final mosaic image from the irregularly sampled point distribution.

**Validation.** We compared our results to results obtained using the mosaicing algorithm as described in [7]. Standard topology inference did not work in a satisfactory way on our large spiral datasets[1]. We therefore used translation mode with no topology inference as the baseline method for comparison.

---

[1] cf. supplemental material at http://hal.archives-ouvertes.fr/hal-00830447

As a ground truth for the paper grid, we acquired an image using a regular benchtop confocal microscope with a motorized platform performing raster scanning and we performed subsequence mosaic reconstruction using built in software from the microscope (see Fig. 3, left). We performed affine registration between the benchtop confocal image and the results of the mosaic reconstruction obtained with the baseline algorithm and our proposed method. We then estimated the correlation coefficient between each frame of the reconstructed mosaic and the confocal image for both methods.

For validation purpose of the chicken breast and pig liver reconstruction, since no benchtop confocal image was available as a reference, we relied on an *oracle* approach by manually infering the topology through visual assessment and we then injected the spatial associations obtained into the mosaicing algorithm. The reconstruction obtained was taken as reference and will be referred to as the *oracle* reconstruction. For both the baseline algorithm and our proposed method, we estimated the displacement between successive frames and compared it to the *oracle* results. More precisely, let $X_i^O$, $X_i^B$, $X_i^V$ be the positions of frame $F_i$ in the final mosaic image obtained using the *oracle*, the baseline algorithm and our proposed Viterbi framework. we computed for each frame $\Delta_i^B = (X_{i+1}^B - X_i^B) - (X_{i+1}^O - X_i^O)$ and $\Delta_i^V = (X_{i+1}^V - X_i^V) - (X_{i+1}^O - X_i^O)$.

## 3   Results

In Fig. 2, we present for the three video sequences the result of the emission probability estimation for all frames versus all frames of the video. We overlaid the Viterbi path in white (for all images) and the *oracle* path in red obtained manually by visual assessment of overlapping frames (for the chicken and liver acquisition only where no ground truth image was available). All estimations were computed using $\sigma_T = 2$ frames for the transition probability. We set $\sigma_d = 15\mu m$ for the industrial robot trajectories (grid and chicken breast) and $\sigma_d = 400\mu m$ for liver acquisition using the in vivo manipulator (where branches can

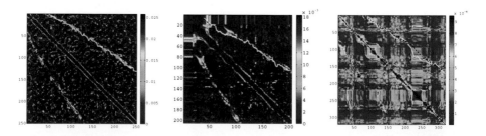

**Fig. 2.** Emission probability matrices for the grid (left), the chicken breast (middle) and the pig liver (right) spiral video sequences. The white line is the Viterbi path found. The red line is the oracle path obtained by visual identification of corresponding frames between successive branches (middle and right images only): the green crosses are the selected associations.

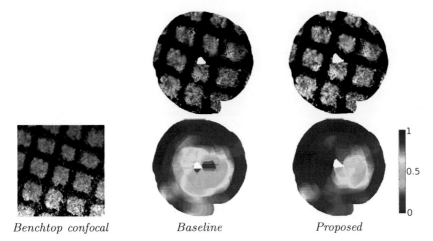

| Benchtop confocal | Baseline | Proposed |

**Fig. 3.** Image representing the value of the correlation coefficient of each frame with the reference benchtop confocal image of the grid for the mosaic reconstruction using the baseline algorithm and using our proposed method

intersect). The selected pairs obtained after the filtering step are indicated with green crosses.

We also compared the mosaic reconstruction of the grid image obtained with the baseline algorithm and our method to the reference image of the grid acquired on a benchtop confocal microscope. For each method, we estimated the correlation coefficient of every frame with the registered reference confocal image. We then compared the sets of correlation coefficients for each frame of the baseline reconstruction and of our method using a sign test. Correlation coefficients proved significantly higher for our method (p-value=4.7037e-20). In Fig. 3,

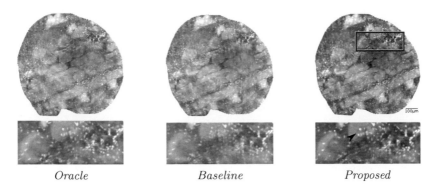

| Oracle | Baseline | Proposed |

**Fig. 4.** Final result of mosaic reconstruction using the *oracle* reconstruction based on visual frame pairing, the baseline algorithm and our proposed method (top row). Magnification of the red frame region: the arrow indicates improvement in the registration with our proposed method.

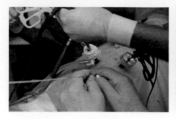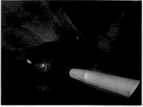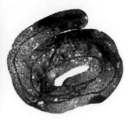

**Fig. 5.** In vivo clinical trial on pig liver: global setup when the probe is inserted (left), laparoscopic view of the robot-probe in contact with the liver (middle), mosaic reconstruction using our framework (right)

next to the confocal image (left), we present images of the mosaic reconstruction (top) and images of the correlation coefficients for each frame (bottom middle and right) for both methods.

The results of mosaic reconstruction obtained for the chicken breast and the pig liver using the baseline algorithm and our method were compared quantitatively to the *oracle* reconstruction: the sign test between populations $\Delta_i^B$ and $\Delta_i^V$ with hypothesis $\Delta_i^B > \Delta_i^V$ showed significant differences (p-value=5.5362e-13 for the chicken and p-value=2.1568e-08 for the pig liver) proving that the relative position of frames in the final mosaic reconstruction were closer to the *oracle* reconstruction using our method compared to the baseline. In Fig. 4, we also display both the mosaic reconstruction and a zoomed region for the chicken breast using the *oracle*, baseline and our method. For the in vivo pig liver dataset, the final mosaic reconstruction can be seen in Fig. 5 (right) using our method.

## 4    Discussion

The intuitive idea of using the equation of the trajectory directly to constrain the pairing and registration of frames could not be effectively used in our problem. In fact, the geometrical precision of the robot was not high enough to be relied on. Moreover, the angular speed of the robot holding the probe is instable due to tissue friction: the consequence of the instability on the position of the frames is amplified at each rotation making the pairing between frames from successive branches non trivially predictable. We thus only used as a priori basic geometrical properties of the spiral we programmed. These properties were 1) there was theoretical overlap between successive branches which meant that from a certain frame number corresponding to the beginning of the second branch, one could always find at least one frame from the previous branch overlapping it and 2) if frame $F_i$ is overlapping frame $F_j$ from next branch, then frame $F_{i+1}$ has very high chances of overlapping a close neighbor of frame $F_{j+1}$. Formulating the problem as a hidden Markov model was a natural choice to implement these properties.

Correlation coefficient proved more robust than the natural sum of squared differences as similarity criterion due to tissue evolution during acquisition. The

Viterbi path providing spatial associations could have been sufficient to reconstruct the mosaic providing we could rely on the transformation estimated between every pair we found. However, in many occasions on real tissue inside the body, texture and features are very homogeneous and similar to one another, making the registration extremely challenging in some regions. Consequently, when the registration between spatial neighbors could not be performed with high confidence, we decided to discard it and to rely only on temporal transformations between frames in these regions. The filtered spatial pairs finally injected to the algorithm play the role of local anchors aiming at stabilizing the mosaic reconstruction. They ought to be regularly reparted along the trajectory: although we do not explicitly enforce the regularity of the pairs we inject, we keep a sufficiently high number of pairs that we can expect a frequency of anchor frames high enough to favorably help the reconstruction.

**Conclusion.** We presented a methodological framework to perform video mosaicing with a weak a priori on the trajectory. Our results showed statistically significant improvements compared to the baseline mosaicing method. Future work includes acquiring longer spiral videos in surgical conditions in vivo, using more flexible transformations to account for tissue deformations and making the mosaic reconstruction fast enough so that it may be used during surgery. We also plan on adapting the proposed framework to groupwise registration problems where images follow a pseudo-periodic pattern such as cardiac images.

# References

1. Brown, M., Lowe, D.: Automatic panoramic image stitching using invariant features. Int. J. Comput. Vis. 74(1), 59–73 (2007)
2. Erden, M., Rosa, B., Szewczyk, J., Morel, G.: Mechanical design of a distal scanner for confocal microlaparoscope: a conic solution. In: Proc. ICRA 2013, pp. 1197–1204 (2013)
3. Gareau, D.S., Li, Y., Huang, B., Eastman, Z., Nehal, K.S., Rajadhyaksha, M.: Confocal mosaicing microscopy in mohs skin excisions: feasibility of rapid surgical pathology. J. Biomed. Opt. 13(5) (2008)
4. Loewke, K.E., Camarillo, D.B., Piyawattanametha, W., Mandella, M.J., Contag, C.H., Thrun, S., Salisbury, J.K.: In vivo micro-image mosaicing. IEEE Trans. Biomed. Eng. 58(1), 159–171 (2011)
5. Rosa, B., Erden, M., Vercauteren, T., Herman, B., Szewczyk, J., Morel, G.: Building large mosaics of confocal endomicroscopic images using visual servoing. IEEE Trans. Biomed. Eng. 60(4), 1041–1049 (2013)
6. Sawhney, H.S., Hsu, S., Kumar, R.: Robust video mosaicing through topology inference and local to global alignment. In: Burkhardt, H., Neumann, B. (eds.) ECCV 1998. LNCS, vol. 1407, pp. 103–119. Springer, Heidelberg (1998)
7. Vercauteren, T., Perchant, A., Malandain, G., Pennec, X., Ayache, N.: Robust mosaicing with correction of motion distortions and tissue deformation for *in vivo* fibered microscopy. Med. Image Anal. 10(5), 673–692 (2006)
8. Wallace, M., Fockens, P.: Probe-based confocal laser endomicroscopy. Gastroenterology 136(5), 1509–1513 (2009)

# Spatially Aware Cell Cluster(SpACCl) Graphs: Predicting Outcome in Oropharyngeal p16+ Tumors

Sahirzeeshan Ali[1], James Lewis[2], and Anant Madabhushi[1,*]

[1] Case Western University, Cleveland, OH USA
[2] Surgical Pathology, Washington University, St Louis, MO USA

**Abstract.** Quantitative measurements of spatial arrangement of nuclei in histopathology images for different cancers has been shown to have prognostic value. Traditionally, graph algorithms (with cell/nuclei as node) have been used to characterize the spatial arrangement of these cells. However, these graphs inherently extract only global features of cell or nuclear architecture and, therefore, important information at the local level may be left unexploited. Additionally, since the graph construction does not draw a distinction between nuclei in the stroma or epithelium, the graph edges often traverse the stromal and epithelial regions. In this paper, we present a new spatially aware cell cluster (SpACCl) graph that can efficiently and accurately model local nuclear interactions, separately within the stromal and epithelial regions alone. SpACCl is built locally on nodes that are defined on groups/clusters of nuclei rather than individual nuclei. Local nodes are connected with edges which have a certain probability of connectedness. The SpACCl graph allows for exploration of (a) contribution of nuclear arrangement within the stromal and epithelial regions separately and (b) combined contribution of stromal and epithelial nuclear architecture in predicting disease aggressiveness and patient outcome. In a cohort of 160 p16+ oropharyngeal tumors (141 non-progressors and 19 progressors), a support vector machine (SVM) classifier in conjunction with 7 graph features extracted from the SpACCl graph yielded a mean accuracy of over 90% with PPV of 89.4% in distinguishing between progressors and non-progressors. Our results suggest that (a) stromal nuclear architecture has a role to play in predicting disease aggressiveness and that (b) combining nuclear architectural contributions from the stromal and epithelial regions yields superior prognostic accuracy compared to individual contributions from stroma and epithelium alone.

* Research reported in this publication was supported by the National Cancer Institute of the National Institutes of Health under Award Numbers R01CA136535-01, R01CA140772-01, R43EB015199-01, and R03CA143991-01. The content is solely the responsibility of the authors and does not necessarily represent the official views of the National Institutes of Health

# 1   Introduction

Graph theory has emerged as a popular method to characterize the structure of large complex networks leading to a better understanding of dynamic interactions that exist between their components [1]. Nodes with similar characteristics tend to cluster together and the pattern of this clustering provides information as to the shared properties, and therefore the function, of those individual nodes [4]. Despite their complex nature, cancerous cells tend to self-organize in clusters and exhibit architectural organization, an attribute which forms the basis of many cancers [2].

In the context of image analysis and digital pathology, some researchers have shown that spatial graphs and tessellations such as those obtained via the Voronoi (VT), Delaunay (DT), and minimum spanning tree (MST), built using nuclei as vertices may actually have biological context and thus be potentially predictive of disease severity [1,3] . These graphs have been mined for quantitative features that have shown to be useful in the context of prostate and breast cancer grading [1]. However, these topological approaches focus only on local-edge connectivity. Moreover, these graphs inherently extract only global features and, therefore, important information involving local spatial interaction may be left unexploited. Additionally, since no distinction is made between the nuclear vertices lying in either the stroma or epithelium, the graph edges often traverse the stromal and epithelial regions (see Figure 1 and 2).

Until recently morphology of the stroma has been largely ignored in characterizing disease aggressiveness [7]. However, there has been recent interest in looking at possible interactions between stromal and epithelial regions and the role of this interaction in disease aggressiveness [6]. However, constructing global Voronoi and Delaunnay graphs which connect all the nuclei (involved in the stroma and epithelium) may not allow for capturing of local tumor heterogeneity. Additionally these global graph constructs do not allow for evaluating contributions of the stromal or epithelial regions alone. Consequently there is a need for locally connected graphs which are spatially aware which will allow for quantitative characterization of spatial interactions within the stroma and epithelial regions separately and hence for combining attributes from both the stromal and epithelial graphs.

Human papillomavirus-related (p16 positive) oropharyngeal squamous cell carcinoma (oSCC) represents a steadily increasing proportion of head and neck cancers and has a favorable prognosis [4]. However, approximately 10% of patients develop recurrent disease, mostly distant metastasis, and the remaining patients often have major morbidity from treatment. Hence, identifying patients with more aggressive (rather than indolent) tumor is critical. In this work we seek to develop an accuracy, image based predictor to identify new features in oSCC cancer, thereby providing new insights into the biological factors driving the progression of oSCC disease. This paper presents a new Spatially Aware Cell Cluster(SpACCl) graph that can efficiently and accurately model local nuclear architecture within the stromal and epithelial regions alone. The novel contributions of this work include,

1. Unlike global graphs (where the vertices are not spatially aware), SpACCl is built locally on nodes that are defined on groups/clusters of nuclei rather than individual nuclei. Consequently, SpACCl can be mined for local topological information, such as clustering and compactness of nodes (nuclei), which we argue may provide image biomarkers for distinguishing between indolent and progressive disease.

2. SpACCl allows for implicit construction of two separate graphs within each of the stromal and epithelial regions to extract features from both the regions. To distinguish epithelium nodes from stromal nodes to individually extract graph features from the two regions, a super-pixel based support vector machine classifier is employed to separate out the regions in the image into stromal and epithelial compartments. Stromal and epithelial interactions are explored by combining graph features extracted from the two regions and using these features to train a classifier to identify progressors (poor prognostic tumors) in p16+ oropharyngeal cancers.

## 2    Constructing Spatially-Aware Cell Cluster Graphs

The intuition behind SpACCl is to capture clustering patterns of nuclei in histologic tissue images and extracting topological properties and attributes that can quantify tumor morphology efficiently. Formally, SpACCl is defined as $G_i = (V_i, E_i)$, where $i \in \{\text{epithelium}, \text{stroma}\}$, $V_i$ and $E_i$ are the set of nodes and the edges respectively. Construction of SpACCl is illustrated in Figure 1 and described in detail below.

### 2.1    Distinguishing Stromal and Epithelial Compartments

The entire image is partitioned into small, spatially coherent cells known as super-pixels [8]. Nuclei within these super-pixels were identified by performing dendogram clustering of the mean intensity values (RGB) of each superpixel, within which we measured the intensity and texture (local binary patterns and harlick) of the superpixel and its neighbors. We then classified superpixels as being either within the epithelium or stroma by training a Support Vector Machine (SVM) classifier on these measurements with hand-labelled superpixels from 100 images.

### 2.2    Cluster Node Identification

The second step is to identify closely spaced (clusters) of nuclei for node assignment. High concavity points are characteristic of contours that enclose multiple objects and represent junctions where object intersection occurs. We leverage a concavity detection algorithm [9] in which concavity points are detected by computing the angle between vectors defined by sampling three consecutive points $(c_{w-1}, c_w, c_{w+1})$ on the contour. The degree of concavity/convexity is proportional to the angle $\theta(c_w)$, which can be computed from the dot product relation: $\theta(c_w) = \pi - \arccos \left( \frac{(c_w - c_{w-1}) \cdot (c_{w+1} - c_w)}{||(c_w - c_{w-1})|| \ ||(c_{w+1} - c_w)||} \right)$. A point is considered to be

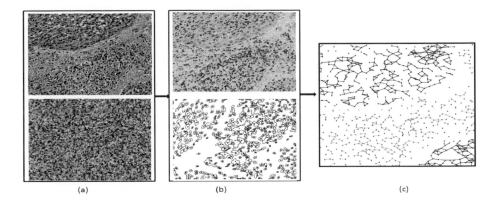

**Fig. 1.** (a) Original image with superpixel based partition of the entire image scene in the bottom panel, (b) (top panel) superpixels are classified as stromal and epithelial regions (cyan being epithelial, yellow being stroma and blue are nuclei), (bottome panel) nuclei clusters identified in the stroma and epithelial regions, and (c) establishing probabilistic links (edges) between identified nodes (third panel),where green edges are within stromal graphs and red edges are within epithelial graphs.

concavity point if $\theta(c_w) > \theta_t$, where $\theta_t$ is an empirically set threshold degree. Number of detected concavity points, $c_w \geq 1$, indicates presence of multiple overlapping/touching nuclei. In such cases, we consider the contour as one node, effectively identifying a cluster node. On each of the segmented cluster, the center of mass is calculated to represent the nuclear centroid.

## 2.3   Edge Connection

The last step is to build the links between the nodes that belong to the same group, i.e. epithelium or stroma, where the pairwise spatial relation between the nodes is translated to the edges (links) of SpACCl with a certain probability. The probability for a link between the nodes $u$ and $v$ reflects the Euclidean distance $d(u,v)$ between them and is given by

$$P(u,v) = d(u,v)^{-\alpha}, \tag{1}$$

where $\alpha$ is the exponent that controls the density of a graph. Probability of 2 nodes being connected is a decaying function of the relative distance. Since the probability of distant nuclei being connected is less, we can probabilistically define the edge set $E_i$ such that

$$E_i = \{(u,v) : r < d(u,v)^{-\alpha}, \forall u, v \in V_i\}, \tag{2}$$

where $r$ is a real number between 0 and 1 that is generated by a random number generator. In establishing the edges of SpACCl, we use a decaying probability function with an exponent of $-\alpha$ with $0 \leq \alpha$. The value of $\alpha$, set empirically (10-fold cross validation process), determines the density of the edges in the graph;

larger values of $\alpha$ produce sparser graphs. On the other hand as $\alpha$ approaches to 0 the graphs become densely connected and approach to a complete graph. Within each tissue region,$i$, there will be $i$ SpACCl graphs, which in turn are comprised of multiple sub-graphs as illustrated in Figure 1(c).

## 2.4   Subgraph Construction

SpaCCl's topological space decomposes into its connected components. The connectedness relation between two pairs of points satisfies transitivity, i.e., if $u \sim v$ and $v \sim w$ then $u \sim w$, which means that if there is a path from $u$ to $v$ and a path from $v$ to $w$, the two paths may be concatenated together to form a path from $u$ to $w$. Hence, being in the same component is an equivalence relation (defined on the vertices of the graph) and the equivalence classes are the connected components. In a nondirected graph $G_i$, a vertex $v$ is reachable from a vertex $u$ if there is a path from $u$ to $v$. The connected components of $G_i$ are then the largest induced subgraphs of $G_i$ that are each connected.

# 3   Feature Mining from SpACCl

Within each image, two separate graphs, $G^e$ and $G^s$ corresponding to the stromal and epithelial regions are obtained. We then extract both global and local graph metrics (features) from the subgraphs. These measurements are then averaged over the entire graph, $G^e$ and $G^s$ respectively. Table 1 summarizes the features we extract, along with their governing equations, and their histological significance and motivation.

# 4   Experimental Design and Results

## 4.1   Data Description

Using a tissue microarray cohort of 160 p16+ oSCC (punched twice with either 0.6 mm or 2 mm cores) with clinical follow up, digitally scanned H&E images at 400X magnification were annotated by an expert pathologist based on whether or not disease progression had occurred. There were 160 p16+ patients on the array – 141 cases of non-progressors and 19 progressors.

## 4.2   Classifier Training and Comparative Evaluation

We extract an identical set of features (listed in Table 1) from $G^e$ and $G^s$, $\mathbf{F} = \{F^e, F^s\}$ from $G_i$. The optimal feature set $\mathbf{Q}^{opt}$ was identified via mRMR feature selection scheme presented in [10], where *clustering D* and *average eccentricity* from $F^e$ and *number of central points* from $F^s$ were identified as the top most performing features. We then evaluated the accuracy of each of $G^s$ and

**Table 1.** Description of the features extracted from SpACCl. Identical features are extracted from each of $G^s$ and $G^e$ respectively.

| SpACCl Feature | Description | Relevance to Histology |
|---|---|---|
| Clustering Coeff C | Ratio of total number of edges among the neighbors of the node to the total number of edges that can exist among the neighbors of the node per node. $\tilde{C} = \frac{\sum_{u=1}^{|V|} C_u}{|V|}$, where $C_u = \frac{|F_u|}{\binom{k_u}{2}} = \frac{2|F_u|}{k_u(k_u-1)}$ | Nuclei Clustering |
| Clustering Coeff D | Ratio of total number of edges among the neighbors of the node and the node itself to the total number of edges that can exist among the neighbors of the node and the node itself per node. $\tilde{D} = \frac{\sum_{u=1}^{|V|} D_u}{|V|}$, where $D_u = \frac{k_u | |E_u|}{\binom{k_u+1}{2}} = \frac{2(k_u | |E_u|)}{k_u(k_u+1)}$ | |
| Giant Connected Comp | Ratio between the number of nodes in the largest connected component in the graph and the total number of nodes (Global) | |
| Average Eccentricity | $\frac{\sum_u^V \epsilon_u}{|V|}$ where eccentricity of the $u^{th}$ node $\epsilon_u$, $u = 1 \cdot |V|$, is the maximum value of the shortest path length from node $u$ to any other node in the graph. | Compactness of Nuclei |
| Percent of Isolated Points | Percentage of the isolated nodes in the graph, where an isolated node has a degree of 0 | |
| Number of Central Points | Number of nodes within the graph whose eccentricity is equal to the graph radius | |
| Skewness of Edge Lengths | Statistics of the edge length distribution in the graph | Spatial Uniformity |

$G^e$ in distinguishing progressors and non-progressors in oropharyngeal SCC by employing a SVM classifier trained on $\mathbf{Q}^{opt}$. We further trained SVM on $F^e$ and $F^s$ separately. A randomized 3 fold cross-validation involving 10 runs was used for mRMR feature selection and training the SVM. To demonstrate that class imbalance did not affect our classifier, we reported accuracy and positive predictive value (PPV) for the classifier for both the progressor and non-progressor cases.

To investigate the significance of encoding pairwise spatial relation between the nodes, we compared SpACCl against Voronoi and Delaunay graph based features (see [1]). Figure 2 illustrates tissue images of p16+ oropharyngeal progressor and non-progressor cases with associated of VT and SpACCl results. SpACCl provides a sparser and more localized representation of nuclear architecture compared to VT. SpACCl also prohibits the traversal of epithelium and stroma by constructing separate graphs for each region. The SVM classifier based of $\mathbf{F}^{opt}$ achieved a maximum accuracy of $90.2 \pm 1.2\%$ (Table 2). Our findings also suggest that the stromal SpACCl graph features, $F^s$, can independently distinguish progressors and non-progressors in this population with an accuracy of 68% which suggests that stromal nuclear architecture is indeed informative in terms of predicting disease aggressiveness.

418     S. Ali, J. Lewis, and A. Madabhushi

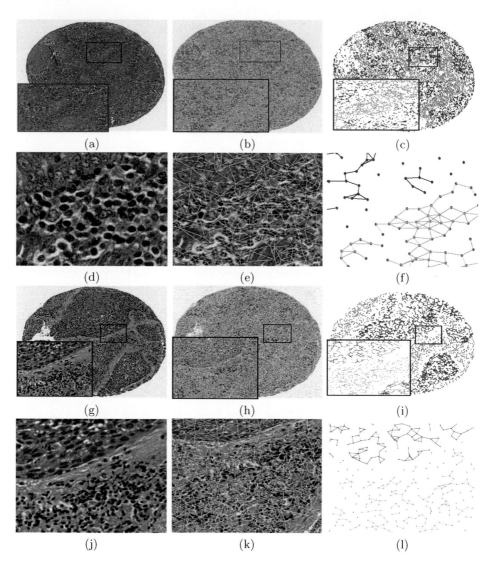

**Fig. 2.** Representative TMA core images of (a) progressor OSCC with enlarged ROIs in (d) and (g) Non-Progressor image. (b) and (h) represent the Delauny graphs of (a) and (g) with enlarged ROIs in (e) and (k). SpACCl graphs for (a) and (g) are shown in (c) and (i) with enlarged ROIs in (f), (l) respectively.

**Table 2.** Accuracies compared against the Voronoi and Delauny graphs, and PPV values for Progressors (p) and Non-Progressor (NP)

| | Tradiational Graphs | | SpACCl | | |
|---|---|---|---|---|---|
| | Voronoi | Delauny | $F^e$ | $F^s$ | $Q^{opt}$ |
| Accuracy | $74.4 \pm 0.6\%$ | $76.7 \pm 0.7\%$ | $86.2 \pm 1.2\%$ | $68.1 \pm 0.2$ | $\mathbf{90.1 \pm 1.5}$ |
| PPV (P) | $77.9 \pm 1.6\%$ | $74.3 \pm 0.5\%$ | $85.2 \pm 1.6\%$ | $76.1 \pm 0.2$ | $89.4 \pm 0.2$ |
| PPV (NP) | $76.9 \pm 0.9\%$ | $76.3 \pm 1.5\%$ | $82.5 \pm 2.6\%$ | $78.7 \pm 0.2$ | $86.5 \pm 0.5$ |

## 5   Concluding Remarks

In this work we presented a new sptially-aware Cell Cluster (SpACCl) graph algorithm and showed its application in the context of predicting disease aggressiveness in p16+ oropharyngeal cancers. SpACCl allows for implicit construction of two separate nuclear graphs within each of the stromal and epithelial regions, which enabled us to independently explore contribution of nuclear architecture within the two regions. It also allowed us to explore the combined contributions of stromal and epithelial nuclear architecture in predicting disease aggressiveness. The results obtained in this work with SpACCl suggest that (a) stromal nuclear architecture has a role to play in predicting patient outcome for this class of tumors and that (b) combining stromal and epithelial nuclear architecture results in better prognostic accuracy compared to graph measures obtained from either the stromal or epithelial graphs alone.

## References

1. Doyle, S., et al.: Cascaded discrimination of normal, abnormal, and confounder classes in histopathology: Gleason grading of prostate cancer. BMC Bioinformatics, 1284–1287 (2012)
2. Epstein, J., et al.: The 2005 international society of urological pathology (isup) consensus conference on gleason grading of prostatic carcinoma. American J. Surgical Path. 29(9), 1228–1242 (2005)
3. Tabesh, A., et al.: Multifeature prostate cancer diagnosis and gleason grading of histological images. IEEE TMI 26(10), 1366–1378 (2007)
4. Lewis, et al.: Tumor cell anaplasia and mutinucleation are predictors of disease recurrence in oropharyngeal cancers. Am. J. Path. (2012)
5. Gunduz, et al.: The cell graphs of cancer. Bioinformatics 20, i145–i155 (2004)
6. Liu, E.T., et al.: N. Engl. J. Med. 357, 2537–2538 (2007)
7. Beck, et al.: Systematic analysis of Breast Cancer morphology uncovers stromal features associated with survival. Sci. Transl. Med. (2011)
8. Ren, X., et al.: Learning a classification model for segmentation. In: ICCV, vol. 1, pp. 10–17 (2003)
9. Fatakdawala, H., et al.: Expectation Maximization driven Geodesic Active Contour with Overlap Resolution (EMaGACOR). IEEE TBME 57(7), 1676–1689 (2010)
10. Peng, H., et al.: Feature selection based on mutual information criteria of max-dependency, max-relevance, and min-redundancy. PAMI 27, 1226–1238 (2005)

# Efficient Phase Contrast Microscopy Restoration Applied for Muscle Myotube Detection

Seungil Huh[1,2], Hang Su[2,3], Mei Chen[4], and Takeo Kanade[1,2]

[1] Lane Center for Computational Biology
[2] Robotics Institute, Carnegie Mellon University
[3] Department of Electronic Engineering, Shanghai Jiaotong University
[4] Intel Science and Technology Center on Embedded Computing

**Abstract.** This paper proposes a new image restoration method for phase contrast microscopy as a mean to enhance the quality of images prior to image analysis. Compared to state-of-the-art image restoration algorithms, our method has a more solid theoretical foundation and is orders of magnitude more efficient in computation. We validated the proposed method by applying it to automated muscle myotube detection, a challenging problem that has not been tackled without staining images. Results on 300 phase contrast microscopy images from three different culture conditions demonstrate that the proposed restoration scheme improves myotube detection, and that our approach is far more computationally efficient than previous methods.

## 1 Introduction

Vision-based analysis adopting phase contrast microscopy often has advantages over the use of fluorescent microscopy for the task of cell behavior and fate analysis; it enables continuous monitoring of intact cells in culture and it reduces the expenditure of consumable reagents as well as human labor. However, the analysis of phase contrast microscopy is not trivial because of the properties of the images: cells often lack distinctive textures, and artifacts, such as bright halos, often appear when cells form a cluster or undergo a certain process.

To address these issues, several image restoration methods have been proposed based on the image formation process of a phase contrast microscope [1,2,3]. These methods were devised to restore phase retardations at each point of a given image, based on which image analysis, such as cell region detection, can be more effectively performed. However, these restorations are often inaccurate due to the strong assumptions [1,2] or unable to generate restored images but can only produce features used for image analysis [3]. Furthermore, the high computational cost limits their applicability.

In this paper, we propose a new phase contrast microscopy image restoration algorithm that has a more solid theoretical foundation and is far more efficient than previous methods. More specifically, our method does not introduce any assumption in the modeling step and minimizes the computation complexity by employing the Wiener deconvolution algorithm [4]. As a result, our method

K. Mori et al. (Eds.): MICCAI 2013, Part I, LNCS 8149, pp. 420–427, 2013.

produces more accurate restored images—not just features—and significantly outperforms previous methods in terms of computational efficiency.

We validated the restoration method by applying it to muscle myotube detection. Detection of muscle myotubes is important in two folds. First, it helps better understanding on the mechanism of muscle differentiation, which is required to improve the treatment of various muscular disorders associated with muscle loss, such as spinal muscular atrophy and muscular dystrophy [5]. In addition, precise detection of muscle myotubes that result from cell differentiation can automate the process of finding the optimal condition to keep stem cells from differentiating and thus losing self-renewal capability. To the best of our knowledge, there has not been published work on vision-based muscle myotube detection in phase contrast microscopy images.

## 2    Previous Work

Phase contrast microscopy is a popular optical microscopy technique that enhances the phase shift in light passing through a specimen and converts it into brightness change in images. According to [1], phase-contrast imaging can be modeled by two waves: the unaltered surround wave $l_S(x)$ and the diffracted wave $l_D(x)$, computed as

$$l_S(x) = i\zeta_p A e^{i\beta} \tag{1}$$

$$l_D(x) = \zeta_c A e^{i(\beta+\theta(x))}\delta(R) + (i\zeta_p - 1)\zeta_c A e^{i(\beta+\theta(R_x))} * Airy(R) \tag{2}$$

where $i^2 = -1$; $A$ and $\beta$ are the illuminating wave's amplitude and phase before hitting the specimen plate, respectively; $\zeta_p$ and $\zeta_c$ are the amplitude attenuation factors by the phase ring and the specimen, respectively; $\theta(x)$ and $\theta(R_x)$ are the phase shifts caused by the specimen at location $x$ and its neighboring region $R_x$ with size $R$, respectively; $\delta(\cdot)$ is a 2D Dirac delta function; and $Airy(R)$ is an obscured Airy pattern [6] with size $R$. A phase-contrast microscopy image $g$ can then be analytically modeled as a function of $\theta$:

$$g(x) = |l_S(x) + l_D(x)|^2 \tag{3}$$

$$= |(i\zeta_p A e^{i\beta} + \zeta_c A e^{i(\beta+\theta(x))})\delta(R) + (i\zeta_p - 1)\zeta_c A e^{i(\beta+\theta(R_x))} * Airy(R)|^2.$$

To restore $\theta$ from $g$, so as to use $\theta$ instead of $g$ for image analysis, [1] applied the approximation $e^{i\theta(x)} \approx 1 + i\theta(x)$ on the assumption that $\theta(x)$ is close to zero. Since this assumption is not valid for thick (and thus bright) cells, cells undergoing mitosis or apoptosis are often missed in the restored images [2]. Later, [2] generalized this model by assuming that $\theta(x)$ is close to a constant, which is not necessarily zero. This method is useful for the detection of particular cell regions, e.g., bright cell regions or dark cell regions; however, it cannot precisely restore phase retardations because the assumption that all phase retardations are close to one value is still generally not true.

Recently, [3] applied the approximation

$$e^{i\theta(x)} \approx \sum_{k=1}^{K} \psi_k(x) e^{i\theta_k} \tag{4}$$

and showed that a phase contrast microscopy image $g$ can be modeled as a linear combination of $K$ diffraction patterns after flat-field correction, as follows:

$$g = \sum_{k=1}^{K} \Psi_k * \left( \sin\theta_k \delta(R) + (\zeta_p \cos\theta_{m_k} - \sin\theta_k) * Airy(R) \right) \tag{5}$$

where $\theta_k$ is the $k$-th representative phase retardation, which is one of the $M$ equally distributed phases within $2\pi$, i.e., $\{0, \frac{2\pi}{M}, \cdots, \frac{2(M-1)\pi}{M}\}$. Given a phase contrast image $g$, by solving Eq. (5), $K$ coefficient matrices $(\Psi_1, \cdots, \Psi_K)$ are obtained. Although these coefficients can be used for image analysis, actual phase retardations may not be accurately estimated because solving for $\theta$ in Eq. (4) with obtained coefficients does not yield a right answer unless $|\sum_{k=1}^{K} \psi_k(x) e^{i\theta_k}| = 1$, which is not guaranteed. In addition, Eq. (5) is an overdetermined system with $K$ times as many unknowns as equations. These unnecessarily many unknowns make the optimization problem difficult, but with little benefit.

## 3    Restoration of Phase Contrast Microscopy

In this section, we propose an effective and efficient restoration method for phase contrast microscopy and discuss the advantages of our method over the previous methods.

### 3.1    Modeling of Phase Contrast Microscopy Imaging

Eq. (3), the original phase-contrast model, can be expanded as follows:

$$
\begin{aligned}
g(x) =& |l_S + l_D|^2 = (l_S + l_D) \cdot (l_S + l_D)^* \\
=& A^2 \Big[ (\zeta_p{}^2 + \zeta_c{}^2)\delta(R) - 2\zeta_c^2 Airy(R) + (\zeta_p^2 + 1)\zeta_c^2 Airy(R) * Airy(R) + \\
& i\zeta_p\zeta_c (e^{-i\theta(x)} - e^{i\theta(x)})\delta(R) + \zeta_p\zeta_c \big( (\zeta_p - i)e^{-i\theta(R_x)} + (\zeta_p + i)e^{i\theta(R_x)} \big) * Airy(R) \Big] \\
=& C_1 + C_2 \Big[ i(e^{-i\theta(x)} - e^{i\theta(x)})\delta(R) + \big( (\zeta_p - i)e^{-i\theta(R_x)} + (\zeta_p + i)e^{i\theta(R_x)} \big) * Airy(R) \Big]
\end{aligned}
\tag{6}
$$

where $C_1$ and $C_2$ are values that are not relevant to $\theta(x)$. Since $e^{i\theta(x)} = \cos(x) + i\sin(x)$, $e^{i\theta(x)}$ can be replaced with $\alpha(x) + i\beta(x)$ on the condition $\alpha(x)^2 + \beta(x)^2 = 1$, and then $g$ is reexpressed as:

$$g(x) = C_1 + C_2 \Big( 2\beta(x)\delta(R) + 2\big(\zeta_p\alpha(R_x) - \beta(R_x)\big) * Airy(R) \Big) \tag{7}$$

$$\text{s.t. } \alpha(x)^2 + \beta(x)^2 = 1.$$

After flat-field correction, we obtain the following model for the entire image.

$$g = C\Big(\zeta_p \alpha * Airy(R) + \beta * \big(\delta(R) - Airy(R)\big)\Big) \quad \text{s.t. } \alpha \otimes \alpha + \beta \otimes \beta = \mathbb{1} \quad (8)$$

where $\alpha$ and $\beta$ are matrices with the same size of $g$ whose values at position $x$ are $\alpha(x)$ and $\beta(x)$, respectively, $\otimes$ is the element-wise matrix multiplication operator, $\mathbb{1}$ is the matrix with all 1, and $C$ is a constant.

## 3.2 Optimization Process for the Restoration

Given $g$, in order to infer $\alpha$ and $\beta$ from this equation, we minimize the following objective:

$$\min_{\alpha,\beta,C} ||g - Cf||_F^2, \quad f = \zeta_p \alpha * Airy(R) + \beta * \big(\delta(R) - Airy(R)\big) \quad (9)$$

$$\text{s.t. } \alpha \otimes \alpha + \beta \otimes \beta = \mathbb{1}$$

where $|| \cdot ||_F$ denotes the Frobenius norm. Note that we also infer $C$ rather than manually setting it because all the parameters that required to determine $C$ are often not given. Once $\alpha$ and $\beta$ are obtained, phase retardation $\theta$ can be computed based on $e^{i\theta(x)} = \alpha(x) + i\beta(x)$.

In order to solve this optimization problem, we propose an iterative scheme using the Wiener deconvolution algorithm [4], which is an efficient way to perform deconvolution and has been popularly used for image deconvolution applications. The optimization procedure is as follows:

- Step 1. Initialize $\alpha$ and $\beta$ at random to satisfy $\alpha \otimes \alpha + \beta \otimes \beta = \mathbb{1}$.
- Step 2. Update $\alpha$ to minimize $||g - Cf||_F^2$ with fixed $\beta$ by solving the following deconvolution problem via Wiener deconvolution.

$$g - \beta * \Big(C\big(\delta(R) - Airy(R)\big)\Big) = \alpha * \big(C\zeta_p Airy(R)\big). \quad (10)$$

- Step 3. Project $\alpha$ and $\beta$ onto the constraint space by multiplying $1/\sqrt{\alpha^2 + \beta^2}$.
- Step 4. Recalculate $C$ to minimize $||g - Cf||_F^2$.

$$C \leftarrow \frac{vec(f) \cdot vec(g)}{vec(f) \cdot vec(f)}. \quad (11)$$

  where $vec(\cdot)$ is the vectorization operator.
- Step 5. Update $\beta$ to minimize $||g - Cf||_F^2$ with fixed $\alpha$ by solving the following deconvolution problem via Wiener deconvolution.

$$g - \alpha * \big(C\zeta_p Airy(R)\big) = \beta * \Big(C\big(\delta(R) - Airy(R)\big)\Big). \quad (12)$$

- Step 6. Project $\alpha$ and $\beta$ in the same way as Step 3.
- Step 7. Recalculate $C$ in the same way as Step 4.
- Step 8. Repeat Steps 2 through 7 until $||g - Cf||_F^2$ is not reduced any more.

Wiener deconvolution requires a parameter that indicates the signal-to-noise ratio of the original data [4]. In our experiments, we tested several values, namely $\{0, 0.01, \cdots, 0.05\}$, and determined the parameter as the one that minimizes the final objective function value simply on the first image.

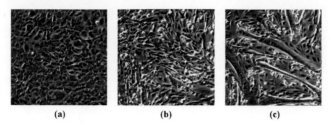

**Fig. 1.** The process of myotube formation: (a) single-nucleated myoblasts; (b,c) nascent and mature myotubes formed by the fusion of myoblasts, respectively

### 3.3   Discussion on the Proposed Restoration Method

The advantages of our method over the previous methods are in three folds:

First, our method can precisely restore phase retardations caused by cells without introducing any unreasonable approximation. On the other hand, previous methods either assume that phase retardations are close to a certain value [1,2] or adopt a linear approximation without appropriate constraints [3].

Second, our method is far more efficient than the previous methods in terms of computation time (time complexity of Wiener deconvolution vs. that of iterative deconvolution; in practice, a few seconds vs. several minutes for processing one image in a typical setting) and memory use (a few MB vs. a few GB). This is an important quality towards enabling real-time processing of time-lapse images.

Third, our method is theoretically more sound than the previous methods, particularly [3]. Since the model involves a lot more unknowns than equations, it might not be theoretically sound to infer the model via an iterative greedy scheme that alternates basis selection and coefficient calculation. In fact, the greedy scheme often selects different sets of bases in a different order (with repetition) for different images, when they do not show similar levels of cell density and maturity, so that feature sets from different images may not be consistent. On the other hand, our optimization is conducted in a standard manner.

One drawback of our method lies in fact that Wiener deconvolution cannot explicitly handle spatial or temporal smoothness terms incorporated into the objective function, unlike iterative deconvolution methods. This issue might be implicitly dealt with by applying smoothing during iterations.

## 4   Muscle Myotube Detection

This section introduces muscle myotube detection task as a testbed of our restoration method. During the differentiation of muscle stem cells, muscle myotubes are formed by the fusion of mononucleated progenitor cells known as myoblasts (See Fig 1.). Given a phase contrast image containing both myoblasts and myotubes, the goal of muscle myotube detection is to identify the area where myotubes are located. This information is useful for measuring how far differentiation has proceeded and provides guidance for human intervention.

## 4.1   Myotube Detection Algorithm

We examined two methods: pixel- and superpixel-based methods.

For the pixel-based method, after image restoration, we extract visual feature around each pixel in the restored image. We use rotation invariant local binary pattern ($LBP^{riu2}$) [7], which is one of the most popular and effective texture features at present. For each pixel, we compute the distribution of different $LBP^{riu2}$ in its neighboring region and use it as visual features of the pixel.

For the superpixel-based method, after image restoration, we perform superpixel segmentation using the entropy rate superpixel segmentation method [8]. Then for each superpixel, we compute the visual feature vector by computing the distribution of different $LBP^{riu2}$ within the superpixel.

After feature computation, we train a linear support vector machine over pixels or superpixels. For the superpixel-based method, given ground truth, the superpixels that contain more positive pixels than negative ones are used as positive samples and the rest as negative samples in the training phase. Testing is also conducted over superpixels; i.e., the pixels belonging to the same superpixel are determined to have the same label.

## 5   Experiment

### 5.1   Data and Comparison

Three sets of phase contrast images of mouse C2C12 myoblasts were acquired under culture conditions with different amount (100, 500, and 1000ng/mL) of IGF2, which accelerates differentiation. Each set contains 100 images; i.e., 300 images were obtained in total. Each image contains $640 \times 640$ pixels.

For comparison, immunofluorescence staining images capturing myotubes were acquired. Each staining image was reduced to a binary image by intensity thresholding. Note that binarized images include most of information on cell differentiation that biologists currently want to obtain via high-throughput screening. It is also worth mentioning that staining images are not the ground truth in that nuclei of myotubes are often not stained and the myotube boundary is not precise. Although imperfect, using staining images is a standard way for comparison since manual annotation is too time-consuming and often subjective.

The data and staining images will be available on the first author's home page (www.cs.cmu.edu/~seungilh).

### 5.2   Experiments and Results

We compare results of our myotube detection methods with those of the methods that do not adopt the restoration process. In these baseline methods, feature extraction was performed on phase contrast images, not the restored images. We perform 10-fold evaluation; for each set of images, we used 1 fold of images (10 images) for testing in turn and the rest for training. For each image, we compare the detection result with the staining image to compute precision and recall.

**Table 1.** Myotube detection results in terms of F-measure. Our restoration method enhances myotube detection accuracy.

|  | IGF2-100 | IGF2-500 | IGF2-1000 |
|---|---|---|---|
| Phase contrast image+pixel | 0.32±0.06 | 0.53±0.11 | 0.67±0.10 |
| Restored image+pixel | 0.44±0.08 | 0.68±0.09 | 0.79±0.07 |
| Phase contrast image+superpixel | 0.61±0.07 | 0.73±0.08 | 0.80±0.08 |
| Restored image+superpixel | **0.65±0.06** | **0.76±0.04** | **0.86±0.05** |

**Table 2.** Performance comparison between our restoration method and the previous restoration method [3]. Computational time is computed for restoration methods.

|  | IGF2-100 | IGF2-500 | IGF2-1000 | Time |
|---|---|---|---|---|
| Our restoration+superpixel | 0.65±0.06 | 0.76±0.04 | 0.86±0.05 | 2 sec |
| Restoration [3]+superpixel | 0.63±0.08 | 0.76±0.07 | 0.86±0.06 | 262 sec |

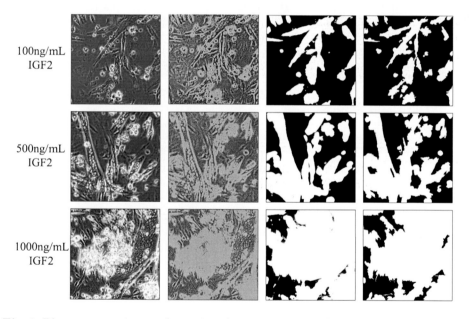

**Fig. 2.** Phase contrast images (1st column), restored images (2nd column), thresholded staining image (3rd column), and myotube detection results with the restoration and superpixel segmentation (4th column)

Over the entire 100 images for each set, we compute the average F-measure, which is the harmonic mean of precision and recall.

As shown in Table 1, when compared with the staining image, the method adopting both the restoration and superpixel segmentation achieves 65% to 86% accuracy in terms of F-measure.[1] Myotube detection is more accurate under the

---

[1] It is reasonable to expect increased performance when the ground truth is used rather than staining images, which are imperfect so can possibly confuse the training model.

condition with more amount of IGF2 because additional IGF2 leads to more mature myotubes the texture of which is more distinct from that of myoblasts. Applying the restoration scheme results in 12% to 15% gain in accuracy for the pixel-based method and 3% to 6% gain in accuracy for the superpixel-based method compared to the baseline methods. Fig. 2 shows examples of restoration images and myotube detection results.

Table 2 demonstrates that the proposed restoration method is considerably more efficient than the state-of-the-art restoration method [3]. Although the performances for myotube detection are comparable on these data sets, our method has advantages over the previous method including computational efficiency, capability to obtain restored images, and a more solid theoretical foundation.

## 6   Conclusions

In this paper, we propose a new image restoration method for phase contrast microscopy, which is theoretically more sound and computationally more efficient than previous methods. We also present a method for myotube detection that adopts the proposed restoration scheme and empirically validate the effectiveness and efficiency of the proposed restoration and myotube detection methods.

The next goal will be to monitor myotube formation over time. Though in this work, we focused on individual images, temporal information can be incorporated in several ways and it will result in a better performance for continuous monitoring of cell fate. We leave the empirical validation as future work.

## References

1. Yin, Z., Kanade, T., Chen, M.: Understanding the phase contrast optics to restore artifact-free microscopy images for segmentation. Med. Image Anal. 16(5), 1047–1062 (2012)
2. Huh, S., Ker, D.F.E., Su, H., Kanade, T.: Apoptosis Detection for Adherent Cell Populations in Time-Lapse Phase-Contrast Microscopy Images. In: Ayache, N., Delingette, H., Golland, P., Mori, K. (eds.) MICCAI 2012, Part I. LNCS, vol. 7510, pp. 331–339. Springer, Heidelberg (2012)
3. Su, H., Yin, Z., Kanade, T., Huh, S.: Phase contrast image restoration via dictionary representation of diffraction patterns. In: Ayache, N., Delingette, H., Golland, P., Mori, K. (eds.) MICCAI 2012, Part III. LNCS, vol. 7512, pp. 615–622. Springer, Heidelberg (2012)
4. Gonzalez, R.C., Woods, R.E.: Digital Image Prcessing. Addison-Wesley Publishing Company, Inc. (1992)
5. Tedesco, F.S., Dellavalle, A., Diaz-Manera, J., Messina, G., Cossu, G.: Repairing skeletal muscle: regenerative potential of skeletal muscle stem cells. J. Clin. Invest. 120(1), 11–19 (2010)
6. Born, M., Wolf, E.: Principles of Optics, 6th edn. Pergamon Press (1980)
7. Ojala, T., Pietikäinen, M., Mäenpää, T.T.: Multiresolution gray-scale and rotation invariant texture classification with local binary pattern. IEEE Trans. Pattern. Anal. Mach. Intell. 24(7), 971–987 (2002)
8. Liu, M.-Y., Tuzel, O., Ramalingam, S., Chellappa, R.: Entropy Rate Superpixel Segmentation. In: Proc. CVPR, pp. 2097–2104 (2011)

# A Generative Model for OCT Retinal Layer Segmentation by Integrating Graph-Based Multi-surface Searching and Image Registration

Yuanjie Zheng[1], Rui Xiao[2], Yan Wang[1], and James C. Gee[1]

[1] Penn Image Computing and Science Laboratory (PICSL), Department of Radiology
[2] Department of Biostatistics and Epidemiology, Perelman School of Medicine at the University of Pennsylvania, Philadelphia, PA, USA

**Abstract.** We proposed a generative probabilistic modeling framework for automated segmentation of retinal layers from Optical Coherence Tomography (OCT) data. The objective is to learn a segmentation protocol from a collection of training images that have been manually labeled. Our model results in a novel OCT retinal layer segmentation approach which integrates algorithms of simultaneous searching of multiple interacting layer interfaces, image registration and machine learning. Different from previous work, our approach combines the benefits of constraining spatial layout of retinal layers, using a set of more robust local image descriptors, employing a mechanism for learning from manual labels and incorporating the inter-subject anatomical similarities of retina. With a set of OCT volumetric images from mutant canine retinas, we experimentally validated that our approach outperforms two state-of-the-art techniques.

## 1 Introduction

The major cause of adult blindness in developed countries is the progressive dysfunction and death of retinal photoreceptors [1]. Photoreceptors, located in the outer nuclear layer (ONL), function cooperatively with the retinal pigment epithelium (RPE). They catch and generate signals that are relayed to the second order neurons in the inner nuclear layer (INL) before being transmitted via ganglion cells to higher visual centers in the brain. The unique laminar organization of the vertebrate retina coupled with the development of novel non-invasive optical coherence topography (OCT) has revolutionized the ability to diagnose and follow the progression of photoreceptor diseases.

However, quantitative analysis of ONL and INL thickness throughout the entire accessible surface of the retina is rarely being done other than for preclinical or clinical investigation purposes. The reason for this limitation is due to the need to perform manual segmentation of the retinal layers, an effort that is extremely time-consuming as it can take up to one week [2] for a single imaged retina! This has clearly hampered the ability to translate such analysis from a research to a clinical setting, and prevented it to become a routine procedure.

Automated segmentation of retinal layers can help to provide an objective, quantitative and sensitive method for thickness analysis of retinal layers imaged non-invasively by OCT. Currently, commercially-available OCT imaging and analysis software are

K. Mori et al. (Eds.): MICCAI 2013, Part I, LNCS 8149, pp. 428–435, 2013.

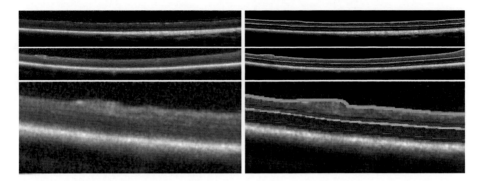

**Fig. 1.** Top two rows, from left to right: OCT cross-sectional scans of mutant dog retina and layer interfaces specified manually (top row) and automatically (2nd row) with the proposed algorithm, indicated with color "red" for ELM, "green" for ILM, "blue" for IPL1, "cyan" for OPL1 and "magenta" for OPL2. ELM-ILM, ELM-OPL1 and OPL2-IPL1 define the full retinal thickness, the ONL layer (thickest dark band) and the INL layer (thinner dark band), respectively. The bottom row shows an enlarged view of a local patch of the second-row images.

limited to offering measurements of either the full retinal thickness and/or that of the nerve fiber layer (NFL), incapable of segmenting other layers such as the ONL and INL. Several automated retinal layer segmentation approaches [3,4,5,6] were recently proposed to segment more retinal layers. They exploit a set of local image descriptors chosen manually or by a learning process to distinguish retinal layer's region or interfaces from other tissues, and optimally locate layers with certain optimization techniques. However, most of them are limited in accuracy and infeasible for a clinical setting due to the subtle differences between certain layers (e.g. IPL1, OPL1 and OPL2 as shown in Fig. 1) and large inter/intra-subject variations of photometric or geometric properties of OCT retinal layers.

In this paper, we propose a generative probabilistic modeling framework in order to develop automatic segmentation of OCT retinal layers. The objective is to learn a segmentation protocol from a collection of manually labeled images. Different from previous work, our framework exploits not only the discrimination ability of a set of local image descriptors learned to distinguish retinal layer interfaces from other tissues but also the anatomical similarity between the labeled image and test image (as shown in Fig. 1). Our approach combines algorithms of graph-based simultaneous searching of multiple interacting surfaces, image registration and machine learning.

This paper is novel in sense of not only a newly proposed generative model which integrates segmentation, registration and learning to more comprehensively make use of image information derived from training images, training labels and test image, but also an early attempt to apply image registration to OCT retinal layer segmentation.

## 2   The Generative Model

Let us use $S$ to represent a set of layer interfaces to be automatically estimated in the test OCT image $I$, $S_n$ to denote those manually delineated layers for each of the training

OCT images $\{I_n\}$, and $T_n$ to stand for the spatial mapping field between the training image $I_n$ and the test image $I$.

Our retinal layer segmentation algorithm is designed to maximize the conditional probability of $S, \{T_n\}$ given $I, \{I_n\}, \{S_n\}$, i.e. find the mode of the posterior distribution $p(S, T_n|I, \{I_n\}, \{S_n\})$. This form of Bayesian estimation is known as a *maximum a posteriori* (MAP) estimation and written as

$$\hat{S}, \{\hat{T}_n\} = \arg \max_{S, \{T_n\}} p(S, \{T_n\}|I, \{I_n\}, \{S_n\}). \tag{1}$$

With Bayesian inference, Eq. (1) is reformulated as

$$\hat{S}, \{\hat{T}_n\} = \arg \max_{S, \{T_n\}} p(I|S) \, p(\{S_n\}|S, \{T_n\}) \, p(S) \atop p(\{I_n\}, I|\{T_n\}, \{S_n\}, S) \, p(\{T_n\}). \tag{2}$$

In Eq. (2), the first term denotes the probability of producing the test image given layer interface segmentation. The second term represents the likelihood of training labels mapped to the coordinate space of the test image, and its maximization constraints the layer interface segmentation to be adherent to the transformed manual labels. The third term means the prior probability of $S$. The fourth term represents the conditional likelihood related to registering the intensities of the training images and test image given their retinal layer segmentations. The last term denotes the prior probability of the transformation field of registering training image to the test image.

The MAP estimation problem of Eq. (2) is in general difficult to solve due to the need to simultaneously solve multiple unknown parameters $\{S, \{T_n\}\}$. For simplicity, we employ an iterative optimization strategy as in [7]. Apparently, the former three terms of Eq. (2) are related to retinal layer segmentation while the fourth and fifth terms are associated with retinal image registration. Following the Bayesian inference theory, the segmentation module is represented as

$$\hat{S}^k = \arg \max_{S^k} p(S^k|T_n^k(S_n), I) = \arg \max_S p(I|S^k) \cdot p(\{T_n^k(S_n)\}|S^k) \cdot p(S^k) \tag{3}$$

where $k$ indexes each iterative step, and the registration module is expressed by

$$\{\hat{T}_n^{k+1}\} = \arg \max_{\{T_n^{k+1}\}} p(\{T_n^{k+1}\}|S^k, \{S_n\}, \{I_n\}, I) = \atop \arg \max_{\{T_n^{k+1}\}} p(\{I_n\}, I|\{T_n^{k+1}\}, \{S_n\}, S^k) \cdot p(\{T_n\}). \tag{4}$$

The MAP problem of Eq. (2) is then resolved by iteratively solving the segmentation formulation in Eq. (3) and registration formulation in Eq. (4) until convergence or over a certain number (e.g. 4 in practice) of times.

## 2.1    Segmentation

We assume that the training images are independent from each other in terms of the mapping fields $\{T_n\}$ and the retinal layers' manual labels $\{S_n\}$. By removing the iteration index, Eq. (3) is rewritten as

$$\hat{S} = \arg \max_S p(I|S) \cdot \left( \prod_{n=1}^{N} p(\{T_n(S_n)\}|S) \right) \cdot p(S) \tag{5}$$

where $N$ denotes the number of training images.

To define a mathematical representation of retinal layer interfaces, suppose the layer segmentation $S$ contains $L$ layer interfaces denoted by a set $\{\varsigma^i | 1 \leq i \leq L\}$. Similarly, the manually labeled retinal layer interfaces for $S_n$ are represented by a set $\{\varsigma_n^i | 1 \leq i \leq L\}$. In the volumetric image $I(x, y, z)$, a layer interface $\varsigma^i$ is a function mapping $(x, y)$ to $z$-values, i.e. $\varsigma^i(x, y) \to z$. Treating $I(x, y, z)$ as a multicolumn model which consists of a set of columns defined by their $(x, y)$ coordinates, $(x, y, \varsigma^i(x, y))$ is the intersection point of column $(x, y)$ with the $i$th interface. As a retinal layer interface, $\varsigma^i$ is commonly assumed to intersect with each column of $I$ exactly once [3].

**Learn from Manual Delineations:** To solve $p(I|S)$ in Eq. (5), for each of the $L$ retinal layer interfaces, we trained an AdaBoost classifier [8] using the self-similarities (SS) image descriptors [9] computed from the training images $\{I_n\}$ and with the corresponding manual segmentations $\{S_n\}$. These trained classifiers are then applied to the test image $I$ to get the probability $p(x, y, z, i)$ of each pixel $(x, y, z)$ belonging to the $i$th retinal layer interface.

**Transform Manual Delineations:** In the second term of Eq. (5), $T_n(S_n)$ transforms the manual segmentation $S_n$ of layer interface for the $n$th training image into the coordinate space of the test image. Suppose the shortest distance of a pixel $(x, y, z)$ in the test image to the $i$th transformed layer interface is $D_{ni}$. Then, we set the probability of $(x, y, z)$ belonging to the $i$th layer interface as $p'_{ni}(x, y, z, i) \propto \exp(-D_{ni}^2/\sigma_m^2)$. Considering all training images, we have

$$p'_i(x, y, z, i) \propto \prod_{n=1}^{N} \exp(-D_{ni}^2/\sigma_m^2), \tag{6}$$

where $p'_i(x, y, z, i)$ denotes the probability of $(x, y, z)$ belonging to $i$th layer interface based on the transformed layer interfaces from all training images.

**Constrain Layer Interfaces:** We incorporate constraints on smoothness of layer interfaces and range of distance between layers in the third term of Eq. (5):

$$p(S) \propto \prod_i \prod_{(x,y)} \prod_{(x',y') \in \mathcal{N}(x,y)} \exp\left(- \left(\varsigma^i(x, y) - \varsigma^i(x', y')\right)^2 / \sigma_s^2\right) \\ \prod_{i,j \neq i} \prod_{(x,y)} \exp\left(- \left(\varsigma^i(x, y) - \varsigma^j(x, y) - m_{d(i,j)}\right)^2 / \sigma_{d(i,j)}^2\right) \tag{7}$$

where $i$ and $j$ index layer interface, $\mathcal{N}(x, y)$ denotes the neighboring pixels of $(x, y)$, $\sigma_s$ is a constant controlling the smoothness degree, $m_{d(i,j)}$ and $\sigma_{d(i,j)}^2$ are the mean and variance of the distances between the $i$th and $j$th layer interfaces.

With above equations, the probability maximization in Eq. (5) can be carried out by a minimization of the following objective function

$$\mathcal{O}(S) = \sum_{(x,y,z)} - \ln p\left(x, y, z, S(x, y, z)\right) + c_1 \sum_{(x,y,z)} \sum_{n=1}^{N} D_{nS(x,y,z)}^2 \\ + c_2 \sum_i \sum_{(x,y)} \sum_{(x',y') \in \mathcal{N}(x,y)} \left(\varsigma^i(x, y) - \varsigma^i(x', y')\right)^2 \tag{8} \\ + \sum_{i,j \neq i} \sum_{(x,y)} \left(\varsigma^i(x, y) - \varsigma^j(x, y) - m_{d(i,j)}\right)^2 / \sigma_{d(i,j)}^2$$

where $c_1$ and $c_2$ are determined by $\sigma_m$ in Eq. (6) and $\sigma_s$ in Eq. (7), respectively.

We employ an optimization approach similar to the techniques in [3,4,6], which tries to transform the optimal and simultaneous segmentation of multiple layer interfaces into a layered-graph-theoretical problem and solve it by finding a minimum-cost s-t cut. We empirically set up the parameters of Eq. (8) as $c_1 = 3.5$, $c_2 = 2.7$, $m_d/\sigma_d$ (in unit of millimicron) being $86.9/12, 35/8, 35/8$, and $158/90$ for layer interfaces of "ELM-OPL1", "OPL1-OPL2", "OPL2-IPL1" and "IPL1-ILM", respectively.

## 2.2    Registration

If we assume the registration of one training image is independent from other training images and remove the iteration index, Eq. (4) is rewritten as

$$\{\hat{T}_n\} = \arg\max_{\{T_n\}} \prod_n p(I_n, I|T_n, S_n, S) \cdot p(\{T_n\}. \tag{9}$$

To practically accomplish the maximization of Eq. (9), we ignore $p(\{T_n\}$ in order for simplicity. We first performed a global registration between each training image and test image by ignoring all segmentations and using the FSL FLIRT tool [10] with six degrees of freedom and the default parameters. Then, deformable registration was conducted using the ANTS Symmetric Normalization (SyN) algorithm [11], with the cross-correlation similarity metric (with radius 2) and a Gaussian regularizer with variance being 9. To register a training image to the test image, we ran the ANTS algorithm on each of the divided image regions by the segmented retinal layer interfaces, including the "outer-ELM", "ELM-OPL1", "OPL1-OPL2", "OPL2-IPL1" and "IPL1-ILM" regions, as shown in Fig. 1. The way we employed to get a smooth deformation field from the registration results for all divided regions is to linearly combine the velocity field outputs. After registration, reference segmentations from each of the training images were warped into the test image space.

## 2.3    Algorithm Overview

Our algorithm from the MAP estimation in Eq. (1) for OCT retinal layer interface segmentation is summarized as below.

**Algorithm** - OCT Retinal Layer Segmentation

1. Train AdaBoost classifiers with $\{I_n\}$ and $\{S_n\}$
2. Run AdaBoost classifiers on $I$ to get $p(x, y, z, i)$ denoting each pixel's probability belonging to a layer interface
3. Minimize Eq. (8) (removing the second term) with the graph-based multi-surface searching algorithm to get an initial segmentation
4. Run FSL FLIRT tool to globally register each of $\{I_n\}$ to $I$
5. Divide each of $\{I_n\}$ into subregions with manual labels
6. Repeat following steps until convergence or over four times
   (a) Divide test image into subregions with current layer segmentation
   (b) Register each of $\{I_n\}$ to $I$ with ANTS and combine with the results of FSL FLIRT
   (c) Minimize Eq. (8) with the graph-based multi-surface searching algorithm to get a refined segmentation

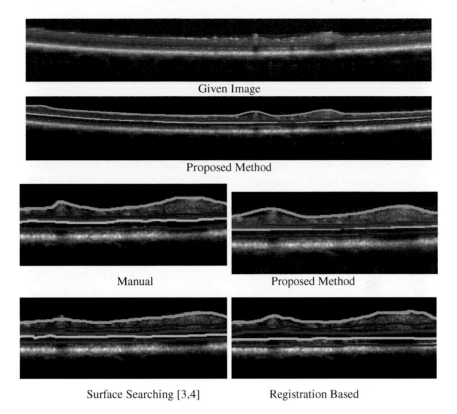

**Fig. 2.** Segmentation results of five retinal layer interfaces shown with different colors on one OCT cross-sectional scan of mutant dog's retina from three segmentation methods

## 3    Experimental Results

We employed a set of Heidelberg Engineering Spectralis OCT raw datap containing 5 volumetric images in format of ".vol", size of $1536 \times 496 \times 49$ and resolution of $5.8 \mu m \times 3.9 \mu m \times 123.9 \mu m$. This data set was acquired from the retinas of research mutant dogs with naturally-occurring inherited retinal degeneration. A trained rater manually delineated the layer interfaces of ELM, OPL1, OPL2, IPL1 and ILM for 3 images.

We first exploited these three manually labeled images to experimentally compare the accuracies of the proposed method which integrates learning, surface searching and image registration as shown in Eq. (2), Eq. (3) and Eq. (4), a pure surface searching method similar to the techniques in [3,4] with an on-surface cost determined by image gradient as in [4] and a set of intra-/inter-surface constraints same to the ones in Eq. (7), and a registration based segmentation technique accomplished by using the FSL FLIRT tool for a global registration followed by the ANTS algorithm for a nonrigid registration as described in Sec. 2.2 and by exploiting the Majority Voting based label fusion strategy [12]. For our method and the registration based segmentation method, a leave-one-out strategy is exploited. Mean and standard deviation of the unsigned retinal layer positioning errors are computed.

**Table 1.** Mean±standard deviation in millimicron of the unsigned positioning errors (shortest distance of a point on an algorithm-produced interface to a manually-specified interface) of three methods on three retinal layers

| Method | ILM | IPL1 | OPL2 | OPL1 | ELM |
|---|---|---|---|---|---|
| Proposed Method | 24.3±12.9 | 14.5±8.8 | 9.3±6.5 | 9.6 ± 5.5 | 18.4± 13.7 |
| Surface Searching | 27.4±14.3 | 25.7±19.9 | 24.9±18.3 | 24.2±19.5 | 18.9±14.6 |
| Registration Based | 23.8±14.5 | 30.1±22.3 | 34.4±25.0 | 32.9±24.2 | 30.3±14.8 |

From the results in Table. 1 and Fig. 2, we got three findings. First, the proposed method accomplishes significant improvements in detection accuracy of the layer interfaces of IPL1, OPL2 and OPL1. Second, the proposed method generates accuracies comparable with the surface searching technique and better than the image registration based approach for ELM segmentation. Third, the proposed method performs comparably with other techniques in segmentation of ILM. We found that our method achieved an average thickness accuracy improvement of 13 millimicron compared to the surface searching technique and 21 millimicron with the registration based technique, over the layers of full retina, ONL and INL. This accuracy improvement is of much more practical importance compared with the need of more computational cost by our algorithm compared with other two methods.

We also visually compared the retinal layer interface segmentation results of these three segmentation algorithms on the left two OCT images for which the manual labels are unavailable. For the proposed method, we used all the manually labeled images as the training set. Similar finding were obtained: the proposed method outperforms other techniques in segmentation of IPL1, OPL2 and OPL1 and performs comparably with other techniques on ILM and ELM segmentations.

## 4   Conclusion

In this paper, we proposed a generative probabilistic model for automated segmentation of retinal layers from OCT image (our model is also extendable to other segmentation tasks, e.g. [13,14]). With Bayesian theories, we proved that our model can be practically approached with existing algorithms on simultaneous searching of interacting surfaces, image registration and learning. Our model integrates the benefits of employing certain prior knowledge on the layout of retinal layer interfaces, a set of effective self-similarity descriptors, mechanism of learning from manual labels and incorporation of inter-subject similarity of retinal anatomies. We experimentally validated that our algorithm outperforms two state-of-the-art techniques in or even outside the field of OCT retinal layer segmentation.

Our future work would focus on validation with a larger data set, segmentation of other retinal layers and clinical studies on retinal degenerations.

**Acknowledgement.** Thanks to Dr. William A. Beltran and Dr. Gustavo D. Aguirre at UPenn Veterinary Medicine for providing the OCT data sets. Thanks to Dr. David Brainard at Department of Psychology of UPenn for his instructive suggestions. This work was made possible by support from National Institute of Health (NIH) via grant P30-EY001583.

# References

1. Wright, A.F., Chakarova, C.F., Abd El-Aziz, M.M., Bhattacharya, S.S.: Photoreceptor degeneration: genetic and mechanistic dissection of a complex trait. Nature Reviews Genetics 11, 273–284 (2010)
2. Beltrana, W.A., et al.: Gene therapy rescues photoreceptor blindness in dogs and paves the way for treating human x-linked retinitis pigmentosa. PNAS 109, 2132–2137 (2012)
3. Garvin, M.K., Abramoff, M.D., Wu, X., Russell, S.R., Burns, T.L., Sonka, M.: Automated 3-d intraretinal layer segmentation of macular spectral-domain optical coherence tomography images. IEEE Trans. Medical Imaging 28, 1436–1447 (2009)
4. Dufour, P.A., Ceklic, L., Abdillahi, H., Schroder, S., Dzanet, S.D., Wolf-Schnurrbusch, U., Kowal, J.: Graph-based multi-surface segmentation of oct data using trained hard and soft constraints. IEEE Trans. Medical Imaging (2012)
5. Yazdanpanah, A., Hamarneh, G., Smith, B.R., Sarunic, M.V.: Segmentation of intra-retinal layers from optical coherence tomography images using an active contour approach. IEEE Trans. Medical Imaging 30, 484–496 (2011)
6. Xu, L., Stojkovic, B., Zhu, Y., Song, Q., Wu, X., Sonka, M., Xu, J.: Efficient algorithms for segmenting globally optimal and smooth multi-surfaces. In: Székely, G., Hahn, H.K. (eds.) IPMI 2011. LNCS, vol. 6801, pp. 208–220. Springer, Heidelberg (2011)
7. Lu, C., Chelikani, S., Papademetris, X., Knisely, J.P., Milosevic, M.F., Chen, Z., Jaffray, D.A., Staib, L.H., Duncan, J.S.: An integrated approach to segmentation and nonrigid registration for application in image-guided pelvic radiotheraphy. Medical Image Analsis 15, 772–785 (2011)
8. Freund, Y., Schapire, R.E.: A decision-theoretic generalization of on-line learning and an application to boosting. Journal of Computer and System Sciences 55(1), 119–139 (1997)
9. Shechtman, E., Irani, M.: Matching local self-similarities across images and videos. In: CVPR (June 2007)
10. Smith, S.M., et al.: Advances in functional and structural mr image analysis and implementation as fsl. Neuroimage 23, S208–S219 (2004)
11. Avants, B., Epstein, C., Grossman, M., Gee, J.: Symmetric diffeomorphic image registration with cross-correlation: Evaluating automated labeling of elderly and neurodegenerative brain. Medical Image Analysis 12, 26–41 (2008)
12. Aljabar, P., Heckemann, R.A., Hammers, A., Hajnal, J.V., Rueckert, D.: Multi-atlas based segmentation of brain images: atlas selection and its effect on accuracy. Neuroimage 46, 726–738 (2009)
13. Zhang, S., Zhan, Y., Metaxas, D.N.: Deformable segmentation via sparse representation and dictionary learning. Medical Image Analysis 16(7), 1385–1396 (2012)
14. Zhang, S., Zhan, Y., Dewan, M., Huang, J., Metaxas, D.N., Zhou, X.S.: Towards robust and effective shape modeling: Sparse shape composition. Medical Image Analysis 16(1), 265–277 (2012)

# An Integrated Framework for Automatic Ki-67 Scoring in Pancreatic Neuroendocrine Tumor

Fuyong Xing[1,2], Hai Su[1,2], and Lin Yang[1,2]

[1] Division of Biomedical Informatics, Department of Biostatistics
[2] Department of Computer Science, University of Kentucky, KY 40506, USA

**Abstract.** The Ki-67 labeling index is a valid and important biomarker to gauge neuroendocrine tumor cell progression. Automatic Ki-67 assessment is very challenging due to complex variations of cell characteristics. In this paper, we propose an integrated learning-based framework for accurate Ki-67 scoring in pancreatic neuroendocrine tumor. The main contributions of our method are: a novel and robust cell detection algorithm is designed to localize both tumor and non-tumor cells; a repulsive deformable model is applied to correct touching cell segmentation; a two stage learning-based scheme combining cellular features and regional structure information is proposed to differentiate tumor from non-tumor cells (such as lymphocytes); an integrated automatic framework is developed to accurately assess the Ki-67 labeling index. The proposed method has been extensively evaluated on 101 tissue microarray (TMA) whole discs, and the cell detection performance is comparable to manual annotations. The automatic Ki-67 score is very accurate compared with pathologists' estimation.

## 1 Introduction

Pancreatic neuroendocrine tumor (NET) cancer is one of the most common cancers worldwide. The Ki-67 labeling index, defined as the ratio between the numbers of immunopositive tumor cells and all tumor cells, has been considered as a valid biomarker to evaluate tumor cell progression and predict therapy responses. Manual Ki-67 assessment is subject to a low throughput processing rate and pathologist-dependent bias. Automatic Ki-67 assessment can provide more objective, high throughput, and reproducible results [6,10]. Automated cell detection can also provide access to computer-aided Ki-67 scoring. Parvin *et al.* [13] proposed an iterative radial voting algorithm based on oriented kernels to localize cell nuclei, in which the voting direction and areas are dynamically updated within each consecutive iteration. This algorithm has outstanding noise immunity and scale invariance. A computationally efficient single-pass voting for cell detection is reported in [15], which applies mean shift clustering instead of iterative voting to seed localization. Other methods [9,11,2,7,8] are also proposed for touching cell detection and segmentation. However, none of these methods addresses the automatic Ki-67 counting problem, which requires an accurate differentiation between tumor and non-tumor cells.

K. Mori et al. (Eds.): MICCAI 2013, Part I, LNCS 8149, pp. 436–443, 2013.

In this paper, we propose a novel integrated learning-based algorithm for automatic scoring of pancreatic NET with Ki-67 staining. In order to accurately detect cells in dense clusters, a robust and efficient region-based hierarchical voting algorithm is proposed to detect cell seeds (geometric centers). These seeds will be used to initialize a repulsive deformable model to extract touching cell boundaries with known object topology constraints. Next, a two stage learning-based scheme is employed to differentiate tumor from non-tumor cells. The algorithm combines both the cellular features and regional structure information. The Ki-67 labeling index is finally calculated using a color histogram to separate immunopositive (brown cells in Ki-67 staining) and immunonegative (blue cells in Ki-67 staining) tumor cells.

## 2   Methodology

### 2.1   Hierarchical Voting-Based Seed Detection

Robust cell detection is achieved by finding the geometric centers (seeds) of the cells. Let $T(x, y)$ denote the original image, and $\nabla T(x, y)$ be the gradient. For those pixels with relatively large magnitude $\|\nabla T(x, y)\|$, single-pass voting [15] defines a cone-shape voting area $A$ with vertex at $(x, y)$ and votes along the negative gradient direction: $\frac{-\nabla T(x,y)}{\|\nabla T(x,y)\|} = -(\cos(\theta(x, y)), \sin(\theta(x, y)))$, where $\theta$ represents the angle of the gradient direction with respect to $x$ axis. A voting image $V(x, y)$ is initialized as zeros and then updated by weighting the gradient magnitude with a Gaussian kernel $g(m, n, \mu_x, \mu_y, \sigma)$:

$$V(x, y) = V(x, y) + \sum_{(m,n) \in A} \|\nabla T(x, y)\|\, g(m, n, \mu_x, \mu_y, \sigma), \qquad (1)$$

where the voting area $A$ is defined by the radial range $(r_{min}, r_{max})$ and angular range $\Delta$. The isotropic Gaussian kernel is parametrically defined with $(\mu_x, \mu_y) = (x + \frac{(r_{max} - r_{min}) \cos\theta}{2}, y - \frac{(r_{max} - r_{min}) \sin\theta}{2})$ and scalar $\sigma$. After the voting map is generated, mean shift [4] is employed to calculate the final seed for each individual cell.

Single-pass voting is computationally efficient, but it is not able to efficiently handle cell size and shape variations. Considering these challenges, in our algorithm, we introduce a region-based hierarchical voting in the distance transform map. A Gaussian pyramid is applied to both the voting procedure and the mean shift clustering step. The hierarchical voting is formulated as:

$$V_{RH}(x, y) = \sum_{l=0}^{L} \sum_{(m,n) \in S} I((x, y) \in A_l(m, n)) M_l(x, y) g(m, n, \mu_x, \mu_y, \sigma), \quad (2)$$

where $V_{RH}(x, y)$ is the confidence map, $S$ represents the set of all voting pixels, $A_l(m, n)$ denotes the cone-shape voting area with vertex $(m, n)$ at layer $l$, $M_l(x, y)$ represents the Euclidean distance transform map at layer $l$, and

$I(\mathbf{x}) = I((x, y) \in A_l(m, n))$ is the indicator function. The pixels with higher $M_l(x, y)$ values near the geometric center of a cell will enhance their contributions in Equation (2). For each pixel $(x, y)$, Equation (2) provides a weighted sum of all the voting values created by its neighboring pixels whose voting areas contain $(x, y)$, instead of only those created by its own. In comparison with single-pass voting, hierarchical voting is more robust with respect to the detection of cells with relatively large size variations.

## 2.2   Repulsive Deformable Model

The proposed cell detection algorithm indiscriminately detects both tumor and non-tumor cells, and therefore the results cannot be directly used to calculate the Ki-67 scoring index. Differentiation between tumor and non-tumor cells is the critical step for automatic Ki-67 scoring. In order to extract discriminative morphological features to separate tumor from non-tumor cells, accurate cellular segmentation is a prerequisite. This is challenging due to the complex color and intensity variations exhibited inside cells, especially within touching cell clumps. Based on the results obtained from Section 2.1, we propose to segment each individual cell using an improved deformable model. Motivated by Zimmer and Olivo-Marin's work [18], we introduce a contour-based repulsive term into the deformable model [3] to prevent evolving contours from crossing and merging with one another. In [3], the original pressure force is designed to deform contour $v(s)$ until the internal $F^{int}(v)$ and external $F^{ext}(v)$ forces achieve a balance:

$$F^{int}(v) = \alpha v''(s) - \beta v''''(s), \quad F^{ext}(v) = \gamma \boldsymbol{n}(s) - \lambda \frac{\nabla E_{ext}(v(s))}{||E_{ext}(v(s))||}, \quad (3)$$

where $\boldsymbol{n}(s)$ together with weight $\gamma$ represents the pressure force, and $\nabla E_{ext}(v(s))$ denotes the image force where $E_{ext}(v(s)) = -||\nabla T(x(s), y(s))||^2$. $\alpha, \beta$, and $\lambda$ are weight parameters. Without a repulsive term, active contours guided by (3) will move independently and may cross with one another within touching cell clumps. In order to prevent contour overlapping, we introduce an external force:

$$F_R^{ext}(v_i) = \gamma \boldsymbol{n}_i(s) - \lambda \frac{\nabla E_{ext}(v_i(s))}{||E_{ext}(v_i(s))||} + \omega \sum_{j=1, j \neq i}^{N} \int_0^1 d_{ij}^{-2}(s, t) \boldsymbol{n}_j(t) dt, \quad (4)$$

where $N$ is the number of cells, $d_{ij}(s, t) = ||v_i(s) - v_j(t)||_2$ is the Euclidean distance between contour $v_i(s)$ and $v_j(t)$. The last term (with parameter $\omega$) in Equation (4) models the repulsion schema: as the contours move closer ($d_{ij}^{-2}(s, t)$ becomes larger), they receive stronger repulsive forces from each other until stop evolving. Using the detected seed as initialization (Section 2.1), this repulsive deformable model can handle touching cells effectively. Compared with [18] that introduces an area-based penalty term to avoid contour overlapping, our model is computationally efficient and requires less memory. Meanwhile, as a parametric model, the proposed repulsive deformable model can preserve known object topology, and therefore each contour represents one cell without splitting or merging. This topology preserving property is significantly different from the widely used geometric repulsive deformable methods [17,12,5].

## 2.3   Two Stage Learning-Based Classification

In order to calculate the final Ki-67 labeling index, a two stage learning-based scheme combining cellular features and regional structure information is designed to differentiate tumor from non-tumor cells.

**Stage I:** Based on the results of cellular segmentation, a SVM classifier is trained to predict the probabilities of segmented cells (tumor or non-tumor cells) using the following cellular features: 1) Geometric descriptors: area, perimeter, circularity, axis ratio (length ratio between estimated major and minor axes), solidity; 2) Color intensity: mean, standard deviation ($\sigma$), smoothness ($1 - 1/(1 + \sigma^2)$), skewness, kurtosis, entropy, contrast, correlation, homogeneity; 3) Cell shapes with Fourier descriptor. In total we have extracted $5 + 9 \times 3 + 80 = 112$ features, where 3 represents R, G, and B color channels, and 80 denotes the first 20 harmonics (each corresponds to 4 coefficients) that are chosen in the Elliptical Fourier transformation. A sparse representation model is used to select a set of most discriminative features by solving:

$$\min_{b} ||Db - a||_2^2, \ s.t. \ ||b||_1 \leq \eta, b \succeq 0, \tag{5}$$

where $D \in \mathbb{R}^{(N^+ + N^-) \times W}$ represents the features extracted from $N^+$ tumor and $N^-$ non-tumor cells, and $W = 112$ denotes the original dimension of the feature vector. The $\eta$ is a parameter controlling the sparsity of $b$. The binary vector $a \in \mathbb{R}^{(N^+ + N^-) \times 1}$ represents the labels of cells used for training in $D$: $a_i = +1$ for tumor and $a_i = -1$ for non-tumor. Due to the $l_1$ norm constraint, the solution $b^* \in \mathbb{R}^{W \times 1}$ to (5) is sparse with nonzero elements corresponding to the selected discriminative features. Based on $b^*$ with $L$ nonzero elements, we can project all the features onto a low-dimensional, discriminative subspace. A SVM classifier is learned to predict the cell category in the transformed feature space. All the cells with low probabilities (usually representing typical non-tumor cells) will be removed before entering Stage II such that the second classifier would be able to focus on a reduced dataset containing more difficult cases.

**Stage II:** In Stage I, only cellular features are considered. The classification accuracy will be improved by introducing the local structure information. This image structural pattern can be described with texture, and modeled with texton [16] feature. A multiple scale Schmid filter bank [16] is used for image filtering:

$$F(r, \sigma, \tau) = F_0(\sigma, \tau) + \cos\left(\frac{\pi r \tau}{\sigma}\right) e^{-\frac{r^2}{2\sigma^2}}, \tag{6}$$

where $\tau$ is the number of cycles of the harmonic function within the Gaussian envelop of the filter and $r = \sqrt{x^2 + y^2}$. A texton library is constructed using the training pancreatic NET TMA specimens. For computational efficiency, the integral histogram [14] is utilized to calculate the multiscale windowed texton histogram. Finally, the logistic boosting is employed to calculate the probability map using the multiscale texton histograms as features.

Using the texture classification-based probability map, each individual cell will obtain a score to evaluate its probability belonging to tumor or non-tumor cells.

In addition, the ratio between the probability of one cell and the probability average for all its neighbouring cells provides a measurement of cell category distribution. Based on these observations, the mean/standard deviation of pixel probabilities in each cell, and the percentage of probability summation of one cell over the probability average for all cells in its local region are calculated. These statistical features are concatenated with the previously predicted cellular probabilities in Stage I to train a second SVM classifier. The output will produce the final labels to differentiate tumor from non-tumor cells. In order to calculate the Ki-67 labeling index, a color histogram is used to separate immunopositive from immunonegative tumor cells since immunopositive/immunonegative ones are usually stained as brown/blue.

## 3    Experimental Results

The proposed algorithm is tested with 101 whole slide scanned pancreatic NET tissue microarray (TMA) images, which are captured at 20× magnification. Several representative image patches (3 or 4) are cropped from each whole disc scanned image slide (in total over 300 image patches). Each slide corresponds to thousands of mixed tumor and non-tumor cells. In total 20 slides are used for training and 81 slides are reserved for testing. The annotations are created by two pathologists and one pathology resident. The subjective nature is handled using a weighted majority voting considering experience. The cell detection algorithm is implemented with C++ for efficiency, while Matlab is used for cell segmentation and classification on a PC machine with $3.3GHz$ CPU and $16Gb$ memory. A rough estimate of cell diameter needs to be provided to the cell detection algorithm, and we set $\sigma = 0.3, l = 2$ in Equation (2), $\alpha = 0.05, \beta = 0, \gamma = 0.5, \lambda = 5, w = 0.7$ in Equation (4), and $\eta = 8$ in Equation (5). The parameters are selected based on cross-validation and fixed during the testing stage.

### 3.1    Cell Detection

Both qualitative and quantitative analyses are conducted for the proposed cell detection algorithm. In Figure 1, thousands of cells are correctly detected and segmented in one TMA disc with several zoomed-in patches for better illustration. The computational time for a digitized $2310 \times 2150$ pixels TMA disc is 96.5 seconds, compared with more than thirty-minute labor intensive work even for manual counting of 3-4 representative patches from the whole disc. We present the detection results using the proposed method on several small randomly selected patches extracted from the whole dataset in Figure 2 compared with three recent state-of-the-art methods: Laplacian-of-Gaussian filters (LoG) [1], iterative radial voting (IRV) [13], and single-pass voting (SPV) [15]. The proposed algorithm is more robust with respect to the variations of cell scale, shape, and intensity. This can be attributed to the region-based hierarchical voting in the distance map.

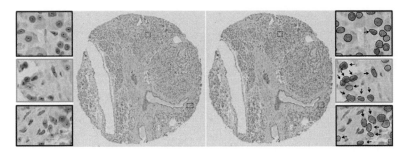

**Fig. 1.** Cell detection (left panel) and segmentation (right panel) using the proposed method. Several patches are zoomed in for better illustration. The cells pointed out by black arrows in each patch of the right panel are non-tumor cells, and the other segmented cells are tumor cells.

To quantitatively evaluate seed detection accuracy, we present the mean value (MV) and standard deviation (STD) of the Euclidean distances between manually located seeds and those created by automatic algorithms in Table 1, where the missing rate ($MR$), over-detection rate (OR), and effective rate (ER) are also presented. The missing or over-detection means no seeds or more than one seed are detected for one ground-truth cell, respectively. These two cases are excluded when we compute the $MV$ for fair comparison. The effective rate is to calculate a ratio between the number

**Table 1.** Seed detection accuracy compared with ground truth

|  | $MV \pm STD$ | $MR$ | $OR$ | $ER$ |
|---|---|---|---|---|
| LoG [1] | $3.23 \pm 1.84$ | 0.03 | 0.09 | 1.28 |
| IRV [13] | $2.62 \pm 2.11$ | 0.12 | 0.16 | 1.2 |
| SPV [15] | $2.59 \pm 2.04$ | 0.10 | 0.02 | 0.91 |
| Proposed | $2.39 \pm 2.0$ | 0.06 | 0.01 | 0.99 |

of detected seeds and ground truth seeds, which measures the methods' robustness to background clutter. $ER = 1$ indicates the strongest robustness. LoG is sensitive to image background, IRV and PSV miss or over-detect some seeds, while the proposed method produces the best performance.

## 3.2   Ki-67 Scoring

In the experiments at Stage I, circularity, axis ratio, color mean, standard deviation, kurtosis, contrast, correlation, and homogeneity are selected by the sparse representation model as the most discriminative features to separate tumor from non-tumor cells. This is reasonable since in our dataset tumor cells usually appear more circular than non-tumor cells with a more inhomogeneous texture and relatively lighter staining. The first SVM classifier applies a Gaussian kernel (the parameter $\sigma = 0.3$ and the penalty $c = 1$) with these selected discriminative features. Combined with the texton histogram-based probabilities, the second SVM classifier with the same set of parameters is trained to produce the final classification of tumor and non-tumor cells. Compared with manual annotations by pathologists, we have achieved 87.68% classification accuracy with 87.12%

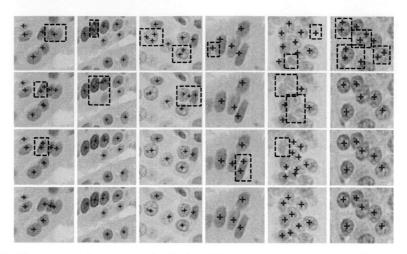

**Fig. 2.** The geometric centers of cells (seeds) detection on several randomly selected image patches. Rows 1, 2, 3, and 4 denote results created by LoG [1], IRV [13], SPV [15], and the proposed algorithm, respectively. The missing or false seeds are surrounded with black dashed rectangles.

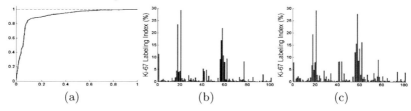

**Fig. 3.** ROC curve (a) of the classification of tumor cells and lymphocytes, automatic Ki-67 score (b), and manual Ki-67 score (c) for 101 patients ($x$-axis)

specificity and 88.01% sensitivity. The ROC curve is displayed in Figure 3(a). The Ki-67 indexing numbers for 101 pancreatic NET patients obtained by our method are shown in Figure 3(b), and they are very close to human manual evaluation of Ki-67 scoring (Figure 3(c)). The absolute mean error rate between automatic and manual Ki-67 scores is 0.88%.

## 4   Conclusion

In this paper, we have introduced an automatic algorithm for Ki-67 scoring on pancreatic NET TMA images. The novel cell detection and Ki-67 scoring system can efficiently and accurately detect thousands of cells in the whole TMA discs and provide accurate Ki-67 score.

**Acknowledgement.** The project described is supported by the National Center for Research Resources, UL1RR033173, and the National Center for Advancing Translational Sciences, UL1TR000117.

## References

1. Al-Kofahi, Y., Lassoued, W., Lee, W., Roysam, B.: Improved automatic detection and segmentation of cell nuclei in histopathology images. TBME 57(4), 841–852 (2010)

2. Arteta, C., Lempitsky, V., Noble, J.A., Zisserman, A.: Learning to detect cells using non-overlapping extremal regions. In: Ayache, N., Delingette, H., Golland, P., Mori, K. (eds.) MICCAI 2012, Part I. LNCS, vol. 7510, pp. 348–356. Springer, Heidelberg (2012)

3. Cohen, L.D.: On active contour models and balloons. CVGIP: Image Understanding 53(2), 211–218 (1991)

4. Comaniciu, D., Meer, P.: Mean shift: A robust approach toward feature space analysis. PAMI 24(5), 603–619 (2002)

5. Dzyubachyk, O., van Cappellen, W.A., Essers, J., Niessen, W.J., Meijering, E.: Advanced level-set-based cell tracking in time-lapse fluorescence microscopy. TMI 29(3), 852–867 (2010)

6. Funel, N., Denaro, M., Faviana, P., Pollina, L.E., Perrone, V.G., Lio, N.D., Boggi, U., Basolo, F., Campani, D.: The new fully automated system for ki67 evaluation in pancreatic neuroendocrine tumors (pnets). Would it be possible to obtain a standard to grade evaluation? J. of Pancreas 13(5S), 562 (2012)

7. Kong, H., Gurcan, M., Belkacem-Boussaid, K.: Partitioning histopathological images: An integrated framework for supervised color-texture segmentation and cell splitting. TMI 30(9), 1661–1677 (2011)

8. Liu, X., Harvey, C.W., Wang, H., Alber, M.S., Chen, D.Z.: Detecting and tracking motion of myxococcus xanthus bacteria in swarms. In: Ayache, N., Delingette, H., Golland, P., Mori, K. (eds.) MICCAI 2012, Part I. LNCS, vol. 7510, pp. 373–380. Springer, Heidelberg (2012)

9. Lou, X., Koethe, U., Wittbrodt, J., Hamprecht, F.: Learning to segment dense cell nuclei with shape prior. In: CVPR, pp. 1012–1018 (2012)

10. Mohammed, Z.M., Elsberger, B., McMillan, D.C., Going, J.J., Orange, C., Mallon, E., Edwards, J., Doughty, J.C.: Comparison of visual and automated assessment of Ki-67 proliferative activity and their impact on outcome in primary operable invasive ductal breast cancer. Br. J. Cancer 106(2), 383–388 (2012)

11. Monaco, J., Hipp, J., Lucas, D., Smith, S., Balis, U., Madabhushi, A.: Image segmentation with implicit color standardization using spatially constrained expectation maximization: detection of nuclei. In: Ayache, N., Delingette, H., Golland, P., Mori, K. (eds.) MICCAI 2012, Part I. LNCS, vol. 7510, pp. 365–372. Springer, Heidelberg (2012)

12. Mosaliganti, K., Gelas, A., Gouaillard, A., Noche, R., Obholzer, N., Megason, S.: Detection of spatially correlated objects in 3D images using appearance models and coupled active contours. In: Yang, G.-Z., Hawkes, D., Rueckert, D., Noble, A., Taylor, C. (eds.) MICCAI 2009, Part II. LNCS, vol. 5762, pp. 641–648. Springer, Heidelberg (2009)

13. Parvin, B., Yang, Q., Han, J., Chang, H., Rydberg, B., Barcellos-Hoff, M.H.: Iterative voting for inference of structural saliency and characterization of subcellular events. TIP 16, 615–623 (2007)

14. Porikli, F.M.: Integral histogram: A fast way to extract histograms in cartesian spaces. In: CVPR, pp. 829–836 (2005)

15. Qi, X., Xing, F., Foran, D.J., Yang, L.: Robust segmentation of overlapping cells in histopathology specimens using parallel seed detection and repulsive level set. TBME 59(3), 754–765 (2012)

16. Schmid, C.: Constructing models for content-based image retrieval. In: CVPR, pp. 39–45 (2001)

17. Yan, P., Zhou, X., Shah, M., Wong, S.T.C.: Automatic segmentation of high-throughput RNAi fluorescent cellular images. TITB 12(1), 109–117 (2008)

18. Zimmer, C., Olivo-Marin, J.C.: Coupled parametric active contours. PAMI 27(11), 1838–1842 (2005)

# A Linear Program Formulation for the Segmentation of *Ciona* Membrane Volumes

Diana L. Delibaltov[1], Pratim Ghosh[1], Volkan Rodoplu[1], Michael Veeman[2,3], William Smith[2], and B.S. Manjunath[1,*]

[1]Department of Electrical and Computer Engineering
[2] Department of Molecular, Cellular and Developmental Biology
[2,1] University of California, Santa Barbara, CA - 93106
[3] Division of Biology, Kansas State University, Manhattan, KS - 66506

**Abstract.** We address the problem of cell segmentation in confocal microscopy membrane volumes of the ascidian *Ciona* used in the study of morphogenesis. The primary challenges are non-uniform and patchy membrane staining and faint spurious boundaries from other organelles (e.g. nuclei). Traditional segmentation methods incorrectly attach to faint boundaries producing spurious edges. To address this problem, we propose a linear optimization framework for the joint correction of multiple over-segmentations obtained from different methods. The main idea motivating this approach is that multiple over-segmentations, resulting from a pool of methods with various parameters, are likely to agree on the correct segment boundaries, while spurious boundaries are method- or parameter-dependent. The challenge is to make an optimized decision on selecting the correct boundaries while discarding the spurious ones. The proposed unsupervised method achieves better performance than state of the art methods for cell segmentation from membrane images.

**Keywords:** Cell segmentation, Linear program, Joint segmentation.

## 1 Introduction

Embryonic morphogenesis involves the emergence of shape at the cell, tissue, organ and organismal levels. A quantitative, systems-level understanding of this process will require a set of robust methods for segmentation and cell specific measurements (volume, shape analysis, etc). Ascidians are invertebrate chordates with particularly small, simple embryos. The major tissues in the ascidian are illustrated in Fig. 1(a). The images used here are confocal microscopy volumes of *Ciona* embryos where the cell peripheries have been stained [10]. [1]

This work addresses the problem of cell segmentation, which is necessary to quantify biologically important parameters of the cell (size, shape, etc) [3]. This

---

[*] This work was supported by NIH HD059217 and NSF III-0808772.
[1] The *Ciona* embryos were fixed, stained with Bodipy-FL phallicidin to label the cortical actin cytoskeleton, cleared in Murray's Clear (BABB), and imaged on an Olympus FV1000 LSCM using a 40x 1.3NA oil immersion objective.

K. Mori et al. (Eds.): MICCAI 2013, Part I, LNCS 8149, pp. 444–451, 2013.
© Springer-Verlag Berlin Heidelberg 2013

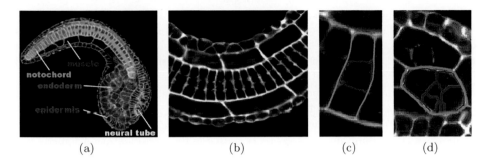

**Fig. 1.** Best viewed in color. (a) The major tissues of the ascidian tadpole. [9] (b) Detail of a confocal section. Notice the faint nuclei boundaries in the string of notochord cells. (c) Subjective surface [13] segmentation method attached to the faint nucleus boundary (red contour). (d) Watershed method [6] (red contour) initialized at local minima incorrectly fragments the cell. The correct segmentations are marked in green.

is a challenging dataset due to varying cortical intensity and faint staining of other organelles. As seen in Fig. 1(c) and 1(d), segmentation methods incorrectly attach to the faint nucleus boundaries captured by the staining. Furthermore, state of the art segmentation methods developed for confocal microscopy membrane volumes, such as [13], require the initialization with a seed point inside each cell of interest, as well as manually cropping the volume around each cell. For high-throughput analysis, it is preferable to have minimal or no human interaction.

Towards this, we tackle the task of 3-D segmentation of the *Ciona* volumes by simultaneously correcting multiple over-segmentations in a principled manner. We start out with the results of multiple segmentation methods resulting from a pool of methods, referred to as the *bag of methods*. The methods could differ in their segmentation scheme or in the choice of parameters for a single algorithm. We assume that all of these are tuned for over-segmentation, thus resulting in super-pixels, and containing more boundaries than necessary. Tuning a method for over-segmentation is a much easier task than searching for the narrow range of parameters which result in the desired boundaries. Furthermore, over-segmentations can be produced efficiently and in parallel, with a method such as [6], which is extremely suitable for edge data. The intuition is that the boundaries of interest are present in all the over-segmentations, along with many other spurious edges which are method- or parameter-dependent. We introduce a linear program framework for simultaneously correcting these over-segmented results in order to achieve consensus among the detected boundaries.

The problem of fusing multiple segmentations has caught interest in recent years in the computer vision community. Vitaladevuni et al., in [14], address the problem of jointly clustering two over-segmentations modelled as a quadratic semi-assignment program, which is relaxed to a linear program. Unlike this work, our method handles multiple over-segmentations and has fewer triangular inequalities. Warfield et. el [11] also combine a set near perfect segmentations from trained raters into one consensus segmentation. The method we propose solves a more challenging problem where the over-segmented inputs are far from correct. The authors of [8] propose a segmentation algorithm which learns a combination of weak segmenters and builds a strong one. The works of [12] and [7] propose label fusion methods where expert-segmented training images are registered to the target image. Unlike these methods, the proposed algorithm achieves a consensus in an unsupervised manner.

We propose a novel method which consists of a linear program optimization framework that simultaneously corrects multiple over-segmentations, such that the agreement between them is maximized. As a result of the convex formulation we can compute a globally optimal solution. The method is generalizable to two- or three-dimensional data. We present results on a 3-D confocal microscopy volume of the membrane stained ascidian *Ciona*. Our method achieves better performance than state of the art segmentation methods for this type of data.

## 2    Joint Correction of Multiple Over-Segmentations

We assume that $N$ over-segmentations of the image $\mathcal{I}$ are available. These over-segmentations, denoted as $S_1 - S_N$ can differ in their methodology or in the parameters of a single algorithm. Every label-map $S_p$ has a total of $N_p$ segments. We consider correcting these $N$ over-segmentations by merging segments with similar characteristics within each label map, while simultaneously obtaining the maximum agreement across the $N$ corrections (Fig. 2(f)). The dissimilarity between neighboring segments within each label-map is characterized by a cost of merging. The agreement between two overlapping segments across two label-maps is characterized by a reward for connecting segments across two consecutive over-segmentations. We formulate the problem as a binary integer program, which minimizes the total cost of merging segments within each label map, while maximizing the total reward for agreement across the segmentations. The binary integer program is further relaxed to a linear program.

The spatial relationship between the super-pixels in each segmentations is modelled as nodes in a graph. The initial over-segmentations are considered in arbitrary order, and every pair of consecutive over-segmentations are connected in the graph as shown in Fig. 2(f).

### 2.1    Binary Integer Program Formulation

We introduce the parameter $C^p$, an $N_p \times N_p$ dimensional matrix whose entries $C_{ij}^p$ represent the penalty (cost) for merging segments $i$ and $j$ within label-map $S_p$. The connectivity parameter $E^{p,p}$ is an $N_p \times N_p$ binary matrix whose entries $E_{ij}^{p,p}$ are 1 if segments $i$ and $j$ both from label-map $S_p$ are in contact by at least one pixel, and 0 otherwise.

We take the $N$ segmentations in arbitrary order and consider every two consecutive label-maps. The connectivity parameter across two consecutive label-maps $E^{p,p+1}$, is defined as $N_p \times N_{p+1}$ matrix, where $E_{ij}^{p,p+1}$ indicates if segment $i$

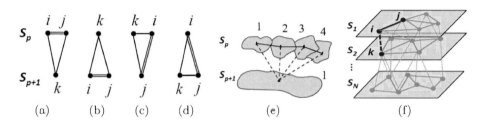

**Fig. 2.** (a)-(d) Given the black single line connections, the red double line connections result from transitivity constraints similar to Eq. (6). (e): Transitivity constraints are only active for neighboring segments, otherwise the LP is infeasible. This diagram shows an example where the transitivity and the connectivity constraints cannot both be satisfied. (f) Graph representation of the multiple over-segmentations. The solid dark line represents $m_{i,j}^{1,1}$, while the dotted dark line represents $m_{i,k}^{1,2}$.

from label-map $S_p$ and segment $j$ from label-map $S_{p+1}$ share at least one pixel. Consequently, the reward parameter, $R^{p,p+1}$, is represented by a $N_p \times N_{p+1}$ matrix, whose entries $R_{ij}^{p,p+1}$ quantify the agreement between segment $i \in S_p$ and $j \in S_{p+1}$.

Next, we introduce the decision variables. Variable $m^{p,p}$ is a $N_p \times N_p$ binary matrix whose entries $m_{ij}^{p,p}$ are non-zero if the two segments $i$ and $j$ from label-map $S_p$ should be merged. Furthermore, variable $m^{p,p+1}$ is a $N_p \times N_{p+1}$ binary matrix whose entries $m_{ij}^{p,p+1}$ indicate whether segment $i \in S_p$ and segment $j \in S_{p+1}$ are likely to be part of the same object from the original image.

Thus, for every pair of consecutive label maps, we can identify two objectives: minimizing the total cost of merging within each label-map $S_p$, and maximizing the total reward for agreement across label map $S_p$ and label map $S_{p+1}$. Fig. 2(f) illustrates this concept. Next, we discuss the objective function and the constraints associated with this program, which verify that the solutions for the three sub-problems are in agreement with each other.

The objective function of the proposed optimization program is represented by equation (1). The first summation indicates the total cost of merging within each label-map. The second summation represents the reward for agreement (merging/connecting) across two consecutive label-maps. Note that minimizing the negative total reward is equivalent to maximizing the positive total reward. The real valued parameter $\lambda$ is used to balance the total cost and total reward, and bias the final result towards more or less merging.

We now introduce the constraints needed to ensure the validity of the resulting segmentations. The range constraint (2) specifies that this is a binary program, for which the decision variables can only take 0, 1 values. The connectivity constraint (3) does not permit the merging of segments which are not neighbors, within each label-map $m^{p,p}$, or across the two consecutive label-maps $m^{p,p+1}$. Constraint (4) handles symmetry: if segment $i$ is merged with segment $j$, this implies that segment $j$ is merged with segment $i$ as well. Note that there is no such constraint for the $m^{p,p+1}$ variables, which are neither square, nor symmetric matrices. Next, equation (5) introduces the self-merger constraint, which implies that every segment is merged with itself. This forces the diagonals of the resulting matrices $m^{p,p}$ to be 1. Again, note that this constraint does not hold for the $m^{p,p+1}$ variables.

minimize:

$$f = \sum_{p=1}^{N} \sum_{i=1}^{N_p} \sum_{j=1}^{N_p} m_{ij}^{p,p} C_{ij}^{p} - \lambda \sum_{p=1}^{N-1} \sum_{i=1}^{N_p} \sum_{j=1}^{N_{p+1}} m_{ij}^{p,p+1} R_{ij}^{p,p+1} \qquad (1)$$

subject to:

- Range: $(\forall i, j, p)$   $\qquad m_{ij}^{p,p}, m_{ij}^{p,p+1} \in \{0, 1\}$   $\qquad\qquad (2)$
- Connectivity: $(\forall i, j, p)$   $\qquad m_{ij}^{p,p} \leq E_{ij}^{p,p} \quad m_{ij}^{p,p+1} \leq E_{ij}^{p,p+1}$   $\qquad (3)$
- Symmetry: $(\forall i, j, p)$   $\qquad\qquad m_{ij}^{p,p} = m_{ji}^{p,p}$   $\qquad\qquad (4)$
- Self-merge: $(\forall i, p)$   $\qquad\qquad\qquad m_{ii}^{p,p} = 1$   $\qquad\qquad\qquad (5)$
- Transitivity: $(\forall i, j, k, p)$   $\quad m_{ij}^{p,p} \geq m_{ik}^{p,p+1} m_{jk}^{p,p+1} E_{ij}^{p,p} E_{ik}^{p,p+1} E_{jk}^{p,p+1}$   $\qquad (6)$

The constraints thus far ensure the validity of the results. However the two sub-problems are still independent of each other: the minimization of the total cost within the label-maps $S_p$ is only affected by the cost parameters, and the maximization of the reward across two consecutive label-maps is only affected by the reward parameters. Thus, the optimization program, with the constraints thus far, will result in the trivial solution: merge nothing within each label-map $S_p$, merge everything across consecutive label-maps.

Therefore, we need to ensure that the two sub-problems match each other, meaning that the decision to merge segments in one label map will affect the result of the other label maps. We introduce the following transitivity constraints. As explained in Fig. 2(a), (6) implies that if segments $i$ and $j$ from label-map $S_p$ are both merged with segment $k$ from label-map $S_{p+1}$, then $i$ and $j$ must also be merged within $S_p$. This ensures that $m^p$ and $m^{p+1}$ are in agreement, through $m^{p,p+1}$. Note that we only enforce this constraint for neighboring segments: $E_{ij}^{p,p}$, $E_{ik}^{p,p+1}$, and $E_{jk}^{p,p+1}$ must be 1 for the constraint to be active. This is because, for situations like Fig. 2(e), the connectivity constraint from (3) will not permit the merging of two segments which do not share a pixel, leading to an infeasible program. Similarly, we consider the situations described in Fig. 2(b), 2(c), and 2(d). Note that transitivity constraints for three nodes pertaining to the same label-map, $i, j, k \in S_p$ are implicit.

The number of constraints is of order $O(n^3)$ in the total number of segments, due to the transitivity constraints. Since the transitivity constraints are only active for neighboring segments, the size of the problem can be bounded by $O(n^2)$ as in [14].

We have thus formulated a Binary Integer Program (BIP) which simultaneously corrects $N$ over-segmentations of an image, while maximizing the agreement between the resulting segmentations. However, this program is an NP-hard problem and cannot be solved in polynomial time. In the following sub-section we describe its relaxation to a Linear Program (LP).

## 2.2   Linear Relaxation

We note that the constraints of (3), (4) and (5) are linear. However the transitivity constraints (6) (and symmetric equivalents) are not linear, and the range constraint of (2) does not form a convex set.

We linearize the transitivity constraints as in (7). The first step results from De Morgan's law, and the second step results from negating and reordering the variables. The remaining three transitivity constraints are linearized similarly.

$$m_{ij}^{p,p} \geq m_{ik}^{p,p+1} m_{jk}^{p,p+1} \cdot E_{ij}^{p,p} E_{ik}^{p,p+1} E_{jk}^{p,p+1}$$
$$= \left(1 - \left(\overline{m_{ik}^{p,p+1}} + \overline{m_{jk}^{p,p+1}}\right)\right) \cdot E_{ij}^{p,p} E_{ik}^{p,p+1} E_{jk}^{p,p+1} \tag{7}$$
$$= \left(m_{ik}^{p,p+1} + m_{jk}^{p,p+1} - 1\right) \cdot E_{ij}^{p,p} E_{ik}^{p,p+1} E_{jk}^{p,p+1}$$

Further, we relax the values of the variables $m^{p,p}$, and $m^{p,p+1}$, defined in the range constraint of (2), from $\{0,1\}$ to $[0,1]$. Occasionally $m^{p,p}$, and $m^{p,p+1}$ may result in fractional values, for which we consider the values above a threshold (0.5). This converts the feasibility set into a convex set, relaxing the BIP to an LP, whose global solution is an approximation of the original BIP.

## 3   Experimental Results

We evaluate the performance of our method on a 3-D confocal volume, as well as analyze its stability using a 2-D example. The comparison metric is the $F$-measure, which is a volume based error metric and is defined as: $F = \frac{2\mathcal{P}\mathcal{R}}{\mathcal{P}+\mathcal{R}}$, where $\mathcal{P}$ and $\mathcal{R}$ are the precision and the recall for a given ground truth volume.

**Performance Evaluation:** Numerical results are reported on the forty cylindrical cells of the notochord tissue in a 3-D dataset for which manually traced ground truth is available. Two over-segmentations are used for this experiment: (1) the Watershed method [6] applied to the image data, and (2) Watershed applied to the filtered image (3-D mean-filter). To solve the optimization program we used CVX, a package for specifying and solving convex programs [5,4].

We construct a cost function which compares the intensity histograms on the border of two neighboring segments, to that of the interior of the segments. This is given by $C_{ij}^p = \max(0, \bar{\mathcal{B}}_{ij}^p - \bar{\mathcal{S}}_{ij}^p)$, where $\bar{\mathcal{B}}_{ij}^p$ and $\bar{\mathcal{S}}_{ij}^p$ represent the mean intensity on the border and the interior, respectively, of two neighboring segments $i, j \in S_p$. A large positive value indicates the presence of a membrane, while a low value suggests a spurious boundary. The reward function for two segments $i \in S_p$ and $j \in S_{p+1}$ is the percentage area of overlap, expressed as $\max(\frac{\mathcal{A}_{ij}^{p,p+1}}{\mathcal{A}_i^p}, \frac{\mathcal{A}_{ij}^{p,p+1}}{\mathcal{A}_j^{p+1}})$.

We compare our work to the following methods relevant to confocal membrane image segmentation. The Subjective Surface variant in [13] is a level-set method specifically designed for membrane image segmentation. It requires initialization with a seed point in every cell. The method in [2] also corrects an over-segmentation by merging segments, however this method requires training

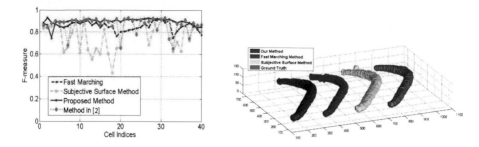

**Fig. 3.** Left: $F$-measure per notochord cell. Right: 3-D rendering of the segmented cells

**Table 1.** $F$-measure statistics on forty notochord cells in 3-D

| Method | Avgerage | Median | Standard Dev. |
|---|---|---|---|
| *Proposed* | *89.36%* | *90.13%* | *3.19%* |
| Method in [2] | 86.25% | 88.91% | 7.30% |
| Fast Marching [1] | 85.58% | 85.95% | 4.18% |
| Subj. Surf. [13] | 77.87% | 82.78% | 13.63% |
| Over-Segmentation #1 | 80.01% | 81.02% | 6.37% |
| Over-Segmentation #2 | 61.62% | 64.18 % | 8.73% |

data. Lastly, the Fast Marching Method [1] computes geodesic distances in the discrete image domain from a seed-point in every cell.

As seen in Fig. 3 and Table 1, the proposed algorithm started out with two over-segmentations with $F$-scores of 80.01% and 61.62%. By combining them, it achieves a score of 89.36% and outperforms the manually initialized methods in [1] and [13], and the trained method in [2], which often leak through broken boundaries and get attached to spurious edges. The lack of manual interaction is essential when handling 3-D data with a very large number of cells. The 3-D rendering of the segmented notochord tissue is presented in Fig. 3.

**Stability Analysis:** Here we investigate the impact of the input segmentations on the performance of the method. In order to evaluate this, three over-segmentations of the confocal section in Fig. 1(b) are obtained using randomly

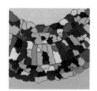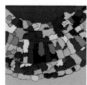

**Fig. 4.** Segmentation of the confocal section in Fig. 1(b). From left to right: Three randomly initialized watershed over-segmentations. Joint correction using proposed method. Ground truth segmentation.

seeded Watershed. The proposed method is used to simultaneously correct these three over-segmentations, as shown in Fig. 4. In an unsupervised manner, the optimization framework correctly segments out the cells from the notochord and muscle tissues, which are relevant in the study of morphogenesis. The $F$-measure is computed and this process is repeated twenty times. The observed scores average to 80.32% and the standard deviation is 3.12%. This indicates that the method is robust to randomized input segmentations. Furthermore, the final values of the approximately 100,000 decision variables involved in this experiment are all binary. This indicates that the LP relaxation is tight and the global solution is in fact the solution to the original BIP from section 2.1. The solver took 4s on a graph of approx. 700 nodes / 7000 edges on a single core i5 at 2.5GHz.

**Conclusion:** We addressed the problem of cell segmentation for 3-D confocal microscopy volumes of the *Ciona*. We introduced an unsupervised method that combines two or more over-segmentations in a linear optimization framework.

# References

1. Cohen, L., et al.: Fast marching the global min. of active contours. In: ICIP 1996 (1996)
2. Delibaltov, D., et al.: An automatic feature based model for cell segmentation from confocal microscopy volumes. In: IEEE ISBI (2011)
3. Delibaltov, D., et al.: Robust biological image sequence analysis using graph based approaches. In: Asilomar Conference on Signals, Systems and Computers (2012)
4. Grant, C.M., Boyd, S.P.: Graph implementations for nonsmooth convex programs. In: Recent Advances in Learning and Control. LNCIS, vol. 371, pp. 95–110. Springer, Heidelberg (2008)
5. Grant, M., et al.: CVX: Matlab software for disciplined convex (2011), http://cvxr.com/cvx
6. Meyer, F., et al.: Morphological segmentation. Journal of Visual Communication and Image Representation (1990)
7. Sabuncu, M.R., et al.: A generative model for image segmentation based on label fusion. IEEE Trans. on Medical Imaging (2010)
8. Chen, T., Vemuri, B.C., Rangarajan, A., Eisenschenk, S.J.: Mixture of segmenters with discriminative spatial regularization and sparse weight selection. In: Fichtinger, G., Martel, A., Peters, T. (eds.) MICCAI 2011, Part III. LNCS, vol. 6893, pp. 595–602. Springer, Heidelberg (2011)
9. Veeman, M., et al.: Chongmague reveals an essential role for laminin-mediated boundary formation in chordate convergence and extension movements. Development Genes and Evolution (2008)
10. Veeman, M.T., et al.: Whole-organ cell shape analysis reveals the developmental basis of ascidian notochord taper. Developmental Biology (2013)
11. Warfield, et al.: Simultaneous truth and performance level estimation (STAPLE): an algorithm for the validation of image segmentation. IEEE TMI (2004)
12. Artaechevarria, X., et al.: Combination strategies in multi-atlas image segmentation: Application to brain MR data. IEEE Trans. on Med. Img. (2009)
13. Zanella, C., et al.: Cells segmentation from 3-D confocal images Of early zebrafish embryogenesis. In: IEEE TIP 2010 (2010)
14. Vitaladevuni, S.N., Basri, R.: Co-clustering of image segments using convex optimization applied to EM neuronal reconstruction. In: CVPR 2010 (2010)

# Automated Nucleus and Cytoplasm Segmentation of Overlapping Cervical Cells

Zhi Lu[1,*], Gustavo Carneiro[2], and Andrew P. Bradley[3,**]

[1] Department of Computer Science, City University of Hong Kong, China
[2] ACVT, The University of Adelaide, Australia
[3] School of Information Technology & Electrical Engineering,
The University of Queensland, Australia

**Abstract.** In this paper we describe an algorithm for accurately segmenting the individual cytoplasm and nuclei from a clump of overlapping cervical cells. Current methods cannot undertake such a complete segmentation due to the challenges involved in delineating cells with severe overlap and poor contrast. Our approach initially performs a scene segmentation to highlight both free-lying cells, cell clumps and their nuclei. Then cell segmentation is performed using a joint level set optimization on all detected nuclei and cytoplasm pairs. This optimisation is constrained by the length and area of each cell, a prior on cell shape, the amount of cell overlap and the expected gray values within the overlapping regions. We present quantitative nuclei detection and cell segmentation results on a database of synthetically overlapped cell images constructed from real images of free-lying cervical cells. We also perform a qualitative assessment of complete fields of view containing multiple cells and cell clumps.

**Keywords:** Overlapping cell segmentation, Pap smear image analysis.

## 1 Introduction

The Pap smear is a screening test used to detect pre-cancerous changes in a sample of cells from the uterine cervix and deposited onto a microscope slide for visual examination. The automated segmentation of overlapping cells in Pap smears remains one of the most challenging problems in image analysis. The main factors affecting the sensitivity of the Pap smear test are the number and type of cells sampled and the presence of mucus, blood and inflammatory cells [2], which affects both the intra- and inter-observer variability and leads to a large variation in false negative rates. [8]. These issues have motivated the development of both automated cell deposition and slide analysis techniques. The advantages of automated cell deposition techniques, such as mono-layer preparations, are that they remove a large portion of blood, mucus, and other

---

* Zhi Lu contributed to this work when he was a visiting student at the University of Adelaide.
** Andrew P. Bradley is the recipient of an Australian Research Council Future Fellowship (FT110100623).

K. Mori et al. (Eds.): MICCAI 2013, Part I, LNCS 8149, pp. 452–460, 2013.

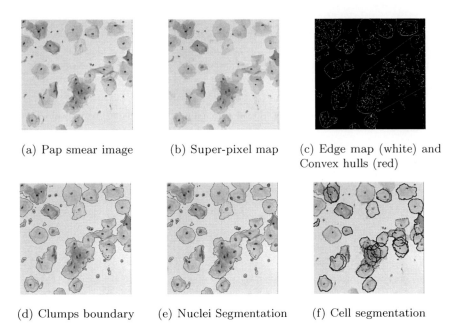

(a) Pap smear image     (b) Super-pixel map     (c) Edge map (white) and
                                                Convex hulls (red)

(d) Clumps boundary     (e) Nuclei Segmentation     (f) Cell segmentation

**Fig. 1.** (a) Typical Pap smear image; (b) Over-segmented super-pixel map is generated by Quick Shift; (c) super-pixel edge map and the convex hull of each clump; (d) Accurate clump boundary; (e) Nuclei detection and segmentation;(f) Overlapping cell segmentation

debris, reduce cell overlap and produce a mono-layer of easily focused cells. Automated slide analysis techniques attempt to improve both sensitivity and specificity by detecting, segmenting and then classifying all of the cells present on a slide [9,17,5,4,3].

The classification of cervical cells is typically based on features, such as shape and area, extracted from the cytoplasm and nucleus of individual cells. This means that an accurate segmentation is critical to automated screening methods. Nevertheless, segmentation is complicated by the fact that they often form overlapping clumps on the glass slide, which means that cells in an upper layer can partially obscure cells lying underneath [10]. Current systems can segment the nucleus and cytoplasm of isolated cervical cells [5] (i.e., free-lying cells without any overlap with other cells); segment overlapping nuclei [3,10]; and segment nuclei and the whole region representing overlapping cytoplasm [4,2]. However, currently segmenting both the individual cytoplasm and nuclei from overlapping cells in Pap smear images is still a challenging problem due to the presence of overlapping cells and the poor contrast of cytoplasm [2] (see Fig. 1(a)).

In this paper, we propose a novel algorithm to segment both the cytoplasm and nucleus of each overlapping cell. The proposed methodology can be divided into two steps. First *scene segmentation*, comprising two sub-stages: 1) cell clump detection using unsupervised classification [14] and 2) nuclei detection using the maximally stable extremal regions (MSER) algorithm [7]. Second, *cell segmentation*, which is the main contribution of this paper, assumes that each nucleus detected in step 1 represents an individual cell that forms a separate level set function. The optimization that generates the final overlapping cell segmentation minimizes an energy function that is constrained by the individual contour area and length [6], an ellipsoidal shape prior [13], and finally the area [18] and gray values within the overlapping regions. We quantitatively evaluate our methodology using a database of 18 synthetically constructed images consisting 60 real free-lying cell images. The results on this dataset show that we obtain a Jaccard index > 0.8 with a near zero false negative rate. We also show encouraging qualitative results using a small set of real Pap smear images. Furthermore, we demonstrate that the performance of our nuclei detection produces state of the art results [2].[1]

## 2    Literature Review

There are three primary approaches to cervical cell segmentation. Traditional methods segment nuclei from single or overlapping cells. For instance, Wu et al. [16] detect the boundary of nuclei by solving an optimal thresholding problem. Morphological analysis is also used to detect overlapping nuclei from cervical cell images [9]. Other approaches segment the nucleus and cytoplasm of single isolated cervical cells. Yang-Mao et al. [17] adapt the gradient vector flow (GVF) to cervical cell segmentation by estimating the orientation of the GVFs in the pixels near an edge. The GVF is also explored in the detection of nucleus and cytoplasm boundaries in a radiating field [5]. This approach produces competitive results, but can analyse only free-lying cells (and thus, a fraction of the cells present on a specimen). Finally, the segmentation of overlapping nuclei can be performed by identifying the nucleus and cytoplasm from candidate regions via a classification algorithm [4,2]. However, instead of accurate boundaries for each overlapping cell, these methods generate a contour of the whole cell clump, which reduces the number of features available for subsequent cellular analysis, i.e., each cell has its own nucleus, but not its own cytoplasm. In the above, the detection of overlapping nuclei is facilitated by their homogeneous texture, ellipsoidal shape and high-gradient boundaries. Unfortunately, none of these characteristics can be associated with the segmentation of overlapping cytoplasm. Furthermore, some of the important features extracted from nuclei are based on optical density and texture, which may be contaminated when nuclei overlap.

The segmentation of overlapping cells has been explored in other types of microscope images. For instance, Wahlby et al. [15] use a watershed segmentation algorithm and a statistical analysis to segment multiple CHO-cells stained with calcein. Furthermore, Quelhas et al. [11] explores a sliding band filter to segment nuclei and cytoplasm of overlapping cells using the Drosophila melanogaster Kc167 dataset. Although relevant to our paper, these works are applied to images

---

[1] Our code & data set are available at GitHub: `github.com/luzhi/miccai2013.git`

where the cells present smaller overlapping areas, when compared to the case of Pap smear images. Therefore, we believe that these approaches would need significant adaptation in order to segment cervical cell images.

# 3   Methods

## 3.1   Extended Depth of Field

A one-pass extended depth of field (EDF) algorithm [1], based on an over-complete discrete wavelet transform, was applied to a "stack" of focal plane images to produce a single EDF image where all cellular objects are in focus. The advantage of this approach is that the scene segmentation, described below, need only be applied to a single (EDF) image rather than a set of images from different focal planes.

## 3.2   Scene Segmentation

Scene segmentation consists of two stages: 1) the segmentation of cell clumps, which facilitates 2) the detection and segmentation of nuclei.

**Segmentation of Cell Clumps.** The segmentation of cell clumps facilitates the detection of nuclei by constraining the search space to clumps only. For instance, in the image of Fig. 1(a), the goal is to segment the six free-lying cells and the set of overlapping cells in different clumps. This segmentation process involves three stages. First, we run the quick shift algorithm [14] in order to find local maxima of a density function that takes into account gray value similarities and spatial proximity. The outcome of this step is a map of super-pixels (Fig. 1(b)), which are labeled with gray values in the range $[0, 1]$, representing the mode of the respective super-pixel. The second stage consists of running an edge detector on this super-pixel map, resulting in a clean edge map that detects the most prominent super-pixel edges and removes most of the background information (Fig. 1(c)). In order to find candidate cell clumps, the third stage utilises an unsupervised binary classifier, where the classes are "background" and "cell clump". The initial assignment is provided by building a convex hull around the connected components of the edge map computed in stage 2 (Fig. 1(c)). Hence, pixels inside the convex hull initially belong to the cell clump class and pixels outside belong to the background. Using maximum likelihood estimation, we learn a Gaussian mixture model (GMM) for each class, based on the gray value of each pixel (Fig. 1(d)).

**Detection and Segmentation of Nuclei.** This is a critical step of our algorithm because each nucleus represents one cell. Nuclei can be characterized by relatively low gray values, homogeneous texture, and well defined, almost circular borders. If we assume that the nuclei do not overlap, then we can use the Maximally Stable Extremal Regions (MSER) algorithm [7] using the cell clumps as the input. The MSER algorithm uses pixel gray value and proximity to detect stable connected components, which are characterized by blobs that represent the candidate nuclei. We filter out some of these candidates if the eccentricity of the blob detected is larger than a threshold (i.e., keeping only the most circular blobs).

## 3.3    Joint Level Set Segmentation of Overlapping Cells

The joint level set optimisation presented in this section is the main contribution of this paper. The segmentation of overlapping cells uses the set of nuclei described in Sec. 3.2 as the initial guess for each level set function. Consider that $\phi : \Omega \to \mathbb{R}$ denotes a level set function (LSF) ($\Omega$ represents the image domain), and that $N$ nuclei have been detected, then the set of LSF's are available is denoted by $\{\phi_i\}_{i=1}^{N}$. The energy functional to be minimized is defined as:

$$\mathcal{E}(\{\phi_i\}_{i=1}^{N}) = \sum_{i=1}^{N} \mathcal{E}_u(\phi_i) + \sum_{i=1}^{N} \sum_{j \in \mathcal{N}(i)} \mathcal{E}_b(\phi_i, \phi_j), \tag{1}$$

where $\mathcal{E}_u(.)$ denotes the unary energy functional defined for each LSF independently, $\mathcal{E}_b(.,.)$ represents the binary function defined over pairs of LSF's, and $\mathcal{N}(i)$ represents the level set functions $\phi_j$ such that their zero level set intersects the zero level set of $\phi_i$. The unary functional is defined by:

$$\mathcal{E}_u(\phi_i) = \mu \mathcal{R}(\phi_i) + \lambda \mathcal{L}(\phi_i) + \alpha \mathcal{A}(\phi_i) + \rho \mathcal{P}_p(\phi_i), \tag{2}$$

where $\mu, \lambda > 0$, $\alpha, \rho \in \mathbb{R}$, $\mathcal{R}(\phi)$ is a regularization term [6] that maintains the signed distance property $| \bigtriangledown \phi_i| = 1$ (guaranteeing that the LSF is smooth), $\mathcal{L}(\phi_i) = \int_{\Omega} g\delta(\phi_i)| \bigtriangledown \phi_i| d\mathbf{x}$ measures the length of the zero level set (with $\delta(.)$ denoting the Dirac delta function, $g = \frac{1}{1+|\nabla G_\sigma * I|}$, and $G_\sigma$ the Gaussian kernel with standard deviation $\sigma$), $\mathcal{A}(\phi_i) = \int_{\Omega} gH(-\phi_i)d\mathbf{x}$ measures the area of $\phi_i < 0$ (H(.) is the Heaviside function), and the shape prior term is defined by [13]:

$$\mathcal{P}_p(\phi_i) = \int_{\Omega} gH(-p(\phi_i))d\mathbf{x}, \tag{3}$$

where $p(\phi_i)$ returns an ellipsoidal shaped LSF estimated from the covariance matrix of the coordinates $\mathbf{x}$ for which $\phi_i(\mathbf{x}) < 0$. The binary functional in (1) is defined as:

$$\mathcal{E}_b(\phi_i, \phi_j) = \zeta f_a \left( \frac{\int_{\Omega} gH(-\phi_i)H(-\phi_j)d\mathbf{x}}{\int_{\Omega} gH(-\phi_i)d\mathbf{x}} \right) + \\ \omega f_g \left( \frac{\int_{\Omega} vH(-\phi_i)d\mathbf{x}}{\int_{\Omega} gH(-\phi_i)d\mathbf{x}} - \frac{\int_{\Omega} vH(-\phi_i)H(-\phi_j)d\mathbf{x}}{\int_{\Omega} gH(-\phi_i)H(-\phi_j)d\mathbf{x}} \right), \tag{4}$$

where the first term in (4) denotes the ratio between the areas of $(\phi_i < 0) \bigcap (\phi_j < 0)$ and $\phi_i < 0$ (with $f_a(y)$ defined as $y$ for $y > \tau_a$ and 0 otherwise, where $\tau_a$ is the maximum overlapping area accepted by the optimisation) [18], and the second term represents the difference between the average gray value in $\phi_i < 0$ subtracted by the average gray value in the intersection $(\phi_i < 0) \bigcap (\phi_j < 0)$ (with $f_g(y)$ defined as $y$ for $y < 0$ and 0 otherwise, and $v$ returns the gray value of position $\mathbf{x}$). The minimization of the energy functional in (1) follows that defined by $\frac{\partial \phi}{\partial t} = -\frac{\partial \mathcal{E}(\{\phi_i\}_{i=1}^N)}{\partial \phi}$. The derivation of these functions is presented in the supplemental material.[2]

# 4   Material and Experimental Setting

Our dataset consists of four Pap smear images with extended depth of field (EDF) [1]. Four non-overlapping fields of view (FOVs) were captured from a single specimen consisting of Papanicolaou-stained cervical cells, prepared using the AutoCyte PREP technology. The specimen was approximately $20\mu m$ "thick" in the focal-dimension. The numerical aperture of the microscope's $\times 40$ objective was 0.75, which gives a depth of field of approximately $1\mu m$. Therefore, for each FOV, a stack of twenty focal plane images were acquired with a separation of $1\mu m$. In these images, all 135 nuclei were manually annotated, with the 13 free-lying cells being fully annotated with nucleus and cytoplasm delineations.

We assess our methodology both qualitatively and quantitatively. The qualitative experiment consists of a visual inspection of the result of our algorithm using the four EDF images. For the quantitative assessment, we generated 18 synthetic Pap smear images (of size $512 \times 512$) containing 2 to 5 cells with different degrees of overlap. In order to generate these synthetic images, we divide the aforementioned set of 13 manually annotated cells, into: 1) a training set of 5 cells that is used to build 3 synthetic training images, and 2) a test set of 8 cells to form 15 test images[3]. In order to build these synthetic images, we take samples from the background of the original EDF images, and place them in the $512 \times 512$ image, using mirror transformation to smooth the transitions between the background patch borders. Then, we pick one of the cells from the training/test set, apply a random rigid transform and random linear brightness transform, and place them on the synthetic image, using a random value (from 0 to 1) for the alpha channel to simulate the partial transparency effect observed in real Pap smear images. Note that the training images are used to assess the best combination of the level set parameters in (1), while the testing images are used to verify the generalization ability of the method with respect to the level set parameters found on the training images. Finally, this quantitative performance is assessed with the average Jaccard index (JI) computed over the "good" cell segmentations [12], where the cell segmentation has a JI above a threshold of $\{0.5, 0.6, 0.7, 0.8\}$. We also report the object based false negative rate (FNR) obtained as the proportion of cells having a JI below this threshold. In addition, pixel based evaluation through true positive rate (TPR) and false positive rate (FPR) for both training and test set are also shown.

---

[2] Appendix at www.cs.cityu.edu.hk/~luzhi/publications/app_MICCAI13.pdf
[3] Early experiments showed results stabilise when at least 13 test images are used.

We also compare our nuclei detection methodology from Pap smear images with that in [2] using the following measurements. First, we compute the precision and recall of nuclei detection by considering the detection region A and annotation B, and noting that a correct detection is defined by $(A \bigcap B)/A > 0.6$ and $(A \bigcap B)/B > 0.6$. Second, we compute the pixel-based precision and recall values of the correct detections above, in addition to the Dice coefficient.

## 5    Experimental Results

We first show the influence of the parameters $\lambda$, $\alpha$, $\rho$ in the unary functional (2), and $\zeta$ and $\omega$ in the binary functional (4). The parameter $\mu$ is fixed at 0.2 per time step [6], where time step is 5. The JI and corresponding FNR for each parameter combination and the best parameters combination for training are shown in Table 1. This table shows the results on the test set using the best parameter combination obtained on the training set. Moreover, in Table 2 we show the pixel-based TPR and FPR on the training and test sets for the "good" segmentations. In Fig. 2, we show examples of the synthetic and real Pap smear image segmentations.

**Table 1.** Qualitative evaluation to show training process and test results in terms of the JI for "good" segmentations

| | | | | | Training set | | | |
|---|---|---|---|---|---|---|---|---|
| $\alpha$ | $\lambda$ | $\rho$ | $\zeta$ | $\omega$ | JI> 0.5 | JI> 0.6 | JI> 0.7 | JI> 0.8 |
| -5 | 4 | 0.15 | 3 | 4.1 | 0.91 (FNR=0) | 0.91 (FNR=0) | 0.91 (FNR=0) | 0.93 (FNR=0.08) |
| -5 | 0 | 0 | 0 | 0 | 0.87 (FNR=0) | 0.87 (FNR=0) | 0.87 (FNR=0) | 0.92 (FNR=0.3) |
| 0 | 4 | 0 | 0 | 0 | 0.93 (FNR=0.67) | 0.93 (FNR=0.67) | 0.93 (FNR=0.67) | 0.93 (FNR=0.67) |
| 0 | 0 | 0.15 | 0 | 0 | 0.77 (FNR=0.25) | 0.83 (FNR=0.42) | 0.86 (FNR=0.5) | 0.93 (FNR=0.67) |
| 0 | 0 | 0 | 3 | 0 | 0.91 (FNR=0) | 0.91 (FNR=0) | 0.91 (FNR=0) | 0.92 (FNR=0.08) |
| 0 | 0 | 0 | 0 | 4.1 | 0.91 (FNR=0) | 0.91 (FNR=0) | 0.91 (FNR=0) | 0.92 (FNR=0.08) |
| | | | | | Test set | | | |
| -5 | 4 | 0.15 | 3 | 4.1 | 0.83 (FNR=0.02) | 0.85(FNR=0.09) | 0.88(FNR=0.21) | 0.91(FNR=0.34) |

We compare our nuclei detection with the approach by Aksoy et al. [2], but this comparison is not ideal as they are run on different data sets[4]. Specifically, Aksoy et al.'s approach is tested on Hacettepe data set (which has 139 nuclei), while ours are the Pap smear images described above (with 135 nuclei). In terms of object-based nuclei detection, we achieve a precision of .69 and recall .90, while [2] has precision of .74 and recall .93. Furthermore, the pixel-based result for our method consists of a precision of .97($\pm$.04), recall .88($\pm$.08) and Dice .92 ($\pm$.04); while [2] has precision of .91($\pm$.08), recall .88($\pm$.07) and Dice .89 ($\pm$.04).

Finally, our algorithm shows an average running time of 56 seconds per cell through the test set using an unoptimized Matlab code on a PC with 2.7GHz Intel Xeon processor and 128 GB RAM.

---

[4] As the database in [2] is not publicly available.

**Table 2.** Pixel-based TPR/FPR on training & test sets for "good" segmentations

| α λ ρ ζ ω | JI> 0.5 | JI> 0.6 | JI> 0.7 | JI> 0.8 |
|---|---|---|---|---|
| Training set (TPR/FPR) | | | | |
| -5 4 0.15 3 4.1 | 0.92/0.0005 | 0.92/0.0005 | 0.92/0.0005 | 0.94/0.0005 |
| -5 0   0   0   0 | 0.94/0.0038 | 0.94/0.0038 | 0.94/0.0038 | 0.94/0.0013 |
|  0 4   0   0   0 | 0.93/0.0001 | 0.93/0.0001 | 0.93/0.0001 | 0.93/0.0001 |
|  0 0 0.15 0   0 | 0.77/0.0001 | 0.84/0.0001 | 0.87/0.0001 | 0.93/0.0001 |
|  0 0   0   3   0 | 0.93/0.0011 | 0.93/0.0011 | 0.93/0.0011 | 0.94/0.0011 |
|  0 0   0   0 4.1 | 0.93/0.0010 | 0.93/0.0010 | 0.93/0.0010 | 0.94/0.0009 |
| Test set (TPR/FPR) | | | | |
| -5 4 0.15 3 4.1 | 0.88/0.0032 | 0.89/0.0025 | 0.92/0.0023 | 0.93/0.0017 |

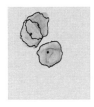 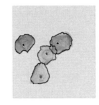 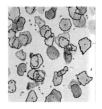 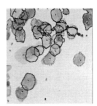

(a) Synthetic images                (b) Real Pap smear images

**Fig. 2.** Qualitative assessment of results

# 6    Discussion and Conclusion

In the results, we can see that on the test set our methodology produces a JI = 0.83 with a nearly zero FNR, which in general can be considered to be an acceptable result, if the "good" cell segmentations has the minimal JI > 0.5. Indeed, the qualitative results in Fig. 2 demonstrate that for all the isolated cells and most of the overlapping cells, our approach successfully segments the individual cytoplasm and nuclei. According to the results in Table 1, it is possible to conclude that both binary terms have a strong positive influence on the results. The main failures observed are caused by the weak transitions between the cytoplasm and background that make the segmentation border move either outside or inside the cytoplasm. Moreover, our nuclei detection produces quantitative results on par with the state of the art [2].

The methodology proposed in this paper provides reasonably accurate results on the challenging problem of segmenting both nuclei and cytoplasm from overlapping cervical cells. Nevertheless, there are a few points that need to be addressed to improve the effectiveness of our approach. The most important issue is that the system still misses the boundary of the cytoplasm on some overlapping cells in regions of poor contrast. Also, to obtain more robust results the system should be extended to process the original stack of multi-focal plane images (see Sec. 4) as per manual analysis.

# References

1. Bradley, A., Bamford, P.: A one-pass extended depth of field algorithm based on the over-complete discrete wavelet transform. In: IVCNZ 2004, pp. 279–284 (2004)
2. Gençtav, A., Aksoy, S., Önde, S.: Unsupervised segmentation and classification of cervical cell images. Pat. Recognition 45, 4151–4168 (2012)
3. Jung, C., Kim, C., Chae, S., Oh, S.: Unsupervised segmentation of overlapped nuclei using bayesian classification. IEEE TBE 57(12), 2825–2832 (2010)
4. Kale, A., Aksoy, S.: Segmentation of cervical cell images. In: ICPR (2010)
5. Li, K., Lu, Z., Liu, W., Yin, J.: Cytoplasm and nucleus segmentation in cervical smear images using Radiating GVF Snake. Pat. Recognition 45, 1255–1264 (2012)
6. Li, C., Xu, C., Gui, C., Fox, M.: Distance regularized level set evolution and its application to image segmentation. IEEE TIP 19(12), 3243–3254 (2010)
7. Matas, J., et al.: Robust wide baseline stereo from maximally stable extremal regions. In: Proc. BMVC, pp. 384–396 (2002)
8. Noorani, H.: Assessment of techniques for cervical cancer screening. CCOHTA 1997: 2E, Canadian Coordinating Office for Health Technology Assessment (1997)
9. Plissiti, M., et al.: Automated detection of cell nuclei in pap smear images using morphological reconstruction and clustering. IEEE TITB 15, 233–241 (2011)
10. Plissiti, M., Nikou, C.: Overlapping cell nuclei segmentation using a spatially adaptive active physical model. IEEE TIP 21(11), 4568–4580 (2012)
11. Quelhas, P., et al.: Cell nuclei and cytoplasm joint segmentation using the sliding band filter. IEEE TMI 29(8), 1463–1473 (2010)
12. Radau, P.: Evaluation framework for algorithms segmenting short axis cardiac MRI. The MIDAS J. - Cardiac MR Left Ventricle Segmentation Challenge (2009)
13. Rousson, M., Paragios, N.: Shape priors for level set representations. In: Heyden, A., Sparr, G., Nielsen, M., Johansen, P. (eds.) ECCV 2002, Part II. LNCS, vol. 2351, pp. 78–92. Springer, Heidelberg (2002)
14. Vedaldi, A., Soatto, S.: Quick Shift and Kernel Methods for Mode Seeking. In: Forsyth, D., Torr, P., Zisserman, A. (eds.) ECCV 2008, Part IV. LNCS, vol. 5305, pp. 705–718. Springer, Heidelberg (2008)
15. Wahlby, C., et al.: Algorithms for cytoplasm segmentation of fluorescence labelled cells. Analytical Cellular Pathology 24(3), 101–111 (2002)
16. Wu, H.-S., Gil, J., Barba, J.: Optimal segmentation of cell images. IEE Proc. on Vision, Image and Signal Processing. 145, 50–56 (1998)
17. Yang-Mao, S.-F., et al.: Edge enhancement nucleus and cytoplast contour detector of cervical smear images. IEEE TSMC, Part B: Cybernetics 38, 353–366 (2008)
18. Zimmer, C., Olivo-Marin, J.-C.: Coupled parametric active contours. IEEE TPAMI 27(1), 1838–1842 (2005)

# Segmentation of Cells with Partial Occlusion and Part Configuration Constraint Using Evolutionary Computation

Masoud S. Nosrati and Ghassan Hamarneh

Medical Image Analysis Lab., Simon Fraser University, BC, Canada
{smn6,hamarneh}@sfu.ca

**Abstract.** We propose a method for targeted segmentation that identifies and delineates only those spatially-recurring objects that conform to specific geometrical, topological and appearance priors. By adopting a "tribes"-based, global genetic algorithm, we show how we incorporate such priors into a faithful objective function unconcerned about its convexity. We evaluated our framework on a variety of histology and microscopy images to segment potentially overlapping cells with complex topology. Our experiments confirmed the generality, reproducibility and improved accuracy of our approach compared to competing methods.

## 1 Introduction

Histology and microscopy image analysis plays a crucial role in studying diseases such as cancer and in obtaining reference diagnosis (e.g. biopsy histopathology). Automatically segmenting cells in such images is one of the preliminary steps toward automatic image analysis and computer-aided diagnosis. In spite of recent advances in segmenting cells based on some homogeneity and smoothness characteristics, segmenting complex cells with a non-homogeneous appearance (with multiple internal regions) remains challenging. This problem becomes even more challenging when these complex cells overlap. Previous works addressed cell overlapping, for single-region cells, using post-processing [14,15,11] (e.g. finding connected components and using parameter sensitive morphological operations [11]). However, cells in histology and microscopy images typically consist of multiple regions (e.g. membrane, nucleus, nucleolus), each with a unique appearance model (intensity, color or texture) and unique geometric characteristics (e.g. cell size and shape prior). Furthermore, well defined spatial interactions usually exist between different regions of a cell (e.g. membrane contains nucleus, and nucleus contains nucleolus). Most existing methods have only considered simple structured cells and ignored their complex composition [1,3,2].

There are many types of priors that benefit the segmentation of spatially-recurring cells with appearance inhomogeneity along with cell-overlapping. Many state-of-the-art image segmentation methods are formulated as optimization problems, which are capable of incorporating multiple criteria (or priors) as energy terms in the objective function and examining the relative performance of different solutions. Incorporating several energy terms enables us to describe

K. Mori et al. (Eds.): MICCAI 2013, Part I, LNCS 8149, pp. 461–468, 2013.

the problem in more detail and thus obtain a more accurate formulation. On the other hand, adding more terms to the objective function generally makes it more complicated and harder to optimize.

In this work, we opt for ensuring the objective function is flexible enough (even if it is nonconvex) to accurately capture the intricacies of the cell segmentation problem. To optimize such objective function and to deal with imminent problems like initialization and local optima, we adopt a global optimization evolutionary computation method, genetic algorithm (GA), which can attain solutions close to the global optimum, does not require Euler Lagrangian or energy gradient calculations, is generally parallelizable, and allows for arbitrarily complex objective functions. Our framework allows us to leverage a variety of expert knowledge or priors by adding them as additional terms in the objective function without being overly concerned about convexification. Finally, to deal with the spatially recurring aspect in cell segmentation, we use genetic algorithms with *tribes* [13] to obtain multiple distinct solutions for our framework.

## 2    Problem Formulation

Given an $n$-channel 2D image $I : \Omega \subset \mathbb{R}^2 \to \mathbb{R}^n$, the goal is to segment the objects of interest (cells) in $I$. We represent the boundary of each object (or each part of a multi-region object) by $\boldsymbol{X}_i \in \Omega$, where $i$ indicates the $i^{th}$ part/region. Next, we review the useful priors in microscopy images that we can leverage.

- **Shape:** When an object has a specific geometrical shape (e.g. circle, ellipse, rectillipse, etc.) we model it by shape parameters such as $\boldsymbol{b} = \{$radius, major axis, eccentricity, etc.$\}$. When no clear geometrical representation exists, we model a shape (e.g. $i^{th}$ region's shape) by its statistical (from $m$ training samples) and vibrational properties as $\boldsymbol{X}_i \approx \bar{\boldsymbol{X}}_i + \boldsymbol{S}_i^c \boldsymbol{b}_i$, where $\bar{\boldsymbol{X}}_i$ is the average of a set of pose-normalized training shapes and $\boldsymbol{S}_i^c = \boldsymbol{S}_{stat} + \beta \boldsymbol{S}_{vib}$ is the combined (statistical $\boldsymbol{S}_{stat}$ and vibrational $\boldsymbol{S}_{vib}$) covariance matrix [8,4], $\beta \propto 1/m$ is the balancing parameter and $\boldsymbol{b}_i = (b_i^1, \cdots, b_i^t)^T$ is a vector of shape parameters. We use the Mahalanobis distance to measure the validity of a novel shape $\boldsymbol{X}_j$ by $F_i^{sh}(\boldsymbol{X}_j) = e^{-\sqrt{(\boldsymbol{X}_j - \bar{\boldsymbol{X}}_i)^T (\boldsymbol{S}_i^c)^{-1} (\boldsymbol{X}_j - \bar{\boldsymbol{X}}_i)}}$.

- **Appearance:** Histology/microscopy images typically have different discriminative **color** channels, $\boldsymbol{c} = \{c_1, \cdots, c_q\}$, where $c_i$ is a color channel, e.g. R, G, B, etc. Further, cells (and their constitutive regions) might also have different discriminative **texture**, $\boldsymbol{t} = \{t_1, \cdots, t_r\}$, where $t_i$ is a texture channel, e.g. multi-scale Gabor or Haar-like features. To leverage cell appearance (color+texture), we concatenate $\boldsymbol{c}$ and $\boldsymbol{t}$ into a regional appearance vector $\boldsymbol{r}$ calculated within inner and outer bands around $\boldsymbol{X}_j$, $\Omega_{in,d}^j$ and $\Omega_{out,d}^j$, with thickness $d$. This band-localization is important since cells can contain inner parts (e.g. nucleus) and can be adjacent to other objects (e.g. other cells), both of which can pollute the regional appearance measures if a band is not used. In addition, by using an inner versus outer band, we are encoding the boundary polarity (e.g. dark to bright). We define the appearance fitness function for object $i$ as

$$F_i^{ap}(\boldsymbol{X}_j) = \frac{1}{2}\left(\frac{1}{|\Omega_{in,d}^j|}\int_{\Omega_{in,d}^j} p(\boldsymbol{x}\in O_i)d\boldsymbol{x} + \frac{1}{|\Omega_{out,d}^j|}\int_{\Omega_{out,d}^j} p(\boldsymbol{x}\in B_i)d\boldsymbol{x}\right) \quad (1)$$

where $p(\boldsymbol{x}\in O_i)$ and $p(\boldsymbol{x}\in B_i)$ are the probabilities of a given pixel $\boldsymbol{x}\in \Omega_{in,d}^j\cup\Omega_{out,d}^j$, belonging to object $i$ ($O_i$) and its background ($B_i$), respectively, and are estimated by training a random forest (RF) consisting of $N_b$ binary decision trees. To segment an $R$-region object in $I$, $R+1$ patches within $R$ different regions of the object plus background are selected (i.e. regions $\mathcal{L}=\{0,\cdots,R\}$) to train the RF. After training, for each pixel $\boldsymbol{x}$, the feature channels, $\boldsymbol{r}(\boldsymbol{x})$, are propagated through each tree resulting in the probability $p_j(\boldsymbol{x}\in k|\boldsymbol{r}(\boldsymbol{x}))$, for the $j^{th}$ tree, where $k\in\mathcal{L}$. These probabilities are combined into a forest's joint probability $p(\boldsymbol{x}\in k|\boldsymbol{r}(\boldsymbol{x}))=\frac{1}{N_b}\sum_{j=1}^{N_b}p_j(\boldsymbol{x}\in k|\boldsymbol{r}(\boldsymbol{x}))$ to determine the probability of $\boldsymbol{x}$ belonging to class $k$. Note that $O_i, B_i\in\mathcal{L}$.

- **Edge:** Since boundaries of cells and their parts exhibit appearance discontinuities, we incorporate edge information in the image by defining the following edge fitness term $F^{ed}(\boldsymbol{X}_j)=\frac{1}{|\boldsymbol{X}_j|}\oint_{\boldsymbol{X}_j}e^{-g(\boldsymbol{X}_j)}$, where $g(.)=1/(\epsilon+\lambda)$, $\lambda$ is the maximum eigenvalue of the structure tensor $J^TJ$ (generalizes scalar field gradients to those of vector fields), where $J$ is the Jacobian matrix of the weighted feature channels, $\boldsymbol{w}^T\boldsymbol{r}$, and the vector $\boldsymbol{w}$, resulting from training the RF, is the importance of each feature channel in discriminating inside versus outside of an object (i.e. maximizes boundary edge response).

- **Pose:** Each cell has a specific size, orientation and position in the image. Given the training data, we estimate the average area ($\bar{A}$) and the principal orientation ($\bar{\theta}$) of cells and use them for imposing constraints on the solutions. We use a cell's centroid, $\boldsymbol{p}=(p^x,p^y)$, to specify its position.

- **Topological constraints:** In addition to the geometrical and appearance properties of an object (color, texture, edge, shape and pose), in multi-region objects, meaningful topological relationships typically exist between different object's regions, e.g. regions *contain/exclude* others. To enforce containment and exclusion between two regions, e.g. $\boldsymbol{X}_j$ is contained in $\boldsymbol{X}_i$, or, $\boldsymbol{X}_i$ and $\boldsymbol{X}_j$ are excluded from one another, the following constraints are imposed:

$$D(\boldsymbol{x}_j) \overset{contain}{\underset{exclude}{\gtrless}} 0 ,\quad \forall \boldsymbol{x_j}\in\boldsymbol{X}_j ,\quad D(x)=SDM(\boldsymbol{X}_i), \quad (2)$$

where $SDM(\boldsymbol{X}_i)$ is the signed distance map of $\boldsymbol{X}_i$ and is positive inside and negative outside $\boldsymbol{X}_i$. Eq. (2) is a general constraint for convex and non-convex shapes. However, for convex shapes, as we typically have in microscopy images, we adopt the following simplification for containment: $||\boldsymbol{p}_j-\boldsymbol{x}_i||-||\boldsymbol{p}_j-\boldsymbol{x}_j'||\geq 0$, and exclusion: $||\boldsymbol{p}_j-\boldsymbol{x}_i||-||\boldsymbol{p}_j-\boldsymbol{x}_j'||\leq 0$, $\forall\boldsymbol{x}_i\in\boldsymbol{X}_i$, for faster computation, where $\boldsymbol{x}_j'\in\overrightarrow{\boldsymbol{p}_j\boldsymbol{x}_i}\cap\boldsymbol{X}_j$ and $\boldsymbol{p}_j=(p_j^x,p_j^y)$ is the spatial position of $\boldsymbol{X}_j$.

- **Inter-part adjacency:** In biomedical applications, the minimum ($d^{min}$) and maximum ($d^{max}$) distances between two adjacent regions of an object are sometimes known. Bounding the minimal and maximal distances between two

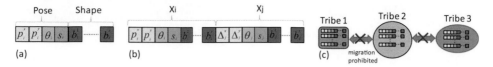

**Fig. 1.** Chromosome structure for (a) a single-region and (b) a two-region object. The position of the second region, $(\Delta_j^x, \Delta_j^y)$, is computed relative to the first object's position. (c) Tribe-based GA. No migration is allowed between tribes.

adjacent boundaries (e.g. $i$ and $j$) from below and above, respectively, prevents segmentation leakage and improves the results. We impose these constraints by:

$$\min(f_{ij}, f_{ji}) \geq d_{ij}^{min} \quad , \quad \max(g_{ij}, g_{ji}) \leq d_{ij}^{max}, \tag{3}$$

where $f_{ij} = \min_{\boldsymbol{x}_i \in \boldsymbol{X}_i} \min_{\boldsymbol{x}_j \in \boldsymbol{X}_j} \|\boldsymbol{x}_i - \boldsymbol{x}_j\|$ and $g_{ij} = \max_{\boldsymbol{x}_i \in \boldsymbol{X}_i} \min_{\boldsymbol{x}_j \in \boldsymbol{X}_j} \|\boldsymbol{x}_i - \boldsymbol{x}_j\|$. For efficiency, we only calculate and restrict $f_{ij}$ and $g_{ij}$ (not $f_{ji}$ and $g_{ji}$).

- **User interaction:** User interaction is another useful prior. This prior can be applied on the boundary and/or the region of an object by providing corresponding seed points, $\boldsymbol{s}_i^b$ and $\boldsymbol{s}_i^r$, and force the solution to satisfy the following constraints $\boldsymbol{s}_i^r \in \Omega_{in,d=\infty}^i$ and $\boldsymbol{s}_i^b \in \Omega_{in,d=\epsilon}^i \cup \Omega_{out,d=\epsilon}^i$.

**Fitness Function:** The overall fitness function (for an $R$-region cell) is constructed by integrating all above mentioned information as

$$F_{total}(\boldsymbol{X}) = \sum_{i=1}^{R} \left( F_i^{sh}(\boldsymbol{X}) + F_i^{ap}(\mathcal{M}_i(\boldsymbol{X})) + F^{ed}(\mathcal{M}_i(\boldsymbol{X})) \right), \text{ subject to} \tag{4}$$

$$\boldsymbol{geometry:} \quad |b_i^j| \leq 3\sqrt{\lambda_i^j} \quad |\theta_i - \bar{\theta}_i| \leq 3\sqrt{\lambda_i^\theta} \quad |\text{Area}(\boldsymbol{X}_i) - \bar{A}_i| \leq 3\sqrt{\lambda_i^A}$$

$$\boldsymbol{user\ interaction:} \quad \boldsymbol{s}_i^r \in \Omega_{in,\infty}^i \quad \boldsymbol{s}_i^b \in \Omega_{in,\epsilon}^i \cup \Omega_{out,\epsilon}^i$$

$$\boldsymbol{topology:} \quad eq.(2) \quad \boldsymbol{adjacency:} \quad eq.(3)$$

where $\boldsymbol{X} = \overline{\boldsymbol{X}} + \boldsymbol{S}^c \boldsymbol{b}$, $\mathcal{M}_i(\boldsymbol{X}) = s_i \mathcal{R}_i \boldsymbol{X} + \mathcal{T}_i$ is a similarity transformation with rotation $\mathcal{R}$, scaling $s$, and translation $\mathcal{T}$, $\lambda_i^j$ is the $j^{th}$ eigenvalue of $i^{th}$ region's covariance matrix and $\lambda_i^A$ and $\lambda_i^\theta$ are the area and orientation variance of $i^{th}$ region, respectively, obtained from the training data.

To find the best fit for such a complex fitness function (4), we adopt GA as a global optimization tool. Although GA does not strictly guarantee the global solution, our results confirm the ability of this approach to accurately segment the spatially-recurring, multi-region cells with partial overlap. In GA, each individual solution is represented by a chromosome consisting of several genes (Fig. 1(a)). The first four genes describe the individual's pose information, $p_i^x$ and $p_i^y$ are the spatial position of $i^{th}$ region and $\theta_i$, $s_i$ and $b_i^1, \cdots, b_i^t$ are its orientation, scale and shape parameters.

**Encoding Multi-region Object's Information into GA:** For simplicity and to conserve space, here we consider a two-region object scenario. Assuming

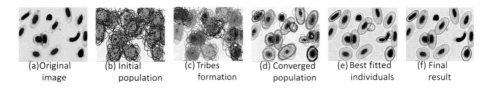

| (a)Original image | (b) Initial population | (c) Tribes formation | (d) Converged population | (e) Best fitted individuals | (f) Final result |

**Fig. 2.** Fish blood cells segmentation

a cell consists of two regions: $X_1$ and $X_2$, where $X_1$ contains $X_2$, we compute $\bar{A}$ and $\bar{\theta}$, as well as the shape parameters, $b$, for $X_1$ and $X_2$, separately, as described before. We represent the cell while encoding the interaction between its regions by concatenating the two chromosomes of $X_1$ and $X_2$. However, the position of $X_2$, $(p_2^x, p_2^y)$, is computed relative to $X_1$'s position, $(p_1^x, p_1^y)$, and its corresponding genes are replaced by $\Delta_x$ and $\Delta_y$ (Fig. 1(b)). $\Delta_x$ and $\Delta_y$ allow $X_2$ to move in small distances around its relative position to $(p_1^x, p_1^y)$. The average relative distance between $X_1$ and $X_2$ as well as limits on $\Delta_x$ and $\Delta_y$ are learned from the training data.

Each object (cell) typically recur in different parts of the image domain. To deal with such spatially recurring aspect of cell segmentation, we use GA with *tribes* to obtain multiple distinct solutions (i.e. cells). In tribes-based GA, the whole population is grouped into several tribes. During the GA evolution and in the gene crossover phase, any two selected parents must be from the same tribe. In fact, tribes are too choosy about who is allowed to join them (Fig. 1(c)); they do not accept any stranger (no migration is allowed) and even children who are not similar to the tribe's population are rejected. This tribes-based GA allows for the desired multiple distinct solutions. We choose the tribes' membership based on the spatial position of each member (cell), i.e. $(p^x, p^y)$.

**Initialization and Implementation:** We used 6 channels of colors (RGB+ HSV) and 3-channel Gabor features as our regional cues. Gabor filters were calculated in 8 different orientations and 3 different scales and were summed up across orientations to obtain rotational-invariance texture features. For RF, we used $N_b = 50$ binary trees. We randomly spread $10,000$ random chromosomes over the image wherever the probability of existing cells obtained from RF is large enough, i.e. $p(x \in O|r(x)) > 0.6$ (Fig. 2(b)). $d_{ij}^{min}$ and $d_{ij}^{max}$ were set based on the training dataset. Although our method can handle user interaction, none was used in our experiments. The crossover and mutation rates were fixed to 0.7 and 0.01, respectively, in all of our experiments. Individuals that are within a distance of $\ell$ pixels from each other establish a tribe (Fig. 2(c)). We implemented our method in MATLAB in a way that all individuals are evaluated simultaneously in parallel. After convergence, Fig. 2(d), the best solution in each tribe is examined (Fig. 2(e)). We use the final fitness measure as a confidence measure, where the user can request displaying e.g. the top 10% confident segmentation. According to our fitness function, the ideal fitness score is 3. In all of our experiments we kept the solutions that are higher than 2.4 (top 20% confident segmentation) as the final solution (Fig. 2(f)).

## 3   Experiments

In our **first experiment**, we evaluated our method on stained breast cancer tissue images used in ICPR 2010's HIMA contest on 'Counting Lymphocytes on Histopathology Images' [7]. We benchmarked our results against the state-of-the-art methods, including the contest's finalists. We used the centroid of the segmented cells to compare our results against the expert annotated ground truth (GT). Fig. 3(a) quantitatively compares our results against the competing methods. The evaluation criteria are based on the Euclidean distance, $d_E$, between the GT and segmented lymphosytes, as well as the absolute difference, $N$, between the true number of cells in GT and detected cells. $m$ and $s$ in Fig. 3(a) are mean and standard deviation, respectively. In Fig. 3(a), Bernardis et al. [2] reported results for different thresholds, $\rho$, on the same dataset. While for some cases (e.g. $\rho = 2$) they achieved better distance accuracy, $d_E$, than our method, they found less true cells (bigger $N$). On the other hand, they obtained better detection rate (smaller $N$) for $\rho = 5$ but with less accuracy, $d_E$. We emphasize that their method has been designed for single-region cells only. Fig. 3(b) demonstrates how our method distinguishes the merged cells. Our method can not only detect and segment the single-region cells but also delineate the different boundaries of a multi-region cell.

To further showcase our method, we ran a **second experiment** on another dataset, MICR, consisting of 20 different histology and microscopy images with multi-region cells. Our results in Fig. 4 verify the use of proposed constraints (topology, thickness and shape) as compared to ubiquitous unconstrained image segmentation methods; graph cuts (GC), and constrained methods; Delong and Boykov [5] (DB). While GC is not designed to segment cells, its results show the issues and difficulties involved in segmenting complex, multi-region cells. Delong and Boykov's method incorporates containment constraint in the GC framework, however, their method is unable to segment the targeted objects solely (Fig. 4). Fig. 3(c) quantitatively compares our method with watershed (WS), GC and DB on both HIMA and MICR datasets using Dice similarity coefficient (DSC).

Due to the random initialization and evolution in GA, they may not always produce the same result. To examine the reproducibility of the proposed approach, in our **third experiment**, we ran our method 20 times on sample images and monitored the fitness and DSC vs. generation (Fig. 5). The results confirm that our method converges to almost similar results (similar DSC) although we randomly initialized the population at each run. From Fig. 5, the fitness values for the $1^{st}$ and $2^{nd}$ cells are lower than the $3^{rd}$ simply because the first two cells overlap. The variations between different runs can be reduced by increasing the size of initial population but at the cost of computational complexity. **Runtime:** Using non-optimized MATLAB code on standard 2.3 GHz CPU, the running time of our algorithm ranged between 60-300 s/image, which depended primarily on the number of cells per image, which varied between 2-60 for both HIMA and MICR.

| Method | $m_{d\varepsilon}$ | $s_{d\varepsilon}$ | $m_N$ | $s_N$ |
|--------|------|------|-------|------|
| Kuse [9] | 3.04 | 3.40 | 14.01 | 4.4 |
| Panagiotakis [12] | 2.87 | 3.80 | 14.23 | 6.3 |
| Graf [6] | 7.60 | 6.30 | 24.50 | 16.2 |
| Kuse [10] | 3.14 | 0.93 | 4.30 | 3.09 |
| Bernardis [2] | | | | |
| $(\rho = 5)$ | 3.22 | 3.92 | 5.40 | 3.68 |
| $(\rho = 4)$ | 2.84 | 2.89 | 8.20 | 4.75 |
| $(\rho = 2)$ | 1.12 | 0.71 | 16.75 | 7.47 |
| Our method | 1.40 | 0.77 | 6.30 | 4.20 |

(a)

(b)

| Dataset | HIMA | MICR |
|---------|------|------|
| WS | 0.68 ± 0.12 | 0.65 ± 0.13 |
| GC | 0.72 ± 0.09 | 0.69 ± 0.20 |
| DB | 0.72 ± 0.08 | 0.76 ± 0.18 |
| Ours | 0.81 ± 0.03 | 0.91 ± 0.01 |

(c)

**Fig. 3.** (a) Comparison against state-of-the-art methods on HIMA dataset [7]. (b) Sample results. Red contours: our segmentation result; small gold + sign: our segmentation centroid; green dots: ground truth. (c) Accuracy comparison with WS, GC and DB methods using DSC (*mean ± std*).

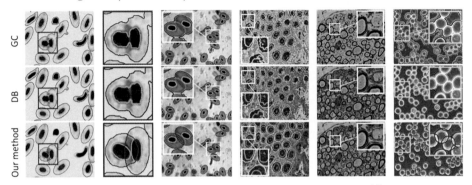

**Fig. 4.** Sample results on MICR dataset. Note how the proposed method segments only the targeted cells. Same data term was used for all experiments.

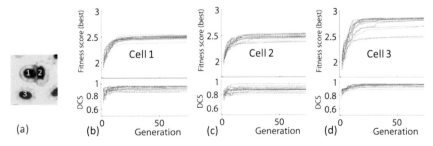

**Fig. 5.** Sample segmentation shown in Fig. 4. (b-d) Fitness and DSC of the best individual of each tribe vs. generation number for the three tribes ($1^{st}$, $2^{nd}$ and $3^{rd}$) corresponding to the three cells in (a), for 20 different runs on (a).

## 4  Conclusion

Segmenting spatially recurring complex objects consisting of different regions with varying shapes, colors and textures remains a challenging problem in biomedical image segmentation. Another layer of complexity is added once these multi-region objects overlap. In this paper we showed how to address this complexity holistically by incorporating several intuitive priors into an objective function without being overly concerned about its optimization. The proposed high level priors help us to segment only the targeted objects (cells) in an image. Fully parallelizing the proposed method is in our agenda as future work.

## References

1. Ali, S., Veltri, R., Epstein, J.I., Christudass, C., Madabhushi, A.: Adaptive energy selective active contour with shape priors for nuclear segmentation and gleason grading of prostate cancer. In: Fichtinger, G., Martel, A., Peters, T. (eds.) MICCAI 2011, Part I. LNCS, vol. 6891, pp. 661–669. Springer, Heidelberg (2011)
2. Bernardis, E., et al.: Pop out many small structures from a very large microscopic image. MedIA 15(5), 690–707 (2011)
3. Cheng, L., Ye, N., Yu, W., Cheah, A.: Discriminative segmentation of microscopic cellular images. In: Fichtinger, G., Martel, A., Peters, T. (eds.) MICCAI 2011, Part I. LNCS, vol. 6891, pp. 637–644. Springer, Heidelberg (2011)
4. Cootes, T.F., et al.: Combining point distribution models with shape models based on finite element analysis. Image Vis. Comp. 13(5), 403–409 (1995)
5. Delong, A., et al.: Globally optimal segmentation of multi-region objects. In: ICCV, pp. 285–292 (2009)
6. Graf, F., Grzegorzek, M., Paulus, D.: Counting lymphocytes in histopathology images using connected components. In: Ünay, D., Çataltepe, Z., Aksoy, S. (eds.) ICPR 2010. LNCS, vol. 6388, pp. 263–269. Springer, Heidelberg (2010)
7. Gurcan, M.N., Madabhushi, A., Rajpoot, N.: Pattern recognition in histopathological images: An ICPR 2010 contest. In: Ünay, D., Çataltepe, Z., Aksoy, S. (eds.) ICPR 2010. LNCS, vol. 6388, pp. 226–234. Springer, Heidelberg (2010)
8. Hamarneh, G., Jassi, P., Tang, L.: Simulation of ground-truth validation data via physically-and statistically-based warps. In: Metaxas, D., Axel, L., Fichtinger, G., Székely, G. (eds.) MICCAI 2008, Part I. LNCS, vol. 5241, pp. 459–467. Springer, Heidelberg (2008)
9. Kuse, M., Sharma, T., Gupta, S.: A classification scheme for lymphocyte segmentation in H&E stained histology images. In: Ünay, D., Çataltepe, Z., Aksoy, S. (eds.) ICPR 2010. LNCS, vol. 6388, pp. 235–243. Springer, Heidelberg (2010)
10. Kuse, M., et al.: Local isotropic phase symmetry measure for detection of beta cells and lymphocytes. J. Pathol. Inf. 2 (2011)
11. Mao, K.Z., et al.: Supervised learning-based cell image segmentation for p53 immunohistochemistry. IEEE TBE 53(6), 1153–1163 (2006)
12. Panagiotakis, C., Ramasso, E., Tziritas, G.: Lymphocyte segmentation using the transferable belief model. In: Ünay, D., Çataltepe, Z., Aksoy, S. (eds.) ICPR 2010. LNCS, vol. 6388, pp. 253–262. Springer, Heidelberg (2010)
13. Turner, A., et al.: Obtaining multiple distinct solutions with genetic algorithm niching methods. In: Ebeling, W., Rechenberg, I., Voigt, H.-M., Schwefel, H.-P. (eds.) PPSN 1996. LNCS, vol. 1141, pp. 451–460. Springer, Heidelberg (1996)
14. Wu, X., et al.: Embedding topic discovery in conditional random fields model for segmenting nuclei using multispectral data. IEEE TBE 59(6), 1539–1549 (2012)
15. Yang, L., Tuzel, O., Meer, P., Foran, D.J.: Automatic image analysis of histopathology specimens using concave vertex graph. In: Metaxas, D., Axel, L., Fichtinger, G., Székely, G. (eds.) MICCAI 2008, Part I. LNCS, vol. 5241, pp. 833–841. Springer, Heidelberg (2008)

# A Metamorphosis Distance for Embryonic Cardiac Action Potential Interpolation and Classification

Giann Gorospe, Laurent Younes, Leslie Tung, and René Vidal

Johns Hopkins University

**Abstract.** The use of human embryonic stem cell cardiomyocytes (hESC-CMs) in tissue transplantation and repair has led to major recent advances in cardiac regenerative medicine. However, to avoid potential arrhythmias, it is critical that hESC-CMs used in replacement therapy be electrophysiologically compatible with the adult atrial, ventricular, and nodal phenotypes. The current method for classifying the electrophysiology of hESC-CMs relies mainly on the shape of the cell's action potential (AP), which each expert subjectively decides if it is nodal-like, atrial-like or ventricular-like. However, the classification is difficult because the shape of the AP of an hESC-CMs may not coincide with that of a mature cell. In this paper, we propose to use a *metamorphosis distance* for comparing the AP of an hESC-CMs to that of an adult cell model. This involves constructing a family of APs corresponding to different stages of the maturation process, and measuring the amount of deformation between APs. Experiments show that the proposed distance leads to better interpolation and classification results.

## 1 Introduction

Stem cells present a new frontier in cardiology. Since the seminal work of [1], advances have been made in the purification of cardiomyocytes (heart muscle cells) from stem cells [2], its comparison to mature cardiomyocyte analogs [3], and its application in cell therapy and regenerative medicine [4]. A key step to future applications in medicine and drug discovery is the ability to isolate and purify populations of cardiomyocytes that are precursors to the adult phenotypes (atrial, ventricular, nodal). To achieve this, discriminative criteria are necessary. While current work approaches this problem chemically [5], in this work we approach it electrophysiologically using the cardiac action potential.

The current standard [6–8] for assessing cardiomyocyte phenotype is by making measurements of certain indicative features of the action potential. As illustrated in Figure 1, such features include upstroke velocity (max $\frac{\partial V}{\partial t}$), which indicates the rate of membrane depolarization, action potential amplitude (APA), which indicates the total change in membrane potential during depolarization, action potential duration $x$ (APD$_x$), which is the amount of time it takes the membrane to reach $x\%$ repolarization after depolarization, and maximum diastolic potential (MDP), which is the minimum membrane potential achieved following repolarization. The discrimination of phenotype is then based on combinations of these features. However, the criterion for classification is often subjective, which makes it difficult to translate to other data sets and scale to larger populations. In addition, the use of these features effectively discards the action potential waveform itself, making it nearly impossible to visualize an action potential near the decision boundary. This additional concern is of importance in

K. Mori et al. (Eds.): MICCAI 2013, Part I, LNCS 8149, pp. 469–476, 2013.
© Springer-Verlag Berlin Heidelberg 2013

the hESC-CM domain where an immature cardiomyocyte may not have decided on its phenotype yet.

We believe that methods based on the action potential waveform itself will lead to more effective ways of assessing cardiomyocyte phenotypes. One approach is to use the Euclidean distance to compare two action potentials, as suggested in [9] for EMG data. However, this is not an ideal measure because, unless two signals are very similar to begin with, Euclidean interpolation of two action potentials leads to intermediary shapes that do not resemble the shape of a prototypical action potential. Another approach is to use dynamic time warping (DTW) to align

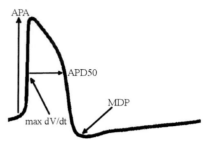

**Fig. 1.** Sample action potential with common biological measurements

two action potentials in time before comparing them with a Euclidean distance [10, 11]. However, DTW does not capture variations in the amplitude of the action potential, hence the shape of a warped action potential may still not resemble that of a prototypical one.

In this paper, we propose to use a *metamorphosis distance* [12, 13] for interpolation and classification of action potentials. A metamorphosis between two action potentials is a sequence of intermediate action potentials obtained by a morphing action and the distance between two action potentials measures the amount of morphing. Our experiments show that this distance leads to intermediate action potentials whose shape resembles that of prototypical action potentials. Moreover, this distance leads to improved classification results on existing datasets.

## 2    Metamorphosis of Cardiac Action Potentials

Let $f_1 : \Omega \to \mathbb{R}$ be an action potential, such as that in Figure 1. We assume that the space of action potentials, $\mathcal{M}$, is the space of periodic, continuously differentiable and square integrable functions, i.e., $\mathcal{M} = L^2(\Omega)$, where $\Omega = \mathbb{S}^1$ is the unit circle.

Let $f_0, f_1 \in \mathcal{M}$ be two action potentials corresponding to an immature and a mature cell, respectively. The Euclidean distance between the two action potentials is defined as $d_{L^2}^2(f_0, f_1) = \int_\Omega (f_0(t) - f_1(t))^2 dt$. This distance is not suitable for comparing two action potentials because the shape of the Euclidean average of two action potentials need not resemble that of the individual action potentials. Our goal is to define a distance $d_{\mathcal{M}}(f_0, f_1)$ that captures the differences in the shapes of the action potentials.

To that end, we define a family of action potentials $f(\cdot, \tau)$ that interpolates between $f_0$ and $f_1$, i.e., $f(t, 0) = f_0(t)$ and $f(t, 1) = f_1(t)$, where the parameter $\tau \in [0, 1]$ captures the stage of differentiation of the cell, i.e., $\tau = 0$ corresponds to an immature cell and $\tau = 1$ corresponds to a mature cell. In constructing $f(\cdot, \tau)$, our goal is to preserve the shape of the action potential as much as possible. One possible approach [14, 15] to constructing $f$ is to find a deformation $\phi : \Omega \to \Omega$ that warps the domain of the action potential of a mature cell $f_1$ to produce the action potential of an immature cell $f_0$, i.e., $f_0(t) = f_1(\phi(t))$. The deformation $\phi$ is assumed to belong to the space of diffeomorphisms in $\Omega$, $\mathcal{G} = \text{Diff}(\Omega)$, a Lie group that acts on the manifold $\mathcal{M}$ by right composition with the inverse [12], i.e., $\phi \cdot f = f(\phi^{-1}(t))$, where $f \in \mathcal{M}$, $\phi \in \text{Diff}(\Omega)$ and $t \in \Omega$. To preserve the shape of the action potential as much as possible, the diffeomorphism that is "closest" to the identity deformation $id \in \mathcal{G}$ is chosen. That is, the distance between $f_0$ and $f_1$ is defined as $d_{\mathcal{M}}(f_0, f_1) = \inf_{\phi \in \mathcal{G}} d_{\mathcal{G}}(\phi, id)$, such that $f_1 \approx \phi \cdot f_0$, where $d_{\mathcal{G}}$ is some distance in $\mathcal{G}$.

The above approach accounts for most of the temporal variations between the two action potentials. However, it does not capture variations in their amplitude (e.g., maximum or minimum). To account for both temporal and amplitude variations, we propose to use a *metamorphosis* [12, 13] to interpolate between the action potentials $f_0$ and $f_1$. A metamorphosis is a family of action potentials $f(\cdot, \tau)$, parameterized by $\tau \in [0, 1]$, such that $f(t, 0) = f_0(t)$ and $f(t, 1) = f_1(t)$. The curve $f(\cdot, \tau) \in \mathcal{M}$ is obtained by the action of a deformation path $\phi(\cdot, \tau) \in \text{Diff}(\Omega)$ onto a template path $i(\cdot, \tau) \in \mathcal{M}$ as $f(\cdot, \tau) = \phi(\cdot, \tau) \cdot i(\cdot, \tau)$. The curve $\phi(\cdot, \tau) \in \text{Diff}(\Omega)$ is such that $\phi(\cdot, 0) = id$ and represents the deformation part of the metamorphosis, while the curve $i(\cdot, \tau) \in \mathcal{M}$ represents the residual, or template evolution, part. Notice that when $i(t, \tau)$ does not depend on $\tau$, the metamorphosis is a pure deformation.

To find a metamorphosis that preserves the shape of the action potentials as much as possible, we need to define an appropriate distance in the space of metamorphoses so that we can choose the metamorphosis closest to the identity. We use the arc length of the curve $f(\cdot, \tau)$, $\sqrt{\int_0^1 \left\| \frac{\partial f}{\partial \tau} \right\|_{T\mathcal{M}}^2 d\tau}$ along the tangent space $T\mathcal{M}$ to define such a distance. Taking the derivative of $f(t, \tau) = i(\phi^{-1}(t, \tau), \tau)$ with respect to $\tau$ leads to:[1]

$$
\begin{aligned}
\frac{\partial f}{\partial \tau}(t, \tau) &= \frac{\partial i}{\partial t}(\phi^{-1}(t, \tau), \tau) \frac{\partial \phi^{-1}}{\partial \tau}(t, \tau) + \frac{\partial i}{\partial \tau}(\phi^{-1}(t, \tau), \tau) \\
&= -\frac{\partial f}{\partial t}(\phi^{-1}(t, \tau), \tau) \frac{\partial \phi}{\partial \tau}(\phi^{-1}(t, \tau), \tau) + \frac{\partial i}{\partial \tau}(\phi^{-1}(t, \tau), \tau).
\end{aligned}
\tag{1}
$$

When $\tau = 0$, we have $\phi(t, 0) = id$ and (1) simplifies to:

$$
\frac{\partial f}{\partial \tau}(t, 0) = \frac{\partial i}{\partial \tau}(t, 0) - \frac{\partial f}{\partial t}(t, 0) \frac{\partial \phi}{\partial \tau}(t, 0).
\tag{2}
$$

This equation allows us to decompose an infinitesimal change in $f$, $\frac{\partial f}{\partial \tau}$, in terms of an infinitesimal change in the template, $\delta = \frac{\partial i}{\partial \tau}$ and an infinitesimal change in the deformation, $v = \frac{\partial \phi}{\partial \tau}$. The Euclidean distance is a reasonable choice to measure $\delta$ because the infinitesimal change in the template is approximately linear. To measure $v$, recall that $v$ represents the instantaneous flow field induced by the diffeomorphism $\phi(t, 0)$. Since we want this flow to be smooth, we can impose a Sobolev norm on the space $V$ of flow fields. For example, we can choose $\| \cdot \|_V = \|T(\cdot)\|_{L^2}$, where $T$ is a linear operator (one example of $T$ is $T(\cdot) = id(\cdot) - \alpha \Delta(\cdot)$). Now, notice from (2) that different combinations of infinitesimal changes $v$ and $\delta$ could lead to the same change $\frac{\partial f}{\partial \tau}$. To remove this ambiguity and define a proper Riemannian metric, we take the minimum length over all such combinations. The measure on $\frac{\partial f}{\partial \tau}$ is then defined as:

$$
\left\| \frac{\partial f}{\partial \tau} \right\|_{T\mathcal{M}}^2 = \inf_{v, \delta} \left\{ \|v\|_V^2 + \frac{1}{\sigma^2} \|\delta\|_{L^2}^2 : \frac{\partial f}{\partial \tau} = \delta - \frac{\partial f}{\partial t} v \right\},
\tag{3}
$$

where $\sigma > 0$ is a balancing parameter.

We can use this infinitesimal evolution to define a distance between two action potentials by summing the collection of infinitesimal changes connecting the two signals. Specifically, let $f_0(t)$ and $f_1(t)$ be two action potentials. The *metamorphosis distance* between the two waveforms in $\mathcal{M}$ is hence defined as:

$$d_{\mathcal{M}}^2(f_0, f_1) = \inf_{v,f} \int_0^1 \|v(t,\tau)\|_V^2 + \frac{1}{\sigma^2}\left\|\frac{\partial f}{\partial \tau}(t,\tau) + \frac{\partial f}{\partial t}(t,\tau)\, v(t,\tau)\right\|_{L^2}^2 d\tau, \quad (4)$$

where $f(t,0) = f_0(t)$, $f(t,1) = f_1(t)$, and $\delta = \frac{\partial i}{\partial \tau}$ is substituted for using (2).

## 3  Numerical Computation of the Metamorphosis Distance

The computation of the metamorphosis distance requires finding $v$ and $f$ that minimize (4). This problem is non-convex, and its solution, if it exists, need not be unique, as multiple velocity and template evolutions paths may connect the two action potentials with the same energy. Regardless, we proceed to solve this problem by discretizing $\tau$ into $N + 1$ timesteps, $\tau_n = (n-1)/N$, $n = 1, \ldots, N + 1$. To discretize the residual evolution term $\frac{\partial f}{\partial \tau} + \frac{\partial f}{\partial t}v$, we follow [16] and make the following approximation:

$$\int_0^1 \left\|\frac{\partial f}{\partial \tau}(t,\tau) + \frac{\partial f}{\partial t}(t,\tau)v(t,\tau)\right\|_{L_2}^2 d\tau \approx \sum_{n=0}^{N-1} \|f(t+v(t,\tau_n), \tau_{n+1}) - f(t,\tau_n)\|_{L_2}^2, \quad (5)$$

which holds as the number of time steps approaches infinity because

$$\lim_{\epsilon \to 0} \frac{f(t+\epsilon v(t,\tau), \tau + \epsilon) - f(t,\tau)}{\epsilon} = \frac{\partial f}{\partial t}v(t,\tau) + \frac{\partial f}{\partial \tau}(t,\tau). \quad (6)$$

Since we also discretize the signal in the time domain, we need to resample $f(t,\tau_n)$ and $f(t + v(t,\tau), \tau_{n+1})$ accordingly. Let $N_{v(t,\tau_n)}$ be the linear operator that acts on $f(t,\tau_{n+1})$ and represents the sampling of $f(t + v(t,\tau_n), \tau_{n+1})$ onto the original grid. In our experiments, $N_{v(t,\tau_n)}$ is generated using linear interpolation. There are $N$ such operators, one for each of the $v(t,\tau_n)$ required in the energy, but each can be updated independently from the others. This operator transforms the residual evolution term into something amenable for vector analysis:

$$\sum_{n=0}^{N-1} \|f(t+v(t,\tau_n), \tau_{n+1}) - f(t,\tau)\|_{L_2}^2 = \sum_{n=0}^{N-1} \|N_{v(t,\tau_n)}f(t,\tau_{n+1}) - f(t,\tau_n)\|_{L_2}^2. \quad (7)$$

Finally, to discretize the deformation energy, we discretize the linear differential operator $T$ over the sampled grid of our signal. Let this discretized differential operator be denoted by $L$. Further, we follow [12] and introduce a smoothing kernel $K = L^{-1}$ and the following substitution: $w = L^{1/2}v$. Minimizing over $w$ instead of $v$ leads to a speed up in computational time [12]. This differential operator $L$ and kernel matrix $K$ can be calculated using the Fourier Transform.

The resulting discrete objective function to be minimized is given by:

$$U(w(t,\tau), f(t,\tau)) = \sum_{n=0}^{N-1} \|w(t,\tau_n)\|_{L_2} + \frac{1}{\sigma^2}\|N_{v(t,\tau_n)}f(t,\tau_{n+1})) - f(t,\tau_n)\|_{L_2}, \quad (8)$$

where $v = K^{1/2}w$, $f(t,\tau_0 = 0) = f_0(t)$, and $f(t,\tau_N = 1) = f_1(t)$. The minimization

**Algorithm 1.** Discrete Metamorphosis Optimization

Given a Template Signal $f_0(t)$, a Target Signal $f_1(t)$, a balance parameter $\sigma$, the number of evolution time steps $N$, and a Sobolev Operator $L$.

1. Initialization.
   a. Set $d_{-1} = \infty$. Calculate $K = L^{-1}$.
   b. Set $w(t, \tau_n) \equiv 0$, $v(t, \tau_n) = K^{1/2} w(t, \tau_n) \equiv 0$, and $N_{v(t,\tau_n)} = I$ for all $\tau_n$.
   c. For $n = 0, \ldots, N$: Set $f(t, \tau_n) = \frac{N-n}{N} f_0(t) + \frac{n}{N} f_1(t)$
   d. Calculate distance $d_0^2 = \sum_{n=0}^{N-1} \|w(t, \tau_n)\|_{L_2}^2 + \frac{1}{\sigma^2} \|N_{v(t,\tau_n)} f(t, \tau_{n+1})) - f(t, \tau_n)\|_{L_2}^2$
2. Until $d_{i-1} - d_i$ converges
   a. Set $d_i \to d_{i-1}$
   b. For $n = 0, \ldots, N-1$, Update $w(t, \tau_n)$ using (9).
      Calculate $v(t, \tau_n) = \mathbb{R}(K^{1/2} w(t, \tau_n))$, Update $N_{v(t,\tau_n)}$.
   c. For $n = 1, \ldots, N-1$, Update $f(t, \tau_n)$ using (10).
   d. Calculate distance $d_i = \sum_{n=0}^{N-1} \|w(t, \tau_n)\|_{L_2} + \frac{1}{\sigma^2} \|N_{v(t,\tau_n)} f(t, \tau_{n+1})) - f(t, \tau_n)\|_{L_2}$

can be done using alternating gradient descent over the substituted velocity $w$ and the metamorphosis $f$. The process is described in Algorithm 1. We initialize the algorithm by making all the velocity fields $w(t, \tau_n) = 0$ for all $t, \tau_n$, and the subsequent interpolation matrices $N_{v(t,\tau_n)} = I$ for all $\tau_n$, where $I$ is the identity. The initial metamorphosis is the Euclidean interpolation: $f(t, \tau_n) = \frac{N-n}{N} J_0(t) + \frac{n}{N} J_1(t), n = 0 \ldots N$.

**Velocity Update.** Differentiating the objective w.r.t. to the transformed velocity gives:

$$\frac{\partial U}{\partial w(t, \tau_n)} = 2w(t, \tau_n) + \frac{2}{\sigma^2} K^{1/2}(f(\bar{t}, \tau_{n+1}) - f(t, \tau_n)) \frac{\partial f(\bar{t}, \tau_{n+1})}{\partial t}, \quad (9)$$

where $\bar{t} = t + K^{1/2} w(t, \tau_n)$. From (9), we see that the kernel ensures that each update of the transformed velocity leads to a smooth velocity field. This appears to speed up the descent process by allowing for larger steps. The original velocity field $v$ can be realized by multiplying $w$ by $K^{1/2}$ and taking the real component.

**Metamorphosis Update.** The update of the intermediary action potentials $f(t, \tau_n)$, $n = 1, \ldots, N-1$, can be calculated from $N_i = N_{v(t,\tau_i)}$ and (8):

$$\frac{\partial U}{\partial f(t, \tau_n)} = 2N_{n-1}^T(N_{n-1} f(t, \tau_n) - f(t, \tau_{n-1})) - 2(N_n f(t, \tau_{n+1}) - f(t, \tau_n)). \quad (10)$$

## 4   Experiments

**Synthetic Data.** We first evaluated how well the shape of the action potential is preserved when using metamorphosis interpolation. We used the model of [17] to generate five mature ventricular action potentials, each one corresponding to a different percentage (80–120%) of the standard value of one of the model parameters (conductance of the potassium rectifier channel). We interpolated between the action potentials at 80% and 120% using metamorphosis with the following parameters: $\sigma = 0.1$, $N = 4$ and a Sobolev norm operator $T(\cdot) = id(\cdot) - \alpha \Delta(\cdot)$ with $\alpha = 8$. Figure 2 compares the Euclidean (blue) and metamorphosis (green) interpolations to the ground truth (red). We

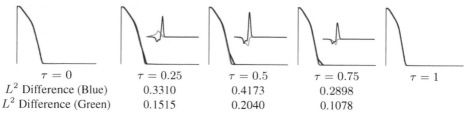

| | $\tau = 0$ | $\tau = 0.25$ | $\tau = 0.5$ | $\tau = 0.75$ | $\tau = 1$ |
|---|---|---|---|---|---|
| $L^2$ Difference (Blue) | | 0.3310 | 0.4173 | 0.2898 | |
| $L^2$ Difference (Green) | | 0.1515 | 0.2040 | 0.1078 | |

**Fig. 2.** A family of ventricular action potentials (red) used as ground truth, Euclidean interpolation (blue), and metamorphosis interpolation (green) between the left and right most potentials, differences between interpolation and ground truth (inset), and the $L^2$ errors in interpolation

see that the Euclidean evolution deviates from the action potential shape (inset of interpolation figures), while the metamorphosis evolution preserves the shape and matches the changing parameter better. While the differences appear to be minor, it is these types of differences that can affect the calculated distances and assignment.

**Real Data.** We performed classification of embryonic cardiomyocytes into mature phenotypes using metamorphosis interpolation from their action potentials to those of mature cell models. The mature signals were synthesized using a mature atrial [18] and a mature ventricular [17] cell model. The embryonic signals were obtained from the dataset of [6], which consists of 16 atrial and 36 ventricular cells, which were manually labeled using biological characteristics of the APs, as described in [6]. Since the embryonic signals were spontaneously paced, we used [19] to adjust their cycle length to 1 second to match the cell models. We also normalized the signals so that they have a baseline voltage of 0 and an amplitude of 1 to concentrate on the shape differences and not on scale/translation differences. These are both constraints we hope to remove in future work.

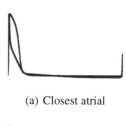

(a) Closest atrial

(b) Closest ventricular

**Fig. 3.** Misclassified embryonic atrial AP (blue) and closest mature model APs (red)

Table 1 shows classification results of 1-NN and 3-NN with Euclidean and metamorphosis distances using $\sigma = 0.3$, $N = 15$ and the same Sobolev norm operator from the synthetic experiment. Notice that the metamorphosis distance improves the classification results for 7-9 ventricular cells, and deteriorates them for two atrial cells. However, we believe this is an artifact of the manual labeling. Specifically, notice from Figure 3 that the shape of one of the misclassified atrial cells resembles more a ventricular shape than an atrial one. We observed a similar result for the other misclassified atrial cell. Figure 4 shows interpolation results from an embryonic ventricular cell (first column) to an atrial or ventricular model (final column) using both distances. $L^2$ interpolation produces intermediate signals whose shape does not resemble that of a prototypical action potential and gives a smaller distance to the wrong model. On the other hand, metamorphosis better preserves the shape during

---

[1] The last step follows from $\frac{\partial f}{\partial t}(t,\tau) = \frac{\partial i}{\partial t}(\phi^{-1}(t,\tau),\tau)\frac{\partial \phi^{-1}}{\partial t}(t,\tau)$ and from taking the derivatives of the relationship $\phi(\phi^{-1}(t,\tau),\tau) = t$ with respect to $t$ and $\tau$ to show that $\frac{\partial \phi^{-1}}{\partial \tau}(t,\tau) = -\frac{\partial \phi}{\partial \tau}(\phi^{-1}(t,\tau),\tau)\frac{\partial \phi^{-1}}{\partial t}(t,\tau)$.

**Table 1.** Number of correctly classified embryonic cardiomyocytes by nearest neighbors

| Method | $L_2$ 1-NN | $L_2$ 3-NN | Metamorphosis 1-NN | Metamorphosis 3-NN |
|---|---|---|---|---|
| Atrial Scoring | **16**/16 | **16**/16 | 14/16 | 14/16 |
| Ventricular Scoring | 29/36 | 27/36 | **36**/36 | **36**/36 |
| Total | 45/52 | 43/52 | **50**/52 | **50**/52 |

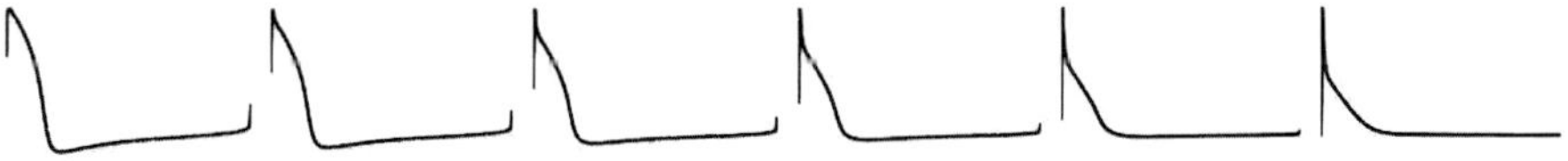

(a) Euclidean interpolation from ventricular to atrial cell: $d_{L^2} = 11.9834$

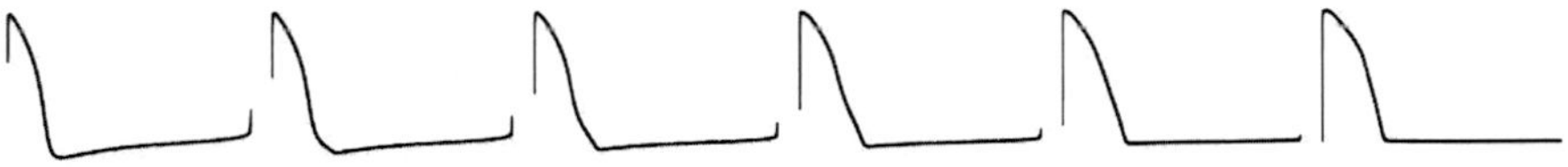

(b) Euclidean interpolation from ventricular to ventricular cell: $d_{L^2} = 12.6498$

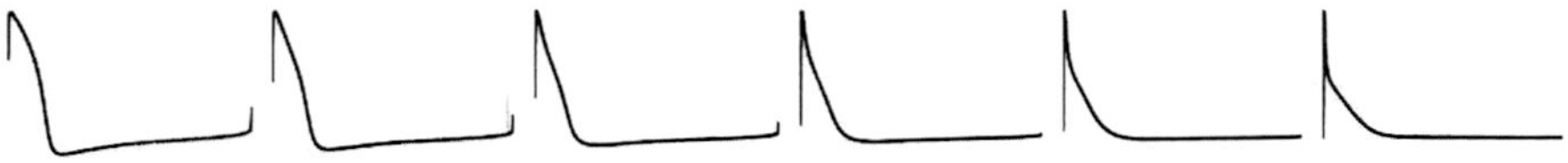

(c) Metamorphosis interpolation from ventricular to atrial cell: $d_{\mathcal{M}} = 5.4423$

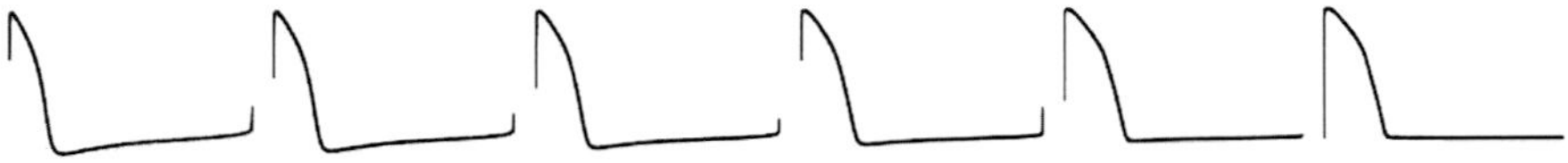

(d) Metamorphosis interpolation from ventricular to ventricular cell: $d_{\mathcal{M}} = 1.6484$

**Fig. 4.** Interpolation from an embryonic ventricular cell to atrial and ventricular models

interpolation and gives a much smaller distance to the correct model than to the incorrect model.

## 5   Conclusion

We have introduced a distance between action potential waveforms based on deformable template theory. The proposed distance aims to preserve the waveform shape and is successful in classifying embryonic cardiomyocytes. The framework could be adapted to other domains where shape preservation is a primary objective. Future work involves extending the framework to unnormalized and unpaced action potentials.

**Acknowledgments.** The authors thank Dr. Jia-Qiang He and Dr. Timothy Kamp for providing the embryonic cardiomyocyte dataset. This work was supported by the Sloan Foundation.

## References

1. Kehat, I., Kenyagin-Karsenti, D., Snir, M., Segev, H., Amit, M., Gepstein, A., Livne, E., Binah, O., Itskovitz-Eldor, J., Gepstein, L.: Human embryonic stem cells can differentiate into myocytes with structural and functional properties of cardiomyocytes. Journal of Clinical Investigation 108(3), 407–414 (2001)

2. Burridge, P.W., Thompson, S., Millrod, M.A., Weinberg, S., Yuan, X., Peters, A., Mahairaki, V., Koliatsos, V.E., Tung, L., Zambidis, E.T.: A universal system for highly efficient cardiac differentiation of human induced pluripotent stem cells that eliminates interline variability. PloS One 6(4) (2011)

3. Asp, J., Steel, D., Jonsson, M., Améen, C., Dahlenborg, K., Jeppsson, A., Lindahl, A., Sartipy, P.: Cardiomyocyte clusters derived from human embryonic stem cells share similarities with human heart tissue. Journal of Molecular Cell Biology 2(5), 276–283 (2010)

4. Laflamme, M.A., Chen, K.Y., Naumova, A.V., Muskheli, V., Fugate, J.A., Dupras, S.K., Reinecke, H., Xu, C., Hassanipour, M., Police, S., O'Sullivan, C., Collins, L., Chen, Y., Minami, E., Gill, E.A., Ueno, S., Yuan, C., Gold, J., Murry, C.E.: Cardiomyocytes derived from human embryonic stem cells in pro-survival factors enhance function of infarcted rat hearts. Nature Biotechnology 25(9), 1015–1024 (2007)

5. Zhang, Q., Jiang, J., Han, P., Yuan, Q., Zhang, J., Zhang, X., Xu, Y., Cao, H., Meng, Q., Chen, L., Tian, T., Wang, X., Li, P., Hescheler, J., Ji, G., Ma, Y.: Direct differentiation of atrial and ventricular myocytes from human embryonic stem cells by alternating retinoid signals. Cell Research 21(4), 579–587 (2011)

6. He, J.Q., Ma, Y., Lee, Y., Thomson, J.A., Kamp, T.J.: Human embryonic stem cells develop into multiple types of cardiac myocytes: action potential characterization. Circulation Research 93(1), 32–39 (2003)

7. Moore, J.C., Fu, J., Chan, Y.C., Lin, D., Tran, H., Tse, H.F., Li, R.A.: Distinct cardiogenic preferences of two human embryonic stem cell (hESC) lines are imprinted in their proteomes in the pluripotent state. Biochemical and Biophysical Research Communications 372(4), 553–558 (2008)

8. Fu, J.D., Rushing, S., Lieu, D., Chan, C., Kong, C.W., Geng, L., Wilson, K., Chiamvimonvat, N., Boheler, K., Wu, J., Keller, G., Hajjar, R., Li, R.: Distinct roles of microRNA-1 and -499 in ventricular specification and functional maturation of human embryonic stem cell-derived cardiomyocytes. PloS One 6(11) (2011)

9. McGill, K.: Optimal resolution of superimposed action potentials. IEEE Transactions on Biomedical Engineering 49(7), 640–650 (2002)

10. Syeda-Mahmood, T., Beymer, D., Wang, F.: Shape-based matching of ECG recordings. International Conference of the IEEE Engineering in Medicine and Biology Society 2007, 2012–2018 (2007)

11. Raghavendra, B.: Cardiac arrhythmia detection using dynamic time warping of ECG beats in e-healthcare systems. In: World of Wireless, Mobile and Multimedia Networks, pp. 1–6 (2011)

12. Younes, L.: Shapes and Diffeomorphisms. Springer (2010)

13. Trouvé, A., Younes, L.: Metamorphoses Through Lie Group Action. Foundations of Computational Mathematics 5(2), 173–198 (2005)

14. Sakoe, H., Chiba, S.: Dynamic programming algorithm optimization for spoken word recognition. IEEE Trans. on Acoustics, Speech, and Signal Processing 26(1), 43–49 (1978)

15. Piccioni, M., Scarlatti, S., Trouvé, A.: A variational problem arising from speech recognition. SIAM Journal on Applied Mathematics 58(3), 753–771 (1998)

16. Garcin, L., Younes, L.: Geodesic image matching: A wavelet based energy minimization scheme. Energy Minimization Methods in Comp. Vision and Pattern Recog., 349–364 (2005)

17. O'Hara, T., Virág, L., Varró, A., Rudy, Y.: Simulation of the undiseased human cardiac ventricular action potential: model formulation and experimental validation. PLoS Computational Biology 7(5) (2011)

18. Nygren, A., Fiset, C., Firek, L., Clark, J., Lindblad, D., Clark, R., Giles, W.: Mathematical model of an adult human atrial cell: The role of K+ currents in repolarization. Circulation Research 82(1), 63–81 (1998)

19. Iravanian, S., Tung, L.: A novel algorithm for cardiac biosignal filtering based on filtered residue method. IEEE Transactions on Biomedical Engineering 49(11), 1310–1317 (2002)

# Segmentation of the Left Ventricle Using Distance Regularized Two-Layer Level Set Approach

Chaolu Feng[1,2], Chunming Li[2,*], Dazhe Zhao[1], Christos Davatzikos[2], and Harold Litt[3]

[1] Key Laboratory of Medical Image Computing of Ministry of Education, Northeastern University, Shenyang, LiaoNing 110819, China
[2] Center for Biomedical Image Computing and Analytics, University of Pennsylvania, Philadelphia, PA 19104, USA
Chunming.Li@uphs.upenn.edu
[3] Department of Radiology, University of Pennsylvania, Philadelphia, PA 19104, USA

**Abstract.** We propose a novel two-layer level set approach for segmentation of the left ventricle (LV) from cardiac magnetic resonance (CMR) short-axis images. In our method, endocardium and epicardium are represented by two specified level contours of a level set function. Segmentation of the LV is formulated as a problem of optimizing the level set function such that these two level contours best fit the epicardium and endocardium. More importantly, a distance regularization (DR) constraint on the level contours is introduced to preserve smoothly varying distance between them. This DR constraint leads to a desirable interaction between the level contours that contributes to maintain the anatomical geometry of the endocardium and epicardium. The negative influence of intensity inhomogeneities on image segmentation are overcome by using a data term derived from a local intensity clustering property. Our method is quantitatively validated by experiments on the datasets for the MICCAI grand challenge on left ventricular segmentation, which demonstrates the advantages of our method in terms of segmentation accuracy and consistency with anatomical geometry.

## 1 Introduction

Non-invasive assessment of left ventricular function is an important part of the diagnosis and management of cardiovascular disease. Cine MRI has been proven to be an accurate and reproducible modality for quantitative evaluation of left ventricular function [1–6]. Relevant measurements include ventricular volume, mass, and cavity ejection fraction (EF), which are based on the results of delineation of endocardial and epicardial boundaries by segmentation techniques. However, LV segmentation is still a open problem and is challenging due to poor contrast between tissues around the epicardium and intensity inhomogeneities in cine CMR images.

---

[*] Corresponding author.

K. Mori et al. (Eds.): MICCAI 2013, Part I, LNCS 8149, pp. 477–484, 2013.
© Springer-Verlag Berlin Heidelberg 2013

Active contour models and level set methods have been extensively applied to image segmentation because they can provide smooth and closed contours as segmentation results and achieve sub-pixel accuracy for identification of object boundaries [7]. They have also been used to segment the LV in [3–6]. Zeng *et al.* proposed a coupled surfaces propagation method to extract the LV myocardium [3]. This method was further developed in [4] and [5]. In these methods, a hard constraint was imposed to force the distance between endocardium and epicardium to be within a given interval. Chung and Vese proposed a multilayer level set method to segment images by representing object boundaries as multiple level sets of a single level set function [6]. However, there is no constraint on the distance between level contours of the level set function in their method. In addition, none of the above-mentioned level set methods is able to deal with intensity inhomogeneities in the images.

In this paper, we propose a novel two-layer level set approach for segmentation of the LV from cine CMR short-axis images. In our method, the endocardium and epicardium are represented by two specified level contours of a level set function. The anatomical geometry of the LV is preserved by a distance regularization constraint on the level contours. The data term of our method, derived from a local intensity clustering property, is able to segment the images in the presence of intensity inhomogeneities [8].

## 2    Distance Regularized Two-Layer Level Set Method

### 2.1    Energy Formulation

We consider an image $I$ as a function $I : \Omega \to \Re$ defined on a continuous domain $\Omega$. Let $\phi : \Omega \to \Re$ be a *level set function*. We denote by $C_0$ and $C_k$ the 0-level and $k$-level contours of $\phi$, i.e. $C_0 \triangleq \{\mathbf{x} : \phi(\mathbf{x}) = 0\}$ and $C_k \triangleq \{\mathbf{x} : \phi(\mathbf{x}) = k\}$. We use the 0-level contour and $k$-level contour to represent the endocardium and epicardium. The contours $C_0$ and $C_k$ separate the image domain $\Omega$ into three regions: $\Omega_1 \triangleq \{\mathbf{x} : \phi(\mathbf{x}) < 0\}$, $\Omega_2 \triangleq \{\mathbf{x} : 0 < \phi(\mathbf{x}) < k\}$, and $\Omega_3 \triangleq \{\mathbf{x} : \phi(\mathbf{x}) > k\}$. According to the heart anatomy, the regions $\Omega_1$ and $\Omega_2$ represent the cavity and myocardium, respectively, and $\Omega_3$ the region outside the epicardium. Let $H$ be the Heaviside function, then the membership functions of these regions can be expressed as $M_1(\phi(\mathbf{x})) = 1 - H(\phi(\mathbf{x}))$, $M_2(\phi(\mathbf{x})) = H(\phi(\mathbf{x})) - H(\phi(\mathbf{x}) - k)$, and $M_3(\phi(\mathbf{x})) = H(\phi(\mathbf{x}) - k)$, with $M_i(\phi(\mathbf{x})) = 1$ for $\mathbf{x} \in \Omega_i$ and $M_i(\phi(\mathbf{x})) = 0$ for $\mathbf{x} \notin \Omega_i$.

In the ideal case that the thickness of the myocardium is a constant, the distance between the 0-level and the $k$-level contours of the level set function that represent the endocardial and epicardial contours is a constant. The equal distance between these two level contours can be ensured by the constraint that $|\nabla\phi(\mathbf{x})|$ is a constant. However, the actual thickness of myocardium is primarily smoothly varying. In this case, we force $|\nabla\phi(\mathbf{x})|$ to be a smooth function $\alpha(\mathbf{x})$ by imposing a constraint on $\phi$ as an energy functional, defined by

$$\mathcal{R}(\phi, \alpha) = \mu \int \frac{1}{2}(|\nabla\phi(\mathbf{x})| - \alpha(\mathbf{x}))^2 dx + \omega \int |\nabla\alpha(\mathbf{x})|^2 dx, \qquad (1)$$

where $\mu > 0$, $\omega > 0$ are the weighting coefficients. The first term forces $|\nabla\phi|$ to be a smooth function $\alpha(\mathbf{x})$, and the smoothness of $\alpha(\mathbf{x})$ is ensured by the second term. This energy $\mathcal{R}(\phi, \alpha)$ is used as the distance regularization term in conjunction with a data term and a length term, as defined below, in the proposed variational framework. It is worth noting that this DR term with $\alpha = 1$ was originally used by Li *et al.* in [9] to force the level set function to be close to a signed distance function, thereby eliminating the need for re-initialization in conventional level set methods. In this paper, the DR term is used for a different purpose, namely, to maintain smoothly varying distance between two level contours.

Note that, the distance between the 0-level and $k$-level contours depends on the values of $k$ and $|\nabla\phi|$. For a given value of $k$, the values of $|\nabla\phi|$ can be adaptively changed in the energy minimization process, such that the distance between the 0-level and $k$-level contours matches the actual distance between the endocardium and epicardium. Therefore, the choice of the level $k$ is flexible, and the result of our method is not sensitive to the choice of $k$. We set $k = 15$ for all the images in the experiments presented in this paper.

Due to the intensity inhomogeneities in CMR, the distributions of the intensities in the regions $\Omega_1$, $\Omega_2$, and $\Omega_3$ often overlap, which is a major challenge when using intensity based segmentation methods. To overcome this difficulty, we exploit the property of intensities in a relatively small circular neighborhood, in which the slowly varying bias can be ignored. This neighborhood can be defined by $\mathcal{O}_\mathbf{y} \triangleq \{\mathbf{x} : |\mathbf{x} - \mathbf{y}| \leq \rho\}$. The partition $\{\Omega_i\}_{i=1}^3$ of the entire domain $\Omega$ induces a partition of the neighborhood $\mathcal{O}_\mathbf{y}$, i.e., $\{\mathcal{O}_\mathbf{y} \cap \Omega_i\}_{i=1}^3$ forms a partition of $\mathcal{O}_\mathbf{y}$. For the slowly varying bias, image intensities in $\mathcal{O}_y \cap \Omega_1$, $\mathcal{O}_y \cap \Omega_2$, and $\mathcal{O}_y \cap \Omega_3$ can be approximated by three constants, denoted by $f_1(\mathbf{y})$, $f_2(\mathbf{y})$, and $f_3(\mathbf{y})$. Therefore, the intensities in the set $\mathbf{I}_i^\mathbf{y} = \{I(\mathbf{x}) : \mathbf{x} \in \mathcal{O}_y \cap \Omega_i\}$ form a cluster with cluster center $m_i \approx f_i(\mathbf{y}), i = 1, 2, 3$. This property of local intensities directs us to apply K-means clustering to classify these local intensities. Therefore, as in [8], we define a clustering criterion for classifying the intensities in $\mathcal{O}_y$ as follows

$$\mathcal{E}_\mathbf{y} = \sum_{i=1}^3 \lambda_i \int_{\mathcal{O}_y \cap \Omega_i} K_\rho(\mathbf{x} - \mathbf{y})|I(\mathbf{x}) - f_i(\mathbf{y})|^2 d\mathbf{x} \tag{2}$$

where $\lambda_1$, $\lambda_2$, and $\lambda_3$ are the weighting coefficients and $K_\rho$ is a kernel function $K_\rho : \Re^n \to [0, +\infty)$, defined by $K_\rho(\mathbf{u}) = a$ for $|\mathbf{u}| \leq \rho$ and $K_\rho(\mathbf{u}) = 0$ for $|\mathbf{u}| > \rho$, where $a > 0$ is a normalization factor such that $\int_{|\mathbf{u}| \leq \rho} K_\rho(\mathbf{u}) = 1$. A desired segmentation can be achieved by seeking an optimal partition $\{\Omega_i\}_{i=1}^3$ and optimal fitting functions $f_1(\mathbf{y})$, $f_2(\mathbf{y})$, and $f_3(\mathbf{y})$, such that $\mathcal{E}_\mathbf{y}$ is minimized for all $\mathbf{y} \in \Omega$. Since $K_\rho(\mathbf{x} - \mathbf{y}) = 0$ for $\mathbf{x} \notin \mathcal{O}_y$, we can rewrite $\mathcal{E}_\mathbf{y}$ as

$$\mathcal{E}_\mathbf{y} = \sum_{i=1}^3 \lambda_i \int K_\rho(\mathbf{x} - \mathbf{y})|I(\mathbf{x}) - f_i(\mathbf{y})|^2 M_i(\phi(\mathbf{x}))d\mathbf{x}, \tag{3}$$

where $M_i(\phi(\mathbf{x}))$ is the membership functions of the region $\Omega_i$ as defined earlier.

As mentioned earlier, the energy $\mathcal{E}_{\mathbf{y}}$ should be minimized for all $\mathbf{y} \in \Omega$. This can be achieved by minimizing the integral of $\mathcal{E}_{\mathbf{y}}$ with respect to the neighborhood center $\mathbf{y}$, which is the energy functional $\mathcal{E}$ defined by

$$\mathcal{E}(\phi, f_1, f_2, f_3) = \sum_{i=1}^{3} \lambda_i \int \left( \int K_\rho(\mathbf{x} - \mathbf{y}) |I(\mathbf{x}) - f_i(\mathbf{y})|^2 M_i(\phi(\mathbf{x})) d\mathbf{x} \right) d\mathbf{y}. \quad (4)$$

As in most active contour models, we smooth the contours by penalizing their lengths. Therefore, we define

$$\mathcal{L}(\phi) = \nu_1 \int |\nabla H(\phi(\mathbf{x}))| d\mathbf{x} + \nu_2 \int |\nabla H(\phi(\mathbf{x}) - k)| d\mathbf{x}, \quad (5)$$

where the first term and the second term compute the arc lengths of the 0-level and $k$-level contours, respectively.

With the energy terms $\mathcal{R}(\phi, \alpha)$, $\mathcal{E}(\phi, f_1, f_2, f_3)$, and $\mathcal{L}(\phi)$ defined above, we propose to minimize the following energy functional:

$$\mathcal{F}(\phi, \alpha, f_1, f_2, f_3) = \mathcal{R}(\phi, \alpha) + \mathcal{E}(\phi, f_1, f_2, f_3) + \mathcal{L}(\phi). \quad (6)$$

## 2.2    Energy Minimization

Minimization of the energy $\mathcal{F}(\phi, \alpha, f_1, f_2, f_3)$ can be achieved by alternately minimizing $\mathcal{F}$ with respect to each of its variables. The energy minimization process starts with an initialization of the level set function $\phi$ and the smooth function $\alpha$. The smooth function $\alpha$ can be initialized as a constant function, i.e. $\alpha = c$ with $c > 0$ being a constant. After a number of iterations of the level set function, the function is updated as the minimizer of the energy $\mathcal{R}(\phi, \alpha)$ given the updated $\phi$ in previous iteration. The minimization of $\mathcal{R}(\phi, \alpha)$ with respect to $\alpha$ can be achieved by solving the gradient flow equation derived from the energy $\mathcal{R}(\phi, \alpha)$, which is a standard heat equation. The heat equation can be solved approximately by a convolution of the function $|\nabla \phi|$ with a Gaussian kernel. For a fixed level set function $\phi$, we minimize $\mathcal{F}(\phi, \alpha, f_1, f_2, f_3)$, or equivalently minimize $\mathcal{E}(\phi, f_1, f_2, f_3)$, with respect to $f_1$, $f_2$, and $f_3$, since the energy $\mathcal{R}(\phi, \alpha)$ and $\mathcal{L}(\phi)$ are independent of $f_1$, $f_2$, and $f_3$. It can be shown that the energy $\mathcal{E}$ is minimized by

$$f_i = \frac{K_\rho(\mathbf{x}) * [M_i(\phi(\mathbf{x})) I(\mathbf{x})]}{K_\rho(\mathbf{x}) * M_i(\phi(\mathbf{x}))} \qquad i = 1, 2, 3. \quad (7)$$

For fixed $f_1$, $f_2$, and $f_3$, we minimize the energy functional $\mathcal{F}$ with respect to $\phi$ using the standard gradient descent method and obtain

$$\frac{\partial \phi}{\partial t} = \lambda_1 e_1(\mathbf{x}) \delta(\phi(\mathbf{x})) - \lambda_2 e_2(\mathbf{x})(\delta(\phi(\mathbf{x})) - \delta(\phi(\mathbf{x}) - k)) - \lambda_3 e_3(\mathbf{x}) \delta(\phi(\mathbf{x}) - k)$$

$$+ (\nu_1 \delta(\phi(\mathbf{x})) + \nu_2 \delta(\phi(\mathbf{x}) - k)) \operatorname{div}\left( \frac{\nabla \phi(\mathbf{x})}{|\nabla \phi(\mathbf{x})|} \right)$$

$$+ \mu \left( \nabla^2 \phi(\mathbf{x}) - \alpha(\mathbf{x}) \operatorname{div}\left( \frac{\nabla \phi(\mathbf{x})}{|\nabla \phi(\mathbf{x})|} \right) \right) \qquad (8)$$

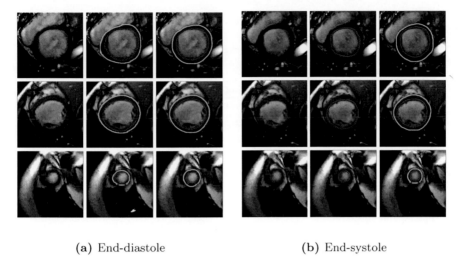

(a) End-diastole                    (b) End-systole

**Fig. 1.** Results of our method (right column) and ground truth (middle column) for the images from case SC-HF-NI-11 at end-diastole shown in (a) and end-systole in (b). Each row shows one of three slices in an 3D image in the left column.

where $e_i(\mathbf{x}) = \int K_\sigma(\mathbf{y} - \mathbf{x})|I(\mathbf{x}) - f_i(\mathbf{y})|^2 dy$, $i = 1, 2, 3$ and $\delta$ is the Dirac delta function, which is the derivative of $H$. In the implementation, we use the smooth function $H_\epsilon(x) = [1 + (2/\pi)arctan(x/\epsilon)]/2$ to approximate the Heaviside function $H$ with $\epsilon = 1$ and use $\delta_\epsilon(x) = (\epsilon/(\epsilon^2 + x^2))/\pi$ to approximate the Dirac delta function $\delta$ as in [8].

## 3    Results and Discussions

We implemented the level set evolution in Eq. (8) by using standard finite difference scheme as in [8]. Time step $\triangle t$ used in the approximation of temporal derivative is set to $\triangle t = 0.1$. For the data used in this paper, we set the other parameters $\rho = 6$, $\mu = 1$, $\omega = 1$, $\lambda_1 = 0.25$, $\lambda_2 = 1.5$, $\lambda_3 = 0.1$, and $\nu_1 = \nu_2 = 0.05 \times 255 \times 255$.

Our method has been validated on the datasets from the MICCAI challenge on left ventricular segmentation (http://smial.sri.utoronto.ca/LV_Challenge/Home.html), which consist of 15 training datasets and 15 validation datasets from a mix of patients and pathologies: healthy (SC-N), hypertrophy (SC-HYP), heart failure with infarction (SC-HF-I), and heart failure with nonischemic disease (SC-HF-NI). Fig. 1 shows our segmentation results and the ground truth for case SC-HF-NI-11 from the datasets. Note that there is no ground truth provided in the challenge for epicardial contour at end-systole. The obtained contours appear to be quite close to the ground truth.

We compared our segmentation results with the ground truth provided by the MICCAI challenge. The metrics for quantitative evaluation include average

**Table 1.** Detected and good percentages from the results of different methods

| | Training | | | | Validation | | | |
|---|---|---|---|---|---|---|---|---|
| | detected (%) | | good (%) | | detected (%) | | good (%) | |
| Method | endo | epi | endo | epi | endo | epi | endo | epi |
| [11] | - | - | - | - | 77.8±17.4 | 85.7±14.1 | 72.5±19.5 | 81.1±14.0 |
| [12] | - | - | - | - | 99.7±1.4 | 100 | 86.4±11.0 | 94.2±7.0 |
| [13] | - | - | 88.4±10.2 | 92.9±6.5 | - | - | 92.3±6.1 | 92.2±5.0 |
| [10] | 100 | 100 | 96.9±7.6 | 99.1±3.6 | 100 | 100 | 94.3±9.9 | 95.6±6.9 |
| Ours | 100 | 100 | 95.4±5.9 | 100 | 100 | 100 | 92.8±9.2 | 96.6±8.1 |

'-' means no value was reported in this paper.

**Table 2.** Comparison of contour accuracy in terms of average perpendicular distance and dice coefficient

| | Training | | | | Validation | | | |
|---|---|---|---|---|---|---|---|---|
| | APD (mm) | | DM | | APD (mm) | | DM | |
| Method | endo | epi | endo | epi | endo | epi | endo | epi |
| [11] | - | - | - | - | 2.07±0.61 | 1.91±0.63 | 0.89±0.03 | 0.94±0.02 |
| [12] | - | - | - | - | 2.29±0.57 | 2.28±0.39 | 0.89±0.03 | 0.93±0.01 |
| [13] | 2.04±0.47 | 2.35±0.57 | 0.89±0.04 | 0.92±0.02 | 2.04±0.47 | 2.35±0.57 | 0.89±0.04 | 0.92±0.02 |
| [10] | 2.09±0.53 | 1.88±0.40 | 0.88±0.06 | 0.93±0.01 | 2.44±0.62 | 2.05±0.59 | 0.88±0.03 | 0.93±0.02 |
| [14] | 2.03±0.34 | 2.28±0.42 | 0.90±0.04 | 0.93±0.02 | 2.10±0.44 | 1.95±0.34 | 0.89±0.04 | 0.94±0.01 |
| [15] | 3.00±0.59 | 2.60±0.38 | 0.86±0.04 | 0.93±0.01 | 3.00±0.59 | 2.60±0.38 | 0.86±0.04 | 0.93±0.01 |
| Ours | 1.82±0.48 | 1.73±0.43 | 0.89±0.06 | 0.94±0.02 | 1.93±0.37 | 1.64±0.42 | 0.89±0.04 | 0.94±0.02 |

'-' means no value reported in this paper; in [13] and [15], only one APD and one DM were provided and there was no clarification about the datasets: training, validation, or together.

perpendicular distance (APD) and the dice metric (DM). In the evaluation criterion, if the APD between the ground truth and the detected contour is less than 5mm, the detected contour is graded as *good*. The quotient formed by dividing the number of detected contours by the number of contours from the ground truth is named as *detected percentage*. Division of the number of good contours by the number of detected contours is called the *good percentage*. Although eight methods were evaluated in the challenge, only four provided the detected and good percentage statistic for their methods. These results are shown together with ours in Table 1. We obtained the highest detected percentage, which is exactly 100% both for endocardial (endo) and epicardial (epi) contours on the training and validation datasets. Although the good percentage for our endocardial contours is 1.5 percent lower than the method in [10], we achieved the highest good percentage for the epicardial contour.

Six out of the eight methods in the challenge provided APDs and DMs for their methods, shown in Table 2 together with these measurements obtained using our method. The statistics of the DMs for our method are similar to the other methods in both the training and validation datasets; however, the statistics of the APDs for our method are the smallest: 1.82±0.48 mm and 1.73±0.43 mm for

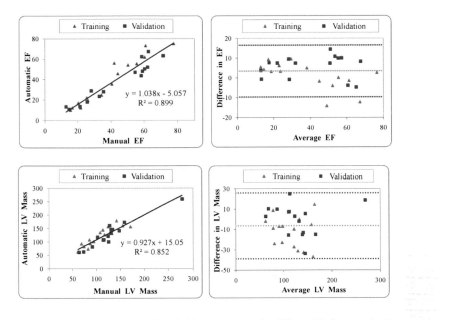

**Fig. 2.** Regression curves and Bland-Altman plots for EF and left ventricular mass

the training datasets and 1.93±0.37 mm and 1.64±0.42 mm for the validation datasets. This demonstrates that our contours are closest to the ground truth.

Linear regression and Bland-Altman plots for the EF and LV mass obtained by our method are shown in Fig. 2. In this challenge, the linear regression and Bland-Altman plots for EF and LV mass are provided in [10], in which the slope, regression coefficient, and bias on Bland-Altman plots were 1.17, 0.92, -5.22% for EF and 0.77, 0.72, 18.38 grams for LV mass. The corresponding metrics for our method are overall better than those provided in [10].

## 4   Conclusion

We have proposed a distance regularized two-layer level set model for segmentation of LV from CMR short-axis images. The distance regularization term in our method has a desirable effect of maintaining the smoothly varying distance between the two specified level contours that represent the endocardium and epicardium. We have validated our method on the MICCAI challenge datasets. Quantitative evaluation and comparison with other state-of-the-art methods demonstrate the advantages of our method in terms of segmentation accuracy and the ability to preserve the anatomical geometry of the extracted endocardial and epicardial contours.

# References

1. Petitjean, C., Dacher, J.N.: A review of segmentation methods in short axis cardiac MR images. Med. Image Anal. 15(2), 169–184 (2011)
2. Lorenzo-Valdés, M., Sanchez-Ortiz, G.I., Elkington, A.G., Mohiaddin, R.H., Rueckert, D.: Segmentation of 4-D cardiac MR images using a probabilistic atlas and the EM algorithm. Med. Image Anal. 8(3), 255–265 (2004)
3. Zeng, X., Staib, L.H., Schultz, R.T., Duncan, J.S.: Volumetric layer segmentation using coupled surfaces propagation. In: IEEE Conference on Computer Vision and Pattern Recognition (CVPR), pp. 708–715 (1998)
4. Paragios, N.: A variational approach for the segmentation of the left ventricle in cardiac image analysis. Int. J. Comput. Vis. 50(3), 345–362 (2002)
5. Lynch, M., Ghita, O., Whelan, P.F.: Left-ventricle myocardium segmentation using a coupled level-set with a priori knowledge. Comput. Med. Imaging Graph. 30(4), 255–262 (2006)
6. Chung, G., Vese, L.A.: Energy minimization based segmentation and denoising using a multilayer level set approach. In: Rangarajan, A., Vemuri, B.C., Yuille, A.L. (eds.) EMMCVPR 2005. LNCS, vol. 3757, pp. 439–455. Springer, Heidelberg (2005)
7. Li, C., Xu, C., Gui, C., Fox, M.D.: Distance regularized level set evolution and its application to image segmentation. IEEE Trans. Image Processing 19(12), 3243–3254 (2010)
8. Li, C., Kao, C., Gore, J.C., Ding, Z.: Minimization of region-scalable fitting energy for image segmentation. IEEE Trans. Image Processing 17(10), 1940–1949 (2008)
9. Li, C., Xu, C., Gui, C., Fox, M.D.: Level set evolution without re-initialization: a new variational formulation. In: IEEE Conference on Computer Vision and Pattern Recognition (CVPR), pp. 430–436 (2005)
10. Jolly, M.P.: Fully automatic left ventricle segmentation incardiac cine MR images using registration and minimum surfaces. The MIDAS Journal - Cardia MR Left Ventricle Segmentation Challenge (2009)
11. Lu, Y., Radau, P., Connelly, K., Dick, A., Wright, G.: Automatic image-driven segmentation of left ventricle in cardiac cine MRI. The MIDAS Journal - Cardia MR Left Ventricle Segmentation Challenge (2009)
12. Wijnhout, J., Hendriksen, D., Assen, H.V., der Geest, R.V.: LV challenge LKEB contribution: fully automated myocardial contour detection. The MIDAS Journal - Cardia MR Left Ventricle Segmentation Challenge (2009)
13. Constantinides, C., Chenoune, Y., Kachenoura, N., Roullot, E., Mousseaux, E., Herment, A., Frouin, F.: Semi-automated cardiac segmentation on cine magnetic resonance images using GVF-Snake deformable models. The MIDAS Journal - Cardia MR Left Ventricle Segmentation Challenge (2009)
14. Huang, S., Liu, J., Lee, L.C., Venkatesh, S.K., Teo, L.L.S., Au, C., Nowinski, W.L.: Segmentation of the left ventricle from cine MR images using a comprehensive approach. The MIDAS Journal - Cardia MR Left Ventricle Segmentation Challenge (2009)
15. Marák, L., Cousty, J., Najman, L., Talbot, H.: 4D morphological segmentation and the MICCAI LV-Segmentation grand challenge. The MIDAS Journal - Cardia MR Left Ventricle Segmentation Challenge (2009)

# Automated Segmentation and Geometrical Modeling of the Tricuspid Aortic Valve in 3D Echocardiographic Images

Alison M. Pouch[1], Hongzhi Wang[2], Manabu Takabe[1], Benjamin M. Jackson[1,3],
Chandra M. Sehgal[2], Joseph H. Gorman III[1,3], Robert C. Gorman[1,3],
and Paul A. Yushkevich[2]

[1] Gorman Cardiovascular Research Group
[2] Department of Radiology
[3] Department of Surgery,
University of Pennsylvania, Philadelphia, PA, USA

**Abstract.** The aortic valve has been described with variable anatomical definitions, and the consistency of 2D manual measurement of valve dimensions in medical image data has been questionable. Given the importance of image-based morphological assessment in the diagnosis and surgical treatment of aortic valve disease, there is considerable need to develop a standardized framework for 3D valve segmentation and shape representation. Towards this goal, this work integrates template-based medial modeling and multi-atlas label fusion techniques to automatically delineate and quantitatively describe aortic leaflet geometry in 3D echocardiographic (3DE) images, a challenging task that has been explored only to a limited extent. The method makes use of expert knowledge of aortic leaflet image appearance, generates segmentations with consistent topology, and establishes a shape-based coordinate system on the aortic leaflets that enables standardized automated measurements. In this study, the algorithm is evaluated on 11 3DE images of normal human aortic leaflets acquired at mid systole. The clinical relevance of the method is its ability to capture leaflet geometry in 3DE image data with minimal user interaction while producing consistent measurements of 3D aortic leaflet geometry.

**Keywords:** medial axis representation, deformable modeling, multi-atlas segmentation, aortic valve, 3D echocardiography.

## 1 Introduction

The aortic valve regulates blood flow from the left ventricle to the ascending aorta and is an integral component of physiological cardiac function. In elderly populations, the valve is frequently affected by degenerative pathology, generally manifesting as stenosis or narrowing of the valve orifice. Aortic valve replacement is a commonly performed and preferred surgical treatment for aortic stenosis [1], and the emergence of transcatheter implantation has increased the patient population eligible for surgical intervention. For accurate prosthesis selection, these procedures require precise

K. Mori et al. (Eds.): MICCAI 2013, Part I, LNCS 8149, pp. 485–492, 2013.

knowledge of aortic valve dimensions, which are conventionally specified by 2D manual measurement of echocardiographic or fluoroscopic images. However, agreement between multi-modal measurements has been equivocal [2-4], most likely because manually derived 2D metrics are limited in their capability to characterize complex 3D valvular geometry. Moreover, there is a surprising lack of consensus in the description of aortic valve geometry, particularly the annulus, which has been defined in markedly different ways [5]. Given the importance of quantitative metrics for diagnostics and treatment planning, there is need for a standardized framework for pre-operative image-based guidance of aortic valve surgery.

Limited work has been devoted to studying in vivo aortic valve geometry, most of which has been performed in ovine subjects [6] or in humans with manual 2D analysis of echocardiographic and multislice computed tomography (MSCT) images [2-4,7]. A few automated methods have been developed to segment the aortic root in MSCT data [8-9], but they do not delineate the aortic leaflets (also referred to as cusps). One proposed segmentation method parametrically represents both the 3D aortic root and leaflet geometry in MSCT images [10]. Thus, the algorithm presented here is one of few methods for automated 3D aortic leaflet shape analysis. The novelty of our work is in the generation of a volumetric segmentation from 3DE data that represents the aortic leaflets as structures with locally varying thickness. The advantage of using 3DE is that it facilitates 3D in vivo measurement of the aortic leaflets, is practical for routine use in the operating room, and does not require radiation exposure or contrast injection. Our method is a unique integration of multi-atlas segmentation and deformable medial modeling techniques, which incorporate expert knowledge of leaflet image appearance in the image analysis task. The algorithm is tested on systolic 3DE images acquired from normal subjects, a challenging application given the user-dependence of ultrasound image acquisition.

## 2     Materials and Methods

### 2.1     Materials

Electrocardiographically gated 3DE images of the aortic valve were acquired from 11 human subjects with normal aortic valve structure and function. The image data were acquired with the iE33 platform (Philips Medical Systems, Andover, MA) using a 2 to 7 MHz matrix-array transesophageal transducer over several consecutive cardiac cycles. The image acquisition protocol did not specify constraints on image orientation or field of view. From each subject's data set, a 3DE image of the open aortic valve at mid systole was selected for analysis. The images were exported in Cartesian format with an approximate size of 224 x 208 x 208 voxels with nearly isotropic resolution ranging between 0.4 to 0.8 mm.

### 2.2     Manual Segmentation

The 11 3DE images of the aortic valve were manually segmented in ITK-SNAP [11]. An expert observer identified the left coronary, non-coronary, and right coronary cusps, associating each with a separate label. In addition, three landmarks were

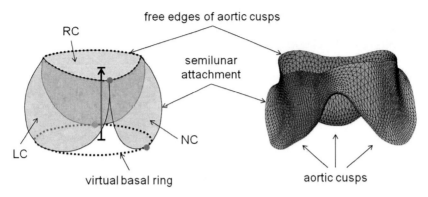

**Fig. 1.** (Left) Schematic of the aortic cusps at systole. The valve orifice is the area enclosed by the cusp free edges, and the virtual basal ring connects the basal attachments of the cusps. Valve height is the distance between the virtual basal ring and valve orifice, shown by the black arrow pointing in the direction of blood flow. Three manually identified landmarks are shown in blue. (Right) The triangulated medial template of the aortic cusps used to initialize deformable modeling. (RC = right coronary cusp, LC = left coronary cusp, NC = non-coronary cusp)

identified: the basal attachment of the non-coronary cusp, the basal attachment of the right coronary cusp, and the non-coronary commissure, illustrated in Fig. 1.

### 2.3    Automated Image Analysis

Automated segmentation and geometrical modeling of the aortic valve in a target image requires a deformable template of the aortic cusps and a set of probability maps, which assign each voxel in the target image a probability of having a given label. The deformable model is a medial axis representation of the aortic leaflets, and the probability maps are derived from multi-atlas joint label fusion, a technique that uses a set of expert-labeled 3DE images (atlases) of the aortic valve to generate a probabilistic segmentation of the target image. To represent aortic leaflet shape in the target image, the template is deformed to optimize a posterior probability in which the Bayesian likelihood is a function of the probability maps obtained by joint label fusion. In the segmentation process, multi-atlas label fusion and deformable medial modeling are complementary techniques: label fusion uses expert knowledge of aortic valve image appearance to estimate voxel-wise label probabilities in the target image, and deformable medial modeling ensures the topological consistency of the segmentations and identifies correspondences on different instances of the aortic valve. The combination of these capabilities facilitates standardized automated measurements of aortic cusp morphology in 3DE image data.

**Multi-atlas Segmentation.** Multi-atlas segmentation uses a small number of expert-labeled images, referred to as atlases, to make separate guesses at the segmentation of the target image. While the guesses are not accurate on their own, they are combined into a more robust segmentation result using a consensus-seeking scheme called label fusion. The present study makes use of *joint* label fusion, an extension of multi-atlas label fusion with spatially-varying weighted voting that reduces segmentation errors produced by redundancies in the atlas set. To perform multi-atlas segmentation, intensity-based registration is performed between all reference atlases and the target image. Registration consists of two stages. First, a global affine registration with six degrees of freedom is obtained by aligning the three landmarks identified during manual segmentation. Second, a B-spline free-form deformable registration is performed [12]. Cross-correlation is the similarity metric used for registration, and a Gaussian regularizer with sigma = 3 is applied. Finally, each atlas is warped into the target image space to generate a candidate segmentation of the target image. A probabilistic consensus segmentation of the three aortic cusps is generated using the joint label fusion method described in [13].

**Deformable Medial Modeling.** The anatomical shape model used in this work is 3D continuous medial representation (cm-rep), which describes the geometry of an object in terms of its medial axis (or morphological skeleton) [14]. The medial axis is defined as the locus of centers of maximally inscribed balls of the object. In this framework, an object is parameterized by $\{\mathbf{m}, R\} \in \mathbb{R}^3 \times \mathbb{R}^+$, where $\mathbf{m}$ is one or a combination of continuous medial manifolds and $R$ is a radial thickness field defined over the medial manifold(s). Each point $\mathbf{m}$ on the medial axis is associated with a scalar value $R$, the radius of the maximally inscribed ball centered at that point. The template-based approach to medial modeling involves first explicitly defining the object's skeletal topology in a deformable model or template. The template parameters $\{\mathbf{m}, R\}$ are modified to obtain the skeleton of an instance of the anatomic structure in a target image. Then the boundary of the structure, defined as the envelope of its maximally inscribed balls, is derived analytically from the medial axis according to the inverse skeletonization equations given in [14]. The medial model imposes a shape-based coordinate system on the anatomic structure that associates each point on the medial manifold $\mathbf{m}$ with one or more profiles of length $R$ that extend from the medial axis to unique surface patches on the object boundary.

In this work, the three aortic valve cusps are modeled as a single object with a non-branching medial manifold. The manifold is discretely represented as a triangulated mesh, which can be sequentially Loop subdivided to a continuous limit. The medial template is generated using a method similar to that described in [15]. The 2D domain of the 3D medial mesh is homeomorphic to an annulus, in which the inner contour maps to the leaflet free edges and the outer contour maps to the semilunar attachments. The medial model of the aortic valve (Fig. 1) has 95 nodes on the leaflet free edges, 163 on the semilunar attachment curve, 1784 on the interior of the medial manifold, and 3824 total nodes on the model boundary. Each medial node is associated with five parameters: $(m_x, m_y, m_z, R, l)$, where $(m_x, m_y, m_z)$ refer to the 3D coordinates of a point on the medial axis and $R$ is the distance between that point and the leaflet's arterial and ventricular surfaces. The parameter $l$ refers to the leaflet label: $l = 1$ is the left coronary cusp, $l = 2$ is the non-coronary cusp, and $l = 3$ is the right coronary cusp. The medial template is initialized with a constant radial thickness: $R = 2$ mm.

Given a target 3DE image $I(x)$ of the aortic valve, a deformable medial template $M$, and a set of probability maps $\{P^l(x): l = 0,1,2,3\}$ obtained by multi-atlas joint label fusion, the medial template is deformed to minimize the negative log of the posterior probability $p(M|I)$, which is proportional to a likelihood function $p(I|M)$ and prior probability $p(M)$. The negative log of the Bayesian likelihood is a probability integral term given by

$$-\log(p(I|M)) \sim 1 - \frac{\Sigma_l P^l(x)|_{M_l}}{I_{volume}},$$
(1)

where $l$ indexes through each label, $x$ indexes through the image voxels, $I_{volume}$ is the target image volume, and $M_l$ represents the part of the model $M$ associated with label $l$. $M_0$ refers to the exterior of the model (background). The Bayesian prior probability is modeled as a sum of validity constraints on medial geometry ($T_{validity}$, detailed in [15]), and a regularization component that acts on the model's two medial edges:

$$-\log(p(M)) \sim T_{validity} + \Sigma_i(1 - \cos(\theta_i)) + \Sigma_j(1 - \cos(\phi_j))$$
(2)

Here, $\theta_i$ is the angle between the outward normals of adjacent nodes $\mathbf{m}_i$ and $\mathbf{m}_{i+1}$ on the leaflet free edges, and $\phi_j$ is the angle between adjacent line segments formed by nodes $\mathbf{m}_{j-1}$ and $\mathbf{m}_j$ and nodes $\mathbf{m}_j$ and $\mathbf{m}_{j+1}$ on the leaflet attachment sites. In effect, the first regularization term encourages the leaflet free edges to point away from the ventricle into the aortic outflow tract, while the second term prevents rippling of the crown-shaped semilunar attachments during model deformation. The deformable model is rigidly initialized by aligning the three manually identified landmarks in the target image to those labeled on the deformable model. Optimization is performed by conjugate gradient descent.

## 3    Results

Segmentation and geometric modeling were evaluated in a leave-one-out cross-validation experiment using manual image segmentation for comparison. The Dice overlap and mean boundary displacement metrics were used for comparison. The accuracy of each step in the segmentation process is given in Table 1, and an example of aortic leaflet segmentation is given in Fig. 2.

**Table 1.** The accuracy of each segementation step. The 95th percentile distance indicates the maximum distance of 95 percent of boundary points on the deformed model from the surface of the manual segmentation. The fourth column indicates the accuracy of model fitting directly to the manual segmentation.

|  | Candidate segmentation (average) | Consensus segmentation | Model-based segmentation | Model fitted to manual segmentation |
|---|---|---|---|---|
| Dice overlap | $0.46 \pm 0.08$ | $0.74 \pm 0.3$ | $0.74 \pm 0.3$ | $0.84 \pm 0.02$ |
| Displacement (mm) | | | | |
| Mean | $0.9 \pm 0.4$ | $0.4 \pm 0.1$ | $0.5 \pm 0.1$ | $0.3 \pm 0.1$ |
| Maximum | $6.9 \pm 4.5$ | $3.5 \pm 0.7$ | $3.2 \pm 0.8$ | $2.7 \pm 0.7$ |
| 95$^{th}$ percentile | $3.5 \pm 1.7$ | $0.9 \pm 0.3$ | $1.0 \pm 0.2$ | $0.7 \pm 0.1$ |

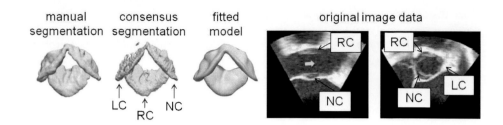

**Fig. 2.** A manual segmentation, consensus segmentation generated by label fusion, and fitted medial model. The model-based segmentation is shown in red (right). The yellow arrow points in the direction of blood flow. (LC, RC, NC = left, right, and non-coronary cusps).

Table 2 lists a number of clinically relevant measurements that were automatically derived from the model-based segmentation. The measures were compared to those computed when the deformable model was fitted directly to the manual segmentation, the accuracy of which is presented in Table 1. For each measurement, the mean ± standard deviation, the bias and limits of agreement given by Bland-Altman analysis, and the Pearson correlation coefficient are provided.

**Table 2.** Comparison of measurements obtained from the automated segmentation and from model fitting to the manual segmentation. (stdev = standard deviation, $R_{coeff}$ = Pearson coefficient, VOA = valve orifice area, BROA = basal ring orifice area, $VOD_{mean}$ = mean valve orifice diameter, $BRD_{mean}$ = mean basal ring diameter, AH = aortic valve height, $SA_{LC}$ = surface area of the left coronary cusp, $SA_{NC}$ = surface area of the non-coronary cusp, $SA_{RC}$ = surface area of the right coronary cusp, $R_{mean}$ = mean radial thickness).

| | Manual (mean ± stdev) | Automated (mean ± stdev) | Bias | Limits of agreement | $R_{coeff}$ |
|---|---|---|---|---|---|
| VOA | $2.63 \pm 0.47$ cm$^2$ | $2.91 \pm 0.71$ cm$^2$ | 0.27 cm$^2$ | -0.55 to 1.09 cm$^2$ | 0.828 |
| BROA | $5.27 \pm 0.69$ cm$^2$ | $5.38 \pm 1.04$ cm$^2$ | 0.11 cm$^2$ | -1.17 to 1.39 cm$^2$ | 0.791 |
| $VOD_{mean}$ | $18.2 \pm 1.7$ mm | $19.2 \pm 2.3$ mm | 1.0 mm | -1.7 to 3.7 mm | 0.808 |
| $BRD_{mean}$ | $25.9 \pm 1.7$ mm | $26.1 \pm 2.5$ mm | 0.2 mm | -3.0 to 3.5 mm | 0.749 |
| AH | $19.0 \pm 2.3$ mm | $17.9 \pm 1.6$ mm | -1.1 mm | -4.7 to 2.5 mm | 0.612 |
| $SA_{LC}$ | $3.93 \pm 0.92$ cm$^2$ | $3.47 \pm 0.61$ cm$^2$ | -0.46 cm$^2$ | -1.75 to 0.82 cm$^2$ | 0.703 |
| $SA_{NC}$ | $3.61 \pm 0.45$ cm$^2$ | $3.36 \pm 0.60$ cm$^2$ | -0.25 cm$^2$ | -1.04 to 0.54 cm$^2$ | 0.746 |
| $SA_{RC}$ | $3.87 \pm 0.53$ cm$^2$ | $3.78 \pm 0.69$ cm$^2$ | -0.09 cm$^2$ | -1.01 to 0.82 cm$^2$ | 0.732 |
| $R_{mean}$ | $0.8 \pm 0.3$ mm | $1.1 \pm 0.3$ mm | 0.3 mm | -0.04 to 0.75 mm | 0.715 |

## 4     Discussion

The proposed 3D aortic valve segmentation method combines the attractive properties of multi-atlas segmentation and deformable medial modeling to generate quantitatively descriptive representations of aortic leaflet anatomy in 3DE images. The algorithm begins by generating candidate segmentations of the target image, each produced by warping an individual atlas to the target image. Based on the metrics presented in

Table 1, the candidates on their own poorly approximate the manual segmentation. Joint label fusion, a robust consensus-seeking scheme, produces a more accurate segmentation of the target image, indicated by a dramatic improvement in the Dice overlap and boundary displacement metrics. While multi-atlas label fusion can segment the target image without the use of deformable modeling, it does not guarantee the topological consistency of different instances of the aortic leaflets. This is evidenced by the extraneous artifact and leaflet hole that can be seen in Fig. 2. Nor does multi-atlas segmentation establish correspondences on different aortic valve segmentations, which makes it difficult to automatically compute standardized measurements of aortic leaflet geometry. Deformable medial modeling complements label fusion by mapping each segmented aortic valve to a common shape-based coordinate system, imposing validity and regularization constraints during Bayesian optimization, and by explicitly encoding the topology of the aortic cusps in the deformable model. With the probability maps generated by joint label fusion, the cm-rep can accurately capture leaflet shape, which is demonstrated by a mean boundary displacement from the manual segmentation on the order of 1 voxel.

Since the measurements presented in Table 2 could not be manually computed with the software used for manual tracing, the measurements derived from the automated segmentation were compared to those obtained by fitting the model directly to the manual segmentation. The advantage of such a comparison is that all measurements are made in 3D using the same software and consistent anatomical definitions. The disadvantage is that the comparison may be affected by the error in model fitting to the manual segmentation presented in Table 1. The results in Table 2 demonstrate consistency between the measurements derived from the automated and manual segmentations. Our measurements of $BRD_{mean}$, BROA, and VOA are comparable to analogous measurements in normal subjects made by MSCT planimetry in [2] and [7].

Unlike most existing methods for aortic valve assessment, the only requisite user interaction of the algorithm is the identification of three landmarks, which are used to initialize deformable registration and model fitting. Although the algorithm has not yet been tested on diseased subjects, the goal of the study is to demonstrate the feasibility of applying the method to a normal population before extending the methodology to pathological assessment. Given our previous success in using cm-rep to model both normal and diseased mitral valves [15] and the parallels between mitral and aortic valve disease processes, we expect the proposed method to characterize normal and pathological aortic cusp geometry equally well. The development of this automated technique is a step towards creating a practical, informative tool for preoperative assessment of patient-specific aortic valve morphology.

**Acknowledgement.** This research was supported by an American Heart Association pre-doctoral fellowship (10PRE3510014) and the National Institutes of Health: HL063954, HL073021, and HL103723 from the NHLBI; AG037376 from the NIA; and EB014346 from the NIBIB.

# References

1. Bonow, R.O., Carabello, B.A., Chatterjee, K., de Leon Jr., A.C., Faxon, D.P., Freed, M.D., Gaasch, W.H., Lytle, B.W., Nishimura, R.A., O'Gara, P.T., O'Rourke, R.A., Otto, C.M., Shah, P.M., Shanewise, J.S., Smith Jr., S.C., Jacobs, A.K., Adams, C.D., Anderson, J.L., Antman, E.M., Fuster, V., Halperin, J.L., Hiratzka, L.F., Hunt, S.A., Nishimura, R., Page, R.L., Riegel, B.: ACC/AHA 2006 Guidelines for the Management of Patients with Valvular Heart Disease. J. Am. Coll. Cardiol. 48(3), e1–e148 (2006)
2. Akhtar, M., Tuzcu, E.M., Kapadia, S.R., Svensson, L.G., Greenberg, R.K., Roselli, E.E., Halliburton, S., Kurra, V., Schoenhagen, P., Sola, S.: Aortic Root Morphology in Patients Undergoing Percutaneous Aortic Valve Replacement: Evidence of Aortic Root Remodeling. J. Thorac. Cardiovasc. Surg. 137(4), 950–956 (2009)
3. Messika-Zeitoun, D., Serfaty, J.M., Brochet, E., Ducrocq, G., Lepage, L., Detaint, D., Hyafil, F., Himbert, D., Pasi, N., Laissy, J.P., Iung, B., Vahanian, A.: Multimodal Assessment of the Aortic Annulus Diameter: Implications for Transcatheter Aortic Valve Implantation. J. Am. Coll. Cardiol. 55(3), 186–194 (2010)
4. Moss, R.R., Ivens, E., Pasupati, S., Humphries, K., Thompson, C.R., Munt, B., Sinhal, A., Webb, J.G.: Role of Echocardiography in Percutaneous Aortic Valve Implantation. JACC Cardiovasc. Imaging. 1(1), 15–24 (2008)
5. Anderson, R.H.: The Clinical Anatomy of the Aortic Root. Heart 84, 670–673 (2000)
6. Dagum, P., Green, G.R., Nistal, F.J., Daughters, G.T., Timek, T.A., Foppiano, L.E., Bolger, A.F., Ingels Jr., N.B., Miller, D.C.: Deformational Dynamics of the Aortic Root: Modes and Physiologic Determinants. Circulation 100(19 suppl.), II54–II62 (1999)
7. Tops, L.F., Wood, D.A., Delgado, V., Schuijf, J.D., Mayo, J.R., Pasupati, S., Lamers, F.P., van der Wall, E.E., Schalij, M.J., Webb, J.G., Bax, J.J.: Noninvasive Evaluation of the Aortic Root with Multislice Computed Tomography Implications for Transcatheter Aortic Valve Replacement. JACC Cardiovasc. Imaging. 1(3), 321–330 (2008)
8. Wang, Q., Book, G., Contreras Ortiz, S.H., Primiano, C., McKay, R., Kodali, S., Sun, W.: Dimensional Analysis of Aortic Root Geometry during Diastole using 3D Models Reconstructed from Clinical 64-Slice Computed Tomography Images. Cardiovasc. Eng. Technol. 2(4), 324–333 (2011)
9. Zheng, Y., John, M., Liao, R., Nottling, A., Boese, J., Kempfert, J., Walther, T., Brockmann, G., Comaniciu, D.: Automatic Aorta Segmentation and Valve Landmark Detection in C-arm CT for Transcatheter Aortic Valve Implantation. IEEE Trans. Med. Imaging. 31(12), 2307–2321 (2012)
10. Ionasec, R.I., Tsymbal, A., Vitanovski, D., Georgescu, B., Zhou, S.K., Navab, N., Comaniciu, D.: Shape-Based Diagnosis of the Aortic Valve. In: Proc. SPIE Med. Imaging, vol. 7259 (2009)
11. Yushkevich, P.A., Piven, J., Hazlett, H.C., Smith, R.G., Ho, S., Gee, J.C., Gerig, G.: User-Guided 3D Active Contour Segmentation of Anatomical Structures: Significantly Improved Efficiency and Reliability. Neuroimage 31(3), 1116–1128 (2006)
12. Tustison, N.J., Avants, B.B., Gee, J.C.: Directly Manipulated Free-Form Deformation Image Registration. IEEE Trans. Image Process. 18(3), 624–635 (2009)
13. Wang, H., Suh, J.W., Das, S., Pluta, J., Craige, C., Yushkevich, P.: Multi-Atlas Segmentation with Joint Label Fusion. IEEE Trans. Pattern Anal. Mach. Intell. 35(3), 611–623 (2013)
14. Yushkevich, P.A., Zhang, H., Gee, J.C.: Continuous Medial Representation for Anatomical Structures. IEEE Trans. Med. Imaging. 25(12), 1547–1564 (2006)
15. Pouch, A.M., Yushkevich, P.A., Jackson, B.M., Jassar, A.S., Vergnat, M., Gorman III, J.H., Gorman, R.C., Sehgal, C.M.: Development of a Semi-Automated Method for Mitral Valve Modeling with Medial Axis Representation using 3D Ultrasound. Med. Phys. 39(2), 933–950 (2012)

# Cardiac Motion Estimation by Optimizing Transmural Homogeneity of the Myofiber Strain and Its Validation with Multimodal Sequences

Zhijun Zhang[1], David J. Sahn[1,2], and Xubo Song[1]

[1] Department of Biomedical Engineering
[2] Department of Pediatric Cardiology
Oregon Health and Science University
20000 NW Walker Road, Beaverton, OR 97006, USA
{zhangzhi,sahn,songx}@ohsu.edu

**Abstract.** Quantitative motion analysis from cardiac imaging is important to study the function of heart. Most of existing image-based motion estimation methods model the myocardium as an isotropically elastic continuum. We propose a novel anisotropic regularization method which enforces the transmural homogeneity of the strain along myofiber. The myofiber orientation in the end-diastolic frame is obtained by registering it with a diffusion tensor atlas. Our method is formulated in a diffeomorphic registration framework, and tested on multimodal cardiac image sequences of two subjects using 3D echocardiography and cine and tagged MRI. Results show that the estimated transformations in our method are more smooth and more accurate than those in isotropic regularization.

**Keywords:** Cardiac motion estimation, diffeomorphic registration, cardiac strain, myofiber orientation.

## 1 Introduction

Cardiac motion estimation is important to study the heart function and its disease mechanism. Cardiac images such as 3D echocardiography, cine-MRI and cardiac CT have been widely used for quantitative motion analysis. However, due to the low spatial and temporal resolution and the complexity of the cardiac biomechanics, accurate cardiac motion estimation is still a challenging problem.

Cardiac motion estimation is generally solved by using nonrigid registration methods. To make the deformation unique, various regularization methods have been proposed to utilize the prior knowledge of the myocardium shape and dynamics. Spatiotemporal smoothness has been used to regularize the deformations [1–3]. Particle trajectory smoothness, transformation symmetry and transitivity have been used to constrain the temporal smoothness [4, 5]. Diffeomorphic image registration has been proposed to estimate transformation as the end of a smoothly evolving process constrained by a differential equation [6] and it has been extended to motion estimation from multiple frames [7, 8]. Anatomical constraint such as myocardium incompressibility has also been used in [8, 9].

K. Mori et al. (Eds.): MICCAI 2013, Part I, LNCS 8149, pp. 493–500, 2013.
© Springer-Verlag Berlin Heidelberg 2013

In reality the myocardium has a fibrous structure and the myocardium motion are closely related to the myofiber orientation [10, 11]. Little effort has been made to incorporate the myofiber orientation as a constraint for motion estimation. Papademetris *et al.* [12] registered the consecutive frames by using a regularization term consisting of a strain energy of the transversely isotropic myofiber model. In our previous work [13], an anisotropic regularization is proposed to make the velocity field more smooth in the myofiber direction.

In this paper, we propose a regularization term to enforce the transmural homogeneity of myofiber strain. It is deduced from the knowledge that the mechanical load is distributed uniformly in the myocardium of healthy subjects [14]. Experiments have shown that optimization of the myofiber strain homogeneity can lead to reasonable myofiber orientations [15]. Tseng *et al.* [16] has shown reversely that the myofiber strain is transmurally uniform. We implement the proposed method in a diffeomorphic registration framework in which the velocity field is regularized to make the myofiber strain transmurally uniform. The myofiber orientation is obtained by registering the reference frame of the sequence with a diffusion tensor (DTI) myofiber atlas. We validate the proposed method with echocardiography and cine-MRI images of two healthy subjects. Results show that our method can derive transformations with more smooth transmural strain and higher tracking accuracy than isotropic regularization methods.

## 2   Method

### 2.1   Diffeomorphic Motion Estimation

We adopt a diffeomorphic registration for our motion estimation method. The deformation between time zero to $t$ is defined by a velocity field using a differential equation of $\frac{d\phi}{dt} = v(\phi(x,t),t), \phi(x,0) = x$, with $x \in \Omega \subset R^3, t \in [0,T]$ and $T = N_s - 1$ where $N_s$ is the number of frames. The motion estimation problem is stated as an optimization of a variational energy of the velocity field $v(x,t)$:

$$\hat{v} = arg \inf_{v \in V} \lambda \int_0^T E_{reg}(v)dt + \sum_{n=1}^{n=T} E_{SSD}(I_{n-1}(x), I_n(\phi_{n-1,n})). \qquad (1)$$

The first term is a regularizer to evaluate the spatiotemporal smoothness. The second term is a similarity measurement which evaluates the summed squared difference (SSD) between $I_{n-1}$ and the unwarped frame $I_n(\phi_{n-1,n})$, with $\phi_{n-1,n}$ being the deformation between $(n-1)$th and $n$th frames. $\lambda$ is the weighting to balance these two energy terms.

We parameterize the velocity field [8] and the solution of Eqn.(1) is obtained by numerical optimization. The velocity field is defined by a series of 3D B-spline functions at time $t_k(k = 0, 1, ..., N_t, t_k = k\Delta t, \Delta t = 1/N_f)$, with $N_f$ being the number of time steps between two consecutive frames, $N_t = N_f \times T$ being the total number of B-spline functions. The velocity field function at time point $t_k$ is defined as $v(x, t_k) = \sum c_{m;k}\beta(x - x_m)$, with $c_{m;k}$ being the control vectors located on a uniform grid of $x_m$ at $t_k$, $\beta(x - x_m)$ being the 3D B-spline kernel function at $\boldsymbol{x}_m$. The transformation $\boldsymbol{\phi}(\boldsymbol{x}, t)$ is expressed as the forward Euler integral of the velocity field $\boldsymbol{v}(\boldsymbol{x}, t)$ by assuming that the velocity of each point is piecewise constant within a time step. The diffeomorphism $\boldsymbol{\phi}_{n-1,n}$ is estimated by composition of all the small deformation defined by the velocity field between time $t_{(n-1)*N_f}$ and $t_{n*N_f}$:

$$\boldsymbol{\phi}_{n-1,n} = \prod_{(n-1)N_f}^{nN_f - 1} (\mathbf{Id} + \boldsymbol{v}_k), \tag{2}$$

with $\mathbf{Id}$ the identity transformation and $\boldsymbol{v}_k = \boldsymbol{v}(\boldsymbol{x}, t_k)$ the velocity field at $t_k$. By using Eqn.(2), each SSD term in Eqn.(1) only depends on the control vectors within the time of consecutive frames. Thus the derivative of the SSD with respect to the control vectors can be evaluated independently.

## 2.2   Regularization of Myofiber Strain along Transmural Direction

The regularization energy consists of spatial and temporal terms. We denote the displacement field with $\boldsymbol{u}(\boldsymbol{x}) = (u_1(\boldsymbol{x}), u_2(\boldsymbol{x}), u_3(\boldsymbol{x}))^t$ and $\boldsymbol{x} = (x_1, x_2, x_3)^t$. Infinitesimal strain is used in our motion analysis because the deformation between two consecutive frames is usually small. The strain tensor $\boldsymbol{\epsilon}$ is defined as:

$$\boldsymbol{\epsilon} = \begin{pmatrix} \frac{\partial u_1}{\partial x_1} & \frac{1}{2}(\frac{\partial u_1}{\partial x_2} + \frac{\partial u_2}{\partial x_1}) & \frac{1}{2}(\frac{\partial u_1}{\partial x_3} + \frac{\partial u_3}{\partial x_1}) \\ \frac{1}{2}(\frac{\partial u_2}{\partial x_1} + \frac{\partial u_1}{\partial x_2}) & \frac{\partial u_2}{\partial x_2} & \frac{1}{2}(\frac{\partial u_2}{\partial x_3} + \frac{\partial u_3}{\partial x_2}) \\ \frac{1}{2}(\frac{\partial u_3}{\partial x_1} + \frac{\partial u_1}{\partial x_3}) & \frac{1}{2}(\frac{\partial u_3}{\partial x_2} + \frac{\partial u_2}{\partial x_3}) & \frac{\partial u_3}{\partial x_3} \end{pmatrix}, \tag{3}$$

with $\epsilon_{i,j} = \frac{1}{2}(\frac{\partial u_i}{\partial x_j} + \frac{\partial u_j}{\partial x_i})$ being the $(i, j)$th component of $\boldsymbol{\epsilon}$. Given the myofiber orientation at point $\boldsymbol{x}$ as $\boldsymbol{f} = (f_1, f_2, f_3)^t$, the myofiber strain at $\boldsymbol{x}$ is evaluated as:

$$\epsilon_f = \boldsymbol{f}^t \boldsymbol{\epsilon} \boldsymbol{f} = \sum_{i,j} \epsilon_{i,j} f_i f_j. \tag{4}$$

We define a function which evaluates the myofiber strain variation along transmural direction $\boldsymbol{\tau} = (\tau_1, \tau_2, \tau_3)^t$ by using the directional derivative:

$$V_{\epsilon_f, \tau} = \frac{\partial \epsilon_f}{\partial \boldsymbol{x}} \boldsymbol{\tau} = \sum_{i,j,p} \frac{\partial^2 u_p}{\partial x_i \partial x_j} f_i f_j \tau_p. \tag{5}$$

Eqn.(5) defines a general form of the strain variation along any direction. We can see that each of the isotropic bending energy term used in [1] evaluates the variation of normal and shear strains along $x_1, x_2, x_3$ directions. We define a regularization term which minimizes the anisotropic myofiber strain variation transmurally on the myocardium ($\boldsymbol{x} \in \Omega_M$), and the isotropic strain variations at points outside the myocardium ($\boldsymbol{x} \in \bar{\Omega}_M$) by:

$$E_{sr} = 27 \int_{\Omega_M} \sum_{i,j,p} (\frac{\partial^2 u_p}{\partial x_i \partial x_j} f_i f_j \tau_p)^2 d\boldsymbol{x} + \int_{\bar{\Omega}_M} \sum_{i,j,p} (\frac{\partial^2 u_p}{\partial x_i \partial x_j})^2 d\boldsymbol{x}, \tag{6}$$

where 27 is used to weight the anisotropic term since the isotropic term has 27 combinations of the strains and directions of derivative. $\Omega_M$ is domain of myocardium points. We apply the spatial regularization to each velocity field $\boldsymbol{v}_k$ to maximize the homogeneity of myofiber strain along transmural direction in the whole cardiac cycle.

The temporal regularization term evaluates the magnitude of first order derivative of the point velocity with respect to time, which is defined as:

$$E_{tr} = \int_{\Omega} |\boldsymbol{v}_k(\boldsymbol{x} + \boldsymbol{v}_{k-1}\Delta t) - \boldsymbol{v}_{k-1}|^2 d\boldsymbol{x}. \tag{7}$$

The total regularization energy in Eqn.(1) is defined as a weighted sum of the spatial and temporal regularization energy at all time points:

$$E_R = \int_0^T E_{reg}dt = \sum_{k=0}^{N_t} E_{sr}(\boldsymbol{v}) + w_t \sum_{k=1}^{N_t} E_{tr}(\boldsymbol{v}). \tag{8}$$

## 2.3 Optimization

We use a steepest descent method to optimize the parameterized function. The derivative of $E_{SSD}(I_{n-1}(\boldsymbol{x}), I_n(\boldsymbol{\phi}_{n-1,n}))$ with respect to the control vectors $\mathbf{c}_{m;k}, ((n-1) * N_f \leq k < n * N_f)$ is:

$$\frac{\partial E_{SSD}}{\partial \mathbf{c}_{m;k}} = \int_{\Omega_s} (I_n(\boldsymbol{\phi}_{n-1,n}) - I_{n-1}) \nabla I_n(\boldsymbol{\phi}_{n-1,n}) \frac{\partial \boldsymbol{\phi}_{n-1,n}}{\partial \mathbf{c}_{m;k}} d\boldsymbol{x}, \tag{9}$$

with $\Omega_s$ being the domain which is controlled by $\mathbf{c}_{m;k}$ and for other value of $k$ the gradient is zero. For the derivative of the spatial regularization with respect to the $p$th component of $\mathbf{c}_{m;k}$, we have:

$$\frac{\partial E_{sr}}{\partial c_{m,p;k}} = \int_{\Omega_s} \sum_{i,j} V_{\epsilon_{i,j,p}}^k \frac{\partial^2 \beta_p(\boldsymbol{x} - \boldsymbol{x}_m)}{\partial x_i \partial x_j} d\boldsymbol{x}, \tag{10}$$

with $V_{\epsilon_{i,j,p}}^k$ being one summand of myofiber strain variation along transmural direction in Eqn.(5) at time point $k$ and $\beta_p(\cdot)$ being the $p$th component of the B-spline function. The derivative of the temporal regularization term is approximated by assuming small displacement between two time steps:

$$\frac{\partial E_{tr}}{\partial c_{m,p;k}} = \int_{\Omega_s} (2 * v_{m,p;k} - v_{m,p;k-1} - v_{m,p;k+1})\beta_p(\boldsymbol{x} - \boldsymbol{x}_m)d\boldsymbol{x}. \tag{11}$$

## 2.4 Myofiber and Transmural Directions on Myocardium

We use a human diffusion tensor image (DTI) [1] as the myofiber atlas. The myofiber direction at each DTI voxel is defined as the eigenvector of the diffusion tensor corresponding to the largest eigenvalue. The myofiber orientation is then mapped into the reference frame by using a transformation estimated from a nonrigid registration with the anatomical image of the DTI. The transmural direction at each myocardium point is estimated from the myofiber orientation. It is defined as a vector in the short axis plane and is perpendicular to the myofiber. The myofiber and transmural directions in the reference frame are propagated to each of the following frames by using the recovered deformation.

---

[1] http://www.ccbm.jhu.edu/research/dSets.php

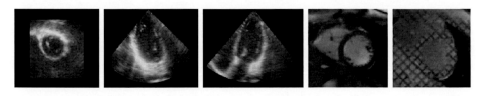

**Fig. 1.** The ED frame of echocardiography and MRIs of one subject. The first three images are orthogonal view of the echocardiography. The last two images are short axis ROIs from the cine MRI and the tagged MRI images.

## 3     Datasets and Experiments

We validated our method using multimodal image sequences of two healthy subjects. In the first experiment, an echocardiographic sequence of each subject was acquired with a Philips IE33 system. The number of frames is 26 and the frame size was $135 \times 126 \times 106$ with voxel size $1.12mm^3$. In the second experiment, both cine MRI and tagged MRI of each subject were acquired with a Siemens system. The number of frames in both sequences was 30 and the frame size was $256 \times 256 \times 10$ with voxel size $1.25mm \times 1.25mm \times 8mm$. Fig.1 shows the images of one subject. In both experiments, we compared the proposed method with a method using isotropic regularization [1]. In first experiment, we evaluated the strains in the 16 AHA segments [17] (apex segment was excluded). Both epicardial and endocardial surface meshes in the end-diastole (ED) frame were generated by automatically labeling the short axis contours and connecting the points into triangle meshes. Eight meshes of intermediate layers were interpolated from the endocardial and epicardial meshes. The radial, circumferential and longitudinal directions in each vertices were automatically calculated as did in [8] and the myofiber direction was estimated by using the transformation from the ED frame to the DTI atlas. The cross-fiber direction was defined as the cross product of the radial and myofiber directions. The myofiber, cross-fiber, circumferential and longitudinal strains were evaluated and their variations along the ten transmural layers in each segments are plotted and compared.

In the second experiments, the cine-MRI images were used to estimate the cardiac motion. The estimated transformation was used to deform the grid crossing points extracted from the ED frame of the tagged MRI. The affine transformation between the tagged MRI and the cine MRI was acquired from the DICOM file headers. We compared the two methods by overlaying the deformed ED tagging grid on the ES frames.

## 4     Results

We use a series of 3D B-spline functions with spatial spacing of 6 and temporal spacing of 1. The weightings $\lambda$ and $w_t$ for the regularization terms are set to 0.1 and 0.005 for both methods.

The results for both subjects are similar and we show the results of first subject as an example. We first show the strain estimation in the echocardiography sequence in Fig.2. By comparing the first two rows, we can see that the strains in our proposed method are more temporally smooth than the method with isotropic regularization. It indicates that the estimated myocardium motion is more uniform in our method. It is more consistent with the cardiac motion of a healthy subject. The errorbars in the bottom row show the average and transmural variance of the myofiber strains in four mid cavity segments. We can see that our estimated motion can lead to transmural homogeneity of the myofiber strain (in blue). Similar result can be seen in the cine MRI experiment (Fig.3). The result of the second experiment is shown in Fig.4. We overlay the deformed tagging grids in both apical and basal planes of ED frame on the end-systolic frame. We can see the improvement of our method over the isotropic regularization method.

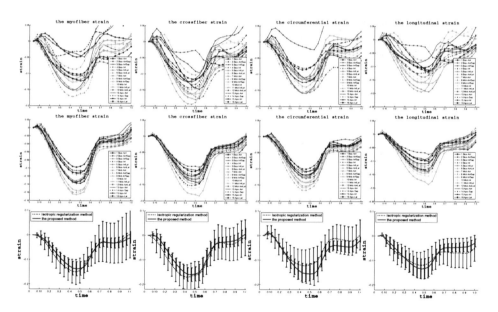

**Fig. 2.** The strains in the echocardiography sequence. (Top row) Strains in the isotropic regularization method. (Middle row) Strains in our method. (Bottom row) Average and transmural variance of the myofiber strains in four segments using isotropic regularization method (red) and our method (blue). The four segments are the anterior, anteriorseptal, inferior and anteriorlateral segments, respectively.

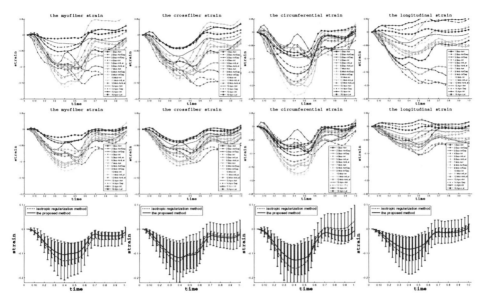

**Fig. 3.** The strains in the cine MRI sequence. (Top row) Strains in the isotropic regularization method. (Middle row) Strains in our method. (Bottom row) Average and transmural variance of the myofiber strains in four segments using isotropic regularization method (red) and our method (blue). Same segments are used as in Fig.2.

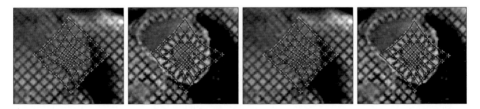

**Fig. 4.** The deformed ED frame grid overlaid on the ES frame in apex and basal slices in isotropic regularization method (left two) and our method (right two)

## 5  Conclusion

We proposed a diffeomorphic cardiac motion estimation method with transmurally myofiber strain homogeneity. We validated our method by using 3D echocardiography and MRI sequences of two healthy subjects. Experiments show that our method can obtain result which is more transmurally smooth and performs better in tracking myocardium points. Our method can be applied to pathological subjects whose myofiber alternation is not significant if given the pathological myofiber orientation. The method may have limitation in cases of the subjects with severe pathology such as infarct, in these cases, our method can be applied to the non-infarct regions.

**Acknowledgement.** This paper is supported by a NIH/NHLBI grant 1R01HL102407-01 awarded to Xubo Song and David Sahn.

# References

1. Elen, A., Choi, H.F., Loeckx, D., Gaom, H., Claus, P., Suetens, P., Maes, F., D'hooge, J.: Three-dimensional cardiac strain estimation using spatiotemporal elastic registration of ultrasound images: a feasibility study. IEEE Trans. Med. Imag. 27(11), 1580–1591 (2008)
2. Ledesma-Carbayo, M.J., Mah-Casado, P., Santos, A., Prez-David, E., GarMA, D.M.: Spatio-Temporal Nonrigid Registration for Ultrasound Cardiac Motion Estimation. IEEE Trans. Med. Imag. 24(9), 1113–1126 (2005)
3. Metz, C.T., Klein, S., Schaap, M., Walsum, T., Niessen, W.J.: Nonrigid registration of dynamic medical imaging data using nD+t B-splines and a groupwise optimization approach. Med. Imag. Anal. 15(2), 238–249 (2011)
4. Castillo, E., Castillo, R., Martinez, J., Shenoy, M., Guerrero, T.: Four-dimensional deformable image registration using trajectory modeling. Physics in Medicine and Biology 55(1), 305–327 (2010)
5. Skrinjar, O., Bistoquet, A., Tagare, H.: Symmetric and Transitive Registration of Image Sequences. International Journal of Biomedical Imaging. (2008)
6. Beg, M.F., Miller, M.I., Trouve, A., Younes, L.: Compute Large Deformation Metric Mappings via Geodesic Flows of Diffeomorphisms. IJCV 61(2), 139–157 (2005)
7. Khan, A.R., Beg, M.F.: Representation of time-varying shapes in the large deformation diffeomorphic framework. In: ISBI 2008, pp. 1521–1524 (2008)
8. Craene, M.D., Piella, G., Camaraa, O., Duchateaua, N., Silvae, E., Doltrae, A., D'hooge, J., Brugadae, J., Sitgese, M., Frangi, A.F.: Temporal diffeomorphic freeform deformation: application to motion and strain estimation from 3D echocardiography. Med. Imag. Anal. 16(1), 427–450 (2012)
9. Mansi, T., Pennec, X., Sermesant, M., Delingette, H., Ayache, N.: iLogDemons: A Demons-Based Registration Algorithm for Tracking Incompressible Elastic Biological Tissues. IJCV 92(1), 92–111 (2011)
10. Ubbink, S.W.J., Bovendeerd, P.H.M., Delhaas, T., Arts, T., Vosse, F.N.: Towards model-based analysis of cardiac MR tagging data: Relation between left ventricular shear strain and myofiber orientation. Med. Imag. Anal. 10(4), 632–641 (2006)
11. Kroon, W., Delhaas, T., Bovendeerd, P., Arts, T.: Computational analysis of myocardial structure: Adaptation of cardiac myofiber orientation through deformation. Med. Imag. Anal. 13(2), 346–353 (2009)
12. Papademetris, X., Sinusas, A.J., Dione, D.P., Duncan, J.S.: Estimation of 3D left ventricular deformation from echocardiography. Med. Imag. Anal. 5(1), 17–28 (2001)
13. Zhang, Z.J., Sahn, D.J., Song, X.B.: Diffeomorphic cardiac motion estimation with anisotropic regularization along myofiber orientation. In: Dawant, B.M., Christensen, G.E., Fitzpatrick, J.M., Rueckert, D. (eds.) WBIR 2012. LNCS, vol. 7359, pp. 199–208. Springer, Heidelberg (2012)
14. Geerts-Ossevoort, L.: Cardiac myofiber reorientation: a mechanism for adaptation? Ph.D thesis. Eindhoven University of Technology, Eindhoven, The Netherlands (2002)
15. Rijcken, J., Bovendeered, P.H.M., Schoofs, A.J.G., Van Campen, D.H., Arts, T.: Optimization of cardiac fiber orientation for homogeneous fiber strain beginning of ejection. Journal of Biomechanics 30(10), 1041–1049 (1997)
16. Tseng, W.Y.I., Reese, T.G., Weisskoff, R.M., Brady, T.J., Wedeen, V.J.: Myocardial Fiber Shortening in Humans: Initial Results of MR Imaging. Radiology 216(7), 128–139 (2000)
17. Partridge, J.B., Anderson, R.H.: Left Ventricular Anatomy: Its Nonmenclature Segmentation, and Planes of Imaging. Clinical Anatomy 22(1), 77–84 (2009)

# A Novel Total Variation Based Noninvasive Transmural Electrophysiological Imaging

Jingjia Xu, Azar Rahimi Dehaghani , Fei Gao, and Linwei Wang

Computational Biomedicine Laboratory, Golisano College of Computing and Information Sciences, Rochester Institute of Technology, Rochester, NY, 14623, USA

**Abstract.** While tomographic imaging of cardiac structure and kinetics has improved substantially, electrophysiological mapping of the heart is still restricted to the body or heart surface with little or no depth information beneath. The progress in reconstructing transmural action potentials from surface voltage data has been hindered by the challenges of intrinsic ill-posedness and the lack of a unique solution in the absence of prior assumptions. In this work, we propose to exploit the unique spatial property of transmural action potentials that it is often piecewise smooth with a steep boundary (gradient) separating the depolarized and repolarized regions. This steep gradient could reveal normal or disrupted electrical propagation wavefronts, or pinpoint the border between viable and necrotic tissue. In this light, we propose a novel adaption of the total-variation (TV) prior into the reconstruction of transmural action potentials, where a variational TV operator is defined instead of a common discrete operator, and the TV-minimization is solved by a sequence of weighted, first-order L2-norm minimizations. In a large set of phantom experiments performed on image-derived human heart-torso models, the proposed method is shown to outperform existing quadratic methods in preserving the steep gradient of action potentials along the border of infarcts, as well as in capturing the disruption to the normal path of electrical wavefronts. The former is further attested by real-data experiments on two post-infarction human subjects, demonstrating the potential of the proposed method in revealing the location and shape of the underlying infarcts when existing quadratic methods fail to do so.

**Keywords:** Electrophysiological imaging, inverse problems, total-variation.

## 1 Introduction

The heart is an electromechanical organ. Its efficient contraction must be coordinated by a steady electrical flow spreading three-dimensionally throughout the myocardium. Disruptions to this electrical propagation can directly predispose the heart to mechanical catastrophe and lead to sudden cardiac death. However, while methods for noninvasive imaging and analysis of 3D structure, kinetics, and mechanics of an individual's heart have substantially improved in recently years, methods for assessing the electrophysiological (EP) aspects have

K. Mori et al. (Eds.): MICCAI 2013, Part I, LNCS 8149, pp. 501–508, 2013.

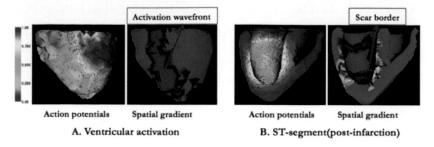

**Fig. 1.** Illustration of the transmural action potential and its spatial gradient

not. In practice, common observations of cardiac electrical activities are voltage data either sensed on the body-surface as noninvasive electrocardiograms (ECG), or mapped on heart surfaces by catheters introduced into the cavity in a minimally-invasive manner. Both data provide a poor surface surrogate for intramural electrical activities that occur deep beneath the surface of the heart.

The critical gap in experimental methods has motivated many computational methods for *EP imaging* that, analogous to tomographic imaging, solve an inverse problem to quantitatively reconstruct transmural action potentials from body-surface voltage data, the forward relationship of which is governed by the *quasi-static electromagneticism* [8]. Unfortunately, in addition to mathematic ill-posed caused by limited number of data that is common to many inverse problems, this biophysical principle determines that there may be an infinite number of solutions that fit the same surface measurement [8]. For a unique solution, a common assumption restricts to the surface of the heart [9]. This guarantees a unique surface solution as a surrogate for the intramural electrical dynamics, and various regularization methods have been applied to reduce the mathematical ill-posedness. Transition to intramural EP imaging has been very limited, and existing methods [7,13] again all essentially amount to a weighted quadratic regularization that imposes either the spatial and/or temporal smoothness of the solution or the conforming to a complex physiological prior [14]. Due to the heuristic model of smoothness, these solutions are observed to be diffused and lose sharp details that are physiologically and clinically critical [14,13].

Our fundamental hypothesis is that, while quadratic methods are suitable for alleviating the mathematical ill-posedness of this problem caused by limited data, sparse methods are further needed for the physically-included non-uniqueness of solutions. In particular, we propose a fresh perspective to view the transmural action potential $u(t)$ as a time-varying 3D image. As illustrated in Fig 1, the edge of this image (*i.e.*, spatial gradient $\nabla u(t)$) is always localized and steep in space. During the depolarization and repolarization, it represents the steep *wavefront* between active and resting regions (Fig. 1 A), revealing potential disruptions to the path of normal electrical flow in diseased hearts. Between the two phases (the ST-segment of an ECG cycle), $\nabla u(t)$ is expected to be close to zero everywhere in a normal heart and appearance of high gradient would again indicate underlying diseases, such as the border of an infarct that divides regions of depolarized viable tissue and necrotic infarct core (Fig. 1 B). This unfolds the importance to preserve the unique spatial feature of $\nabla u(t)$ during the reconstruction of $u(t)$, which is in line with the essence of total-variation (TV) minimization to promote a solution with sharp boundaries/gradients between piecewise smooth regions. Since its original development, TV minimization has been applied to preserve the sharp edge of an image in a variety of applications such as image de-noising [11] and blind de convolution [2].

In this paper, we propose a novel adaptation of the spatial TV-prior into transmural EP imaging. We first define a variational form of TV-prior to approximate the continuous TV form by a numerical integration, so as to overcome the weakness of a common discrete TV-prior in being error-prone to calculate on the irregular mesh of the heart. The concept of iteratively re-weighted norm (IRN) method is then coupled with this TV-prior to solve the TV minimization. In a set of 137 phantom experiments, the proposed method was shown to deliver significantly higher accuracy (paired $t$-test) over existing quadratic methods in preserving the steep gradient of action potentials that is distributed along the border of an infarct during the ST-segment. It is also shown to outperform existing quadratic methods in preserving the structure of electrical propagation wavefronts, and in capturing the change of these wavefronts caused by the existence of an infarct. Real-data experiments on two post-infarction patients further verify the potential of the proposed method in detecting the abnormally steep gradient and thus revealing the shape of the infarct border.

## 2    Methodology

Cardiac electrical flow produces time-varying voltage data, easily accessible on the body-surface, as if our torso were a *quasi-static* electromagnetic field [8]. With different numerical methods and discrete representation of the heart-torso anatomy of a given subject [7,14], this biophysical relationship can be represented in a matrix form: $\phi(t) = \mathbf{H}\mathbf{u}(t)$, where $\phi(t)$ is the discrete field of voltage data sensed on the body surface, $\mathbf{u}(t)$ the discrete filed of transmural action potential across the depth of the myocardium, and the transfer matrix $\mathbf{H}$ is specific to each individual's torso anatomy and typically considered time-invariant. The condition number of $\mathbf{H}$ was shown to be typically at the order of $10^{-14}$ [14]. We propose to incorporate the TV-prior into the reconstruction of transmural action potentials and, at this stage, we exclude the temporal factor and focus on the reconstruction with a spatial TV-prior at separate time instants:

$$\hat{\mathbf{u}} = \min_{\mathbf{u}}\{||\mathbf{H}\mathbf{u} - \phi||_2^2 + \lambda TV(\mathbf{u})\} \tag{1}$$

**Variational TV-form:** The first challenge comes from the need of a proper definition of $TV(\mathbf{u})$. In image-processing applications, a discrete version of $TV(\mathbf{u})$ is calculated as the *L1-norm of the discrete gradient field of* $\mathbf{u}$: $TV(\mathbf{u}) = ||\nabla\mathbf{u}||_1 = \sum_{i=1}^n \sqrt{\nabla_x\mathbf{u}_i^2 + \nabla_y\mathbf{u}_i^2 + \nabla_z\mathbf{u}_i^2}$. However, it is not possible to formulate an explicit gradient operator for the entire discrete field without separately employing directional gradient operators. Furthermore, the gradient field is highly affected by the resolution of the discrete field **u**, and is much more difficult and error-prone to calculate on the complex mesh of the heart than a regular image. Therefore, we define an approximation of the continuous form of TV as:

$$TV(\mathbf{u}) = \int_{\Omega_h} |\nabla u| d\Omega_h \approx \Sigma_{i=1}^{N} |\nabla\varphi_i \mathbf{u}| \tag{2}$$

where a numerical integration is performed over the myocardial field $\Omega_h$, involving a summation of $\nabla u$ over N (at the order of $10^5$) Gaussian quadrature points. Based on the discretization method used (meshfree method used in our study), $\nabla u$ on each Gauss point is approximated by a linear combination of its neighboring points in the discrete field **u** based on the $1 \times n$ shape functions $\varphi_i$ ($\nabla\varphi_i$ being the $3 \times n$ spatial gradients of $\varphi_i$). Because each Gauss point has a small set of support nodal points, $\varphi_i$ and $\nabla\varphi_i$ are sparse with a small number of non-zero values. This definition of $TV(\mathbf{u})$ is also consistent with the data-fidelity term in equation (1), where the biophysical model **H** is calculated from numerical approximations of integrals involved in the *quasi-static* Maxwell equations.

**TV-minimization with Iteratively Re-weighted Norm (TVIRN):** To solve the L1-norm penalty function in equation (1), we adopt the concept of IRN [10], so that variational form of TV (2) is approximated as a sequence of L2 norm of the weighted gradient; each weight is the square root of the gradient value in the previous $(k-1)$-th iteration for $k = 1, 2, \cdots$ until convergence. In this way, a small spatial gradient in previous iterations will generate a large penalty in the current iteration, while a large gradient will be promoted until the final solution exhibits a piecewise smooth pattern with steep gradient in between:

$$\int_{\Omega_h} |\nabla u^{(k)}| d\Omega_h \approx \int_{\Omega_h} |\frac{\nabla u^{(k)}}{\sqrt{\nabla u^{(k-1)}}}|^2 d\Omega_h \approx \mathbf{u}^{(k)T} (\sum_{i=1}^{N} \frac{(\nabla\varphi_i^T \nabla\varphi_i)}{|\nabla\varphi_i \mathbf{u}^{(k-1)}|}) \mathbf{u}^{(k)} \tag{3}$$

The weight matrix is calculated over $N$ Gaussian quadrature points. Each sparse matrix $\nabla\varphi_i^T \nabla\varphi_i$ on each Gauss point is constant once the discretization of the ventricular model is established and only needs to be computed once for the entire recursive procedure. At each iteration, it is weighted by action potential of the same Gauss point $|\nabla\varphi_i \mathbf{u}^{(k-1)}|$ calculated from $\mathbf{u}^{(k-1)}$. Therefore, the TV-minimization (1) can be solved by a set of weighted L2-minimizations:

$$\hat{\mathbf{u}}^{(k)} = \min_{\mathbf{u}} ||\mathbf{H}\mathbf{u}^{(k)} - \phi||_2^2 + \lambda^{(k)} \mathbf{u}^{(k)T} (\sum_{i=1}^{N} \frac{(\nabla\varphi_i^T \nabla\varphi_i)}{|\nabla\varphi_i u^{(k-1)}|}) \mathbf{u}^{(k)} \tag{4}$$

$$\rightarrow \hat{\mathbf{u}}^{(k)} = (\mathbf{H}^T \mathbf{H} + \lambda^{(k)} \sum_{i=1}^{N} \frac{\nabla\varphi_i^T \nabla\varphi_i}{|\nabla\varphi_i \mathbf{u}^{(k-1)}| + \beta})^{-1} \mathbf{H}^T \phi \tag{5}$$

where $\lambda^{(k)}$ is the regularization parameter used at iteration $k$. $\beta$ is a small positive value to reduce numerical errors when $|\nabla\varphi_i \mathbf{u}^{(k-1)}|$ at the $i$-th Gauss point is close to zero. As explained above, at each iteration the optimization (5) involves only a weighted summation of the set of $N$ pre-stored matrices, and the matrix inversion is calculated by *Conjugate Gradient* method in this study.

---

**Algorithm 1.** Total-Variation Iteratively Re-weighted Norm (TVIRN)

---

**Initialization:** $\mathbf{u}^{(0)} = (\mathbf{H}^T\mathbf{H} + \lambda_0\mathbf{W}^T\mathbf{W})^{-1}\mathbf{H}^T\mathbf{\Phi}$, $k = 1$

**while** $(||TV(\mathbf{u}^{(k)}) - TV(\mathbf{u}^{(k-1)})||_2 \leq tol$, tol $= 10^{-5})$

$\lambda^{(k)} = \dfrac{||\mathbf{H}^T\mathbf{H}||_\infty}{||\sum_{i=1}^{N} \frac{\nabla\varphi_i^T\nabla\varphi_i}{|\nabla\varphi_i\mathbf{u}^{(k-1)}|+\beta}||_\infty}$, $\hat{\mathbf{u}}^{(k)} = (\mathbf{H}^T\mathbf{H} + \lambda^{(k)}\sum_{i=1}^{N} \frac{\nabla\varphi_i^T\nabla\varphi_i}{|\nabla\varphi_i\mathbf{u}^{(k-1)}|+\beta})^{-1}\mathbf{H}^T\mathbf{\Phi}$

$k = k + 1$

**end**

---

**Algorithm Summary:** A summary of the algorithm is provided in Algorithm 1. First, an existing weighted quadratic method [7] is used to overcome the mathematical ill-posedness of the problem and to obtain an initial solution of $\mathbf{u}^{(0)}$. The regularization parameter $\lambda^{(0)}$ is calculated by the L-curve method [5]. After initialization, the iteration as described above (5) repeats until the convergence criterion, *i.e.*, the difference between two successive gradients of solutions is smaller than a pre-defined tolerance. There is currently no established method for determining regularization parameter in L1-based problems, and most works rely on an empirical procedure to select an optimal value of $\lambda$ after a large set of experiments. Here we use a more objective method [12] to automatically update the magnitude of $\lambda^{(k)}$ at each iteration based on the infinity norm of the matrices involved in the data-fidelity and the regularization terms (see Algorithm 1).

## 3   Experiments and Results

Phantom and real-data experiments are both used in this study. Phantom experiments are conducted on four realistic human heart-torso models derived from CT images, where we test the proposed method in preserving: 1) steep $\nabla\mathbf{u}$ along the border of infarcts during the ST-segment, and 2) propagation wavefronts in normal versus infarcted hearts. Two real-data experiments are further performed on post-infarction human subjects to detect the steep gradient of action potentials distributed along the border of infarcts. The accuracy is measured by the *consistency metric* $CoM = \frac{S_1\cap S_2}{S_1\cup S_2}$ between the region of steep gradients $(S_1)$ in reconstructed action potentials and the *true* region of steep gradients$(S_2)$. In current study, a threshold value is automatically calculated from the mean and standard deviation of result. Comparison studies are performed between TVIRN and existing quadratic methods for transmural EP imaging, including the 1-order [13] and 0-order [7] Tikhonov regularization.

**Steep Potential Gradients Along Infarct Border:** In this set of phantom experiments, action potentials during the ST-segment are set to be 0 for the infarct core, and 1 for the health region(normalized physiological range(-20-90)). 370-lead or 120-lead body-surface ECG are simulated and corrupted with 20-dB Gaussian noise as inputs for transmural *EP imaging*. We consider infarcts of different sizes and locations according to the 17 standard AHA segments of LV. In total we consider 137 cases of infarcts of different locations and sizes from 0.5% to 50% of LV. On average the TVIRN takes 8.5 iterations to converge.

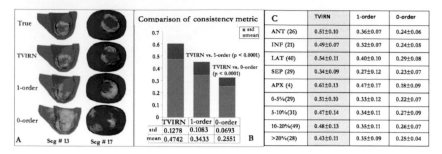

**Fig. 2.** Reconstruction accuracy in preserving the steep gradient of transmural action potentials during the ST-segment of an ECG cycle in infarcted hearts. A. Two examples of steep action potential gradients along the infarcts. B and C. Quantitative analysis.

Fig 2 (A) shows two examples of the *true* steep spatial gradients of action potentials along border of infarcts located at anterior (segment 13) and apical (segment 17) regions of the LV, respectively. This spatial structure of the steep gradient is well preserved in the reconstructed action potentials by TVIRN method. In comparison, gradient of the action potential reconstructed by the 0-order quadratic method is diffused and does not reveal the location or the shape of the underlying infarcts. The 1-order quadratic regularization shows improved accuracy over its 0-order counterpart but the reconstructed gradient is still blurred and loses the topology of the infarct border.

Fig 2 (B) lists the *consistency metric* for 137 cases, where paired student's $t$-test shows that the accuracy of TVIRN at the steep action potential gradients is significantly higher than that of the other two quadratic methods ($p < 0.0001$). Fig 2 (C) lists the *COM* with respect to the locations and sizes of the infarcts, respectively. As shown, TVIRN has the best performance when the infarcts are located at apical and lateral regions of the heart. It is the most difficult to correctly capture the gradient of action potentials when the infarct is at the septal area of the LV, the region most hidden from body-surface data. The accuracy of TVIRN is similar dealing with infarcts of different sizes.

**Activation/repolarization Wavefronts:** We continue to consider whether TVIRN can capture disruptions to electrical propagation wavefronts (steep gradient of action potentials) caused by the existence of infarcts. In this set of experiments, transmural propagation of ventricular action potentials is simulated with the *Aliev-Panfilov* model [1] with parameter $a$ (representing tissue excitability) set to be 0.5 for infarcts and 0.15 for healthy tissue. Time sequences of 120-lead ECGs are simulated and corrupted with 20-db white Gaussian noise. Selected time frames during activation or repolarization are used for reconstructions.

Depolarization: Fig 3 (A,C) shows an example of the activation wavefront in a normal heart when the electrical flow propagates from the RV to LV (purple arrow), and that at the same time instant on the same heart model but with an infarct localized at the mid-basal anterior region of the LV (labeled by red line). It is evident that the infarct works as a structural obstacle and re-routes

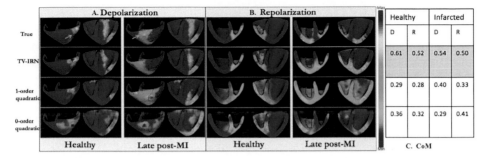

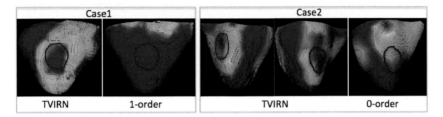

**Fig. 3.** Change of propagation wavefronts in normal and infarcted hearts. The proposed TVIRN faithfully captures the change of path while quadratic methods fail to do so.

**Fig. 4.** Spatial gradients of transmural action potentials reconstructed from TVIRN and quadratic methods on two post-infarction human hearts. The red cycles represent the core of the MRI-delineated infarcts.

the activation wavefront. The proposed method captures the steep wavefront in the reconstructed action potential in both normal and disrupted electrical flow. In comparison, the 0-order quadratic method fails to distinguish the depolarized region from the resting region in both cases. The 1-order quadratic method partially captures the wavefront but not on the endocardium, and it also fails to accurately reflect the disruption caused by the infarct.

Repolarization: Fig 3 (B,C) shows the repolarization wavefront of the same normal and infarcted hearts, where the infarct both disrupts the repolarization wavefront and changes the action potential gradients around the infarct border. Again, TVIRN method is able to capture both the normal and disrupted spatial gradients of the reconstructed action potentials. In comparison, the other two quadratic methods fail to reveal the abnormal repolarization wavefront related to the location or structure of the infarct.

**Real-data Study of Steep Gradient Along Infarct Border:** We consider MRI and body-surface ECG data on two post-infarction patients made available to this study by the *2007 PhysioNet / Computers in Cardiology Challenges* [4]. MRI data are used to construct the patient-specific heart-torso model. Body-surface ECG data were recorded by standard 120-lead Dalhousie protocol [6]. Gold standards of infarct quantification were obtained form Gadolinium-enhanced MRI by cardiologists, revealing that the core regions of the infarct are labeled by the red cycle in Fig 4. As shown in Fig 4, both of reconstructed action potentials of TVIRN exhibit a steep gradient that are localized and distributed along the infarct cores, even in case 2 with two separate infarct regions. In comparison, action potentials reconstructed from neither of the other two quadratic methods reveal any physiological meaningful information regarding the existence, location, or structure of the infarct. These observations are consistent with the findings in our phantom experiments.

**Conclusion:** This paper presents a novel approach to transmural EP imaging based on a spatial TV-prior, and demonstrates its superiority over existing quadratic methods in a set of phantom and real-data experiments. The adaption of TV-prior was also recently considered for potential reconstruction on the epicardium [3]. In comparison, our method is first proposed to reconstruct transmural action potential with a close tie its spatial property. The next immediate step is to integrate temporal constraints with the spatial TV-prior to improve the accuracy and temporal consistency of the proposed method.

# References

1. Aliev, R.R., et al.: A simple two-variable model of cardiac excitation. Chaos, Solitions & Fractals 7(3), 293–301 (1996)
2. Chan, T., Wong, C.K.: Total variation blind deconvolution. IEEE Transactions on Image Processing 7(3), 370–375 (1998)
3. Ghosh, S., Rudy, Y.: Application of l1-norm regularization to epicardial potential solutions of the inverse electrocardiography problem. Annals of Biomedical Engineering 37(5), 902–912 (2009)
4. Goldberger, A.L., et al.: Physiobank, physiotoolkit, and physionet: Components of a new research resource for complex physiological signals. Circulation 101, e215–e220 (2000)
5. Hansen, P., O'Leary, D.: The use of the l-curve in the regularization of discrete ill-posed problems. SIAM Journal on Scientific Computing 14(6), 1487–1503 (1993)
6. Hubley-Kozey, C.L., Mitchell, L.B., Gardner, M.J., et al.:
7. Liu, Z., Liu, C., He, B.: Noninvasive reconstruction of three-dimensional ventricular activation sequence from the inverse solution of distributed equivalent current density. IEEE Transactions on Medical Imaging 25(10), 1307–1318 (2006)
8. Plonsey, R.: Bioelectric phenomena. Wiley Online Library (1999)
9. Ramanathan, C., Ghanem, R., et al.: Noninvasive electrocardiographic imaging for cardiac electrophysiology and arrhythmia. Nature Medicine 10(4), 422–428 (2004)
10. Rodríguez, P., Wohlberg, B.: Efficient minimization method for a generalized total variation functional. IEEE Transactions on Image Processing 18(2), 322–332 (2009)
11. Rudin, L., Osher, S., Fatemi, E.: Nonlinear total variation based noise removal algorithms. Physica D 60, 259–268 (1992)
12. Schmidt, M., Fung, G., Rosales, R.: Optimization methods for l1-regularization. University of British Columbia, Technical Report TR-2009-19 (2009)
13. Wang, D., Kirby, R., MacLeod, R., Johnson, C.: Identifying myocardial ischemia by inversely computing transmembrane potentials from body-surface potential maps. In: International Symposium on NFSIBH, pp. 121–125 (2011)
14. Wang, L., Wong, K., Zhang, H., Liu, H., Shi, P.: Noninvasive computational imaging of cardiac electrophysiology for 3-d infarct. IEEE Transactions on Biomedical Engineering 58(4), 1033–1043 (2011)

# Right Ventricle Segmentation with Probability Product Kernel Constraints

Cyrus M.S. Nambakhsh[1,3], Terry M. Peters[1,3], Ali Islam[1,3], and Ismail Ben Ayed[1,2]

[1] The University of Western Ontario, London, ON, Canada
[2] GE Healthcare, London, ON, Canada
[3] Robarts Research Institute, London, ON, Canada
[4] St. Joseph's Health Care, London, ON, Canada

**Abstract.** We propose a fast algorithm for 3D segmentation of the right ventricle (RV) in MRI using shape and appearance constraints based on probability product kernels (PPK). The proposed constraints remove the need for large, manually-segmented training sets and costly pose estimation (or registration) procedures, as is the case of the existing algorithms. We report comprehensive experiments, which demonstrate that the proposed algorithm (i) requires only a single subject for training; and (ii) yields a performance that is not significantly affected by the choice of the training data. Our PPK constraints are non-linear (high-order) functionals, which are not directly amenable to standard optimizers. We split the problem into several surrogate-functional optimizations, each solved via an efficient convex relaxation that is amenable to parallel implementations. We further introduce a scale variable that we optimize with fast fixed-point computations, thereby achieving pose invariance in real-time. Our parallelized implementation on a graphics processing unit (GPU) demonstrates that the proposed algorithm can yield a real-time solution for typical cardiac MRI volumes, with a speed-up of more than 20 times compared to the CPU version. We report a comprehensive experimental validations over 400 volumes acquired from 20 subjects, and demonstrate that the obtained 3D surfaces correlate with independent manual delineations.

## 1 Introduction

Quantification of right ventricle (RV) function, including ejection fraction, ventricular enlargement, aneurysms, wall motion and contraction/motion analysis can be useful in the diagnosis of various cardiovascular abnormalities. RV segmentation in 3D magnetic resonance images (MRI) is an essential step towards such quantifications, yielding RV dynamics which translate into extensive clinical information [1]. However, manual segmentation of 4D (3D+time) cardiac volumes is tedious and time-consuming. As pointed out in the recent cardiac-segmentation review in [2], RV segmentation in MRI is still acknowledged to be a difficult and completely unsolved problem, unlike left ventricle (LV) segmentation which has been intensively researched during the last decade [2]. The main difficulties arise from the complex deformations of the RV chamber in 3D, its highly variable, crescent-shaped structure and the presence of papillary muscles.

K. Mori et al. (Eds.): MICCAI 2013, Part I, LNCS 8149, pp. 509–517, 2013.

Most of the existing RV/LV segmentation algorithms, for instance, those based on statistical shape models [3], registration [4], and probabilistic-atlas classification [5], require an intensive learning from a large, manually-segmented training set. Although they can lead to outstanding performance in cases that befit the training set, these algorithms may have difficulty in capturing the substantial variations in a clinical context, with the results often being dependent on the choice of a specific training set. Furthermore, most of the existing shape-based algorithms require additional costly pose optimization procedures (rotation, translation, and scaling), which are often based on slow gradient-descent techniques. To remove the dependence on a training set, several recent cardiac image segmentation studies have attempted to build subject-specific models from a user-provided segmentation of a single 2D frame in a cardiac sequence [6,7,8,9]. Unfortunately, these solutions are designed for LV segmentation, and require an intensive user input, e.g., the algorithm in [7] uses manual segmentations of several 2D slices in one subject data. Moreover, these approaches are difficult to extend beyond the 2D case.

This study investigates rapid 3D segmentation of the right ventricle (RV) in cardiac MRI with shape and appearance constraints based on probability product kernels (PPK), which relax the need for large, manually-segmented training sets and costly pose estimation (or registration) procedures. We report comprehensive experiments, which demonstrate that the proposed algorithm (i) requires only a single subject for training; and (ii) yields a performance that is not significantly affected by the choice of the training data. Our PPK constraints are non-linear (high-order) functionals, which are not directly amenable to standard optimizers. We split the problem into several surrogate-functional optimizations, each solved via an efficient convex relaxation that is amenable to parallel implementation. We further introduce a scale variable which we optimize with fast fixed-point computations, thereby achieving scale-invariance in real-time. Our parallelized implementation on a graphics processing unit (GPU) demonstrates that the proposed algorithm can yield a real-time solution for a typical cardiac MRI volume, with a speed-up of more than 20 times in comparison to the CPU version. We report a performance evaluation over 400 volumes acquired from 20 subjects, and demonstrate that the obtained 3D surfaces correlate with independent manual delineations.

## 2    Formulation

**The Functional:** Let $I : \Omega \subset \mathbb{R}^3 \to \mathcal{Z}_I \subset \mathbb{R}$ be an image function which maps 3D domain $\Omega$ to a finite set of intensity values $\mathcal{Z}_I$. Let $D : \Omega \to \mathcal{Z}_D \subset \mathbb{R}$ be a function that measures the distance between each point $\mathbf{x} = (x, y, z) \in \Omega$ and a given anatomical landmark (i.e., a point) $\mathcal{O} \in \Omega$, which will be used to build a translation-invariant shape prior and to learn an intensity prior. $D(\mathbf{x}) = \|\mathbf{x} - \mathcal{O}\|$, with $\|\cdot\|$ the standard L2 norm. $\mathcal{Z}_D$ is a finite set of distance values. $\mathcal{O}$ is obtained from a very simple user input that amounts to the manual identification of the centroid of the RV cavity within a middle slice with a single mouse click. Let $A : \Omega \to \mathcal{Z}_A \subset \mathbb{R}$ be a function measuring the angle between the vector pointing from each point $\mathbf{x} \in \Omega$ to $\mathcal{O}$ and the fixed $x$-axis unit vector $v$: $A(\mathbf{x}) = \frac{<\mathbf{x}\mathcal{O}, v>}{\|\mathbf{x}\mathcal{O}\|\|v\|}$. Our objective functional is:

$$\hat{u} = \arg \min_{u \in \{0,1\}} \mathcal{E}(u) \text{ with}$$

$$\mathcal{E}(u) := \underbrace{- \left\langle \mathbf{P}^I(u,.), \mathbf{M}^I \right\rangle_\rho}_{Intensity \ Prior} \underbrace{-\alpha_D \left\langle \mathbf{P}^D(u,.), \mathbf{M}^D \right\rangle_\rho \underbrace{-\alpha_A \left\langle \mathbf{P}^A(u,.), \mathbf{M}^A \right\rangle_\rho}_{Angle \ prior}}_{Shape \ prior}$$

$$+ \underbrace{\gamma \int_\Omega C |\nabla u| \, d\mathbf{x}}_{Smoothness/Edges} \qquad (1)$$

The following is a detailed description of the notations and variables that appear in the optimization problem we define in equation (1):

- $u : \Omega \to \{0,1\}$ is a binary function, which defines a variable partition of $\Omega$: $\{\mathbf{x} \in \Omega / u(\mathbf{x}) = 1\}$, corresponding to the target RV segment, and $\{\mathbf{x} \in \Omega / u(\mathbf{x}) = 0\}$, corresponding to the complement of the target segment in $\Omega$.
- For image data $J \in \{I, D, A\} : \Omega \subset \mathbb{R}^3 \to \mathcal{Z}_J$, and for any binary function $u : \Omega \to \{0,1\}$, $\mathbf{P}^J(u,.)$ is a vector encoding the probability density function (pdf) of data $J$ within the segment defined by $\{\mathbf{x} \in \Omega / u(\mathbf{x}) = 1\}$:

$$\mathbf{P}^J(u, z) = \frac{\int_\Omega \mathcal{K}_z(J) u \, d\mathbf{x}}{\int_\Omega u \, d\mathbf{x}} \qquad \forall z \in \mathcal{Z}_J \qquad (2)$$

with $\mathcal{K}_z$ a Gaussian window: $\mathcal{K}_z(y) = \frac{1}{(2\pi\sigma^2)^{(1/2)}} \exp\left(-\frac{\|z-y\|^2}{2\sigma^2}\right)$, with $\sigma$ the width of the window.

- $\langle f, g \rangle_\rho$ is the *probability product kernel* [10], which evaluates the affinity between two pdfs $f$ and $g$:

$$\langle f, g \rangle_\rho = \sum_{z \in \mathcal{Z}} [f(z)g(z)]^\rho \quad \rho \in ]0,1], \mathcal{Z} \in \{\mathcal{Z}_I, \mathcal{Z}_D, \mathcal{Z}_A\} \qquad (3)$$

The higher $\langle f, g \rangle_\rho$, the better the affinity between $f$ and $g$. Notice that the PPk in (3) can be viewed as a generalization of the Bhattacharyya coefficient [7]. Minimization of the PPKs in (1) aims at finding a target region whose shape and intensity pdfs most closely match *a priori* learned models:

- $\mathbf{M}^I$ is a model of intensity. We learn $\mathbf{M}^I$ from intensity data within a cylinder centered at $\mathcal{O}$. The radius of the cylinder, $d$, is a free parameter which has to be fixed experimentally.
- $\mathbf{M}^D$ and $\mathbf{M}^A$ are models of distances and angles respectively, describing a RV shape invariant with respect to translation. We learn these models from a single training subject different from the testing subject.
- $C : \Omega \to \mathbb{R}$ is an edge-indicator function given by $C(\mathbf{x}) = \frac{1}{1+\nabla I(\mathbf{x})}$. $\gamma$, $\alpha_D$ and $\alpha_A$ are positive constants that balance the contribution of each constraint in (1).

**Introducing a Scale Variable:** The shape prior in (1) is not invariant with respect to scale (or size) of the RV regions. To illustrate this, we plotted in Fig. 2 (c) the distance pdfs corresponding to the ground-truth segmentations of 20 different subjects (two different volumes for each subject). The figure demonstrates that the distance pdfs have similar Gaussian shapes, but shifted supports. This shift is due to inter-subject variations in scale (or size). To account for such shifts, we further introduce a scale variable in the model of distances: $\mathbf{M}^D(.,s) : \mathcal{Z}_D \times \mathbb{R} \to [0,1] / \mathbf{M}^D(z,s) = \mathbf{M}^D(z+s), s \in \mathbb{R}$. Thus, to account for this new variable ($s$), we replace the distance-based prior in (1) by a scale-dependent prior: $\langle \mathbf{P}^D(u,.), \mathbf{M}^D \rangle_\rho \to \langle \mathbf{P}^D(u,.), \mathbf{M}^D(.,s) \rangle_\rho$. Therefore, $s$ becomes a variable which has to be optimized along with the segmentation region. With this new variable, our problem becomes: $\{\hat{u}, \hat{s}\} = \min_{u,s} \mathcal{E}(u,s)$.

**Two-step Optimization:** Our model has two different types of variables, the target region described by indicator function $u$ and the scale variable $s$. We therefore adopt an iterative two-step procedure, by first fixing the scale variable and optimizing the proposed functional with respect to $u$ via convex relaxed surrogate functionals, and then optimizing over the scale variable via fixed-point computations, with $u$ fixed.

**Step 1–Optimization with Respect to the Segment Via Surrogate Functionals and Convex Relaxation:** To simplify further development, let us assume that our functional contains only one probability product kernel and has the following general form:

$$\min_{u(x)\in\{0,1\}} \left\{ \mathcal{E}(u) := -\langle \mathbf{P}(u,.), \mathbf{M} \rangle_\rho + \gamma \int_\Omega C \left| \nabla u \right| d\mathbf{x} \right\} \tag{4}$$

Observe that we omitted the superscripts that we defined previously for the pdfs to simplify further presentation and notations. Once the problem in (4) is solved, extension to a weighted sum of probability product kernels, as is the case in (1), becomes straightforward. Unfortunately, the probability product kernel in (4) is a non-linear (high-order) functional, which results in a difficult (non-convex) optimization problem that is not directly amenable to standard solvers. We split the problem into several surrogate-functional optimizations, each solved via an efficient convex relaxation.

**Surrogate Functionals:** We proceed by constructing and optimizing iteratively surrogate functionals of $\mathcal{E}$ (whose optimization is easier than the original functional):

**Definition 1.** *Given a fixed labeling $u^i$ ($i$ is the iteration number), $\mathcal{S}(u,u^i)$ is a surrogate functional of $\mathcal{E}$ if it satisfies the following conditions [11]:*

$$\mathcal{E}(u) \leq \mathcal{S}(u,u^i) \tag{5a}$$

$$\mathcal{E}(u) = \mathcal{S}(u,u) \tag{5b}$$

Rather than optimizing directly $\mathcal{E}$, we optimize the surrogate functional over the first variable at each iteration:

$$u^{i+1} = \min_u \mathcal{S}(u,u^i), \quad i = 1,2,\dots \tag{6}$$

Using the constraints in (5a) and (5b), and by the definition of minimum in (6), we can show that the solutions in (6) yield a decreasing sequence of $\mathcal{E}$: $\mathcal{E}(u^i) = \mathcal{S}(u^i, u^i) \geq \mathcal{S}(u^{i+1}, u^i) \geq \mathcal{E}(u^{i+1})$. Therefore, if $\mathcal{E}$ is lower bounded, sequence $\mathcal{E}(u^i)$ converges to a minimum of $\mathcal{E}$. Now, consider the following proposition [1] :

**Proposition 1.** *Given a fixed* $u^i : \Omega \to \{0,1\}$, *the following functional is a surrogate of functional* $\mathcal{E}$ *defined in (4):*

$$\mathcal{S}(u, u^i) = - \langle \mathbf{P}(u^i, .), \mathbf{M} \rangle_\rho + \int_\Omega f^i u^- \, d\mathbf{x} + \int_\Omega g^i u^+ \, d\mathbf{x} + \int_\Omega C \, |\nabla u| \, d\mathbf{x} \quad (7)$$

*where*

$$u^-(\mathbf{x}) := \begin{cases} 1 - u(\mathbf{x}), & \text{for } u^i(\mathbf{x}) = 1 \\ 0, & \text{otherwise} \end{cases} , u^+(\mathbf{x}) := \begin{cases} u(\mathbf{x}), & \text{for } u^i(\mathbf{x}) = 0 \\ 0, & \text{otherwise} \end{cases} \quad (8)$$

*and*

$$f^i = \sum_{z \in \mathcal{Z}} \frac{\mathcal{D}_{z,i,\rho} \mathcal{T}_{\mathbf{M},z}}{\int_\Omega \mathcal{T}_{\mathbf{M},z} u^i \, d\mathbf{x}} \; ; \; \mathcal{T}_{\mathbf{M},z} = \mathcal{K}_z(J)\mathbf{M}(z) ; \quad (9)$$

$$\mathcal{D}_{z,i,\rho} = \left[ \frac{\int_\Omega \mathcal{T}_{\mathbf{M},z} u^i \, d\mathbf{x}}{\int_\Omega u^i \, d\mathbf{x}} \right]^\rho \; ; g^i = \sum_{z \in \mathcal{Z}} \frac{\mathcal{D}_{z,i,\rho}}{\rho \int_\Omega u^i \, d\mathbf{x}} \quad (10)$$

**Convex Relaxation:** Now, note that $\mathcal{S}(u, u^i)$ has a linear form, which is amenable to powerful global solvers. At each iteration, we optimize $\mathcal{S}(u, u^i)$ with the convex-relaxation technique recently developed in [12]. The optimizer in [12] is amenable to parallel implementations on graphics processing units (GPU). Therefore, it can yield real-time solutions for 3D grids.

**Step 2–Fixed-point Optimization with Respect to the Scale Variable:** We fix labeling variable $u$ and optimize $\mathcal{E}$ with respect $s$. Considering a variable change $z \leftarrow z - s$ and the fact that only the distance-distribution prior depends on $s$, we have:

$$\frac{\partial \mathcal{E}}{\partial s} = -\alpha_D \frac{\partial \langle \mathbf{P}^D(u, .), \mathbf{M}^D(., s) \rangle_\rho}{\partial s}$$

$$= -\rho \alpha_D \sum_{z \in \mathcal{Z}_D} \frac{\partial \mathbf{P}^D(u, z - s)}{\partial s} \left[ \mathbf{M}^D(z) \right]^\rho \left[ \mathbf{P}^D(u, z - s) \right]^{\rho-1} \quad (11)$$

Using the pdf expression in (2), we also have:

$$\frac{\partial \mathbf{P}^D(u, z - s)}{\partial s} = \frac{\int_\Omega \frac{\partial \mathcal{K}_z(s+D)}{\partial s} u \, d\mathbf{x}}{\int_\Omega u \, d\mathbf{x}} = \frac{\int_\Omega (z - s - D) \mathcal{K}_z(s + D) d\mathbf{x}}{\sigma^2 \int_\Omega u \, d\mathbf{x}} \quad (12)$$

---

[1] The proof of proposition 1 is given in the supplemental material available at: http://externe.emt.inrs.ca/users/benayedi/BenAyed-Miccai13-Supp.pdf

**Table 1.** Quantitative evaluations over 400 volumes acquired from 20 subjects. The statistics are expressed as mean ± std.

| RMSE (mm) | DM | GPU time/volume | CPU time/volume |
|---|---|---|---|
| 2.30 ± 0.12 | 0.84 ± 0.07 | 0.129 sec | 2.72 sec |

Embedding (12) in (11), setting the obtained expression to zero, and after some manipulations, we obtain the following necessary condition for a minimum of $\mathcal{E}$ with respect to $s$:

$s - g(s) = 0$ where

$$g(s) = \frac{\sum_{z \in \mathcal{Z}_D} \int_\Omega (z - D) \mathcal{K}_z(D + s) \left[\mathbf{M}^D(z)\right]^\rho \left[\mathbf{P}^D(u, z - s)\right]^{\rho-1} u d\mathbf{x}}{\sum_{z \in \mathcal{Z}_D} \int_\Omega \mathcal{K}_z(D + s) \left[\mathbf{M}^D(z)\right]^\rho \left[\mathbf{P}^D(u, z - s)\right]^{\rho-1} u d\mathbf{x}}$$

(13)

Note that since the necessary condition in (13) has the form of a fixed-point equation, the solution can be obtained by fixed-point iterations:

$$s^{n+1} = g(s^n), \ n = 1, 2, \ldots$$

(14)

Let $s^{opt}$ be the limit of sequence $s^n$ at convergence. We have: $s^{opt} = lim_{n \to +\infty} s^{n+1} = lim_{n \to +\infty} g(s^n) = g(lim_{n \to +\infty} s^n) = g(s^{opt})$. Consequently, $s_{opt}$ is a solution of the necessary condition obtained in (13).

## 3  Experiments

We evaluated the algorithm over a data set containing short axis cardiac cine MRI volumes of 20 subjects (20 volumes per subject, each corresponding to a cardiac phase, i.e., we used 400 volumes in total). We performed three of types of experiments (The parameters were invariant for all the subjects $\alpha_D = 0.2; \alpha_A = 0.1; \gamma = 65$):

- Standard quantitative evaluations, which compare the results with independent manual segmentations approved by an expert;
- Comprehensive evaluations which demonstrate: (i) the performance of the proposed algorithm is not significantly affected by the choice of the training subject and (ii) the shape description we propose does not change significantly from one subject to another; and
- Computational evaluations, which demonstrate that the parallelized computations can bring a significant speed-up of more than 20 times.

**Example:** Fig. 1 depicts a typical example of the results, and demonstrates a high conformity between the manual and automatic segmentation.

**Computational Evaluations:** The parallelized implementation was run on an NVIDIA Tesla C1600 GPU, and the non-parallelized version on a 2.13 GHz Xeon (E5506), with 6 GB of RAM. Table 1 reports the average GPU/CPU times per volume. The parallelized implementation requires about 0.129 seconds for a typical volume, a speed-up of more than 20 times compared to the CPU version.

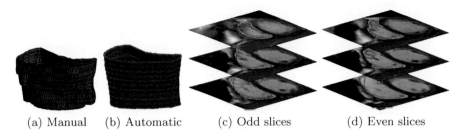

(a) Manual    (b) Automatic    (c) Odd slices    (d) Even slices

**Fig. 1.** An typical example using a 125 x 125 x 6 volume. (a-b): Manual and automatic surfaces; (c-d): The corresponding 2D contours/slices.

**Quantitative Performance Evaluations:** We proceeded to a leave-one-out validation, where one subject was used for training and the rest of the subjects were used for testing. We assessed the similarities between the ground truth and the obtained segmentations using a surface-based measure, the Root Mean Squared Error ($RMSE$), and a region-based measure, the Dice Metric ($DM$). Here following an description of these measures.

- *Dice Metric (DM):* Let $V_m$ and $V_a$ be the automated and manually segmented volumes, respectively. $DM$ is given by $DM = 2\frac{V_a \cap V_m}{V_a + V_m}$, and is always in [0 1], 1 indicating a perfect match and 0 a total mismatch.
- *RMSE:* $RMSE$ evaluates a distance between automated surfaces and the corresponding manual ones. The $RMSE$ over $N$ points is given by: $RMSE = \sqrt{\frac{1}{N}\sum_{i=1}^{N}(\hat{x}_i - \tilde{x}_i)^2 + (\hat{y}_i - \tilde{y}_i)^2}$ where $(\hat{x}_i, \hat{y}_i)$ is a point on the automatically detected surface and $(\tilde{x}_i, \tilde{y}_i)$ is the corresponding point on the manually traced surface. The lower $RMSE$, the better the conformity of the results to the ground truth.

Table 1 reports the results, and demonstrates that the obtained 3D surfaces correlate with manual delineations. Note that a $DM$ higher than 0.80 indicates an excellent agreement between manual and automatic segmentations [7].

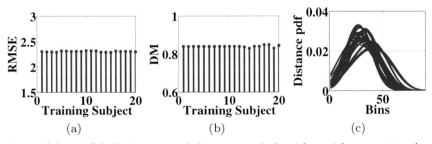

(a)    (b)    (c)

**Fig. 2.** (a) and (b): Robustness of the proposed algorithm with respect to the choice of the training subject, (c): Invariance of the distance-based shape model.

**Robustness with Respect to the Choice of Training Subject:** We proceeded to a comprehensive leave-one-in evaluation method consisting of 20 tests, each corresponding to the choice of a different training subject. Then, we segmented the entire dataset and measured the corresponding average $DM$ and $RMSE$. Figs. 2 (a) and (b) plot the obtained average $DM$ and $RMSE$ as functions of the index of the training subject, demonstrating a very low variation.

**Invariance of the Shape-prior Models:** Using ground-truth segmentations, we plotted in Fig.2 (c) the distance distributions corresponding to the 20 subjects in the dataset (We used two volumes for each subject). The figure demonstrates that the distributions have very similar shapes, but slightly different supports. These slight shifts, which are due to inter-subject variations in scale (or size), are handled efficiently with the proposed fixed-point computations.

## 4 Conclusion

We proposed a real-time 3D MRI segmentation of the right ventricle based on probability product kernel constraints. The proposed algorithm removes the need for large, manually-segmented training sets and costly pose estimation procedures. We reported comprehensive experiments, which support the fact that a single subject is sufficient for training our algorithm and demonstrate that the obtained performance is independent of the choice of training data.

## References

1. Grothues, F., Moon, J.C., Bellenger, N.G., Smith, G.S., Klein, H.U., Pennell, D.J.: Inter-study reproducibility of right ventricular volumes, function, and mass with cardiovascular magnetic resonance. Am. Heart. J. 147(2), 218–223 (2004)
2. Petitjean, C., Dacher, J.N.: A review of segmentation methods in short axis cardiac mr images. Medical Image Analysis 15, 169–184 (2011)
3. Zhang, H., Wahle, A., Johnson, R.K., Scholz, T.D., Sonka, M.: 4-D cardiac MR image analysis: left and right ventricular morphology and function. IEEE Transactions on Medical Imaging 29(2), 350–364 (2010)
4. Zhuang, X., Rhode, K.S., Arridge, S.R., Razavi, R.S., Hill, D., Hawkes, D.J., Ourselin, S.: An atlas-based segmentation propagation framework using locally affine registration – application to automatic whole heart segmentation. In: Metaxas, D., Axel, L., Fichtinger, G., Székely, G. (eds.) MICCAI 2008, Part II. LNCS, vol. 5242, pp. 425–433. Springer, Heidelberg (2008)
5. Lorenzo-Valdés, M., Sanchez-Ortiz, G.I., Elkington, A.G., Mohiaddin, R.H., Rueckert, D.: Segmentation of 4d cardiac mr images using a probabilistic atlas and the em algorithm. Medical Image Analysis 8(3), 255–265 (2004)
6. Ben Ayed, I., Lu, Y., Li, S., Ross, I.: Left ventricle tracking using overlap priors. In: Metaxas, D., Axel, L., Fichtinger, G., Székely, G. (eds.) MICCAI 2008, Part I. LNCS, vol. 5241, pp. 1025–1033. Springer, Heidelberg (2008)
7. Ben Ayed, I., Chen, H.M., Punithakumar, K., Ross, I., Li, S.: Max-flow segmentation of the left ventricle by recovering subject-specific distributions via a bound of the bhattacharyya measure. Medical Image Analysis 16, 87–100 (2012)

8. Zhu, Y., Papademetris, X., Sinusas, A.J., Duncan, J.S.: Segmentation of the left ventricle from cardiac mr images using a subject-specific dynamical model. IEEE Transactions on Medical Imaging 29(4), 669–687 (2010)

9. Hautvast, G., Lobregt, S., Breeuwer, M., Gerritsen, F.: Automatic contour propagation in cine cardiac magnetic resonance images. IEEE Transactions on Medical Imaging 25(11), 1472–1482 (2006)

10. Jebara, T., Kondor, R.I., Howard, A.: Probability product kernels. Journal of Machine Learning Research 5, 819–844 (2004)

11. Zhang, Z., Kwok, J.T., Yeung, D.Y.: Surrogate maximization/minimization algorithms and extensions. Machine Learning 69, 1–33 (2007)

12. Yuan, J., Bae, E., Tai, X.C.: A study on continuous max-flow and min-cut approaches. In: CVPR, pp. 2217–2224 (2010)

# A Learning-Based Approach for Fast and Robust Vessel Tracking in Long Ultrasound Sequences

Valeria De Luca*, Michael Tschannen, Gábor Székely, and Christine Tanner

Computer Vision Laboratory, ETH Zürich, 8092 Zürich, Switzerland

**Abstract.** We propose a learning-based method for robust tracking in long ultrasound sequences for image guidance applications. The framework is based on a scale-adaptive block-matching and temporal realignment driven by the image appearance learned from an initial training phase. The latter is introduced to avoid error accumulation over long sequences. The vessel tracking performance is assessed on long 2D ultrasound sequences of the liver of 9 volunteers under free breathing. We achieve a mean tracking accuracy of 0.96 mm. Without learning, the error increases significantly (2.19 mm, p<0.001).

**Keywords:** tracking, block-matching, learning, real-time, ultrasound.

## 1 Introduction

During conformal radiation therapies, motion in the treatment region needs to be compensated to ensure accuracy of the dose delivery. For the thorax and abdomen, motion due to respiration is substantial and can not be neglected [11,21]. Image-guided radiation therapies use image information gathered during therapy for adjusting the treatment plan. Tracking the respiratory motion on such images requires an accuracy in the millimeter range and real-time feedback. Potential imaging techniques for guidance include CT, MRI and ultrasound (US). The latter represents the only modality that is real-time, non-ionizing and cheap.

Structures on US sequences of the abdomen have been tracked using optical flow [5], speckle tracking algorithms [8], intensity-based registration [22], active contours [23], hybrid methods [6,13,3] and US imaging models [12]. Block-matching algorithms (BMAs) compute the local displacements from interpolating the translations that provide the best match of image regions in two consecutive frames. Many BMAs have been proposed (e.g. [1,19,14,2,8]), yet their performance has so far only been assessed on relative short sequences (<1 min). Therapy guidance requires the tracking of long sequences, which poses a special challenge for BM due to its iterative nature. Moreover, our sequences suffer from noise, interferences, low SNR and frame dropouts. To create a robust framework for feature tracking in long sequences, we propose an algorithm, which combines several BM components and includes a novel adaptation of the block size to

---

* We thank the Swiss National Science Foundation (CRSII2 127549) for funding.

K. Mori et al. (Eds.): MICCAI 2013, Part I, LNCS 8149, pp. 518–525, 2013.
© Springer-Verlag Berlin Heidelberg 2013

the feature scale. In addition, we exploit the approximate periodicity of breathing motion for learning image appearance and corresponding motion behavior (extracted by accurate but slow image registration) to allow frequent temporal realignment of the BMA for drift-free real-time tracking.

## 2   Material

US liver sequences of 9 volunteers during free breathing were acquired at the Geneva University Hospital [17]. To evaluate US tracking performance for hybrid US and MR guided treatments [17], an Acuson clinical scanner (Antares; Siemens Medical Solutions, Mountain View, CA) was modified to be MR compatible, and US and MR images were simultaneously acquired. The US images (real-time second harmonic images with 1.8-2.2 MHz center frequency) were exported on-the-fly using a frame grabber device. 2D US images were acquired at a fixed location (longitudinal or intercostal plane) over 5:21, 5:28 and 10:08 min for 1, 7 and 1 volunteer(s), respectively. The resulting 2650 to 14516 frames had a temporal and spatial resolution of 14-25 Hz and 0.3-0.7 mm, respectively.

## 3   Method

### 3.1   Scale-adaptive Block-matching

The key components of our proposed scale-adaptive BMA (SA-BMA) are a novel adaptation of the block size to the feature scale and the new combination of the interpolation function from [14] with the temporal realignment from [19].

**Block Configuration.** Traditionally the size of the blocks is chosen empirically [16,7] or equal to the US speckle size [10]. We adapt the block size to the feature size to ensure that every block contains a part of the feature, which limits the aperture problem and avoids ambiguities due to homogeneous blocks.

The position of features to track, e.g. $P_j(t_0)$ for vessel $j$, are manually selected in $I(t_0)$, see Fig. 1. BM is performed for a region of interest ($ROI_j(t_0)$) around feature $j$, which covers a $M \mathrm{x} N$ grid of equally sized squares (called blocks) $B_{i,j}$ of size $\Delta b_j$ with center points $G_{i,j}$, $i \in [1, \ldots, MN]$, defined at $t_0$. $\Delta b_j$ is determined from the feature size. In detail, as vessel cross sections have elliptic shape, we search for blob-like features centered at $P_j$. A scale-space approach (local maxima of a Difference-of-Gaussian (DoG)) [15,20] is used to detect the most likely blob in $ROI_j(t_0)$. The resulting scale $s$ is related to the minor semi-axis $r_j$ of an ellipse fitted to the vessel section by $r_j = \sqrt{2s}$ and $\Delta b_j = \lceil r_j \rceil$.

**Displacement Calculation.** We compute the motion field in each $ROI_j$ by determining the displacement at $G_{i,j}$ via BM, and use weighted interpolation [14] to obtain the displacement of $P_j$. At time step $t^*$ the displacement of $G_{i,j}(t^{ref})$ in the reference frame $t^{ref}$ to $G_{i,j}(t^*)$, denoted as $\mathbf{d}_{G_{i,j}}(t^*)$, is determined by the displacement $\mathbf{v}$ which maximized the normalized cross-correlation (NCC) between $B_{i,j}(t^{ref})$ and the block from $I(t^*)$ centered at $G_{i,j}(t^{ref})+\mathbf{v}$. The values of $\mathbf{v}$ are restricted to cover only a certain search region. The reference frame is generally the previous frame ($t^* - 1$). Other strategies for $t^{ref}$ are described in the next paragraph. The displacement of the tracked point from $t^{ref}$ to $t^*$ ($\mathbf{d}_j(t^*)$) is deduced from the block displacements $\mathbf{d}_{G_{i,j}}(t^*)$ by weighted interpolation:

$$\mathbf{d}_j(t^*) = \sum_{\hat{i}} w_{\hat{i}} \mathbf{d}_{G_{\hat{i},j}}(t^*), \tag{1}$$

where $w_{\hat{i}}$ are the weights and $\hat{i} = \{i|Q(i,t^*) = 1\}$. $Q(i,t^*)$ is the filtering mask for $ROI_j$ at time $t^*$, which is defined by $Q(i,t^*) = 1$ for the 9 $G_{i,j}(t^{ref})$ closest to $P_j(t^{ref})$, and $Q(i,t^*) = 0$ otherwise. We consider the weights $w_{\hat{i}}$ [14]:

$$w_{\hat{i}} = 0.5 \frac{1}{D_{\hat{i}}^2 + 1} \frac{1}{\sum_{\hat{i}} \frac{1}{D_{\hat{i}}^2 + 1}} + 0.5 \frac{\alpha_{\hat{i}}}{\sum_{\hat{i}} \alpha_{\hat{i}}}, \tag{2}$$

with $D_{\hat{i}}$ the Euclidean distance from $G_{\hat{i},j}(t^{ref})$ to $P_j(t^{ref})$, and $\alpha_{\hat{i}} = \sigma_{\hat{i}}^2/\mu_{\hat{i}}$ the ratio between the variance ($\sigma_{\hat{i}}^2$) and the mean ($\mu_{\hat{i}}$) of the pixel intensities in $B_{\hat{i},j}(t^*)$. This interpolation scheme has the advantage that it incorporates regularization (first term) and accounts for the relative image content (second term) [14]. The position of the tracked point is $P_j(t^*) = P_j(t^{ref}) + \mathbf{d}_j(t^*)$.

**Reference Frame Definition.** BMAs can generally only cope with small deformations and appearance changes, as they are based on the translations of local regions. Hence BM is applied to temporally consecutive frames (i.e. $t^{ref} = t^* - 1$) for tracking. However, this strategy is subject to error accumulation leading to drift. Such errors are particularly relevant in long sequences. Yet the approximate periodic nature of respiratory motion provides frequently frames which are similar to the initial frame and BM is again applicable for aligning these [19]. Errors occur also due to the quantization of $\mathbf{d}_{G_{i,j}}$. Hence we introduce the following strategy:

> if NCC($ROI_j(t_0), ROI_j(t^*)$) > $\theta_{NCC,j}$ then $t^{ref} = t_0$
> else if $\|\mathbf{d}_j(t^*)\| \leq \epsilon_d$ then $t^{ref} = t^{ref}_{prev}$
> else $t^{ref} = t^* - 1$ end

where NCC($A, B$) is the NCC between image region $A$ and $B$, $\theta_{NCC,j}$ is the 84th percentile of the NCC values gathered from an initial subset of the sequence, $\epsilon_d = 0.01$ pixel, and $t^{ref}_{prev}$ denotes $t^{ref}$ from the previous image pair.

## 3.2 Learning-based Tracking

During therapy, images are acquired continuously over several minutes. Hence temporal realignment of the images is crucial to ensure robust tracking and to avoid error accumulation. For repetitive motion, such as breathing, redundancy within the images can be exploited [4]. Following a similar strategy, we divide the method into a training and tracking phase. During training we learn the relationship between image appearance and the corresponding displacements, from a slower, but more robust tracking method. During the clinical application, the displacements are computed by the proposed SA-BMA (see Sec. 3.1), with the reference frame given by the closest frame from the training set. This strategy allows temporal realignment over many more breathing states than previously.

**Training Phase.** In the training phase we acquire a sequence covering 10 breathing cycle, resulting in $T_{10C}$ images $I(t_i)$, $t_i \in [t_0, \ldots, T_{10C}]$.

The images $I(t_i)$ are registered to $I(t_0)$, to obtain spatial correspondence. The registration optimizes the parameters of an affine transformation with respect to NCC over a manually selected region around $P_j(t_0)$ and is initialized by the result from $I(t_{i-1})$ to $I(t_0)$.

To store the image appearance efficiently, we embed the images $I(t_i) \in \mathbb{R}^D$ into a low-dimensional representation $\mathbf{S}(t_i) = [s_1(t_i); \ldots; s_L(t_i)] \in \mathbb{R}^L$, with $L \ll D$, using Principal Component Analysis (PCA) [4]. We select $L$ such that the cumulative energy of the first $L$ eigenvectors just exceeds 95%. In addition, we select the PCA component $s_B$ in $\mathbf{S}$ that captures the main breathing motion, by computing the FFT of each $s_i$ and choosing the one that has a power spectral density maximum at 0.15-0.4 Hz (2.5-6 s, common breathing). $\mathbf{S}$ and the corresponding registration results (e.g. $P_j$) are stored $\forall t_i$.

**Tracking Phase.** New images are continuously acquired during treatment. Given the current image $I(t^*)$, we first project it into the PCA space ($\mathbf{S}(t^*) = [s_1(t^*); \ldots; s_L(t^*)]$). Then, depending on its similarity to the training data and the previous frame, a reference frame is chosen. The logic is as follows:

    outlierFlag = false
    if $||\mathbf{S}(t^*) - \mathbf{S}(t_0)||_2 < \theta_1$ then $t^{ref} = t_0$
    else if $argmin_{t_x \in [t_0,\ldots,T_{10C}]}||\mathbf{S}(t^*) - \mathbf{S}(t_x)||_2 < \theta_2$ then $t^{ref} = t_x$
    else if $||\mathbf{S}(t^*) - \mathbf{S}(t^* - 1)||_2 < \theta_2$ then $t^{ref} = t^* - 1$
    else outlierFlag = true end
    if (outlierFlag == false) then do SA-BMA
    else do affine registration and update $\mathbf{S}$ end

The threshold $\theta_1$ is the 5th percentile of the Euclidean distance between $\mathbf{S}(t_0)$ and $\mathbf{S}(t_i)$ $\forall t_0 < t_i \leq T_{10C}$. $\theta_2$ is the 95th percentile of the distribution of the minimum Euclidean distances between the $\mathbf{S}(t_i)$ in the training set [4].

## 3.3   Evaluation

We compared the performance of SA-BMA (Sec. 3.1) and LB-BMA (Sec. 3.2). As baseline BMA, we modified the SA-BMA to have fixed block size $\Delta b_j = 16$. The methods were tested for a total of 25 vessels in 9 sequences, see Fig. 1. We visually inspected the tracking quality for all vessels. We quantitatively evaluated the tracking error for the 15 vessels, which appeared to allow reliable annotations. We randomly selected 10% of the tracking phase images and manually annotated the position (denoted as $\bar{P}_j$) corresponding to $P_j(t_0)$. For the annotated frame $(\hat{t})$, we calculated the tracking error $TE_j(\hat{t}) = ||P_j(\hat{t}) - \bar{P}(\hat{t})||$. We summarize the results by the mean (MTE), standard deviation (SD) and 95th percentile of all $TE(\hat{t})$, considering all landmarks as a single distribution. We computed the

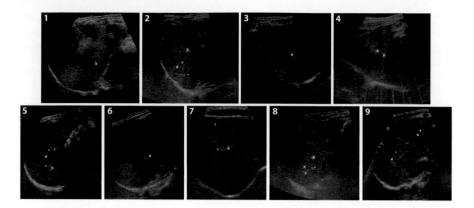

**Fig. 1.** $I(t_0)$ of the 9 sequences and manual annotation of the tracked vessel centers $P_j(t_0)$, $j \in [1, \ldots, 25]$. Quantitative evaluation was based on the 15 $P_j$ marked by 'x'. Visible artifacts include MR-RF interferences (4), and small acoustic windows (2,3,6,8).

MTE for each landmark $j$ ($MTE_j$) and report the range for the 15 vessels. We included the motion magnitude of the vessels, i.e. $\left\| P_j(t_0) - \bar{P}(\hat{t}) \right\|$.

We estimated the inter-observer variability of the annotations. Two additional experts annotated 3% of randomly selected images from the tracking phase. We then defined as ground truth the mean position over the 3 annotations and calculated the tracking error as before.

## 4    Results

We tracked a total of ~50000 frames, acquired over a total of ~50 min. $\Delta b_j$ ranges in [4, 22] pixels and the size of the tracked vessels varies from 2 to 9 mm. The PCA space is characterized by $L$ in the range of [86, 287], vs. $D > 3660$.

We firstly evaluated the registration error for the training images. The affine registration achieves an accuracy of $0.63 \pm 0.36$ mm (1.30 mm) on average (MTE $\pm$ SD (95th percentile of TE)), with a $MRE_j$ range of [0.42, 0.84] mm.

Table 1 lists the results for the proposed approaches, SA-BMA and LB-BMA. We compared LB-BMA considering **S** (LB-BMA$_{95}$) and $\mathbf{s}_B$ (LB-BMA$_B$). The best performance is achieved by LB-BMA$_{95}$ with a MTE of 0.96 mm. Fig. 2 illustrates the benefit of the proposed methods for the worst case of BMA. For LB-BMA$_{95}$ (LB-BMA$_B$) and all 25 tracked vessels, $t^{ref}$ is picked from the training set for 68.3% (99.0%) of the frames, while 1.4% (1.0%) require affine registration.

The inter-observer MTE varies from 0.30 to 0.34 mm (95th TE from 0.63 to 0.68 mm, $MTE_j$ range [0.16, 0.70]). For the inter-observer data set, the median $TE_j$ of BMA and SA-BMA, SA-BMA and LB-BMA$_B$, and SA-BMA and LB-BMA$_{95}$ were statistically significantly different at the 0.001 level (Wilcoxon sign-rank test), while LB-BMA$_B$ and LB-BMA$_{95}$ were not (p=0.53). No other statistical tests were performed.

**Table 1.** Tracking results (in mm) for the different methods w.r.t. manual annotation from one and three observers. Best results are in bold face.

|  | 1 Obs - 10%, ~7500 images | | 3 Obs - 3%, ~2500 images | |
|---|---|---|---|---|
|  | MTE ±SD ($95^{th}$TE) | rangeMTE$_j$ | MTE ±SD ($95^{th}$TE) | rangeMTE$_j$ |
| VesselMotion | 5.17 ± 3.21 (10.59) | [2.81, 11.48] | 5.22 ± 3.23 (10.57) | [3.00, 11.30] |
| BMA | 3.22 ± 2.26 (7.24) | [1.25, 12.35] | 3.20 ± 2.26 (7.17) | [1.26, 12.16] |
| SA-BMA | 2.19 ± 1.46 (4.90) | [1.20, 5.79] | 2.18 ± 1.45 (4.83) | [1.22, 5.78] |
| LB-BMA$_B$ | 1.24 ± 1.41 (3.81) | [1.04, **1.49**] | 1.21 ± 1.39 (3.67) | [0.98, **1.49**] |
| LB-BMA$_{95}$ | **0.96 ± 0.64 (2.26)** | [**0.38**, 2.34] | **0.97 ± 0.65 (2.20)** | [**0.36**, 2.24] |

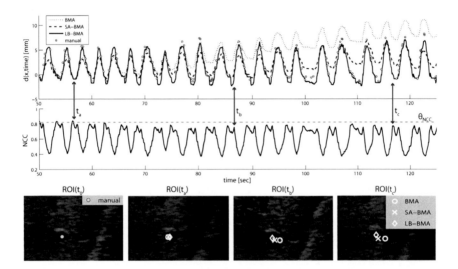

**Fig. 2.** Comparison of the tracking performance for a sequence where BMA failed (MTE$_j$=12.4 mm). (Top) Main motion component of manual annotation and $d_j$ from 3 methods for a temporal subset. (Middle) Corresponding NCC to first image. (Bottom, left to right) First image with annotation ($P(t_0)$), image with tracking results at last realignment ($t_a$) of (SA-)BMA, at $t_a + 30$ s and $t_a + 60$ s. Drift occurs in a significant (moderate) way for BMA (SA-BMA) for $t > t_a$, while LB-BMA remains robust.

The average time to compute the motion of the tracked vessel per frame was 100 ms (range [30, 350] ms). The PCA projection in LB-BMA required ~13 ms per frame. These measures were obtained using non-optimized Matlab software and no GPU parallel computing (single PC with Intel®Core™i7-920 at 2.66 GHz processor and 8 GB RAM), and exclude outliers, i.e. images that required affine registration. The latter was computed in approximately 0.8-2.5 s per image region, using the Insight Segmentation and Registration Toolkit (ITK).

## 5    Conclusion

We proposed a novel and robust framework for vessel tracking in long US sequences. The method is based on learning the relationship between image appearance and feature displacements to allow frequent reinitialization of a scale-adaptive block-matching algorithm. The method was evaluated on long US sequences of the liver of 9 volunteers under free breathing and achieved a mean accuracy of 0.96 mm for tracking vessels for 5-10 min. To our knowledge, this is the first evaluation for tracking such long US sequences. Our performance also improves the state-of-the-art in 2D US tracking of the human liver (1.6 mm [23]). The proposed method is robust to interference, noise (see Fig. 1), and frame dropouts. Moreover, it is potentially real-time [9,18,4].

Standard BMA might fail in long sequences, due to an inappropriate block size, changes in the image similarity values and error accumulation. The introduction of scale-adaptive blocks and the learning strategy were both significant for the improvement of the results. While adaption to the feature size reduces the error caused by ambiguous matches, the use of NCC for measuring the feasibility of temporal realignment can be misleading. Even with adaptation to the individual US sequence, temporal realignment of the tracking was often too sparse. In contrast, the proposed learning based approach enables more frequent realignments to relevant images by exploiting the repetition in the images and learning the main variation in image appearance. This allows us to detect outliers and then adapt to these previously unseen variations by affine registration, which is slow but able to handle larger displacements.

Reducing computational costs by using only the breathing signal for measuring image similarity increased mean errors slightly (0.96 vs. 1.24 mm). While affine registration performed well on the training set, it was only applied to outliers (1%) during real-time tracking due to its computational complexity [4].

The achieved accuracy and robustness of the proposed tracking method for long and very difficult US sequences makes us confident of its success for real-time US guidance during radiation therapy under free-breathing.

## References

1. Boukerroui, D., Noble, J.A., Brady, J.M.: Velocity Estimation in Ultrasound Images: A Block Matching Approach. In: Taylor, C.J., Noble, J.A. (eds.) IPMI 2003. LNCS, vol. 2732, pp. 586–598. Springer, Heidelberg (2003)
2. Byram, B., Holley, G., Giannantonio, D., Trahey, G.: 3-D phantom and in vivo cardiac speckle tracking using a matrix array and raw echo data. IEEE Trans. Ultrason. Ferroelectr. Freq. Control 57(4), 839 (2010)
3. Cifor, A., Risser, L., Chung, D., Anderson, E.M., Schnabel, J.A.: Hybrid feature-based Log-Demons registration for tumour tracking in 2-D liver ultrasound images. In: Proc. IEEE Int. Symp. Biomed. Imaging, p. 724 (2012)
4. De Luca, V., Tanner, C., Szekely, G.: Speeding-up Image Registration for Repetitive Motion Scenarios. In: Proc. IEEE Int. Symp. Biomed. Imaging, p. 1355 (2012)
5. Demi, M., Bianchini, E., Faita, F., Gemignani, V.: Contour tracking on ultrasound sequences of vascular images. Pattern Recognition and Image Anal. 18, 606 (2008)

6. Foroughi, P., Abolmaesumi, P., Hashtrudi-Zaad, K.: Intra-subject elastic registration of 3D ultrasound images. Med. Image Anal. 10(5), 713 (2006)
7. Harris, E.J., Miller, N.R., Bamber, J.C., Evans, P.M., Symonds-Tayler, J.R.N.: Performance of ultrasound based measurement of 3D displacement using a curvilinear probe for organ motion tracking. Phys. Med. Biol. 52(18), 5683 (2007)
8. Harris, E.J., Miller, N.R., Bamber, J.C., Symonds-Tayler, J.R.N., Evans, P.M.: Speckle tracking in a phantom and feature-based tracking in liver in the presence of respiratory motion using 4D ultrasound. Phys. Med. Biol. 55(12), 3363 (2010)
9. Hsu, A., Miller, N.R., Evans, P.M., Bamber, J.C., Webb, S.: Feasibility of using ultrasound for real-time tracking during radiotherapy. Med. Phys. 32(6), 1500 (2005)
10. Kaluzynski, K., Chen, X., Emelianov, S.Y., Skovoroda, A.R., O'Donnell, M.: Strain rate imaging using two-dimensional speckle tracking. IEEE Trans. Ultrason. Ferroelectr. Freq. Control 48(4), 1111 (2001)
11. Keall, P.J., Mageras, G.S., Balter, J.M., Emery, R.S., Forster, K.M., Jiang, S.B., Kapatoes, J.M., Low, D.A., Murphy, M.J., Murray, B.R., Ramsey, C.R., Van Herk, M.B., Vedam, S.S., Wong, J.W., Yorke, E.: The management of respiratory motion in radiation oncology report of AAPM Task Group 76. Med. Phys. 33, 3874 (2006)
12. King, A.P., Rhode, K.S., Ma, Y., Yao, C., Jansen, C., Razavi, R., Penney, G.P.: Registering preprocedure volumetric images with intraprocedure 3-D ultrasound using an ultrasound imaging model. IEEE Trans. Med. Imaging 29(3), 924 (2010)
13. Leung, C., Hashtrudi-Zaad, K., Foroughi, P., Abolmaesumi, P.: A Real-Time Intrasubject Elastic Registration Algorithm for Dynamic 2-D Ultrasound Images. Ultrasound. Med. Biol. 35(7), 1159 (2009)
14. Lin, C.H., Lin, M.C.J., Sun, Y.N.: Ultrasound motion estimation using a hierarchical feature weighting algorithm. Comput. Med. Imaging Graph. 31(3), 178 (2007)
15. Lindeberg, T.: Feature detection with automatic scale selection. Int. J. Comput. Vision 30, 79 (1998)
16. Morsy, A.A., Von Ramm, O.T.: FLASH correlation: a new method for 3-D ultrasound tissue motion tracking and blood velocity estimation. IEEE Trans. Ultrason. Ferroelectr. Freq. Control 46(3), 728 (1999)
17. Petrusca, L., Cattin, P., De Luca, V., Preiswerk, F., Celicanin, Z., Auboiroux, V., Viallon, M., Arnold, P., Santini, F., Terraz, S., Scheffler, K., Becker, C.D., Salomir, R.: Hybrid Ultrasound/Magnetic Resonance Simultaneous Acquisition and Image Fusion for Motion Monitoring in the Upper Abdomen. Invest. Radiol. 48, 333 (2013)
18. Pinton, G.F., Dahl, J.J., Trahey, G.E.: Rapid tracking of small displacements with ultrasound. IEEE Trans. Ultrason. Ferroelectr. Freq. Control 53(6), 1103 (2006)
19. Revell, J., Mirmehdi, M., McNally, D.: Computer Vision Elastography: Speckle Adaptive Motion Estimation for Elastography Using Ultrasound Sequences. IEEE Trans. Med. Imaging 24(6), 755 (2005)
20. Schneider, R.J., Perrin, D.P., Vasilyev, N.V., Marx, G.R., del Nido, P.J., Howe, R.D.: Real-time image-based rigid registration of three-dimensional ultrasound. Med. Image Anal. 16, 402 (2012)
21. Shirato, H., Shimizu, S., Kitamura, K., Onimaru, R.: Organ motion in image-guided radiotherapy: lessons from real-time tumor-tracking radiotherapy. Int. J. Clin. Oncol. 12, 8 (2007)
22. Wein, W., Cheng, J.Z., Khamene, A.: Ultrasound based Respiratory Motion Compensation in the Abdomen. In: MICCAI Workshop on Image Guidance and Computer Assistance for Soft-Tissue Interventions (2008)
23. Zhang, X., Günther, M., Bongers, A.: Real-Time Organ Tracking in Ultrasound Imaging Using Active Contours and Conditional Density Propagation. In: Liao, H., "Eddie" Edwards, P.J., Pan, X., Fan, Y., Yang, G.-Z. (eds.) MIAR 2010. LNCS, vol. 6326, pp. 286–294. Springer, Heidelberg (2010)

# Supervised Feature Learning for Curvilinear Structure Segmentation

Carlos Becker*, Roberto Rigamonti, Vincent Lepetit, and Pascal Fua

CVLab, École Polytechnique Fédérale de Lausanne, Switzerland
{name.surname}@epfl.ch

**Abstract.** We present a novel, fully-discriminative method for curvilinear structure segmentation that simultaneously learns a classifier and the features it relies on. Our approach requires almost no parameter tuning and, in the case of 2D images, removes the requirement for hand-designed features, thus freeing the practitioner from the time-consuming tasks of parameter and feature selection. Our approach relies on the Gradient Boosting framework to learn discriminative convolutional filters in closed form at each stage, and can operate on raw image pixels as well as additional data sources, such as the output of other methods like the Optimally Oriented Flux. We will show that it outperforms state-of-the-art curvilinear segmentation methods on both 2D images and 3D image stacks.

## 1 Introduction

Linear structures, such as blood vessels, bronchial networks, or dendritic arbors are pervasive in biological images and their modeling is critical for analysis purposes. Thus, automated delineation techniques are key to exploiting the endless streams of image data that modern imaging devices produce. Among such delineation techniques, there is a whole class of approaches such as [1–3] that take as input image segmentations in which pixels or voxels within linear structures are labeled as one and others as zero. The better the initial segmentation, the more effective these methods are. To generate them, most approaches compute a local *linearity measure* and threshold the resulting scores. This linearity measure can be postulated *a priori* [4, 5], optimized to find specific patterns [6, 7], or learned [8–10] from training data.

In this paper, we propose a novel approach to computing linearity, which yields better segmentations than using state-of-the-art methods such as [5, 10]. We introduce an original fully-discriminative method that relies on the Gradient Boosting framework [11, 12] to simultaneously compute optimal filters and boosting weights at each iteration.

Our weak classifiers rely on convolutional filters whose kernels are learned during boosting. Arguably, this could be described as learning the classifier parameters as it is often done by boosting algorithms. However, because the parameter space is so large, a standard boosting approach, such as a grid search, would

---

* This work was supported in part by the ERC grant MicroNano.

K. Mori et al. (Eds.): MICCAI 2013, Part I, LNCS 8149, pp. 526–533, 2013.

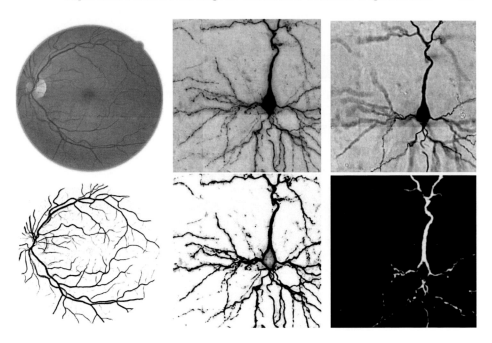

**Fig. 1.** Raw images **(top)** and probability maps $p(y = 1|x)$ **(bottom)** obtained with our approach on retinal scans **(left)** and brightfield microscopy in 2D **(center)** and 3D **(right)**(slice cut)

be impractical. Instead, we compute the kernels in closed form, which allows us to handle the enormous size of the parameter space. Convolutional Neural Networks [13] and Deep Belief Networks (DBNs) [14] also simultaneously learn convolutional features and classification weights. DBNs in particular do so in an unsupervised way and only use discriminative information for fine-tuning. The latter may not be ideal since it has recently been shown that fully-supervised versions of these approaches have a large unexploited potential and can significantly outperform competing methods in challenging tasks [15]. However, the neural network architecture adopted in [15] requires specialized set-up and careful design, and it is computationally expensive to train, even on GPUs. By contrast, our approach is much less computationally demanding and involves just few, easily-tunable parameters. The low computational burden is particularly relevant in that it allows us to deal with 3D image stacks which, despite the prominency they are gaining in the medical domain, cannot be handled by competing algorithms such as [15] due to the high computational cost.

In the remainder of this paper, we first review briefly the standard Gradient Boosting framework, and then introduce our approach for jointly learning the filters our weak learners rely on and the parameters of the classifier that uses them. Finally, we demonstrate superior performance on several very different kinds of images that feature linear structures.

## 2   Gradient Boosting

Gradient Boosting [11, 12] is a an approach to approximating a function $\varphi^*$ : $\mathbb{R}^n \to \mathbb{R}$ by a function $\varphi$ of the form $\varphi(\mathbf{x}) = \sum_{j=1}^{M} \alpha_j h_j(\mathbf{x})$ , where the $\alpha_j \in \mathbb{R}$ are real-valued weights, $h_j : \mathbb{R}^n \to \mathbb{R}$ are weak learners, and $\mathbf{x} \in \mathbb{R}^n$ is the input vector. Gradient Boosting can be seen as a generalization of AdaBoost that can make use of real-valued weak learners and minimize different loss functions [11]. Gradient Boosting has shown significant performance improvements in many classification problems with respect to classic AdaBoost [16].

Given training samples $\{(\mathbf{x}_i, y_i)\}_{i=1,...,N}$, where $\mathbf{x}_i \in \mathbb{R}^n$ and $y_i = \varphi^*(\mathbf{x}_i)$, $\varphi(\cdot)$ is constructed in a greedy manner, iteratively selecting weak learners and their weights to minimize a loss function $\mathcal{L} = \sum_{i=1}^{N} L(y_i, \varphi(\mathbf{x}_i))$. We use the quadratic approximation introduced in [12]. Commonly used classification loss functions are the exponential loss $L = e^{-y_i \varphi(\mathbf{x}_i)}$ and the log loss $L = \log(1 + e^{-2y_i \varphi(\mathbf{x}_i)})$.

The weak learners $h_j(\cdot)$ are generally either decision stumps or regression trees [11]. Regression trees are a generalization of decision stumps and usually yield significantly better performance [11], achieving state-of-the-art in many classification problems [16]. Regression trees are typically learned in a greedy manner, building them one split at a time, starting from the root [11].

## 3   Proposed Approach

Assume that we are given training samples $\{(\mathbf{x}_i, y_i)\}_{i=1...N}$, where $\mathbf{x}_i \in \mathbb{R}^n$ represents an image, a patch, or the output of a pre-processing filter —in practice we use OOF [5] for 3D data— and $y_i \in \{-1, 1\}$ its label. Our goal is to simultaneously learn both the features and a function $\varphi(\mathbf{x}) : \mathbb{R}^n \to \mathbb{R}$ based on these features to predict the value of $y$ corresponding to previously unseen $\mathbf{x}$.

We first recall below how decision stumps and regression trees can be built to optimize a Gradient Boosting classifier. We then describe how we learn relevant features while growing the trees.

### 3.1   Growing Regression Trees

Typically, Gradient Boosting implementations search through sets of weak learners that rely on a fixed set of features, such as Haar wavelets. At each iteration $j$, it selects the $h_j(\cdot)$ that minimizes

$$h_j(\cdot) = \underset{h(\cdot)}{\operatorname{argmin}} \sum_{i=1}^{N} w_i^j \left( h(\mathbf{x}_i) - r_i^j \right)^2 \tag{1}$$

where weight-response pairs $\{w_i^j, r_i^j\}$ are computed by differentiating $L(y_i, \varphi)$ [12].

We consider here weak learners that are regression trees based on convolutions of $\mathbf{x}$ with a set of learned convolution kernels $\mathcal{K}_j$. We write them as $h_j(\mathbf{x}) = T(\theta_j, \mathcal{K}_j, \mathbf{x})$ where $\theta_j$ denotes the tree parameters. Standard approaches learn only the $\theta_j$, while we also learn the kernels $\mathcal{K}_j$.

---

**Algorithm 1.** Split Learning

---

**Input:** Training samples $\{\mathbf{x}_i\}_{i=1,..,N}$. Number $P$ of kernels to explore.
Weights and responses $\{w_i, r_i\}_{i=1,..,N}$. at boosting iteration $j$, as in [12].
Set $\mathbb{W}$ of window locations and sizes, and set $\mathbb{L}$ of regularization factors.

// *Phase I: kernel search*
1: **for** $p = 1$ to $P$ **do**
2:     Pick $N_{T_1}$ random samples from training set into $T_1$
3:     Pick random window $W_{\mathbf{c}_p, a_p} \in \mathbb{W}$, random regularization factor $\lambda_p \in \mathbb{L}$
4:     Find kernel $\mathbf{k}_p$:

$$\mathbf{k}_p = \underset{\mathbf{k}}{\operatorname{argmin}} \sum_{i \in T_1} w_i \left( \mathbf{k}^\top W_{\mathbf{c}_p, a_p}(\mathbf{x}_i) - r_i \right)^2 + \lambda_p \sum_{(m,n) \in \mathcal{N}} \left( \mathbf{k}^{(m)} - \mathbf{k}^{(n)} \right)^2$$

5: **end for**

// *Phase II: split search*
6: Pick $\frac{N}{2}$ random samples from training set into $T_2$
7: **for** $p = 1$ to $P$ **do**
8:     Let $W_p(\cdot) = W_{\mathbf{c}_p, a_p}(\cdot)$
9:     Find $\tau_p, \eta_{1,p}, \eta_{2,p}$ for $\mathbf{k}_p$ through exhaustive search on $T_2$:

$$\tau_p, \eta_{1,p}, \eta_{2,p} = \underset{\tau, \eta_1, \eta_2}{\operatorname{argmin}} \sum_{i | \mathbf{k}_p^\top W_p(\mathbf{x}_i) < \tau} w_i \left( r_i - \eta_1 \right)^2 + \sum_{i | \mathbf{k}_p^\top W_p(\mathbf{x}_i) \geq \tau} w_i \left( r_i - \eta_2 \right)^2$$

10:     Compute split cost on $T_2$:

$$\epsilon_p = \sum_{i | \mathbf{k}_p^\top W_p(\mathbf{x}_i) < \tau_p} w_i \left( r_i - \eta_{1,p} \right)^2 + \sum_{i | \mathbf{k}_p^\top W_p(\mathbf{x}_i) \geq \tau_p} w_i \left( r_i - \eta_{2,p} \right)^2$$

11: **end for**

12: **return** $(\mathbf{k}_p, \tau_p, \eta_{1,p}, \eta_{2,p})$ that yields the smallest $\epsilon_p$.

---

The tree learning procedure is performed one split at a time, as in [11]. A split consists of a test function $t(\cdot) \in \mathbb{R}$, a threshold $\tau$, and return values $\eta_1$ and $\eta_2$. Its prediction function can be written as

$$s(\cdot) = \begin{cases} \eta_1 & \text{if } t(\cdot) < \tau \\ \eta_2 & \text{otherwise.} \end{cases} \tag{2}$$

Given $t(\cdot)$, the optimal root split at iteration $j$ is found by minimizing

$$\sum_{i | t(\mathbf{x}_i) < \tau} w_i^j \left( r_i^j - \eta_1 \right)^2 + \sum_{i | t(\mathbf{x}_i) \geq \tau} w_i^j \left( r_i^j - \eta_2 \right)^2, \tag{3}$$

where $\tau$, $\eta_1$, and $\eta_2$ are typically found through exhaustive search [11].

In our approach, we introduce a test function that operates on the results of $\mathbf{x}_i$ and a kernel $\mathbf{k}$, namely $t(\mathbf{x}_i) = \mathbf{k}^\top \mathbf{x}_i$. Therefore, learning a split in our framework involves searching for a kernel $\mathbf{k}$, leaf values $\eta_1$ and $\eta_2$, and split point $\tau$ that minimize Eq. (3) with $t(\mathbf{x}_i) = \mathbf{k}^\top \mathbf{x}_i$.

Since the space of all possible kernels is enormous, we perform this minimization in stages. Our approach is described in Alg. 1: we first construct a set of kernel candidates, then for each candidate we find the optimal $\tau$ through exhaustive search. For a given pair of kernel $\mathbf{k}$ and threshold $\tau$, the optimal values for $\eta_1$ and $\eta_2$ are then simply found as the weighted average of the $r_i^j$ values of the $\mathbf{x}_i$ samples that fall on the corresponding side of the split.

This parameter selection step for $\eta_1, \eta_2$, and $\tau$ is standard [11] but the kernel learning is not, as we consider a much more general form for the kernels $\mathbf{k}$ than is usually done. We now describe this step in detail.

## 3.2   Learning Convolution Kernels

To make computations tractable, we restrict the kernels $\mathbf{k}$ to being square windows within $\mathbf{x}$. This remains more general than most previous methods while reducing the dimensionality of the problem and allowing our splits to focus on local image features.

Let us introduce an operator $W_{\mathbf{c},a}(\mathbf{x})$ that returns, in vector form, the pixel values of $\mathbf{x}$ within a square window centered at $\mathbf{c}$ with side length $a$. The criterion of Eq. (1) becomes

$$\sum_{i=1}^{N} w_i^j \left( \mathbf{k}^\top W_{\mathbf{c},a}(\mathbf{x}_i) - r_i^j \right)^2 , \tag{4}$$

where $\mathbf{k}$ is now restricted to a square window parametrized by $\mathbf{c}$ and $a$. Given $\mathbf{c}$ and $a$, we can compute the optimal $\mathbf{k}$ in closed form by solving the least-squares problem of Eq. (4). To avoid overfitting, we introduce two refinements:

1. **Regularization.** We favor smooth kernels by introducing a regularization term into the criterion of Eq. (4), which becomes:

$$\sum_i w_i^j \left( \mathbf{k}^\top W_{\mathbf{c},a}(\mathbf{x}_i) - r_i^j \right)^2 + \lambda \sum_{(m,n)\in\mathcal{N}} \left( \mathbf{k}^{(m)} - \mathbf{k}^{(n)} \right)^2 , \tag{5}$$

   where $(m,n) \in \mathcal{N}$ are pairs of indexes that correspond to neighboring pixels and $\mathbf{k}^{(m)}$ is the $m^{\text{th}}$ pixel of kernel $\mathbf{k}$. The second term in Eq. (5) imposes a smooth kernel, controlled by $\lambda \geq 0$. Note that Eq. (5) can be minimized in closed form using least squares.

2. **Splitting the training set.** Filters and splits are learned on a subset of random samples from the training set, namely $T_1$ and $T_2$, as shown in Alg. 1.

As described in Alg. 1, we repeat this operation for many randomly selected values of $W_{\mathbf{c},a}(\mathbf{x})$, $\lambda$, $T_1$, and $T_2$ to select the split that returns the smallest value for the criterion of Eq. (3). The recursive splitting procedure of Alg. 1 then produces trees that are used as weak learners in Gradient Boosting.

Note that with the exponential loss we have $r_i^j \in \{-1,1\}$ [12]. In this case and when no regularization is imposed ($\lambda = 0$), the $\mathbf{k}$ that minimizes Eq. (4) is identical to the solution of LDA [11] up to a scale factor. However, this is a particular case of our formulation, which instead allows for smoothing as well as more outlier-robust losses such as the log loss. Smoothing yields higher generalization, while outlier-robust losses are essential to deal with noisy annotations.

# 4    Experiments and Results

We evaluated our approach[1] on three curvilinear structure delineation tasks, considering both a 2D dataset composed by retinal scans, and a set of 3D brightfield images. The first one, called **DRIVE** [18], is a publicly-available set of 40 RGB retinal scans and the aim is to segment blood vessels for automated diagnosis purposes. Since we have two different ground truth sets from two different ophthalmologists, it is possible to estimate the score a human expert achieves in the segmentation task. We preserved the original splitting between train and test images. The second dataset is composed by four **brightfield micrographs of dyed neurons**. We used both the original 3D image stacks and their 2D minimum-intensity projections. The projected images are particularly complex in that both staining and projection processes introduce significant structured and unstructured noise. Also, the images are quite small compared with, for example, those of [10, 19], although the ground truth is very accurate in our case. These factors make this task particularly challenging, and therefore a good test. Furthermore, the scarcity of training samples makes learning algorithms prone to overfitting. For the 2D experiments we used two images for training and the other two for testing. For 3D we used two fully-labeled large stacks, one of size $620 \times 1300 \times 135$ for training and another one of size $768 \times 1436 \times 77$ for testing.

We compare our method against the Optimally Oriented Flux (OOF) filter [5] and [10]. [5] is a handcrafted filter, widely acknowledged as being very good for delineating tubular structures, while [10] is a hybrid approach that complements hand-crafted features with features learned in an unsupervised fashion, which outperforms [5] on both 2D datasets. The parameters of the baselines were tuned to achieve their best performance, in order to provide a fair comparison. For [10] we tried Random Forests [11] and Boosted Trees, choosing the one that yields the highest performance (Random Forests for the DRIVE dataset, Boosted Trees for the brightfield images).

In all our experiments we set $N_{T_1} = 10000$ and use the log loss to increase robustness to outliers [11], with $M = 2000$, $P = 100$ and maximum kernel size $19 \times 19 \times (19)$ 2D/(3D). We used two-level trees, $\alpha = 0.1$ [11], and $\mathbb{L} = \{500, 1000, 1500, 2000\}$ for all experiments. The only parameter varied between datasets is patch size, chosen according to the scale of the structures of interest.

Learning supervised filters in 3D is computationally intensive, so we restricted the search to symmetric separable filters, learning one component at a time with Eq. (5). This reduces training and testing time considerably. Rotation invariance in the 3D case is also a major challenge, as learning it directly from the data would require impractically many training samples. One option to solve this issue is to introduce artificial rotations of the data, but this would imply an extremely high computational burden. We therefore employed the OOF score as an additional channel, given that it incorporates the invariance we seek. This is conceptually similar to what was done in [10], where unsupervised filters are

---

[1] See [17] for a more detailed description of our approach and parameters. Source code available at http://cvlab.epfl.ch.

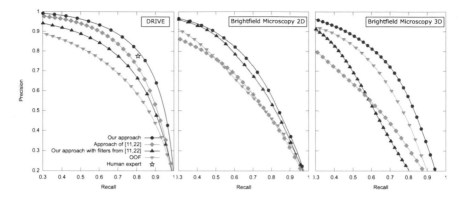

**Fig. 2. (a-c)** Precision-recall curves for pixel classification, obtained for different thresholds on $p(y = 1|x)$. Our approach outperforms all baselines in the 2D and 3D datasets, without the need for parameter tuning.

complemented with additional features. To reduce computational complexity further, we use stumps instead of trees for this task.

To compute the probability of each pixel in the input image of being part of a linear structure $p(y = 1|\mathbf{x})$, we take the sample vectors $\mathbf{x}$ to be image patches centered on individual pixels. Once our classifier is trained, we can compute $p(y = 1|\mathbf{x}) = (1 + e^{-2\varphi(\mathbf{x})})^{-1}$ [11]. Fig. 1 depicts some of the resulting probability maps for each dataset. Total training time was 4 hours for the 2D datasets and 6 hours for the 3D one on a 32-core 64-bit architecture.

Fig. 2 shows that our approach not only outperforms the baselines, but also outperforms human performance on DRIVE in terms of pixel error. It also yields high performance on 2D and 3D brightfield images, in spite of the inherent difficulty of this data.

To assess the importance of the supervised filter learning procedure we used the full filter banks of [10, 19], composed by 121 filters, in the context of our architecture. This was done by using the pre-computed filters as sub-patches in random positions, and then performing the usual procedure of Alg. 1. The resulting curves are labeled "*Our approach with filters from [10]*". The gap between this curve and the one for our approach shows that the supervised filter learning component of our method is largely responsible for its success.

## 5   Conclusion

We presented a new approach for curvilinear structure segmentation in 2D and 3D images, which automatically learns features and the classifier that uses them simultaneously. Our method outperforms current state-of-the-art curvilinear segmentation techniques, requiring almost no parameter tuning, relieving the practitioner from the time-consuming tasks of parameter and feature selection.

In future work, we will endeavor to extend our approach to textured features such as organelles in EM imagery.

# References

1. Lee, T., Kashyap, R., Chu, C.: Building Skeleton Models via 3D Medial Surface Axis Thinning Algorithms. Graphical Models and Image Processing (1994)
2. Vasilkoski, Z., Stepanyants, A.: Detection of the Optimal Neuron Traces in Confocal Microscopy Images. Journal of Neuroscience Methods 178(1) (2009)
3. Chothani, P., Mehta, V., Stepanyants, A.: Automated tracing of neurites from light microscopy stacks of images. Neuroinformatics 9(2-3) (2011)
4. Frangi, A.F., Niessen, W.J., Vincken, K.L., Viergever, M.A.: Multiscale vessel enhancement filtering. In: Wells, W.M., Colchester, A.C.F., Delp, S.L. (eds.) MICCAI 1998. LNCS, vol. 1496, pp. 130–137. Springer, Heidelberg (1998)
5. Law, M.W.K., Chung, A.C.S.: Three Dimensional Curvilinear Structure Detection Using Optimally Oriented Flux. In: Forsyth, D., Torr, P., Zisserman, A. (eds.) ECCV 2008, Part IV. LNCS, vol. 5305, pp. 368–382. Springer, Heidelberg (2008)
6. Jacob, M., Unser, M.: Design of steerable filters for feature detection using canny-like criteria. IEEE Transactions on Pattern Analysis and Machine Intelligence 26(8) (2004)
7. Meijering, E., Jacob, M., Sarria, J.C.F., Steiner, P., Hirling, H., Unser, M.: Design and Validation of a Tool for Neurite Tracing and Analysis in Fluorescence Microscopy Images. Cytometry Part A 58A(2) (April 2004)
8. Santamaría-Pang, A., Colbert, C.M., Saggau, P., Kakadiaris, I.A.: Automatic centerline extraction of irregular tubular structures using probability volumes from multiphoton imaging. In: Ayache, N., Ourselin, S., Maeder, A. (eds.) MICCAI 2007, Part II. LNCS, vol. 4792, pp. 486–494. Springer, Heidelberg (2007)
9. González, G., Aguet, F., Fleuret, F., Unser, M., Fua, P.: Steerable features for statistical 3D dendrite detection. In: Yang, G.-Z., Hawkes, D., Rueckert, D., Noble, A., Taylor, C. (eds.) MICCAI 2009, Part II. LNCS, vol. 5762, pp. 625–632. Springer, Heidelberg (2009)
10. Rigamonti, R., Lepetit, V.: Accurate and efficient linear structure segmentation by leveraging ad hoc features with learned filters. In: Ayache, N., Delingette, H., Golland, P., Mori, K. (eds.) MICCAI 2012, Part I. LNCS, vol. 7510, pp. 189–197. Springer, Heidelberg (2012)
11. Hastie, T., Tibshirani, R., Friedman, J.: Introduction. In: The Elements of Statistical Learning. Springer Series in Statistics. Springer, New York (2009)
12. Zheng, Z., Zha, H., Zhang, T., Chapelle, O., Sun, G.: A General Boosting Method and Its Application to Learning Ranking Functions for Web Search. In: NIPS (2007)
13. LeCun, Y., Bottou, L., Bengio, Y., Haffner, P.: Gradient-Based Learning Applied to Document Recognition. PIEEE (1998)
14. Hinton, G.: Learning to Represent Visual Input. Philosophical Transactions of the Royal Society (2010)
15. Cireşan, D., Giusti, A., Gambardella, L., Schmidhuber, J.: Deep Neural Networks Segment Neuronal Membranes in Electron Microscopy Images. In: NIPS (2012)
16. Caruana, R., Niculescu-Mizil, A.: An Empirical Comparison of Supervised Learning Algorithms. In: ICML (2006)
17. Becker, C.J., Rigamonti, R., Lepetit, V., Fua, P.: KernelBoost: Supervised Learning of Image Features For Classification. Technical report (2013)
18. Staal, J., Abramoff, M., Niemeijer, M., Viergever, M., van Ginneken, B.: Ridge Based Vessel Segmentation in Color Images of the Retina. TMI (2004)
19. Rigamonti, R., Sironi, A., Lepetit, V., Fua, P.: Learning Separable Filters. In: CVPR (2013)

# Joint Segmentation of 3D Femoral Lumen and Outer Wall Surfaces from MR Images

Eranga Ukwatta[1], Jing Yuan[1], Wu Qiu[1], Martin Rajchl[1], Bernard Chiu[2],
Shadi Shavakh[1], Jianrong Xu[3], and Aaron Fenster[1]

[1] Robarts Research Institute, Western University, London, ON, Canada
[2] Department of Electronic Engineering, City University of Hong Kong, Hong Kong
[3] Renji Hospital, Shanghai Jiao Tong University, Shanghai 200127, China
{eukwatta,jyuan,wqiu,mrajchl,afenster}@robarts.ca, bcychiu@cityu.edu.hk

**Abstract.** We propose a novel algorithm to jointly delineate the femoral
artery lumen and outer wall surfaces from 3D black-blood MR images,
while enforcing the spatial consistency of the reoriented MR slices along
the medial axis of the femoral artery. We demonstrate that the resulting optimization problem of the proposed segmentation can be solved
globally and exactly by means of convex relaxation, for which we introduce a novel *coupled continuous max-flow (CCMF) model* based on an
Ishikawa-type flow configuration and show its duality to the studied convex relaxed optimization problem. Using the proposed *CCMF model*, the
exactness and globalness of its dual convex relaxation problem is proven.
Experiment results demonstrate that the proposed method yielded high
accuracy (i.e. Dice similarity coefficient $> 85\%$) for both the lumen and
outer wall and high reproducibility (intra-class correlation coefficient of
0.95) for generating vessel wall area. The proposed method outperformed
the previous method, in terms of computation time, by a factor of $\sim 20$.

**Keywords:** Femoral artery segmentation, convex optimization.

## 1 Introduction

Peripheral arterial disease (PAD) is inflammatory, occluding the arteries with a
long term accumulation of plaque. Although PAD may cause morbidity ranging
from leg pain to critical limb ischemia, it has long been underestimated and
may have been overshadowed by cardio- and cerebro-vascular events and mortality [1,2]. The ankle-brachial index (ABI) is currently used for the diagnosis of
PAD, but it is limited in its utility for assessing the progression of the disease and
prediction of clinical events. With this regard, MR imaging has been investigated
to assess PAD [1] plaque burden and facilitates thickness and volumetric measurements, which are more sensitive to the clinical outcomes than ABI. It is of
great interest to efficiently generate an accurate delineation of the femoral lumen
and outer wall surfaces (see Fig. 1(a) and (b)) from 3D black-blood femoral MR
images (comprising of about 500 - 1000 slices per dataset), which is, however,
challenging due to the thin-and-elongated shape of the superficial femoral arteries (SFA) (see Fig. 1(a)) and strong overlapping of the intensity distributions

K. Mori et al. (Eds.): MICCAI 2013, Part I, LNCS 8149, pp. 534–541, 2013.

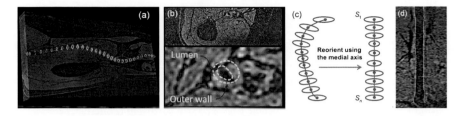

**Fig. 1.** (a) An example 3D femoral MR image with manual delineations; (b) A transverse slice of a 3D femoral MR image with manual delineations; (c) Reorientation of the femoral MR image using the medial axis of the artery. The reorientation procedure is described in Section 3; and (d) Long axis view of reoriented 3D MR image.

of the outer wall and its surrounding region. Typically, manual segmentation of the femoral lumen and outer wall requires about 80 min [2]. To our knowledge, there is only one study [2] describing a semi-automated segmentation of both the femoral lumen and outer wall surfaces from femoral MR images. Chiu *et al.* [2] proposed a 2D slice-by-slice B-spline snake segmentation procedure, where the segmentation of each slice is propagated as initialization for the subsequent slice to assist segmenting its succeeding slice. Their approach [2] explored sequential segmentation procedures of the femoral lumen and outer wall, which required about 8-10 min of time with extensive user interactions. In addition, such slice-by-slice technique does not globally enforce the inherent spatial coherence of the contours along the medial axis of artery, thus segmentation errors of one slice can be propagated and accumulated in segmentation of its following slices.

**Contributions** We propose a novel and efficient global optimization-based algorithm to jointly segment the outer wall and lumen of the SFA from 3D black-blood MR images, while globally enforcing the spatial consistency of the re-oriented slice sequence (see Fig. 1(d)) along the medial axis of the artery. We demonstrate that the resulting combinatorial optimization problem can be solved globally and exactly by means of convex relaxation, for which we introduce a new *coupled continuous max-flow (CCMF) model* and present its duality to the studied convex relaxation model. The proposed *CCMF* formulation directly derives a fast dual optimization algorithm.

## 2   Method

We propose a novel global optimization approach to simultaneously segment the SFA lumen and outer wall surfaces from the input 3D femoral MR image $\mathcal{V}$. Let $\mathcal{S}_1 \ldots \mathcal{S}_n$ be $n$ 2D transverse slices of $\mathcal{V}$ translated along the medial axis of the femoral artery (see Fig. 1(c) and (d) for illustration), where the tubular-like shape of the femoral artery entails spatial consistency along the specified medial axis of the segmented lumen and outer wall regions between every two adjacent reoriented slices. The algorithm simultaneously segments the $n$ MR slices into background, outer wall, and lumen by properly enforcing such prior knowledge.

## 2.1   Joint Segmentation of Lumen and Outer Wall

**Slice-wise Multi-Region Segmentation Model.** Let $\mathcal{R}_i^B$, $\mathcal{R}_i^W$ and $\mathcal{R}_i^L$, $i = 1 \ldots n$, denote the three regions of background, outer wall and lumen, within the 2D slice $\mathcal{S}_i$, respectively; $u_i^W(x), u_i^L(x) \in \{0,1\}$, $i = 1 \ldots n$, be the corresponding indicator labeling functions of $\mathcal{R}_i^W$ and $\mathcal{R}_i^L$. Since the outer wall region $\mathcal{R}_i^W$ contains the lumen region $\mathcal{R}_i^L$ [3](see Fig. 1(b)) within each slice $\mathcal{S}_i$, $i = 1 \ldots n$,

$$u_i^L(x) \leq u_i^W(x), \quad \forall x \in \mathcal{S}_i; \quad i = 1 \ldots n. \tag{1}$$

The segmentation of each slice $\mathcal{S}_i$, $i = 1 \ldots n$, into the three regions of $\mathcal{R}_i^B$, $\mathcal{R}_i^W$, and $\mathcal{R}_i^L$ can be formulated as a coupled continuous min-cut problem [4], which minimizes the following energy function

$$E_i(u_i^W, u_i^L) := \Big\{ \int (1 - u_i^W) C_i^B \, dx + \int (u_i^W - u_i^L) C_i^W \, dx + \int u_i^L C_i^L \, dx \Big\}$$

$$+ \Big\{ \int_{\Omega} g_i(x) |\nabla u_i^W| \, dx + \int_{\Omega} g_i(x) |\nabla u_i^L| \, dx \Big\} \tag{2}$$

over the binary labeling functions $u_i^{W,L}(x) \in \{0,1\}$, subject to constraint (1).

In (2), the functions $C_i^B(x)$, $C_i^W$, and $C_i^L(x)$ evaluate the cost to label pixel $x \in \mathcal{S}_i$, $i = 1 \ldots n$, as the background region $\mathcal{R}_i^B$, the complementary region $\mathcal{R}_i^W \backslash \mathcal{R}_i^L$ and the lumen region $\mathcal{R}_i^L$ respectively; hence, the sum of the first three terms gives the total cost of labeling each pixel with the slice $\mathcal{S}_i$. Moreover, the two weighted total-variation functions of (2) measure the smoothness of the two regions $\mathcal{R}_i^W$ and $\mathcal{R}_i^L$ w.r.t. the labeling functions $u_i^W(x), u_i^L(x) \in \{0,1\}$, where $g_i(x) = \lambda_1 + \lambda_2 \exp(-\lambda_3 |\nabla I(x)|)$ is a function of the image gradient.

**Spatial Consistency Prior between Adjacent Slices.** The $n$ slices $\mathcal{S}_1 \ldots \mathcal{S}_n$ are aligned along the medial axis of the femoral artery (see the blue dotted line in Fig. 1(c)). The tubular shape of the femoral artery enables a strong spatial consistency between every two adjacent slices. With this regard, we propose to enforce such consistency prior of the segmented regions $\mathcal{R}_i^W$ and $\mathcal{R}_i^L$, $i = 1 \ldots n$, by penalizing the total spatial differences of the extracted regions between two neighbouring slices, i.e. minimizing

$$\pi_i(u) := \int_{\Omega} |u_{i+1}^W - u_i^W| \, dx + \int_{\Omega} |u_{i+1}^L - u_i^L| \, dx, \quad i = 1 \ldots n-1. \tag{3}$$

**Optimization Formulation.** In view of (2) and (3), we propose to segment the 3D coupled femoral artery surfaces of the outer wall and lumen by segmenting the $n$ 2D image slices while incorporating inter-slice consistency (3), which can be formulated with a balancing weight $\alpha > 0$ as

$$\min_{u^{L,W}(x) \in \{0,1\}} \sum_{i=1}^{n} E_i(u_i) + \alpha \sum_{i=1}^{n-1} \pi_i(u); \quad \text{s.t. } u_i^L(x) \leq u_i^W(x), \quad i = 1 \ldots n. \tag{4}$$

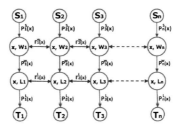

**Fig. 2.** Flow configurations of the proposed *coupled continuous max-flow model*

## 2.2 Convex Relaxation and Coupled Continuous Max-Flow Model

In this study, we show that the proposed optimization problem (4) can be globally and exactly solved by its convex relaxation

$$\min_{u^{L,W}(x)\in[0,1]} \sum_{i=1}^{n} E_i(u_i) + \alpha \sum_{i=1}^{n-1} \pi_i(u); \quad \text{s.t. } u_i^L(x) \leq u_i^W(x), \ i = 1\ldots n, \quad (5)$$

where the binary-valued constraints $u_i^{L,W}(x) \in \{0,1\}$ in (4) are replaced by their convex relaxation $u_i^{L,W}(x) \in [0,1]$. Note that, (5) amounts to a convex optimization problem with a global optimum. Here, we study (5) by introducing its dual formulation, i.e. the novel *CCMF model*, and show the thresholding of the computed optimum of the convex relaxation problem (5) solves its original combinatorial optimization problem (4) globally and exactly.

**Coupled Continuous Max-Flow (CCMF) Model.** We introduce the new flow configuration based on the studies in [4] (as illustrated in Fig. 2). For each image slice $\mathcal{S}_i$, $i = 1\ldots n$, we add two image copies $\Omega_i^W$ and $\Omega_i^L$ w.r.t. the regions $\mathcal{R}_i^W$ and $\mathcal{R}_i^L$; two additional flow terminals: the source $s_i$ and the sink $t_i$, are added; link the source $s_i$ to each pixel $x$ in $\Omega_i^W$, along which the directed source flow $p_i^s(x)$ is defined; link each pixel $x \in \Omega_i^W$ to the same pixel $x$ at $\Omega_i^L$, along which the directed outer wall flow $p_i^W(x)$ is defined; link each pixel $x \in \Omega_i^L$ to the sink $t_i$, along which the directed lumen flow $p_i^L(x)$ is defined; within $\Omega_i^W$ and $\Omega_i^L$, the local vector flow fields $q_i^W(x), q_i^L(x) \in \mathbb{R}^2$ are given around each pixel $x$. Between two adjacent $\Omega_i^W$ and $\Omega_{i+1}^W$, $i = 1\ldots n-1$, we link $x \in \Omega_i^W$ to the same position $x \in \Omega_{i+1}^W$, along which a coupled flow $r_i^W(x)$ streaming in both directions is defined. Between two adjacent $\Omega_i^L$ and $\Omega_{i+1}^L$, $i = 1\ldots n-1$, we link $x \in \Omega_i^L$ to the same position $x \in \Omega_{i+1}^L$, along which a coupled flow $r_i^L(x)$ streaming in both directions is defined.

With the above flow configuration, we introduce the novel *CCMF model*, which maximizes the total flow streaming from the $n$ sources:

$$\max_{p^s,p^t,q,r} \sum_{i=1}^{n} \int_\Omega p_i^s(x)\, dx \quad (6)$$

subject to the flow capacity constraints

$$p_i^s(x) \leq C_i^B(x), \ p_i^W(x) \leq C_i^W(x), \ p_i^L(x) \leq C_i^L(x); \ i = 1\ldots n; \quad (7)$$

$$\left|q_i^W(x)\right| \le g_i(x), \ \ \left|q_i^L(x)\right| \le g_i(x); \ \ i = 1 \dots n; \tag{8}$$

$$\left|r_i^W(x)\right| \le \alpha, \ \ \left|r_i^L(x)\right| \le \alpha; \ \ i = 1 \dots n-1; \tag{9}$$

and the flow conservation constraints within each $\Omega_i^{W,L}$, $i = 1 \dots n$:

$$\rho_1^W(x) := \left( \operatorname{div} q_1^W - p_1^s + p_1^W + r_1^W \right)(x) = 0; \tag{10}$$

$$\rho_1^L(x) := \left( \operatorname{div} q_1^L - p_1^W + p_1^L + r_1^L \right)(x) = 0; \tag{11}$$

$$\rho_i^W(x) := \left( \operatorname{div} q_i^W - p_i^s + p_i^W + r_i^W - r_{i-1}^W \right)(x) = 0; \ \ i = 2 \dots n-1; \tag{12}$$

$$\rho_i^L(x) := \left( \operatorname{div} q_i^L - p_i^W + p_i^L + r_i^L - r_{i-1}^L \right)(x) = 0; \ \ i = 2 \dots n-1; \tag{13}$$

$$\rho_n^W(x) := \left( \operatorname{div} q_n^W - p_n^s + p_n^W - r_{n-1}^W \right)(x) = 0; \tag{14}$$

$$\rho_n^L(x) := \left( \operatorname{div} q_n^L - p_n^W + p_n^L - r_{n-1}^L \right)(x) = 0. \tag{15}$$

**Global and Exact Optimization of** (4)**.** By introducing the multiplier functions $u_i^{W,L}(x)$, $i = 1 \dots n$, to the linear equalities (10) - (15), we then have the equivalent primal-dual model of (6) such that

$$\min_{u^{W,L}} \max_{p,q,r} \sum_{i=1}^n \int_\Omega p_i^s(x)\,dx + \sum_{i=1}^n \langle u_i^W, \rho_i^W \rangle + \sum_{i=1}^n \langle u_i^L, \rho_i^L \rangle \tag{16}$$

subject to the flow capacity constraints (7) - (9). By variational analysis, we can prove the following results:

**Proposition 1.** *The coupled continuous max-flow model* (6)*, the convex relaxation model* (5) *and the primal-dual model* (16) *are equivalent to each other:*

$$(6) \iff (5) \iff (16). \tag{17}$$

**Proposition 2.** *Let* $(u_1^{W,L}(x), \dots u_n^{W,L}(x))^* \in [0,1]$ *be the global optimum of the convex relaxation problem* (5)*, the thresholds* $\tilde{u}_i^{W,L}(x) \in \{0,1\}$*,* $i = 1 \dots n$*, by any* $\gamma \in [0,1)$*, where*

$$\tilde{u}_i^W(x) = \begin{cases} 1, & (u_i^W)^*(x) > \gamma \\ 0, & (u_i^W)^*(x) \le \gamma \end{cases}, \ \ \tilde{u}_i^L(x) = \begin{cases} 1, & (u_i^L)^*(x) > \gamma \\ 0, & (u_i^L)^*(x) \le \gamma \end{cases} \ \ i = 1 \dots n, \tag{18}$$

*solves the original combinatorial optimization problem* (4) *globally and exactly.*

**Coupled Continuous Max-Flow Model.** By Prop. 2, the global optimum of the proposed challenging segmentation problem (4) can be achieved by thresholding the optimum of its convex relaxation (5) with any $\gamma \in [0,1)$. However, Prop. 1 shows that the optimum of such convex relaxation problem (5) is given by the optimal multipliers to the corresponding linear equality conditions (10)-(15). Indeed, this directly derives the *CCMF model* based on the the modern augmented Lagrangian algorithm [5,6]; see also [4,7] for detailed algorithmic scheme. The proposed *CCMF algorithm* avoids directly solving the non-smooth function terms in (5) and achieves high efficiency in practice.

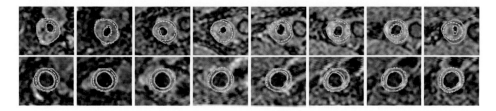

**Fig. 3.** Slice-wise comparison of the computation results (cyan) to the manual segmentation (yellow) for the femoral wall and lumen boundaries for three 3D MR images

## 3  Experiments and Results

**Segmentation Pipeline.** Initially, the user identifies approximately a 300 mm section of the SFA and then samples some seed points on the lumen, outer wall, and background regions in the first and the last slices to generate the corresponding model probability density functions (PDFs) of intensities $Pr(I(x))$, $j = L, W, B$, which are applied to segment the first and last slices using the introduced 2D segmentation algorithm [8]. The 2D segmentations of the first and last slices are further utilized to refine the approximation of the model PDFs for the lumen, outer wall, and background regions of the 3D MR image.

In parallel, an approximate medial axis of the femoral artery is computed to align and reorient the stack of slices for segmentation. Using multi-planar reformatting software, the observer approximately chooses the mid points on transverse cross-sections of the artery with an inter-slice distance of 30 mm (about 11 points in total). These points are then connected by the live-wire algorithm [9], which computes the minimum cost path linking the user-marked points and generates the rest of the points on the medial axis. The Frangi vesselness filter [10] is applied to the 3D MR image and its output is used as the cost map for the live-wire algorithm. The transverse slices are then reoriented along the computed medial axis, as shown in Fig. 1(c) and (d).

The 2D segmentation result of the first slice is used as initialization of the 3D algorithm. We then apply the proposed *CCMF* algorithm to jointly segment the 3D femoral lumen and outer wall surfaces from the reoriented 3D MR image, where the intensity log-likelihood terms [11] $C_i^j(x) = -\ln(Pr(I(x)))$, $j = L, W, B$, are used as the data costs of (2). The femoral lumen and outer wall surfaces generated using the algorithm are then mapped to the original space using the inverse transformation, which can be used for further analysis of the vessel wall boundaries. In addition, the parameters (i.e., $\alpha = 18, \lambda_{1,2,3} = 0.1, 1.7, 3$) were optimized sequentially by varying one parameter at a time. The optimized parameters were fixed during the experiments for the entire dataset.

**Data and Acquisition.** Our data set comprises of ten 3D motion-sensitized driven equilibrium (MSDE) prepared rapid gradient echo sequence (3D MERGE) images from seven subjects. Five of these subjects were symptomatic with intermittent claudication. The MR images were acquired using two stations with

**Table 1.** Performance results of the proposed algorithm for 10 3D femoral MR images

| Metric | DC (%) | AO (%) | MAD (mm) | MAXD (mm) | $VWA_{AVG}$ (mm$^2$) | $VWA_{RMSE}$ (mm$^2$) |
|---|---|---|---|---|---|---|
| Wall | 89.14±3.70 | 81.16±3.88 | 0.44±0.10 | 0.97±0.23 | 6.18±5.11 | 7.8 |
| Lumen | 85.43±3.39 | 80.42±10.74 | 0.40±0.08 | 0.87±0.13 | | |

**Table 2.** Intra-observer variability results of the algorithm using five repetitions of the same observer for 6 femoral MR images

| Metric | Lumen | Wall | VWA | Metric | Lumen | Wall | VWA | Metric | Lumen | Wall | VWA |
|---|---|---|---|---|---|---|---|---|---|---|---|
| CV(%) | 6.43 | 4.88 | 6.69 | ICC | 0.969 | 0.937 | 0.949 | SD (mm$^2$) | 1.9 | 2.6 | 2.3 |

**Table 3.** Comparison of the algorithm to Chiu *et al.* [2] using the same data set

| Metric | AO (%) | AD (%) | MAD (mm) | MAXD (mm) | $VWA_{AVG}$ (mm$^2$) | $VWA_{RMSE}$ (mm$^2$) |
|---|---|---|---|---|---|---|
| Proposed method Wall | 82.87±4.72 | 23.54±8.21 | 0.43±0.13 | 0.89±0.16 | 4.77±5.12 | 6.29 |
| Lumen | 81.35±8.46 | 24.95±9.32 | 0.42±0.09 | 0.86±0.16 | | |
| Chiu *et al.* [2] Wall | 84.75±9.46 | 12.90±12.95 | 0.32±0.23 | 0.77±0.52 | 4.58±7.10 | 8.45 |
| Lumen | 85.60±9.36 | 9.77±9.78 | 0.20±0.17 | 0.55±0.48 | | |

field-of-view of $400 \times 40 \times 250$ mm to cover up to 500 mm longitudinally with isotropic voxel size of 1.0 mm. The imaging parameters were TR = 10 ms, TE = 4.8 ms, flip angle = 6°, turbo factor = 100 and one excitation (NEX).

**Results.** The experiments were performed on a Windows PC with a Intel Core i7 CPU and 3GB RAM. The proposed *CCMF* algorithm was implemented in C++ with an interface in Matlab (Natick, MA) and required only 10 s to segment each 3D image, in addition to about 98 s for initialization and pre-processing. The final reconstructed 3D lumen and outer wall surfaces are compared to the manual segmentations on a slice-by-slice basis; some example reconstructed slice-wise results are shown for three subjects in Fig. 3. For the slice-by-slice validation, our data set consisted of 355 2D slices extracted from 10 3D femoral MR images.

To assess the accuracy, we used Dice similarity coefficient (DSC), area overlap (AO), area difference (AD), average and root mean square vessel wall area (VWA) errors [2] and mean and maximum absolute distance errors (MAD and MAXD). Table 1 shows the accuracy evaluation of the proposed algorithm, which yielded a DSC $\geq$ 85% for both the lumen and outer wall and sub-millimeter errors in MAD and MAXD. The user repeatedly segmented six femoral MR images five times to assess the reproducibility of the algorithm in generating VWA using coefficient of variation (CV), intra-class correlation coefficient (ICC), and standard deviation (SD) (as shown in Table 2). Table 3 shows the comparison of the proposed algorithm to the 2D slice-based method [2] using the same data set. Our algorithm yielded comparably accurate results to [2] while requiring much fewer user interactions and less computation time ($\sim$ 10 s vs. 230 - 290 s).

# 4    Discussion and Conclusions

Our algorithm yielded high accuracy (i.e. DSC $\geq$ 85% and sub-millimeter error values for MAD and MAXD as shown in Table 1) for the segmentation of both the SFA lumen and outer wall. The algorithm also yielded high reproducibility (i.e. ICC of 0.95 and CV as low as 6.69%) for generating VWA, which is the most important aspect of the algorithm for longitudinal monitoring of PAD plaque burden, because a systematic bias may cancel out when VWA change is measured from baseline to follow-up. The algorithm required much less computing time (10 s vs. 230 - 290 s) and user interactions, comparing to Chiu et al. [2], while achieving a comparable accuracy in AO, MAD and MAXD. Currently, most of the observer time is used for identifying the medial axis of the artery, which may be further improved by using an automated centerline detection algorithm.

**Acknowledgements.** The authors are grateful for the funding support from the Canadian Institutes of Health Research (CIHR) and the Canada Research Chairs (CRC) Program. B. Chiu acknowledges the support of City University of Hong Kong start-up Grant #7200245.

# References

1. Isbell, D., Meyer, C., Rogers, W., Epstein, F., et al.: Reproducibility and reliability of atherosclerotic plaque volume measurements in peripheral arterial disease with cardiovascular magnetic resonance. J. Cardiov. Magn. Reson. 9(1), 71–76 (2007)
2. Chiu, B., Sun, J., Zhao, X., Wang, J., Balu, N., Chi, J., Xu, J., Yuan, C., Kerwin, W.: Fast plaque burden assessment of the femoral artery using 3d black-blood mri and automated segmentation. Medical Physics 38, 5370–5384 (2011)
3. Ukwatta, E., Yuan, J., Rajchl, M., Fenster, A.: Efficient global optimization based 3D carotid AB-LIB MRI segmentation by simultaneously evolving coupled surfaces. In: Ayache, N., Delingette, H., Golland, P., Mori, K. (eds.) MICCAI 2012, Part III. LNCS, vol. 7512, pp. 377–384. Springer, Heidelberg (2012)
4. Bae, E., Yuan, J., Tai, X.C., Boycov, Y.: A fast continuous max-flow approach to non-convex multilabeling problems. Technical report CAM-10-62, UCLA (2010)
5. Bertsekas, D.P.: Nonlinear Programming. Athena Scientific (September 1999)
6. Yuan, J., Bae, E., Tai, X.: A study on continuous max-flow and min-cut approaches. IEEE CVPR, 2217–2224 (2010)
7. Yuan, J., Bae, E., Tai, X.-C., Boykov, Y.: A continuous max-flow approach to potts model. In: Daniilidis, K., Maragos, P., Paragios, N. (eds.) ECCV 2010, Part VI. LNCS, vol. 6316, pp. 379–392. Springer, Heidelberg (2010)
8. Ukwatta, E., Yuan, J., Rajchl, M., Tessier, D., Fenster, A.: 3D carotid multi-region MRI segmentation by globally optimal evolution of coupled surfaces. IEEE Transactions of Medical Imaging 32(4), 770–785 (2013)
9. Barrett, W.A., Mortensen, E.N.: Interactive live-wire boundary extraction. Medical Image Analysis 1(4), 331–341 (1997)
10. Frangi, A.F., Niessen, W.J., Vincken, K.L., Viergever, M.A.: Multiscale vessel enhancement filtering. In: Wells, W.M., Colchester, A.C.F., Delp, S.L. (eds.) MICCAI 1998. LNCS, vol. 1496, pp. 130–137. Springer, Heidelberg (1998)
11. Rajchl, M., Yuan, J., Ukwatta, E., Peters, P.: Fast interactive multi-region cardiac segmentation with linearly ordered labels. In: IEEE ISBI, pp. 1409–1412 (2012)

# Model-Guided Directional Minimal Path for Fully Automatic Extraction of Coronary Centerlines from Cardiac CTA

Liu Liu[1], Wenzhe Shi[2], Daniel Rueckert[2], Mingxing Hu[3],
Sebastien Ourselin[3], and Xiahai Zhuang[4,*]

[1] Shanghai Jiaotong Universiy, Shanghai, China
[2] Biomedical Image Analysis Group, Imperial College London, UK
[3] Centre for Medical Image Computing, University College London, UK
[4] Shanghai Advanced Research Institute, Chinese Academy of Sciences, China
zhuangxh@sari.ac.cn

**Abstract.** Extracting centerlines of coronary arteries is a challenging but important task in clinical applications of cardiac CTA. In this paper, we propose a model-guided approach, the directional minimal path, for the centerline extraction. The proposed method is based on the minimal path algorithm and a prior coronary model is used. The model is first registered to the unseen image. Then, the start point and end point for the minimal path algorithm are provided by the model to automate the centerline extraction process. Also, the direction information of the coronary model is used to guide the path tracking of the minimal path procedure. This directional tracking improves the robustness and accuracy of the centerline extraction. Finally, the proposed method can automatically recognize the branches of the extracted coronary artery using the prior information in the model. We validated the proposed method by extracting the three main coronary branches. The mean accuracy of the 56 cases was 1.32±0.81 mm and the detection ratio was 88.7%.

## 1 Introduction

Cardiac Computer Tomography Angiography (CTA) is widely used in clinical routine for coronary artery studies. Extracting centerlines of the coronary artery is important in the coronary related clinical applications. Since manual extraction and annotation can be time-consuming and skill-demanding, automating this process is becoming increasingly desirable. Many works [1-4, 8] focused on extracting the complete tree of the coronary artery. However, it is difficult to automatically recognize and discriminate the branches of the coronary tree without manual interactions. The methods [5-7] based on the minimal path have been used to extract the centerline of a specific vessel or a coronary branch, but the start point and end point, also known as seed points, are commonly manually selected. The detection methods also tend to fail when the seed points are off the

---

* Corresponding author.

K. Mori et al. (Eds.): MICCAI 2013, Part I, LNCS 8149, pp. 542–549, 2013.

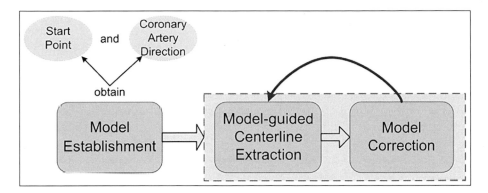

**Fig. 1.** The flowchart of the proposed directional minimal path

coronary or when the branch has discontinues segments due to bypass surgeries or image artifacts.

In this paper, we propose a new method, the model-guided directional minimal path (DMP), for extracting centerlines of the main branches of the coronary artery. The path tracking in the DMP incorporates the direction information of a prior coronary model, to achieve fast and robust coronary tracking. The start point and the end point required in the minimal path framework are also provided from the prior model. Finally, with the prior information in the model, the branches of the extracted coronary centerlines are automatically recognized, resulting in a fully automated centerline extraction method.

## 2    Proposed Method

The proposed directional minimal path method incorporates a prior model into the framework of the traditional minimal path method [5-7], to extract the centerlines of the coronary artery. The model consists of a cardiac CTA volume, referred to as the CTA model, and the coronary centerlines, referred to as the coronary model. The directional minimal path extraction framework has three key stages: model establishment, model-guided centerline extraction, and model correction, as Fig. 1 shows:

a) In the model establishment, the model is registered to the unseen image, to provide the start point as well as the initial direction for the minimal path.

b) In the model-guided centerline extraction, the start point and the direction from the prior model is incorporated into the framework.

c) The model correction is used to optimize the direction for the model-guided centerline extraction.

The model-guided centerline extraction and model correction are repeated iteratively until the algorithm reaches the neighbor region of the end point of the coronary model or maximal iteration steps.

## 2.1   Model Establishment

In model establishment, the CTA model is first registered to the unseen image using a deformable registration scheme [11,12]. The registration consists of three steps, i.e. global affine registration for localization of the whole heart, locally affine registration method for initialization of substructures such as the four chambers and great vessels, and the active control point status free-form deformation registration for refinement of local details. The resultant transformation is then used to map the coronary model onto the image space of the unseen image. The established model provides the start point and the initial direction of the coronary artery for the following directional minimal path procedure. The ideal start point should be the ostia for coronary artery extraction. However, the volumetric registration algorithm tends to produce mismatch of ostia due to its relative small size of volume in the whole heart structure, resulting in less robust coronary extraction. We therefore propose to define the start point to the mean position of the left ostium and the right ostium, for extracting both the left coronary artery and the right coronary artery.

## 2.2   Model-Guided Centerline Extraction

The model-guided centerline extraction is implemented in the framework of the minimal path method, where the cost function of path incorporates the directional information of the coronary model. This is why we call the method the directional minimal path.

In the minimal path framework, the path of the coronary artery is extracted by finding the minimal accumulated cost between the start and end points. The energy function of the path (or curve) $C$ can be define as follows:

$$E(C) = \int_\Omega (P(C(t)) + \omega)dt. \tag{1}$$

where $P(\boldsymbol{x})$ denotes the potential or cost at the location $\boldsymbol{x}$, $\omega$ is a regularization factor, and $t$ is the arch length.

In the directional minimal path, we propose the cost function to include three terms: vesselness [9] $v(\boldsymbol{x})$ based on eigenvalues of the Hessian, similarity [10] $s(\boldsymbol{x})$ based on intensity, and direction $d(\boldsymbol{x})$ based on the prior coronary model. We redefine the cost function $P(\boldsymbol{x})$ as follows:

$$P(\boldsymbol{x}) = \frac{1}{v(\boldsymbol{x})^\alpha * s(\boldsymbol{x})^\beta * d(\boldsymbol{x})^\gamma + \varepsilon}. \tag{2}$$

where $\varepsilon$ is a small positive value to prevent the singularities, and the parameters $\alpha$, $\beta$, and $\gamma$, which all set to 1 in our experiments, are used to control the cost contrast. The similarity term $s(\boldsymbol{x})$ can be defined as follows:

$$s(\boldsymbol{x}) = \begin{cases} e^{-\frac{1}{2}(\frac{I(\boldsymbol{x})-\mu_{ca}}{\sigma_{ca}})^2}, I < \mu_{ca} \\ 1, I \geq \mu_{ca}. \end{cases} \tag{3}$$

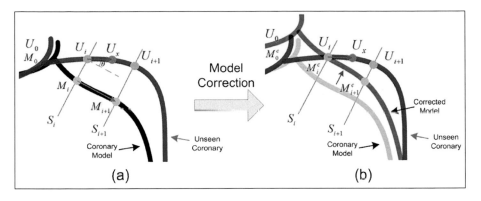

**Fig. 2.** The model-guided centerline extraction and model correction

where $\mu_{ca}$ and $\sigma_{ca}$ are the intensity mean and standard deviation of the coronary lumen. As the intensity information of the coronary lumen in the unseen image is unknown, we propose to estimate them using the intensity information of the prior model and the intensity information of the contrast enhanced chambers in the unseen image. In the prior model, the mean intensity of the coronary artery, $\mu_{mca}$, and the enhanced chambers, $\mu_{me}$, can be accurately computed before the extraction. The contrast enhanced chambers in the unseen image can be identified in the model establishment, where the enhanced chambers in the CTA model were mapped onto the unseen image by the registration. Given the intensity mean of the enhanced chambers of the unseen image, $\mu_{ue}$, is computed, by assuming a constant linear relationship between the intensity value of the contrast enhanced chambers and that of the coronary artery segments, the intensity mean of the coronary artery in the unseen image, $\mu_{uca}$, is then estimated as follows:

$$\mu_{ca} = \mu_{ue} + (\mu_{mca} - \mu_{me}). \tag{4}$$

In Eq. (2), $d(\boldsymbol{x})$ is determined by the angle $\theta(\boldsymbol{x})$ between the coronary model and the current path in the minimal path method:

$$d(\boldsymbol{x}) = e^{-\frac{1}{2}(\frac{G(\boldsymbol{x})-\mu_d}{\sigma_d})^2},$$
$$G(\boldsymbol{x}) = \begin{cases} \cos(\theta(\boldsymbol{x})), if \cos(\theta(\boldsymbol{x})) > 0 \\ 0, else. \end{cases} \tag{5}$$

where $\mu_d = 1$, and $\sigma_d = 0.5$ in our experiments.

The angle between the coronary model and the current path is obtained by the piecewise method as illustrated in Fig. 2 (left), where a coronary artery branch of interest is divided into several segments. In a coronary segment, $U_i$ and $U_{\boldsymbol{x}}$ denote the start point and the current point in the minimal path process. $M_i$ and $M_{i+1}$ denote the start point and the end point of the current segment in the coronary model. The length of each segment $S_i S_{i+1}$ can be set as a fixed value. The end point of current segment is regarded as the start point in the next segment. Also, to compute the direction information for each candidate path point $x$, one needs to obtain the corresponding segment from the coronary model and employs the direction information of the model for the computation of $\theta(x)$. This is achieved by the model correction process.

### 2.3   Model Correction

The prior model gives a good initial estimation after its establishment. However, due to the registration error and the variance of the cardiac anatomy, it is difficult to achieve an accurate match between the coronary model and the corresponding coronary branches in the unseen image. Model correction is embedded with the model-guided centerline extraction to optimize the direction information provided from the model, as follows:

a) For current start point $U_i$, search a point on the coronary model, which is the closest point to $U_i$. This closest point is referred to as $M_i^c$.

b) Remap (correct) the coronary model to the unseen image space by aligning $M_i^c$ to current start point $U_i$.

c) Search along the coronary model to find a point $M_{i+1}^c$ whose geodesic distance to $M_i^c$ is the predefined length of a segment.

For each candidate path point $x$, $\theta(x)$ is then defined to the included angle between vector, $\overrightarrow{M_i^c M_{i+1}^c}$, and vector, $\overrightarrow{U_i U_x}$ as illustrated in Fig. 2 (right). It should be noted that this realignment in model correction does not change the orientation of the coronary model. Instead, it helps to select a better segment from the model to provide more accurate direction for the next iteration, as this selected segment is expected to be more similar to the current coronary segment in the unseen image.

## 3   Experimental Results

We tested the proposed DMP method on eight cardiac CTA volumes, to extract the three main branches of the coronary artery, including the right coronary artery (RCA), left anterior descending artery (LAD), and left circumflex artery (LCX). The centerlines of the coronary branches of interest had been manually annotated in each subject, providing the gold standard for the evaluation.

### 3.1   Evaluation Using Synthetic Models

In this experiment, ten synthetic coronary models are generated for each subject, resulting in 80 cases. The synthetic models were generated by moving the start and end points of the gold standard centerlines, and then deforming the whole coronary. The moving distance was random values between 0-15 mm, and the deformation is computed as follows:

$$F_M(i) = V_S \frac{n-1-i}{n-1} + V_E \frac{i}{n-1}, i \in (0, n-1). \tag{6}$$

**Table 1.** The results of the two compared methods using synthetic models

| Methods | Mean(mm) | Std(mm) | Max(mm) | Detect Ratio |
|---|---|---|---|---|
| Directional Minimal Path | 0.904 | 0.524 | 2.273 | 97.5% |
| Vesselness Minimal Path | 1.093 | 0.555 | 2.332 | 50.0% |

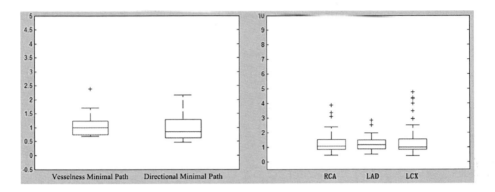

**Fig. 3.** Box-whisker plots of the centerline extraction results (mm)

where $n$ is the number of points of a gold standard centerline, $i$ is the index of centerline points, $V_S$ and $V_E$ are the displacements of the start and end points. The deformed coronary was then used as the established coronary model for the DMP algorithm.

The vesselness-based minimal path (VMP) method [7] was also evaluated for comparisons with the proposed DMP method. The start point for the VMP method was manually labeled on the ostia, while the end point was given by the same way as the DMP method. This is because the VMP failed in most of the cases when the start points were the random values as the DMP used. The mean distance between the gold standard and the final results of the successful cases [8] were presented in Table 1, and the box-whisker plots of the two groups of results were given in Fig. 3 (left). Compared with the VMP method, the proposed DMP achieved no worse mean distance on the successful cases, but the detection ratio (success rate of extraction process) was much higher, 97.5% VS 50%. It should also be noted that the DMP was fully automatic, while the compared VMP required manual input of the start points.

## 3.2   Evaluation Using Real Models

In this experiment, we employed the leave-one-out strategy, by considering one of the eight subjects as the prior model and the rest as the test dataset, resulting in 56 cases. Fig. 4 provides the visualization result of an extraction result. Table 2 provides the quantitative results and Fig. 3 (right) shows the box-whisker plots of the mean accuracies. The overall extraction accuracy was promising, thought it was slightly worse than the synthetic experiment due to the large difference

**Table 2.** The results of directional minimal path method using deformable registration

| Branches | Mean(mm) | Std(mm) | Max(mm) | Detect Ratio |
|---|---|---|---|---|
| Right Coronary Artery | 1.217 | 0.662 | 2.966 | 92.9% |
| Left Anterior Descending | 1.245 | 0.787 | 3.285 | 82.1% |
| Left Circumflex Artery | 1.490 | 0.980 | 3.776 | 91.1% |

**Table 3.** The results of directional minimal path method using affine registration

| Branches | Mean(mm) | Std(mm) | Max(mm) | Detect Ratio |
|---|---|---|---|---|
| Right Coronary Artery | 1.081 | 0.557 | 2.564 | 85.7% |
| Left Anterior Descending | 1.085 | 0.595 | 2.518 | 83.9% |
| Left Circumflex Artery | 1.416 | 0.922 | 3.660 | 87.5% |

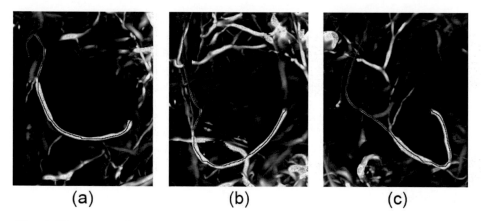

**(a)**    **(b)**    **(c)**

**Fig. 4.** The maximal intensity projection of the vesselness with extracted centerlines

of shapes (direction information) between the model and the unseen cases. Also, the maximal errors were generally within the maximal lumen diameters. Finally, the DMP method also demonstrated good robustness against the real cases, as the detection ratios were 92.9%, 82.1%, and 91.1% for the three branches respectively.

Meanwhile, in order to evaluate the effects under the different register methods, the original registration scheme, including affine and nonrigid registration, was replaced by an affine registration method, for the model establishment. The extraction results of this method were presented in Table 3. The detect ratios of the method only using affine registration were worse in RCA and LCA extraction, and marginally better in LAD extraction, compared to the original method which used the deformable registration. However, the accuracy of the centerline extraction of the two methods was not significantly different, as the p-values of them were 0.284 (RCA), 0.095 (LAD), and 0.741 (LCX).

# 4    Conclusions

In this paper, we presented a novel coronary extraction algorithm, the model-guided directional minimal path (DMP). This approach allows fully automatic extraction of coronary arteries, including the labeling of the main branches. The experiments showed the proposed DMP was robust and accurate in extracting the three main branches. The future work includes extending the DMP for whole coronary tree extraction and validating the algorithm using more clinical datasets.

# References

1. Bouraoui, B., Ronse, C., Baruthio, J., Passat, N., Germain, P.: Fully automatic 3D segmentation of coronary arteries based on mathematical morphology. In: International Symposium on Biomedical Imaging: From Nano to Macro, pp. 1059–1062 (2008)
2. Carrillo, J., Hoyos, M., Davila, E., Orkisz, M.: Recursive tracking of vascular tree axes in 3d medical images. Int. J. Comput. Assist. Radiol. Surg. 1(6), 331–339 (2007)
3. Gülsün, M.A., Tek, H.: Robust vessel tree modeling. In: Metaxas, D., Axel, L., Fichtinger, G., Székely, G. (eds.) MICCAI 2008, Part I. LNCS, vol. 5241, pp. 602–611. Springer, Heidelberg (2008)
4. Castro, C., Luengo-Oroz, M., Santos, A., Ledesma-Carbayo, M.: Coronary artery tracking in 3D cardiac CT images using local morpho-logical reconstruction operators. The Midas Journal. In: MICCAI Workshop - Grand Challenge Coronary Artery Tracking (2008)
5. Zhu, N., Chung, A.C.S.: Minimum average-cost path for real time 3D coronary artery segmentation of CT images. In: Fichtinger, G., Martel, A., Peters, T. (eds.) MICCAI 2011, Part III. LNCS, vol. 6893, pp. 436–444. Springer, Heidelberg (2011)
6. Deschamps, T., Cohen, L.D.: Minimal paths in 3D images and application to virtual endoscopy. In: Vernon, D. (ed.) ECCV 2000. LNCS, vol. 1843, pp. 543–557. Springer, Heidelberg (2000)
7. Wink, O., Frangi, A., Verdonck, B., Viergever, M., Niessen, W.: 3D MRA coronary axis determination using a minimum cost path approach. Magn. Reson. Med. 47(6), 1169–1175 (2002)
8. Schaap, M., Metz, C., Walsum, T., et al.: Standardized evaluation methodology and reference database for evaluating coronary artery centerline extraction algorithms. Medical Image Analysis 13(5), 701–714 (2009)
9. Frangi, A.F., Niessen, W.J., Vincken, K.L., Viergever, M.A.: Multiscale vessel enhancement filtering. In: Wells, W.M., Colchester, A.C.F., Delp, S.L. (eds.) MICCAI 1998. LNCS, vol. 1496, pp. 130–137. Springer, Heidelberg (1998)
10. Tang, H., Walsum, T., Onkelen, R., et al.: Semiautomatic carotid lumen segmentation for quantification of lumen geometry in multispectral MRI. Medical Image Analysis 16(6), 1202–1215 (2012)
11. Rueckert, D., Sonoda, L., Hayes, C., Hill, D., Leach, M., Hawkes, D.: Nonrigid registration using free-form deformations: application to breast MR images. IEEE Transactions on Medical Imaging 18(8), 712–721 (1999)
12. Zhuang, X., Rhode, K., Razavi, R., Hawkes, D., Ourselin, S.: A registration-based propagation framework for automatic whole heart segmentation of cardiac MRI. IEEE Transactions on Medical Imaging 29(9), 1612–1625 (2010)

# Globally Optimal Curvature-Regularized Fast Marching for Vessel Segmentation

Wei Liao, Karl Rohr, and Stefan Wörz

University of Heidelberg, BIOQUANT, IPMB, and DKFZ Heidelberg
Dept. Bioinformatics and Functional Genomics, Biomedical Computer Vision Group

**Abstract.** We introduce a novel fast marching approach with *curvature* regularization for vessel segmentation. Since most vessels have a smooth path, curvature can be used to distinguish desired vessels from short cuts, which usually contain parts with high curvature. However, in previous fast marching approaches, curvature information is not available, so it cannot be used for regularization directly. Instead, usually *length* regularization is used under the assumption that shorter paths should also have a lower curvature. However, for vessel segmentation, this assumption often does not hold and leads to short cuts. We propose an approach, which integrates curvature regularization directly into the fast marching framework, independent of length regularization. Our approach is *globally optimal*, and numerical experiments on synthetic and real retina images show that our approach yields more accurate results than two previous approaches.

## 1 Introduction

Vessel segmentation plays an essential role in medical image analysis. For example, segmentation of retinal vessels is important for the analysis of retina images, which is crucial for the diagnosis of diseases such as diabetes. Using minimal path approaches, vessel segmentation can be formulated elegantly as *energy minimization* problems. To solve such problems, there exist *efficient algorithms*, such as Dijkstra's Algorithm ([1]) or the fast marching method (e.g., [2]), which usually allow finding the *global optimum*. Furthermore, the vessel centerlines (comprising the coordinates and order of the points) are obtained *directly*, which is an advantage compared to indirect approaches where an additional step is required after, for example, a binary segmentation. Therefore, minimal path approaches are particularly interesting for vessel segmentation.

Usually, the essential step of minimal path approaches is the outward propagation of a wavefront $\mathcal{W}$ from a start point to an end point. To determine the speed $\mathcal{F}$ of $\mathcal{W}$, there exist different strategies. In classical minimal path approaches, $\mathcal{F}$ relies on simple image features like edges (e.g., [2]), while later approaches use more elaborate intensity models (e.g., [3]). Also, additional key points can be used to adjust $\mathcal{F}$ iteratively in order to avoid problems like short cuts (e.g., [4, 5]). However, none of these approaches exploits the important geometric property that the vessels should have a smooth path. To account for the smoothness,

K. Mori et al. (Eds.): MICCAI 2013, Part I, LNCS 8149, pp. 550–557, 2013.

manually inserted key points can be used (e.g., [6]), which is time-consuming and depends strongly on the accuracy of the human operator. Alternatively, oriented filters (e.g., [7]) can be used to incorporate the smoothness automatically, but the filter orientation is quantized and integrated as additional dimension of $\mathcal{F}$, which inevitably introduces quantization errors and increases the computational effort. In [8], an iterative approach is used, where in each iteration, paths which deviate significantly from a predicted direction within a region-of-interest (ROI) are discarded. However, there is no guarantee to reach the end point. Alternatively, the approach in [9] uses the optimally oriented flux (OOF) [10] to estimate the local vessel orientation, but the OOF filter relies on image gradients, without considering the actual path geometry. In some approaches, $\mathcal{F}$ is updated dynamically to control the propagation of $\mathcal{W}$. For example, in [11, 12], the geometry of the path is used to update $\mathcal{F}$. However, there only the normal of $\mathcal{W}$ is considered. On the other hand, in [13] a longer locally back-traced path is considered, but only the appearance of the path is used to update $\mathcal{F}$, not the geometry. In addition, some of the above mentioned methods, e,g., [4, 5, 8], are not globally optimal.

In this contribution, we present a novel curvature-regularized fast marching approach for vessel segmentation. For the first time, curvature is taken into account using the *actual geometry* of vessels, instead of using the response of local filters as in [7, 9]. Furthermore, the curvature regularization is independent of length regularization. Our approach combines and extends previous approaches [11–13]: Instead of using only the normal of $\mathcal{W}$ as in [11, 12], we extract for each pixel on $\mathcal{W}$ a longer locally back-traced path $\gamma_{\text{local}}$. In addition, instead of using the appearance of $\gamma_{\text{local}}$ as in [13], we compute the curvature $\kappa$ of $\gamma_{\text{local}}$. The further propagation of $\mathcal{W}$ is controlled by *dynamically* updating $\mathcal{F}$ according to $\kappa$. Our approach is *globally optimal*, and the experiments show that we obtain significantly improved results compared to two previous approaches.

## 2    Classical Fast Marching for Vessel Segmentation

In this section, we first briefly review the classical fast marching scheme for vessel segmentation, and then we discuss the problem of length regularization.

**Energy Function.** Fast marching approaches aim at finding a path $\gamma$ between a given start point $\mathbf{x}_s$ and end point $\mathbf{x}_e$ such that an energy function is minimized. In classical approaches, the *energy function* is usually formulated as:

$$E(\gamma) := \int_{\gamma} \Big( \mathcal{P}(\gamma(s)) + w \Big) ds = \underbrace{\int_{\gamma} \mathcal{P}(\gamma(s)) ds}_{\text{data term}} + \underbrace{w \cdot \int_{\gamma} 1 ds}_{\text{regularization term}}, \quad (1)$$

where $\mathcal{P}$ is a *potential function* defined based on image data, $s$ is the arc length parameter, and $w$ is a regularization constant. For many problems, it is more convenient to consider $\mathcal{P}$ as the inverse of a speed function $\mathcal{F}$, i.e., $\mathcal{P} = \frac{1}{\mathcal{F}}$. Let a wavefront $\mathcal{W}$ start at $\mathbf{x}_s$ and keep propagating outwards at the speed $\mathcal{F}$. At each

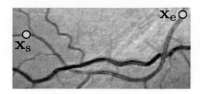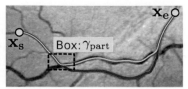

**Fig. 1.** Left: Retinal vessels crossing each other (image from DRIVE dataset [14]). Right: Segmentation results. Yellow and red colors indicate the results of a length-regularized approach [2] and our curvature-regularized approach, respectively.

position $\mathbf{x}$, the arrival time of $\mathcal{W}$ is recorded as $\mathcal{U}_{\mathbf{x}_s}(\mathbf{x})$. Upon reaching $\mathbf{x}_e$, the propagation stops, and then the minimal path $\hat{\gamma}_{\mathbf{x}_s,\mathbf{x}_e}$ is obtained with *subpixel accuracy* by a gradient descent of $\mathcal{U}_{\mathbf{x}_s}$ from $\mathbf{x}_e$ back to $\mathbf{x}_s$.

**Problem of Length Regularization.** Since $\int_\gamma 1 ds$ is the length of the path $\gamma$ [2], the regularization term in (1) assigns lower energy to shorter paths. Usually, shorter paths are assumed to have a lower curvature, so previous approaches employ *length regularization* to indirectly control the curvature of the path. However, this assumption is not always true, especially for vessels, since they often cross each other, and the shortest path found using length regularization may belong to different vessels. This problem is shown in Fig. 1: Although the red path is correct, an approach with length regularization [2] yields the yellow path, since it is shorter. With *curvature regularization*, the curvature (smoothness) of vessels can be exploited *independently* of the length regularization, so shorter paths with wrong sharp turns can be avoided. Obviously, the geometry of the path is necessary to compute the curvature. However, with previous approaches, the path geometry is usually not known until the propagation of $\mathcal{W}$ is *finished*, so a curvature regularization cannot be used with these approaches.

## 3    Curvature-Regularized Fast Marching

In this section, we first introduce a *new energy function* of minimal paths with curvature regularization, and then we show how to incorporate the curvature using a novel fast marching approach with dynamic speed.

### 3.1    New Energy Function with Curvature Regularization

Our new energy function is formulated as:

$$E(\gamma) := \int_\gamma \Big( \mathcal{P}(\gamma(s)) + \mathcal{C}(\gamma(s)) + w \Big) ds. \tag{2}$$

Compared to the energy function of the classical fast marching approaches (1), our approach includes a new term $\mathcal{C}$ which represents the curvature regularization, and which is independent of the length regularization $w$. The curvature is *not* computed over the entire path $\gamma$, but over local paths $\gamma_{\text{local}}$ of a *fixed length*

$\Gamma$ and starting at the position $\gamma(s)$ (see Fig. 2b). The function $\mathcal{C}$ can be defined using the curvature $\kappa$ of $\gamma_{\text{local}}$:

$$\mathcal{C}(\mathbf{x}) := \begin{cases} \mathcal{C}_0, & \text{if } \kappa(\gamma_{\text{local}}(\mathbf{x})) > T_\kappa, \\ 0, & \text{otherwise,} \end{cases} \tag{3}$$

where $\mathcal{C}_0$ is a large constant, and $T_\kappa$ is a threshold. Using the new energy func-tion (2), it is now possible to avoid paths containing parts with high curvature, even if such paths may be shorter than the correct paths. For example, in Fig. 1, our approach avoids the yellow path, because it contains a part $\gamma_{\text{part}}$ with high curvature (dashed box). On the other hand, the red path does *not* contain highly curved parts. Consequently, our approach correctly finds the red path.

## 3.2   Incorporating Curvature with Dynamic Speed

**Necessity of Dynamic Speed.** As mentioned in Sec. 2, previous fast marching approaches cannot incorporate the curvature information because the geometry of the path is unknown during the propagation of $\mathcal{W}$. Furthermore, once $\mathcal{W}$ starts to propagate, $\mathcal{F}$ cannot change anymore. In order to use curvature regularization, the geometry of a local path $\gamma_{\text{local}}$ must be computed *during* the propagation of $\mathcal{W}$, and the speed $\mathcal{F}$ must be updated *dynamically* according to the curvature $\kappa(\gamma_{\text{local}})$. In other words, the propagation of $\mathcal{W}$ and the extraction of $\gamma_{\text{local}}$ must take place in an alternating manner. This can be realized by extending a fast marching approach with dynamic speed [13].

**Initial Speed.** To initialize our dynamic speed $\mathcal{F}$, we apply a commonly used speed based on the response of a multiscale vesselness filter ([15]), i.e. $\mathcal{F}(\mathbf{x}) := \mathcal{V}(\mathbf{x}) = \max_{\sigma_{\min} \leq \sigma \leq \sigma_{\max}} \mathcal{V}_\sigma(\mathbf{x})$, with

$$\mathcal{V}_\sigma(\mathbf{x}) = \begin{cases} 0, & \text{if } \lambda_2 > 0 \\ \exp\left(-\frac{1}{\beta^2} \cdot \frac{\lambda_1^2}{\lambda_2^2}\right)\left(1 - \exp\left(-\frac{1}{2c^2} \cdot (\lambda_1^2 + \lambda_2^2)\right)\right), & \text{otherwise,} \end{cases} \tag{4}$$

where the filter has the scale $\sigma \in [\sigma_{\min}, \sigma_{\max}]$ and its sensitivity is controlled by $\beta$ and $c$. $\lambda_1$ and $\lambda_2$ are the eigenvalues of the Hessian matrix at $\mathbf{x}$.

**Computing the Dynamic Speed.** In classical fast marching approaches, the pixel $\mathbf{x}_{\min}$ on $\mathcal{W}$ with *minimum* arrival time $\mathcal{U}_{\mathbf{x}_s}(\mathbf{x})$ is the position of wave propa-gation, i.e., $\mathcal{W}$ advances to the neighbors of $\mathbf{x}_{\min}$ outside $\mathcal{W}$. In our approach, we decide during the iteration whether to advance $\mathcal{W}$ or not. At $\mathbf{x}_{\min}$, we compute the curvature $\kappa(\gamma_{\text{local}})$ of a local path $\gamma_{\text{local}}$, which is extracted using gradient descent of $\mathcal{U}_{\mathbf{x}_s}$ inside $\mathcal{W}$. If $\kappa(\gamma_{\text{local}}) > T_\kappa$, then the speed $\mathcal{F}(\mathbf{x}_{\min})$ is reduced, which corresponds to the case $\mathcal{C}(\mathbf{x}_{\min}) = \mathcal{C}_0$ in (3). Consequently, $\mathcal{U}_{\mathbf{x}_s}(\mathbf{x}_{\min})$ is increased to a high value. In other words, the propagation through $\mathbf{x}_{\min}$ is slowed down. If $\kappa(\gamma_{\text{local}}) \leq T_\kappa$, then $\mathcal{W}$ advances as in classical fast marching approaches, which corresponds to the case $\mathcal{C}(\mathbf{x}_{\min}) = 0$ in (3). The update *dur-ing* the propagation of $\mathcal{W}$ is the *dynamic* aspect of our speed $\mathcal{F}$. Since the new speed is not larger than the original speed, our approach satisfies the optimality criterion in [13], so the path found using our approach is *globally optimal*.

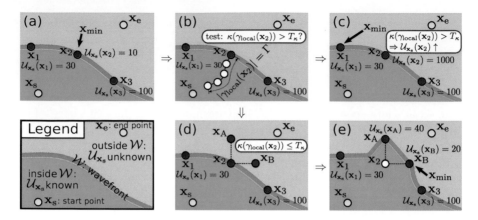

**Fig. 2.** One iteration of the wave propagation incorporating curvature regularization. (a) Select the pixel $\mathbf{x}_{\min}$ on $\mathcal{W}$ with minimum arrival time. (b) For $\gamma(s) = \mathbf{x}_2$, extract $\gamma_{\text{local}}(\mathbf{x}_2)$ with length $\Gamma$, test $\kappa(\gamma_{\text{local}})$. (c) $\kappa(\gamma_{\text{local}})$ too large: $\mathcal{F}(\mathbf{x}_2)$ is reduced and therefore $\mathcal{U}_{\mathbf{x}_s}(\mathbf{x}_2)$ increases. Select another pixel on $\mathcal{W}$. (d) $\kappa(\gamma_{\text{local}})$ small: Compute arrival time for neighbors. (e) $\mathcal{W}$ advances.

One iteration of this scheme is illustrated in Fig. 2. The wavefront $\mathcal{W}$ is shown as an orange stripe. Inside $\mathcal{W}$ (green region), $\mathcal{U}_{\mathbf{x}_s}$ is known since $\mathcal{W}$ has already visited all pixels there, but outside $\mathcal{W}$ (blue region), $\mathcal{U}_{\mathbf{x}_s}$ is unknown. Let $\mathbf{x}_1, \mathbf{x}_2, \mathbf{x}_3$ be pixels on $\mathcal{W}$ (Fig. 2a). The pixel $\mathbf{x}_{\min}$ with minimum $\mathcal{U}_{\mathbf{x}_s}$, i.e. $\mathbf{x}_2$, is considered. The steps shown in Fig. 2b and 2c are the main difference to classical fast marching approaches. Starting at $\mathbf{x}_2$, a local path $\gamma_{\text{local}}(\mathbf{x}_2)$ with a fixed length $\Gamma$ is extracted (Fig. 2b). This is possible since $\mathcal{U}_{\mathbf{x}_s}$ is known inside $\mathcal{W}$. After that, the curvature $\kappa(\gamma_{\text{local}}(\mathbf{x}_2))$ is compared with $T_\kappa$ (Fig. 2b). If $\kappa(\gamma_{\text{local}}(\mathbf{x}_2)) > T_\kappa$, then $\mathcal{F}(\mathbf{x}_2)$ should be reduced, and $\mathcal{U}_{\mathbf{x}_s}(\mathbf{x}_2)$ re-computed, while $\mathcal{W}$ does *not* change (Fig. 2c). Obviously, $\mathcal{U}_{\mathbf{x}_s}(\mathbf{x}_2)$ increases, so the propagation through $\mathbf{x}_2$ (with $\gamma_{\text{local}}(\mathbf{x}_2)$ having high curvature) is slowed down. If $\kappa(\gamma_{\text{local}}(\mathbf{x}_2)) \leq T_\kappa$, then we proceed as in classical fast marching approaches: The neighbors of $\mathbf{x}_2$ outside $\mathcal{W}$, i.e., $\mathbf{x}_A$ and $\mathbf{x}_B$, are found (Fig. 2d) and $\mathcal{W}$ advances to $\mathbf{x}_A$ and $\mathbf{x}_B$, while $\mathbf{x}_2$ is moved into the inside of $\mathcal{W}$ (Fig. 2e). In either case, the pixel on $\mathcal{W}$ with minimum $\mathcal{U}_{\mathbf{x}_s}$ value, i.e., $\mathbf{x}_{\min}$, will be considered in the next iteration.

## 4   Experimental Results

We carried out experiments using synthetic images and retina images on a PC with a 2.27 GHz CPU and 3 GB memory, and compared our approach with two previous approaches: The classical fast marching approach using the vesselness measure [15] as speed (Classical FM), and the intensity-based approach in [3] (Li-Yezzi FM). Most parameter values are fixed for all data, empirically determined based on one image: $w = 1, \mathcal{C}_0 = 10^7, \sigma_{\min} = 1, \sigma_{\max} = 2, \beta = 0.5, c = 0.5$. $\Gamma$ and $T_\kappa$ typically have values of 10 and 0.2, respectively. Our algorithm is relatively robust to the choice of parameter values.

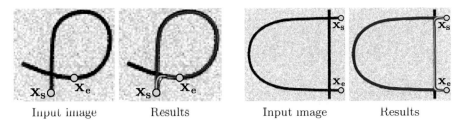

| Input image | Results | Input image | Results |

**Fig. 3.** Results on synthetic images. The yellow, blue and red lines show the results of Classical FM, Li-Yezzi FM, and our approach, respectively.

**Synthetic Images.** We tested our approach with different synthetic images. For example, Fig. 3 shows a loop, as well as a curve which crosses a straight line. In both cases, our approach yields the paths with low curvature (red lines), even though these paths are much longer than the short cuts. In contrast, both Classical FM and Li-Yezzi FM result in short cuts.

**Retina Images.** We have used all 40 retina images of the DRIVE dataset [14] for evaluation. For *each* image, one to three vessels which *cross* other vessels are selected, resulting in 81 vessels in total. Such vessels are very common in retina images. The results for four vessels are shown in Fig. 4. In the first row, the vessel crosses another vessel which has a similar radius. There, Classical FM results in a short cut with high curvature, while our approach finds the correct path. Li-Yezzi FM also finds the correct path, because the intensity of the vessel is quite different from the other vessel. However, as shown in the second row, the intensity is not a good feature, since the intensities inside the vessel vary significantly. As a result, the Li-Yezzi FM approach runs into a neighboring vessel, while Classical FM and our approach yield the correct path. For the vessel in the third row, Classical FM and Li-Yezzi FM both yield short cuts. In contrast, our approach achieves the correct path in this case, as well as in the fourth row, which shows an even more difficult case: The correct vessel is much longer than the short cuts.

For a quantitative evaluation, we compared the results of our approach and the two previous approaches with the ground truth provided in the DRIVE dataset. The ground truth is a binary segmentation of all pixels corresponding to vessels, while the results from fast marching approaches are centerlines with subpixel accuracy. To enable a comparison, we determine the set $S_0$ of pixels which lie on the path of the segmented centerline, and the set $S_1$, which is given by the pixels of $S_0$ inside the vessel in the binary segmentation. The quotient $Q_{\text{inside}} = \frac{|S_1|}{|S_0|}$ is used to measure the accuracy of the segmented centerlines. The results and run time for the four vessels in Fig. 4 as well as the mean values for all 81 vessels are summarized in Table 1. It can be seen that our approach yields significantly higher values for $Q_{\text{inside}}$ compared to Classical FM and Li-Yezzi FM (e.g., 99.13% on average, compared to 45.27% and 48.18% for previous approaches). Additionally, a lower mean run time of 0.68 s compared to 0.79 s (Li-Yezzi FM) is achieved.

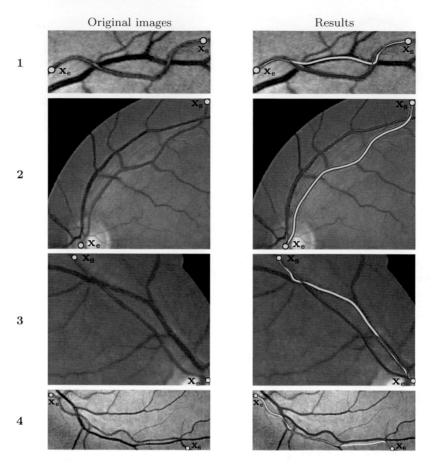

**Fig. 4.** Results for four vessels from the DRIVE dataset. The yellow, blue and red lines show the results of Classical FM, Li-Yezzi FM, and our approach, respectively.

**Table 1.** Comparison of quantitative results for retinal vessels

| Vessel | Classical FM | | Li-Yezzi FM | | **Our approach** | |
|---|---|---|---|---|---|---|
| | $Q_{\text{inside}}$ | Time | $Q_{\text{inside}}$ | Time | $Q_{\text{inside}}$ | Time |
| 1 | 54.90% | 0.08 s | 94.04% | 0.17 s | 94.55% | 0.26 s |
| 2 | 100.00% | 0.39 s | 11.49% | 2.76 s | 100.00% | 0.88 s |
| 3 | 26.42% | 0.19 s | 67.49% | 0.79 s | 99.61% | 0.63 s |
| 4 | 31.96% | 0.31 s | 42.78% | 1.41 s | 99.42% | 0.96 s |
| Mean for all 81 | 45.27% | 0.22 s | 48.18% | 0.79 s | 99.13% | 0.68 s |

## 5    Discussion and Conclusions

We presented a novel globally optimal fast marching approach for vessel segmentation with curvature regularization. The fast marching method can be interpreted as the propagation of a wavefront. *During* the propagation, we dynamically update the speed of the wavefront according to the curvature of local paths, in order to avoid erroneous segmentation results which are shorter but have higher curvature. Experimental results on synthetic and retina images show that using our approach, short cuts with high curvature can be effectively avoided, and therefore our approach yields better results, in particular, for vessels which cross other vessels. Although our approach involves additional computation of the curvature, it is more efficient than a previous approach [3].

**Acknowledgment.** Support of the Deutsche Forschungsgemeinschaft (DFG) within the project QuantVessel (RO 2471/6) is gratefully acknowledged.

# References

1. Dijkstra, E.: A Note on Two Problems in Connection with Graphs. Numerische Mathematik, 269–271 (1959)
2. Cohen, L., Kimmel, R.: Global Minimum for Active Contour Models: A Minimal Path Approach. Internat. J. of Computer Vision 24, 57–78 (1997)
3. Li, H., Yezzi, A.: Vessels as 4-D Curves: Global Minimal 4-D Paths to Extract 3-D Tubular Surfaces and Centerlines. IEEE TMI 26, 1213–1223 (2007)
4. Benmansour, F., Cohen, L.: Fast Object Segmentation by Growing Minimal Paths from a Single Point on 2D or 3D Images. J. of Math. Imag. Vis. 33, 209–221 (2009)
5. Kaul, V., Yezzi, A., Tsai, Y.: Detecting Curves with Unknown Endpoints and Arbitrary Topology Using Minimal Paths. IEEE TPAMI 34, 1952–1965 (2012)
6. Poon, K., Hamarneh, G., Abugharbieh, R.: Live-Vessel: Extending Livewire for Simultaneous Extraction of Optimal Medial and Boundary Paths in Vascular Images. In: Ayache, N., Ourselin, S., Maeder, A. (eds.) MICCAI 2007, Part II. LNCS, vol. 4792, pp. 444–451. Springer, Heidelberg (2007)
7. Pechaud, M., Keriven, R., Peyre, G.: Extraction of Tubular Structures Over an Orientation Domain. In: Proc. CVPR 2009, Miami, FL/USA, vol. 1, pp. 336–342 (2009)
8. Lo, P., van Ginneken, B., de Bruijne, M.: Vessel Tree Extraction Using Locally Optimal Paths. In: Proc. ISBI 2010, Rotterdam, The Netherlands, pp. 680–683 (2010)
9. Benmansour, F., Cohen, L.D.: Tubular Structure Segmentation Based on Minimal Path Method and Anisotropic Enhancement. Int. J. of Computer Vision 92, 192–210 (2011)
10. Law, M., Chung, A.: Three Dimensional Curvilinear Structure Detection Using Optimally Oriented Flux. In: Forsyth, D., Torr, P., Zisserman, A. (eds.) ECCV 2008, Part IV. LNCS, vol. 5305, pp. 368–382. Springer, Heidelberg (2008)
11. Parker, G., Wheeler-Kingshott, C., Barker, G.: Estimating Distributed Anatomical Connectivity Using Fast Marching Methods and Diffusion Tensor Imaging. IEEE Trans. on Medical Imaging 21, 505–512 (2002)
12. Joshi, V., Garvin, M., Reinhardt, J., Abramoff, M.: Identification and Reconnection of Interrupted Vessels in Retinal Vessel Segmentation. In: Proc. ISBI 2011, Chicago, IL/USA, pp. 1416–1420 (2011)
13. Liao, W., Wörz, S., Rohr, K.: Globally Minimal Path Method Using Dynamic Speed Functions Based on Progressive Wave Propagation. In: Lee, K.M., Matsushita, Y., Rehg, J.M., Hu, Z. (eds.) ACCV 2012, Part II. LNCS, vol. 7725, pp. 25–37. Springer, Heidelberg (2013)
14. Staal, J., Abramoff, M., Niemeijer, M., Viergever, M., van Ginneken, B.: Ridge based vessel segmentation in color images of the retina. IEEE Trans. on Medical Imaging 23, 501–509 (2004)
15. Frangi, A., Niessen, W., Vincken, K., Viergever, M.: Multiscale vessel enhancement filtering. In: Wells, W.M., Colchester, A.C.F., Delp, S.L. (eds.) MICCAI 1998. LNCS, vol. 1496, pp. 130–137. Springer, Heidelberg (1998)

# Low-Rank and Sparse Matrix Decomposition for Compressed Sensing Reconstruction of Magnetic Resonance 4D Phase Contrast Blood Flow Imaging (LoSDeCoS 4D-PCI)

Jana Hutter[1,2], Peter Schmitt[4], Gunhild Aandal[3], Andreas Greiser[4], Christoph Forman[1,2], Robert Grimm[1], Joachim Hornegger[1,2], and Andreas Maier[1,2]

[1] Pattern Recognition Lab, University Erlangen-Nuremberg, Germany
[2] School of Advanced Optical Technologies, Erlangen, Germany
[3] University Hospital Cleveland, Cleveland, Ohio, USA
[4] Siemens AG Healthcare Sector, Magnetic Resonance, Erlangen, Germany

**Abstract.** Blood flow measurements using 4D Phase Contrast blood flow imaging (PCI) provide an excellent fully non-invasive technique to assess the hemodynamics clinically in-vivo. Iterative reconstruction techniques combined with parallel MRI have been proposed to reduce the data acquisition time, which is the biggest drawback of 4D PCI. The novel LoSDeCoS technique combines these ideas with the separation into a low-rank and a sparse component. The high-dimensionality of the PC data renders it ideally suited for this approach. The proposed method is not limited to a single body region, but can be applied to any 4D flow measurement. The benefits of the new method are twofold: It allows to significantly accelerate the acquisition; and generates additional images highlighting temporal and directional flow changes. Reduction in acquisition time improves patient comfort and can be used to achieve better temporal or spatial resolution, which in turn allows more precise calculations of clinically important quantitative numbers such as flow rates or the wall shear stress. With LoSDeCoS, acceleration factors of 6-8 were achieved for 16 in-vivo datasets of both the carotid artery (6 datasets) and the aorta (10 datasets), while decreasing the Normalized Root Mean Square Error by over 10 % compared to a standard iterative reconstruction and by achieving similarity values of over 0.93. Inflow-Outflow phantom experiments showed good parabolic profiles and an excellent mass conservation.

## 1 Introduction

Knowledge about patient-specific hemodynamics is important in the diagnosis and treatment planning of various cardiovascular diseases such as stenoses or aneurysms in the carotid arteries or in the aorta. Dynamic 3D flow information allows to visualize not only the flow rate, but also turbulent flow as well as the hemodynamics in complex or pathologic vessel systems. Standard clinically used

K. Mori et al. (Eds.): MICCAI 2013, Part I, LNCS 8149, pp. 558–565, 2013.

techniques including Doppler ultrasound or Digital Substraction Angiography have the drawbacks of user-dependent results or the exposure to ionizing radiation. 4D PCI provides a fully non-invasive alternative to assess three-directional blood flow. The acquisition time for this technique, especially if high temporal and spatial resolution or an extended anatomic coverage are desired, tends to be very high, limiting its wider clinical use at present. With recently proposed combinations of compressed sensing algorithms and parallel MRI techniques using data simultaneously acquired by multiple coils, significant reductions of the acquisition time were achieved.

## 1.1   PCI Acquisition

The data for an MR volume is acquired by successive $k$-space scans until the full $k$-space $\mathbf{Y}$ is covered. Reconstruction using the matrix $\mathbf{A}$ leads to the final volume $\mathbf{X} = \mathbf{AY}$ with $\mathbf{Y} \in \mathbb{C}^{N_k}$ and $\mathbf{X} \in \mathbb{C}^{N}$ with $N = N_x \times N_y \times N_z$. The traditional reconstruction is done by simple inverse Fourier Transform $\mathbf{A} = \mathbf{F}^{-1}$.

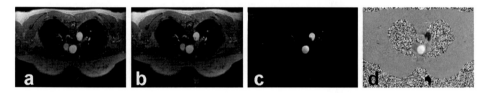

**Fig. 1.** Aortic Phase Contrast dataset: (a) Flow compensated image, (b) Magnitude of velocity sensitive image, (c) Phase Contrast image and (d) Phase Difference image

The technique typically uses ECG triggering to acquire $N_p$ phases in the cardiac cycle. As the data is collected over multiple heart cycles until $k$-space coverage is complete, reduction of the number of required $k$-space lines leads to a direct decrease in acquisition time. To visualize the flow dynamics in three directions, four MR scans are needed: one velocity-compensated scan $\mathbf{Y_{v0}}$; and three scans sensitive to the velocity $\mathbf{Y_{v1}}, \mathbf{Y_{v2}}$ and $\mathbf{Y_{v3}}$ [1] (see Fig. 1a,b). For a final series of images with $N_p$ temporal phases which are sensitive to flow in three directions, $4N_p$ full 3D datasets have to be acquired and reconstructed from the same spatial field of view. Combining all three encodings leads to the typical PCI image: $\mathbf{PC} = \sum (\mathbf{X_{v0}} - \mathbf{X_{vs}})^2$. (Fig. 1c) The velocity information is obtained by calculating the phase difference between the velocity compensated and each of the velocity encoded scans: $\Delta_s = \arg(\mathbf{X_{v0}}) - \arg(\mathbf{X_{vs}})$ (Fig. 1d).

## 1.2   Spatial Redundancy

Compressed sensing algorithms rely on sampling only $\bar{N}_k << N_k$ $k$-space samples. In order to achieve good image quality with data sampled below the Nyquist criteria, dedicated reconstruction techniques are required, which rely on prior knowledge as regularization. Commonly used regularization terms include Wavelet Transforms, Total Variation or temporal smoothness.

The 4D flow dataset contains a high degree of anatomical redundancy between the $4N_p$ different volumes, as they are all acquired from the same spatial region. Particularly important for this acquisition technique are the flow changes across the different temporal phases, appearing in a small fraction of the volume. The final volume can thus be split into a shared anatomical- structural part and the regions with directionally and spatially varying flow characteristics. This separation agrees well with a mathematical separation into a low-rank and a sparse component. The reconstruction of the images (zoom to the ICA/ECA) using 48/5/2 singular values (Fig. 2) shows well the separation possibilities. The image quality concerning the vascular structures and the surrounding tissue is preserved with less singular values, while the temporal and spatial flow variations over time are lost.

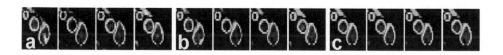

**Fig. 2.** Reconstruction with (a) 48, (b) 5 and (c) 2 singular values

### 1.3   State of the Art

Iterative reconstruction algorithms have been recently applied to PCI using different regularizations and algorithms [2,3,4]. Employed algorithms include Lagrangian based alternating direction [5] and Split Bregman, successfully applied to MRI by Aeltermann et al. [6]. Splitting the problem into a sparse and a low-rank part was discussed by Candès et al.[7] and recently introduced for brain, multi-slice breast and dynamic MRI [8,9,10]. The novel LoSDeCoS algorithm exploits the special properties of 4D Phase Contrast data for the division into a low-rank and sparse component and solves for that using a specially adapted Split Bregman solver able to deal with Total Variation, $L_1$ and the nuclear norm.

## 2   Iterative Reconstruction Using LoSDeCoS

Each volume $\mathbf{X}$ is transformed into a vector $\boldsymbol{x}$ containing all image pixels. This allows to significantly enlarge the vector space used for low-rank estimation. All 4D flow volumes, both the temporal phases and the velocity encodings are used to form a common matrix $\mathbf{M} \in \mathbb{C}^{N \times 4N_p}$.

$$
\mathbf{M} = \begin{bmatrix} \boldsymbol{x}_0^{v0,0} & \boldsymbol{x}_0^{v1,0} & \boldsymbol{x}_0^{v2,0} & \boldsymbol{x}_0^{v3,0} & & \boldsymbol{x}_0^{v0,N_p} & \boldsymbol{x}_0^{v1,N_p} & \boldsymbol{x}_0^{v2,N_p} & \boldsymbol{x}_0^{v3,N_p} \\ \vdots & \vdots & \vdots & \vdots & \cdots\cdots & \vdots & \vdots & \vdots & \vdots \\ \boldsymbol{x}_N^{v0,0} & \boldsymbol{x}_N^{v1,0} & \boldsymbol{x}_N^{v2,0} & \boldsymbol{x}_N^{v3,0} & & \boldsymbol{x}_N^{v0,N_p} & \boldsymbol{x}_N^{v1,N_p} & \boldsymbol{x}_N^{v2,N_p} & \boldsymbol{x}_N^{v3,N_p} \end{bmatrix} \tag{1}
$$

## 2.1   Division into a Low-Rank and a Sparse Matrix

$\mathbf{M}$ consists of a low rank part $\mathbf{L}$, representing stationary tissue, and a sparse matrix $\mathbf{S}$ of the same dimensions. The sparse part includes the highly varying but sparse regions, which contain moving magnetization (flow).

The low rank requirement rank($\mathbf{L}$) $< r$ is due to computational efforts relaxed to the convex nuclear norm $||\mathbf{L}||_* = \sum \omega$, where $\omega$ are the singular values of $\mathbf{S}$, as calculated by the complex SVD. The sparse component should fulfill $||\Phi S||_{L_0} < c$, with $\Phi$ being an operator that transforms the data into a sparse domain. The LoSDeCoS method uses both Wavelet ($\Psi$) and isotropic TV norm as sparsifying transforms. The calculated minimization therefore equals to $\min_S \alpha_1 ||\mathbf{S}||_{TV} + \alpha_2 ||\psi \mathbf{S}||_{L_1}$.

## 2.2   Iterative Reconstruction with the Split Bregman Algorithm

The parallel MRI reconstruction algorithm requires coil profiles $\mathbf{C_c}$ describing the sensitivity information of the $N_c$ spatially varying coils. Those profiles, the discrete Fourier transform $\mathbf{F}$ as well as the undersampling projection $\mathbf{P}$ form the iterative reconstruction matrix $\mathbf{A} = \mathbf{PFC}$, which is used to fit the calculated image $\mathbf{M}$ to the acquired undersampled data $\mathbf{y}$ by minimizing the data fidelity term $||\mathbf{AM} - \mathbf{y}||_{L_2}^2$. The final objective function used in the minimization problem reads as follows:

$$\min_{\mathbf{S},\mathbf{L}} ||\mathbf{A}(\mathbf{S} + \mathbf{L}) - \mathbf{y}||_{L_2}^2 + \alpha_1 ||\mathbf{S}||_{TV} + \alpha_2 ||\psi \mathbf{S}||_{L_1} + \alpha_3 ||\mathbf{L}||_* . \qquad (2)$$

The combination of different norms makes the problem hard to solve in the form of an unconstrained minimization problem (2). The Split Bregman algorithm is better suited, as it splits the problem into its different components, which are then minimized each with an adapted strategy. Additional variables $\mathbf{d}_\nabla = (\nabla \mathbf{S})$, $d_w = \psi \mathbf{S}$, $d_n = \mathbf{L}$ and the residual errors $\boldsymbol{\mu}$ are used to combine the actual solutions of all steps in a common $L_2$ minimization step. The algorithm is initialized with $\mathbf{S} = \mathbf{L} = 0$ as well as $\boldsymbol{\mu} = 0$ (residual variables) and consists of three substeps in every iteration.

$$
\begin{cases}
(\mathbf{S}^{k+1}, \mathbf{L}^{k+1}) = & \text{argmin}_{\mathbf{S}^k, \mathbf{L}^k} ||\mathbf{A}(\mathbf{L}^k + \mathbf{S}^k) - \mathbf{y}||_{L_2}^2 + \alpha_3 ||d_n^k - \mathbf{L}^k - \mu_n^k||_{L_2}^2 \\
& +\alpha_1 ||\mathbf{d}_\nabla^k - \nabla \mathbf{S}^k - \mu_\nabla^k||_{L_2}^2 + \alpha_2 ||d_w^k - \psi \mathbf{S}^k - \mu_w^k||_{L_2}^2 \quad (3a) \\
(\mathbf{d}_\nabla^{k+1}) = & \text{argmin}_{\mathbf{d}_\nabla^k} ||\mathbf{d}_\nabla^k - \nabla \mathbf{S}^{k+1} - \mu_\nabla^k||_{L_2}^2 + ||\nabla \mathbf{S}^{k+1}||_{2,1} \quad (3b) \\
(d_w^{k+1}) = & \text{argmin}_{d_w} ||d_w^k - \psi \mathbf{S}^{k+1} - \mu_w^k||_{L_2}^2 + ||\psi d_w^k||_{L_1} \quad (3c) \\
(d_n^{k+1}) = & \text{argmin}_{d_n^k} ||d_n^k - \mathbf{L}^{k+1} - \mu_n^k||_{L_2}^2 + ||d_n^k||_* \quad (3d)
\end{cases}
$$

First, the $L_2$ problem (3a) is minimized using a limited-memory Quasi-Newton algorithm with three iterations. The obtained results $\mathbf{S}^{k+1}, \mathbf{L}^{k+1}$ are used in the next step, which successively minimizes the regularization terms using adapted methods for each of them: The isotropic TV (3b) was minimized using adapted shrinkage [11], Wavelet (3c) with soft thresholding. The nuclear norm minimization is done with singular value thresholding. The complex SVD for $\mathbf{L}$ results in

$\mathbf{L} = \mathbf{U}\Sigma\mathbf{V}^*$. The nuclear norm is equal to $\sum tr(\Sigma)$. The new $\mathbf{L}$ is computed as $\mathbf{L}^{k+1} = \mathbf{U}\bar{\Sigma}\mathbf{V}^*$ with $\bar{\Sigma} = diag(\bar{\sigma}_{i,i})|\bar{\sigma}_{i,i} = \sigma_{i,i}$ if $\sigma_{i,i} \geq \epsilon_n$ and $\bar{\sigma}_{i,i} = 0$ if $\sigma_{i,i} \leq \epsilon_n$. $\epsilon_n$ is chosen fixed for all datasets as $0.1\sigma_{i,i}$.

The last step is the update of the residual variables $\mu$ as follows: $\mu_\nabla^{k+1} = \mu_\nabla^k + \nabla\mathbf{S}^{k+1} - \mathbf{d}_\nabla^{k+1}$, $\mu_w^{k+1} = \mu_w^k + \psi\mathbf{S}^{k+1} - d_w^{k+1}$ and $\mu_n^{k+1} = \mu_n^k + \mathbf{L}^{k+1} - d_n^{k+1}$.

# 3  Experiments and Results

## 3.1  Experimental Setup

Volunteer data (10 aortic datasets, 6 carotid datasets) was acquired on a clinical 3T scanner (MAGNETOM Skyra, Siemens Healthcare, Erlangen). In addition, phantom data was acquired using an MR compatible pump (Compu-Flow 1000, Shelley). Further evaluation was done on the phantom data. The inflow-outflow setup used for this study with two connected tubes of diameter 1.9mm and a regulated parabolic flow with 150 ml/s allows to study quantitative values such as the flow and the conservation of mass. The parameters for the carotid/aortic/phantom data were TR 49.8/41.9/49.6 ms, TE 3.5/2.7/3.4 ms, flip angle 20° and slice thickness 4/5/3.1mm. The FOV was 200×200×40mm for carotids (matrix $256^2$), 340×230×25mm for the aorta (matrix 416×288) and 190×130mm for the phantom (matrix 176×256). Temporal phases and velocity sensitivity range (venc) were chosen patient specific, between 10 and 16 phases and venc $\in [60, 150]$cm/s.

The whole $k$-space was acquired for all datasets and retrospectively undersampled using sampling patterns $\mathbf{U}$ incoherent in both temporal phase and velocity encoding direction. An acceleration factor of 8, corresponding to 32 lines out of 256 was applied to the carotid datasets and the phantom data. For the aortic data the acceleration factor was 6. The fully sampled directly reconstructed data $\mathbf{X}_{REF}$ is used for evaluation purposes. The undersampled data was reconstructed three times. Using an iterative SENSE approach without regularization $\mathbf{X}_{IS}$, a compressed sensing SENSE approach involving both TV and $L_1$ regularization $\mathbf{X}_{IRS}$ and with the proposed novel LoSDeCoS method $\mathbf{X}_{LOS}$. The parameters were chosen identical for all datasets as $\alpha_1 = 0.00005, \alpha_2 = 0.005, \alpha_3 = 0.05$, ten LBFGS iterations and six outer iterations.

## 3.2  Quantitative Evaluation

The normalized root mean square error $NRMSE(\mathbf{R}, \mathbf{X}) = ||\mathbf{R} - \mathbf{X}||_2^2 / ||\mathbf{X}||_2^2$, as well as the structured similarity measure SSIM [12] were used to evaluate the LoSDeCoS results against the reference and the standard reconstruction methods. To assess the image quality, angiography specific Contrast-to-Noise-Ratios (CNR) were used.

$$\text{SSIM}(\mathbf{R}, \mathbf{X}) = \frac{2\mu_R\mu_X + c_1}{\mu_X^2 + \mu_R^2 + c_1} + \frac{\sigma\sigma_{XR} + c_2}{\sigma_R^2 + \sigma_X^2 + c_2} \quad \text{CNR}(\mathbf{X}) = \frac{\mu_{\mathbf{X_{T1}}} - \mu_{\mathbf{X_{T2}}}}{\sqrt{0.5(\sigma_{\mathbf{X_{T1}}}^2 + \sigma_{\mathbf{X_{T2}}}^2)}}. \quad (4)$$

For the phantom data, the deviation from mass conservation, involving total inflow $F_i$ and outflow $F_o$ was evaluated: $DM = |F_i - F_o| / F_i$ (0 in ideal settings).

## 4    Results

The upper row of Fig. 3 shows the results for the fully sampled reference against different reconstruction results using the same acceleration of 8. The influence of separating low-rank and sparse components is illustrated in the lower row of Fig. 3 showing the **L, S** and **M** for the temporal phases $t_1 = 100\,ms$, and $t_2 = 250\,ms$. Especially the filling of the internal carotid artery is well visualized in **S** as indicated by the arrow. The quantitative results in Table 1 show that the SSIM and NRMSE values are significantly higher for the new approach. A SSIM could be increased from 0.81 for the best compared method to 0.94 for LoSDeCoS in the aorta. For the higher accelerated carotids the increase is even more evident, 0.82 instead of 0.65. The $CNR_{VB}$ values for LoSDeCoS are superior to the compared as well as to the reference dataset, which is due to the higher suppression of background noise by exploiting the low rank. The $CNR_{VT}$ was in the range of the reference, but lower than the compared methods. This result, combined with the significantly better SSIM and NRMSE, shows that LoSDeCoS preserves the vascular and tissue contrast better than the regularized SENSE method which tends to suppress the tissue more.

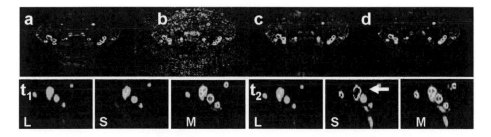

**Fig. 3.** Upper row: Carotid results for (a) reference, (b) IS, (c) IRS and (d) LoSDeCoS Lower row: Low-rank, sparse and combined result for phases $t_1$ and $t_2$

**Table 1.** Quantitative evaluation of the human data

|  | Aorta (acceleration 6.0) | | | | Carotids (acceleration 8.0) | | | |
|---|---|---|---|---|---|---|---|---|
|  | $\mathbf{X}_{REF}$ | $\mathbf{X}_{IS}$ | $\mathbf{X}_{IRS}$ | $\mathbf{X}_{LOS}$ | $\mathbf{X}_{REF}$ | $\mathbf{X}_{IS}$ | $\mathbf{X}_{IRS}$ | $\mathbf{X}_{LOS}$ |
| $SSIM$ | 1.00 | 0.79 | 0.81 | 0.94 | 1.00 | 0.30 | 0.65 | 0.82 |
| $NRMSE$ | 0.00 | 118.51 | 115.63 | 93.84 | 0.00 | 183.91 | 144.29 | 138.50 |
| $CNR_{VT}$ | 11.46 | 14.72 | 17.91 | 14.18 | 15.87 | 10.47 | 16.12 | 15.97 |
| $CNR_{VB}$ | 26.27 | 14.03 | 16.32 | 27.06 | 24.14 | 11.83 | 22.10 | 29.25 |

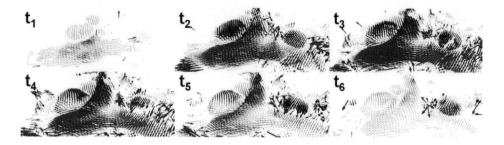

**Fig. 4.** Representation of the flow patterns in the aorta in 6 consecutive timesteps

In summary, the results show that LoSDeCoS achieves even at higher acceleration factors excellent results for the reconstructed volumes. The accuracy of this data is essential for the calculation of any meaningful physiological value calculation. Representative 3D velocity fields over time are shown in Fig. 4, the absolute flow values of the ascending aorta over the cardiac cycle obtained from the LoSDeCoS results (Fig. 5a) in comparison with the reference values illustrate that LoSDeCoS is very well suited to calculate accurate 4D flow results. A manual segmentation of the aorta done by an experienced radiologist was used to calculate the total flow $F$. Figure 5b,c illustrate the parabolic in-/outflow profiles obtained from phantom experiments using LoSDeCoS. The mass conservation deviation $DM$ for LoSDeCoS equals $0.86\%$, compared to $4.5\%$ for iterative regularized SENSE and $1.3\%$ for iterative SENSE (Reference: $0.63\%$).

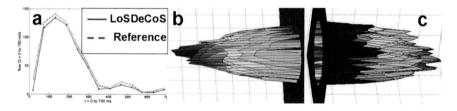

**Fig. 5.** (a) Aortic flow over time. (b-c) Parabolic In- and Outflow profiles

## 5    Discussion and Conclusions

The proposed LoSDeCoS algorithm has been proven to yield very good reconstruction results for 4D PCI data by enabling a significant reduction in acquisition time from roughly 10 min. for a 4D scan of the aortic arch down to under 2 min. While being successfully applied to both the carotid bifurcation region and the aortic arch, it has further shown its generalization capabilities to different body regions. In addition, the proposed reconstruction framework is, due to the splitting, well adapted to incorporate further regularizations such as phase corrections [13] or divergence terms.

**Acknowledgements.** The authors gratefully acknowledge funding of the Erlangen Graduate School in Advanced Optical Technologies (SAOT) by the German Research Foundation in the framework of the German excellence initiative.

# References

1. Chai, P., Mohiaddin, R.: How we perform cardiovascular magnetic resonance flow assessment using phase-contrast velocity mapping. J. Cardiovasc. Magn. Reson. 7, 705–716 (2005)
2. Kim, D., Dyvorne, H.A., Otazo, R., Feng, L., Sodickson, D.K., Lee, V.S.: Accelerated phase-contrast cine MRI using k-t SPARSE-SENSE. Magn. Reson. Med. 67, 1054–1064 (2011)
3. Joseph, A.A., Merboldt, K.D., Voit, D., Zhang, S., Uecker, M., Lotz, J., Frahm, J.: Real-time phase-contrast MRI of cardiovascular blood flow using undersampled radial fast low-angle shot and nonlinear inverse reconstruction. NMR Biomed. 25, 917–924 (2011)
4. Tao, Y., Rilling, G., Davies, M., Marshall, I.: Compressed sensing reconstruction with retrospectively gated sampling patterns for velocity measurement of carotid blood flow. In: Proc. Joint Annual Meeting ISMRM- ESMRMB, Stockholm, Sweden, p. 4866 (2010)
5. Esser, E.: Applications of Lagrangian based alternating direction methods and connections to split Bregman. CAM Report 09-31, UCLA (2009)
6. Aelterman, J., Luong, H., Goossens, B., Piurica, A., Philips, W.: COMPASS: a Joint Framework for Parallel Imaging and Compressive Sensing in MRI. In: IEEE Int. Conf. on Image Processing (ICIP), Hong Kong, China, pp. 1653–1656 (2010)
7. Candes, E.J., Li, X., Ma, Y., Wright, J.: Robust principal component analysis? J. ACM 58, 11:1–11:37 (2011)
8. Majumdar, A., Ward, R.: Exploiting rank deficiency and transform domain sparsity for MR image reconstruction. Magn. Reson. Imaging. 30, 9–18 (2012)
9. Yin, X., Ng, B., Ramamohanarao, K., Baghai-Wadji, A., Abbott, D.: Exploiting sparsity and low-rank structure for the recovery of multi-slice breast MRIs with reduced sampling error. Med. Biol. Eng. Comput. (2012)
10. Tremoulheac, B., Atkinson, D., Arridge, S.R.: Motion and Contrast Enhancement Separation Model Reconstruction from Partial Measurements in Dynamic MRI. In (Proceedings) MICCAI Workshop on Sparsity Techniques in Medical Imaging, Nice, France (2012)
11. Goldstein, T., Osher, S.: The Split Bregman Method for L1-Regularized Problems. SIAM J. Img. Sci. 2, 323–343 (2009)
12. Wang, Z., Bovik, A.C., Sheikh, H.R., Simoncelli, E.P.: Image Quality Assessment: From Error Visibility to Structural Similarity. IEEE Transactions on Image Processing 13, 600–612 (2004)
13. Zhao, F., Noll, D.C., Nielsen, J.F., Fessler, J.A.: Separate Magnitude and Phase Regularization via Compressed Sensing. IEEE Trans. Med. Imaging 31, 1713–1723 (2012)

# Anatomical Labeling of the Circle of Willis Using Maximum A Posteriori Graph Matching

David Robben[1,*], Stefan Sunaert[2], Vincent Thijs[3], Guy Wilms[2],
Frederik Maes[1], and Paul Suetens[1]

[1] iMinds - Medical Image Computing (ESAT/PSI), KU Leuven, Belgium
[2] Department of Radiology, University Hospitals Leuven, KU Leuven, Belgium
[3] Department of Neurology, University Hospitals Leuven, KU Leuven, Belgium
david.robben@esat.kuleuven.be

**Abstract.** A new method for anatomically labeling the vasculature is presented and applied to the Circle of Willis. Our method converts the segmented vasculature into a graph that is matched with an annotated graph atlas in a maximum a posteriori (MAP) way. The MAP matching is formulated as a quadratic binary programming problem which can be solved efficiently. Unlike previous methods, our approach can handle non tree-like vasculature and large topological differences. The method is evaluated in a leave-one-out test on MRA of 30 subjects where it achieves a sensitivity of 93% and a specificity of 85% with an average error of 1.5 mm on matching bifurcations in the vascular graph.

**Keywords:** Graph matching, vasculature, anatomical labeling, Circle of Willis, MAP.

## 1 Introduction

The Circle of Willis (CoW) is a circle of arteries in the skull base that connects the left and right side of the anterior cerebral circulation with the posterior cerebral circulation. This structure is highly variable: only 42% of the population has a complete circle [2] and in the other cases, one or more arteries are missing. In the past years, several research papers addressed the problem of segmenting the CoW and the cerebral vasculature in general, without labeling them. Having an algorithm that can anatomically label the vasculature, however, can be important for many applications. In clinical settings, it can give an interventional radiologist additional guidance when navigating through the vasculature of a patient, or it can provide automatic measurements of the diameter of certain vessels. In a research context, it can be used to detect patterns in the vasculature of subpopulations (e.g. geometric risk factors for vascular pathologies) in a more accurate fashion. Despite these applications, literature is very limited. Since a similar problem is encountered in the labeling of the bronchial segments in the lungs, we also consider this in our literature study.

* David Robben is supported by a Ph.D. fellowship of the Research Foundation - Flanders (FWO).

K. Mori et al. (Eds.): MICCAI 2013, Part I, LNCS 8149, pp. 566–573, 2013.

Most methods first transform the segmented image into a graph, and then label this graph. Tschirren et al. [9] use atlas-based graph matching to label the bronchi of a patient. Although a probabilistic graph atlas is created - containing the average and standard deviation of certain properties - the matching has no probabilistic interpretation. Mori et al. published several works about bronchial labeling. Their latest approach [6] uses multiclass AdaBoost to assign a probability to each branch and label. Subsequently, a depth-first search finds the global optimal assignment of branch names taking into account topological constraints. In another line of work, Mori et al. [5] label the abdominal arteries, which they consider more difficult than labeling bronchi due to the larger variation. They state that their approach is expected not to work on vasculature of other organs. Bogunovic et al. [1] label 5 bifurcations in the anterior circulation of the CoW. They are the first to introduce a maximum a posteriori approach to the matching problem. All possible isomorphisms between the target graph and the atlas are explicitly enumerated and for each mapping the likelihood is calculated to find the maximum. The likelihood term only compares the bifurcations but not the branches in between. Although the performance of the method is very good, it is not computationally scalable: a preprocessing step is required to prune the graph to about 20 candidate vertices. It should be noted that all of the previous methods assume that the graph is a tree and allow limited or even no topological variations.

Takemura et al. [8] propose a method that does not use graphs. They label the CoW by rigidly registering the to-be-labeled image to an atlas. Due to the large variability in the shape of the vasculature, the quality of results varies enormously between the different subjects and for the different arteries. They report voxel-wise classification rates as high as 86% for large vessels as the Internal Carotid Artery (ICA) and as low as 0.5% for small vessels such as the Posterior Communicating Artery (PcomA).

This paper introduces a novel and generic approach to anatomically label vessels, and demonstrates its performance on the CoW and its adjacent vessels. In this paper, we label 24 Points of Interest (PoI): 15 bifurcations and 9 endpoints of the cerebral vasculature (Fig. 1).

## 2  Methodology

### 2.1  Creation of a Vascular Graph

The first step in our algorithm is the conversion of a vascular image into an attributed graph $G = (V_G, E_G, A_G)$ with $V_G$ the set of vertices, $E_G$ the set of edges and $A_G$ the attributes of the vertices and edges. The vertices $V_G$ represent the bifurcations and endpoints of the vessels and the edges $E_G$ represent the vascular trajectories between the – both directly and indirectly connected – vertices. In case multiple paths connect two points, the shortest is used to calculate the attributes. Segmentation of the MRA images is done with region growing and this segmented image is subsequently thinned using Palagyi's thinning algorithm [7]. The resulting skeleton image is converted into a graph and

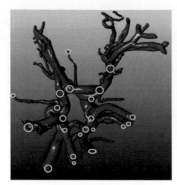
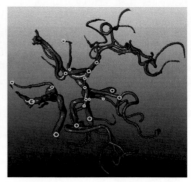

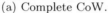

(a) Complete CoW.        (b)   Missing first segment of the
Anterior Cerebral Artery (ACA1)
and missing PcomA.

**Fig. 1.** Two (clipped views of the) CoW and our points of interest

the attributes are calculated. The attributes of an edge $e_G = (v_G, v'_G)$ are: the Euclidean and geodesic length, the average radius and the relative position of $v_G$ to $v'_G$. The only attributes for the vertices are the position and a rotation invariant bifurcation descriptor which is a vector that contains the fraction of vessel-to-background on a sphere centered around the vertex for six different radii.

## 2.2   Atlas Construction

The creation of an atlas requires a training set of vascular graphs and the ground truth annotation of the PoI on these graphs. Note that not every PoI will be present in each vascular graph. The atlas itself is a probabilistic attributed graph $A = (V_A, E_A, A_A)$. The vertices $V_A$ are the PoIs, the edges $E_A$ the relations between those PoIs and $A_A$ the attributes. The attributes of a vertex $v_A$ are: the probability that this point exists in an image $P_{exist,v}$ and the probability distribution of its position and feature vector. The attributes of an edge $e_A = (v_A, v'_A)$ are: the probability of existence of a branch between $v_A$ and $v'_A$, called $P_{exist,e}$, the probability distribution of its Euclidean length $P_{lE}$, geodesic length $P_l$ and radius $P_r$, the probability distribution of the relative position of $v_A$ to $v'_A$, called $P_{\Delta xyz}$, and the probability that another PoI $v''_A$ lies on this edge $P_{on\,(v_A,v'_A)}(v''_A)$. The atlas also contains the prior distribution for all these attributes, that is the distribution taken over all vertices or edges in the images. All probability distributions are calculated using one-dimensional kernel density estimation.

## 2.3   MAP Graph Matching

Labeling an image corresponds to finding a match between the vascular graph $G$ and the atlas $A$ (see Fig. 2). The match $M$ is a subset of the candidate

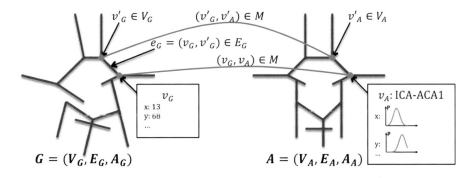

**Fig. 2.** The terminology used in graph matching

correspondences $CC = \{(v_G, v_A)|v_G \in V_G, v_A \in V_A\}$, with the additional constraint that every vertex $v_A$ or $v_G$ can only occur once in the match $M$. We are interested in the match $M^*$ with the maximum a posteriori probability:

$$M^* = argmax_M P(M|G, A) = argmax_M P(G|M, A)P(M|A). \qquad (1)$$

We derive a general formulation to efficiently solve this problem taking into account information about both the bifurcations and the edges.

To simplify the notation, we introduce two additional sets. The set of vertices of $A$ that occur in match $M$ will be called $V_{A,M} = \{v_A|(v_G, v_A) \in M\}$ and the set of vertices of $A$ that do not occur in match $M$ will be called $V_{A,\bar{M}} = \{v_A|v_A \in V_A, v_A \notin V_{A,M}\}$. The set of vertices of $G$ that occur in match $M$ will be called $V_{G,M} = \{v_G|(v_G, v_A) \in M\}$ and the set of vertices of $G$ that do not occur in match $M$ will be called $V_{G,\bar{M}} = \{v_G|v_G \in V_G, v_G \notin V_{G,M}\}$.

**Matching Prior.** The prior term $P(M|A)$ states how likely a certain match a priori is: not every PoI has an equal probability to exist in $G$ and thus to be matched. Assuming independency:

$$P(M|A) = \prod_{v_A \in V_{A,M}} P_{exist,v}(v_A) \cdot \prod_{v_A \in V_{A,\bar{M}}} (1 - P_{exist,v}(v_A)) \qquad (2)$$

where $P_{exist}(v_A)$ is the probability that $v_A$ is present in an image. By taking the logarithm, this term can be rewritten as a sum of a constant term and a term depending on $M$:

$$logP(M|A) = \sum_{v_A \in V_A} log(1 - P_{exist,v}(v_A)) + \sum_{v_A \in V_{A,M}} log \frac{P_{exist,v}(v_A)}{1 - P_{exist,v}(v_A)}. \qquad (3)$$

**Matching Likelihood.** The likelihood term $P(G|M, A)$ expresses the probability that graph $G$ exists, given the atlas and the match:

$$P(G|M, A) = \prod_{(v_G,v_A)\in M} \left[ P_{att}(v_G|v_A) \cdot \prod_{(v'_G,v'_A)\in M} \sqrt{P_{att}((v_G, v'_G)|(v_A, v'_A))} \right.$$

$$\left. \cdot \prod_{v'_G\in V_{G,\bar{M}}} \sqrt{P_{att}((v_G, v'_G))} \right]$$

$$\cdot \prod_{v_G\in V_{G,\bar{M}}} \left[ P_{att}(v_G) \cdot \prod_{v'_G\in V_{G,\bar{M}}} \sqrt{P_{att}((v_G, v'_G))} \right] .$$

In this equation $P_{att}(v_G|v_A)$ is the probability that $v_A$ has the attributes of $v_G$, $P_{att}((v_G, v'_G)|(v_A, v'_A))$ is the probability that the edge between $v_A$ and $v'_A$ has the attributes of the edge between $v_G$ and $v'_G$, $P_{att}(v_G)$ is the prior probability that a vertex has the attributes of $v_G$ and $P_{att}((v_G, v'_G))$ is the prior probability that an edge has the attributes of the edge between $v_G$ and $v'_G$. Table 1 states how these terms are calculated for our chosen attributes. By taking the logarithm, the likelihood can be rewritten as a sum of a constant term and a term depending on $M$:

$$log P(G|M, A) = \sum_{v_G\in V_G} \left[ \log P_{att}(v_G) + \frac{1}{2} \sum_{v'_G\in V_G} \log P_{att}((v_G, v'_G)) \right]$$

$$+ \sum_{(v_G,v_A)\in M} \left[ \log \frac{P_{att}(v_G|v_A)}{P_{att}(v_G)} + \frac{1}{2} \sum_{(v'_G,v'_A)\in M} \log \frac{P_{att}((v_G, v'_G)|(v_A, v'_A))}{P_{att}((v_G, v'_G))} \right]$$

**Quadratic Binary Programming.** Now we introduce $x$, a binary vector of length $|CC|$ that is equivalent to $M$ by $x[i] == 1 \Leftrightarrow CC[i] \in M$. The MAP problem can be written as a Quadratic Binary Programming problem $x^T Q x$. $Q$ is a symmetric matrix of size $|CC| \times |CC|$ with its elements determined by the previous equations:

$$Q_{i,i} = \log \frac{P_{exist,v}(v_A)}{1 - P_{exist,v}(v_A)} + \log \frac{P_{att}(v_G|v_A)}{P_{att}(v_G)} \qquad Q_{i,j} = \frac{1}{2} \log \frac{P_{att}((v_G, v'_G)|(v_A, v'_A))}{P_{att}((v_G, v'_G))}$$

with $(v_G, v_A) = CC[i]$ and $(v'_G, v'_A) = CC[j]$. Additionally, to prevent double assignment of a certain label, if $CC[k]$ and $CC[l]$ contain the same graph or atlas vertex, $Q_{k,l} = -\infty$. The a posteriori probability is (up to a constant) equivalent to $x^T Q x$ and thus: $M^* \equiv x^* = argmax_x x^T Q x$.

## 2.4   Matching

Once $Q$ is formed, matching is equivalent to finding the binary vector $x^*$ with highest score $x^T Q x$. The largest eigenvector of $Q$ serves as an initialization [3] and randomized greedy search [4] optimizes the result further. Then we check for every three found correspondences $(v_G, v_A)$, $(v'_G, v'_A)$, $(v''_G, v''_A)$ if the connectivity

**Table 1.** Example of how $P_{att}$ is defined, with $e_G = (v_G, v_G')$ and $e_A = (v_A, v_A')$. The posterior distribution is described in the first column, the prior distribution in the second column. The probability calculation depends on the connectivity in $G$: if $v_G$ and $v_G'$ are connected, the first row is considered, otherwise the second.

| | $P_{att}(e_G\|e_A)$ | $P_{att}(e_G)$ |
|---|---|---|
| | $P_{exist,e}(e_G\|e_A)$ | $P_{exist,e}(e_G)$ |
| $(v_G, v_G') \in E_G$ | $. P_r(e_G\|e_A) . P_l(e_G\|e_A)$ | $. P_r(e_G) . P_l(e_G)$ |
| | $. P_{lE}(e_G\|e_A) . P_{\Delta xyz}(e_G\|e_A)$ | $. P_{lE}(e_G) . P_{\Delta xyz}(e_G)$ |
| $(v_G, v_G') \notin E_G$ | $(1 - P_{exist,e}(e_G\|e_A))$ | $(1 - P_{exist,e}(e_G))$ |
| | $. P_{lE}(e_G\|e_A) . P_{\Delta xyz}(e_G\|e_A)$ | $. P_{lE}(e_G) . P_{\Delta xyz}(e_G)$ |

of $v_G$, $v_G'$ and $v_G''$ in $G$ is allowed according to $P_{on\,(v_A, v_A')}(v_A'')$. The most violating correspondence is removed from $x$, $CC$ and $Q$ and the search continues. This process is repeated until there are no more violations.

# 3   Evaluation

The evaluation used a dataset of 30 TOF-MRA images acquired on three different scanners (Philips Intera, Philips Ingenia and Philips Achieva). Both males and females are included and the age varies between 20 and 82. The dataset contains both healthy and diseased vasculature, with the latter having stenosis or aneurisms. Six topological variants of the CoW are present: there are CoW with the Anterior Communicating Artery (AComA), the left and/or right PComA and/or the right ACA1 missing. The voxel size is 0.39x0.39x0.5 mm$^3$. All images were segmented using region growing and converted to annotated vascular graphs. On average, one vascular graph contains 197 vertices. An observer (D.R.) manually indicated the Points of Interest (PoI) on each vascular graph, which serves as ground truth. In total a maximum of 30 images × 24 PoI/image = 720 PoI could be present in those 30 images, but only 575 PoI were present.

A leave-one-out cross-validation was performed to asses the performance of the proposed method. This means that every image was matched once, using an atlas that is constructed using the other 29 images. The construction of an atlas based on the annotated vascular graphs takes about 5 minutes using single-threaded Python code on an Intel Core i5 at 2.7 Ghz. The running time for matching a graph with the atlas depends on $|CC|$, the number of candidate correspondences considered. Using $CC = \{(v_G, v_A)|P_{att}(v_G|v_A) > 0\}$, on average 1000 candidate correspondences are considered and matching requires 2 minutes running time on the same computer. Every matching succeeded and the results are summarized in Fig. 3. In total, there are 540 true positives with an average error of 1.5 mm, 21 false positives (PoI that do not exist in the image but are assigned), 124 true negatives and 35 false negatives (PoI that are in the image but are not assigned). Two labeled images are shown in Fig. 4. We notice that the large majority of the correspondences is correct, and the label is placed on the exact same place as in the ground truth. The larger errors are without exception caused by the PoI that

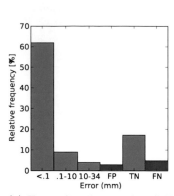

| PoI | %TP | %FP | %TN | %FN | error(mm) |
|---|---|---|---|---|---|
| ICA-OA | 65 | 17 | 13 | 5 | 0.40 |
| PCA2 End | 93 | 0 | 3 | 3 | 1.78 |
| PCA1-PComA | 7 | 0 | 82 | 12 | 0.00 |
| ACA1-AComA | 87 | 8 | 2 | 3 | 0.99 |
| VBA-PCA1 | 97 | 0 | 0 | 3 | 0.46 |
| VBA End | 100 | 0 | 0 | 0 | 1.31 |
| ICA End | 100 | 0 | 0 | 0 | 0.94 |
| M1-M2 | 95 | 0 | 0 | 5 | 3.72 |
| ICA-PCoA | 10 | 0 | 82 | 8 | 0.00 |
| ICA-ACA1 | 88 | 2 | 2 | 8 | 0.65 |
| SCA End | 98 | 0 | 0 | 2 | 4.45 |
| OA End | 60 | 8 | 23 | 8 | 0.21 |
| VBA-SCA | 98 | 0 | 0 | 2 | 0.35 |

(a) Error distribution for all PoI. (b) Results for each PoI (left and right combined). Error is the average error of the TP.

**Fig. 3.** Results of the leave-one-out test

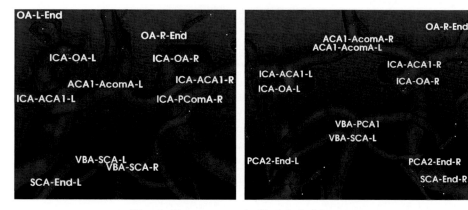

**Fig. 4.** Two automatically labeled images

are endpoints in the atlas: these points are directly connected to only one other PoI and are thus less well defined than PoI that are connected to three other PoI. If the endpoints are not considered, the maximum error is 12 mm and the average error 0.6 mm. Usage of better feature vectors for the bifurcations should probably minimize this problem, as was demonstrated by Bogunovic [1]. For 26 out of the 30 matchings, the score $x^{*T}Qx^*$ is greater than the ground truth score, which also suggests that better features are the key to better labeling.

## 4    Conclusion

A new vascular labeling algorithm is introduced. To our best knowledge it is the first graph-based algorithm that does not require a tree structure of the vasculature. As such, it is capable to label the complete Circle of Willis. The problem is formulated as a maximum a posteriori formulation that can be solved efficiently using Quadratic Binary Programming. The approach was evaluated in a leave-one-out test on 30 MRA images. In future work, we will use better feature vectors for the bifurcations. Additionally, we expect that a rigid registration of the vascular images prior to creation of the vascular graphs will result in an atlas with more sharply defined probability distributions for the attributes and thus better matching. We also intend to enlarge the dataset to support even more variations of the CoW. Finally, although the segmentation itself is good, the thinning is not optimal as kissing vessels can form spurious, topology changing bifurcations that cause additional variability and make labeling more challenging. We are exploring centerline segmentation algorithms and combined segmentation/labeling to alleviate this problem.

# References

1. Bogunović, H., Pozo, J.M., Cárdenes, R., Frangi, A.F.: Anatomical labeling of the anterior circulation of the Circle of Willis using maximum a posteriori classification. In: Fichtinger, G., Martel, A., Peters, T. (eds.) MICCAI 2011, Part III. LNCS, vol. 6893, pp. 330–337. Springer, Heidelberg (2011)
2. Krabbe-Hartkamp, M., Van der Grond, J., de Leeuw, F., de Groot, J., Algra, A., Hillen, B., Breteler, M., Mali, W.: Circle of Willis; morphologic variation on three-dimensional time-of-flight MR angiograms. Radiology 207(1), 103–111 (1998)
3. Leordeanu, M., Hebert, M.: A spectral technique for correspondence problems using pairwise constraints. In: ICCV, vol. 2, pp. 1482–1489 (2005),
   http://www.ri.cmu.edu/publication_view.html?pub_id=5161
4. Merz, P., Freisleben, B.: Greedy and local search heuristics for unconstrained binary quadratic programming. Journal of Heuristics 8(2), 197–213 (2002)
5. Mori, K., Oda, M., Egusa, T., Jiang, Z., Kitasaka, T., Fujiwara, M., Misawa, K.: Automated nomenclature of upper abdominal arteries for displaying anatomical names on virtual laparoscopic images. In: Liao, H., Edwards, P.J., Pan, X., Fan, Y., Yang, G.-Z. (eds.) MIAR 2010. LNCS, vol. 6326, pp. 353–362. Springer, Heidelberg (2010)
6. Mori, K., Ota, S., Deguchi, D., Kitasaka, T., Suenaga, Y., Iwano, S., Hasegawa, Y., Takabatake, H., Mori, M., Natori, H.: Automated anatomical labeling of bronchial branches extracted from CT datasets based on machine learning and combination optimization and its application to bronchoscope guidance. In: Yang, G.-Z., Hawkes, D., Rueckert, D., Noble, A., Taylor, C. (eds.) MICCAI 2009, Part II. LNCS, vol. 5762, pp. 707–714. Springer, Heidelberg (2009)
7. Palágyi, K., Sorantin, E., Balogh, E., Kuba, A., Halmai, C., Erdohelyi, B., Hauseg-ger, K.: A sequential 3D thinning algorithm and its medical applications. In: Insana, M.F., Leahy, R.M. (eds.) IPMI 2001. LNCS, vol. 2082, pp. 409–415. Springer, Heidelberg (2001)
8. Takemura, A., Suzuki, M., Harauchi, H., Okumura, Y.: Automatic anatomical labeling method of cerebral arteries in MR-angiography data set. Japanese Journal of Medical Physics 26(4), 187–198 (2006)
9. Tschirren, J., McLennan, G., Palágyi, K., Hoffman, E.A., Sonka, M.: Matching and anatomical labeling of human airway tree. IEEE Transactions on Medical Imaging 24(12), 1540–1547 (2005)

# Normalisation of Neonatal Brain Network Measures Using Stochastic Approaches

Markus Schirmer[1,*], Gareth Ball[1], Serena J. Counsell[1], A. David Edwards[1],
Daniel Rueckert[2], Joseph V. Hajnal[1], and Paul Aljabar[1]

[1] Division of Imaging Sciences & Biomedical Engineering, King's College London, UK
[2] BioMedIA Group, Dept. of Computing, Imperial College London, UK
`markus.schirmer@kcl.ac.uk`

**Abstract.** Diffusion tensor imaging, tractography and the subsequent derivation of network measures are becoming an established approach in the exploration of brain connectivity. However, no gold standard exists in respect to how the brain should be parcellated and therefore a variety of atlas- and random-based parcellation methods are used. The resulting challenge of comparing graphs with differing numbers of nodes and uncertain node correspondences necessitates the use of normalisation schemes to enable meaningful intra- and inter-subject comparisons. This work proposes methods for normalising brain network measures using random graphs. We show that the normalised measures are locally stable over distinct random parcellations of the same subject and, applying it to a neonatal serial diffusion MRI data set, we demonstrate their potential in characterising changes in brain connectivity during early development.

**Keywords:** neonatal, MRI, diffusion, connectivity, network analysis.

## 1 Introduction

Over the last two decades, applications of network theory to a variety of fields have become more prevalent. Neuroimaging applications of network and graph theoretical techniques are comparatively recent (for an overview see e.g. [1]) and have demonstrated their utility in exploring the relations among regions in the brain and how these are affected by neural diseases [2,3].

In the brain, one often distinguishes between structural and functional connectivity. Functional connectivity is typically represented by correlations among the activations of different regions in the brain. By contrast, structural connectivity is based on estimation of neural pathways inferred from diffusion properties of cerebral white matter. It is possible to estimate this connectivity with diffusion tensor imaging [4]. The work we present is generic and can be applied to any type of brain network data, although it will be described with a focus on structural connectivity in the developing neonatal brain.

Understanding the development and formation of structural connectivity after pre-term birth is highly desirable, as it has been shown that pre-term birth is

---

* Corresponding author.

K. Mori et al. (Eds.): MICCAI 2013, Part I, LNCS 8149, pp. 574–581, 2013.

associated with adverse neurocognitive and behavioural outcome in later life [5]. Apart from practical difficulties in acquiring diffusion data from neonatal subjects, further challenges to neonatal connectivity analysis lie in the absence of an established set of regions with which to define the nodes of a network or graph. In adult data, network analysis of tractography data often relies on standard parcellations of the brain into a number of what are assumed to be functionally coherent regions. These define the nodes of a graph in which edges represent connected regions, which may be weighted by connection strength [6,7].

In neonates however, the lack of a standard set of regions has led to the adoption of approaches based on randomly generated parcellations of the brain as these rely on fewer assumptions regarding the presence of functionally defined regions. Ball et al. [8] apply a random parcellation approach to the cortical masks of a neonatal diffusion MRI (dMRI) dataset in a study of changes to cortical and thalamic connectivity in preterm infants. In their work, Poisson disk sampling [9] was used to generate around 500 region centres with a constraint on the minimum distance between each pair. In a tractography analysis streamlines were propagated from every region and the connection strength between the thalamus and each target region was calculated as integrated anisotropy along the path [8,11]. Streamlines connecting a region with itself were removed. Repeating this for different random parcellations generates multiple connectivity matrices for a single subject, which provide per-node network measures that can be propagated back to provide voxel-wise maps.

**Challenges of Stochastic Parcellations.** Defining the regions stochastically means that the number of regions can vary across parcellations of the same brain. For example, Poisson disk sampling specifies a target number of regions but this can vary from the number of regions generated due to the distance constraint. It is also important to note that some network measures have been shown to be highly dependent on the number of regions [12].

This motivates the need to address potential biases in network measures derived from randomised parcellations of dMRI data. It is important both for generating summary measures for an individual brain from multiple connectivity matrices and for making meaningful inter- and intra-subject comparisons of network-based measures, particularly across different studies. The dependence of measures on the number of regions/nodes is illustrated in Fig. 1 for a particular network measure (clustering coefficient) obtained from a set of connectivity matrices based on random parcellations of the same subject.

This work presents techniques for removing the number of region dependence from network measures. Our methods normalise a measure $m(G)$ on a directed and weighted graph $G$ against the value of $m(G')$, where $G'$ is obtained by randomly perturbing the structure of $G$, by modifying its edge structure and/or edge weights. These randomised networks may not represent physiologically plausible networks, however, they may be seen as 'white noise' used to identify the significance and change of network measures obtained from imaging data. The process is schematically illustrated in Fig. 2. We show that established random graph approaches can yield unsuitable normalisations for measures such as the

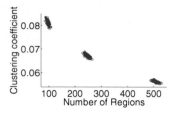 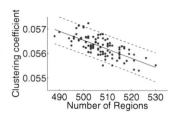

**Fig. 1.** The dependence of the clustering coefficient on the number of regions in different parcellations of the same subject. Left: Sets of parcellations with around 100, 250 and 500 regions. Right: Detailed view around 500 regions.

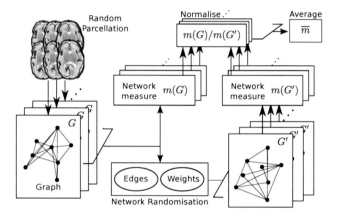

**Fig. 2.** Processing pipeline used for removing the number of region dependence

clustering coefficient and present a novel approach which allows for a better comparison. Furthermore, we validate our method by applying it to serial dMRI data of 16 neonates and show the evolution of their network measures over time.

## 2    Methods and Materials

The methods for generating a random realisation of a graph obtained from the random parcellations of the cortical mask are described below. We emphasise the distinction of the stochastic step for generating a random network during normalisation and the one used to generate the initial parcellations on which an observed network is defined.

**Edge Structure.** Two established algorithms to create random networks for comparison use either an Erdös-Rényi model (ER) or pairwise switching of the edges (PS), an algorithm which keeps the number of outgoing edges of each node constant. In this section we will briefly review both approaches. Not altering the edge structure will be referred to as edge preserving (EP).

We denote a graph $G = \{V, E, W\}$, where $V$ and $E$ are the vertex and edge sets and $W = \{w_{ij}\}$ the set of edge weights, which represent the connectivity matrix derived from the tractography. We denote the neighbourhood $N_i$ of node $i$ to be the set of edge-wise neighbours $\{j \in V : ij \in E\}$ and $G$ is assumed to be simple, i.e. without multiple edges or self-loops.

For $PS$, nodes $r$ and $s$ are randomly selected from $V$ and $t$ and $u$ are randomly chosen from $N_r$ and $N_s$ respectively. If the graph remains simple, remove the edge $rt$ and $su$ from $E$ and add $ru$ and $st$ [13]. In order to amplify the perturbation of the graph, we modified PS to maximise its effect. For each node $v \in V$, we iterate over all nodes $r \in N_v$, select $s \in V \backslash \{r\}$ and apply PS to $r$ and $s$. This is repeated for all nodes. By contrast, ER starts with the same number of nodes $N$ as the observed graph. Edges are then randomly assigned to node pairs until the number of edges equals the number in the observed graph.

**Weight Assignment.** The white matter connectivity networks studied are weighted by the integrated anisotropy, necessitating a method for assigning weights to the edges of the derived random graphs. We applied three types of methods for achieving this: The *original weights* set may be redistributed naturally in case of PS by switching them along with the edges, or randomly permuted in EP/ER. We also draw weights *uniformly* from the interval [0,max], where max is the maximum weight in the original graph. Finally we draw weights at random from the weight set based on the shortest path distances between all node pairs in the original graph, which are calculated using the *Dijkstra* algorithm. For the last method, distances along each edge $ij$ are converted as $1/w_{ij}$. Subsequently calculated shortest distances between all node pairs are then converted back to weights, again as reciprocals, to generate a complete weighted graph matrix. The entries in this matrix are then drawn for assignment to the perturbed graph.

**Network Measures.** There is a vast literature on measures for characterising networks. A good summary of measures commonly used for brain networks is given by Rubinov and Sporns [14].

Betweenness centrality (BC) relates to the amount of information passing through a particular node, assuming that information travels along the shortest paths. A node $s$ in a graph has $BC(s)$ given by $BC(s) = \sum_{r,t:r\neq s\neq t} \frac{\lambda_{rt}(s)}{\lambda_{rt}}$, where $\lambda_{rt}$ is the number of shortest paths from $r$ to $t$ and $\lambda_{rt}(s)$ is the number that pass through $s$. The BC of the network can be characterised by the mean of $BC(s)$ over all nodes.

The out-degree $k_{out}(s)$ of a node $s$ in a weighted network is defined as the sum of the weights of all outgoing connections. It represents a measure of how well a node is connected within a network. We calculated the mean out-degree, $k_{out}$, over all nodes in order to compare this measure across networks.

The clustering coefficient, $C(s)$ of a node $s$, is a commonly used measure which represents the ratio of triangles containing $s$ to the maximum number possible. $C(s)$ is given by [15]

$$C(s) = \frac{t_s^{\rightarrow}}{k(s)\,(k(s)-1) - 2\sum_{r \in V} e_{sr}e_{rs}},$$

where $t_s^{\rightarrow}$ is the number of directed triangles around node $s$, $k(s) = k_{out}(s) + k_{in}(s)$ is the total degree and $e_{ij} = 1$, if $ij \in E$ and zero otherwise. The clustering coefficient $C$ of a network can then be calculated as the average of $C(s)$ over all nodes $s$. It can be interpreted as the predominance of clustered components around nodes. It is also used in determining small-worldness, as small-world networks tend to have higher clustering coefficients.

The characteristic path-length, $\lambda(s)$, of a node $s$ is defined as average shortest path-length between $s$ and all other nodes in the network. It can be interpreted as a measure of integration of a particular node in the network and is given by $\lambda(s) = \frac{1}{|V|-1} \sum_{t \neq s} d_{st}$, where $d_{st}$ is the shortest distance between nodes $s, t \in V$ and $|V|$ is the total number of nodes. The mean measure, $\lambda$, is referred to as global characteristic path-length. It also relates to small-worldness, as small-world networks tend to have lower values of $\lambda$.

The efficiency $E(s)$ of node $s$ is computed similarly to the characteristic path-length. In this case, however, the average is taken over the reciprocals of the shortest paths. The advantage of the efficiency over the characteristic path-length lies in the meaningful computation for multi-component networks, as infinite paths between nodes in disconnected components have zero efficiency. The overall efficiency of a network can be expressed by the mean of $E(s)$ over all nodes $s$, where $E(s)$ is given by $E(s) = \frac{1}{|V|-1} \sum_{t \neq s} d_{st}^{-1}$.

The diameter of a network is given by the longest of all the shortest paths in the network and is representative of the size of the network. In case of information flow it can therefore represent the longest path (or time) for a signal to flow from any node to any other node.

**Data.** Serial dMRI data was acquired from 16 infants born at less than 32 weeks gestational age and recruited as part of ongoing studies at Queen Charlotte's and Chelsea Hospital. Mean gestational age at birth was $28.0 \pm 2.4$ weeks and the mean age at scan was $30.8 \pm 2.1$ and $41.1 \pm 1.0$ weeks at the first and second scans respectively. Each infant successfully underwent 32-direction dMRI. Single shot echo planar imaging dMRI was acquired in the transverse plane in 32-non-collinear directions using the following parameters: TR: 8000 msec; TE: 49 msec; slice thickness: 2 mm; field-of-view: 224 mm; matrix: $128 \times 128$ (voxel size: $1.75 \times 1.75 \times 2$ mm; b-value: $750$ sec/mm$^2$; SENSE factor of 2. Random cortical parcellations were obtained using Poisson disk sampling [9] and a probabilistic diffusion tractography algorithm was applied [10]. Diffusion MRI data were pre-processed using the FSL's Diffusion Toolkit and corrected for geometric distortions. For more details the reader is referred to [8].

## 3    Results

In a series of experiments, we assessed the performance of the different normalisation schemes, each consisting of a method for determining edge structure and a method of assigning edge weights as described above. The results of comparing the different schemes for parcellations with around 500 regions are summarised in Table 1. The variance explained by the number of regions was used to assess each measure and the mean explained variance over 12 runs for each of 8 different subjects was recorded for each measure. On average, the best performance (largest reduction in explained variance) was obtained by schemes that drew the weights of the randomised graph uniformly from an interval between zero and the maximum weight of the original matrix. In particular, Table 1 shows that the established ER and PS methods, with weights drawn from the original graph, performed badly with respect to the clustering coefficient. The approach based on Dijkstra performed particularly poorly with respect to the clustering coefficient and introduced a higher out-degree correlation than originally present. We will therefore focus further analyses on the subcategory of altering the edge weights with the uniformly drawn weights.

**Table 1.** The variance (%) of each measure explained by the number of regions in a network before and after each normalisation scheme (original weights (OW), uniform (UNI), Dijkstra (D), Erdös-Rényi (ER), pairwise switching (PS), edge preserving (EP)) for all measures. Stars mark the lowest value for each measure. In case of the missing values (OW) the measures stayed the same after normalisation.

| | Before | ER | | | PS | | | EP | | |
|---|---|---|---|---|---|---|---|---|---|---|
| | | OW | UNI | D | OW | UNI | D | OW | UNI | D |
| $BC$ | 76.7 | 10.1 | 2.9 | 9.6 | 10.8 | 2.6 | 5.6 | — | 2.7 | 1.1* |
| $k_{out}$ | 7.8 | — | 2.2* | 33.3 | — | 2.2* | 33.6 | — | 2.2* | 34.0 |
| $C$ | 49.3 | 43.4 | 7.7 | 45.1 | 42.7 | 3.8 | 52.9 | — | 2.2* | 32.5 |
| $\lambda$ | 28.6 | 11.4 | 2.2 | 8.1 | 7.7 | 2.1 | 10.1 | 0.7* | 2.1 | 21.2 |
| $E$ | 36.0 | 12.3 | 2.2 | 18.0 | 6.6 | 2.2 | 22.5 | 1.0* | 2.2 | 32.0 |
| $dia$ | 2.8 | 2.0 | 2.1 | 1.2 | 1.9 | 1.7 | 1.2 | — | 1.1* | 0.8 |

In order to decide on the edge structure method, we considered their performance over a wider range of regions. For this, we parcellated a data set with target numbers of 100, 250 and 500 regions, creating 100 networks in each case. This analysis showed that EP outperformed ER and MPS by reducing the explained variance on average the most for both the 100 and 250 region parcellations.

Based on these results, we selected the combination of EP with uniformly drawn weights. We applied this scheme to the serial dMRI data of all subjects with around 500 region parcellations by generating one random realisation of the observed network for normalisation. Repeating the process multiple times did not yield major improvements. Figure 3 shows the change over time of the resulting normalised measures. We assessed the normalised measures in terms of the consistency of their change with time. In almost all the cases, the clustering coefficient increases with age at scan, while the characteristic path-length decreases. This suggests that the degree to which the brain represents a small-world network increases with age. The out-degree and efficiency both increase with time, indicating improved connectivity in the brain with age. The results for BC and network diameter are not conclusive, showing no consistent change over time. However, the average betweenness centrality is consistently much lower than in each corresponding random network ($\approx 0.22$). This suggests an increased resilience to node failure or 'attacks' on the network. We performed paired t-tests for the normalised serial measures of all subjects. These were significant ($p < 0.001$) for all measures, except for BC and diameter.

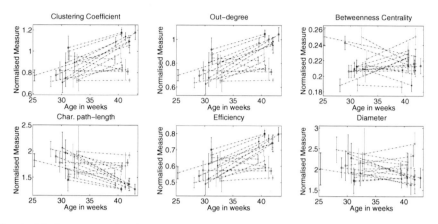

**Fig. 3.** Median normalised values of network measures determined from 100 parcellations per subject. Each colour-marker combination represents one infant with the distribution of measures from multiple randomly parcellated networks at two time points (connected by a dashed line). Four of six measures show a distinct tendency in their evolution in time (see text).

## 4     Conclusion

We presented novel approaches for generating random graphs from neural connectivity graphs for the purpose of normalising network measures. The results indicate that edge preserving with uniformly drawn weights between zero and the maximum of the original weights outperforms established approaches. Although some dependence on the number of regions remained over the larger scale of 100-500 regions, it allowed for a better local comparison of measures for networks with around 500 regions. It should be noted that, with fewer regions, there was greater variation in both the normalised and raw network measures. This highlights the difficulty of comparing network measures across the different scales that are commonly used in atlas-based methods [16]. In future work, we will focus on eliminating the number of region dependence on a wider scale and on determining the optimal number of regions for representing brain networks. We note that the benefit of the presented random graph approach over regression-based models is that only one observed network is required to carry out the normalisation, while a number of networks would be needed for regression. In comparison with trend analysis, our method therefore provides a comparatively cheap approach for normalising against the number of regions and it enables network measures to be compared across subjects and over time.

**Acknowledgments.** This research was supported by the National Institute for Health Research (NIHR) Biomedical Research Centre at Guy's and St Thomas' NHS Foundation Trust and King's College London. The views expressed are those of the author(s) and not necessarily those of the NHS, the NIHR or the Department of Health. Medical Research Council (MRC) Centre for Transplantation, King's College London, UK — MRC grant no. MR/J006742/1.

# References

1. Sporns, O.: The human connectome: a complex network. Ann. N.Y. Acad. Sci. 1224, 109–125 (2011)
2. Bullmore, E., Sporns, O.: Complex brain networks: graph theoretical analysis of structural and functional systems. Nat. Rev. Neurosci. 10(3), 186–198 (2009)
3. Supekar, et al.: Network analysis of intrinsic functional brain connectivity in Alzheimer's disease. PLoS Comput. Biol. 4(6), 1–11 (2008)
4. Alexander, et al.: Diffusion tensor imaging of the brain. Neurotherapeutics 4(3), 316–329 (2007)
5. Delobel-Ayoub, et al.: Behavioral problems and cognitive performance at 5 years of age after very preterm birth: the EPIPAGE Study. Pediatrics 123(6), 1485–1492 (2009)
6. Sporns, O., Tononi, G., Kötter, R.: The human connectome: A structural description of the human brain. PLoS Comput. Biol. 1(4), 245–251 (2005)
7. Hagmann, et al: Mapping the structural core of human cerebral cortex. PLoS Biol. 6(7), 1479–1493 (2008)
8. Vall, et al.: The influence of preterm birth on the developing thalamocortical connectome. Cortex, 1–11 (2012)
9. Bridson, R.: Fast poisson disk sampling in arbitrary dimensions. In: ACM SIGGRAPH, vol. 2007 (2007)
10. Behrens, et al.: Probabilistic diffusion tractography with multiple fibre orientations: What can we gain? Neuroimage 34(1), 144–155 (2007)
11. Robinson, et al.: Identifying population differences in whole-brain structural networks: a machine learning approach. NeuroImage 50(3), 910–919 (2010)
12. Zalesky, et al.: Whole-brain anatomical networks: does the choice of nodes matter? NeuroImage 50(3), 970–983 (2010)
13. Maslov, S., Sneppen, K.: Specificity and stability in topology of protein networks. Science 296(5569), 910–913 (2002)
14. Rubinov, M., Sporns, O.: Complex network measures of brain connectivity: uses and interpretations. NeuroImage 52(3), 1059–1069 (2010)
15. Fagiolo, G.: Clustering in complex directed networks. Phys. Rev. E 76(2), 026107 (2007)
16. Van Wijk, et al.: Comparing brain networks of different size and connectivity density using graph theory. PloS one 5(10), 13701 (2010)

# Localisation of the Brain in Fetal MRI Using Bundled SIFT Features

Kevin Keraudren[1], Vanessa Kyriakopoulou[2], Mary Rutherford[2],
Joseph V. Hajnal[2], and Daniel Rueckert[1]

[1] Biomedical Image Analysis Group, Imperial College London
[2] Centre for the Developing Brain & Department Biomedical Engineering Division of
Imaging Sciences, King's College London

**Abstract.** Fetal MRI is a rapidly emerging diagnostic imaging tool. Its
main focus is currently on brain imaging, but there is a huge potential
for whole body studies. We propose a method for accurate and robust
localisation of the fetal brain in MRI when the image data is acquired as
a stack of 2D slices misaligned due to fetal motion. We first detect possible brain locations in 2D images with a Bag-of-Words model using SIFT
features aggregated within Maximally Stable Extremal Regions (called
bundled SIFT), followed by a robust fitting of an axis-aligned 3D box
to the selected regions. We rely on prior knowledge of the fetal brain
development to define size and shape constraints. In a cross-validation
experiment, we obtained a median error distance of 5.7mm from the
ground truth and no missed detection on a database of 59 fetuses. This
2D approach thus allows a robust detection even in the presence of substantial fetal motion.

## 1 Introduction

Fetal Magnetic Resonance Imaging (MRI) has had great successes in the last
years with the development of motion correction methods providing high quality
isotropic volumes of the brain [7,11], thus enabling a better understanding of
the fetal brain development. Such reconstruction methods typically rely on data
acquired as stacks of 2D slices of real-time MRI, freezing in-plane motion. In
order to reduce the scan time while avoiding slice cross-talk artefacts, contiguous
slices are not acquired sequentially but in an interleaved manner. Slices are
quite often misaligned due to fetal motion and form an inconsistent 3D volume
(Figure 1). Motion correction is the registration of 2D slices of the fetal brain
to an ideal 3D volume. Cropping a box around the brain is a prerequisite to
exclude maternal tissues that can make the registration fail. We thus propose a
method to automatically find a precise bounding box around the brain in order
to speed-up the preprocessing steps of the motion correction procedure.

**Related Work.** Regression Forests perform the task of organ detection by
learning a regression between image features, such as 3D Haar-like features, and
the offset to the corners of the bounding boxes of organs [10]. By treating the

K. Mori et al. (Eds.): MICCAI 2013, Part I, LNCS 8149, pp. 582–589, 2013.

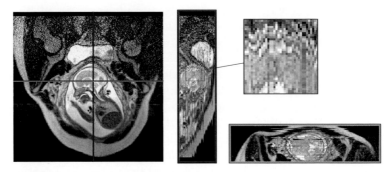

**Fig. 1.** Example scan with the native 2D slices in sagittal orientation. A zoomed patch of the coronal section highlights interleaving artefacts due to fetal motion.

localisation problem as a regression problem, it implies some rough alignment between part of the training database and the new data. An adult patient usually lies inside the scanner in a standard orientation, but this is not the case of a fetus. Moreover, the fetus is surrounded by maternal tissues instead of air, thus hindering a straightforward application of such a method.

Marginal Space Learning (MSL) is a more general framework that can be described as an optimized sliding window search with a hierarchy of coarse-to-fine boosting-based organ detectors [15]. Learning is performed on affinely registered datasets, and the search covers all locations, scales and orientations. Steerable features apply a rotated grid over the image to sample features in order to perform local rotation and scaling without transforming the whole volume, thus making the search more computationally feasible. MSL has been successfully applied to various problems, such as the localisation of the four heart chambers in adult CT scans [15], semantic browsing of the fetal body in 2D ultrasound [2], or automatic fetal face detection in 3D ultrasound [4].

To the best of our knowledge, only two fully automated localisation methods of the fetal brain in MRI have been proposed so far in the literature: Anquez et al. [1] proposed to start from detecting the eyes with 3D template matching, followed by a segmentation of the brain using a 2D graph-cut segmentation of the mid-sagittal slice rotated at several angles. The best matching segmentation is selected and used to initialise a 3D graph-cut segmentation. Ison et al. [6] proposed a more general method based on a two-stage Random Forest classifier: the first stage distinguishes maternal tissues from fetal head tissues, while the second stage classifies fetal head tissues into 6 classes. The last step uses a Markov Random Field appearance model to establish an orientation of the brain based on the centroids of the previously identified fetal tissues.

**Overview.** In this paper, we chose to focus on the task of finding an axis-aligned bounding box for the fetal brain. This is in contrast with [6] which aimed at finding an oriented bounding box, and [1] which aimed at segmenting the skull bone content. This relaxation of the problem enables us to focus on positioning a tight bounding box on the brain while dealing with 2D slices misaligned or corrupted due to fetal motion. Although acquisitions are carried out in conventional orientations, there is unpredictability in the positioning of the fetus. Hence, similarly to Marginal Space Learning, we decided to decompose the search space by performing a 2D detection process before accumulating the votes in 3D, and we removed the scale component by inferring it from the gestational age.

In a first stage, Maximally Stable Extremal Regions (MSER [9]) are extracted from the 2D slices and approximated by ellipses. Then, the regions whose size and aspect ratio conform with prior knowledge of the fetal development are classified into brain or not-brain based on histograms of the SIFT features found within the fitted ellipses (bundled SIFT [14]), following a Bag-of-Words model (BOW [3]). Finally, a RANdom SAmple Consensus procedure (RANSAC [5]) is performed to find a best fitting 3D cube whose dimensions are inferred from prior knowledge. This localisation pipeline is summarised in Figure 2. In the remainder of this paper, we will describe in more details our proposed method and evaluate it in a 10-fold cross validation, comparing it to a sliding window BOW using 2D or 3D SIFT features.

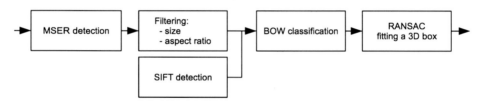

**Fig. 2.** Proposed pipeline for localising the fetal brain

## 2   Method

### 2.1   Detection and Selection of MSER Regions

Maximally Stable Extremal Regions (MSER), introduced by Matas et al. [9], are a common feature detection method in computer vision. MSER regions can be defined as sets of connected pixels stable over a large range of intensity thresholds. Such regions can be characterised by homogeneous intensity distributions and high intensity differences at their boundary. Each region is defined by a seed pixel and a lower and upper intensity thresholds, the whole region resulting from a floodfill operation. In the case of fetal T2 MR images, MSER regions are well suited to the task of selecting candidate regions for the brain as the skull content appears much brighter than the surrounding bone and skin tissues.

In its first stages, our localisation pipeline proceeds slice by slice, working on 2D images, and starts by detecting candidate MSER regions $\mathcal{R}_i$ which are sets of connected pixels. An ellipse $\mathbf{E}_i$ is then fitted to each $\mathcal{R}_i$ with a least-squares minimization. As the shape of the brain is well approximated by an ellipsoid, the ellipses $\mathbf{E}_i$ have the ability to recover the shape of the brain even if the detected $\mathcal{R}_i$ only corresponds to a segment of cerebrospinal fluid (CSF, Figure 3.b), or amniotic fluid surrounding the fetal head (Figure 3.c). The ellipses $\mathbf{E}_i$ are then filtered by size and aspect ratio using the gestational age combined with prior knowledge of the fetal development, namely the *occipitofrontal diameter*, *OFD*, and the *biparietal diameter*, *BPD* [12]. This prior knowledge is obtained from 2D ultrasound studies [12] and is discussed in more details in Section 3.

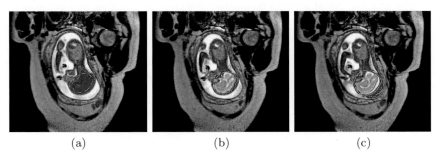

(a)                    (b)                    (c)

**Fig. 3.** Example MSER regions $\mathcal{R}_i$ (red overlay) and their fitted ellipses $\mathbf{E}_i$ (green dashes): (a) skull bone content, (b) cerebrospinal fluid, (c) amniotic fluid

## 2.2   Classification of Selected MSER Regions Using Bundled SIFT Features

MSER regions alone do not provide a descriptor that can be used for classification. As a versatile rotation invariant classification framework, we chose to use a Bag-of-Words model by computing for each region $\mathcal{R}_i$ the histogram of the SIFT features (*Scale-Invariant Feature Transform* [8]) within the ellipse $\mathbf{E}_i$, similarly to the bundled SIFT features of Wu et al. [14]. In the Bag-of-Words method for image classification presented by Csurka et al. [3], SIFT features are extracted from training images and a set of words $\mathcal{V}$ (*visual vocabulary*) is obtained through k-means clustering, each word being the centroid of a cluster. Each SIFT feature $f_{\text{SIFT}}$ can then be associated to its nearest neighbour $f_{\text{NN}} \in \mathcal{V}$ to build a histogram of words. A Support Vector Machine (SVM) classifier is then used to assign a class to this histogram.

SIFT features are the association of a keypoint corresponding to a local extrema in a scale-space Gaussian pyramid (*blob*) and a descriptor built from histograms of gradient orientations. The blob detection process provides scale invariance to the descriptor, whereas rotation invariance is obtained from the main gradient orientation over the blob. Rotation invariance helps accommodate the unknown orientation of the fetal brain, while scale invariance attenuates the variations due to gestational age.

In the **learning stage** of our pipeline, all SIFT features are extracted from the 2D slices of all training scans and clustered using a k-means algorithm. The $N$ cluster centers form the vocabulary $\mathcal{V}$. Then, MSER regions $\mathcal{R}_i$ are detected and selected (Section 2.1). The ellipses $\mathbf{E}_i$ centered on the brain are kept as positive examples, while those further than $OFD/2$ are kept as negative examples. For each $\mathbf{E}_i$, a histogram of bundled SIFT features is computed. After an $L_2$ normalisation, the histograms are used to train an SVM classifier. As in [3], a linear kernel SVM has been used. In the **detection stage**, for each MSER region selected, a normalised histogram of SIFT features is computed, and the previously trained SVM is used to classify regions as brain or not-brain. Figure 4.a shows an example slice with all the candidate MSER regions, while Figure 4.b shows the result of the selection and classification processes.

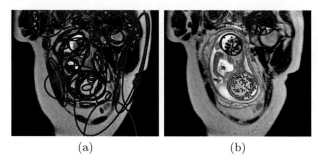

(a)                               (b)

**Fig. 4.** (a) All detected MSER regions. (b) MSER regions are filtered based on their size and aspect ratio, then classified according to their histograms of SIFT features (green for brain regions, red for not-brain)

## 2.3   RANSAC Fitting of a Cube

The 2D detection works reliably in mid-brain slices but not in peripheral slices of the brain. Estimating a 3D box is thus important for a reliable estimate of the entire brain region. As the set of candidate regions classified as brain by the SVM classifier may still contain outliers, we perform a RANSAC procedure [5] to find a best fitting position for a 3D axis-aligned bounding cube. We thus randomly select a small set of ellipses $\mathbf{E}_i$ and use their centroid to define a bounding cube of width $OFD$. For a region $\mathcal{R}_i$ to be considered an *inlier*, it must be completely included in this cube and the center of the ellipse $\mathbf{E}_i$ must be at a small distance from the cube center. The cube position is then refined by taking the centroid of these inliers. This process is repeated a predefined number of times, typically 1000 times, and the cube with the largest number of inliers is selected.

## 3   Experiments

**Implementation.** To gain prior knowledge on the expected size of the brain knowing the gestational age, we used a 2D ultrasound study from Snijders and

Nicolaides [12] performed on 1040 normal singleton pregnancies. The $5^{th}$ and $95^{th}$ centile values of *OFD* and *BPD* have been used to define the acceptable size and aspect ratio for the selected MSER regions (Section 2.1). The size of the detected bounding box in the robust fitting procedure (Section 2.3) has been set to the $95^{th}$ centile of *OFD* in order to contain the whole fetal brain. The size $N$ of the BOW vocabulary (Section 2.2) has been set to 400. The automated detection process takes less than a minute on a normal PC.

**Data.** Fetal MRI was performed on a 1.5T MRI system, T2-weighted dynamic ssTSE images were obtained with the following scanning parameters: TR 15000ms, TE 160ms, slice thickness of 2.5mm, slice overlap of 1.5mm, flip angle $90°$. The in-plane resolution varies between 0.94 and 1.25mm, with the number of interleaved packets ranging from 4 to 6. Our database includes 59 healthy fetuses whose gestational age range from 22 to 39 weeks, with 5 fetuses scanned twice and 1 three times, amounting to a total of 66 datasets. Each dataset consists of 3 to 8 scans acquired in three standard orthogonal planes, representing a total of 117 sagittal, 113 coronal and 228 transverse scans. We performed a 10-fold cross validation, with 39 training subjects and 20 testing subjects for each fold. For the ground truth, bounding boxes have been tightly drawn around the brain.

**Results.** The brain localisation results are summarised in Table 1, whereas examples of detected bounding boxes and their corresponding ground truth are shown in Figure 5 and in the supplementary material.[1] We compared our method against sliding a window of fixed size *OFD* with a Random Forest classifier on histograms of 2D or 3D SIFT features, using the extension to 3D of SIFT proposed in [13]. For each stack of slices, we measured the distance between the center of the ground truth bounding box and the detected bounding box. Similarly to [6], we defined a correct detection as 70% of the brain being included in the detected box. 2D SIFT features performed better than 3D SIFT features, which can be attributed to the inconsistency of the 3D data, whereas the bundled SIFT drastically improved the localisation accuracy with an error below 5.7mm in more than 50% of cases. This greater precision comes from applying a classifier only at specific locations (MSER regions) instead of all pixels, thus resulting in a more localised probability map. This localisation of the center of the brain shows improved results compared to [6] who reported a median error of 10mm in the detection of 6 landmarks corresponding to centroids of fetal head tissues. However, contrary to [6], the orientation of the brain is not determined. Our method is more general than [1] as it does not rely on localising the eyes. There has been no false detection or missed detection with bundled SIFT, with a worst case error of 25mm presented in Figure 5.e. In 85% of cases, the detected bounding box contains entirely the ground truth bounding box.

The prior knowledge gained from the gestational age plays an important role in disregarding most of the detected MSER regions. Indeed, on average during

---

[1] www.doc.ic.ac.uk/~kpk09/MICCAI-451.mp4

**Table 1.** Detection results averaged over the cross validation, all orientations combined

| Centiles | Error (mm) | | |
|---|---|---|---|
| | *2D SIFT* | *3D SIFT* | *Bundled SIFT* |
| $25^{th}$ | 10.9 | 14.8 | **4.0** |
| $50^{th}$ | 15.5 | 20.8 | **5.7** |
| $75^{th}$ | 20.5 | 30.4 | **8.4** |
| Detection | 98% | 85% | 100% |
| Complete brain | 38% | 23% | 85% |

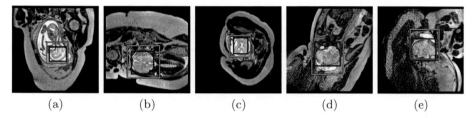

(a)              (b)              (c)              (d)              (e)

**Fig. 5.** Examples of detected bounding boxes (green) and ground truth (red). a), b) and c) are respectively sagittal, coronal and transverse acquisitions of different subjects. d) and e) show detections with the largest error, which can be attributed to the presence of the maternal bladder near the fetal head.

the 10-fold cross validation, 98% of the candidate regions are disregarded in the first stage of the pipeline. As a comparison, the SVM classifier further disregards 41% of the remaining candidates, and the RANSAC procedure removes 18% outliers. No distinction has been made between sagittal, transverse or coronal acquisitions, which is another advantage of the proposed method.

When using normal growth charts to define a realistic range of sizes of the brain, our goal is to remove improbable detections while still allowing a large variation in brain size. From standard growth charts, extending to include 99.6% of subjects corresponds to a 1 week error. Simulating extreme growth restriction by adding a 5 weeks error in all gestational ages, the detection rate is still 91%.

## 4   Conclusion

We presented a novel automatic localisation method for the fetal brain in MRI. Proceeding slice by slice, MSER regions are first detected and filtered by size and aspect ratio before being classified using histograms of SIFT features. An expected size of the brain is inferred from the gestational age and prior knowledge of the fetal development. Finally, a 3D bounding cube is fitted to the selected regions with a RANSAC procedure. The method is not specific to the scan orientation, with a median distance error of 5.7mm from the ground truth. Further work will be required to integrate this brain localisation method in a motion correction pipeline, such as automatically masking out maternal tissues.

# References

1. Anquez, J., Angelini, E., Bloch, I.: Automatic Segmentation of Head Structures on Fetal MRI. In: ISBI, pp. 109–112. IEEE (2009)
2. Carneiro, G., Georgescu, B., Good, S., Comaniciu, D.: Detection and Measurement of Fetal Anatomies from Ultrasound Images using a Constrained Probabilistic Boosting Tree. IEEE Transactions on Medical Imaging 27(9), 1342–1355 (2008)
3. Csurka, G., Dance, C., Fan, L., Willamowski, J., Bray, C.: Visual Categorization With Bags of Keypoints. In: Workshop on Statistical Learning in Computer Vision, ECCV, vol. 1, p. 22 (2004)
4. Feng, S., Zhou, S., Good, S., Comaniciu, D.: Automatic Fetal Face Detection from Ultrasound Volumes via Learning 3D and 2D Information. In: CVPR, pp. 2488–2495. IEEE (2009)
5. Fischler, M., Bolles, R.: Random Sample Consensus: A Paradigm for Model Fitting with Applications to Image Analysis and Automated Cartography. Communications of the ACM 24(6), 381–395 (1981)
6. Ison, M., Donner, R., Dittrich, E., Kasprian, G., Prayer, D., Langs, G.: Fully Automated Brain Extraction and Orientation in Raw Fetal MRI. In: Workshop on Paediatric and Perinatal Imaging, MICCAI, pp. 17–24. Springer (2012)
7. Jiang, S., Xue, H., Glover, A., Rutherford, M., Rueckert, D., Hajnal, J.: MRI of Moving Subjects using Multislice Snapshot Images with Volume Reconstruction (SVR): Application to Fetal, Neonatal, and Adult Brain Studies. IEEE Transactions on Medical Imaging 26(7), 967–980 (2007)
8. Lowe, D.: Object Recognition from Local Scale-invariant Features. In: ICCV, vol. 2, pp. 1150–1157. IEEE (1999)
9. Matas, J., Chum, O., Urban, M., Pajdla, T.: Robust Wide Baseline Stereo from Maximally Stable Extremal Regions. In: BMVC, pp. 384–393 (2002)
10. Pauly, O., Glocker, B., Criminisi, A., Mateus, D., Möller, A.M., Nekolla, S., Navab, N.: Fast Multiple Organ Detection and Localization in Whole-body MR Dixon Sequences. In: Fichtinger, G., Martel, A., Peters, T. (eds.) MICCAI 2011, Part III. LNCS, vol. 6893, pp. 239–247. Springer, Heidelberg (2011)
11. Rousseau, F., Glenn, O., Iordanova, B., Rodriguez-Carranza, C., Vigneron, D., Barkovich, J., Studholme, C., et al.: Registration-based Approach for Reconstruction of High Resolution In Utero Fetal MR Brain Images. Academic Radiology 13(9), 1072–1081 (2006)
12. Snijders, R., Nicolaides, K.: Fetal Biometry at 14–40 Weeks' Gestation. Ultrasound in Obstetrics & Gynecology 4(1), 34–48 (2003)
13. Toews, M., Wells III, W.M.: Efficient and Robust Model-to-Image Alignment using 3D Scale-Invariant Features. Medical Image Analysis (2012)
14. Wu, Z., Ke, Q., Isard, M., Sun, J.: Bundling Features for Large Scale Partial-duplicate Web Image Search. In: CVPR, pp. 25–32. IEEE (2009)
15. Zheng, Y., Barbu, A., Georgescu, B., Scheuering, M., Comaniciu, D.: Four-chamber Heart Modeling and Automatic Segmentation for 3D Cardiac CT Volumes using Marginal Space Learning and Steerable Features. IEEE Transactions on Medical Imaging 27(11), 1668–1681 (2008)

# Surface Smoothing: A Way Back in Early Brain Morphogenesis

Julien Lefèvre[1,2,*], Victor Intwali[3], Lucie Hertz-Pannier[4,5], Petra S. Hüppi[6], Jean-Francois Mangin[5], Jessica Dubois[7], and David Germanaud[4,5]

[1] Aix-Marseille Univ, Département d'Informatique et Interractions, Marseille, France
[2] CNRS, LSIS, UMR 7296, Marseille, France
julien.lefevre@univ-amu.fr
[3] Ecole Centrale Marseille, France
[4] UMR 663, INSERM, Université Paris Descartes, Paris, France
[5] CEA, I2BM, DSV, NeuroSpin, Gif/Yvette, France
[6] Geneva University Hospitals, Department of Pediatrics, Switzerland
[7] U992, INSERM, NeuroSpin, Gif/Yvette, France

**Abstract.** In this article we propose to investigate the analogy between early cortical folding process and cortical smoothing by mean curvature flow. First, we introduce a one-parameter model that is able to fit a developmental trajectory as represented in a Volume-Area plot and we propose an efficient optimization strategy for parameter estimation. Second, we validate the model on forty cortical surfaces of preterm newborns by comparing global geometrical indices and trajectories of central sulcus along developmental and simulation time.

## 1 Introduction

The onset and rapid extension of cortical folds between 20 and 40 weeks of human gestation has been long known from ex vivo examination and observed in vivo since the early days of MRI [10]. Recently reconstruction and segmentation techniques have allowed to study more quantitatively normal developmental trajectories of premature newborns [6] or foetus [15,4] as well as abnormal trajectories in diseases such as ventriculomegaly [16].

Nevertheless the normal and abnormal gyrification process is still suffering from a lack of comprehensive biological mechanisms. In this context several numerical models have been proposed recently with different underlying hypotheses such as mechanical tensions along white matter fibers [8], genetic determination of future gyri [18,13] or tissue growth [19] that can be modulated by skull constraints [14]. However there is no real consensus on this issue and validations are often focused on a limited number of parameters.

Other approaches have modeled cortical folding process in a less biologically explicit but maybe more pragmatic way. Harmonic analysis has been proposed through spherical wavelets [20] or manifold harmonics (Laplace-Beltrami eigenfunctions) [9]. They both make an analogy between the appearance of new folds

---

* This work is funded by the Agence Nationale de la Recherche (ANR-12-JS03-001-01, 'Modegy').

K. Mori et al. (Eds.): MICCAI 2013, Part I, LNCS 8149, pp. 590–597, 2013.

and the addition of new non-vanishing components in the spectral decomposition of surface coordinates. A related approach was found before in [2] where a scale-space of the mean curvature was used to recover the early steps of gyrogenesis and identify "sulcal roots" - putative elementary atoms of cortical folds. This last theory has been used to study the issue of cortical folding variability but to our knowledge it has never been confronted to real developmental data.

That is why this article aims at going beyond a strict visual analogy by testing in which extent some geometric flows can play backward the gyrification process. Our contributions are twofold: first we propose a 1 parameter model derived from mean curvature flow as well as an optimization procedure to fit the parameter on any brain developmental sequence. Second, we present validation tools based on global geometric indices and sulci, tested on 40 preterm newborns.

## 2   Methodology

### 2.1   Mathematical Preliminaries

In the following we will consider $\mathcal{M}_0$ a compact surface of $\mathbb{R}^3$, without boundaries, which will be a left hemisphere in our applications. $\mathcal{M}_0$ can be represented by local mappings around open sets $U$, $Q : U \subset \mathbb{R}^2 \to Q(U) \subset \mathcal{M}_0 \subset \mathbb{R}^3$. The surface is supposed to be smooth enough to define a normal vector $N(\mathbf{x})$, oriented from the outside to the inside and principal curvatures $\kappa_1 \geq \kappa_2$ at each point $\mathbf{x}$. The mean curvature $H(\mathbf{x})$ is given by $(\kappa_1 + \kappa_2)/2$. Thus the mean curvature flow equation can be defined by two equivalent ways :

$$\partial_t P(\mathbf{x}, t) = H(\mathbf{x}, t)N(\mathbf{x}, t) \quad (1) \qquad \partial_t P(\mathbf{x}, t) = \Delta_{\mathcal{M}_t} P(\mathbf{x}, t) \quad (2)$$

with initial condition $P(\mathbf{x}, 0) = Q(\mathbf{x})$. For each time $t$, $P(\mathbf{x}, t)$ represents a local mapping or equivalently coordinates associated to an evolving surface $\mathcal{M}_t$ whose $\Delta_{\mathcal{M}_t}$ is the Laplace-Beltrami operator and $H(\mathbf{x}, t)$ the mean-curvature. There are several numerical implementations of mean curvature flow using (normalized or not) umbrella operator [5] or finite element methods [3]. It is known that the mean curvature equation has a solution on a finite time interval and if $\mathcal{M}_0$ is convex it shrinks to a single point becoming asymptotically spherical [11].

It is also important to briefly recall that Laplace-Beltrami operator of a surface $\mathcal{M}$ is a functional $\Delta_{\mathcal{M}} : f \to \Delta_{\mathcal{M}}f$ that acts as a classical Laplacian (or second derivative) on a function $f : \mathcal{M} \to \mathbb{R}$. This operator has important spectral properties (see [17,9]) since for the functional space of square integrable functions on $\mathcal{M}$ equipped with the scalar product $< f, g >= \int_{\mathcal{M}} fg$ there exists an orthonormal basis $\Phi_i$ and positive integers $0 = \lambda_0 < \lambda_1 \leq \lambda_2 \leq ... \leq \lambda_i$ such as $\Delta_{\mathcal{M}}\Phi_i = -\lambda_i\Phi_i$. Those manifold harmonics $\Phi_i$ represent brain shapes with slightly better sparsity than with spherical harmonics [17].

Last the volume inside the surface $\mathcal{M}$ can be efficiently computed by discretizing the following equality that is a consequence of Green-Ostrogradski formula:

$$\text{Vol}(\mathcal{M}) = \int_{\mathcal{M}} F(\mathbf{x}) \cdot N(\mathbf{x})d\mathbf{x} \quad (3)$$

provided that $F$ is a vector field whose divergence is 1 (e.g. $F(x, y, z) = (x, 0, 0)$).

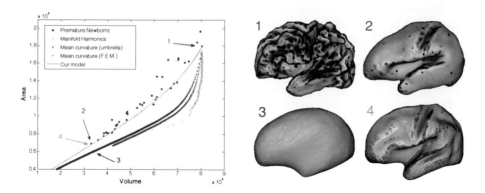

**Fig. 1.** Left: Trajectories in a Volume-Area plot with different techniques: mean curvature flow with two different discretization, manifold harmonics and our optimization method. Circles in blue correspond to Volume-Area measurements on Premature newborns. Right: Surfaces of premature newborns with largest (1) and smallest (2) volume. Mean-curvature flow (3) and our method (4) applied on surface (1) till reaching surface (2). Scales are not preserved for visualization. Only left hemispheres were considered.

## 2.2   Mean Curvature Flow for Retrospective Morphogenesis

It has often been observed that mean curvature flow, Laplacian smoothing or truncation in manifold harmonics reconstruction are offering a striking analogy with a developmental sequence of brains. This analogy can be illustrated by simple visualizations of real cortical surface versus smoothed ones or more objectively by comparing quantitative values such as volume or areas (see Fig. 1). In the case of mean curvature flow, the surface areas in the smoothed sequence are lower than expected from data. This supports that the shrinking process during smoothing is too fast and therefore we may compensate this effect by an "anti-shrinking" force, for instance proportional to $N(\mathbf{x}, t)$. When this proportionality factor equals the average of the mean curvature on $\mathcal{M}$, the volume is preserved [7] which is not the case in the developmental process. Thus we have adopted a pragmatic approach by adding a simple linear term $-aP(\mathbf{x}, t)$ to Eq. (1) and (2). In the case of a sphere this quantity has the same direction as the inward normal and one can consider that it is a crude approximation of normal direction for closed shapes. This leads to consider the following one-parameter model:

$$\partial_t P_a(\mathbf{x}, t) = \Delta_{\mathcal{M}_t} P_a(\mathbf{x}, t) - aP_a(\mathbf{x}, t) \tag{4}$$

This partial differential equation is non-linear and we can also propose a linear version by taking the laplacian $\Delta_{\mathcal{M}_0}$ on the original surface $\mathcal{M}_0$ instead of $\Delta_{\mathcal{M}_t}$. The following proposition will simplify optimization in the next part:

**Proposition 1.** *For each $a \in \mathbb{R}$, Eq. (4) and the equivalent with $\Delta_{\mathcal{M}_0}$ have an unique solution given by:*

$$P_a(\mathbf{x}, t) = e^{-at} P_0(\mathbf{x}, t) \tag{5}$$

*Proof.* Given the formula it is easy to compute $\partial_t P_a(\mathbf{x}, t)$ and to check that $P_a(\mathbf{x}, t)$ is solution of both PDE (4). We give in appendix a more constructive proof of this result in the linear case which involves Manifold Harmonics.

## 2.3  Parameter Estimation

We consider a collection of surfaces $\mathcal{S} = \{S_1, ..., S_d\}$ that represents a reversed developmental sequence from a final surface $S_1$. Each surface $S_i$ correspond to a gestational age (G.A.) $t_i$ and $t_d \leq ... \leq t_1$. We have to define a criterion that measures the error between a real developmental sequence and a simulated one starting from a surface $S_k$ with G.A. $t_k$ through one of our two models. In the case of brain development, we only consider global quantities that are the volume (Vol$(S)$) inside the surface and the total area (Area$(S)$), respectively normalized by $\max_i \text{Vol}(S_i)$ and $\max_i \text{Area}(S_i)$. We can therefore define an error attached to a sequence $\mathcal{S}$, a starting surface $S_k$ and a parameter $a$:

$$E(\mathcal{S}, t_k, a) = \sum_{i \leq k} d_i(a, t_i^*) \text{ with } t_i^* = \arg\min_t d_i(a, t) \tag{6}$$

where $d_i(a, t) = \left[\text{Area}(S_i) - \text{Area}\big(P_a(\cdot, t)\big)\right]^2 + \left[\text{Vol}(S_i) - \text{Vol}\big(P_a(\cdot, t)\big)\right]^2$. This error can be easily interpreted as the sum of distances between each data and the simulations $P_a(\cdot, t)$ obtained from $S_k$ in a Volume-Area plot such as on Fig. 1. Our criterion to be minimized is defined in the Volume-Area space to avoid a direct identification of a simulation time $t_i^*$ - that depends also on $a$ - and a developmental time $t_i$.

Proposition 1 yields a trick to avoid a systematic computation of simulated surfaces for each value of $a$. Namely volumes and areas $P_a$ are given by:

$$\text{Vol}\big(P_a(\cdot, t)\big) = \text{Vol}\big(P_0(\cdot, t)\big)e^{-3at}, \ \text{Area}\big(P_a(\cdot, t)\big) = \text{Area}\big(P_0(\cdot, t)\big)e^{-2at} \tag{7}$$

since Eq. (5) can be simply understood as an homothety. To simplify notations we will denote them as $\text{Vol}_a(t)$ and $\text{Area}_a(t)$ in the following. Optimization of parameter $a$ can then be done by using a classical low-dimensional approach such as Nelder-Mead Simplex Method.

When $a = 0$, we have classical formulas [7] that we will use at initial time

$$\frac{d\text{Area}_0(t)}{dt} = -\int_{\mathcal{M}_t} H(\mathbf{x}, t)^2 \qquad \frac{d\text{Vol}_0(t)}{dt} = -\int_{\mathcal{M}_t} H(\mathbf{x}, t) \tag{8}$$

Thus we can choose $dt$, discretization step of the mean curvature flow such as

$$A(S_k) - A(S_{k-1}) \geq \alpha dt \widehat{H_k^2} \text{ and } V(S_k) - V(S_{k-1}) \geq \alpha dt \widehat{H_k} \tag{9}$$

for any starting surface $S_k$. The hat denotes an average of the mean curvature on the surface. For $\alpha = 10$ it guarantees to have a good sampling of the simulations in the Volume-Area domain. All the previous results can be summarized in:

---

**Algorithm 1.** Optimize Trajectory

---

**Require:** $\{S_1, ..., S_d\}$, $k \in \{1, .., d\}$
 1: $\mathcal{M} := S_0$, i=0, Bool=TRUE
 2: Compute biggest dt satisfying (9)
 3: **while** Bool **do**
 4:    Compute A[i]:=Area($\mathcal{M}$) and Compute V[i]:=Vol($\mathcal{M}$) with Eq. (3)
 5:    Bool=A[i] > min Area($S_i$) OR V[i] > min Vol($S_i$)
 6:    Compute $\mathcal{M}$ at (i+1)dt with discretized Eq. (4)
 7:    i++
 8: **end while**
 9: Define objective function f($\cdot$)=$E(\mathcal{S}, t_k, \cdot)$ through Eq. (6) and (7)
10: a*=Nelder Mead Simplex Method (f)
11: **return** a*

---

## 3    Validation

### 3.1    Quantitative Tools

*Global Geometric Indices.* In a first attempt to validate our retrospective model we compared visual aspects of simulations to real data by using geometric measurements that can be done on the cortical surface. Rather than using directly principal curvatures we transformed these quantities in a more interpretable way thanks to *curvedness* and *shape index* (see [1] for a recent application in neuroimaging):

$$C(\mathbf{x}) = \sqrt{\kappa_1^2 + \kappa_2^2} \qquad SI(\mathbf{x}) = \frac{2}{\pi} \arctan \frac{\kappa_1 + \kappa_2}{\kappa_1 - \kappa_2} \qquad (10)$$

Curvedness encodes the degree of folding whereas Shape Index that varies between -1 and +1 is scale invariant and only represents changes in local configurations at $\mathbf{x}$ from cusp (-1) to casp (1) through saddle (0) or cylinder (0.5). We compute three global indices $(\overline{C}, \overline{SI}_+, \overline{SI}_-)$ from these two quantities by taking a) the median of $C(\mathbf{x})$, b) the median of $SI(\mathbf{x})$ for $\mathbf{x}$ such as $SI(\mathbf{x}) > 0$, c) the same for $SI(\mathbf{x}) < 0$.

*Sulcus-Based Validation.* A second validation of our model was done by considering very early developing sulci such as the central one. Lines of central sulcus (CS) fundi were delineated semi-automatically [12]. Then evolution of these lines were followed through the developmental sequence and the simulations, provided that a matching process exists to register the surfaces. For a given surface $\mathcal{M}_t$ we defined the following mapping based on the three first manifold harmonics:

$$\mathbf{x} \to \left(\Phi_1(\mathbf{x})^2 + \Phi_2(\mathbf{x})^2 + \Phi_3(\mathbf{x})^2\right)^{-1/2} \left(\Phi_1(\mathbf{x}), \Phi_2(\mathbf{x}), \Phi_3(\mathbf{x})\right) \qquad (11)$$

By construction it transforms each point of $\mathcal{M}_t$ to a point of the sphere of $\mathbb{R}^3$. Empirical properties of the 3 harmonics guarantee the transformation to be an homeomorphism, in particular the fact that $(\Phi_i)_{i=1,2,3}$ have always 2 nodal domains on the studied surfaces. If necessary we flip the sign of $\Phi_i$ by considering coordinates of their extremal points in a common 3D referential.

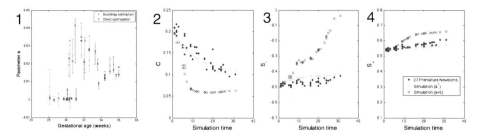

**Fig. 2.** 1: Sensibility analysis of parameter $a$ for 35 largest brains: bootstrap estimation of mean and confidence intervals (blue) vs direct optimization (red). 2-4: Comparison of the three global indices ($C$, $SI_+$, $SI_-$) between data (blue), our model (green) and mean curvature flow (red).

## 3.2   Results

*Data.* We considered 40 T2-weighted images of preterm newborns with no apparent anatomical abnormalities and whose gestational age ranges from 26.7 to 35.7 weeks. They were segmented according to the method exposed in [6].

*Sensibility Analysis.* Our method allows a fast bootstrap estimation of the mean and confidence intervals of $a_k^*$ (for the 35 largest brains to keep at least 5 points to estimate $a$) by applying algorithm (1) to different resampled sets $\{S_1^*, ..., S_d^*\}$ taken from $\mathcal{S}$ (45 s for 1000 bootstrapped samples). Comparison of $a$ through direct optimization and through resampling is shown on Fig. 2 with respect to G.A. It seems that one can distinguish three different temporal periods ($28-31$, $31-34$, $34-36$) where the values of $a$ are different as well as the sensibility.

*Geometric Measurements.* We compared the three global geometric indices between premature newborns, simulations with optimal parameter $a^*$ and $a = 0$ starting from the largest brain $S_1$ (see Fig. 2). For each subject $i$ we obtain a time $t_i^*$ from Eq. (6) that can be located on the x-axis. The behavior of the different curves is reproducible with different initial brains $S_k$ (not shown): one can observe that the median curvedness is decreasing from larger to smaller brains, whereas $\overline{SI_+}$ and $\overline{SI_-}$ are relatively more stable. It is quite remarkable to note the good fit of the optimal model and the divergence of mean curvature flow for the three different measurements that are not surrogates of volume and areas.

*Trajectory of Central Sulcus.* On Fig. 3 we have a direct comparison of the evolution of CS fundi on original surfaces and on corresponding smoothed surfaces with our model starting from the largest brain. The spherical mapping allows to see clearly a translation of CS lines when we start from older brains (yellow in the middle) to younger ones (black) and similarly from initial (yellow) to final (black) ones in the simulation.

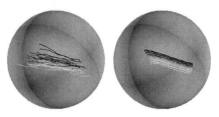

**Fig. 3.** Lines of CS fundi on real data (left) and on our simulations (right). See text for color code. North pole corresponds to frontal lobe.

## 4   Discussion

Our results demonstrate the feasibility of simulating the reversed cortical folding process observed on a cross-sectional study of premature newborns through a one parameter model derived from the mean curvature flow. Our model is only constrained by two global quantities, volume and area but it is able to predict evolution of geometrical quantities related to the shape of the cortical surfaces. Even if global, these quantities are not surrogates of those to optimize. More locally our model reproduces also a translation of central sulcus observed in the data that suggests a faster growth in frontal area than in parietal one that may be consistent with results in [15] for fetal brains from 24 to 28 G.A. Sensibility analysis on the parameter $a$ reveals 3 different periods where its values and confidence intervals are fluctuating. Since $a$ can be interpreted as the amplitude of an "anti-shrinking" force, this result suggests possible different scenarios in the cortical folding process with different kinetics. However larger confidence intervals in the interval $31 - 34$ G.A. may also come from a bias resulting from less time points to estimate the parameter.

In future works we intend to apply our method on fetal brains and compare their developmental trajectories to those of premature newborns such as in [4]. Longitudinal studies would also be an ideal application of our framework to compare more accurately in space the relevance of our model.

## References

1. Awate, S.P., Win, L., Yushkevich, P.A., Schultz, R.T., Gee, J.C.: 3D cerebral cortical morphometry in autism: Increased folding in children and adolescents in frontal, parietal, and temporal lobes. In: Metaxas, D., Axel, L., Fichtinger, G., Székely, G. (eds.) MICCAI 2008, Part I. LNCS, vol. 5241, pp. 559–567. Springer, Heidelberg (2008)
2. Cachia, A., Mangin, J.F., Riviere, D., Kherif, F., Boddaert, N., Andrade, A., Papadopoulos-Orfanos, D., Poline, J.B., Bloch, I., Zilbovicius, M., Sonigo, P., Brunelle, F., Régis, J.: A primal sketch of the cortex mean curvature: a morphogenesis based approach to study the variability of the folding patterns. IEEE Transactions on Medical Imaging 22(6), 754–765 (2003)
3. Clarenz, U., Diewald, U., Rumpf, M.: Anisotropic geometric diffusion in surface processing. In: Proceedings of the Conference on Visualization 2000, pp. 397–405. IEEE Computer Society Press (2000)
4. Clouchoux, C., Kudelski, D., Gholipour, A., Warfield, S.K., Viseur, S., Bouyssi-Kobar, M., Mari, J.L., Evans, A.C., du Plessis, A.J., Limperopoulos, C.: Quantitative in vivo mri measurement of cortical development in the fetus. Brain Structure and Function 217(1), 127–139 (2012)
5. Desbrun, M., Meyer, M., Schröder, P., Barr, A.H.: Implicit fairing of irregular meshes using diffusion and curvature flow. In: Proceedings of the 26th Annual Conference on Computer Graphics and Interactive Techniques, pp. 317–324 (1999)
6. Dubois, J., Benders, M., Cachia, A., Lazeyras, F., Ha-Vinh Leuchter, R., Sizonenko, S.V., Borradori-Tolsa, C., Mangin, J.F., Hüppi, P.S.: Mapping the early cortical folding process in the preterm newborn brain. Cereb. Cort. 18(6), 1444–1454 (2008)
7. Escher, J., Simonett, G.: The volume preserving mean curvature flow near spheres. Proceedings American Mathematical Society 126, 2789–2796 (1998)

8. Geng, G., Johnston, L.A., Yan, E., Britto, J.M., Smith, D.W., Walker, D.W., Egan, G.F.: Biomechanisms for modelling cerebral cortical folding. Medical Image Analysis 13(6), 920–930 (2009)
9. Germanaud, D., Lefèvre, J., Toro, R., Fischer, C., Dubois, J., Hertz-Pannier, L., Mangin, J.-F.: Larger is twistier: Spectral analysis of gyrification (spangy) applied to adult brain size polymorphism. NeuroImage 63(3), 1257–1272 (2012)
10. Girard, N., Raybaud, C., Poncet, M.: In vivo mr study of brain maturation in normal fetuses. American Journal of Neuroradiology 16(2), 407–413 (1995)
11. Huisken, G.: Flow by mean curvature of convex surfaces into spheres. Journal of Differential Geometry 20(1), 237–266 (1984)
12. Le Troter, A., Rivière, D., Coulon, O.: An interactive sulcal fundi editor in brainvisa. In: 17th International Conference on Human Brain Mapping, Organization for Human Brain Mapping (2011)
13. Lefèvre, J., Mangin, J.F.: A reaction-diffusion model of human brain development. PLoS Computational Biology 6(4), e1000749 (2010)
14. Nie, J., Guo, L., Li, G., Faraco, C., Miller, L.S., Liu, T.: A computational model of cerebral cortex folding. Journal of Theoretical Biology 264(2), 467–478 (2010)
15. Rajagopalan, V., Scott, J., Habas, P.A., Kim, K., Corbett-Detig, J., Rousseau, F., Barkovich, A.J., Glenn, O.A., Studholme, C.: Local tissue growth patterns underlying normal fetal human brain gyrification quantified in utero. The Journal of Neuroscience 31(8), 2878–2887 (2011)
16. Scott, J.A., Habas, P.A., Rajagopalan, V., Kim, K., Barkovich, A.J., Glenn, O.A., Studholme, C.: Volumetric and surface-based 3d mri analyses of fetal isolated mild ventriculomegaly. In: Brain Structure and Function, pp. 645–655 (2012)
17. Seo, S., Chung, M.K.: Laplace-beltrami eigenfunction expansion of cortical manifolds. In: IEEE International Symposium on Biomedical Imaging (2011)
18. Striegel, D.A., Hurdal, M.K.: Chemically Based Mathematical Model for Development of Cerebral Cortical Folding Patterns. PLoS Comput. Biol. 5(9) (2009)
19. Toro, R.: On the possible shapes of the brain. Evol. Biol. 39(4), 600–612 (2012)
20. Yu, P., Grant, P.E., Qi, Y., Han, X., Ségonne, F., Pienaar, R., Busa, E., Pacheco, J., Makris, N., Buckner, R.L., et al.: Cortical surface shape analysis based on spherical wavelets. IEEE Transactions on Medical Imaging 26(4), 582–597 (2007)

## Appendix: Proof of Proposition 1

We decompose $P_a(\mathbf{x}, t)$ in the basis of eigenfunctions of the operator $\Delta_{\mathcal{M}_0}$:

$$P_a(\mathbf{x}, t) = \sum_{i=0}^{+\infty} \hat{\mathbf{p}}_i(a, t) \Phi_i(\mathbf{x})$$

where $\hat{\mathbf{p}}_i(a, t) \in \mathbb{R}^3$ is given by $\int_{\mathcal{M}_0} P_a(\mathbf{x}, t) \Phi_i(\mathbf{x}) d\mathbf{x}$. Then since $P_a$ satisfies Eq. (4) (with $\Delta_{\mathcal{M}_0}$ instead of $\Delta_{\mathcal{M}_t}$):

$$0 = \partial_t P_a - a\Delta_{\mathcal{M}_0} P_a + aP_a = \sum_{i=0}^{+\infty} \left[ \partial_t \hat{\mathbf{p}}_i(a, t) + \lambda_i \hat{\mathbf{p}}_i(a, t) + a\hat{\mathbf{p}}_i(a, t) \right] \Phi_i(\mathbf{x})$$

So $\hat{\mathbf{p}}_i(a, t) = \hat{\mathbf{p}}_i(a, 0) e^{-\lambda_i t} e^{-at}$. Last we have to notice that $\hat{\mathbf{p}}_i(a, 0)$ is independent of $a$ since they correspond to the coefficients of the initial surface $\mathcal{M}_0$ and that $\hat{\mathbf{p}}_i(a, 0) e^{-\lambda_i t}$ are the coefficients of $\mathcal{M}_t$ for $a = 0$. We conclude that $P_a(\mathbf{x}, t) = e^{-at} P_0(\mathbf{x}, t)$.

# 4D Hyperspherical Harmonic (HyperSPHARM) Representation of Multiple Disconnected Brain Subcortical Structures

Ameer Pasha Hosseinbor[1], Moo K. Chung[1], Stacey M. Schaefer[1],
Carien M. van Reekum[2], Lara Peschke-Schmitz[1], Matt Sutterer[1],
Andrew L. Alexander[1], and Richard J. Davidson[1]

[1] University of Wisconsin-Madison, USA
[2] University of Reading, UK
hosseinbor@wisc.edu

**Abstract.** We present a novel surface parameterization technique using *hyperspherical harmonics* (HSH) in representing compact, multiple, disconnected brain subcortical structures as a single analytic function. The proposed hyperspherical harmonic representation (HyperSPHARM) has many advantages over the widely used spherical harmonic (SPHARM) parameterization technique. SPHARM requires flattening 3D surfaces to 3D sphere which can be time consuming for large surface meshes, and can't represent multiple disconnected objects with single parameterization. On the other hand, HyperSPHARM treats 3D object, via simple stereographic projection, as a surface of 4D hypersphere with extremely large radius, hence avoiding the computationally demanding flattening process. HyperSPHARM is shown to achieve a better reconstruction with only 5 basis compared to SPHARM that requires more than 441.

## 1 Introduction

Many shape modeling frameworks in computational anatomy assume topological invariance between objects and are not applicable for objects with different or changing topology. There are numerous such examples from longitudinal child development to cancer growth. For example, an infant may have about 300-350 bones at birth but an adult has 206 bones. These bones fuse together as the infant grows. This type of topological difference and changes cannot be incorporated directly into the processing and analysis pipeline with existing shape models that assume topological invariance and mainly work on a single connected component. The difficulty is mainly caused by the lack of a single, coherent mathematical parameterization for multiple, disconnected objects.

Probably the most widely applied shape parameterization technique for cortical structures is the spherical harmonic (SPHARM) representation [4,7,10], which has been mainly used as a data reduction technique for compressing global shape features into a small number of coefficients. The main global geometric features are encoded in low degree coefficients while the noise will be in high degree spherical harmonics. The method has been used to model various brain structures such as ventricles [7], hippocampi [10] and cortical surfaces

K. Mori et al. (Eds.): MICCAI 2013, Part I, LNCS 8149, pp. 598–605, 2013.

[4]. SPHARM, however, can't represent multiple disconnected structures with a single parameterization. Since SPHARM requires a smooth map from surfaces to a 3D sphere, various computationally intensive surface flattening techniques have been proposed: diffusion mapping [4], conformal mapping [1], and area preserving mapping [7]. The surface flattening is used to parameterize the surface using two spherical angles. The angles serve as coordinates for representing the surface using spherical harmonics. Then the surface coordinates can be mapped onto the sphere and each coordinate is represented as a linear combination of spherical harmonics.

Note that a 3D volume is a surface in 4D. By performing simple stereographic projection on a 3D volume, it is possible to embed the 3D volume onto the surface of a 4D hypersphere, which bypasses the difficulty of flattening 3D surface to 3D sphere. Extending the concept further, any two or more disconnected 3D objects can be projected onto a single connected surface in 4D hypersphere. Then the disconnected 3D objects can be represented as the linear combination of 4D hyperspherical harmonics (HSH), which are the multidimensional analogues of the 3D spherical harmonics.

The HSH have been mainly confined to quantum chemistry, where their utility first became evident with respect to solving the Schrödinger equation for the hydrogen atom. It had been solved in position-space by Schrödinger, himself, but not in momentum-space, which is related to position-space via the Fourier transform. Sometime later, V. Fock solved the Schrödinger equation for the hydrogen atom directly in momentum-space. In his classic paper [6], Fock stereographically projected 3D momentum-space onto the surface of a 4D unit hypersphere, and after this mapping was made, he was able to show that the eigenfuctions were the 4D HSH. Recently, the HSH have been utilized in a wider array of fields than just quantum chemistry, including computer graphics visualization [3] and crystallography [9]. However, as of yet, they have remained elusive for medical imaging.

In this paper, following the approach of Fock, we model multiple disconnected 3D objects in terms of the 4D HSH by stereographically projecting each object's surface coordinates onto a 4D hypersphere, and label such a representation HyperSPHARM. Significantly, we show that HyperSPHARM can better reconstruct such objects than SPHARM using just a few basis functions. The method is applied to modeling disconnected brain subcortical structures, specifically the left and right hippocampus and amygdala.

## 2    Methods

### 2.1    4D Hyperspherical Harmonics

Consider the 4D unit hypersphere $S^3$ existing in $\mathbb{R}^4$. The Laplace-Beltrami operator on $S^3$ is defined as $\Delta_{S^3} = \frac{1}{\sin^2 \beta} \frac{\partial}{\partial \beta} \sin^2 \beta \frac{\partial}{\partial \beta} + \frac{1}{\sin^2 \beta} \Delta_{S^2}$, where $\Delta_{S^2}$ is the Laplace-Beltrami operator on the unit sphere $S^2$. The eigenfuctions of $\Delta_{S^3}$ are the 4D HSH $Z_{nl}^m(\beta, \theta, \phi)$: $\Delta_{S^3} Z_{nl}^m = -l(l+2)Z_{nl}^m$. The 4D HSH are defined as [5]

**Table 1.** List of a Few HSH

$$
\begin{array}{ll}
Z_{00}^{0}(\beta,\theta,\phi) = \frac{1}{\pi\sqrt{2}} & Z_{10}^{0}(\beta,\theta,\phi) = \frac{\sqrt{2}}{\pi}\cos\beta \\
Z_{11}^{-1}(\beta,\theta,\phi) = \frac{-\sqrt{2}}{\pi}\sin\beta\,\sin\theta\,\sin\phi & Z_{11}^{0}(\beta,\theta,\phi) = \frac{\sqrt{2}}{\pi}\sin\beta\,\cos\theta \\
Z_{11}^{1}(\beta,\theta,\phi) = \frac{-\sqrt{2}}{\pi}\sin\beta\,\sin\theta\,\cos\phi & Z_{20}^{0}(\beta,\theta,\phi) = \frac{1}{\pi\sqrt{2}}(3 - 4\sin^2\beta) \\
Z_{21}^{-1}(\beta,\theta,\phi) = \frac{-\sqrt{3}}{\pi}\sin 2\beta\,\sin\theta\,\sin\phi & Z_{21}^{0}(\beta,\theta,\phi) = \frac{\sqrt{3}}{\pi}\sin 2\beta\,\cos\theta
\end{array}
$$

$$
Z_{nl}^{m}(\beta,\theta,\phi) = 2^{l+1/2}\sqrt{\frac{(n+1)\Gamma(n-l+1)}{\pi\Gamma(n+l+2)}}\,\Gamma(l+1)\sin^l\beta\,C_{n-l}^{l+1}(\cos\beta)\,Y_l^m(\theta,\phi),
$$

(1)

where $(\beta,\theta,\phi)$ obey $(\beta \in [0,\pi], \theta \in [0,\pi], \phi \in [0,2\pi])$, $C_{n-1}^{l+1}$ are the Gegenbauer (ultraspherical) polynomials, and $Y_l^m$ are the 3D spherical harmonics. The index $l$ denotes the degree of the HSH, $m$ is the order, and $n = 0,1,2,...,$ and these three integers obey the conditions $0 \le l \le n$ and $-l \le m \le l$. The number of HSH corresponding to a given value of $n$ is $(n+1)^2$. The first few 4D HSH are shown in Table 1. The HSH form an orthonormal basis on the hypersphere, and the normalization condition reads

$$
\int_0^{2\pi}\int_0^{\pi}\int_0^{\pi} Z_{nl}^{m}(\beta,\theta,\phi)Z_{n'l'}^{m'*}(\beta,\theta,\phi)\sin^2\beta\,\sin\theta d\beta d\theta d\phi = \delta_{nn'}\delta_{ll'}\delta_{mm'} \quad (2)
$$

## 2.2    4D Stereographic Projection of 3D Surface Coordinates onto Hypersphere

Consider a 3D finite, compact object (i.e. has no singularities) comprised of surface coordinates $\mathbf{s} = (s^1, s^2, s^3)$. In order to model the surface coordinates with the HSH, we need to map them onto a 4D hypersphere, which can be achieved via stereographic projection [6]. The surface coordinates in spherical space are $s^1 = r\sin\theta\cos\phi$, $s^2 = r\sin\theta\sin\phi$, and $s^3 = r\cos\theta$, where $r = \sqrt{(s^1)^2 + (s^2)^2 + (s^3)^2}$. Consider a 4D hypersphere of radius $p_o$, whose coordinates are defined as

$$
\begin{aligned}
u_1 &= p_o \sin\beta \sin\theta \cos\phi \\
u_2 &= p_o \sin\beta \sin\theta \sin\phi \\
u_3 &= p_o \sin\beta \cos\theta \\
u_4 &= p_o \cos\beta.
\end{aligned}
$$

The relationship between $(s^1, s^2, s^3)$ and $(u_1, u_2, u_3, u_4)$ is then

$$
u_1 = \frac{2p_o^2 s^1}{r^2 + p_o^2}, \quad u_2 = \frac{2p_o^2 s^2}{r^2 + p_o^2}, \quad u_3 = \frac{2p_o^2 s^3}{r^2 + p_o^2}, \quad u_4 = \frac{p_o(r^2 - p_o^2)}{r^2 + p_o^2} \quad (3)
$$

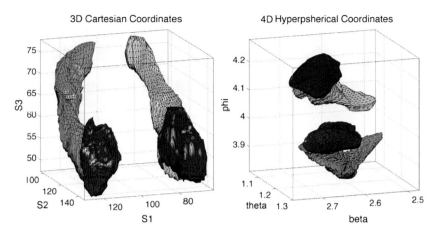

**Fig. 1.** The 3D subcortical structures (left) in the coordinates $(s^1, s^2, s^3)$ went through the 4D stereographic projection that resulted in conformally deformed structures (right) in the 4D spherical coordinates $(\beta, \theta, \phi)$. The 3D subcortical structure is then embedded on the surface of the 4D hypersphere with radius $p_0 = 2000$, which makes the surface of the hypersphere to be almost Euclidean.

According to Eq. (3), the surface coordinate $(0, 0, 0)$ projects onto the south pole $(0, 0, 0, -p_o)$ of the hypersphere. As $r \to \infty$, the projection $(u_1, u_2, u_3, u_4)$ moves closer to the north pole $(0, 0, 0, p_o)$ of hypersphere. Thus, the north pole is not associated with any $(s^1, s^2, s^3)$, but gives us a way of envisioning infinity as a point. Eq. (3) establishes a one-to-one correspondence between the 3D volume and 4D hypersphere (Figure 1). The radius of the hypersphere $p_o$ controls the density of the projected surface coordinates onto the hypersphere's surface.

Stereographic projection exhibits two important properties. First, it is conformal, which means it preserves angles - the angles $(\theta, \phi)$ defining the 3D surface are preserved in 4D hyperspherical space. However, stereographic projection does not preserve volume; in general, the volume of a region in the 3D plane doesn't equal the volume of its projection onto the hypersphere.

## 2.3 HSH Expansion of 3D Surface Coordinates

Stereographically projecting a 3D object's surface coordinates onto a 4D hypersphere results in them existing along the hypersphere's surface. According to Fourier analysis, any square-integrable function defined on a sphere can be expanded in terms of the spherical harmonics. Thus, we can expand each coordinate component $s^i$, where $i = 1, 2, 3$, in terms of the 4D HSH:

$$s_{p_o}^i(\beta, \theta, \phi) \approx \sum_{n=0}^{N} \sum_{l=0}^{n} \sum_{m=-l}^{l} C_{nlm}^i Z_{nl}^m(\beta, \theta, \phi), \qquad (4)$$

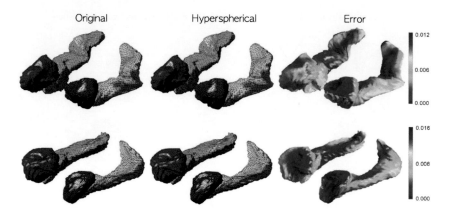

**Fig. 2.** Hyperspherical harmonic representation of amygdala and hippocampus surfaces for subject 10 and 60. The vertex-wise reconstruction errors are also plotted. As expected, most errors are occurring near sharp peaks and corners.

where $s_{p_o}^i$ denotes the $i^{th}$ component of the surface coordinates $\mathbf{s}$ existing on hypersphere of radius $p_o$. The realness of the surface coordinates requires use of the real HSH, and so we employ a modified real basis used in [8] for $Y_l^m$. For a given truncation order $N$, the total number of expansion coefficients is $W = (N+1)(N+2)(2N+3)/6$.

## 2.4   Numerical Implementation

Suppose each $s^i$ of our 3D surface consists of $M$ vertices. This is the total number of mesh vertices for all disconnected surfaces. The task then is to estimate each $s^i$'s coefficients $C_{nlm}^i$ in Eq. (4) from the $M$ surface vertices.

Let $\Omega_j = (\beta_j, \theta_j, \phi_j)$ denote the hyperspherical angles at the $j$-th mesh vertex. Denote $\mathbf{s}^i$ as the $M$ x 1 vector representing each $s^i$'s $M$ vertices, $\mathbf{C}^i$ the $W$ x 1 vector of unknown expansion coefficients $C_{nlm}^i$ for each $s^i$, and $\mathbf{A}$ the $M$ x $W$ matrix constructed with the HSH basis

$$\mathbf{A} = \begin{pmatrix} Z_{00}^0(\Omega_1) & Z_{10}^0(\Omega_1) & Z_{11}^{-1}(\Omega_1) & Z_{11}^0(\Omega_1) & \cdots & Z_{NN}^N(\Omega_1) \\ \vdots & \vdots & \vdots & \vdots & \ddots & \vdots \\ Z_{00}^0(\Omega_M) & Z_{10}^0(\Omega_M) & Z_{11}^{-1}(\Omega_M) & Z_{11}^0(\Omega_M) & \cdots & Z_{NN}^N(\Omega_M) \end{pmatrix}.$$

Thus, the general linear system representing Eq. (4) is described by $\mathbf{s}^i = \mathbf{A}\mathbf{C}^i$. This system of over-determined equations is solved via linear least squares, yielding

$$\widehat{\mathbf{C}^i} = (\mathbf{A}^T\mathbf{A})^{-1}\mathbf{A}^T\mathbf{s}^i \tag{5}$$

The reconstructed $s^i$ is $\widehat{\mathbf{s}^i} = \mathbf{A}\widehat{\mathbf{C}^i}$, and so our reconstructed 3D surface is defined by the $M$ x 3 matrix $\widehat{\mathbf{s}} = (\widehat{s^1}, \widehat{s^2}, \widehat{s^3})$. The mean squared error (MSE) between

**Table 2.** The mean squared error (MSE) and its standard deviation of reconstruction. MSE is computed over all mesh vertices and averaged over 69 subjects. Degree 2, 10 and 20 SPHARM representations require $3^2 = 9, 11^2 = 121$ and $21^2 = 441$ basis functions, respectively. The reconstruction error of HSH expansion of order $N = 1$ is substantially smaller than those of SPHARM, even though only 5 HSH basis functions are used.

| | SPHARM 2 | SPHARM 10 | SPHARM 20 | HSH 1 |
|---|---|---|---|---|
| Left Amygdala | $1.08 \pm 0.17$ | $0.054 \pm 0.010$ | $0.022 \pm 0.005$ | $0.18 \pm 0.04 \times 10^{-5}$ |
| Right Amygdala | $0.60 \pm 0.11$ | $0.052 \pm 0.008$ | $0.023 \pm 0.003$ | $0.27 \pm 0.06 \times 10^{-5}$ |
| Left Hippocampus | $1.77 \pm 0.33$ | $0.127 \pm 0.026$ | $0.043 \pm 0.040$ | $0.90 \pm 0.20 \times 10^{-5}$ |
| Right Hippocampus | $1.08 \pm 0.17$ | $0.054 \pm 0.010$ | $0.022 \pm 0.005$ | $0.18 \pm 0.04 \times 10^{-5}$ |

the original surface and the reconstructed surface can then be computed as $\mathrm{tr}\left[(\mathbf{s} - \widehat{\mathbf{s}})^T (\mathbf{s} - \widehat{\mathbf{s}})\right]/M$.

# 3    Experimental Results and Applications

We collected high-resolution T1-weighted inverse recovery fast gradient echo MRI in 124 contiguous 1.2-mm axial slices (TE=1.8 ms; TR=8.9 ms; flip angle = 10°; FOV = 240 mm; 256 × 256 data acquisition matrix) of 69 middle-age and elderly adults ranging between 38 to 79 years (mean age = 58.0 ± 11.4 years). The data were collected as a part of a national study called MIDUS (Midlife in US; http://midus.wisc.edu) for the health and well-being in the aged population [12]. There are 23 men and 46 women in the study. Brain tissues in the MRI scans were automatically segmented using Brain Extraction Tool (BET) [11] and trained raters manually segmented the parts of limbic system: amygdala and hippocampus. A nonlinear image registration using the diffeomorphic shape and intensity averaging technique with the cross-correlation as the similarity metric through Advanced Normalization Tools (ANTS) [2] was performed and the study specific template is constructed. The isosurfaces of the segmentation were extracted using the marching cube algorithm (Figure 2).

Four brain subcortical structures, specifically the left and right hippocampus and amygdala, were reconstructed for 69 subjects. For each structure, the HSH expansion parameters were $N = 1$ and radius $p_o = 2000$, which results in $W = 5$ HSH expansion coefficients for each $s^i$. So total of 15 HSH coefficients can parameterize a single surface and 60 coefficients all four disconnected surfaces (i.e. left and right hippocampus and amygdala). Figure 2 shows the reconstructed HSH surfaces for two subjects. The length of the residual is computed and plotted on the reconstructed surfaces. As expected, the most reconstruction errors are found near peaks and corners.

## 3.1    Comparison against SPHARM Representation

We have compared the reconstruction errors between HSH and SPHARM representations. Hippocampus and amygdala surface meshes are flattened to a unit

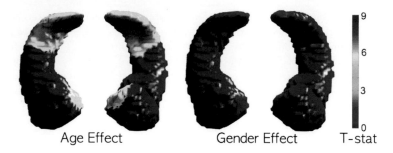

Age Effect          Gender Effect      T-stat

**Fig. 3.** The regions showing statistically significant age effect thresholded at $p < 0.05$ (corrected). There is no gender effect.

sphere and resampled to a uniform grid along the sphere. Then degree 2, 10 and 20 SPHARM representations are constructed. The MSE of each reconstruction is computed within each surface and averaged over 69 subjects (Table 2). Its standard error is also computed over all 69 subjects. The degree $k$ SPHARM representations requires $(k + 1)^2$ SPHARM basis functions.

The degree 2, 10 and 20 SPHARM representations require 9, 121 and 441 basis functions. Even with only 5 basis functions, HSH is achieving substantially low MSE compared with SPHARM reconstruction with 441 basis functions, demonstrating the superior efficiency in the HSH representation.

### 3.2   Influence of Age and Gender

HSH representations were obtained for hippocampus and amygdala surfaces of all 69 subjects. The representation behaves like surface smoothing technique where high frequency noise is removed as shown in Figure 2. The 69 reconstructed surfaces are then averaged to produce the population specific template. The 3D displacement vector field from the template to individual surface is taken as the response vector in the multivariate general linear model (MGLM) [4] and its $T$-statistic is computed and thresholded at $p < 0.05$. The random field based multiple comparisons are performed to give stringent results. We have detected significant influence of age mainly on the tail regions of the hippocampus while there is no influence of gender on any of the structures.

## 4   Conclusion and Discussion

In this paper, we have presented a new analytic approach for representing multiple disconnected shapes using a single analytic function, which is a linear combination of HSH. The method is applied to parameterizing 4 disconnected subcortical structures (two amygdalae and two hippocampi) using only 60 HSH coefficients. The resulting HSH coefficients are global and contain information about all four structures, so they do not provide any local shape information.

Therefore, HyperSPHARM might be better suited to sparse techniques such as wavelets, which will be explored in future. Despite HSH being a global basis, by reconstructing surfaces at each voxel and using HSH as a way to filter out high frequency noise, it was possible to use HSH for local inference at vertex level as shown in our application. Although the individual image volumes are registered to a template using diffeomorphic warping [2], we might only need an affine registration to initially align the structures and simply match the coefficients as in SPHARM [4] but the issue is not explored here and left as a future study.

**Acknowledgements.** This research was supported by the National Institute of Aging (P01-AG20166) and National Institute on Mental Health (R01 MH043454). Seung-Goo Kim of Max Planck Institutes performed image registration.

# References

1. Angenent, S., Hacker, S., Tannenbaum, A., Kikinis, R.: On the laplace-beltrami operator and brain surface flattening. IEEE Transactions on Medical Imaging 18, 700–711 (1999)
2. Avants, B., Epstein, C., Grossman, M., Gee, J.: Symmetric diffeomorphic image registration with cross-correlation: Evaluating automated labeling of elderly and neurodegenerative brain. Medical Image Analysis 12, 26–41 (2008)
3. Bonvallet, B., Griffin, N., Li, J.: 3D shape descriptors: 4D hyperspherical harmonics "An exploration into the fourth dimension". In: IASTED International Conference on Graphics and Visualization in Engineering, pp. 113–116 (2007)
4. Chung, M., Worsley, K., Brendon, M., Dalton, K., Davidson, R.: General multivariate linear modeling of surface shapes using SurfStat. NeuroImage 53, 491–505 (2010)
5. Domokos, G.: Four-dimensional symmetry. Physical Review 159, 1387–1403 (1967)
6. Fock, V.: Zur theorie des wasserstoffatoms. Z. Physik 98, 145–154 (1935)
7. Gerig, G., Styner, M., Jones, D., Weinberger, D., Lieberman, J.: Shape analysis of brain ventricles using spharm. In: MMBIA, pp. 171–178 (2001)
8. Koay, C.G., Ozarslan, E., Basser, P.J.: A signal transformational framework for breaking the noise floor and its applications in MRI. J. Magn. Reson. 197, 108–119 (2009)
9. Mason, J.K., Schuh, C.A.: Hyperspherical harmonics for the representation of crystallographic texture 56, 6141–6155 (2008)
10. Shen, L., Ford, J., Makedon, F., Saykin, A.: surface-based approach for classification of 3d neuroanatomical structures. Intelligent Data Analysis 8, 519–542 (2004)
11. Smith, S.: Fast robust automated brain extraction. Human Brain Mapping 17, 143–155 (2002)
12. Van Reekum, C., Schaefer, S., Lapate, R., Norris, C., Greischar, L., Davidson, R.: Aging is associated with positive responding to neutral information but reduced recovery from negative information. Social Cognitive and Affective Neuroscience 6, 177–185 (2011)

# Modality Propagation:
# Coherent Synthesis of Subject-Specific Scans with Data-Driven Regularization

Dong Hye Ye[1], Darko Zikic[2], Ben Glocker[2], Antonio Criminisi[2], and Ender Konukoglu[3]

[1] Department of Radiology, University of Pennsylvania, Philadelphia, PA, USA
[2] Microsoft Research, Cambridge, UK
[3] Martinos Center for Biomedical Imaging, MGH, Harvard Medical School, MA, USA

**Abstract.** We propose a general database-driven framework for coherent synthesis of subject-specific scans of desired modality, which adopts and generalizes the patch-based label propagation (LP) strategy. While modality synthesis has received increased attention lately, current methods are mainly tailored to specific applications. On the other hand, the LP framework has been extremely successful for certain segmentation tasks, however, so far it has not been used for estimation of entities other than categorical segmentation labels. We approach the synthesis task as a *modality propagation*, and demonstrate that with certain modifications the LP framework can be generalized to continuous settings providing coherent synthesis of different modalities, beyond segmentation labels. To achieve high-quality estimates we introduce a new data-driven regularization scheme, in which we integrate intermediate estimates within an iterative search-and-synthesis strategy. To efficiently leverage population data and ensure coherent synthesis, we employ a spatio-population search space restriction. In experiments, we demonstrate the quality of synthesis of different MRI signals (T2 and DTI-FA) from a T1 input, and show a novel application of modality synthesis for abnormality detection in multi-channel MRI of brain tumor patients.

## 1 Introduction

Medical imaging enjoys a multitude of image modalities, each locally quantifying and mapping different characteristics of the underlying anatomy. For instance, while CT images display local tissue densities, diffusion weighted images quantify the tissue directionality. Even derived quantities such as local fractional anisotropy (FA) can be seen as modalities, as they quantify certain characteristics of the anatomy. There is increased interest in methods which perform subject-specific synthesis of a certain *target modality*, from a given *source modality*. The ability to automatically generate different appearances of the same anatomy, without an actual acquisition, enables various applications such as creating virtual models [1], multi-modal registration [2,3,4], super-resolution [5], atlas construction [6] and virtual enhancement [7]. Most of the current methods are tailored to specific applications. Some approaches perform synthesis using

K. Mori et al. (Eds.): MICCAI 2013, Part I, LNCS 8149, pp. 606–613, 2013.

explicit models, for example for simulating US from CT [2] or modality conversion between T1 and T2 [3]. Explicit modeling is application-dependent and does not generalize easily. Other approaches use existing databases for synthesis. In [8] the FLAIR channel is created from T1 and T2 for brain MRI, the MR inhomogeneity field is estimated in [9], synthesis of an alternative modality to facilitate the registration in correlative microscopy is considered in [4], and in [10,11] synthesis of high resolution images is tackled. Despite being database-driven, the above works focus on specific problems, and propose case-specific approaches that differ significantly from one another. Admittedly, the general synthesis problem poses additional difficulties over the specific versions, due to the multitude of possible scenarios. Different modalities characterize different physical properties, and the target modality might contain richer information than the source.

We propose a general framework for modality synthesis which avoids explicit modeling and operates by utilizing a database of images with arbitrary target and source modalities. For each point in the target image, we perform a local patch-based search in the database and nearest neighbor information is used for estimating the target modality value for this point. The intuition behind our method comes from the observation that local and contextual similarities observed in one modality often extend to other modalities. Our method can be seen as a generalization of so-called label propagation (LP) strategies (cf. [12,13,14]), especially of the recent patch-based approaches [15,16]. LP has been very successful for certain segmentation tasks, being the de facto standard for brain anatomy segmentation. To our best knowledge, LP has so far been exclusively used in the setting of segmentation, with discrete, categorical labels. We show in this work that with certain generalizing modifications, the LP framework can be adapted to continuous non-categorical tasks with high-quality synthesis of arbitrary modalities. We refer to our approach as *modality propagation* (MP).

Label propagation operates in two steps. First, for each location in the target image a set of label candidates is determined from the database. Second, these candidates are fused into a single label based on one of the numerous fusion strategies. Label fusion has been shown to be crucial for achieving high-quality results for segmentation. However, currently available fusion strategies are specific to discrete categorical labels. For our general setting, dealing with continuous values, we replace the fusion step with a data-driven regularization approach. We show that this improves the quality – similar to fusion strategies – while being applicable to general problems, beyond segmentation. Our data-driven regularization is inspired by Image Analogies [17], using both source *and* target modalities within an iterative search-and-synthesis strategy.

After describing our MP framework in the next section, we demonstrate its properties on synthesis of MR-T2 and DTI-FA maps from MRI-T1 in (Sec 3.1). In Sec 3.2, we present the potential of our framework by proposing a novel approach for abnormality detection in multi-channel brain MRI where we synthesize patient-specific pseudo-healthy T2 images from T1, in order to highlight differences to the actual patients' T2 scans.

## 2   Coherent Synthesis via Modality Propagation

In the context of modality propagation, the process of synthesis refers to the following task: Given a source image $I$ with modality-specific information of the underlying anatomy, we seek to generate a corresponding target image $S$ of the same anatomy but from another modality. The new image $S$ is constructed using both subject-specific image $I$ and a population database. This database contains $N$ exemplar image pairs $\mathcal{T} = \{(I_n, S_n)\}_{n=1}^{N}$ where images $I_n$ and $S_n$ are assumed to be spatially aligned. The idea behind MP is that local similarities between structures both visible in $I$ and in the database images $\{I_n\}$ should indicate similarities between $\{S_n\}$ and $S$, the image to-be-synthesized. By finding correspondences between input $I$ and database $\{I_n\}$, information can be transferred from the set $\{S_n\}$ in order to synthesize $S$. This approach can be applied to arbitrary pairs of source and target modality.

For each image point $\mathbf{x}$ the estimate $S(\mathbf{x})$ is determined through patch-based nearest neighbor search within the population database $\mathcal{T}$. Previous works perform this search based on information extracted from images $I$ and $\{I_n\}$ only. In this context, we develop an iterative search-and-synthesis strategy which is inspired by Image Analogies [17]. The key idea is to incorporate the partly synthesized image into the nearest neighbor search.

Our algorithm is based on two main components which aim for improved coherency: 1) patch-based search in a restricted space, 2) iterative synthesis using intermediate results yielding a data-driven regularization.

***Search Space Restriction:*** For each image point $\mathbf{x}$ we perform a patch-based nearest neighbor search within the database images $\mathcal{T}$. The restriction of the search space is achieved on two different layers, a *spatial* and *population* layer. We enforce spatial restriction by assuming affine alignment of all subjects both within the population database and between the database and the input image $I$. Depending on the expected accuracy of the registration, this allows us to restrict the search to a small search window $W_{\mathbf{x}}$ centered at the point $\mathbf{x}$. A search window placed in a particular database image $I_n$ is denoted by $W_{\mathbf{x}}^{I_n}$.

Restriction at the population layer is achieved by obtaining a subset of database images that are most "similar" to $I$. The input image is divided into equally sized cells, and for each cell, the $k$ nearest neighbors in terms of sub-image dissimilarity are determined within the population database. The size of the sub-images is equal to the size of the cells, and the $k$ neighbors can be different for different cells. The patch-based search for all image points within a particular cell is restricted to the same set of $k$ database images. For notational convenience, we define a set of the $k$NN image indices as $\mathcal{N}_{\mathbf{x}}^{k}$ linked to an image point $\mathbf{x}$, instead of a cell.

The search space restriction is important for two reasons. First, a smaller search space yields lower computation times, in particular when dealing with larger databases. Second, and more importantly, the spatial restriction increases correlation between high patch similarity and correct anatomical correspondence.

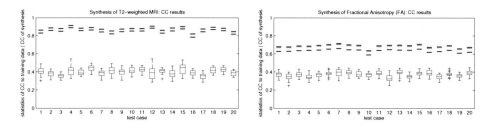

**Fig. 1.** Correlation coefficients between synthesis and ground truth after 1st, 2nd, and 3rd iteration in red, green, and blue for T2 and FA. The box plots summarize the CC distribution between ground truth and all database images.

***Iterative Synthesis:*** The actual task of synthesizing the output image $S$ is performed in an iterative manner. The first iteration is similar to well-known label propagation methods. A patch $P_{\mathbf{x}}^{I}$ centered at the image point $\mathbf{x}$ is extracted from the input image $I$. Based on the restriction strategy mentioned above, we perform a nearest neighbor search by evaluating patch dissimilarities between $P_{\mathbf{x}}^{I}$ and all patches in the spatio-population search space as

$$(\hat{n}, \hat{\mathbf{y}}) = \underset{n \in \mathcal{N}_{\mathbf{x}}^{k}; \mathbf{y} \in W_{\mathbf{x}}^{I_n}}{\arg\min} \; d(P_{\mathbf{x}}^{I}, P_{\mathbf{y}}^{I_n}) \; . \tag{1}$$

For $d$ we consider sum of squared differences (SSD), though other definitions, e.g. based on correlation, are possible. Based on Equation (1), we determine the best matching patch to be the one centered at $\hat{\mathbf{y}}$ in the database image $I_{\hat{n}}$. The synthesis image is then updated by setting $S(\mathbf{x}) := S_{\hat{n}}(\hat{\mathbf{y}})$. Once this is performed for all image points, we obtain a fully synthesized image $S$.

A limitation of this process is that the rich information in $\{S_n\}$ remains unused during search. This might yield inaccurate anatomical coherency and noisier outputs. Coherency of $S$ can be greatly improved when intermediate results are considered in a subsequent refinement. After obtaining an initial estimate of $S$, for subsequent iterations the patch-based nearest neighbor search is performed using a modified version of Equation (1) where we incorporate information from the synthesized modality:

$$(\hat{n}, \hat{\mathbf{y}}) = \underset{n \in \mathcal{N}_{\mathbf{x}}^{k}; \mathbf{y} \in W_{\mathbf{x}}^{I_n}}{\arg\min} \; (1 - \alpha) \, d(P_{\mathbf{x}}^{I}, P_{\mathbf{y}}^{I_n}) + \alpha \, f(P_{\mathbf{x}}^{S}, P_{\mathbf{y}}^{S_n}) \; . \tag{2}$$

Note, this definition covers the one for the first iteration when $\alpha = 0$. The metric $f$ depends on the nature of the target modality. In case of scalar-valued modalities, it can be the same as $d$. Integrating the synthesized data into the search yields a significant improvement on the spatial coherency. One can think of the function $f(P_{\mathbf{x}}^{S}, P_{\mathbf{y}}^{S_n})$ as a data driven regularization term. The effect of this term will be demonstrated in our experiments.

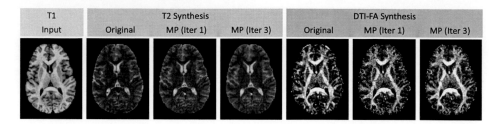

**Fig. 2.** Visual results for synthesis of T2 and FA maps from T1 MRI input. Synthesis is shown for the 1st and 3rd iteration. Note the reduction of noise and improved consistency of structural appearance both in T2 and FA. In particular, the white matter tracts in FA and the ventricle structures in T2 are well synthesized.

## 3    Experiments

Modality Propagation (MP) is a general tool that can be applied to possibly any source-target modality pair. Here we present two different applications of the algorithm: synthesis of T2 and FA MRI signals from T1, and abnormality detection via modality synthesis. We also analyze the impact of individual components, such as the iterative search-and-synthesis strategy.

We use the same parameter settings throughout all experiments. The size of patches $P$ is $3 \times 3 \times 3$ voxels, and the local search window $W$ is set to $9 \times 9 \times 9$. The database sub-image indices $\mathcal{N}^k$ are determined for cells with the same size as the search windows. We determine $k = 5$ nearest neighbors from the database for each cell. Synthesis starts with a weighting factor $\alpha = 0$, as no synthesized information is available initially. In subsequent iterations, the weighting is increased to reach $\alpha = 1$ yielding increased importance of the intermediate synthesis. This has the effect of data driven regularization. We found that 3 iterations are in general sufficient for MP to converge.

### 3.1    Synthesis of T2 and DTI-FA from T1 MRI

The first application is synthesis of T2 and FA from corresponding T1-weighted MR brain images. The goal of this experiment is to demonstrate synthesis of different structures mapping different physical properties, from the same input source. A possible use case for this is modality translation, e.g. for multi-modal registration [3]. We use the NAMIC database which has T1, T2 and Diffusion Tensor images (DTI) for 20 individuals, 10 normal controls and 10 schizophrenia patients (http://hdl.handle.net/1926/1687). We compute FA maps with the 3D Slicer software (http://www.slicer.org). Images are linearly registered, skull-stripped, inhomogeneity corrected, histogram-matched within each modality, and resampled to 2 mm resolution.

We apply a leave-one-out cross-validation, so each synthesis result is based on 19 subjects. This allows us to compute the similarity between the synthesized and the real images. Graphs in Figure 1 show the quantification of this image

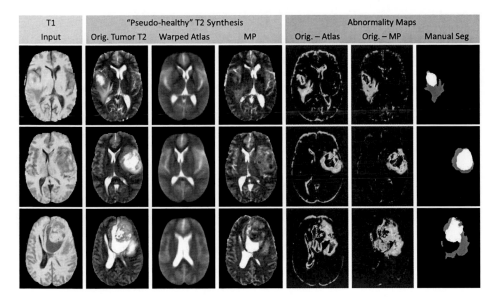

**Fig. 3.** Visual results for the abnormality detection using synthesis of "pseudo-healthy" images. We compare our results with a deformable atlas approach. The abnormality maps are computed by subtracting the warped atlas and the synthesized T2 from the original T2. For comparison, we also show manual tumor segmentations.

similarity. We use correlation coefficient (CC) as its normalized values allow us to compare the different experiments. The horizontal lines shown in red, green and blue indicate the CC after the 1st, 2nd and 3rd iteration of MP, respectively. To provide a comparative context, we also compute the CC between the ground truth and all database images. These values are summarized as box plots in the same figure. We make several observations: 1) The synthesized images are significantly closer to the real one than any other database image. 2) Synthesis for T2 gets closer to ground truth than for FA. We believe this is due to the fact that physical properties quantified by FA are very different from the ones quantified by T1 and T2. T1 and T2 capture more similar structures. Furthermore, FA contains more local information in terms of anisotropy and directionality of the tissue, and synthesizing FA from T1 is less accurate. 3) The improvement obtained by the 2nd and 3rd iteration is higher for FA than for T2. As the type of local information in FA is different, the anatomical coherency is not entirely captured using T1 as input. However, using the synthesized channel in the nearest neighbor search greatly improves the structural coherency.

Visual examples for T2 and FA synthesis after the 1st and 3rd iteration are shown in Figure 2. These images demonstrate the impact of the iterative algorithm. We observe that the prominent structures, such as the ventricles or the large white matter bundles, are accurately constructed. Smaller structures, such as small fiber tracts in the FA maps or thin sulci in T2, are less accurate. A larger training database could yield higher accuracies for smaller structures.

## 3.2   Abnormality Detection in Multi-Channel MRI

In our second application we build a system for abnormality detection which is based on the concept of comparing a suspicious image to an image of a healthy subject. Automatic techniques often make use of an atlas constructed from a healthy population. The atlas is spatially aligned with the test image, and subtraction of the two reveals differences (or abnormalities) in the test image. The main difficulty is the nonlinear registration in the presence of pathologies.

We take a synthesis approach making use of the properties of different MR signals commonly acquired for tumor patients. While for this particular tumor, pathological tissue enhances in T2 yielding a hyper-intense appearance, it does not substantially alter the intensity profile in (non-contrasted) T1. The patient's T1 image serves as input for synthesis of a "pseudo-healthy" T2 image by employing a database of 100 healthy subjects for which both T1 and T2 images are available (IXI database http://biomedic.doc.ic.ac.uk/brain-development/). Abnormality maps are computed by subtracting the synthesized T2 from the original T2 image. We use images of 20 tumor patients from the BRATS dataset (http://www2.imm.dtu.dk/projects/BRATS2012/)[1].

For comparison, we use an atlas constructed from the healthy-subjects and non-linearly registered onto the patients' T1 images. Figure 3 presents the visual results. The first four columns display patients' T1 and T2 images, the aligned atlas and the pseudo-healthy image synthesized using MP. The fifth and sixth column display the abnormality maps obtained by computing the differences between the patient's T2 image and the registered atlas, and the synthesized image. The last column displays manual tumor delineations. The abnormality maps obtained using MP are much cleaner, especially in areas not related to tumor, and abnormal areas are more prominent. Our approach provides a simple alternative which avoids the challenging nonlinear registration problem in presence of pathologies. These maps could be used for further segmentation steps.

## 4   Summary

We propose Modality Propagation, a general algorithm for patient-specific synthesis of arbitrary modalities, which employs population data, and generalizes the patch-based label propagation scheme. As main contributions of our work, we see: 1) Generalization of the LP strategy to arbitrary modalities, and showing that this general framework can obtain high-quality coherent results for applications beyond segmentation; 2) We propose an efficient data-driven regularization scheme for improvement of the result quality, as a general alternative to LP fusion strategies; 3) We propose a novel scheme for abnormality detection in multi-channel brain MRI, which utilizes the proposed MP framework. With increasing availability of population databases we believe our work can be an important component for developing subject-specific analysis tools.

---

[1] BRATS is organized by B. Menze, A. Jakab, S. Bauer, M. Reyes, M. Prastawa, and K. Van Leemput. The database contains fully anonymized images from following institutions: ETH Zurich, Univ. of Bern, Univ. of Debrecen, and Univ. of Utah.

# References

1. Prakosa, A., Sermesant, M., Delingette, H., Marchesseau, S., Saloux, E., Allain, P., Villain, N., Ayache, N.: Generation of Synthetic but Visually Realistic Time Series of Cardiac Images Combining a Biophysical Model and Clinical Images. IEEE TMI 32(1), 99–109 (2013)
2. Wein, W., Brunke, S., Khamene, A., Callstrom, M., Navab, N.: Automatic CT-ultrasound registration for diagnostic imaging and image-guided intervention. MedIA 12(5), 577–585 (2008)
3. Kroon, D., Slump, C.: MRI modalitiy transformation in demon registration. In: IEEE ISBI, pp. 963–966 (2009)
4. Cao, T., Zach, C., Modla, S., Powell, D., Czymmek, K., Niethammer, M.: Registration for correlative microscopy using image analogies. In: Dawant, B.M., Christensen, G.E., Fitzpatrick, J.M., Rueckert, D. (eds.) WBIR 2012. LNCS, vol. 7359, pp. 296–306. Springer, Heidelberg (2012)
5. Zhang, Y., Wu, G., Yap, P.T., Feng, Q., Lian, J., Chen, W., Shen, D.: Hierarchical Patch-Based Sparse Representation - A New Approach for Resolution Enhancement of 4D-CT Lung Data. IEEE TMI 31(11), 1993–2005 (2012)
6. Commowick, O., Warfield, S.K., Malandain, G.: Using frankenstein's creature paradigm to build a patient specific atlas. In: Yang, G.-Z., Hawkes, D., Rueckert, D., Noble, A., Taylor, C. (eds.) MICCAI 2009, Part II. LNCS, vol. 5762, pp. 993–1000. Springer, Heidelberg (2009)
7. Nuyts, J., Bal, G., Kehren, F., Fenchel, M., Michel, C., Watson, C.: Completion of a Truncated Attenuation Image from the Attenuated PET Emission Data. IEEE TMI 32(2), 237–246 (2013)
8. Roy, S., Carass, A., Shiee, N., Pham, D., Prince, J.: MR contrast synthesis for lesion segmentation. In: IEEE ISBI, pp. 932–935 (2010)
9. Roy, S., Carass, A., Bazin, P., Prince, J.: Intensity inhomogeneity correction of magnetic resonance images using patches. In: SPIE Med. Imaging (2011)
10. Rousseau, F.: Brain hallucination. In: Forsyth, D., Torr, P., Zisserman, A. (eds.) ECCV 2008, Part I. LNCS, vol. 5302, pp. 497–508. Springer, Heidelberg (2008)
11. Rueda, A., Malpica, N., Romero, E.: Single-image super-resolution of brain MR images using overcomplete dictionaries. MedIA 17(1), 113–132 (2013)
12. Rohlfing, T., Russakoff, D.B., Maurer, C.R.: Expectation maximization strategies for multi-atlas multi-label segmentation. In: Taylor, C.J., Noble, J.A. (eds.) IPMI 2003. LNCS, vol. 2732, pp. 210–221. Springer, Heidelberg (2003)
13. Wolz, R., Chu, C., Misawa, K., Mori, K., Rueckert, D.: Multi-organ Abdominal CT Segmentation Using Hierarchically Weighted Subject-Specific Atlases. In: Ayache, N., Delingette, H., Golland, P., Mori, K. (eds.) MICCAI 2012, Part I. LNCS, vol. 7510, pp. 10–17. Springer, Heidelberg (2012)
14. Artaechevarria, X., Munoz-Barrutia, A., Ortiz-de Solorzano, C.: Combination strategies in multi-atlas image segmentation: Application to brain MR data. IEEE TMI 28(8), 1266–1277 (2009)
15. Coupé, P., Manjón, J., Fonov, V., Pruessner, J., Robles, M., Collins, D.: Patch-based segmentation using expert priors: Application to hippocampus and ventricle segmentation. NeuroImage 54(2), 940–954 (2011)
16. Rousseau, F., Habas, P., Studholme, C.: A supervised patch-based approach for human brain labeling. IEEE TMI 30(10), 1852–1862 (2011)
17. Hertzmann, A., Jacobs, C., Oliver, N., Curless, B., Salesin, D.: Image Analogies. In: ACM Conference on Computer Graphics and Interactive Techniques (2001)

# Non-Local Spatial Regularization of MRI $T_2$ Relaxation Images for Myelin Water Quantification

Youngjin Yoo[1,3] and Roger Tam[2,3]

[1] Department of Electrical and Computer Engineering
[2] Department of Radiology
[3] MS/MRI Research Group,
University of British Columbia, Vancouver, BC, Canada

**Abstract.** Myelin is an essential component of nerve fibers and monitoring its health is important for studying diseases that attack myelin, such as multiple sclerosis (MS). The amount of water trapped within myelin, which is a surrogate for myelin content and integrity, can be measured *in vivo* using MRI relaxation techniques that acquire a series of images at multiple echo times to produce a $T_2$ decay curve at each voxel. These curves are then analyzed, most commonly using non-negative least squares (NNLS) fitting, to produce $T_2$ distributions from which water measurements are made. NNLS is unstable with respect to the noise and variations found in typical $T_2$ relaxation images, making some form of regularization inevitable. The current methods of NNLS regularization for measuring myelin water have two key limitations: 1) they use strictly local neighborhood information to regularize each voxel, which limits their effectiveness for very noisy images, and 2) the neighbors of each voxel contribute to its regularization equally, which can over-smooth fine details. To overcome these limitations, we propose a new regularization algorithm in which local and non-local information is gathered and used adaptively for each voxel. Our results demonstrate that the proposed method provides more globally consistent myelin water measurements yet preserves fine structures. Our experiment with real patient data also shows that the algorithm improves the ability to distinguish two sample groups, one of MS patients and the other of healthy subjects.

**Keywords:** $T_2$ relaxation, quantitative MRI, brain, white matter, myelin, regularization.

## 1 Introduction

Myelin water fraction (MWF) is an imaging surrogate biomarker for myelin, and is currently the only myelin-specific quantitative MRI measure. Central nervous system (CNS) tissue is inhomogeneous and has two main water environments, one within the myelin, the other being intracellular and extracellular water. MWF is defined as the ratio of myelin water over the total amount of water.

K. Mori et al. (Eds.): MICCAI 2013, Part I, LNCS 8149, pp. 614–621, 2013.

Most MWF studies are done only in white matter (WM), which contains most of the myelin. Normal appearing white matter (NAWM) in MS patients has lower MWF than WM from control subjects, suggesting that myelin loss is a key feature of NAWM pathology in MS. Although multi-echo $T_2$ relaxation with the non-negative least squares (NNLS) algorithm used to fit a $T_2$ decay curve with a $T_2$ distribution [1] is a strong candidate for monitoring demyelination and remyelination in MS patients, one of its current main drawbacks is limited reproducibility due to the instability of the NNLS algorithm. This causes the technique to work well only on data of high SNR; unfortunately, this is often not a practical assumption as $T_2$ relaxation data tend to be noisy. To improve the robustness of MWF computation, applying various denoising methods to the multi-echo images have been studied [2,3,4,5]. Regularization approaches for NNLS have been also studied, ranging from the conventional Tikhonov regularization [6,7], which is non-spatial, to smoothing methods that work by averaging the neighboring spectra to constrain the NNLS of a given voxel [8]. While the spatial regularization methods have been shown to improve MWF reproducibility, the current approaches only use a small local neighborhood for each voxel, and do not take advantage of more distant neighbors that may have similar $T_2$ distributions. In addition, these methods assume that neighboring voxels always have similar $T_2$ distributions, which is not the case in areas with fine details, such as the WM structures near the cortex of the brain, and such details can be lost during regularization.

We present a spatial regularization method that reduces global variability by using information from non-local voxels but also improves fine details by using weighted averaging that avoids combining $T_2$ distributions that are very different. The algorithm starts with an initial $T_2$ distribution estimate using the conventional Tikhonov regularized NNLS algorithm. These distributions are then used in a non-local means algorithm [9], using the symmetric Kullback-Leibler (SKL) divergence [10] to quantify the similarity between distributions, to compute the priors for a spatially regularized NNLS, which produces the final $T_2$ distribution for each voxel. We show that by incorporating non-local means for $T_2$ distributions into a spatially regularized NNLS framework, an accurate and robust MWF map can be produced. We demonstrate on real MRIs that the method improves the consistency of MWF measurements and the ability to distinguish between MS patients and healthy subjects.

## 2   Preliminaries

Whittall and MacKay proposed a multi-exponential analysis for MRI [1,7] based on the NNLS algorithm of Lawson and Hanson [11], which inverts a relaxation decay curve to a relaxation time distribution. A set of exponential basis functions characterizes the measured signal $y_i$

$$y_i = \sum_{j=1}^{M} s_j e^{-t_i/T_{2j}} = \sum_{j=1}^{M} a_{ij} s_j, \quad i = 1, 2, \dots, N, \tag{1}$$

where $t_i$ is the measurement time, $M$ is the number of logarithmically spaced $T_2$ decay times, $N$ represents the total number of data points (number of acquired $T_2$ echoes, 32 in our data), $s_j$ is the relative amplitude for each partitioned $T_2$ time, $T_{2j}$, and $\mathbf{A} = [a_{i,j}]_{N \times M}$. The set of $s_j$ represents the $T_2$ distribution for which we need to solve. The NNLS algorithm [11] is used to minimize

$$\chi^2_{\min} = \min_{s \geq 0} \left[ \sum_{i=1}^{N} \left| \sum_{j=1}^{M} a_{ij} s_j - y_i \right|^2 \right]. \tag{2}$$

Extra constraints can be incorporated into Eq. 2 to provide more robust fits in the presence of noise [7], using the additional term on the right.

$$\chi^2_r = \min_{s \geq 0} \left[ \sum_{i=1}^{N} \left| \sum_{j=1}^{M} a_{ij} s_j - y_i \right|^2 + \mu \sum_{k=1}^{K} \left| \sum_{j=1}^{M} s_j - f_k \right|^2 \right] \tag{3}$$

where $\mathbf{f}$ is the corresponding vector of right-hand side values. With a given target value for the misfit $\chi^2_r$, the parameter $\mu$ is automatically determined by the generalized cross-validation approach. From Eq. 3, the $T_2$ distribution can be estimated as the set of $s_j$ for the decay times $T_{2j}$. If $\mathbf{f}$ is set to 0, Eq. 3 is equivalent to the conventional Tikhonov regularization, which we abbreviate as rNNLS.

In the closest related work [8] to ours, the $T_2$ distribution prior $\mathbf{f}$ in Eq. 3 is estimated by averaging the spectra of nine neighboring voxels of each voxel, which achieves spatial regularization but can smooth over fine details.

## 3   Method

We compute an initial $T_2$ distribution for each voxel using rNNLS. The regularization parameter $\mu$ is selected such that $\chi^2_r$ in Eq. 3 is equal to $1.02\chi^2_{\min}$ where $\chi^2_{\min}$ is the unregularized minimum misfit found in Eq. 2. The constant multiplier is set to 1.02 to be consistent with previously reported works using Tikhonov regularization [8,12]. Given initial $T_2$ distributions $\mathbf{s} = \{\mathbf{s}(i) \mid i \in I\}$ for an image $I$, a $T_2$ distribution prior $\mathbf{f}(i)$, for a voxel position $i$, is computed using the non-local means algorithm [9] as a weighted average of all the $T_2$ distributions in $I$,

$$f_k(i) = \sum_{j \in I} w(i,j) s_k(j), \quad \forall k \in \{1, 2, \ldots, K\}, \tag{4}$$

where the weight $w(i,j)$ depends on the similarity between the distributions at voxel $i$ and $j$, and satisfies the conditions $0 \leq w \leq 1$ and $\sum_j w(i,j) = 1$. $K$ is set to be the number of logarithmically spaced $T_2$ decay times. The similarity between the two distributions at $i$ and $j$ are measured from the $T_2$ distribution vectors $v(D_i)$ and $v(D_j)$, where $D_c$ denotes a square neighborhood of fixed size $D$ and centered at voxel position $c$. By treating each $T_2$ distribution in a voxel as a probability distribution, the similarity between $v(D_i)$ and $v(D_j)$ can be measured by the SKL divergence [10] as follows

$$E(v(D_i), v(D_j)) = \frac{1}{V} \sum_{\substack{\rho \in v(D_i) \\ \varrho \in v(D_j)}} \mathrm{SKL}_{\mathrm{div}}(\mathbf{s}(\rho) \parallel \mathbf{s}(\varrho)) \qquad (5)$$

where $V$ is the number of voxels in a square neighborhood, $\mathbf{s}(\rho)$ and $\mathbf{s}(\varrho)$ are normalized versions of the distributions, and the SKL divergence is defined as

$$\mathrm{SKL}_{\mathrm{div}}(\mathbf{s}(\rho) \parallel \mathbf{s}(\varrho)) = \sum_{k=1}^{K} \left( s_k(\rho) \log \left[ \frac{s_k(\rho)}{s_k(\varrho)} \right] + s_k(\varrho) \log \left[ \frac{s_k(\varrho)}{s_k(\rho)} \right] \right). \qquad (6)$$

The weight $w$ used in Eq. 4 is defined as

$$w(i, j) = \frac{1}{\sum_{j \in I} e^{-\left( \frac{E(v(D_i), v(D_j))}{h} \right)^2}} e^{-\left( \frac{E(v(D_i), v(D_j))}{h} \right)^2} \qquad (7)$$

where the parameter $h$ controls the degree of filtering.

After computation of the spatial $T_2$ distribution prior $\mathbf{f}$, the final regularized $T_2$ distribution is estimated by the NNLS algorithm in Eq. 3. The MWF for each voxel is defined as the percentage of signal having a $T_2$ between 15 and 50 ms. To vary the degree of regularization, the target value for the misfit $\chi_r^2$ is adjusted relative to $\chi_{min}^2$ in Eq. 2 by a multiplier $\eta$, which in turns determines $\mu$. Since the parameters largely depend on noise level, we randomly selected one subject from our data sets for tuning, which should not bias the overall results. We empirically select the parameters $\eta$ and $h$ to produce the most homogeneous MWF maps in the NAWM of the subject, as measured by the coefficient of variation (CoV). The CoV is generally reduced with higher $\eta$ and $h$. We first chose $\eta$, starting with $\eta = 1.02$ and increased by 0.01 until the decrease in CoV stabilized. Next we chose $h$ similarly. We use $\eta = 1.07$ and $h = 1.5$ for all of the experiments. For practical purposes, we use a fixed search window of $21 \times 21$ and set the neighborhood size for computing the SKL divergence to $7 \times 7$, as this has been shown to be effective for non-local denoising of other types of images [9] and structural MRI images [13]. Due to the strong anisotropy of our test data we apply the regularization in 2D on a slice-by-slice basis.

## 4   Results

In this section, we compare three methods of NNLS regularization for MWF computation: Tikhonov regularization (rNNLS), the spatial regularization presented in [8] (srNNLS), and our proposed non-local spatial regularization (nlsrNNLS). The methods are evaluated under three criteria: the visual quality of the MWF maps, CoV within the NAWM of healthy subjects, and the ability to distinguish between healthy subjects and MS patients as measured by Student's $t$-tests and overlapping coefficients (OVLs). All experiments are performed on the NAWM regions of each scan. The $T_2$ relaxation sequence consists of a $90°$ excitation pulse followed by 32 slab-selective refocusing pulses (32 echoes, TR = 1200 ms, TE = 10 ms – 320 ms, echo spacing 10 ms), with voxel size = $0.937 \times 0.937 \times 5$mm and image dimensions $256 \times 256 \times 7$ voxels. All images are acquired on a Philips Achieva 3T scanner. To measure CoV, the MRIs of twenty healthy subjects are used. WM segmentation masks are created from registered $T_1$-weighted images using the FAST software [14]. For the $t$-tests and OVLs, the scans of 18 healthy subjects and 17 MS patients are used. Each subject was scanned at month 0 (baseline) and month 6. Using a C++ GPU implementation, rNNLS, srNNLS and nlsrNNLS take about 10, 16, and 20 mins respectively to process the data for one patient.

## 4.1   Visual Assessment

Figure 2 shows a comparison of the visual quality in the MWF maps of a healthy subject and an MS patient. Both srNNLS and nlsrNNLS appear to reduce spatial variability and noise, but nlsrNNLS produces greater spatial coherence overall and is clearly better than both other methods at reconstructing the finer details in the thin WM structures near the cortex. The MS lesions in the MWF map of the MS patient produced by nlsrNNLS are more clearly visible and have more distinct boundaries.

## 4.2   Coefficient of Variation

In order to compare the variability within the MWF maps produced by each method, we measure the CoV within the WM of each scan of 20 healthy subjects (Figure 1). Both spatial regularization methods significantly improve CoV over rNNLS, with nlsrNNLS being slightly better than srNNLS. The mean CoV values and standard errors are shown in Table 1. There is a statistically significant group difference ($p = 5.12 \times 10^{-5}$) between srNNLS (mean CoV = 1.10) and nlsrNNLS (mean CoV = 0.97).

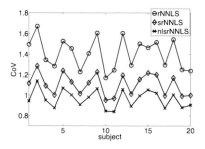

**Fig. 1.** Comparison of CoV measured on MWF maps of 20 healthy subjects

**Table 1.** Mean CoV measured on the WM of 20 healthy subjects. The $p$-value is computed by a two-sample $t$-test between srNNLS and nlsrNNLS.

|  | CoV |
|---|---|
| rNNLS [7] | $1.4060 \pm 0.1498$ |
| srNNLS [8] | $1.1047 \pm 0.1052$ |
| **nlsrNNLS** | **$0.9653 \pm 0.0861$** |
| $p$-value | $5.1240 \times 10^{-5}$ |

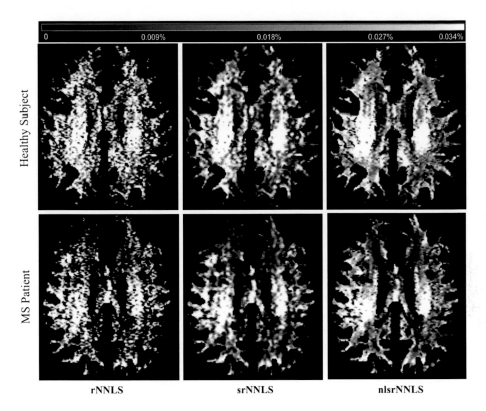

**Fig. 2.** Comparison of MWF maps produced by rNNLS [7] (left), srNNLS [8] (middle) and nlsrNNLS (right) algorithms in WM for healthy subject (top) and MS patient (bottom). The nlsrNNLS shows an improved visibility of the MWF maps with reduced noise and sharp details preserved.

### 4.3   Student's *t*-test and Overlapping Coefficient

The data for 18 healthy subjects and 17 MS patients are used to compare the ability of the three regularization methods to distinguish between these two groups. The three mean MWF values computed from each group are shown in Figure 3. The mean MWF values from the MS patients are significantly lower ($p < 0.05$ for all three regularization methods) than those from the healthy subjects at both month 0 and month 6. The $p$-values computed using $t$-tests between the MS patients and healthy subjects are shown in Table 2. The nlsrNNLS method yields the lowest $p$-values in this data set, which suggests it can produce MWF maps that are more sensitive to the differences between MS and healthy brains. To confirm this result, we construct normal distributions for each group and compute the OVL as a second measure of how well the patients and normals can be distinguished. The results from this test for all three regularization methods are summarized in Table 2. Again, the nlsrNNLS yields the best results by producing the lowest overlap values.

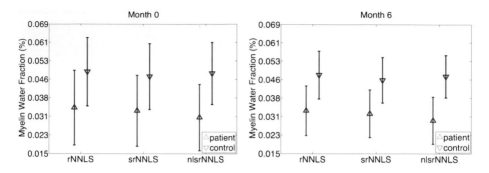

**Fig. 3.** Mean MWF values produced by the three regularization algorithms from 18 healthy and 17 MS patients at baseline (left) and month 6 (right). Error bars are standard errors. The nlsrNNLS shows the most clear difference between the two groups.

**Table 2.** Overlapping coefficients and $t$-test $p$-values for distinguishing between 18 healthy subjects and 17 MS patients computed using the MWF maps produced by the three regularization algorithms. All $p$-values are significant ($< 0.05$), but nlsrNNLS produces MWF values that are most sensitive for distinguishing the two groups.

|  | Month 0 | | Month 6 | |
|---|---|---|---|---|
|  | OVL | $p$-value | OVL | $p$-value |
| rNNLS [7] | 0.6137 | $7.2 \times 10^{-3}$ | 0.4628 | $2.0260 \times 10^{-4}$ |
| srNNLS [8] | 0.6157 | $7.4 \times 10^{-3}$ | 0.4701 | $2.4650 \times 10^{-4}$ |
| **nlsrNNLS** | **0.4915** | **$4.3543 \times 10^{-4}$** | **0.3241** | **$3.7601 \times 10^{-6}$** |

## 5   Conclusion

We have presented a non-local spatial regularization for the NNLS algorithm to reliably measure myelin water in WM *in vivo*. The proposed spatial $T_2$ distribution prior is adaptively estimated based on the SKL divergence, and exploits information from the global WM region. Three different regularization methods have been compared using three main criteria (visual quality, CoV and ability to distinguish between MS patients and normals), and it has been observed that the proposed nlsrNNLS algorithm compares favorably with the other methods. Future work would include further optimization of algorithmic parameters, validation beyond a single scanner, longitudinal/ROIs studies (including lesions), scan-to-scan variability, and investigation of how well nlsrNNLS would work in combination with denoising strategies applied to the multi-echo images [4,5].

**Acknowledgements.** The authors gratefully acknowledge Drs. Irene Vavasour and Alex MacKay for the use of their data and Drs. Anthony Traboulsee and David Li for helpful discussions. This work was supported by funding from the

University of British Columbia and the Natural Sciences and Engineering Research Council of Canada.

# References

1. MacKay, A., Whittall, K., Adler, J., Li, D.K.B., Paty, D., Graeb, D.: In vivo visualization of myelin water in brain by magnetic resonance. Magnetic Resonance in Medicine 31, 673–677 (1994)
2. Jones, C., Whittall, K., MacKay, A.: Robust myelin water quantification: averaging vs. spatial filtering. Magnetic Resonance in Medicine 50, 206–209 (2003)
3. Hwang, D., Chung, H., Nam, Y.: Robust mapping of the myelin water fraction in the presence of noise: Synergic combination of anisotropic diffusion filter and spatially regularized nonnegative least squares algorithm. Journal of Magnetic Resonance Imaging 195, 189–195 (2011)
4. Jang, U., Hwang, D.: High-quality multiple $T_2^*$ contrast MR images from low-quality multi-echo images using temporal-domain denoising methods. Medical Physics 39, 468–474 (2012)
5. Kwon, O., Woo, E., Du, Y., Hwang, D.: A tissue-relaxation-dependent neighboring method for robust mapping of the myelin water fraction. NeuroImage, 1–10 (2013)
6. Tikhonov, A.: Solution of incorrectly formulated problems and the regularization method. Soviet Math. Doklady 4, 1035–1038 (1963)
7. Whittall, K., MacKay, A.: Quantitative interpretation of NMR relaxation data. Journal of Magnetic Resonance 84, 134–152 (1989)
8. Hwang, D., Du, Y.: Improved myelin water quantification using spatially regularized non-negative least squares algorithm. Journal of Magnetic Resonance Imaging 30, 203–208 (2009)
9. Buades, A., Coll, B., Morel, J.: A Non-Local Algorithm for Image Denoising. In: IEEE Computer Society Conference on Computer Vision and Pattern Recognition, vol. 2, pp. 60–65. IEEE, Washington, DC (2005)
10. Johnson, D., Sinanovic, S.: Symmetrizing the Kullback-Leibler distance. IEEE Transactions Information Theory (2001)
11. Lawson, C., Hanson, R.: Solving least squares problems. Prentice-Hall, Englewood Cliffs (1974)
12. Levesque, I., Chia, C., Pike, G.: Reproducibility of in vivo magnetic resonance imaging-based measurement of myelin water. Journal of Magnetic Resonance Imaging 32, 60–68 (2010)
13. Manjón, J., Carbonell-Caballero, J., Lull, J., García-Martí, G., Martí-Bonmatí, L., Robles, M.: MRI denoising using non-local means. Medical Image Analysis 12, 514–523 (2008)
14. Zhang, Y., Brady, M., Smith, S.: Segmentation of brain MR images through a hidden Markov random field model and the expectation-maximization algorithm. IEEE Transactions on Medical Imaging 20, 45–57 (2001)

# Robust Myelin Quantitative Imaging from Multi-echo T2 MRI Using Edge Preserving Spatial Priors

Xiaobo Shen[1], Thanh D. Nguyen[2], Susan A. Gauthier[2], and Ashish Raj[2]

[1] Department of Computer Science, Cornell University, Ithaca, NY
xs83@cornell.edu
[2] Department of Radiology, Weill Cornell Medical College, New York, NY
{tdn2001,sag2015,asr2004}@med.cornell.edu

**Abstract.** Demyelinating diseases such as multiple sclerosis cause changes in the brain white matter microstructure. Multi-exponential T2 relaxometry is a powerful technology for detecting these changes by generating a myelin water fraction (MWF) map. However, conventional approaches are subject to noise and spatial in-consistence. We proposed a novel approach by imposing spatial consistency and smoothness constraints. We first introduce a two-Gaussian model to approximate the T2 distribution. Then an expectation-maximization framework is introduced with an edge-preserving prior incorporated. Three-dimensional multi-echo MRI data sets were collected from three patients and three healthy volunteers. MWF maps ob-tained using the conventional, Spatially Regularized Non-negative Least Squares (srNNLS) algorithm as well as the proposed algorithm are compared. The proposed method provides MWF maps with improved depiction of brain structures and significantly lower coefficients of variance in various brain regions.

**Keywords:** T2 relaxometry, myelin water fraction, edge-preserving priors.

## 1 Introduction

Multi-echo T2 relaxometry is a MR imaging technique in which a series of T2-weighted images are obtained at different echo times. It is a powerful tool to detect tissue damages in various demyelinating diseases such as multiple sclerosis (MS) [1]. By fitting a multi-exponential decay curve to this data, it is possible to deduce the T2 distribution of various water compartments in brain tissues to analyze their contributions separately. In particular, this analysis can provide numerical evaluation of the relative contribution of the myelin water compartment, represented as myelin water fraction (MWF), which can be used to assess the healthiness of white matter (WM).

Conventional approach [2] to extracting MWF can be easily impacted by small amounts of measurement noise and image artifacts. Consequently, diagnostically acceptable quality can only come from greatly increasing the number of sampled echoes [3] or much higher SNR, but these cause clinically unfeasible scan time. To reduce scan time, several authors have proposed alternative methods based on the gradient echo data acquisition with multi-compartmental steady-state signal [4], [5].

K. Mori et al. (Eds.): MICCAI 2013, Part I, LNCS 8149, pp. 622–630, 2013.
© Springer-Verlag Berlin Heidelberg 2013

Recently, spatial smoothing constraints were proposed to improve the stability of the solution [6], [7]; however, these methods nevertheless rely on the single-voxel approach with a strong reliance on a pre-computed reference image. We have recently developed a spatial constrained algorithm parameterizing the T2 distribution into 2 Gaussian peaks and a long T2 component. Not only does this approach reduce the number of unknowns into 8 per voxel, it also allows for efficient, iterative conjugate gradient type algorithms. However, global, convex constraints are subject to tissue boundary blurring.

In this paper, we extend the spatial constrained approach to incorporate an edge-preserving prior (EPP) proposed by Raj et al [8] into a expectation-maximization (EM) style framework. The maximization (energy minimization) part applies EPP to the height parameters of two Gaussian peaks with a Quadratic Pseudo-Binary Optimization (QPBO) algorithm[9]. The expectation part updates other parameters with a nonlinear least square algorithm. We demonstrate the improvements by comparing the proposed method with the conventional and Spatially Regularized Non-negative Least Squares Algorithm (srNNLS method) [6] using visual and numerical assessments on simulated data and in vivo data.

## 2      Theory

### 2.1      Conventional T2 Relaxometry Analysis

At each voxel, given MR signals y measured at echo times $TE_k$ (k = 1,..., K), a set i = 1,...,N of discrete sub-components are hypothesized to exist, each producing an exponentially decaying signal $\alpha_i \exp(-TE_k/T_2(i))$ with a known T2 constant of $T_2(i)$ and an unknown volume fraction of $\alpha_i$ . Assuming a slow exchange regime [10], the signal equation can be written as following:

$$y(TE_k) = \sum_{i=1}^{N} \alpha_i \exp\left(-\frac{TE_k}{T_2(i)}\right) + \varepsilon \qquad (1)$$

or equivalently, $\mathbf{y} = \mathbf{A}\mathbf{x} + \boldsymbol{\varepsilon}$, with $\mathbf{A}_{ki} = \exp(-TE_k/T_2(i))$. Vector $\mathbf{y}$ is a collection of data $y_k$ acquired at echo time $TE_k$, $\mathbf{x}$ is a vector of the unknown $\alpha_i$, and $\boldsymbol{\varepsilon}$ denotes the noise vector. This linear system is typically under-determined (N>K) and ill-posed, making it hard to solve for $\mathbf{x}$ [2], [11]. Voxel-wise Tikhonov regularization [12] was proposed to partially overcome this problem with a non-negative least square (NNLS) algorithm. Unfortunately, the robustness requires extremely high SNR and more sampled echoes [13].

### 2.2      Multi-voxel Iterative Expectation-Maximization (EM) style Algorithm

Our proposed method encodes an EPP that T2 characteristics of the water compartments change smoothly within coherent brain regions but change abruptly across region boundaries. We first model the T2 distribution as a sum of two Gaussian distributions (one for the fast relaxing myelin water pool (T2~20 ms) and the other for the slower intra/extracellular water pool (T2~80 ms)), whose parameters (mean location, height and variance) are unknown. We also add a very long relaxing cerebrospinal fluid (CSF) pool with unknown T2 and strength. Thus in the i-th voxel $v_i$ we have the following set of unknowns: $\theta(v_i) = \{\alpha_1(i), m_1(i), \sigma_1(i), \alpha_2(i), m_2(i), \sigma_2(i), h_{CSF}(i), m_{CSF}(i)\}$, where $\alpha$, m and $\sigma$ stand for the height, mean and variance of the Gaussian peak, and $h_{CSF}$ and $m_{CSF}$ are the height and location for the CSF signal. So the T2 distribution at that voxel is: $x_i(\tau) = G(\theta(v_i), \tau) = \alpha_1(i)\mathcal{N}(\tau | m_1(i), \sigma_1(i)) + \alpha_2(i)\mathcal{N}(\tau | m_2(i), \sigma_2(i)) + h_{CSF}(i)\delta(\tau - m_{CSF}(i))$, where each Gaussian is denoted as $\mathcal{N}(\cdot)$, $\delta$ denotes the delta function, and the T2 distribution is over the variable $\tau$ which is a set of sampled T2. By keeping $\tau$ fixed for all voxels, we have $x_i = G(\theta(v_i))$. Secondly, we collect multi-voxel parameters into a vector $\bar{\theta} = \{\theta(v_i), i = 1, ..., N_v\}$, and map the Gaussian parameters to the resulting vectors of T2 distributions for all voxels by $\bar{x} = G(\bar{\theta})$. Single voxel quantity $y$ is also collected into a multi-voxel vector $\bar{y}$. The expanded matrix is similarly defined as $A_{exp}$. We then use the nonlinear least square (NLS) algorithm to minimize the non-convex function:

$$\hat{\theta} = \arg\min_{\bar{\theta}} \|\bar{y} - A_{exp}G(\bar{\theta})\|^2 + \mu_N\|D_N\bar{\theta}\|^2 \tag{2}$$

Where $D_N$ is a diagonal matrix whose diagonal elements are the normalization factors corresponding to each element in $\theta(v_i)$, and $\mu_N$ is the overall regularization scalar. We also define the residual data cost vector $\bar{C} = \{c(v_i), i = 1, ..., N_v\}$ for all voxels, and it can be simply calculated by substituting $\bar{\theta}$ into the following equation:

$$\bar{C} = \|\bar{y} - A_{exp}G(\bar{\theta})\|^2 + \mu_N\|D_N\bar{\theta}\|^2 \tag{3}$$

Thirdly, we can obtain the optimized $\widehat{\alpha_1}$ and $\widehat{\alpha_2}$ from $\hat{\theta}$ in Eq. 2. The optimized $\hat{C}$ is obtained by substituting $\hat{\theta}$ into Eq. 3. $\hat{C}$, $\widehat{\alpha_1}$ and $\widehat{\alpha_2}$ provide the prior information which can be used for constructing the costs of single-voxel (unary) and pairwise terms for QPBO. Towards the construction, the value ranges of $\widehat{\alpha_1}$ and $\widehat{\alpha_2}$ are first discretized into $n$ levels respectively, and each level is for a candidate $\alpha$-expansion move [8]. The discretization is carried out non-uniformly based on the frequency of values in $\widehat{\alpha_1}$ or $\widehat{\alpha_2}$. After discretization, we have $n$ levels $l_1 = \{min(\widehat{\alpha_1}), ..., max(\widehat{\alpha_1})\}$ for $\overline{\alpha_1}$. For each potential $\alpha$-expansion for $\widehat{\alpha_1}$ where $\alpha \in l_1$, the cost $\bar{C}_{exp}$ can be calculated by replacing $\alpha_1$ of all voxels in $\hat{\theta}$ with the

**Table 1.** Cost definition, where $N_p$ is the number of pixels at slice $s$, and $\hat{C}_s$ and $\bar{C}_{exp_s}$ denote the subset for only slice $s$. Binary label $b_i = 1$ indicates an expansion move to $\alpha$ at pixel i. $\widehat{\alpha_{1_s}}$ denotes the subset for only slice $s$, and $Nei$ is a set of all non-duplicated neighbor pixel index pairs on slice $s$.

| Unary or pairwise term | Cost |
|---|---|
| $B_1(b_i)$  $i \in \{1, ..., N_p\}, b_i = 0$ | $\hat{C}_s(i)$ |
| $B_1(b_i)$  $b_i = 1$ | $\bar{C}_{exp_s}(i)$ |
| $B_2(b_i, b_j)$  $(i,j) \in Nei, i \neq j, b_i = 0, b_j = 0$ | $|\widehat{\alpha_{1_s}}(i) - \widehat{\alpha_{1_s}}(j)|$ |
| $B_2(b_i, b_j)$  $b_i = 0, b_j = 1$ | $|\widehat{\alpha_{1_s}}(i) - \alpha|$ |
| $B_2(b_i, b_j)$  $b_i = 1, b_j = 0$ | $|\alpha - \widehat{\alpha_{1_s}}(j)|$ |
| $B_2(b_i, b_j)$  $b_i = 1, b_j = 1$ | $0$ |

scalar $\alpha$ and then substituting the modified $\hat{\theta}$ into Eq. 3. Since the slice separation of MR data is much larger than slice resolution, we applied QPBO algorithm slice by slice. The unary and pairwise costs for each slice $s$ are defined in Table 1.

Based on Table 1, we minimize the following function for slice $s$ by QPBO (M part):

$$E_s = \arg\min_{b_i, b_j} \sum_{i=1}^{N} D_1(b_i) + \mu_S \sum_{(i,j) \in Nei} B_2(b_i, b_j) \qquad for\ \forall i, \qquad b_i \in \{0, 1\} \qquad (4)$$

where $\mu_S$ is the spatial regularization scalar for all pairwise cost terms. If the resulted binary label $b_i = 1$, we update $\widehat{\alpha_{1_s}}(i) = \alpha$ and $\hat{C}_s(i) = \bar{C}_{exp_s}(i)$, and we do this for all slices. The expansion moves for $\widehat{\alpha_2}$ are achieved in the same manner. After finishing all expansion moves for $\widehat{\alpha_1}$ and $\widehat{\alpha_2}$, we update the remaining 6 parameters in $\hat{\theta}$ by using a NLS algorithm (E part). This can be simply done by minimizing Eq. 4 with fixed $\alpha_1$ and $\alpha_2$ terms. Typically over 2-4 iterations, we can obtain stable results.

# 3     Methods

## 3.1     Data

(1) **Real data.** One healthy volunteer at 1.5T using the conventional 3D multi-echo spin echo (MESE) sequence, two healthy volunteers and three MS patients at 3T using a 3D T2prep spiral sequence were obtained on a commercial MR imager (GE HDxt, GE Healthcare, Waukesha, WI). The imaging parameters were as follows: 3D MESE: axial FOV = 30 cm, matrix size = 256x128, partial phase FOV factor = 0.6, slice thickness = 5 mm, number of slices = 12, TR = 2500 ms, echo spacing = 5 ms, number of TEs = 32, scan time = 38 min; 3D T2prep spiral: axial FOV = 24-30 cm, matrix size = 192x192, slice thickness = 5 mm, number of slices = 32, TR = 2500 ms, flip angle = 10°, number of TEs = 15-26, scan time = 10-26 min. The SNR of a data set was calculated according to [14]. The average SNR of the three healtjy data sets was 339±150. The average SNR of three MS subjects was 456±46.

(2) **Simulated data.** Synthetic image data based on Montreal Neurological Institute (MNI) brain template were generated at SNR level varying from 100 to 1000. We first set the volume fraction weighted by the probabilities of WM and GM from the MNI template. Then Gaussian noise is artificially added to generate different SNR levels.

## 3.2     Algorithm Implementation and Parameter Optimization

Lsqnonlin function in MATLAB (R2011b) was used to solve Eq. 2. QPBO package (Version 1.3) was used. The whole program runs on a PC (Intel core 2 Duo processor at 2.2GHz, 4GB memory). Sparse matrices were adopted for storing voxel indexing used by lsqnonlin and pairwise voxel neighborhood.

We adopted a supervised trial and error method to find the optimal $\mu_N$ and $\mu_S$ with different choices of $\mu_N$ or $\mu_S$ varying logarithmically from $10^{-2}$ to $10^{-4}$.

We assess the spatial quality of the MWF map and the numerical residual of NLS fitting for each choice and we select the value that represents the best compromise between data fidelity and visual quality. The processing duration was collected by running proposed algorithm with optimal parameter sets. The diagonal values of matrix $D_N$ were determined empirically based on our knowledge to the general T2 distribution of brain voxels. For instance, we assign higher values (higher penalty) to its elements corresponding to myelin water pool because this pool accounts for smaller percentage of total signal.

### 3.3     Evaluation criteria

MWF was calculated as the ratio of signal integral from the myelin water signal to the integral of the total signal. For simulated data, mean square errors (MSE) of the algorithm resulted MWF maps with the true MWF maps were calculated at various SNR.

For MR data, Two quantitative criteria were used to compare the proposed algorithm to the conventional algorithm: 1) the spatial variation of MWF map within brain structures, as measured by the coefficient of variance (COV); 2) the ability to distinguish myelin-rich WM from lesion, as measured by the p-value (two-tailed two-sample t-tests) of MWF differences observed between selected normal WM ROI and selected lesion ROI in each patient subject. P-values of less than 0.05 were considered statistically significant.

## 4     Results

Figure 1 compares MSE of MWF maps for brain simulated data, demonstrating the improved accuracy obtained with the proposed method compared to the srNNLS method and the conventional method, particularly at low SNR.

**Fig. 1.** Comparisons of mean square error (MSE) of the MWF map for Brain Simulation among three methods at SNR $\in$ {100, 300, 500, 1000}

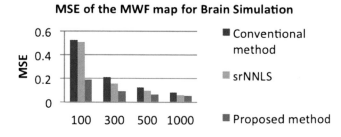

For real data, Figure 2 shows MWF maps obtained from three healthy subjects. The proposed approach provides higher spatial coherence and better depiction of the WM structures. Bottom row of Figure 2 shows anatomical T2-prep spiral images wherein regions of low signal intensity correspond to WM tissues with high myelin content (except CSF regions which also appear dark). Table 2 summarizes mean COVs calculated within various regions for the MWF maps of the three subjects.

**Table 2.** Comparisons of Mean Coefficient of Variance (COV) of MWF in various ROIs

|  | Mean Coefficient of Variance (COV) of MWF maps | | |
|  | Conventional | srNNLS | Proposed |
|---|---|---|---|
| WM | 0.8358 | 0.7638 | 0.1287 |
| GM | 1.1479 | 0.9873 | 0.2023 |
| Genu of corpus callosum | 0.4505 | 0.3702 | 0.0850 |
| Splenium of corpus callosum | 0.4781 | 0.4003 | 0.1084 |
| Internal capsule | 0.2775 | 0.2476 | 0.0629 |

Three patient sets were used for assessing performance of differentiating normal WM and lesion. The average P-values for Conventional, srNNLS and proposed method are 0.086, 0.069 and 0.0018. Figure 3 is the selected visual results for lesion differentiation.

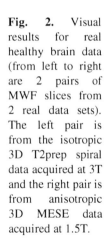

**Fig. 2.** Visual results for real healthy brain data (from left to right are 2 pairs of MWF slices from 2 real data sets). The left pair is from the isotropic 3D T2prep spiral data acquired at 3T and the right pair is from anisotropic 3D MESE data acquired at 1.5T.

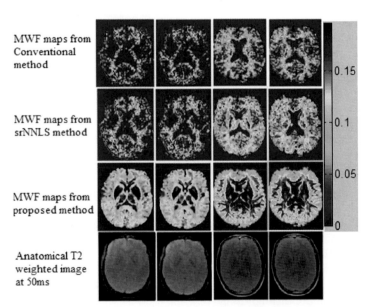

MWF maps from Conventional method

MWF maps from srNNLS method

MWF maps from proposed method

Anatomical T2 weighted image at 50ms

0.15
0.1
0.05
0

We can see that the proposed method differentiated lesions better than the other two, while the conventional and srNNLS methods resulted in almost identical results.

The processing durations for 9 slices of size 192x192 pixels were approximately 4 hours, 6 hours and 2.7 hours with conventional, srNNLS method and proposed methods.

**Fig. 3.** Visual results for real patient brain data (from left to right are 2 pairs of MWF slices from 2 patient data sets). The red arrows in FLAIR images point to the lesions, and the blue arrows in MWF maps point to the corresponding areas. The red circles in FLAIR images represent the selected normal WM ROIs for calculating p-value, and the blue circles in MWFs is the corresponding areas

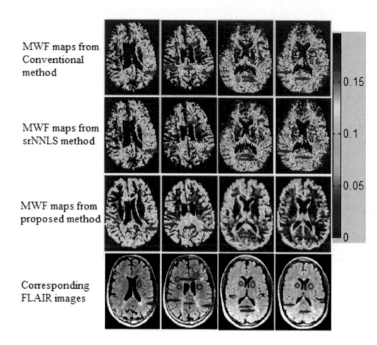

## 5    Discussion

This study demonstrated that the MWF maps obtained with the proposed method are less noise and better spatial consistency. The coverage within the white matter is significantly larger, with clear depiction of even fine and juxtacortical WM structures. The corpus callosum is faithfully depicted, and so are frontal projection fibers. Numerically, for simulated data, the MSEs from the proposed method at various SNRs are significantly lower. For real data, the mean COV of the proposed method demonstrated improved local smoothness at various ROIs. The improvment of the proposed algorithm for distinguishing WM and lesions is substantiated by p-values.

Compared with Kumar et al [14], the MWF maps generated from our algorithm have similar appearance but better visual quality in terms of visual smoothness and delineation of different brain structures. With our proposed method, the MWFs for genu of corpus callosum, splenium of corpus callosum and internal capsules are 17.1±1.8%, 15.5±2.0% and 18.1±1.0% separately over three healthy subjects. The corresponding values reported in [14] are 16.7±1.8%, 14.6±3.1% and 14.2±1.5%, and the corresponding values reported in [15] are 10.2±0.2%, 14.4±0.2% and 17.2±0.2%. The COV values were slightly higher than that Oh et al reported in [16] and lower than that Kumar et al reported in [14]. The above deviations may be due to the use of different modality data, limited number of subjects and the various sizes of the selected ROIs. Compared with mcDESPOT [4], the proposed method is able to infer the T2 distribution rather 2 pure water pools.

The primary clinical goal for this work is to produce whole brain MWF maps for patients with MS. The improved robustness of our algorithm against noise effect may therefore benefit recently developed rapid 3D spiral T2 relaxometry sequences for whole brain coverage, in which SNR was traded for acquisition time.

# References

[1] Laule, C., Vavasour, I.M., Moore, G.R.W., Oger, J., Li, D.K.B., Paty, D.W., MacKay, A.L.: Water content and myelin water fraction in multiple sclerosis. A T2 relaxation study. Journal of Neurology 251(3), 284–293 (2004)

[2] Whittall, K.P., MacKay, A.L.: Quantitative interpretation of NMR relaxation data. Journal of Magnetic Resonance 84(1), 134–152 (1969)

[3] Haacke, E.M., Brown, R.W., Thompson, M.R., Venkatesan, R.: Magnetic Resonance Imaging: Physical Principles and Sequence Design, p. 1008. Wiley-Liss (1999)

[4] Deoni, S.C.L., Rutt, B.K., Arun, T., Pierpaoli, C., Jones, D.K.: Gleaning multicomponent T1 and T2 information from steady-state imaging data. Magnetic Resonance in Medicine: Official Journal of the Society of Magnetic Resonance in Medicine/Society of Magnetic Resonance in Medicine 60(6), 1372–1387 (2008)

[5] Kolind, S.H., Deoni, S.C.: Rapid three-dimensional multicomponent relaxation imaging of the cervical spinal cord. Magnetic Resonance in Medicine: Official Journal of the Society of Magnetic Resonance in Medicine / Society of Magnetic Resonance in Medicine 65(2), 551–556 (2011)

[6] Hwang, D., Du, Y.P.: Improved myelin water quantification using spatially regularized non-negative least squares algorithm. Journal of Magnetic Resonance Imaging: JMRI 30(1), 203–208 (2009)

[7] Bjarnason, T.A., McCreary, C.R., Dunn, J.F., Mitchell, J.R.: Quantitative T2 analysis: the effects of noise, regularization, and multivoxel approaches. Magnetic Resonance in Medicine: Official Journal of the Society of Magnetic Resonance in Medicine/Society of Magnetic Resonance in Medicine 63(1), 212–217 (2010)

[8] Raj, A., Singh, G., Zabih, R., Kressler, B., Wang, Y., Schuff, N., Weiner, M.: Bayesian parallel imaging with edge-preserving priors. Magnetic Resonance in Medicine: Official Journal of the Society of Magnetic Resonance in Medicine/Society of Magnetic Resonance in Medicine 57(1), 8–21 (2007)

[9] Boros, E., Hammer, P.L.: Pseudo-Boolean optimization. Discrete Applied Mathematics 123(1-3), 155–225 (2002)

[10] Lancaster, J.L., Andrews, T., Hardies, L.J., Dodd, S., Fox, P.T.: Three-pool model of white matter. Journal of Magnetic Resonance Imaging: JMRI 17(1), 1–10 (2003)

[11] Haacke, E.M., Brown, R.W., Thompson, M.R., Venkatesan, R.: Magnetic Resonance Imaging: Physical Principles and Sequence Design, p. 1008. Wiley-Liss (1999)

[12] Tychonoff, A.N., Arsenin, V.Y.: Solution of Ill-posed Problems. Winston, New York (1977)

[13] Graham, S.J., Stanchev, P.L., Bronskill, M.J.: Criteria for analysis of multicomponent tissue T2 relaxation data. Magnetic Resonance in Medicine: Official Journal of the Society of Magnetic Resonance in Medicine/Society of Magnetic Resonance in Medicine 35(3), 370–378 (1996)

[14] Kumar, D., Nguyen, T.D., Gauthier, S.A., Raj, A.: Bayesian algorithm using spatial priors for multiexponential T(2) relaxometry from multiecho spin echo MRI. Magnetic Resonance in Medicine: Official Journal of the Society of Magnetic Resonance in Medicine/Society of Magnetic Resonance in Medicine (January 2012)

[15] Meyers, S.M., Laule, C., Vavasour, I.M., Kolind, S.H., Mädler, B., Tam, R., Traboulsee, A.L., Lee, J., Li, D.K.B., MacKay, A.L.: Reproducibility of myelin water fraction analysis: a comparison of region of interest and voxel-based analysis methods. Magnetic Resonance Imaging 27(8), 1096–1103 (2009)

[16] Oh, J., Han, E.T., Pelletier, D., Nelson, S.J.: Measurement of in vivo multi-component T2 relaxation times for brain tissue using multi-slice T2 prep at 1.5 and 3 T. Magnetic Resonance Imaging 24(1), 33–43 (2006)

# Is Synthesizing MRI Contrast Useful for Inter-modality Analysis?

Juan Eugenio Iglesias[1], Ender Konukoglu[1], Darko Zikic[2], Ben Glocker[2], Koen Van Leemput[1,3,4], and Bruce Fischl[1]

[1] Martinos Center for Biomedical Imaging, MGH, Harvard Medical School, USA
[2] Microsoft Research, Cambridge, UK
[3] Department of Applied Mathematics and Computer Science, DTU, Denmark
[4] Departments of Information and Computer Science and of Biomedical Engineering and Computational Science, Aalto University, Finland

**Abstract.** Availability of multi-modal magnetic resonance imaging (MRI) databases opens up the opportunity to synthesize different MRI contrasts without actually acquiring the images. In theory such synthetic images have the potential to reduce the amount of acquisitions to perform certain analyses. However, to what extent they can substitute real acquisitions in the respective analyses is an open question. In this study, we used a synthesis method based on patch matching to test whether synthetic images can be useful in segmentation and inter-modality cross-subject registration of brain MRI. Thirty-nine T1 scans with 36 manually labeled structures of interest were used in the registration and segmentation of eight proton density (PD) scans, for which ground truth T1 data were also available. The results show that synthesized T1 contrast can considerably enhance the quality of non-linear registration compared with using the original PD data, and it is only marginally worse than using the original T1 scans. In segmentation, the relative improvement with respect to using the PD is smaller, but still statistically significant.

## 1 Introduction

Synthesizing MRI contrasts is a computational technique that modifies the intensities of a MRI scan in such a way that it seems to have been acquired with a different protocol. It finds application in several areas of neuroimaging. For example, in multi-site studies, an ideal synthesis method would have (in principle) the potential of making it possible to combine scans from different scanner manufacturers in the analysis without affecting the statistical power to detect population differences [1]. Contrast synthesis can also be used in segmentation: many publicly available methods (especially those based on machine learning, e.g. [2]) are MRI contrast specific and rely on absolute voxel intensities. Synthesis allows us to apply them to data with other types of MRI contrast [3].

Synthesis also has potential benefits for cross-modality image registration, for which metrics based on mutual information (MI) are typically used [4]. While MI suffices to linearly register data, it often fails in the nonlinear case when the

K. Mori et al. (Eds.): MICCAI 2013, Part I, LNCS 8149, pp. 631–638, 2013.

number of degrees of freedom of the transform is high. On the other hand, highly flexible transforms do not represent a big problem in the intra-modality case, for which metrics such as the sum of squared differences (SSD) or normalized cross-correlation (NCC) have been proven successful [5]. Synthesis can be used to convert an ill-posed inter-modality registration problem into an intra-modality problem that is easier to solve, as recently shown in [6] for microscopic images.

Previous work in synthetic MRI can be classified into three major branches. The first family of approaches, such as [7], is based on the acquisition of a set of MRI scans that make it possible to infer the underlying, physical MRI parameters of the tissue (T1, PD, T2/T2*). While these parameters can be used to synthesize any arbitrary MRI contrast, data acquired with such a protocol is scarce, limiting the applicability of this approach. The second branch uses a single scan to estimate the synthetic image by optimizing a (possibly space dependent) transform that maps one MRI contrast to the other, often in conjunction with registration. The transform model can be parametric, such as [8] (a mixture of polynomials), or a non-parametric joint histogram, as in [9].

The third type of approach is exemplar-based. The underlying principle is to use a pre-acquired database of images from different subjects, for which two modalities are available: *source*, which will also be acquired for new subjects, and *target*, that will be synthesized. Given the source of a test subject, the target can be synthesized using patch-matching [10] or dictionary learning approaches [11,6]. Exemplar-based approaches are particularly interesting as they do not model the imaging parameters and they naturally incorporate spatial context (i.e. neighboring voxels) in the synthesis, as opposed to applying a transform to the intensity of each voxel independently. They are extremely general and produce visually attractive results even with image databases of limited size.

While patch-based synthesis can produce results that are visually impressive, it is unclear if the synthesized images are mere "pastiches" or they can substitute real acquisitions for some tasks in multi-modal MRI analysis. To answer this question, we used a patch-matching driven, exemplar-based approach to synthesize T1 data from PD images, for which T1 images were also available. Then, we used a separate dataset of T1 scans to register and segment: 1. the PD images; 2. the synthetic T1 data; and 3. the true T1 data. These experiments allow us to quantitatively assess whether more accurate registration and segmentation can be obtained using the synthesized T1 images rather than the PD data, as well as the decrease in performance when synthesized T1 images replace the true T1 volumes. Finally, we also compare the performance of the exemplar-based approach with two intensity-transform-based synthesis techniques.

## 2   Patch-Based Synthesis Method

Here we use a patch-matching algorithm inspired by the methods in [12,13] and also Image Analogies [10]. Given a source image $I$, the goal is to synthesize a target image $S$ using a pre-acquired database of coupled images $T = \{(I_n, S_n)\}_{n=1}^{N}$ from $N$ different subjects. We define an image patch centered in a spatial location $\mathbf{x}$ as $W^d(\mathbf{x}) = \{y : \|y - x\|_2 \leq d\}$. Our method implements patch-matching:

for every $\mathbf{x}$, we search the database for the patch in source modality $I_n(W^d(\mathbf{y}))$ that best resembles $I(W^d(\mathbf{x}))$. Then we use the information in the corresponding patch in target modality $S_n(W^d(\mathbf{y}))$ to generate the synthesized value $S(W^d(\mathbf{x}))$.

Specifically, the search for the most similar patch is formulated as:

$$(n^*, \mathbf{y}^*) = \underset{n,y}{\text{argmin}} \, \| I \left( W^d(\mathbf{x}) \right) - I_n \left( W^d(\mathbf{y}) \right) \|_2. \tag{1}$$

This minimization problem provides an estimate for the synthesized patch as $S\left( W^d(\mathbf{x}) \right) = S_{n^*}\left( W^d(\mathbf{y}^*) \right)$. Because each $\mathbf{x}$ is included in more than one patch, the method estimates multiple synthesized intensity values for $\mathbf{x}$, one coming from each patch $\mathbf{x}$ is contained in. Let us denote these different estimates with $S^{W^d(\mathbf{x}')}(\mathbf{x})$, i.e., the synthetic value at $\mathbf{x}$ as estimated by the patch centered in $\mathbf{x}'$. Based on this, we compute the final estimate for $S(\mathbf{x})$ as the average:

$$S(\mathbf{x}) = \frac{1}{|\{\mathbf{x}' : \mathbf{x} \in W^d(\mathbf{x}')\}|} \sum_{\{\mathbf{x}' : \mathbf{x} \in W^d(\mathbf{x}')\}} S^{W^d(\mathbf{x}')}(\mathbf{x}), \tag{2}$$

where $|\cdot|$ is the cardinality of the set.

The optimization in Equation 1 can be computationally expensive, considering that it needs to be solved if for each voxel $\mathbf{x}$. Two simple cost reduction methods are used here. First, as done in [12], we assume that all images are linearly aligned, which allows us to restrict the search window for $\mathbf{y}$ as:

$$(n^*, y^*) = \underset{n, \mathbf{y} \in W^D(\mathbf{x})}{\text{argmin}} \, \| I \left( W^d(\mathbf{x}) \right) - I_n \left( W^d(\mathbf{y}) \right) \|_2, \tag{3}$$

where $W^D(\mathbf{x})$ is a patch of size $D$ around $\mathbf{x}$. The second speed-up is to solve the minimization problem in a multi-resolution fashion using a search grid pyramid. At low resolution, a large $D$ can be used. The found correspondences can be carried over to the higher resolution, and the search repeated with a smaller $D$.

## 3    Experiments and Results

### 3.1    MRI Data

We used two datasets in this study, one for training and one for testing. The training dataset consists of 39 T1-weighted scans acquired with a MP-RAGE sequence in a 1.5T scanner, in which 36 structures of interest were labeled by an expert rater with the protocol in [14]. We note that this is the same dataset that was used to build the atlas in FreeSurfer [15]. The test dataset consists of MRI scans from eight subjects acquired with a FLASH sequence in a 1.5T scanner. Images with two different flip angles were acquired, producing PD-weighted and T1-weighted images in the same coordinate frame. The test dataset was labeled using the same protocol; the annotations were made on the T1 data in order to make them as consistent as possible with the training dataset.

The brain MRI scans were skull-stripped, bias-field corrected and affinely aligned to Talairach space with FreeSurfer. The T1 volumes (both training and test) were intensity-normalized using FreeSurfer. The PD volumes were approximately brought to a common intensity space by multiplying them by a scaling factor that matched their medians to a constant intensity value.

## 3.2   Experimental Setup

We performed two sets of experiments to evaluate the use of synthetic MRI on registration and segmentation. For **registration**, we first non-linearly registered the training dataset to the test images, and then used the resulting transform to propagate the corresponding labels. The Dice overlap between the ground truth and deformed labels was used as a proxy for the quality of the registrations. To evaluate the algorithms at different levels of flexibility of the spatial transform, we considered two deformation models: one coarse and one fine. As a coarse deformation model, we used a grid of widely spaced control points (30 mm. separation) with B-spline interpolation as implemented in Elastix [16]. As a more flexible model, we used the symmetric diffeomorphic registration method implemented in ANTS [17], with Gaussian regularization (kernel width 3 mm).

Five approaches were tested in this experiment. First, registering the training data to the PD volumes using MI as a metric (computed with 32 bins); Second, registering the training data to the test T1 volumes using NCC, which works better than MI in intramodality scenarios. The output from this method represents an upper bound on the quality of the registration that can be achieved with synthetic MRI. The other three methods correspond to registering the training data to synthetic T1 volumes (generated with three different approaches) using NCC as cost function. The synthesis was carried out in a leave-one-out fashion such that, when synthesizing the T1 volume corresponding to a PD scan, the remaining seven T1-PD pairs were treated as the corresponding database.

The three contrast synthesis algorithms were: 1. the exemplar-based method described in Section 2 (patch size $d = \sqrt{3}$, i.e., 26 neighborhood, and search window size $D = 16\sqrt{3}$); 2. an in-house implementation of the algorithm in [8]; and 3. an in-house implementation of [9]. In the corresponding original papers, [8] and [9] use the information from the registered image to estimate the gray level transform and the joint histogram, respectively. Instead, we compute the transforms directly from the information in the training dataset. For [8], we used the monofunctional dependence with a ninth-order polynomial.

In the **segmentation** experiments, we fed the real T1 scans as well as their synthetic counterparts (computed with the same three methods) to the FreeSurfer pipeline, which produces an automated segmentation of the brain structures of interest based on an atlas built using the training dataset, i.e. 39 T1 images. As in the registration experiment, the results from the real T1 scans serve as an upper limit of the performance with the synthetic data. As another benchmark, we segmented the PD scans directly as well. Since FreeSurfer requires T1 data, we segmented the PD scans using the sequence-independent method implemented in the software package SPM [18], which is based on a statistical atlas. To make the comparison with FreeSurfer as fair as possible, we used the statistical atlas from this package in the SPM segmentation.

Both in the registration and segmentation experiments, statistical significance was assessed with paired, non-parametric tests (Wilcoxon signed rank). For a more compact presentation of results, we merged right and left labels and used only a representative subset of the 36 labeled structures in the evaluation: white matter (WM), cortex (CT), lateral ventricle (LV), thalamus (TH), caudate (CA), putamen (PT), pallidum (PA), hippocampus (HP) and amygdala (AM).

## 3.3   Results

**Qualitative Synthesis Results:** Figure 1 displays an axial slice of a scan from the test dataset (both in T1 and PD) along with the corresponding T1 images generated from the PD data using the three evaluated synthesis methods. The exemplar-based approach, despite introducing some minimal blurring due to the averaging, produces a visually better synthesis of the ground truth T1 data. In particular, it displays excellent robustness to noise and outliers; for instance, the vessels are interpreted as white matter by the other approaches methods while the exemplar-based method correctly maps them to dark intensities.

**Registration:** Figure 2 show boxplots for the Dice scores achieved by the different approaches using the coarse and fine deformation models. For the coarse model, using T1 data (synthetic or real) has little impact on the accuracy for the white matter, cortex, ventricles, thalamus and caudate. However, it yields a considerable boost for the putamen, pallidum, hippocampus and amygdala. All synthesis approaches outperform directly using the PD volume in non-linear registration. The exemplar-based method produces results as good as the acquired T1, outperforming the other two synthesis approaches.

The flexible model is more attractive in practice because it can produce much more accurate deformation fields. However, MI becomes too flexible in this scenario, making the inter-modal registration problem ill posed. Hence, direct registration of T1 to PD data produces poor results. Combining synthesis and NCC yields much higher performance. Again, the exemplar-based approach stays on par with the real T1, outperforming the other two synthesis approaches.

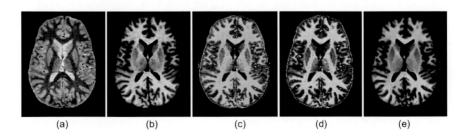

(a)                (b)                (c)                (d)                (e)

**Fig. 1.** Sagittal slice of a sample MRI scan from the test dataset: (a) PD-weighted volue, (b) T1-weighted volume, (c) T1 volume synthesized from the PD data using [8], (d) synthesized with [9], (e) synthesized with the exemplar-based method

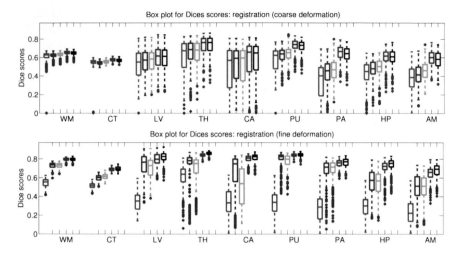

**Fig. 2.** Boxplot of Dice scores in the registration experiment with the coarse (top) and symmetric diffeomorphic (bottom) deformation models. See Section 3.2 for the abbreviations. Color code: magenta = PD registered with MI, red = synthetic T1 from [8], green = synthetic T1 from [9], blue = synthetic T1 from exemplar-based approach, black = ground truth T1. Horizontal box lines indicate the three quartile values. Whiskers extend to the most extreme values within 1.5 times the interquartile range from the ends of the box. Samples beyond those points are marked with crosses. All the differences are statistically significant at p=0.001 (sample size $39 \times 8 = 312$).

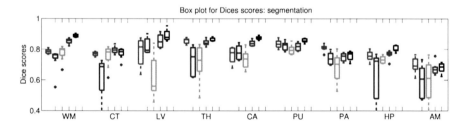

**Fig. 3.** Boxplot of the Dice scores in the segmentation experiment. See caption of Figure 2 for the abbreviations and color code.

**Segmentation:** the boxplot for the Dice scores in the segmentation experiment are show in Figure 3, whereas numerical results and p-values for the statistical tests are displayed in Table 1. The decrease in performance of using exemplar-based synthetic T1 with respect to using the acquired T1 is small. However, considering that scores obtained when directly segmenting PD images are high, we conclude that the potential benefits of synthetic MRI in this application are less than in registration. Still, we note that the patch-based approach is able to significantly outperform the segmentation based on the PD data (2% increment in Dice, $p = 0.04$ despite the small $N = 8$). This suggests that improving the synthesis method has the potential to make synthesis useful for segmentation.

**Table 1.** Mean Dice score (in %) for each method and brain structure and p-values corresponding to a comparison with the proposed approach. Note that many p-values are the same due to the non-parametric nature of the test.

| Method | WM | CT | LV | TH | CA | PT | PD | HP | AM | All combined |
|--------|-----|-----|-----|-----|-----|-----|-----|-----|-----|--------------|
| Proposed | 85.2 | 79.5 | 85.3 | 84.2 | 83.9 | 81.6 | 74.9 | 76.6 | 67.3 | 79.8 |
| PD data [18] | 78.4 | 76.8 | 78.1 | 85.4 | 76.2 | 83.3 | 80.7 | 75.5 | 69.7 | 78.3 |
| p-value | 7.8e-3 | 1.6e-2 | 7.8e-3 | 1.1e-1 | 7.8e-3 | 2.3e-2 | 7.8e-3 | 3.8e-1 | 3.8e-1 | 4.2e-2 |
| Syn. T1 [8] | 73.2 | 62.1 | 72.9 | 66.6 | 68.8 | 72.3 | 65.3 | 58.2 | 53.6 | 65.9 |
| p-value | 7.8e-3 | 7.8e-3 | 2.3e-2 | 7.8e-3 | 1.6e-2 | 9.5e-1 | 7.4e-1 | 7.8e-3 | 2.3e-2 | 4.5e-10 |
| Syn. T1 [9] | 77.5 | 75.7 | 61.6 | 71.3 | 66.5 | 71.2 | 63.4 | 66.2 | 55.9 | 67.7 |
| p value | 7.8e-3 | 7.8e-3 | 7.8e-3 | 7.8e-3 | 7.8e-3 | 3.8e-1 | 2.0e-1 | 7.8e-3 | 1.1e-1 | 3.3e-11 |
| Real T1 | 88.8 | 77.3 | 89.0 | 86.3 | 87.3 | 85.6 | 75.8 | 80.4 | 68.0 | 82.1 |
| p-value | 7.8e-3 | 2.0e-1 | 7.8e-3 | 1.6e-2 | 7.8e-3 | 7.8e-3 | 3.1e-1 | 7.8e-3 | 6.4e-1 | 3.7e-7 |

## 4 Discussion

This article tried to answer the question whether synthesizing MRI contrast, in particular with the generic exemplar-based approach based on simple patch-matching, is useful in inter-modal analysis of brain MRI. Our experiments showed that exemplar-based synthesis outperforms methods based on intensity transforms. We also found that, in cross-modality registration, synthesizing a scan that resembles the moving images and using NCC as a metric produces considerably more accurate deformation fields than directly registering across modalities with MI. In segmentation, synthesizing a T1 volume and segmenting it with FreeSurfer was only marginally better than segmenting the original PD data directly. These results suggest that synthesis can be a poor man's alternative to acquiring new images for cross-subject non-linear registration. Future work will include evaluating how synthesis affects other analyses, e.g., cortical thickness.

**Acknowledgements.** This research was supported by NIH NCRR (P41-RR14075), NIBIB (R01EB013565, R01EB006758), NIA (AG022381, 5R01AG008122-22), NCAM (RC1 AT005728-01), NINDS (R01 NS052585-01, 1R21NS072652-01, 1R01NS070963), Academy of Finland (133611) and TEKES (ComBrain), and was made possible by the resources provided by Shared Instrumentation Grants 1S10RR023401, 1S10RR019307, and 1S10RR023043. Additional support was provided by the NIH BNR (5U01-MH093765), part of the multi-institutional Human Connectome Project.

## References

1. Friedman, L., Stern, H., Brown, G.G., Mathalon, D.H., Turner, J., Glover, G.H., Gollub, R.L., Lauriello, J., Lim, K.O., Cannon, T., et al.: Test–retest and between-site reliability in a multicenter fMRI study. Hum. Brain Mapp. 29, 958–972 (2007)
2. Tu, Z., Narr, K.L., Dollár, P., Dinov, I., Thompson, P.M., Toga, A.W.: Brain anatomical structure segmentation by hybrid discriminative/generative models. IEEE Trans. Med. Im. 27, 495–508 (2008)

3. Roy, S., Carass, A., Shiee, N., Pham, D.L., Prince, J.L.: MR contrast synthesis for lesion segmentation. In: IEEE Int. Symp. Biom. Im. (ISBI), pp. 932–935. IEEE (2010)

4. Maes, F., Collignon, A., Vandermeulen, D., Marchal, G., Suetens, P.: Multimodality image registration by maximization of mutual information. IEEE Trans. Med. Im. 16, 187–198 (1997)

5. Klein, A., Andersson, J., Ardekani, B.A., Ashburner, J., Avants, B., Chiang, M.C., Christensen, G.E., Collins, D.L., Gee, J., Hellier, P., et al.: Evaluation of 14 nonlinear deformation algorithms applied to human brain MRI registration. Neuroimage 46, 786 (2009)

6. Cao, T., Zach, C., Modla, S., Powell, D., Czymmek, K., Niethammer, M.: Registration for Correlative Microscopy Using Image Analogies. In: Dawant, B.M., Christensen, G.E., Fitzpatrick, J.M., Rueckert, D. (eds.) WBIR 2012. LNCS, vol. 7359, pp. 296–306. Springer, Heidelberg (2012)

7. Fischl, B., Salat, D.H., van der Kouwe, A.J., Makris, N., Ségonne, F., Quinn, B.T., Dale, A.M.: Sequence-independent segmentation of magnetic resonance images. Neuroimage 23, S69–S84 (2004)

8. Guimond, A., Roche, A., Ayache, N., Meunier, J.: Three-dimensional multimodal brain warping using the demons algorithm and adaptive intensity corrections. IEEE Trans. Med. Im. 20, 58–69 (2001)

9. Kroon, D.J., Slump, C.H.: Mri modalitiy transformation in demon registration. In: IEEE Int. Symp. Biom. Im (ISBI), pp. 963–966 (2009)

10. Hertzmann, A., Jacobs, C.E., Oliver, N., Curless, B., Salesin, D.H.: Image analogies. In: Proc. Ann. Conf. Comp. Graph. and Interac. Techniques, pp. 327–340 (2001)

11. Roy, S., Carass, A., Prince, J.: A Compressed Sensing Approach for MR Tissue Contrast Synthesis. In: Székely, G., Hahn, H.K. (eds.) IPMI 2011. LNCS, vol. 6801, pp. 371–383. Springer, Heidelberg (2011)

12. Coupé, P., Manjón, J.V., Fonov, V., Pruessner, J., Robles, M., Collins, D.L.: Patch-based segmentation using expert priors: Application to hippocampus and ventricle segmentation. Neuroimage 54, 940–954 (2011)

13. Rousseau, F., Habas, P., Studholme, C.: A supervised patch-based approach for human brain labeling. IEEE Trans. Med. Im. 30, 1852–1862 (2011)

14. Caviness Jr., V., Filipek, P., Kennedy, D.: Magnetic resonance technology in human brain science: blueprint for a program based upon morphometry. Brain Dev. 11, 1–13 (1989)

15. Fischl, B., Salat, D., Busa, E., Albert, M., Dieterich, M., Haselgrove, C., van der Kouwe, A., Killiany, R., Kennedy, D., Klaveness, S., Montillo, A., Makris, N., Rosen, B., Dale, A.: Whole brain segmentation: Automated labeling of neuroanatomical structures in the human brain. Neuron 33, 341–355 (2002)

16. Klein, S., Staring, M., Murphy, K., Viergever, M., Pluim, J.: Elastix: a toolbox for intensity-based medical image registration. IEEE Trans. Med. Im 29, 196–205 (2010)

17. Avants, B.B., Epstein, C., Grossman, M., Gee, J.C.: Symmetric diffeomorphic image registration with cross-correlation: Evaluating automated labeling of elderly and neurodegenerative brain. Med. Im. Anal. 12, 26–41 (2008)

18. Ashburner, J., Friston, K.J.: Unified segmentation. Neuroimage 26, 839–851 (2005)

# Regularized Spherical Polar Fourier Diffusion MRI with Optimal Dictionary Learning

Jian Cheng[1], Tianzi Jiang[2], Rachid Deriche[3], Dinggang Shen[1], and Pew-Thian Yap[1]

[1] Department of Radiology and BRIC, The University of North Carolina at Chapel Hill, USA
[2] CCM, LIAMA, Institute of Automation, Chinese Academy of Sciences, China
[3] Athena Project Team, INRIA Sophia Antipolis, France
{jian_cheng,dgshen,ptyap}@med.unc.edu

**Abstract.** Compressed Sensing (CS) takes advantage of signal sparsity or compressibility and allows superb signal reconstruction from relatively few measurements. Based on CS theory, a suitable dictionary for sparse representation of the signal is required. In diffusion MRI (dMRI), CS methods proposed for reconstruction of diffusion-weighted signal and the Ensemble Average Propagator (EAP) utilize two kinds of Dictionary Learning (DL) methods: 1) Discrete Representation DL (DR-DL), and 2) Continuous Representation DL (CR-DL). DR-DL is susceptible to numerical inaccuracy owing to interpolation and regridding errors in a discretized $q$-space. In this paper, we propose a novel CR-DL approach, called Dictionary Learning - Spherical Polar Fourier Imaging (DL-SPFI) for effective compressed-sensing reconstruction of the **q**-space diffusion-weighted signal and the EAP. In DL-SPFI, a dictionary that sparsifies the signal is learned from the space of continuous Gaussian diffusion signals. The learned dictionary is then adaptively applied to different voxels using a weighted LASSO framework for robust signal reconstruction. Compared with the start-of-the-art CR-DL and DR-DL methods proposed by Merlet et al. and Bilgic et al., respectively, our work offers the following advantages. First, the learned dictionary is proved to be optimal for Gaussian diffusion signals. Second, to our knowledge, this is the first work to learn a voxel-adaptive dictionary. The importance of the adaptive dictionary in EAP reconstruction will be demonstrated theoretically and empirically. Third, optimization in DL-SPFI is only performed in a small subspace resided by the SPF coefficients, as opposed to the **q**-space approach utilized by Merlet et al. We experimentally evaluated DL-SPFI with respect to L1-norm regularized SPFI (L1-SPFI), which uses the original SPF basis, and the DR-DL method proposed by Bilgic et al. The experiment results on synthetic and real data indicate that the learned dictionary produces sparser coefficients than the original SPF basis and results in significantly lower reconstruction error than Bilgic et al.'s method.

## 1 Introduction

Diffusion MRI (dMRI) is a unique non-invasive technique for investigation of white matter microstructure in the human brain. A central problem in dMRI is to estimate the Ensemble Average Propagator (EAP) $P(\mathbf{R})$, which describes fully the probability distribution of water molecule displacement $\mathbf{R}$, from a limited number of measurements of the signal attenuation $E(\mathbf{q})$ in the **q** (wave-vector) space. Under narrow

K. Mori et al. (Eds.): MICCAI 2013, Part I, LNCS 8149, pp. 639–646, 2013.

pulse condition, $E(\mathbf{q})$ and $P(\mathbf{R})$ are related by the Fourier transform, i.e., $P(\mathbf{R}) = \int_{\mathbb{R}^3} E(\mathbf{q}) \exp(-2\pi i \mathbf{q}^T \mathbf{R}) d\mathbf{q}$. Various methods have been proposed for reconstructing the EAP. The most common method is Diffusion Tensor Imaging (DTI). However, due to its Gaussian assumption, DTI is incapable of modeling complex non-Gaussian diffusion resulting from crossing fibers. Diffusion Spectrum Imaging (DSI) acquires measurements for more than 500 discrete points in the $\mathbf{q}$-space and performs Fourier transform numerically to obtain the EAP, followed by an numerical radial integration to estimate the Orientation Distribution Function (ODF) [1]. However, the long scanning time ($\approx$ 1 hour) required by DSI significantly limits its utility, especially in clinical settings. Spherical Polar Fourier Imaging (SPFI), by leveraging a continuous representation of $E(\mathbf{q})$, requires a more moderate number of signal measurements. This continuous representation is based on the Spherical Polar Fourier (SPF) basis and provides closed-form expressions for EAP and ODF computation [2,3].

Recovering a latent function from a small number of samples in Fourier domain is a classic problem in Compressed Sensing (CS) theory [4], where a good basis that allows sparse representation is crucial for the reconstruction. Although some analytic bases, including discrete basis like wavelets [5] and continuous basis like the SPF basis, have been proposed as sparse bases for EAP estimation, based on CS theory, a sparser basis can be learned from well chosen exemplars via Dictionary Learning (DL) techniques [8,9]. Bilgic et al. [10] learns a discrete dictionary via the K-SVD [8] approach and uses it in the FOCal Underdetermined System Solver (FOCUSS) algorithm for EAP estimation. This strategy dramatically reduces the number of samples and scanning time required by DSI. However, Bilgic et al.'s approach suffers from numerical errors similar to DSI because their dictionary is composed of a set of discrete basis vectors. On the other hand, Merlet et al. [7] learns a continuous dictionary, parametrized as a linear combination of some atoms adopted from SPF basis, from synthetic Gaussian signals. The learned basis allows conversion of the diffusion signals to the respective ODFs and EAPs using close-form expressions modified from [3]. However, the method proposed in [7] have some inherent limitations in both theoretical analysis and practical usage. For example, they learned the scale parameter $\zeta$ associated with the SPF basis from the training data, instead of the testing data. We shall show in the current paper that the optimal scale $\zeta$ should be adaptively estimated from testing data. In addition, they have also neglected isotropic exemplars in the training data, causing over-fitting problems in less anisotropic areas such as the grey matter.

In this paper, we propose a novel CR-DL approach, called Dictionary Learning - Spherical Polar Fourier Imaging (DL-SPFI), for effective compressed-sensing reconstruction of the diffusion signal and the EAP. Our approach offers a number of advantages over [7]. First, we dramatically reduce the dimensionality of the optimization problem by working in a small subspace of the SPF coefficients, instead of $\mathbf{q}$-space as done in [7]. Second, the dictionary learned using our approach can be applied optimally and adaptively to each voxel by voxel-dependent determination of the optimal scale parameter. In contrast, both [7] and [10] do not consider inter-voxel variation. Third, we consider the constraint $E(0) = 1$ during both learning and estimation processes. Section 2 provides a brief overview of SPFI and shows how the constraint $E(0) = 1$ can be incorporated in SPFI. Section 3 demonstrates the equivalence between dictionary learning and estimation regularization and provides details on DL-SPFI. Section 4 validates DL-SPFI in comparison with L1-SPFI using the original SPF basis and FOCUSS with/without DL, as implemented in [10].

## 2  Spherical Polar Fourier Imaging (SPFI) Revisited

The SPF basis is a continuous complete basis that can represent sparsely Gaussian-like signals [2,3]. If $E(\mathbf{q})$ is represented by the SPF basis $\{B_{nlm}(\mathbf{q})\} = \{G_n(q)Y_l^m(\mathbf{u})\}$, i.e.,

$$E(q\mathbf{u}) = \sum_{n=0}^{N}\sum_{l=0}^{L}\sum_{m=-l}^{l} a_{nlm}B_{nlm}(\mathbf{q}), \quad B_{nlm}(\mathbf{q}) = G_n(q|\zeta)Y_l^m(\mathbf{u}) \tag{1}$$

where $G_n(q|\zeta) = \left[\frac{2}{\zeta^{3/2}}\frac{n!}{\Gamma(n+3/2)}\right]^{1/2}\exp\left(-\frac{q^2}{2\zeta}\right)L_n^{1/2}(\frac{q^2}{\zeta})$ is the Gaussian-Laguerre polynomial, $Y_l^m(\mathbf{u})$ is the real Spherical Harmonic (SH) basis, and $\zeta$ is the scale parameter, then the EAP $P(\mathbf{R})$ is represented by the Fourier dual SPF (dSPF) basis in Eq. (2), where $B_{nlm}^{dual}(\mathbf{R})$ was proved to be the Fourier transform of $B_{nlm}(\mathbf{q})$. The definition of the dSPF basis can be found in [3].

$$P(R\mathbf{r}) = \sum_{n=0}^{N}\sum_{l=0}^{L}\sum_{m=-l}^{l} a_{nlm}F_{nl}(R)Y_l^m(\mathbf{r}) \qquad B_{nlm}^{dual}(\mathbf{R}) = F_{nl}(R)Y_l^m(\mathbf{r}) \tag{2}$$

The SPF coefficients $\mathbf{a} = (a_{000},\ldots,a_{NLL})^T$ can be estimated from the signal attenuation measurements $\{E_i\}$ via least square fitting with $l_2$-norm or $l_1$-norm regularization, where the constraint $E(0) = 1$ can be imposed by adding artificial samples at $q = 0$ [3,6]. Here we propose an alternative continuous approach to impose this constraint. From $E(0) = 1$, we have $\sum_0^N a_{nlm}G_n(0) = \sqrt{4\pi}\delta_l^0$, $0 \le l \le L$, $-l \le m \le l$. Based on this, we can separate the coefficient vector $\mathbf{a}$ into $\mathbf{a} = (\mathbf{a}_0^T, \mathbf{a}'^T)^T$, where $\mathbf{a}_0 = (a_{000},\ldots,a_{0LL})^T$, $\mathbf{a}' = (a_{100},\ldots,a_{NLL})^T$, and represent $\mathbf{a}_0$ using $\mathbf{a}'$, i.e.,

$$a_{0lm} = \frac{1}{G_0(0)}\left(\sqrt{4\pi}\delta_l^0 - \sum_{n=1}^{N}a_{nlm}G_n(0)\right), \quad 0 \le l \le L, \quad -l \le m \le l \tag{3}$$

Based on Eq. (1), the $l_1$-norm regularized estimation of $\mathbf{a}'$, called $l_1$-SPFI [6], can be formulated as

$$\min_{\mathbf{a}'} \|\mathbf{M}'\mathbf{a}' - \mathbf{e}'\|_2^2 + \|\mathbf{\Lambda}\mathbf{a}'\|_1 \tag{4}$$

$$\mathbf{M}' = \begin{bmatrix} \left(G_1(q_1|\zeta) - \frac{G_1(0|\zeta)}{G_0(0|\zeta)}G_0(q_1|\zeta)\right)Y_0^0(\mathbf{u}_1) & \cdots & \left(G_N(q_1|\zeta) - \frac{G_N(0|\zeta)}{G_0(0|\zeta)}G_0(q_1|\zeta)\right)Y_L^L(\mathbf{u}_1) \\ \vdots & \ddots & \vdots \\ \left(G_1(q_S|\zeta) - \frac{G_1(0|\zeta)}{G_0(0|\zeta)}G_0(q_S|\zeta)\right)Y_0^0(\mathbf{u}_S) & \cdots & \left(G_N(q_S|\zeta) - \frac{G_N(0|\zeta)}{G_0(0|\zeta)}G_0(q_S|\zeta)\right)Y_L^L(\mathbf{u}_S) \end{bmatrix}, \quad \mathbf{e}' = \begin{bmatrix} E_1 - \frac{G_0(q_1)}{G_0(0)} \\ \vdots \\ E_S - \frac{G_0(q_S)}{G_0(0)} \end{bmatrix}, \tag{5}$$

where $\|\cdot\|_p$ denotes the $l_p$-norm, $\{E_i\}_{i=1}^S$ are the $S$ signal attenuation measurements in q-space, and the regularization matrix $\mathbf{\Lambda}$ can be devised as a diagonal matrix with elements $\Lambda_{nlm} = \lambda_l l^2(l+1)^2 + \lambda_n n^2(n+1)^2$ to sparsify the coefficients, where $\lambda_l$ and $\lambda_n$ are the regularization parameters for the angular and radial components. Note that $E(\mathbf{q}) - \frac{G_0(q)}{G_0(0)} = E(\mathbf{q}) - \exp(-\frac{q^2}{2\zeta})$ is the signal with the isotropic Gaussian part removed, and $\left(G_n(q) - \frac{G_n(0)}{G_0(0)}G_0(q)\right)Y_l^m(\mathbf{u})$ is the basis $G_n(q)Y_l^m(\mathbf{u})$ with the isotropic Gaussian part removed. After estimating $\mathbf{a}'$, $\mathbf{a}_0$ can be obtained using Eq. (3), and the estimated EAP $\mathbf{a}$ satisfies $E(0) = 1$.

## 3   Dictionary Learning and Regularization

**Equivalence between Dictionary Learning and Regularization Design.** It was shown in [6] that a well-designed regularization matrix enhances coefficient sparsity for better reconstruction. A better regularization matrix can be learned from a set of given signals $\{e'_i\}$. In fact, learning the regularization matrix from data is equivalent to the so-called dictionary learning, i.e.,

$$\underbrace{\min_{A', \Lambda, \zeta} \sum_i \|\Lambda a'_i\|_1 \text{ s.t. } \|M'a'_j - e'_j\|_2 \leq \epsilon_{DL}, \ \forall j}_{\text{Regularization Design}} \quad \leftrightarrow \quad \underbrace{\min_{C, D, \zeta} \sum_i \|c_i\|_1 \text{ s.t. } \|M'Dc_j - e'_j\|_2 \leq \epsilon_{DL}, \ \forall j}_{\text{Dictionary Learning}} \quad (6)$$

where $A = (a'_1, \ldots, a'_Q)$ is the SPF coefficient matrix. The transform matrix $D$ will result in a transformed SPF basis $M'D$ that can be used for even sparser representation of the signal. $C = (c_1, \ldots, c_Q)$ is the new coefficient matrix in association with the transformed basis. Here, we include the scale parameter $\zeta$ of the SPF basis as a parameter to be learned. More discussion on this in the next section. Our formulation is more general than the formulation in [7] for two reasons. First, it can be proved that all atoms in the dictionary used in [7] can be represented as a finite linear combination of the SPF basis used in Eq. (6); the opposite, however, is not true.[1] Hence, the space spanned by the atoms in [7] is just a subspace of the space spanned by the SPF basis. Second, based on the equivalence in Eq. (6), we can further devise a regularization matrix after DL to weight the atoms differently for more effective reconstruction.

**Efficient, Optimal, and Adaptive Dictionary Learning.** Although it is possible to learn a dictionary from real data, as done in DL-FOCUSS [10], the learned dictionary may be significantly affected by noise and the small sample size. An alternative solution to this is to perform DL using some synthetic data that approximate well the real signal. Similar to [7], we propose to learn a continuous basis using mixtures of Gaussian signals. Compared with the DL strategy in [7], our method introduces several theoretical improvements. **1)** Instead of using the DL formulation in Eq. (6), we propose to solve

$$\min_{C, D, \zeta} \sum_i \|c_i\|_1 \text{ s.t. } \|Dc_j - a'_j\|_2 \leq \epsilon_{DL}, \ \forall j, \qquad (7)$$

which, due to the orthogonality of the SPF basis, is equivalent to Eq. (6) if $N$ and $L$ are large enough. In [7] $\{e_i\}$ was generated using thousands of samples, resulting in a high-dimensional minimization problem. In contrast, Eq. (7) works in the small subspace resided by the SPF coefficients and hence significantly reduces the complexity of the learning problem. Note that $\zeta$ in Eq. (7) is contained inside $\{a'_j\}$. **2)** In [7], a constraint was placed on the sparsity term $\|c_i\|_1$, instead of the fitting error term, as is done Eq. (7). Since there is no prior knowledge on the level of sparsity, it is better to place the constraint on the fitting error. Threshold $\epsilon_{DL}$ can be chosen simply as 0.01 for unit-norm normalized $\{a'_j\}$. **3)** It is not necessary to generate a large sample of signals randomly from the mixture of tensor models, like what is done in [7]. We proved in Theorem 1 that the single tensor model is sufficient to learn a dictionary which sparsifies multi-Gaussian signals. That is, the training data $\{e_j\}$ can be generated simply from $\{E(\mathbf{q}|T) = \exp(-4\pi^2\tau q^2 \mathbf{u}^T T \mathbf{u}) \mid T \in \text{Sym}^3_+\}$, where $\text{Sym}^3_+$ is the space of $3 \times 3$ positive

---

[1] All proofs in this paper are omitted due to space limitation, available upon request.

symmetric matrices, and $\tau$ is the diffusion time. **4)** Compared with the classical DL described in [8,9], the DL formulation in Eq. (6) is more difficult to solve because $\mathbf{M}'$ is dependent on $\zeta$. In [7] $\zeta$ and there $\mathbf{D}$ are iteratively updated using the Levenberg-Marquardt algorithm, which is actually problematic. Theorems 2 and 3 show that $\zeta$ should be determined adaptively from testing signals, not from training signals.

**Theorem 1 (Sparsity of Mixture of Tensors).** *Let $(\mathbf{D}_*, \zeta_*)$ be the optimal dictionary learned in Eq. (7) using signals generated from the single tensor model. Let $\{c'_i\}_{i=1}^p$ be the p sparse coefficients under arbitrarily given p SPF coefficients $\{a'_i\}_{i=1}^p$ and $(\mathbf{D}_*, \zeta_*)$. Let $c'_*$ be the sparse vector corresponding to SPF coefficient $a' = \sum_{i=1}^p w_i a'_i$ and $(\mathbf{D}_*, \zeta_*)$, with $\sum_i w_i = 1$, $w_i \geq 0$. Then we have $\|c'_*\|_1 \leq \max(\|c'_1\|_1, \ldots, \|c'_p\|_1)$.*

**Theorem 2 (Optimal Scale).** *If $\{e_i\}$ is generated from the single tensor model with fixed mean diffusivity (MD) $d_0$, then for large enough N, fixed L, and small enough $\epsilon_{DL}$, the optimal scale $\zeta$ for the DL problem in Eq. (6) is $\zeta_* = (8\pi^2 \tau d_0)^{-1}$.*

**Theorem 3 (Optimal Dictionary).** *For signals generated from the single tensor model using a range of MD value $[d_0, td_0]$, $t \geq 1$, if the dictionary $\{\mathbf{D}_0, \zeta_0\}$ is the optimal solution for (7), then for another range of $[d_1, td_1]$, $\{\mathbf{D}_0, \zeta_1\}$ is still optimal if $\zeta_0 d_0 = \zeta_1 d_1$.*

The above theorems indicate that the optimal dictionary can be learned by using the single tensor model set with a range of MD values. The dictionary can then be applied adaptively to each voxel by adjusting the scale $\zeta$. In this work, we fixed $\zeta_0 = (8\pi^2 \tau d_0)^{-1}$, where $d_0 = 0.7 \times 10^{-3}$ mm$^2$/s, and generated the signals using the single tensor model with MD in range $[0.5, 0.9] \times 10^{-3}$, FA in range $[0, 0.9]$, and with the tensor oriented in 321 directions equally distributed on $\mathbb{S}^2$. The corresponding SPF coefficients $\{a'_j\}$ in Eq. (7) were then computed with $N = 4$, $L = 8$ via numerical inner product. Efficient DL was then performed using the online method in [9] to learn $\mathbf{D}$, which is initialized using the identity matrix. By solving Eq. (7), we learned 250 atoms. Including the isotropic atoms $\{B_{n00}(\mathbf{q})\}_{n=1}^N$, we have a total of 254 atoms. Note that the isotropic atoms are important so that grey matter and the CSF can be sparsely represented; this is not considered in [7]. Given a testing signal vector $e$, which represents a partial sampling of the $\mathbf{q}$-space, our method, called DL-SPFI for brevity, reconstructs the entire $\mathbf{q}$-space by first setting the scale $\zeta$ based on the estimated MD for the signal vector and then computing the signal-space coding coefficients $c$ by solving

$$\min_c \|\mathbf{M}'\mathbf{D}c - e'\|_2^2 + \|\Lambda c\|_1 \tag{8}$$

Note that additional regularization is imposed via $\Lambda$, which is devised as a diagonal matrix with elements $\Lambda_i = \frac{S}{h_i}\lambda$, where $\lambda$ is the regularization tuning parameter, $S$ is the dimension of $e'$, and $h_i$ is the energy of $i$-th atom, which essentially penalizes atoms with low energy. After estimating $c$, the SPF coefficients $a = (a_0^T, a'^T)^T$ are obtained by first computing $a' = \mathbf{D}c$ and then computing $a_0$ using Eq. (3). Finally, the EAP/ODF can be obtained using closed-form expressions [3,11].

## 4   Experiments

We compared the proposed DL-SPFI with $l_1$-FOCUSS (without DL) and DL-FOCUSS, both described in [10]. The DSI dataset and the codes provided by Bilgic[2] were used.

---

[2] http://web.mit.edu/berkin/www/software.html

**Signal Sparsity.** The theorems were first validated. First, fixing MD value $d_1 = 0.6 \times 10^{-3}$ mm²/s and using FA range $[0, 0.9]$, we generated sample signals from the single tensor model and the mixture of tensor model with the tensors orientated in random directions. The coefficients $a'$ for each sample were calculated via numerical integral with $N = 4$, $L = 8$, $\zeta = \zeta_0 = (8\pi^2\tau d_0)^{-1}$. Coefficients $c$ were then obtained via Eq. (7), based on $a'$, $\zeta_0$, and the learned dictionary $\mathbf{D}$. The signal sparsity with respect to the SPF basis and the learned DL-SPF basis was then evaluated by counting the number of coefficients in $a'$ and $c$ with absolute values larger than $0.01\|a'\|$ and $0.01\|c\|$, respectively. The top left subfigure in Fig. 1 shows that signal sparsity associated with the SPF basis decreases as FA increases, whereas sparsity for DL-SPF basis is quite consistent for both single- and multi-tensor samples, if MD value $d_1$ is within the MD range used during DL. This experiment validated Theorem 1. Second, we used MD value $d_2 = 1.1 \times 10^{-3}$ mm²/s and evaluated the signal sparsity of two bases associated with $\zeta_0$ and adaptive scale $\zeta = (8\pi^2\tau d_2)^{-1}$ for the mixture of tensor model using different FA values. The top right subfigure in Fig. 1 shows that even though the MD value $d_2$ of the testing signal is not within the MD range used in the training data, by adaptively setting the scale for the testing data, the signal can still be sparsely represented by the learned DL-SPF basis, thanks to theorem 3. Note that we have shown that it is not necessary to use mixture of tensors to learn the basis, as was done in [7]. Moreover, in [7] sparsity evaluation was performed using the estimated signal from a very limited number of noisy samples, while in fact the evaluation should be done using the original signal.

**RMSE in Cylinder Model.** We also evaluated the DL-SPF basis using the Söderman cylinder model [12] different from the tensor model used in our DL process. Using the same DSI-based sampling scheme described in [10] ($b_{max} = 8000 s/mm^2$, 514 **q**-space signal measurements), we generated a ground truth dataset using the cylinder model with the default parameters in [12]. Utilizing the evaluation method described [10], we estimated the DL-SPF coefficients from the an under-sampled version of the ground truth dataset (generated using a power-law density function $R = 3$ [10]) and reconstructed the **q**-space signals in the all 514 directions. Reconstruction accuracy was evaluated with respect to the ground truth dataset using the root-mean-square error (RMSE). The same evaluations was repeated by adding Rician noise with signal-to-noise ratio (SNR) of 20. For DL-SPFI and $l_1$-SPFI, we set $\lambda = \lambda_l = \lambda_n = 10^{-8}$ for the noise-free dataset and $10^{-5}$ for the noisy dataset. The subfigures in the second row of Fig. 1 indicates that DL-SPFI yields the lowest RMSE in both noiseless and noisy conditions, whereas the RMSE of $l_1$-SPFI increases significantly when the signal is noisy.

**RMSE in Real DSI Data.** We performed a similar evaluation using the real DSI data provided by Bilgic. In [10], the dictionary of DL-FOCUSS was learned from one slice and reconstruction was performed on the other slice. The dictionary of DL-SPFI was learned from the synthetic signals and was applied directly to the testing slice. Due to noise, comparing the estimated signal to the real signal is not a proper way of evaluation. In [10], the RMSE was computed with respect to a dataset with 10 averages, which is however not released. Therefore, we opted to report two types of RMSEs. The first is the RMSE (2.82%) between the signal estimated from the under-sampled data with 170 samples and the signal estimated from the fully-sampled dataset with 514 samples. The second is the RMSE (9.81%) between the signal estimated from under-sampled data and

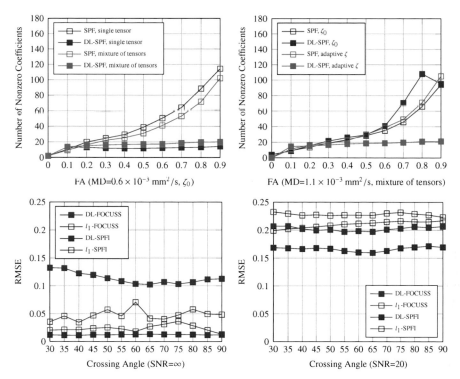

**Fig. 1. Synthetic Experiments.** The first row shows the average number of non-zero coefficients associated with the SPF basis and the DL-SPF basis for the single- and multiple-tensors and with and without adaptive scales. The second row shows the RMSE values of various methods using the Söderman cylinder model with and without noise.

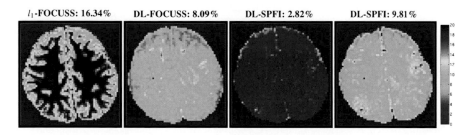

**Fig. 2. Real Data.** From left to right: the RMSE images for $l_1$-FOCUSS [10], DL-FOCUSS [10], DL-SPFI between estimations using the under-sampled dataset and the fully-sampled dataset, and DL-SPFI between the estimation from under-sampled data and the fully-sampled data.

the measured signal. Note that the outcomes for these two types RMSEs are identical for DL-FOCUSS because the estimated signal from the fully-sampled dataset is simply the fully-sampled dataset itself due to the discrete representation. In this sense, the CR-DL is much more difficult than DR-DL. Since the first type of RMSE is small, we can conclude that, by using DL-SPFI, the under-sampled dataset is sufficient for reasonable EAP reconstruction. The scanning time can hence be significantly reduced.

## 5   Conclusion

In this paper, we have demonstrated that DL-SPFI is capable of reconstructing the **q**-space signal accurately using a reduced number of signal measurements. In DL-SPFI, an optimal dictionary is learned from exemplar diffusion signals generated from the single tensor model and can be applied adaptively to each voxel for effective signal reconstruction. Compared with the DR-DL based method in [10], DL-SPFI avoids numerical errors by using a continuous representation of the **q**-space signal, allowing closed-form computation of ODF and EAP. Compared with the CR-DL method in [7], DL-SPFI is significantly more efficient because DL optimization is performed in a small dimensional subspace of SPF coefficients, while DL in [7] is performed in a high dimensional space of fully sampled diffusion signal measurements in **q**-space. Experimental results based on synthetic and real data indicate that DL-SPFI yields superb reconstruction accuracy using data with significantly reduced signal measurements.

**Acknowledgement.** This work was supported in part by a UNC start-up fund and NIH grants (EB006733, EB008374, EB009634, MH088520, AG041721, and MH100217).

## References

1. Wedeen, V.J., Hagmann, P., Tseng, W.Y.I., Reese, T.G., Weisskoff, R.M.: Mapping complex tissue architecture with diffusion spectrum magnetic resonance imaging. Magnetic Resonance In Medicine 54, 1377–1386 (2005)
2. Assemlal, H.E., Tschumperlé, D., Brun, L.: Efficient and robust computation of PDF features from diffusion MR signal. Medical Image Analysis 13, 715–729 (2009)
3. Cheng, J., Ghosh, A., Jiang, T., Deriche, R.: Model-Free and Analytical EAP Reconstruction via Spherical Polar Fourier Diffusion MRI. In: Jiang, T., Navab, N., Pluim, J.P.W., Viergever, M.A. (eds.) MICCAI 2010, Part I. LNCS, vol. 6361, pp. 590–597. Springer, Heidelberg (2010)
4. Donoho, D.: Compressed sensing. IEEE Transactions on Information Theory 52(4) (2006)
5. Menzel, M.I., Tan, E.T., Khare, K., Sperl, J.I., King, K.F., Tao, X., Hardy, C.J., Marinelli, L.: Accelerated diffusion spectrum imaging in the human brain using compressed sensing. Magnetic Resonance in Medicine 66(5), 1226–1233 (2011)
6. Cheng, J., Merlet, S., Caruyer, E., Ghosh, A., Jiang, T., Deriche, R., et al.: Compressive Sensing Ensemble Average Propagator Estimation via L1 Spherical Polar Fourier Imaging. In: Computational Diffusion MRI - MICCAI Workshop (2011)
7. Merlet, S., Caruyer, E., Deriche, R.: Parametric dictionary learning for modeling EAP and ODF in diffusion MRI. In: Ayache, N., Delingette, H., Golland, P., Mori, K. (eds.) MICCAI 2012, Part III. LNCS, vol. 7512, pp. 10–17. Springer, Heidelberg (2012)
8. Aharon, M., Elad, M., Bruckstein, A.: K-SVD: An Algorithm for Designing Overcomplete Dictionaries for Sparse Representation. In: IEEE TSP (2006)
9. Mairal, J., Bach, F., Ponce, J., Sapiro, G.: Online learning for matrix factorization and sparse coding. The Journal of Machine Learning Research 11, 19–60 (2010)
10. Bilgic, B., Setsompop, K., Cohen-Adad, J., Yendiki, A., Wald, L.L., Adalsteinsson, E.: Accelerated diffusion spectrum imaging with compressed sensing using adaptive dictionaries. Magnetic Resonance in Medicine (2012)
11. Cheng, J., Ghosh, A., Deriche, R., Jiang, T.: Model-free, regularized, fast, and robust analytical orientation distribution function estimation. In: Jiang, T., Navab, N., Pluim, J.P.W., Viergever, M.A. (eds.) MICCAI 2010, Part I. LNCS, vol. 6361, pp. 648–656. Springer, Heidelberg (2010)
12. Özarslan, E., Shepherd, T.M., Vemuri, B.C., Blackband, S.J., Mareci, T.H.: Resolution of complex tissue microarchitecture using the diffusion orientation transform (DOT). NeuroImage 31, 1086–1103 (2006)

# On Describing Human White Matter Anatomy: The White Matter Query Language

Demian Wassermann[1], Nikos Makris[2], Yogesh Rathi[1], Martha Shenton[1],
Ron Kikinis[1], Marek Kubicki[1], and Carl-Fredrik Westin[1]

[1] Brigham and Women's Hospital and Harvard Medical School, Boston, MA, USA
demian@bwh.harvard.edu
[2] Massachusetts General Hospital and Harvard Medical School, Boston, MA, USA

**Abstract.** The main contribution of this work is the careful syntactical definition of major white matter tracts in the human brain based on a neuroanatomist's expert knowledge. We present a technique to formally describe white matter tracts and to automatically extract them from diffusion MRI data. The framework is based on a novel query language with a near-to-English textual syntax. This query language allows us to construct a dictionary of anatomical definitions describing white matter tracts. The definitions include adjacent gray and white matter regions, and rules for spatial relations. This enables automated coherent labeling of white matter anatomy across subjects. We use our method to encode anatomical knowledge in human white matter describing 10 association and 8 projection tracts per hemisphere and 7 commissural tracts. The technique is shown to be comparable in accuracy to manual labeling. We present results applying this framework to create a white matter atlas from 77 healthy subjects, and we use this atlas in a proof-of-concept study to detect tract changes specific to schizophrenia.

## 1 Introduction

Diffusion magnetic resonance imaging (dMRI) is a technique that allows to probe the structure of white matter the human brain *in vivo*. dMRI streamline tractography has provided the opportunity for non-invasive investigation of white matter anatomy. Most common methods for isolating fiber bundles based on streamline tractography require the manual placement of multiple regions of interest (ROIs). These methods include an approach that starts from seed points within a predefined region of interest, and then calculates and preserves only tracts that touch other predefined ROIs [1]. A different approach creates seed points throughout the entire brain (whole brain tractography) keeping tracts that pass through conjunctions, disjunctions or exclusions of ROIs either off-line [2] or interactively [3]. An alternative method to manual placement of ROIs is to use a clustering approach [4–6]. Clustering methods are in general fully automatic, unguided, and take advantage of the similarity of fiber paths. However, incorporating precise information about human anatomy into a clustering method is difficult.

The ability to target specific tracts for analyses compared to whole brain studies increases the statistical power and sensitivity of the study, and simplifies the interpretation of results, but requires precise consistent delineation of the tracts across subjects. Although several fascicules, such as the cingulum bundle, are widely recognized

K. Mori et al. (Eds.): MICCAI 2013, Part I, LNCS 8149, pp. 647–654, 2013.

and well defined in field of neuroanatomy, there are others which existence or subdivisions is still a matter of discussion. Examples are the different systems to define and subdivide the superior longitudinal fasciculus (SLF) proposed by Catani [7] and Makris [8], and the discussion regarding existence of the inferior occipito-frontal fasciculus (IOFF) in humans [9]. Three major challenges make it difficult to extend and reproduce tractography-based dissections and tract-specific analyses: 1) the anatomical dissection of the white matter into specific fascicles is currently in discussion; 2) comparing fascicle definitions across atlases is a difficult task due to the lack of a system to unify the definitions; 3) semi-automated approaches are usually based on a fixed set of fascicles difficult to extend due to amount of technical knowledge needed for the task.

The main contribution of this paper is a system to express anatomical descriptions of white matter tracts in a near-to-English textual language, and we believe this work can help address the above challenges. We designed this textual language to be human-readable to make the tract descriptions easy to change and extend without the need of an engineering background and to be used for automated white matter virtual dissections. The white matter query language (WMQL) proposed in this paper has several applications. For example Wakana's and Catani's definition of tracts using regions of interest (ROIs) [10, 2], can readily be represented using WMQL definitions. This will yield an human readable definition that also can be extended by an anatomist for finer division. Another interesting application is to post-process clustering results and automatically label clusters as anatomically known tracts [4–6]. In this paper we present definitions of different tracts from current literature and formulated WMQL descriptions. Our anatomy dictionary currently contains descriptions of 10 association and 8 projection tracts per hemisphere, and 7 commissural tracts. An implementation of WMQL as well as the definitions specified in this publication can be downloaded at
`http://demianw.github.com/tract_querier`

## 2 Methods

We designed the queries in white matter query language (WMQL) to formalize current descriptions in anatomy literature. Such descriptions are constructed in terms of different relationships between gyri, sulci, subcortical structures or white matter areas. The operations of WMQL, can be divided into 3 groups: 1) **anatomical terms** stating if a tract traverses or ends in a certain brain structure, 2) **relative position terms** indicating whether the tracts are, for instance, medial or frontal to a structure like the amygdala, and 3) **logical operations** like conjunction, disjunction or exclusion of the previous two types of clauses. We illustrate these three types of operations in fig. 1.

To apply WMQL queries to dissect dMRI-based tractographies, like in fig. 1, we need to situate gyri, sulci and other structures used for the queries relative to the tractography. For this, we overlay an atlas of the brain structures on top the tractography, in this work we used the cortical and white matter parcellation based on the Desikan atlas as described by [11] and the neuroanatomic structure segmentation by [12] which are readily available in FreeSurfer (http://www.freesurfer.org). We provide the details of this process in the section MRI Data Acquisition and Processing. It is worth noting that WMQL does not depend on a particular atlas.

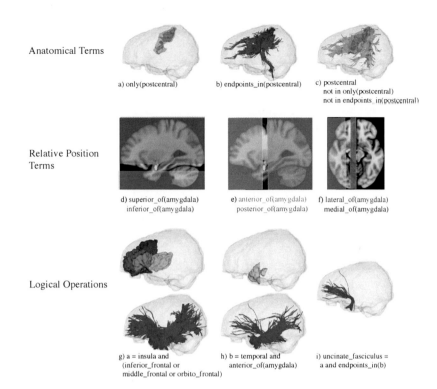

**Fig. 1.** WMQL Terms (a-f) along with an example construction of a WMQL query (g-i). Regions in (g-i): insula (cyan); the orbito-frontal (purple), middle-frontal (brown) and inferior-frontal (dark green) gyri. h) shows the anterior temporal lobe (light green) defined as the section of the temporal lobe anterior to the amygdala (yellow).

To implement the white matter query language, we group the tracts in sets representing whether they have an endpoint in each anatomical label (fig. 1b); traverse anatomical label (fig. 1c); or their position relative to each anatomical label (fig. 1d-f). Then, for each anatomical label, like the amygdala, we have six sets:

1. endpoints_in(amygdala): all tracts with at least an endpoint in the amygdala.
2. amygdala: all the tracts traversing the amygdala.
3. anterior_of(amygdala), posterior_of(amygdala), medial_of(amygdala), lateral_of(amygdala), superior_of(amygdala), inferior_of(amygdala) : containing the tracts traversing brain areas delimited by their relative position to the amygdala

We calculate the endpoint sets (1) by computing which label is the tract touching at each endpoint and adding the tract to the corresponding set. The sets representing label traversals (2) are computed by following each tract and adding it to the set corresponding to a particular label, like the amygdala, if tract traverses it. Finally, we compute the 6 relative positioning sets (3) by checking the points the tract traverses with respect to a label. For instance, every tract that traverses the area anterior to the amygdala, shown in orange in fig. 1e, will be added to the set anterior_of(amygdala). We implement this efficiently using a tree of axis-aligned bounding boxes of the structures as a spatial index of the labels and then computing the relative positions of the tracts with respect to the bounding boxes composing each label [13]. For two sets of tracts a and b and the set of all tracts L, we formalize the WQML logical operations as follows:

$a$ **or** $b := \{tract : tract \in a \cup b\}$    **only**$(a) := \{tract : tract \in a \wedge tract \notin (L \setminus a)\}$

$a$ **and** $b := \{tract : tract \in a \cap b\}$    $a$ **not in** $b := \{tract : tract \in a \wedge tract \notin b\}$

We have illustrated these operations in fig. 1 a), c); and g)-i). Tracts in WMQL are defined by using an assignment operation, for instance, we defined the left UF in fig. 1i as assigning a meaning to UF.left:

*UF.left = insula.**left** and (lateral_frontal.**left** or medial_frontal.**left** or orbito_frontal.**left**) and endpoints_in(temporal.**left** and anterior_of(amygdala.**left**)) not in hemisphere.**right***

To simplify the definitions of tracts in both hemispheres with a single assignment, we included the suffixes .side and .opposite to WMQL. Creating a bihemispheric definition becomes:

*UF.side = insula.**side** and*
*(lateral_frontal.**side** or medial_frontal.**side** or orbito_frontal.**side**) and*
*endpoints_in(temporal.**side** and anterior_of(amygdala.**side**)) not in hemisphere.**opposite***

In this way WMQL allows a single definition for tracts found in both hemispheres simultaneously. The formalization of WMQL as the basic set operations allows us to define white matter tracts using all the flexibility and expressiveness power of set theory and propositional logic. Finally, to implement the WMQL language, we defined the WMQL in Backus normal form; we used an LL(1) parser for this grammar which transforms WMQL expressions into an abstract syntax tree; and we implemented an algorithm to traverse the tree evaluating the WMQL operations.

# 3    Results

## 3.1    Development of WMQL

We are using WMQL to formalize tract descriptions from classic neuroanatomy textbooks and current literature on the anatomy of the white matter [14, 10, 8, 15]. In table 1, we show the queries for 10 association tracts. In the following, for each tract we describe in WMQL, we provide a description derived from anatomy literature and the derived WMQL query. The population results of these queries are shown in fig. 2 along with the commisural and projection tracts whose definitions we did not include for space reasons. Using the WMQL, we have constructed a comprehensive atlas based on high angular MRI (HARDI) tractography [16] . The combination of WMQL with current tractography technologies has enabled us to generalize previous atlases [10, 2] and extend them with white matter tracts not included in these like the middle longitudinal fasciculus (MdLF) or the three different superior longitudinal fasciculi. In total, our atlas includes 10 long association tracts; 8 projection tracts per hemisphere (7 corticostriatal and the Cortico-spinal tract) and the 7 sections of the corpus callosum according to [15].

**Table 1.** Association Tract Definitions in WMQL: Cingulum bundle (CG); Extreme Capsule (EmC); and the fascicules: Superior Longitudinal (SLF) sections I to III; Arcuate (AF); Inferior occipito frontal (IOFF); Middle Longitudinal (MdLF); Uncinate (UF)

| |
|---|
| **CB.side = only(**(cingular.**side** or cingular_cortex.**side**) **and** (middle_frontal.**side** or cuneus.**side** or entorhinal.**side** orsuperior_frontal.**side** or inferior_parietal.**side** or fusiform.**side** or medial_orbitofrontal.**side** or lateral_orbitofrontal.**side** or parahippocampal.**side** or precuneus.**side** or lingual.**side** or centrum_semiovale.**side)**) |
| **EmC.side = (endpoints_in(**inferior_frontal.**side** or middle_frontal.**side**) **andendpoints_in(**inferior_parietal_lobule.**side**) **and**temporal.**side and** insula.**side)not in** hemisphere.**opposite** |
| **SLF_I.side = (**superior_parietal.**side and** precuneus.**side and** superior_frontal.**side) or(**superior_parietal.**side and** precuneus.**side and** superior_frontal.**side and** lateral_occipital.**side) not in** cingular.**side not in** temporal.**side not in** subcortical.**side not in** hemisphere.**opposite** |
| **SLF_II.side =(**inferior_parietal.**side** or supramarginal.**side** or lateral_occipital.**side) and endpoints_in(**middle_frontal.**side)) not in** temporal.**side not in** subcortical.**side not in** hemisphere.**opposite** |
| **SLF_III.side = ((**inferior_parietal.**side** or supramarginal.**side** or lateral_occipital.**side) and endpoints_in(**inferior_frontal.**side)) not in** temporal.**side not in** subcortical.**side not in** hemisphere.**opposite** |
| **AF.side = (**inferior_frontal.**side** or middle_frontal.**side** or precentral.**side) and** (superior_temporal.**side** or middle_temporal.**side) not in medial_of(**supramarginal.**side)not in** subcortical.**side not in** hemisphere.**opposite** |
| **IOFF.side = (**lateralorbitofrontal.**side and** occipital.**side) and** temporal.**side not in** subcortical.**side not in** cingular.**side not in** superior_parietal_lobule.**side not in** hemisphere.**opposite** |
| **ILF.side = only(**temporal.**side and** occipital.**side) and anterior_of(**hippocampus.**side) not in** parahippocampal.**side** |
| **MdLF.side = only(** (temporal_pole.**side** or superior_temporal.**side) and (**inferior_parietal.**side** or superior_parietal.**side** or supramarginal.**side** or precuneus.**side** or (centrum_semiovale.**side and** superior_parietal.**side) or (**centrum_semiovale.**side and** inferior_parietal.**side))** |
| **UF.side = insula.side and (**inferior_frontal.**side** or middle_frontal.**side** or orbito_frontal.**side) and endpoints_in(**temporal.**side and anterior_of(**amygdala.**side))** |

### 3.2   Application of WMQL to Tract Extraction and Statistical Analyses

Diffusion-weighted images (DWI) from 77 healthy subjects (HS) ($32.9 \pm 12.4$ years old of age; 64 males; right handed) and 20 male schizophrenic subjects (SZ) paired with the HS were acquired. DWI data were acquired on a GE Signa HDxt 3.0T (51 directions with b=900 s/mm2, 8 b=0 s/mm2 images, 1.7 mm$^3$ isotropic voxels). A T1 MRI acquisition was also performed (25.6cm2 field of view, 1mm$^3$ isotropic voxels). For each DWI image, we obtained a 2-tensor full-brain tractography placing ten seeds per voxel and obtaining an average of one million tracts per subject. We overlaid a parcellation of the cortical and sub-cortical structures and the white matter on DWI images by processing the T1 images of each subject using FreeSurfer and registering the results to the DWI images using ANTS [17]. For each subject, this resulted in the subcortical structures labeled and the cortex the white matter parcellated [11].

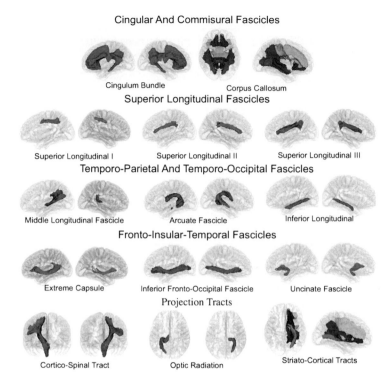

**Fig. 2.** Iso-surfaces in blue (p-value = 0.01, corrected for multiple comparisons) shows 11 association, 8 projection and 7 commissural tracts

**Validation.** To validate our extraction protocol, 2 different experts segmented 5 tracts (IOFF, UF, ILF, CST and AF) in each hemisphere of 10 healthy subjects following the protocol in [10]. Overlap between those and the ones extracted was calculated with the kappa measure [2]. For all tracts $k > .7$ which is considered good agreement, the worse being the left AF ($k = .71$) and the best the left CST ($k = .89$).

**White Matter Atlas Generation with WMQL:** For each subject we extracted 37 white matter tracts using WMQL queries derived from classical and current literature of the human brain white matter. Some of these are detailed in table 1. Processing each full brain tractography took $5 \pm .25$ min. to initialize and $7 \pm .02$ sec. per query.

To generate a tract atlas, we normalized all the FA maps to MNI space, created a population FA template using ANTS and then generated group effect maps for each tract [7]. To obtain the group effect maps, we started by calculating a binary visitation map for each tract of each subject. This map is a mask in MNI space where a voxel has a value of one if the tract traverses that voxel and 0 if it doesn't. We create the group effect map for each tract through voxel-wise statistics. The group effect map assesses the probability that a tract traverses each voxel. For this, we rejected the null hypothesis that that voxel is not traversed by such tract. We first smoothed the visitation maps with a 2mm (FWHM) isotropic Gaussian to approximate the distribution of the data to a Gaussian one [18]. Then, we rejected the hypothesis that the voxel does not belong

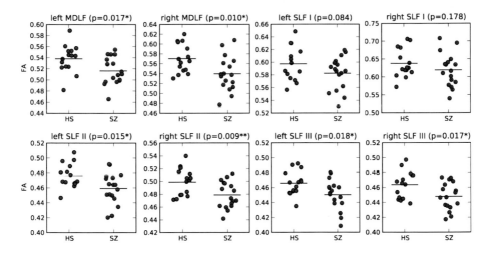

**Fig. 3.** Compared mean FA over different tracts between healthy subjects (HS) and schizophrenic subjects (SZ). The p-value was computed using a t-test correcting for age. We observe significant differences on the left and right MdLF, and the left and right SLF II and III tracts. Notation: the * means p-value $< .05$ and ** p-value $< .01$.

to the tract, i.e. the mean traversal value over all subjects on that voxel is different to 0, by using a voxel wise t-test for a one-sample mean. We calculated the corrected significance using permutation testing (10,000 iterations) to avoid a high dependence on Gaussian assumptions [19]. We set the significance threshold for considering that a voxel belongs to the tract to p-value $< 0.0001$ corrected for multiple comparisons.

**Group Differences in Schizophrenia.** As a proof of concept, we analyzed the tracts that are not included in other atlases, but found in our WM atlas only: MdLF, SLF I, II and III in 20 SZ subjects and controls extracted from the HS paired by age and gender. We used the group maps to obtain a weighted average of FA resulting in one value per subject and performed a t-test for each tract correcting for age. We show these results in fig. 3. Results show agreement with recent discoveries in SZ in the MdLF tract [20]

## 4   Conclusion

In this work we have introduced the White Matter Query Language: a tool to represent anatomical knowledge of white matter tracts and extract them from full-brain tractographies. This tool is a complement to current semi-automated approaches in tract extraction based in clustering and can be used to implement ROI-based approaches. The utility of the tool was illustrated by constructing an atlas of white matter tracts from 77 healthy subjects and then performing a statistical analysis in schizophrenia. The textual descriptions in WMQL add transparency between the conceptualization of white matter fiber tracts and their extraction from a dMRI.

**Acknowledgments.** This work has been supported by NIH grants: R01MH074794, R01MH092862, P41RR013218, R01MH097979, P41EB015902 and Swedish Research Council (VR) grant 2012-3682.

# References

1. Mori, S., van Zijl, P.C.M.: Fiber tracking: principles and strategies-a technical review. NMR in Biomedicine (2002)
2. Wakana, S., Caprihan, A., Panzenboeck, M.M., Fallon, J.H., Perry, M., Gollub, R.L., Hua, K., Zhang, J., Jiang, H., Dubey, P., Blitz, A., van Zijl, P.C., Mori, S.: Reproducibility of quantitative tractography methods applied to cerebral white matter. NImg (2007)
3. Akers, D., Sherbondy, A., Mackenzie, R., Dougherty, R., Wandell, B.: Exploration of the brain's white matter pathways with dynamic queries. In: IEEE Viz. (2004)
4. Wassermann, D., Bloy, L., Kanterakis, E., Verma, R., Deriche, R.: Unsupervised white matter fiber clustering and tract probability map generation: Applications of a Gaussian process framework for white matter fibers. NImg (2010)
5. O'Donnell, L.J., Westin, C.F.: Automatic Tractography Segmentation Using a High-Dimensional White Matter Atlas. TMI (2007)
6. Wang, X., Grimson, W.E.L., Westin, C.F.: Tractography segmentation using a hierarchical Dirichlet processes mixture model. NImg (2011)
7. Thiebaut de Schotten, M., Ffytche, D.H., Bizzi, A., Dell'acqua, F., Allin, M., Walshe, M., Murray, R., Williams, S.C., Murphy, D.G., Catani, M.: Atlasing location, asymmetry and inter-subject variability of white matter tracts in the human brain with MR diffusion tractography. NImg (2010)
8. Makris, N., Kennedy, D.N., McInerney, S., Sorensen, A.G., Wang, R., Caviness, V.S., Pandya, D.: Segmentation of Subcomponents within the Superior Longitudinal Fascicle in Humans: A Quantitative, In Vivo, DT-MRI Study. Cerebral Cortex (2005)
9. Schmahmann, J.D., Pandya, D.: The Complex History of the Fronto-Occipital Fasciculus. Journal of the History of the Neurosciences (2007)
10. Catani, M., Thiebaut de Schotten, M.: A diffusion tensor imaging tractography atlas for virtual in vivo dissections. Cortex (2008)
11. Salat, D.H., Greve, D.N., Pacheco, J.L., Quinn, B.T., Helmer, K.G., Buckner, R.L., Fischl, B.: Regional white matter volume differences in nondemented aging and Alzheimer's disease. NImg (2009)
12. Fischl, B., Salat, D.H., Busa, E., Albert, M., Dieterich, M., Haselgrove, C., van der Kouwe, A., Killiany, R., Kennedy, D., Klaveness, S., Montillo, A., Makris, N., Rosen, B., Dale, A.M.: Whole Brain Segmentation: Automated Labeling of Neuroanatomical Structures in the Human Brain. Neuron (2002)
13. Bergen, G.V.D.: Efficient Collision Detection of Complex Deformable Models using AABB Trees. Journal of Graphic Tools (1997)
14. Parent, A.: Carpenter's Human Neuroanatomy. Williams & Wilkins (1996)
15. Witelson, S.F., Kigar, D.L.: Anatomical development of the corpus callosum in humans: A review with reference to sex and cognition. In: Brain Lateralization in Children: Developmental Implications (1988)
16. Malcolm, J.G., Michailovich, O., Bouix, S., Westin, C.F., Shenton, M.E., Rathi, Y.: A filtered approach to neural tractography using the Watson directional function. TMI (2010)
17. Avants, B., Epstein, C., Grossman, M., Gee, J.C.: Symmetric diffeomorphic image registration with cross-correlation: Evaluating automated labeling of elderly and neurodegenerative brain. MIA (2008)
18. Ashburner, J., Friston, K.J.: Voxel-Based Morphometry—The Methods. NImg (2000)
19. Nichols, T.E., Holmes, A.P.: Nonparametric permutation tests for functional neuroimaging: a primer with examples. In: HBM (2002)
20. Asami, T., Saito, Y., Whitford, T.J., Makris, N., Niznikiewicz, M., McCarley, R.W., Shenton, M.E., Kubicki, M.: Abnormalities of middle longitudinal fascicle and disorganization in patients with schizophrenia. Schizophrenia Research (2013)

# Voxelwise Spectral Diffusional Connectivity and Its Applications to Alzheimer's Disease and Intelligence Prediction[*]

Junning Li[1,**], Yan Jin[1,2,**], Yonggang Shi[1], Ivo D. Dinov[1], Danny J. Wang[3],
Arthur W. Toga[1], and Paul M. Thompson[1,2]

[1] Laboratory of Neuro Imaging
[2] Imaging Genetics Center
[3] Brain Mapping Center UCLA School of Medicine, Los Angeles, CA 90095, USA
{jli,yjin,yshi,idinov,jj.wang,toga,thompson}@loni.ucla.edu

**Abstract.** Human brain connectivity can be studied using graph theory. Many connectivity studies parcellate the brain into regions and count fibres extracted between them. The resulting network analyses require validation of the tractography, as well as region and parameter selection. Here we investigate whole brain connectivity from a different perspective. We propose a mathematical formulation based on studying the eigenvalues of the Laplacian matrix of the diffusion tensor field at the voxel level. This voxelwise matrix has over a million parameters, but we derive the Kirchhoff complexity and eigen-spectrum through elegant mathematical theorems, without heavy computation. We use these novel measures to accurately estimate the voxelwise connectivity in multiple biomedical applications such as Alzheimer's disease and intelligence prediction.

## 1 Introduction

The human brain is a complex network of structurally connected regions that interact functionally. Brain connectivity can be studied from different perspectives. Functional MRI, can reveal correlated activity and even causal relationships that underlie the communication of distributed brain systems. On the other hand, diffusion weighted MRI (DWI) measures the local profile of water diffusion in tissues, yielding information on white matter (WM) integrity and connectivity that traditional structural MRI cannot provide. DWI is non-invasive, and is increasingly used to study macro-scale anatomical connections linking brain regions through fibre pathways.

Brain networks are commonly described as a mathematical graph, consisting of a collection of nodes, representing a parcellation of the brain anatomy or regions of interest (ROIs), and a set of edges between pairs of nodes, describing some property of the connection between that pair of regions. The brain exhibits several organization principles, including "small-worldness", characterized by the coexistence of dense local clustering between neighboring nodes and high global

---

[*] This work is supported by grants K01EB013633, R01MH094343, P41EB015922, RO1MH080892, R01EB008432, and R01EB007813 from NIH.
[**] These two authors contributed equally to this work.

efficiency (short average path length) due to few long-range connections [1]. This property results in a sparse connectivity matrix that can be explored using graph theory. A typical way to construct the connectivity matrix is to group adjacent voxels into ROIs (anatomically meaningful grey matter regions) or nodes, and count the fibres passing through each pair of nodes. Then standard measures of connectivity including small worldness, clustering, path length, and efficiency can be computed to reveal how the brain is affected by genetic factors [2] and neurological diseases such as Alzheimer's disease [3].

However, this classical approach has limitations. First, there is lack of validation of WM fibres generated by tractography. Based on different reconstruction or tracking models (tensor vs. orientation distribution function and deterministic vs. probabilistic), different tractography algorithms and variations in their parameters can lead to large differences in the resulting network measures [4]. Automatic cortical grey matter segmentation from an atlas is also susceptible to registration error. Furthermore, the spatial scale of the parcellation of the grey matter into nodes of the connectivity graph may affect connectivity measures by as much as 95% [5]. Finally, parameter thresholding in graph analysis also influences the interpretation of the results [6].

To avoid these problems, we propose a novel mathematical formulation to explore brain connectivity from a different perspective. Instead of investigating linkages among sub-regions of the brain, we use the tensor information from DWI at the voxel level. In this way, we avoid making further assumptions on tractography that diffusion images do not intrinsically provide. Then we show that the diffusion equation can be characterized by the Laplacian matrix of the tensor field. In graph theory, the Laplacian matrix is a matrix representation of a graph. It can be used to calculate the number of spanning trees for a given graph. We, therefore, circumvent the nodal parcellation problem by studying voxelwise linkage. Although others have studied voxel connectivity in its local neighborhood [7], our work focuses more on studying the brain as a whole entity. Finally, we present two important characteristics of a graph, the number of spanning trees (Kirchhoff complexity) and the eigen-spectrum, both of which can be computed without any parameter tuning. As there may be well over a million voxels in a typical image volume, the Kirchhoff complexity and eigen-spectrum can be challenging to compute. We therefore present an algorithm to calculate them efficiently. In the Experimental Section, we illustrate how to evaluate these measures in two biomedical applications (Alzheimer's disease and intelligence prediction).

## 2    Voxelwise Spectral Diffusional Connectivity

### 2.1    Diffusion Equation and Tensor

DWI yields information on WM fibres by measuring signals sensitive to the directional diffusion of water molecules. A diffusion process is usually described by the diffusion equation, which is a partial differential equation as follows

$$\frac{\partial f(x,t)}{\partial t} = \langle \nabla, T(x)\nabla f(x,t)\rangle,$$

(1)

where $f(x, t)$ is the density of the diffusing material at time $t$ and at location $x$ (in the continuous domain), $T(x)$ is the diffusion tensor at location $x$, and $\nabla$ represents the spatial derivative operator. Here $-T(x)\nabla f(x, t)$ can be understood as the "flux", the amount of diffusing material moving through a unit surface at location $x$, and over a unit time interval starting at time $t$.

$T(x)$ fully characterizes the diffusion properties of a field. The diffusion tensor images reconstructed from DWI are voxel estimates of the diffusion field $T(x)$. To make $T(x)$ reflect the spatial density of WM fibres, we modulate diffusion tensors with its fractional anisotropy (FA).

## 2.2   Laplacian Matrix and Graph

To study $T(x)$ numerically, the spatially and temporally continuous process defined by Eq. (1) should be discretized. As we are interested in $T(x)$ itself, not the diffusion process $f(x, t)$, we discretize it only spatially with the finite difference method. Then the discretized version of Eq. (1) becomes $\frac{\partial f}{\partial t} = -Af$, where $A$ is a square matrix of size $n$, where $n$ is the number of voxels of interest. $A$ should satisfy the following criteria: (1) It is self-adjoint because the diffusivity between two voxels should be independent of the direction of the flux that crosses them. (2) The sum of each row or each column needs to be zero because the total volume of the diffusion material should be preserved . (3) Its off-diagonal elements are non-positive because the molecules diffuse from high concentration to low concentration. Matrices that satisfy all the three properties are called Laplacian matrices.

Laplacian matrices and graphs have a one-to-one mapping relationship. Given the adjacency matrix of an undirected and weighted graph $G$ whose elements $\{g_{ij}\}$ indicate the edge weight between two adjacent vertices $i$ and $j$, its Laplacian matrix $A = \{a_{ij}\}$ is defined as

$$a_{ij} = \begin{cases} -g_{ij}, & \text{if } i \neq j; \\ \sum_{k=1}^{n} g_{ik}, & \text{if } i = j. \end{cases} \tag{2}$$

We can see that how the Laplacian matrix is constructed also implies that a graph can be inversely constructed from its Laplacian matrix. It is worth noting that the Laplacian matrix $A$ of a connected graph is positive semi-definite. There is one and only one zero eigenvalue and the rest of the eigenvalues are all positive.

With this one-to-one correspondence relationship, we claim that a diffusion field can be studied via its Laplacian matrix or its corresponding graph. For example, we can study its connectivity complexity, as addressed in Section 2.3, its eigen-spectrum, as addressed in Section2.4, or its vertex centrality in future work.

## 2.3   Spanning Trees and Kirchhoff Complexity

A spanning tree of a connected graph $G$ is a sub-graph connecting all the vertices in $G$, which does not contain any circular path. Adding one edge to a spanning tree creates a circle and deleting one edge from a spanning tree partitions the tree into two disjoint sets. Spanning trees play important roles in graph theory. It is also related to fundamental circles and fundamental cut sets of a graph. One measurement of the complexity of a graph is the number of its spanning trees, which is called the Kirchhoff complexity [8]. The extended Kirchhoff complexity for weighted graphs is defined as

$$K(G) = \sum_{\pi \in T(G)} w(\pi), \qquad w(\pi) = \prod_{i,j \in \pi} g_{ij}, \tag{3}$$

where $T(G)$ is the set of spanning trees of an undirected weighted graph $G = \{g_{ij}\}$, $\pi$ is a spanning tree, and $w(\pi)$ is the weight associated with $\pi$ by multiplying all the weights of its edges.

We choose $K(G)$ to indicate the complexity of a connectivity network because it enumerates all the possible ways to connect all the vertices in a graph without circles and it also considers the effectiveness of the connection by weighting with its edge weights.

Although $K(G)$ is defined by enumeration, its calculation does not require enumeration. It can be solved with the Kirchhoff Matrix-Tree theorem [9] as follows.

**Kirchhoff's Matrix-Tree Theorem:** Given a connected undirected weighted graph $G$, its Kirchhoff complexity is

$$K(G) = \frac{1}{n}\lambda_1\lambda_2\cdots\lambda_{n-1} = \det(A_{-i}), \tag{4}$$

where $\lambda_1, \lambda_2, \cdots, \lambda_{n-1}$ are the non-zero eigenvalues of the Laplacian matrix of $G$, $A_{-i}$ is the matrix derived by removing the $i$th row and the $i$th column from the Laplacian matrix, and $n$ is the number of vertices of $G$. Interestingly, no matter what value $i$ takes, the result is the same.

Eq. (4) requires the calculation of the matrix determinant, but direct and exact calculation of the determinant of large matrices is not currently feasible, as it may lead to numerical overflow. Fortunately, we can calculate the logarithm of the determinant very efficiently with matrix factorization. Given a symmetric $A_{-i}$, we first decompose it as $A_{-i} = LDL^\mathsf{T}$ by the LDL decomposition where $L$ is a square lower uni-triangular matrix and $D$ is a diagonal matrix with rank $n-1$. Now we have two properties: $\det(A_{-i}) = \det(L)\det(D)\det(L^\mathsf{T}) = \det(D)$ and $\det(D) = \prod_{i=1}^{n-1} d_{ii}$ where $d_{ii}$ is the $i$th diagonal element of $D$. Then we can calculate the logarithm of Kirchhoff complexity as

$$\ln K = \ln\det(A_{-i}) = \sum_{i=1}^{n-1} \ln d_{ii}. \tag{5}$$

### 2.4   Estimation of Eigenvalue Spectrum

The eigenvalues of a Laplacian matrix $A$ not only decide the complexity of a graph (see Eq. (4)) but also convey important information on the temporal responses of the differential equation $\frac{\partial f}{\partial t} = -Af$. However, calculating the eigenvalues of a large sparse matrix demands cumbersome computation and can be impractical. For example, at the 128 x 128 x 128 image volume size, the Laplacian matrix derived from the diffusion tensor images has approximately $2 \times 10^6$ rows and columns. For such a large matrix, direct and exact calculation of their eigenvalues is practically impossible. As we are only interested in the distribution of the eigenvalues instead of their exact values, we can estimate the cumulative distribution function (CDF) of the eigenvalues with Sylvester's Law of Inertia.

**Sylvester's Law of Inertia:** Given a symmetric and real-valued matrix $A$, its transformation $B = SAS^\mathsf{T}$, where $S$ is an invertible square matrix, has the same number of positive/negative eigenvalues as $A$ does.

Let $h(\beta)$ be the number of $A$'s eigenvalues which are equal or smaller than $\beta$, that is, $h(\beta) = |\{\lambda_i \leqslant \beta\}|$ where $\lambda_i$'s are the eigenvalues of $A$. To calculate $h(\beta)$, we first factorize $A_\beta = A - \beta I$ as $A_\beta = LDL^\mathsf{T}$ by the LDL decomposition, where $I$ is the identity matrix, and $L$ and $D$ are denoted as in Section 2.3. Now we have three properties: (1) if $\lambda$ is an eigenvalue of $A$, then $\lambda - \beta$ is an eigenvalue of $A_\beta$; (2) $D$ has the same number of positive/negative eigenvalues as $A_\beta$ does; (3) The eigenvalues of $D$ are its diagonal elements. These properties implies that $h(\beta)$ equals the number of the diagonal elements of $D$ which are less than or equal to 0, even though the diagonal elements of $D$ are not necessarily the eigenvalues of $A_\beta$. The detailed eigen-spectrum computation algorithm is summarized in **Algorithm 1**.

---

**Algorithm 1.** Estimation of Eigen-Spectrum with $m$ Bins

---

1. Calculate the largest eigenvalue $\lambda_{\max}$ of $A$ with the power iteration method.
2. Set bin positions $\{\beta_i = \frac{i}{m}\lambda_{\max}, i = 1, \cdots m\}$ for estimating $h(\beta)$.
3. For each $\beta_i$:
   (a) Decompose $A - \beta_i I$ as $LDL^\mathsf{T}$.
   (b) $h(\beta_i) = |\{d_{kk} \leq 0\}|$ where $d_{kk}$'s are the diagonal elements of $D$.

---

## 3    Experiments

In this section, we show how to apply the theory we derived in Section 2 to two real biomedical problems.

### 3.1    Graph Construction and Connectivity Computation

The raw diffusion images were corrected for eddy-current induced distortions with FMRIB Software Library (FSL) and then skull-stripped using the FSL tool, BET. The FA modulated tensor field was reconstructed using our own C++ diffusion tool package developed with Segmentation & Registration Toolkit (ITK). Negative eigenvalues of the reconstructed tensors were rectified to their absolute values. Next, the FA image of each subject was linearly aligned to a single-subject International Consortium for Brain Mapping (ICBM) FA atlas from Johns Hopkins University [10] (the atlas was downsampled to the 2 x 2 x 2 mm$^3$ resolution to facilitate the computation). The purpose of registration was to reduce the possible bias in graph construction introduced by individual volumetric differences. Tensors were linearly interpolated and re-oriented with the preservation-of-principal-direction method [11] when the affine transformation was applied. The discretized Laplacian matrix of the transformed tensor field was constructed. Finally, the logarithm of Kirchhoff complexity was computed as described in Section 2.3 and the logarithmic eigen-spectrum was estimated according to **Algorithm 1** in Section 2.4. The Laplacian matrices are sparse and it took about 5 minutes to perform one LDL routine for a square matrix of size $2 \times 10^6$ with a 2.8 GHz Xeon CPU.

## 3.2    Alzheimer's Disease

Alzheimer's disease (AD) is an irreversible, progressive brain disease that destroys memory and cognition, and is the most common cause of dementia in older people. All of our subjects were recruited as part of phase 2 of the Alzheimer's Disease Neuroimaging Initiative (ADNI2) - an ongoing, longitudinal, multi-center study designed to find biomarkers for the early detection of AD. 155 subjects were categorized into four groups: normal (sex/average age: 22 male (M)/22 female (F)/72.7 years), early mild cognitive impairment (eMCI) (38M/24F/74.0), late mild cognitive impairment (lMCI) (15M/11F/73.0), and AD (15M/8F/75.8). MCI is an intermediate stage between normal aging and AD. 46 DWI volumes were acquired per subject: 5 T2-weighted $b_0$ image volumes and 41 diffusion-weighted volumes ($b = 1000$ s/mm$^2$). Each volume dimension was 256 x 256 x 59 and the voxel size was 1.37 x 1.37 x 2.7 mm$^3$.

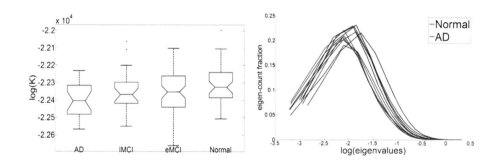

**Fig. 1.** The figure on the left shows the box plot of the logarithm of Kirchhoff complexity of the four groups and the figure on the right illustrates 5 representative normalized logarithmic eigen-spectra for AD patients (in *red*) and normal controls (in *blue*), respectively

Fig. 1 (left) shows a box plot of the logarithm of Kirchhoff complexity of the four groups. The minimum and the maximum of each group are displayed in *black*, the lower quartile and the upper quartile in *blue*, and the median in *red*. All outliers are marked with "+". The median logarithm of Kirchhoff complexity decreases from the normal group to both MCI groups and to the AD group. On the right, we show ten normalized logarithmic eigen-spectra of the AD group and the normal controls (5 people from each group were randomly selected).

The peaks of the spectra are shifted towards the right in the AD patients, relative to the normal controls. After excluding outliers indicated by the box plot, we also performed a $t$-test on the logarithm of Kirchhoff complexity between each pair of groups, and the $t$-statistic between AD and normal group was -3.24 ($p$=0.0019). The trend of decreasing global structural network connectivity from the normal group to the AD group is consistent with similar findings in functional [12] and anatomical connectivity studies [3].

### 3.3 Intelligence

80 pediatric subjects were included in this study, from 7 to 17 years old with an average age of 12.2 years. 30-direction DWI data was collected ($b = 1000$ s/mm$^2$). The voxel dimension was 128 x 128 x 128, with an isotropic voxel size of 2 mm.

Regression analysis was applied to study the correlation between the subjects' performance intelligence quotient (PIQ) and the logarithm of Kirchhoff complexity, in conjunction with their age variability. The response variable was PIQ, and the regressors were the logarithm of Kirchhoff complexity and age. Scatter plots relating the variables are shown in Fig. 2. Both one-factor and two-factor regressions were performed. Statistics from the regression analysis are listed in Table 1. PIQ and the logarithm of Kirchhoff complexity show statistically significant correlation ($r^2 = 0.066$ or 6.6%) at the 5% significance level. Our result is consistent with Cole $et$ $al.$'s study [13] with functional MRI in which measures of global brain connectivity were found to explain about 5% of the normal variance in intellectual function.

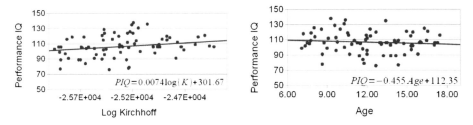

**Fig. 2.** Scatter plots and regression equations of PIQ against the logarithm of Kirchhoff complexity and age, respectively

**Table 1.** Regression statistics. The logarithm of Kirchhoff complexity is statistically significant as a predictor of PIQ in both one-factor and two-factor linear regression models.

| Regression Model | Variable | Coefficient (95% CI) | $r^2$ | $t$-statistic | $p$-value |
|---|---|---|---|---|---|
| One-factor | $\ln(K)$ | 7.41±6.43 ×10$^{-3}$ | 0.066 | 2.30 | **0.0246** |
| | Age | -0.455±1.08 | 0.009 | -0.840 | 0.404 |
| Two-factor | $\ln(K)$ | 7.23±6.48 ×10$^{-3}$ | 0.071 | 2.22 | **0.0292** |
| | Age | -0.361±1.06 | | -0.681 | 0.498 |

## 4    Conclusion and Future Work

Here we presented a new method to study overall brain connectivity at the voxel level instead of defining ROI-based nodes and using fibre guidance from tractography. Laplacian matrix of the diffusion tensor field has been proven to have a one-to-one correspondence with its connectivity graph. The voxelwise matrix is high dimensional - making a brute force solution impossible with normal laboratory computing resources. Instead, our measures, the Kirchhoff complexity and eigen-spectrum, can be computed efficiently without an unreasonable computational burden. We illustrate how to apply our measures to biological and medical questions. In our experiments, our estimates have a reasonable interpretation as indices of brain connectivity for disease characterization and intelligence prediction. Future work on voxelwise diffusion connectivity shows promise. For example, we can study the betweenness centrality of a vertex (voxel) and determine the relative importance of a voxel within the network. Or we can perform eigen-embedding to project voxels to higher-dimensional space and invent a new way to define ROIs.

## References

1. Bassett, D.S., Bullmore, E.: Small-world Brain Networks. Neuroscientist 12(6), 512–523 (2006)
2. Jahanshad, N., Prasad, G., Toga, A.W., McMahon, K.L., de Zubicaray, G.I., Martin, N.G., Wright, M.J., Thompson, P.M.: Genetics of path lengths in brain connectivity networks: HARDI-based maps in 457 adults. In: Yap, P.-T., Liu, T., Shen, D., Westin, C.-F., Shen, L. (eds.) MBIA 2012. LNCS, vol. 7509, pp. 29–40. Springer, Heidelberg (2012)
3. Daianu, M., et al.: Analyzing the Structural $k$-core of Brain Connectivity Networks in Normal Aging and Alzheimer's Disease. In: 15th MICCAI NIBAD Workshop, Nice, France, pp. 52–62 (2012)
4. Bastiani, M., et al.: Human Cortical Connectome Reconstruction from Diffusion Weighted MRI: the Effect of Tractography Algorithm. NeuroImage 62(3), 1732–1749 (2012)
5. Zalesky, A., et al.: Whole-brain Anatomical Networks: Does the Choice of Nodes Matter? NeuroImage 50(3), 970–983 (2010)
6. Dennis, E.L., Jahanshad, N., Toga, A.W., McMahon, K.L., de Zubicaray, G.I., Martin, N.G., Wright, M.J., Thompson, P.M.: Test-Retest Reliability of Graph Theory Measures of Structural Brain Connectivity. In: Ayache, N., Delingette, H., Golland, P., Mori, K. (eds.) MICCAI 2012, Part III. LNCS, vol. 7512, pp. 305–312. Springer, Heidelberg (2012)
7. Zalesky, A., Fornito, A.: A DTI-Derived Measure of Cortico-Cortical Connectivity. IEEE Trans. Med. Imaging 28(7), 1023–1036 (2009)
8. Tutte, W.T.: Graph Theory. Cambridge University Press (2001)
9. Chaiken, S.: A Combinatorial Proof of the All Minors Matrix Tree Theorem. SIAM. J. 3(3), 319–329 (1982)
10. Oishi, K., et al.: Atlas-based Whole Brain White Matter Analysis using Large Deformation Diffeomorphic Metric Mapping. NeuroImage 46(2), 486–499 (2009)
11. Alexander, D.C., et al.: Spatial Transformations of Diffusion Tensor Magnetic Resonance Images. IEEE Trans. Med. Imaging 20(11), 1131–1139 (2001)
12. Supekar, K., et al.: Network Analysis of Intrinsic Functional Brain Connectivity in Alzheimer's Disease. PLoS Comput. Biol. 4(6), e1000100 (2008)
13. Cole, M.C., et al.: Global Connectivity of Prefrontal Cortex Predicts Cognitive Control and Intelligence. J. Neurosci. 32(26), 8988–8999 (2012)

# Auto-calibrating Spherical Deconvolution Based on ODF Sparsity

Thomas Schultz[1] and Samuel Groeschel[2]

[1] University of Bonn, Germany
[2] Experimental Pediatric Neuroimaging and Department of Pediatric Neurology & Developmental Medicine, University Children's Hospital Tübingen, Germany[*]

**Abstract.** Spherical deconvolution models the diffusion MRI signal as the convolution of a fiber orientation density function (fODF) with a single fiber response. We propose a novel calibration procedure that automatically determines this fiber response. This has three advantages: First, the user no longer needs to provide an estimate of the response. Second, we estimate a per-voxel fiber response, which is more adequate for the analysis of patient data with focal white matter degeneration. Third, parameters of the estimated response reflect diffusion properties of the white matter tissue, and can be used for quantitative analysis.

Our method works by finding a tradeoff between a low fitting error and a sparse fODF. Results on simulated data demonstrate that auto-calibration successfully avoids erroneous fODF peaks that can occur with standard deconvolution, and that it resolves fiber crossings with better angular resolution than FORECAST, an alternative method. Parameter maps and tractography results corroborate applicability to clinical data.

## 1  Introduction

Constrained Spherical Deconvolution (CSD) [1] is one of the most widely used methods for inferring fiber distributions from High Angular Resolution Diffusion Imaging (HARDI). It obtains a fiber Orientation Density Function (fODF) by deconvolving the measured HARDI signal with a kernel that describes the response of a single fiber compartment. This single fiber response is a central parameter of the method. It is often assumed to be constant throughout the brain and estimated from voxels that are assumed to contain a single fiber bundle [2].

Recently, it has been pointed out that a mismatch between the true fiber response and the kernel used in CSD can lead to spurious peaks in the fODF [3]. Therefore, a more careful choice of the deconvolution kernel has the potential to improve fODF estimates, especially in cases where white matter degradation is studied, since degraded fibers can have a significantly different MR response.

---

[*] We would like to thank Bernhard Schölkopf (MPI for Intelligent Systems, Tübingen) for discussions about this work. S.G. gratefully acknowledges support through grant IZKF 2103-0-0 of the Medical Faculty of the University of Tübingen.

K. Mori et al. (Eds.): MICCAI 2013, Part I, LNCS 8149, pp. 663–670, 2013.

To the best of our knowledge, the only available method to estimate a per-voxel fiber response is FORECAST (Fiber ORientation Estimated using Continuous Axially Symmetric Tensors) [4]. FORECAST offers a fast estimate of the kernel, but we will demonstrate that it drastically underestimates the anisotropy of the single fiber response in case of crossing fiber compartments, which limits the angular resolution at which they can be resolved.

We propose an alternative way of selecting a kernel, based on balancing fitting error and fODF sparsity. This amounts to the idea that spurious fODF peaks are a result of overfitting to the measurement noise, and that they can be avoided by regularizing with an appropriate sparsity prior. The assumption that fODFs in white matter are sparse has previously been exploited to achieve super-resolved deconvolution [1]. In this work, we use it to determine the local fiber response.

## 2    Related Work

FORECAST models the HARDI signal as arising from a continuous mixture of fiber compartments that are each described by an axially symmetric diffusion tensor [4]. The parameters of those tensors, mean diffusivity $\bar{\lambda}$ and perpendicular diffusivity $\lambda_\perp$, are assumed to be constant within each voxel, but not throughout the brain. This is equivalent to performing spherical deconvolution with a per-voxel response function that corresponds to the axially symmetric tensor model.

In numerical experiments, FORECAST has achieved excellent results [4]. However, these experiments have used the true value of $\bar{\lambda}$, which was known from simulating the data, during analysis. When analyzing in vivo data, that true value is unknown. In this case, FORECAST uses the mean diffusivity *measured in the voxel* as an estimate of $\bar{\lambda}$, the mean diffusivity *of the single fiber response*.

Unfortunately, this heuristic underestimates $\bar{\lambda}$ significantly when two fiber compartments cross. This is why FORECAST exhibits a strong bias in estimated FA and a reduced ability to resolve crossings in our own experiments in Section 4, where we analyze simulated data with the same heuristic that FORECAST would apply to in vivo data. The key advantage of our novel method is that it estimates a per-voxel kernel without assuming prior knowledge of $\bar{\lambda}$.

## 3    Balancing Fitting Error and Sparsity

Given a kernel $\mathbf{R}$, spherical deconvolution [2] obtains the spherical harmonics coefficients $\hat{\mathbf{f}}_\mathbf{R}$ of the corresponding fiber ODF $\hat{F}_\mathbf{R}(\theta, \phi)$ by minimizing

$$\hat{\mathbf{f}}_\mathbf{R} = \arg\min \|\mathbf{QRf}_\mathbf{R} - \mathbf{s}\|_2, \tag{1}$$

where $\mathbf{s}$ is a vector of measured signal attenuations in $n$ gradient directions, $\mathbf{R}$ convolves $\mathbf{f}_\mathbf{R}$ with a kernel representing the single fiber response, and $\mathbf{Q}$ evaluates the spherical harmonics in the $n$ gradient directions.

Even though $\mathbf{f}_\mathbf{R}$ is commonly constrained to represent a non-negative function $F_\mathbf{R}(\theta, \phi)$ [1], it has been pointed out that this does not reliably prevent erroneous peaks in the fODF [5], especially when the kernel $\mathbf{R}$ overestimates the anisotropy of the true single fiber response [3]. We propose to reduce spurious peaks via an additional sparsity constraint on $F_{\mathbf{R}}$, by selecting a kernel $\hat{\mathbf{R}}$ such that

$$\hat{\mathbf{R}} = \arg\min \frac{1}{\sqrt{n}}\|\mathbf{Q}\mathbf{R}\hat{\mathbf{f}}_{\mathbf{R}} - \mathbf{s}\|_2 + \nu\|\hat{F}_{\mathbf{R}}(\theta,\phi)\|_{0.5}, \qquad (2)$$

where $\nu$ controls the tradeoff between fitting error and sparsity. In our experiments, this parameter did not require any tuning; it has been fixed at $\nu = 0.02$.

An ambiguity in Eq. (2) arises from the fact that scaling $\mathbf{R}$ by factor $c$ can be offset by scaling $\hat{\mathbf{f}}_{\mathbf{R}}$ by $c^{-1}$. We avoid this problem by fixing the scale of all candidate kernels $\mathbf{R}$ such that all $\hat{F}_{\mathbf{R}}$ integrate to unity. Since this constrains the $\ell_1$ norm of $\hat{F}_{\mathbf{R}}$ to a constant, we instead use the $\ell_{0.5}$ norm to induce sparsity, which we define as $\|F(\theta,\phi)\|_{0.5} := \iint \sqrt{|F(\theta,\phi)|}$.

## 3.1 The Fiber Response as a Function of cFA

We simplify the problem of finding an optimum of Eq. (2) by only considering kernels that correspond to axially symmetric tensors. Their spherical harmonics coefficients are derived in [4] as a function of $b$ value and parameters $\bar{\lambda}$ and $\lambda_\perp$.

For our purposes, a re-parametrization in terms of parallel diffusivity $\lambda_\parallel$ and Fractional Anisotropy (FA) is more convenient, since FA has a standardized range over which we can optimize. From FA and $\lambda_\parallel$, we compute $\lambda_\perp$ by observing that the difference $\Delta := \lambda_\parallel - \lambda_\perp$ is the unique root of the quadratic function

$$(2\,\mathrm{FA}^2 - 1)\Delta^2 - 4\,\mathrm{FA}^2\lambda_\parallel\Delta + 3\,\mathrm{FA}^2\lambda_\parallel^2 = 0 \qquad (3)$$

that falls within $[0, \lambda_\parallel]$. Since $\bar{\lambda} := (\lambda_\parallel + 2\lambda_\perp)/3$, this easily reduces our preferred parameters to those used in [4].

During optimization, we use FA of the single fiber response as the independent variable that we modify to achieve an optimum of Eq. (2). The second parameter of $\mathbf{R}$, $\lambda_\parallel$, is always chosen such that, for the given value of FA, the fODF $\hat{F}_{\mathbf{R}}$ integrates to unity. As shown in [4], this requires that $\lambda_\parallel$ and $\Delta$ correctly predict the average signal attenuation

$$\frac{\bar{S}}{S_0} = \frac{\sqrt{\pi}}{2}\frac{\mathrm{erf}(\sqrt{b\Delta})}{\sqrt{b\Delta}}e^{-b(\lambda_\parallel - \Delta)}. \qquad (4)$$

For a fixed choice of FA, the attenuation predicted by Eq. (4) is a monotonic function of $\lambda_\parallel$. Therefore, we can use a simple bracketing technique to numerically solve for the value of $\lambda_\parallel$ that predicts the empirical signal attenuation.

Unlike the standard Fractional Anisotropy computed from diffusion tensor MRI, which quantifies the anisotropy of *diffusion within the voxel*, the FA parameter inferred during calibration models the anisotropy *of the individual fiber compartments*. Thus, it is affected far less by fiber crossings or fanning. To emphasize this difference, we will refer to this new measure as *calibration FA* (cFA).

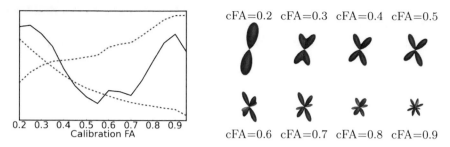

**Fig. 1.** Calibrating deconvolution to higher cFA reduces fitting error (blue dashes), but introduces erroneous fODF peaks. Our method avoids this via an objective function (black line) that combines fitting error with a sparsity term (red dashes).

Selecting a lower cFA amounts to using a smoother convolution kernel. Therefore, fitting residuals increase as calibration FA decreases (cf. blue dashes in Fig. 1). At the same time, fODFs become sparser, eliminating erroneous peaks that are caused by overfitting to the measurement noise when using an overly large cFA. Our method automatically determines a suitable tradeoff.

### 3.2    Finding the Optimal Kernel

For a given candidate $\mathbf{R}$, we evaluate Eq. (2) by first finding the corresponding $\hat{\mathbf{f}}_{\mathbf{R}}$ via a non-negative constrained version of Eq. (1). We then evaluate the fitting error and estimate the $\ell_{0.5}$ norm by taking $m$ samples $F_i$ of $F_{\mathbf{R}}(\theta, \phi)$, distributed uniformly on the hemisphere, and computing

$$\|F(\theta, \phi)\|_{0.5} \approx \frac{4\pi}{m} \sum_{i=1}^{m} \sqrt{F_i}. \tag{5}$$

In practice, we simply use the same $m = 300$ directions that enforce non-negativity in the iterative implementation of CSD by Tournier et al. [1].

Since the dependence of $\hat{\mathbf{f}}_{\mathbf{R}}$ on $\mathbf{R}$ cannot be expressed in closed form, we cannot compute an analytical derivative of Eq. (2) for optimization. Instead, we simply continue to increase or decrease the value of cFA by some stepsize, as long as the steps improve the objective value, and remain within cFA $\in [0.2, 0.95]$. Once no more improvements are possible, we continue with a reduced stepsize, until it falls below 0.01. This easy-to-implement procedure permits auto-calibrated deconvolution of a full brain scan ($> 160,000$ voxels) in around 22 minutes on a standard quad-core 2.67 GHz workstation.

## 4    Results on Simulated Data

To confirm that sparsity-based kernel selection produces useful results, we perform numerical experiments, assuming the same acquisition parameters as the clinical sequence we routinely use for deconvolution-based tractography: 64 uniformly distributed gradient directions, $b = 2000\,\mathrm{s/mm^2}$, plus one image at $b = 0$.

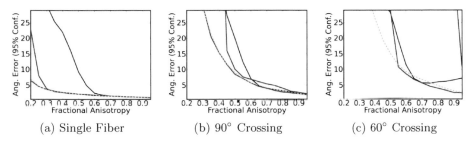

(a) Single Fiber            (b) 90° Crossing            (c) 60° Crossing

**Fig. 2.** In simulated low-noise data, auto-calibration (red) produces more accurate results than deconvolution with a fixed kernel (black) or FORECAST (blue)

### 4.1 Studying Model Assumptions in Low-Noise Data

We focus on the effects of model assumptions by simulating diffusion weighted data with weak Rician noise ($SNR_0 = 50$) from a mixture of axially symmetric diffusion tensors with normally distributed $\bar{\lambda}$ (statistics taken from a white matter ROI in a healthy subject). We report the 95% confidence intervals, over 500 trials, of the angular distance between largest fODF peaks and ground truth fiber directions. If an fODF has too few significant peaks (using 0.1 as a threshold), we assign the maximum error (90°) to the missing ground truth direction.

Fig. 2 compares the performance of constrained spherical deconvolution with a fixed calibration to cFA = 0.75 (black lines) to FORECAST (blue) and our proposed auto-calibration (red). We also provide the accuracy of an "oracle"-based deconvolution that uses the true kernel that was used to simulate the data (dashed yellow line). This is not a practically useful method, since the kernel is unknown for in vivo data. However, it provides a reference which confirms that in many cases, auto-calibration performs close to optimal.

Results confirm a previous finding that even when noise is very low, deconvolution is unreliable when the kernel overestimates the true anisotropy [3]. Auto-calibration effectively ameliorates this problem, especially in the single-fiber case. For a 90° fiber crossing, it performs only marginally better than FORECAST; however, it is able to resolve smaller angles, such as the 60° shown in Fig. 2 (c), which FORECAST only resolves at the highest anisotropies.

Our comparison does not include the damped Richardson-Lucy algorithm, which was proposed as an alternative way of reducing spurious peaks in deconvolution [5]. However, Parker et al. [3] report that this method is not able to deal with low target FA $\leq 0.5$. Our method remains useful beyond that point.

### 4.2 Stability at Lower SNR

Under more realistic noise ($SNR_0 = 20$), auto-calibration continues to provide more reliable estimates than non-adaptive deconvolution, especially in the single fiber case (Fig. 3 (a)). For crossing fibers (in (b): 75° with volume fractions 0.6 : 0.4), it provides better accuracy than FORECAST, and a higher angular resolution: Unlike FORECAST, it continues to reliably resolve 60° crossings.

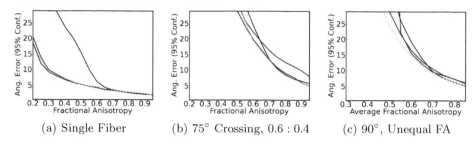

(a) Single Fiber          (b) 75° Crossing, 0.6 : 0.4          (c) 90°, Unequal FA

**Fig. 3.** At $SNR_0 = 20$, auto-calibration (red) continues to provide a clear advantage over standard deconvolution (black), especially for single-fiber voxels (a)

Fig. 3 (c) demonstrates that auto-calibration still performs well when its model assumptions are violated: Even though the crossing fibers do not have the same FAs in this case (simulated FAs are 0.1 larger and smaller than the average value specified in the plot), performance is on par with standard CSD.

Even though a cFA value can also be derived from the FORECAST kernel, we found that it exhibits a strong bias. Given 60- to 90-degree two-fiber crossings with FA in [0.5,0.95], the mean difference between the cFA from FORECAST and the ground truth was $-0.253 \pm 0.064$. This bias is caused by the biased estimate of $\bar{\lambda}$, which is explained in Section 2, and is removed in our method, whose estimated cFA matches the true FA with accuracy $0.030 \pm 0.061$.

### 4.3   Required Number of $b = 0$ Measurements and $b$ Value

Our HARDI acquisition scheme maximizes angular resolution by taking as many different gradient directions as possible within the clinically feasible time budget, leaving just a single image with $b = 0$. In contrast, Anderson takes a much larger number of $b = 0$ images for FORECAST, arguing that via Eq. (4), $S_0$ plays an important role in estimating the kernel [4]. We repeated our simulations with 60 uniform directions plus 5 $b = 0$ images, rather than our default 64+1, as well as with 55+10. For both single and crossing fibers, we found that taking more images at $b = 0$ reduced variance in the estimates of cFA and $\lambda_{\parallel}$ during calibration, and therefore leads to a more reliable estimation of the deconvolution kernel. Unfortunately, the loss of angular resolution that results from having fewer directions still led to a slight increase in angular reconstruction errors.

We also tried several $b$ values in our numerical experiments and found that reconstructing a 75° crossing of fibers with FA $\in [0.5, 0.95]$ with a 95% confidence in orientation of less than 30° at $SNR_0 = 20$, required $b \geq 1400 \, s/mm^2$.

## 5   Results on Measured Data

### 5.1   Mapping Kernel Parameters

Fig. 4 confirms a theoretical advantage of our novel cFA measure: In regions where decrease of traditional FA is known to be due to fiber crossings and spread

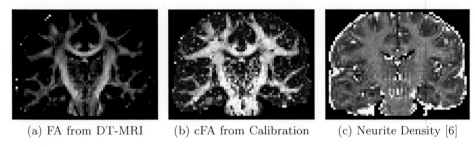

(a) FA from DT-MRI  (b) cFA from Calibration  (c) Neurite Density [6]

**Fig. 4.** Compared to Fractional Anisotropy from the diffusion tensor model (a), our novel cFA parameter (b) depends less on orientation dispersion within the voxel

(marked by arrows in (a)), cFA remains high (b). In this respect, it is similar to the neurite density parameter in the recently proposed NODDI framework [6]. However, unlike NODDI, it does not require diffusion acquisition on a second $b$ shell. We believe that maps of kernel parameters such as cFA could complement recent efforts to derive new quantitative measures from fODFs [7,8].

ODF sparsity is reduced in regions of fanning fibers. Even though Fig. 4 (b) suggests that our method can deal with this violation of its model assumption to some degree, the impact of fanning merits closer investigation in the future.

### 5.2 Reduction of Erroneous Fibers in Tractography

Finally, we have used auto-calibrated deconvolution as a basis of deterministic streamline tractography in a patient with metachromatic leukodystrophy, a demyelinating white matter disorder. Fig. 5 shows that auto-calibration produced a successful tractography without requiring a user-specified single fiber response. Compared to diffusion tensor tractography and CSD with the standard global calibration procedure [2], it reduces the number of streamlines that deviate into

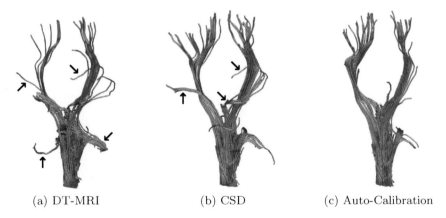

(a) DT-MRI  (b) CSD  (c) Auto-Calibration

**Fig. 5.** Compared to diffusion tensor (a) or constrained deconvolution tractography (b), auto-calibration (c) reduces the number of false positive streamlines

adjacent bundles (arrows in (a) and (b)). All methods start from the same seeds in the brain stem and use the same curvature-based termination criteria.

# 6   Conclusion

We have extended the widely used spherical deconvolution technique with a method for auto-calibration. We have successfully applied it to simulated data with different $b$ values and noise levels, and to measured data from healthy subjects, as well as from patients with white matter degeneration, without having to tune any parameters or providing a global single fiber response.

In numerical experiments, our per-voxel kernel estimates outperform constrained deconvolution with a fixed kernel, and FORECAST, the only other method that estimates a per-voxel deconvolution kernel. Results on measured data indicate a potential for using kernel parameters for quantitative analysis, and for improving the specificity of streamline tractography.

# References

1. Tournier, J.D., Calamante, F., Connelly, A.: Robust determination of the fibre orientation distribution in diffusion MRI: Non-negativity constrained super-resolved spherical deconvolution. NeuroImage 35, 1459–1472 (2007)
2. Tournier, J.D., Calamante, F., Gadian, D.G., Connelly, A.: Direct estimation of the fiber orientation density function from diffusion-weighted MRI data using spherical deconvolution. NeuroImage 23, 1176–1185 (2004)
3. Parker, G.D., Marshall, D., Rosin, P.L., Drage, N., Richmond, S., Jones, D.K.: A pitfall in the reconstruction of fibre ODFs using spherical deconvolution of diffusion MRI data. NeuroImage 65, 433–448 (2013)
4. Anderson, A.W.: Measurement of fiber orientation distributions using high angular resolution diffusion imaging. Magnetic Resonance in Medicine 54(5), 1194–1206 (2005)
5. Dell'Acqua, F., Scifo, P., Rizzo, G., Catani, M., Simmons, A., Scotti, G., Fazio, F.: A modified damped richardson-lucy algorithm to reduce isotropic background effects in spherical deconvolution. NeuroImage 49, 1446–1458 (2010)
6. Zhang, H., Schneider, T., Wheeler-Kingshott, C.A., Alexander, D.C.: NODDI: practical in vivo neurite orientation dispersion and density imaging of the human brain. NeuroImage 61(4), 1000–1016 (2012)
7. Raffelt, D., Tournier, J.D., Rose, S., Ridgway, G.R., Henderson, R., Crozier, S., Salvado, O., Connelly, A.: Apparent fibre density: A novel measure for the analysis of diffusion-weighted magnetic resonance images. NeuroImage 59(4), 3976–3994 (2012)
8. Dell'Acqua, F., Simmons, A., Williams, S.C.R., Catani, M.: Can spherical deconvolution provide more information than fiber orientations? hindrance modulated orientational anisotropy, a true-tract specific index to characterize white matter diffusion. Human Brain Mapping (2012) Early view, doi:10.1002/hbm.22080

# Evaluating Structural Connectomics in Relation to Different Q-space Sampling Techniques

Paulo Rodrigues[1,2], Alberto Prats-Galino[3], David Gallardo-Pujol[2],
Pablo Villoslada[4], Carles Falcon[5], and Vesna Prčkovska[4]

[1] Mint Labs S.L., Barcelona, Spain
[2] Dept. of Personality, Faculty of Psychology, UB, Barcelona, Spain
[3] LSNA, Facultat de Medicina, UB, Barcelona, Spain
[4] Center for Neuroimmunology, Department of Neurosciences, IDIBAPS, Hospital Clinic, Barcelona, Spain
[5] Medical Imaging Platform, IDIBAPS, Barcelona, Spain

**Abstract.** Brain networks are becoming forefront research in neuroscience. Network-based analysis on the functional and structural connectomes can lead to powerful imaging markers for brain diseases. However, constructing the structural connectome can be based upon different acquisition and reconstruction techniques whose information content and mutual differences has not yet been properly studied in a unified framework. The variations of the structural connectome if not properly understood can lead to dangerous conclusions when performing these type of studies. In this work we present evaluation of the structural connectome by analysing and comparing graph-based measures on real data acquired by the three most important Diffusion Weighted Imaging techniques: DTI, HARDI and DSI. We thus come to several important conclusions demonstrating that even though the different techniques demonstrate differences in the anatomy of the reconstructed fibers the respective connectomes show variations of 20%.

## Introduction

Over the last decade, the study of complex networks has expanded dramatically across different scientific fields including Neuroscience. The brain is a complex system whose complex components continuously create complex patterns. Therefore, a natural paradigm for studying the brain is via network analysis. A comprehensive map of neural connections of the brain is called "connectome" [1,2]. At the macroscopic scale, the connectome can be seen as a network, usually represented as a matrix, where each vertex represents well-defined cortical or sub-cortical structures and the edges quantify the structural white matter connectivity as measured with tractography. When this matrix is estimated from Diffusion Weighted MRI (dwMRI) data we speak about structural connectivity. In the process of calculating the connectomes, from the measured data, several parameters are involved that can lead to variations of the connectivity matrices. In the structural connectome however, the most important step is the fibre tractography that depends not only

K. Mori et al. (Eds.): MICCAI 2013, Part I, LNCS 8149, pp. 671–678, 2013.
© Springer-Verlag Berlin Heidelberg 2013

on the acquired dwMRI data but also on the choice for particular reconstruction and fibre-tracking algorithms, as pointed out by Bastiani et al [3]. The most common acquisition model is the Diffusion Tensor Imaging (DTI) [4] which requires modest q-space acquisitions with short scanning time ( 3-5min). However, DTI has been proved to have limitations in complex fibre areas. Therefore, more complex acquisitions models were developed, known as High Angular Resolution Diffusion Imaging (HARDI) [5], with denser q-space sampling on a spherical shell. It has been demonstrated that it is able to give good results even at lower (clinically preferable) b-values [6] resulting in scanning times of about 15 min. The richest q-space sampling technique is Diffusion Spectrum Imaging [7], resolving more complex fibre configurations, however, at a cost of very long acquisition times (>35min). With the arrival of the connectomics many groups have initiated research in this direction, choosing the dwMRI data acquisition technique, however, without knowing how this choice influences the quality of the connectomes. The choice of suitable technique with high reproducibility for the purpose of constructing structural connectomics has not yet been properly addressed in literature, even though some attempts have been done for the functional connectome [8]. In this work, we evaluate the information difference contained in the structural connectomes constructed from the same subject scanned with different dwMRI acquisition techniques (DTI, HARDI and DSI). Since the goal is not evaluating all the possible parameters involved in the process, we acquire the data with the most commonly used parameters in literature. We perform the connectome construction for all the modalities with equal parameter settings. We furthermore test the reproducibility of the connectome and information difference in relation to the acquisition using network analysis. Finally we perform a 'blind' qualitative analysis of different fibre bundles involved in the connectome construction by an experienced Neuroanatomist.

## 1    Methods

***Data:*** MRI acquisitions were performed on 5 healthy volunteers (4 male and 1 female, age:$31.2\pm2.9$ years) using a twice refocused spin-echo echo-planar imaging sequence on a 3T Siemens Trio MRI scanner (Erlangen, Germany). Informed consent was obtained prior to the acquisition. The MRI protocol included the following sequences: a) 3D structural T1-weighted MPRAGE sequence: Repetition Time (TR): $1900ms$, Echo Time (TE): $4.44ms$, Inversion recovery time (TI): $1050ms$, Flip angle: $8°$, FOV: $220\times220mm^2$, isometric $1mm^3$; b)The parameters for the dwMRI sequences are given in the table 1 (top). We have acquired in total 21 datasets from which 7 DTI, 6 HARDI and 8 DSI. For some of the subjects the scans were repeated in the same scanning session or after one month. In table 1 (bottom) we report the subset of data we used for each of the performed tests and the number of subjects involved.

**Connectome Construction:** We calculated the connectomes using publicly available software, the connectome mapper (cmp)[1] [9]. For all imaging modalities

---

[1] http://www.connectomics.org

**Table 1.** *Top*: Scanning parameters used in our dwMRI acquisitions. *Due to technical reasons two DTI datasets were obtained using spatial resolution of $1.25 \times 1.25 \times 2.5 mm^3$. **Due to technical reasons one DSI dataset was obtained using spatial resolution of $3mm^3$ isometric. *bottom*: Data overview per performed test.

| Modality | DTI | HARDI | DSI | |
|---|---|---|---|---|
| $b-val\ (s/mm^2)$ | 1000 | 1500 | $b_{max}{=}8000$ | |
| num. grad. | 30 | 82 | 515 | |
| num. $b_0$ | 1 | 6 | N/A | |
| spatial res. $(mm^3)$ | $2.5 \times 2.5 \times 2.5^*$ | $1.25 \times 1.25 \times 2.5$ | $2.2 \times 2.2 \times 3^{**}$ | |
| $TR/TE$ | 6900/89 | 7600/98 | 8200/164 | |
| acq.time(min) | 3.56 | 11.33 | 35.42 | |
| Evaluation | DTI | HARDI | DSI | #subjects |
| reproducibility | 5 | 4 | 6 | 3 |
| intra-subject | 7 | 6 | 6 | 4 |
| network based | 7 | 6 | 8 | 5 |
| qualitative | 3 | 3 | 3 | 3 |

we used the default settings (re-sampling the dwMRI data to $1mm^3$ isometric voxel size using trilinear interpolation, tracking stopping criteria at angle=60°, number of seeds=32, fibre filtering with enabled spline filter and cut-off filter in the interval of [20;500] mm). For DTI fibre tracking, the cmp uses the standard FACT method and for Qball and DSI FACT-alike algorithm implemented in the Diffusion Toolkit [10]. For two subjects to improve the registration step we performed non-linear registration using the T2 data, and for the rest of the subjects we used linear registration. We employed Lausanne parcellation since it offers 5 hierarchical scales to test and compare the quality of the connectomes. Depending on the imaging modality, DTI, HARDI (Qball) or DSI reconstruction was performed. For network creation, we first apply an absolute threshold in order to discard edges with less than 10 fibres (considered spurious fibres from data observation), and connection matrices are created by either binarizing edge weights, or by normalizing the edge weights with maximum number of found fibres.

**Indices for Connectome Comparison and Quality Assessment:** The simplest way of comparing networks is to assess the difference between their overall matrix representations. We computed the correlation between the graphs as described in Table 2. We computed several other indices (normalized root-mean-square deviation, dot product of the direct embedding of the matrix into a vector-space representation, Hamming distance and Fleiss' kappa reliability of agreement) but since they do not give further insight, we omit them for simplicity of presentation.

**Table 2.** Correlation measure of structural connectome agreement, represented as a matrix where $A_{i,j}$ is the weighted edge between nodes $i$ and $j$

| | |
|---|---|
| covariance | $cov(\mathbf{y_1}, \mathbf{y_2}) = \frac{1}{N(N-1)} \sum_{i \neq j}^{N} \left(A_{i,j}^{(1)} - m_1\right)\left(A_{i,j}^{(2)} - m_2\right)$ <br> where $m_l = \frac{1}{N(N-1)} \sum_{i \neq j}^{N} A_{i,j}^{(l)}$ |
| correlation [11] | $\rho(\mathbf{y_1}, \mathbf{y_2}) = \frac{cov(\mathbf{y_1},\mathbf{y_2})}{\sqrt{var(\mathbf{y_1})var(\mathbf{y_2})}}$ |

***Network-Based Indices:*** To compare certain network features of the matrices we used the brain connectivity toolbox[2]. We considered graph **density**, node **strength, characteristic path length** and **global efficiency** over binary undirected graph representation of the connectomes.

***Track-Based Quality Assessment Indices:*** We extracted 40 fibre bundles that connect different cortical regions in the lowest parcellation scale (33) since it corresponds to the underlying anatomy. The regions were carefully selected spanning the whole brain in order to capture fibres with different neuroanatomical nature: commisural, projection, u-fibres and subcortical fibres. We exported the fibres of each reconstruction technique per subject and grouped in triplets of bundles visualised in the Amira[3] software. This data was presented to a professor in Neuroanatomy in a completely anonymized way (the fibres were only shown with different colors and no reference to the underlying acquisition modality). He was asked to score the accuracy of the fibres to the underlying anatomy as objectively as possible with scores from 1-3, where 3 stands for the most accurate and 1 for the least accurate technique. In case few techniques present similar accuracy they could be scored with the same score. We additionally report percentage of the missing fibre bundles (out of the 40 considered) that each technique fails to reconstruct, i.e., finds no fibers between 2 regions or only aberrant fibers.

## 2   Results

**Reproducibility of the Structural Connectome:** Structural connectome can be seen as a potential imaging marker sensitive to certain pathologies of the white matter (e.g., Multiple Sclerosis, Schizophrenia). If the variability of the connectome is larger than its sensitivity to the pathology then this will alter the accuracy of the experimental design study. Therefore one important analysis that we conducted here is assessing the variability of the connectome constructed from data acquired in the same imaging session, as well as after some period of time (one month) and compare it among connectomes constructed with different acquisitions schemes (DTI, HARDI and DSI) at different scales of parcellation (33-500). For simplicity, we show results for scale 33, since trends are kept across scales. Fig. 1(a,b) shows that highest reproducibility is achieved within same day for DTI and DSI acquisitions (0.95, normalized network). At 1 month time difference, DTI shows the least correlation 0.76. This shows that the connectivity maps can change in healthy subjects for about 20%, within a month (worst case scenario performing DTI acquisition). HARDI shows the highest reproducibility across time, however this might be due to the small sample size. Same trend is observed for binarized connectomes, however the variability change is in the order of 15%.

**Intra-subject Structural Connectome Variability:** To assess the differences between structural connectomes built using different modalities, we calculate the

---

[2] https://sites.google.com/site/bctnet/
[3] http://www.vsg3d.com/amira/overview

similarity between different modalities within each subject. Fig. 1(c,d) demonstrates the biggest agreement in the connectomes between DTI and HARDI (both in normalized and binarized case). Taking the biggest agreement from the previous analysis as reference (same day DSI, normalized 0.95) we can observe that DSI and DTI connectomes disagree in about 23%, DSI and HARDI disagree 19% whereas DTI and HARDI differ in 10%. For binarized connectomes, the minimal agreement is between DSI and HARDI of about 23% difference (reference 0.75). These results should be taken with care given the low amount of subjects involved in the analysis.

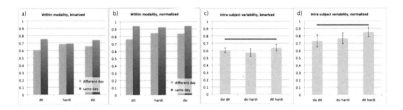

**Fig. 1. left:** Within subject, connectome variability with different modalities, for binarized (a) and normalized (b) networks. **right:** Correlation within intra-subject connectomes for binarized (c) and normalized (d) networks.

**Network-Based Indices Subject Variability:** Network-based indices are typically used to assert pathologies of the brain white matter. A very important fundamental analysis is to evaluate how sensitive and reproducible these indices are w.r.t. different acquisition modalities. As anatomical connectivity becomes increasingly sparse with higher scale, **density** values decrease. As we can observe in Fig. 2, DSI shows higher density values than DTI and HARDI, which may indicate a denser connectome. **Global Efficiency** is the average inverse shortest path length in the network. DSI presents higher global efficiency index, while DTI and HARDI show similar values. **Characteristic path length** is the average shortest path length in the network and it is normally used to compute small-worldness. It increases with scale, DSI showing the lowest values, while DTI and HARDI are similar. **Strength** is the average of the sum of weights of links connected to each node. It is seen as highly predictive of stronger functional

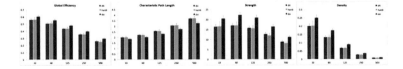

**Fig. 2.** Variability of network-based indices across scales and modality. Overall, DSI shows more distinctive indexes than DTI and HARDI (very similar to each other), however HARDI shows a higher standard deviation. This may suggest that HARDI is more sensitive to inter-subject variability.

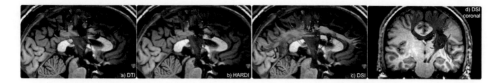

**Fig. 3.** Initial exploration of DTI vs HARDI vs DSI differences. DSI is obviously able to capture complex crossing structures, such as the superior longitudinal fasciculus connecting the frontal, occipital, parietal, and temporal lobes.

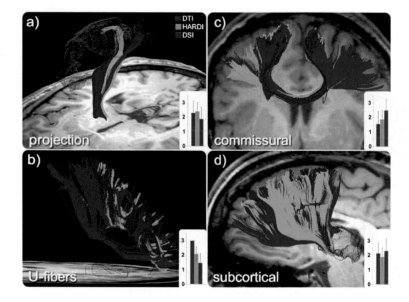

**Fig. 4.** Illustration of fibre bundle quality assessment. Red stands for DTI, green for HARDI and blue for DSI techniques. In each category the corresponding graphs show the average scores and standard deviation. **a)** DSI bundle originates in a different section of the postcentral medial ROI (likely the sensory leg nerves) while DTI and HARDI depict similar bundles, however HARDI bundle is more selective. **b)** Generally U-fibres are very well captured by DTI, whereas DSI does not depict the underlying anatomical shape, and often connects distant regions with additional long straight fibre bundles. HARDI generally has multiple isolated groups of U-fibre bundles. **c)** In the commissural bundles DSI is typically the best technique. It has long, extensive connections from the middle and upper parts of the cortex through the *corpus callosum*. DTI fibre bundles are vertically oriented, only connecting paramedial parts of this region. HARDI stands between the two techniques. **d)** These connections are composed of different fibre bundles connecting different regions of the thalamus with the cortex. In the evaluation some techniques proved better than others in relation to the anatomical correctness. Therefore in these regions when we perform the overall statistic we get similar reconstruction quality by all of the three techniques.

connectivity. Same trend applies here, where DSI shows higher values while DTI and HARDI have similar behaviour. Higher strength values are shown in middles scales (60 and 125), suggesting a stronger depiction of the overall connectivity at these scales.

**Track-Based Quality Assessment:** Fig. 3 gives an illustration of the obvious benefits of DSI as a modelling and ultimately fibre reconstruction technique over DTI and HARDI since it is able to capture long fibre bundles such as the *superior longitudinal fasciculus* that is passing and crossing through complex fibre structures and many other complex configurations in the brain. This has been illustrated by Wedeen et al. [7]. However, in the connectomic approach with the predefined regions of parcellation we observe that these differences are not significantly favourable over DTI and HARDI. The differences have been clearly demonstrated in figure 4 where different techniques, for different fibre groups seem more anatomically correct. Furthermore, each technique missed the following fraction of fibre bundles (out of the analysed 40 bundles): DTI - 24%, HARDI - 18%, DSI - 14%.

## 3   Conclusion

In this paper we have evaluated the characteristics and mutual differences of the structural connectomes constructed over different dwMRI acquisition schemes: DTI, HARDI and DSI. We have done this by employing graph based measures to real data that can quantify the information content and the differences between different techniques, at different scales of hierarchy. From these measures we observed that the connectome does not significantly capture richer information by using locally more accurate acquisition schemes such as DSI. In fact these techniques applied on a clinical scanner (3T) might produce noisier images leading to more aberrant fibres. Therefore in certain cases, such as the short U-fibres, simple techniques as DTI can outperform. Furthermore, in the case of global connectomic approaches, connectivity is typically measured as a function of the number of fibres passing through two ROIs of parcellation or average values of scalar measures such as FA. In certain approaches, the connectivity matrices are binarized, and as such the anatomical properties of the fibres are ignored. This explains the small differences (15-20%) between the connectomes constructed by different acquisition schemes. In the qualitative analysis this is strongly demonstrated showing at times many aberrant fibres in DSI and HARDI approaches that in the connectivity matrices appear as valid connections. Future research should be aimed at capturing anatomical properties of the connectivity fibres as weights of the connectome, such as fibre volume, bundle cohesiveness and cluster based approaches. DSI can be seen as a powerful tool for neurosurgical application since it can detect complex fibre bundles, however it presents more aberrant fibers. In neurosurgery applications there is a direct visualization of the reconstructed fiber tracts, immediately identifiable by the neurosurgeons. However in connectomics, such false positives can be misleading (e.g., Fig. 4b) which implicates wrong connections between sub-regions at a higher scale. This can be wrongly interpreted as differences between two categories of subjects. Given the variation of performance in the qualitative analysis of the different reconstruction techniques, more modest (w.r.t. acquisition time and high b values), such as multi-shell HARDI approaches [12] would give significantly better results, combined with adaptive reconstruction techniques depending on the parts of the brain regions we evaluate. Finally, this study shows only preliminary results done on 5 subjects. To improve the statistic analysis, larger cohort of subjects should be analysed, and the intra-subject variability (20% difference in longitudinal acquisition) must be taken into careful consideration.

# References

1. Hagmann, P.: From Diffusion MRI to Brain Connectomics. PhD thesis, EPFL (2005)
2. Sporns, O., Tononi, G., Kötter, R., Ko, R.: The human connectome: A structural description of the human brain. PLoS Computational Biology 1(4), e42 (2005)
3. Bastiani, M., Shah, N.J., Goebel, R., Roebroeck, A.: Human cortical connectome reconstruction from diffusion weighted MRI: the effect of tractography algorithm. NeuroImage 62(3), 1732–1749 (2012)
4. Pierpaoli, C., Basser, P.J.: Toward a quantitative assessment of diffusion anisotropy. MRM 36, 893–906 (1996)
5. Tuch, D.S., Reese, T.G., Wiegell, M.R., Makris, N.G., Belliveau, J.W., Wedeen, V.J.: High Angular Resolution Diffusion Imaging Reveals Intravoxel White Matter Fiber Heterogeneity. MRM 48(4), 577–582 (2002)
6. Prčkovska, V., Roebroeck, A.F., Pullens, W.L.P.M., Vilanova, A., ter Haar Romeny, B.M.: Optimal Acquisition Schemes in High Angular Resolution Diffusion Weighted Imaging. In: Metaxas, D., Axel, L., Fichtinger, G., Székely, G. (eds.) MICCAI 2008, Part II. LNCS, vol. 5242, pp. 9–17. Springer, Heidelberg (2008)
7. Wedeen, V.J., Wang, R.P., Schmahmann, J.D., Benner, T., Tseng, W.Y.I., Dai, G., Pandya, D.N., Hagmann, P., D'Arceuil, H., de Crespigny, A.J.: Diffusion spectrum magnetic resonance imaging (DSI) tractography of crossing fibers. NeuroImage 41(4), 1267–1277 (2008)
8. Telesford, Q.K., Morgan, A.R., Hayasaka, S., Simpson, S.L., Barret, W., Kraft, R.A., Mozolic, J.L., Laurienti, P.J.: Reproducibility of Graph Metrics in fMRI Networks. Frontiers in Neuroinformatics 4, 10 (2010)
9. Daducci, A., Gerhard, S., Griffa, A., Lemkaddem, A., Cammoun, L., Gigandet, X., Meuli, R., Hagmann, P., Thiran, J.P.: The connectome mapper: an open-source processing pipeline to map connectomes with MRI. PloS one 7(12), e48121 (2012)
10. Wang, R., Benner, T., Sorensen, A.G., Wedeen, V.J.: Diffusion Toolkit: A Software Package for Diffusion Imaging Data Processing and Tractography. In: Proceedings of the 15th ISMRM Conference, p. 3720 (2007)
11. Butts, C.T.: Social network analysis: A methodological introduction. Asian Journal of Social Psychology 11(1), 13–41 (2008)
12. Zhan, L., Leow, A., Aganj, I., Lenglet, C., Sapiro, G., Yacoub, E., Harel, N., Toga, A., Thompson, P.: Differential information content in staggered multiple shell hardi measured by the tensor distribution function. I S Biomd. Imaging, 305–309 (March 30-April 2, 2011)

# Tensor Metrics and Charged Containers for 3D Q-space Sample Distribution

Hans Knutsson[1] and Carl-Fredrik Westin[2]

[1] Linköping University, Sweden
[2] Harvard Medical School, USA
knutte@imt.liu.se, westin@bwh.harvard.edu

**Abstract.** This paper extends Jones' popular electrostatic repulsion based algorithm for distribution of single-shell Q-space samples in two fundamental ways. The first alleviates the single-shell requirement enabling full Q-space sampling. Such an extension is not immediately obvious since it requires distributing samples evenly in 3 dimensions. The extension is as elegant as it is simple: Add a container volume of the desired shape having a constant charge density and a total charge equal to the negative of the sum of the moving point charges. Results for spherical and cubic charge containers are given. The second extension concerns the way distances between sample point are measured. The Q-space samples represent orientation, rather than direction and it would seem appropriate to use a metric that reflects this fact, e.g. a tensor metric. To this end we present a means to employ a generalized metric in the optimization. Minimizing the energy will result in a 3-dimensional distribution of point charges that is uniform in the terms of the specified metric. The radically different distributions generated using different metrics pinpoints a fundamental question: Is there an inherent optimal metric for Q-space sampling? Our work provides a versatile tool to explore the role of different metrics and we believe it will be an important contribution to further the continuing debate and research on the matter.

**Keywords:** diffusion MRI, Q-space sampling, electrostatic forces.

## 1   Introduction

In the effort of extracting meaningful micro-structural properties from diffusion weighted MRI (dMRI) it becomes clear that a large number of acquisitions are required to get the full extent of the information [1]. The discussion concerning optimal q-space sampling strategies has been lively from the very start of diffusion imaging [1–4, 8–10]. Among the most well known approaches is the electrostatic repulsion algorithm suggested by Jones et. al. [5]. Jones' algorithm finds a 'uniform' single-shell distribution of Q-space sample points by finding the lowest electrostatic energy of a system consisting of N antipodal charge pairs on the surface of a sphere. However, when aiming for a full 3-dimensional reconstruction of the diffusion propagator the sample points should be evenly distributed in the targeted 3-dimensional Q-space. Such a solution can not be

K. Mori et al. (Eds.): MICCAI 2013, Part I, LNCS 8149, pp. 679–686, 2013.

attained using the traditional electrostatic repulsion approach since alleviating the single-shell constraint will make the sample distribution expand indefinitely.

Further, it is doubtful if the Euclidean vector difference metric traditionally used is the best possible choice. The Q-space samples actually represent orientation, rather than direction. For this reason it would seem more appropriate to consider charges moving in, for example, an outer product tensor space.

In this paper we present a novel and general framework allowing the generation of full 3-dimensional Q-space sample distributions. Our framework extends the electrostatic charge distribution model in two fundamental ways:

1. Enabling a user specified definition of the 3-dimensional space to be sampled.
2. Enabling a user specified definition of the distance metric to be used.

## 2 Theory

Jones' algorithm finds a 'uniform' distribution of q-space sample points by finding the lowest electrostatic energy of a system consisting of $N$ antipodal equal charge pairs on the surface of a sphere. The system energy takes the form:

$$E = \sum_m \sum_n (\|\hat{\mathbf{x}}_m - \hat{\mathbf{x}}_n\|^{-1} + \|\hat{\mathbf{x}}_m + \hat{\mathbf{x}}_n\|^{-1}) \tag{1}$$

where $n, m \in [1 : N]$. See figure 1 left for our simulation result using 500 sample points. An extension beyond the single-shell is not immediately obvious since a full Q-space sampling requires samples that are evenly distributed in 3 dimensions.

**Charged Containers for 3D Sampling -** To extend the sample distribution generation to cover a full 3d Q-space simply add a volume of the desired shape, having an evenly distributed total charge equal to the negative of the sum of the moving point charges. This volume will then act as a container for the point charges. To add the corresponding energy term we need to find the added potential field. The sphere is the simplest possible container and one of the very few cases for which a simple closed form interior potential function is known:

$$V_c = -N (3 - r^2) \tag{2}$$

where $r$ is the distance from the container center. Note, however, that it is possible to specify any shape of the negatively charged volume as long as a good approximation of the spatial gradient can be found, see section 3. Alleviating the sphere surface requirement and adding the container contribution to the traditional energy function yields:

$$E = \sum_m \sum_{n \neq m} (\|\mathbf{x}_m - \mathbf{x}_n\|^{-1} + \|\mathbf{x}_m + \mathbf{x}_n\|^{-1}) - 2N \sum_m (3 - \|\mathbf{x}_m\|^2) \tag{3}$$

Here the 'self energy' contribution from the individual antipodal pairs have been excluded from the summation ($n \neq m$). This is consistent with the view that the sole purpose of the pair construction is to implement an appropriate metric, i.e. the antipodal pair points do not repel each other. Minimizing this energy function for 500 charge pairs we get the solution shown in figure 1 right.

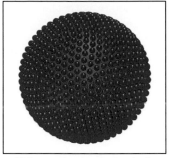
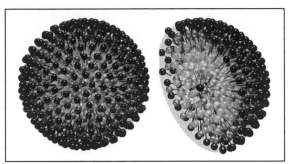

500 samples in single-shell          500 samples in spherical container

**Fig. 1.** Results from optimization of a 500 sample positions in Q-space. Classic Jones single-shell electrostatic repulsion (left). Electrostatic forces with spherical container (right). The rightmost plot shows only half of the sphere to display the interior sampling. Colors indicate distance to the container center, Red = 0, Blue = 1.

**Tensor Metrics for Distribution of Q-space Samples -** While the energy definition of eq (1) works well in the intended single-shell context a different definition is natural for a fully 3-dimensional Q-space sampling system. The Q-space samples represent orientation, rather than direction. For this reason it would seem more appropriate to consider charges moving in an outer product tensor space. To enable the use of different metrics we present a means to employ a generalized metric in the optimization. Thus, each charge act as if positioned in a higher dimensional space that naturally represents the concept of orientation [6]. To this end we introduce the following general tensor related metric:

$$\mathcal{D}^2(\mathbf{x}_m, \mathbf{x}_n) \equiv w_r \underbrace{(r_m^\alpha - r_n^\alpha)^2}_{\mathcal{D}_r^2} + w_\varphi \underbrace{2\,(r_m r_n)^\beta \left[1 - (\hat{\mathbf{x}}_m^T \hat{\mathbf{x}}_n)^\gamma\right]}_{\mathcal{D}_\varphi^2} \tag{4}$$

where $r = \|\mathbf{x}\|$, $\hat{\mathbf{x}} = \frac{\mathbf{x}}{r}$, $w_r$ and $w_\varphi$ are weighting factors. The parameters $\alpha$, $\beta$ and $\gamma$ are exponents controlling radial and angular behavior. For clarity we will in the following sometimes omit the variables $(\mathbf{x}_m, \mathbf{x}_n)$. The following examples demonstrate the generality of the proposed metric. Inserting $w_r = w_\varphi = \alpha = \beta = \gamma = 1$ and using the fact that $\hat{\mathbf{x}}_m^T \hat{\mathbf{x}}_n = \cos(\varphi)$ gives:

$$\mathcal{D}^2 = (r_m - r_n)^2 + 2\,r_m r_n \left[1 - \cos(\varphi)\right] = \|\mathbf{x}_m - \mathbf{x}_n\|^2 \tag{5}$$

which show that this parameter setting corresponds to the standard Euclidean metric. A number of other useful metrics are also instances of this general metric. For example: $w_r = w_\varphi = 1$ and $\alpha = \beta = \gamma = 2$ gives the outer product tensor metric, $\mathcal{D} = \|\mathbf{x}_m \mathbf{x}_m^T - \mathbf{x}_n \mathbf{x}_n^T\|$. $w_r = w_\varphi = 1$ and $\alpha = \beta = \gamma = N$ gives the N:th order outer product tensor metric, $\mathcal{D} = \|\mathbf{x}_m^{\otimes N} - \mathbf{x}_n^{\otimes N}\|$. Using $w_r = 1$, $w_\varphi = 2$ and $\alpha = \beta = \gamma = 2$ gives the double angle metric corresponding to a traceless outer product tensor, $\mathcal{D} = r_m^2 + r_n^2 - 2r_m r_n \cos(2\varphi)$. See figure 2 for visualizations of 4 different metrics. Regardless of the metric used the potential caused by a point charge at position $\mathbf{x}_n$ at a position $\mathbf{x}_m$ can, in analogy with the classic electrostatic potential, be defined in terms of the distance, $\mathcal{D}$, as:

$$V = \mathcal{D}^{-1} = (\mathcal{D}^2)^{-\frac{1}{2}} \tag{6}$$

The electrostatic force acting on the charge at $\mathbf{x}_m$, is calculated by differentiation of the potential field with respect to $\mathbf{x}_m$.

$$F = \frac{\partial V}{\partial \mathbf{x}_m} = \frac{\partial V}{\partial \mathcal{D}^2}\frac{\partial \mathcal{D}^2}{\partial \mathbf{x}_m} \tag{7}$$

From equation (6) we find that the first partial derivative is given by:

$$\frac{\partial V}{\partial \mathcal{D}^2} = -\frac{1}{2}(\mathcal{D}^2)^{-\frac{3}{2}} = -\frac{1}{2}\mathcal{D}^{-3} \tag{8}$$

The second partial derivative can be expressed as a sum of the partial derivatives of the radial and angular parts, $\mathcal{D}_r^2$ and $\mathcal{D}_\varphi^2$.

$$\frac{\partial \mathcal{D}^2}{\partial \mathbf{x}_m} = \frac{\partial \mathcal{D}_r^2}{\partial \mathbf{x}_m} + \frac{\partial \mathcal{D}_\varphi^2}{\partial \mathbf{x}_m} \tag{9}$$

Before carrying out the differentiation it may be helpful to rewrite the distance definition, equation (4), so that standard differentiation rules can be directly applied.

$$\begin{cases} \mathcal{D}_r^2 = \left[(\mathbf{x}_m^T\mathbf{x}_m)^{\frac{\alpha}{2}} - (\mathbf{x}_n^T\mathbf{x}_n)^{\frac{\alpha}{2}}\right]^2 \\ \mathcal{D}_\varphi^2 = 2\,(\mathbf{x}_m^T\mathbf{x}_m)^{\frac{\beta}{2}}(\mathbf{x}_n^T\mathbf{x}_n)^{\frac{\beta}{2}}\left[1 - (\mathbf{x}_m^T\mathbf{x}_m)^{-\frac{\gamma}{2}}(\mathbf{x}_n^T\mathbf{x}_n)^{-\frac{\gamma}{2}}(\mathbf{x}_m^T\mathbf{x}_n)^\gamma\right] \end{cases} \tag{10}$$

The radial part is relatively straightforward and carrying out the differentiation we get:

$$\frac{\partial \mathcal{D}_r^2}{\partial \mathbf{x}_m} = 2\alpha\,(r_m^\alpha - r_n^\alpha)\,r_m^{\alpha-1}\,\hat{\mathbf{x}}_m \tag{11}$$

The angular part requires a bit longer derivation which is left to the devoted reader. The end result expressed in terms of $r$, $\hat{\mathbf{x}}$ and $\cos(\varphi)$ is:

$$\frac{\partial \mathcal{D}_\varphi^2}{\partial \mathbf{x}_m} = 2\,r_n^\beta\,r_m^{\beta-1}\left(\left[\beta + (\gamma-\beta)\cos^\gamma(\varphi)\right]\hat{\mathbf{x}}_m - \gamma\cos^{\gamma-1}(\varphi)\,\hat{\mathbf{x}}_n\right) \tag{12}$$

**Electrostatic Force Field from Charged Container -** The force field caused by a charged container $(\Omega_c)$ with a certain local charge density $(q_c)$ can, in any metric $(\mathcal{D})$, be attained through integration over all charges followed by spatial differentiation. Using the classic electrostatic single charge potential field function, $(r^{-1})$, with the distance given by our generalized metric we get:

$$F_c(\mathbf{x}) = \frac{\partial}{\partial \mathbf{x}}\underbrace{\int_{\mathbf{y}\in\Omega_b} q_c(\mathbf{y})\,\mathcal{D}(\mathbf{x},\mathbf{y})^{-1}\,d\mathbf{y}}_{V_c(\mathbf{x})} \tag{13}$$

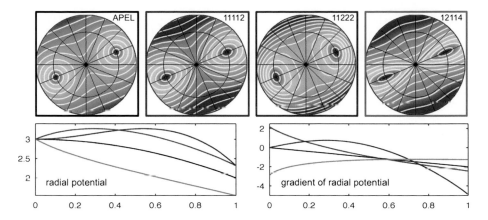

**Fig. 2.** Four distance maps generated by the metrics used in the experiments (top). The plots show distances from a reference point positioned at the center of the red area. Due to symmetry the 3D distance map is rotation invariant, i.e. the distance maps on any plane through the origin and the reference point are identical. The white lines are iso-distance lines (iso-surfaces in 3D). Note the variation in radial/angular metric ratio around the reference point, this ratio links strongly to the shell forming behavior shown in figure 3. The colored curves show container potentials (lower left) and the corresponding gradients (lower right) as a function of radius for the same four metrics. The curves have the same color as the frame of the corresponding distance map: APEL (black), T-11112 (blue), T-11222 (red) and T-12114 (green).

approximation of numerically computed values was found to perform well. Although a spatially varying charge density, $q_c$, can easily be specified the density was, in order to achieve a uniform sample distribution, set to be spatially constant in all experiments reported here. See figure 2 for the results obtained using a spherical container and four different metrics:

| APEL | Antipodal Electrostatic |
|------|--------------------------|
| T-11112 | $w_r = 1,\ w_\varphi = 1,\ \alpha = 1,\ \beta = 1,\ \gamma = 2$ |
| T-11222 | $w_r = 1,\ w_\varphi = 1,\ \alpha = 2,\ \beta = 2,\ \gamma = 2$ |
| T-12114 | $w_r = 1,\ w_\varphi = 2,\ \alpha = 1,\ \beta = 1,\ \gamma = 4$ |

## 3   Results

The energy minimization was performed using a simulated annealing inspired gradient search algorithm. Search times are roughly proportional to the square of the number of tensor charges, higher accuracy will of course require longer search times. Typically finding a low energy point for a 200-samples system can be done in less than a minute using a standard laptop.

**Natural Shells -** A consistent and compelling feature of the container based minimum energy solutions is that the sample point distributions, regardless of the number of charges used, takes the form of shells. The number of shells, the

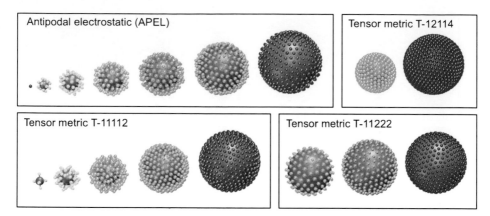

**Fig. 3.** Four examples of the forming of shells that occur using the charged container approach. The shells have been segmented and are shown separately from the center out, left to right. The color indicate sample radius. The upper left result is also shown in a non-segmented version in figure 1 right. All examples have 500 sample points. The plots clearly show that the different metrics gives rise to radically different sample distributions and shell forming behavior. Intuitively it makes sense that if the ratio angular/radial distance increases (see figure 2), i.e. the surface area of a sphere increases relative to it's radius, fewer shells with more samples in each will be formed.

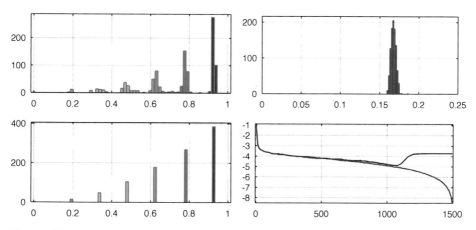

**Fig. 4.** Plots displaying different features of the optimization of a 500 sample point distribution using the antipodal electrostatic metric (APEL). Histogram of number of samples vs radius, the forming of shells is clearly visible (top left). Histogram of samples vs distance to closest neighbors, the narrow peak shows that the distribution is highly uniform in Q-space (top right). Histogram of samples vs radius after the shells have been forced to become radially thin (bottom left). The 10-logarithm of the system energy vs number of iterations for two separate optimization runs (bottom right). The blue curve shows a typical run. The red curve shows a run where a gradually increasing extra force was applied to produce thin shells. Note that the end results has more than 4 orders of magnitude higher energy which shows that adding a 'shelling' forming force will produce precise shells but will increase the system energy considerably, i.e. the 'soft' shells provide a more even sample distribution.

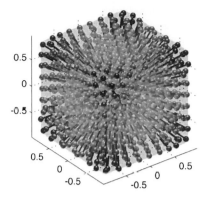 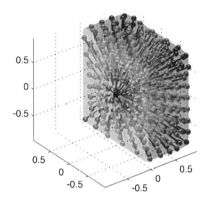

**Fig. 5.** Optimization result using a cubic charge container and the antipodal electrostatic metric (APEL). The rightmost plot shows only half of the cube to display the interior sampling.

radial position and number of charges in each shell is, however, highly dependent on the metric used. Figure 3 shows the resulting distribution of 500 sample points using four different metrics. For each metric case below the number of samples per shell and the mean shell radii are given in brackets.

| | | | |
|---|---|---|---|
| APEL | - 7 shells | # (1, 7, 25, 53, 87, 135, 192) | radii (0, .19, .33, .48, .63, .78, .93) |
| T-11112 | - 5 shells | # (3, 24, 78, 150, 245) | radii (.19, .32, .51, .70, .88) |
| T-11222 | - 3 shells | # (86, 153, 261) | radii (.77, .87, .97) |
| T-12114 | - 2 shells | # (135, 365) | radii (.52, .79) |

The shells are naturally 'soft', i.e. the distribution of radii in each shell has a certain width due to interaction with other shells, see figure 4. Adding a 'shelling' forming force will produce precise shells but will increase the system energy showing that the 'soft' shells provide a more even sample distribution, see figure 4. Figure 4 also includes a histogram of the the distances to closest neighbors, the standard deviation is only 2% of the mean distance showing that the distribution of samples is indeed very uniform. Figure 5 shows an example using a uniformly charged cube as the container. The second term of eq(3) was here replaced by a sixth order polynomial to approximate the interior potential [7]. The cube-ness of the charge distribution is clearly visible. Interestingly, a tendency to form spherical shells is still present for the inner parts of the cube.

## 4    Conclusions

We have presented a novel method for generating Q-space sample distributions that are uniform in a user specified metric and cover a user specified part of q-space. Whether to sample linearly or quadratically in Q-space radius is, for example, determined by one parameter ($\alpha = \beta \in \{1, 2\}$). We have demonstrated the feasibility for a range of different cases. The results are interesting from several points of view. There is a marked tendency for the samples to group in shells. This fact indicates that the present work provides an interesting alternative to recently proposed shell-interaction schemes [4, 8–10]. It may sometimes be preferable to distribute the Q-samples in a cube since much higher Q-values can then in practice be attained towards the corners [11]. We have shown that the charged container approach produces good results also for this case. Further, the distribution attained for the cube case is far from Cartesian, this may be an advantage in a sparse reconstruction, e.g. compressed sensing, setting.

Perhaps the most important aspect of our contribution is that it provides a new and powerful tool in future investigations concerning Q-space sampling. Since scanner time will always be an issue every improvement of sampling efficiency will ultimately be of great clinical value.

**Acknowledgement.** The authors acknowledge the Swedish Research Council grants 2011-5176, 2012-3682 and NIH grants R01MH074794, P41RR013218, and P41EB015902.

# References

1. Assaf, Y., Freidlin, R.Z., Rohde, G.K., Basser, P.J.: New modeling and experimental framework to characterize hindered and restricted water diffusion in brain white matter. Magn. Reson Med. 52(5), 965–978 (2004)
2. Wu, Y.C., Alexander, A.L.: Hybrid diffusion imaging. Neuroimage 36(3), 617–629 (2007)
3. Alexander, D.C.: A general framework for experiment design in diffusion MRI and its application in measuring direct tissue-microstructure features. Magn. Reson Med. 60(2), 439–448 (2008)
4. Westin, C.F., Pasternak, O., Knutsson, H.: Rotationally invariant gradient schemes for diffusion MRI. In: Proc. of the ISMRM Annual Meeting (ISMRM 2012), p. 3537 (2012)
5. Jones, D.K., Simmons, A., Williams, S.C.R., Horsfield, M.A.: Non-invasive assessment of axonal fiber connectivity in the human brain via diffusion tensor MRI. Magn. Reson Med. 42, 37–41 (1999)
6. Knutsson, H.: Representing local structure using tensors. In: SCIA 1989, Oulu, Finland, pp. 244–251 (1989)
7. Hummer, G.: Electrostatic potential of a homogeneously charged square and cube in two and three dimensions 36(3), 285–291 (1996)
8. Caruyer, E., Cheng, J., Lenglet, C., Sapiro, G., Jiang, T., Deriche, R.: Optimal Design of Multiple Q-shells experiments for Diffusion MRI. In: MICCAI Workshop CDMRI (2011)
9. Merlet, S., Caruyer, E., Deriche, R.: Impact of radial and angular sampling on multiple shells acquisition in diffusion MRI. Med. Image Comput. Comput. Assist. Interv. 14(Pt 2), 116–123 (2011)
10. Ye, W., Portnoy, S., Entezari, A., Blackband, S.J., Vemuri, B.C.: An Efficient Interlaced Multi-shell Sampling Scheme for Reconstruction of Diffusion Propagators. IEEE Trans. Med. Imaging 31(5), 1043–1050 (2012)
11. Scherrer, B., Warfield, S.K.: Parametric Representation of Multiple White Matter Fascicles from Cube and Sphere Diffusion MRI. PLoS ONE 7(11), 1–20 (2012)

# Optimal Diffusion Tensor Imaging
# with Repeated Measurements

Mohammad Alipoor[1], Irene Yu Hua Gu[1], Andrew J.H. Mehnert[1,2],
Ylva Lilja[3], and Daniel Nilsson[3]

[1] Department of Signals and Systems, Chalmers University of Technology,
Gothenburg, Sweden
alipoor@chalmers.se
[2] MedTech West, Sahlgrenska University Hospital, Gothenburg, Sweden
[3] Institute of Neuroscience and Physiology, Sahlgrenska University Hospital,
Gothenburg, Sweden

**Abstract.** Several data acquisition schemes for diffusion MRI have been
proposed and explored to date for the reconstruction of the 2nd order
tensor. Our main contributions in this paper are: (i) the definition of
a new class of sampling schemes based on repeated measurements in
every sampling point; (ii) two novel schemes belonging to this class; and
(iii) a new reconstruction framework for the second scheme. We also
present an evaluation, based on Monte Carlo computer simulations, of
the performances of these schemes relative to known optimal sampling
schemes for both 2nd and 4th order tensors. The results demonstrate
that tensor estimation by the proposed sampling schemes and estimation
framework is more accurate and robust.

**Keywords:** diffusion tensor imaging, optimal sampling scheme, tensor
estimation.

## 1   Introduction

Diffusion tensor imaging (DTI) measures the restricted diffusion of water molecules in tissues, thus revealing information about tissue micro-structure. It involves acquiring a series of diffusion-weighted images (DWIs), each acquired
with diffusion sensitization along a particular gradient direction. Six or more
non-collinear directions are needed to reconstruct a 2nd order tensor. The overall acquisition time needs to be compatible with in-vivo measurement. Thus, one
of the most fundamental questions in DTI is how to optimally sample $q$-space.
The classical case, i.e. single-sphere $q$-space sampling with a constant $b$-value
for constructing the second order tensor, has been the subject of much study
over the last decade. Two observations can be drawn from the literature: (i) it
is widely accepted among researchers that sampling points should be uniformly
distributed over the unit sphere (the motivation is that the SNR of the measured
signal is dependent on the orientation and anisotropy of the tensor [1,2]); and
(ii) it is widely accepted that more sampling points leads to more accurate tensor estimation (the motivation for acquiring more measurements is to mitigate

K. Mori et al. (Eds.): MICCAI 2013, Part I, LNCS 8149, pp. 687–694, 2013.

noise and not to capture more directional or spatial information). Nevertheless whilst both of these sampling tenets are intuitively appealing they have not been proved. Higher reconstruction accuracy equates to reducing noise by either making additional measurements in more directions, or repeating measurements in a smaller number of directions. Research to date has been focused on the former strategy. An open question is whether, given the possibility of making $N$ measurements, it is better to make measurements in $N$ unique directions or to repeat measurements over a fewer number of directions. In this paper, the question is addressed for both 2nd and 4th order tensor imaging. In particular, this paper introduces a new class of sampling schemes with $r_i > 1$ repeated measurements in each direction, and proffers two sampling strategies from this class. In addition, for the second scheme, a new tensor estimation framework is proposed. The two approaches are compared to the optimal solutions of the conventional strategy of taking $r_i = 1$. The remainder of this paper is organized as follows. In the next section we discuss related work and present the general evaluation framework that is used to evaluate sampling schemes. Section 3 introduces the proposed sampling schemes and estimation framework. In section 4, Monte Carlo simulation results and comparisons with conventional optimal schemes are presented.

## 2    Related Work

A wide variety of diffusion tensor data sampling schemes have been proposed ranging from electrostatic repulsion (to obtain uniform sampling on the unit sphere) [1], to minimum condition number (MCN) [3] (to minimize the noise effect on the estimated tensor elements, and thus tensor-derived quantities, by minimization of the condition number of the design matrix [3] associated with the linear least squares parametric estimation of the diffusion tensor). The reader is referred to [2] for a comprehensive review of these sampling schemes.

Simulations in [4] showed that the icosahedral sampling scheme is superior to the MCN scheme in terms of rotational invariance of the condition number (CN). Several other criteria have also been proposed to measure the optimality of sampling schemes including total tensor variance [5], interaction energy of identical charges positioned at sampling points [1], signal deviation [6], variance of tensor-derived scalars [4,7], minimum angle between pairs of encoding directions, and SNR of tensor-derived scalars [8]. However, very few studies have considered optimal sampling schemes for 4th order tensor imaging [2]. A common framework [7,9,4,6,3] to evaluate sampling schemes (mainly for the 2nd order tensor) is via Monte Carlo simulations. In particular this involves: (1) defining a diagonal tensor $D_0$ with a prescribed fractional anisotropy (FA) and eigenvalues; (2) rotating this initial tensor, i.e. obtaining $D = R^T D_0 R$ where $R$ is the rotation matrix (corresponding to a rotation by Euler angles $\theta, \phi$ and $\psi$); (3) simulating the diffusion signal at the sampling points defined by the scheme under evaluation using the Stejskal-Tanner [10] equation; (4) adding Rician distributed noise to the synthetic signals (to obtain a prescribed SNR); (5) using the noisy signal to obtain a reconstruction/estimate, $\hat{D}$, of $D$; (6) computing the optimality measure of interest; (7) repeating steps (2)-(6) $N_{MC}$ times (for different realizations of noise); (8) recording the mean value of the optimality measure; and (9) repeating steps (2)-(8) $N_R$ times (for different rotations). This general evaluation framework (GEF) is both well-known and widely used (typically with two 90 degree crossing fibers).

## 3    Proposed Work

Given that the distribution of noise in MRI magnitude images is nearly Gaussian for SNR $> 2$ [11], and that a typical SNR value for DTI is 12.5 [12], this motivates repetition of measurements on the same sampling points followed by averaging. To the authors' knowledge, only two papers have considered sampling schemes with repeated measurements [7,4] (in order to fairly compare with other sampling schemes with more sampling points but not to study noise mitigation by repeated measurements). Let $Name/N_u/r$ denote a gradient encoding scheme (GES) with $N_u$ unique sampling points and $r$ repetitions per point. To study the effect of noise mitigation by repeated measurements one should compare $X/\frac{N}{r}/r$ with $X/N/1$. There is only one such a comparison in [4] with the variance of FA as the only measure of optimality. This implies that in [4,7] the purpose was not to study noise mitigation by repeated measurements. We continue by briefly describing the commonly used reconstruction framework. The basic Stejskal-Tanner equation for diffusion MRI signal attenuation is [10]

$$-\frac{1}{b}\ln\left(\frac{S}{S_0}\right) = d(\mathbf{g}) \tag{1}$$

where $d(\mathbf{g})$ is the diffusivity function, $S$ is the measured signal when the diffusion sensitizing gradient is applied in the direction $\mathbf{g}$, $S_0$ is the observed signal in the absence of such a gradient, and $b$ is the diffusion weighting taken to be constant over all measurements. The diffusivity function $d(\mathbf{g})$ is modeled using even order ($m$) symmetric tensors as follows

$$d(\mathbf{g}) = \sum_{i=0}^{m}\sum_{j=0}^{m-i} t_{ij}\mu_{ijm}g_1^i g_2^j g_3^{m-i-j} \tag{2}$$

where $\mathbf{g} = [g_1\ g_2\ g_3]^T$, $\mu_{ijm} = m!/i!j!(m-i-j)!$, and the $t_{ij}$ denote $n = (m+1)(m+2)/2$ distinct entries of the $m$-th order tensor. The diffusivity function is expressed as the inner product $d(\mathbf{g}) = \mathbf{t}^T\hat{\mathbf{g}}$ where $\hat{\mathbf{g}} = [g_3^m\ mg_2 g_3^{m-1}\ 0.5m(m-1)g_2^2 g_3^{m-2}\cdots g_1^m]^T$ and $\mathbf{t} = [t_{00}\ t_{01}\cdots t_{m0}]$. Note that both vectors $\mathbf{t}$ and $\hat{\mathbf{g}}$ are vectors in $\mathbb{R}^n$ and $d(\mathbf{g},\mathbf{t}) = d(\mathbf{g})$ is used for simplification. Given measurements in $N \geq n$ different directions $\mathbf{g}_k$ the tensor estimation problem is then formulated as

$$\min \sum_{k=1}^{N}(d_k - \hat{d}_k)^2, \quad \text{s.t. } d(\mathbf{g}) \geq 0 \tag{3}$$

where $d_k = d(\mathbf{g}_k)$ are the values predicted by the model, and $\hat{d}_k = -b^{-1}\ln(S_k/S_0)$ are the measured values.

## 3.1   Optimality Measures

$\mathbf{G} = [\hat{\mathbf{g}}_1 \ \hat{\mathbf{g}}_2 \cdots \ \hat{\mathbf{g}}_N]^T$ is the design matrix associated with the least squares (LS) estimation of the diffusion tensor. Its CN, $k(\mathbf{G})$ is widely used to measure the optimality of a sampling scheme. Alternatively the CN of the information matrix $B = \mathbf{G}^T\mathbf{G}$ is used ($k(\mathbf{G}) = \sqrt{k(B)}$) [4]. Nevertheless these CNs do not give the full picture [2]. For this reason herein we use two optimality measures: CN and signal deviation. An interesting property of the CN is that the CN of a scheme consisting of $N_u$ unique directions is the same as that for a scheme in which repeated measurements are made in these $N_u$ directions (the proof is easily obtained by constructing the information matrix). The signal deviation for an estimation procedure is given by [6]

$$S_{\text{dev}} = \frac{1}{N} \sum_{i=1}^{N} |S_i - \hat{S}_i| \tag{4}$$

where $S_i$ is the noise-free synthetic signal and $\hat{S}_i$ is the signal reconstructed from the estimated tensor.

## 3.2   First Scheme

Herein we describe our first solution for determining an optimal sampling scheme. It is based on the idea that if we can only make a fixed number of measurements then we should make repeated measurements in some optimal sampling points instead of seeking to acquire measurements in more unique directions. This strategy is motivated by the following facts: (i) as long as our reconstruction framework has only $n$ free parameters, increasing the number of sampling points does not lead to the acquisition of more directional/spatial information; (ii) the acquisition of more samples and the application of LS estimation methods mitigates noise (as noted above for SNR > 2 the noise is nearly Gaussian and so repeated measurements also leads to improved SNR); and (iii) the CN is invariant under repetitions.

Given that the icosahedral scheme is widely accepted as an optimal sampling scheme for both 2nd and 4th [6] order DTI we used this scheme as a the basis for our experiments. In particular we chose to compare measurement over $N_u$ unique directions with repeated measurements (up to a total of $N_u$) over only 6 directions. Hereinafter this sampling strategy is called 'S1'. We used the algorithm proposed in [13] to estimate diffusion tensors for this strategy.

## 3.3   Second Scheme and Its Reconstruction Framework

Herein we describe our second solution for determining an optimal sampling scheme, applicable for 2nd order tensors. In conventional tensor estimation frameworks, all tensor elements are estimated at the same time. We propose a new estimation framework by splitting the tensor estimation into two steps as follows. From (2) it can be seen that we can directly measure the diagonal elements of the

2nd order tensor by applying only three gradient directions. This defines the first step of our second scheme

$$\text{GES}_{\text{step1}} : \{d([1\,0\,0]) = t_{20},\ d([0\,1\,0]) = t_{02},\ d([0\,0\,1]) = t_{00}\}.\qquad(5)$$

The motivation for these choices is to obtain CN=1. These directions can of course be repeated several times. Once the diagonal elements of the diffusion tensor are obtained (from above), another set of three sampling points are measured to estimate the off-diagonal elements. The $\mathbf{G}$ matrix for estimation of the off-diagonal elements is

$$\mathbf{G}_{\text{step2}} = \begin{bmatrix} g_{x1}g_{y1} & g_{x1}g_{z1} & g_{y1}g_{z1} \\ g_{x2}g_{y2} & g_{x2}g_{z2} & g_{y2}g_{z2} \\ g_{x2}g_{y2} & g_{x2}g_{z2} & g_{y2}g_{z2} \end{bmatrix}.\qquad(6)$$

We minimized the condition number of (6) using particle swarm optimization [14] to obtain the sampling points for this step. We acknowledge that other optimization schemes could be used at this step. The outcome is that many solutions lead to a CN equal to one. One example is

$$\text{GES}_{\text{step2}} = \{[0.10\ -0.75\ -0.65],[-0.65\ -0.10\ -0.75],[-0.75\,0.65\ -0.10]\}$$

that is used in our experiments. Hereinafter we call this scheme 'S2'. For a DTI data acquisition scheme with $N = 30$ measurements this implies that one may sample these six points five times (denoted as S2/6/5). Other repetition variations are also possible. For example, if $N = 21$ then four repetitions of $\text{GES}_{\text{step1}}$ and three repetitions of $\text{GES}_{\text{step2}}$ is a possibility (S2/6/4,3). Let $r_{\text{s1}}$ and $r_{\text{s2}}$ be the number of repetitions for each step respectively. First we simply average the measured signal to estimate the diagonal elements of the diffusion tensor (averaging is done over signals acquired by $\text{GES}_{\text{step1}}$). Substituting in the known diagonal elements yields a system of linear equations in three unknowns (off-diagonal elements). The system is overdetermined (because $r_{\text{s2}} > 1$) and is solved using LS. The motivation for this scheme is to keep CN=1 all the way through, and to employ the repetition idea from 'S1'.

## 4    Simulations

### 4.1    Simulation Setup

The measurements of diffusion signal magnitude can be modeled as [15]: $S(\mathbf{g}_i) = |A(\mathbf{g}_i) + w|,\ i = 1,\dots,N$ where $w$ is Rician distributed random noise with standard deviation $\sigma$, $A(\mathbf{g}_i) = \sum_{j=1}^{u} \frac{S_0}{u} \exp(-b\mathbf{g}_i^T D_j \mathbf{g}_i)$ is the ideal signal (without noise) from a voxel containing $u$ fiber bundles and $D_j$ is the 2nd order diffusion tensor for the $j$-th fiber. Synthetic data were generated using this model with the the following setup: $N \in \{6,\dots,321\}$, $b = 1500\,\text{sec}/(\text{mm}^2)$, $D_1 = \text{diag}(17,1,1) \times 10^{-4}\ (\text{mm}^2)/\text{sec}$, $D_2 = \text{diag}(1,17,1) \times 10^{-4}\ (\text{mm}^2)/\text{sec}$, $u \in \{1,2\}$, SNR $= 12.5$ (a typical level of noise [12]) and $N_{\text{MC}} = 100$. In all

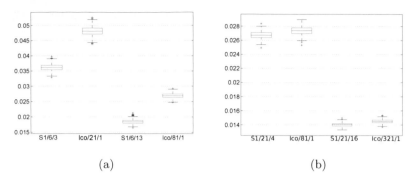

**Fig. 1.** A comparison between our proposed scheme 'S1' and 'Ico' based on signal deviation statistics. (a) 2nd order tensor and one fiber bundle ($m = 2, u = 1$); (b) 4th order tensor and two fiber bundles ($m = 4, u = 2$). Our proposed 'S1' outperforms 'Ico' in terms of accuracy and robustness.

experiments the optimality measure was computed for $N_R = 441$ different rotations. Given the axial symmetry of the diffusion ellipsoid rotation angle, $\psi$ was set to zero in all simulations [9]. The space of possible rotations over $\theta$ and $\phi$ was uniformly sampled with 21 steps (both in the interval $[0, 2\pi]$).

## 4.2    Simulation Results

As mentioned earlier, repetitions do not change the CN. The CN of the icosahedral scheme for 2nd order tensor reconstruction is rotationally invariant and equal to 1.5811 [4]. In the case of the 4th order tensor the CN is not rotationally invariant but has a mean less than 7 (dependent on $N_u$) [6].

Following the GEF introduced in section 2, we report summary statistics for the optimality measure at step (9); i.e. statistics summarizing the mean signal deviation ($S_{\mathrm{dev}}$) over all possible rotations of the tensor. Figure 1 shows a comparison of the signal deviation statistics for our proposed 'S1' relative to the icosahedral (denoted 'Ico') sampling scheme [4]. Figure 1(a) shows that 'S1' yields more accurate and robust reconstruction compared to 'Ico' for the 2nd order tensor ($m = 2$) and one fiber bundle ($u = 1$). Notably these results are obtained in a shorter scanning time (fewer measurements). Figure 1(b) shows that 'S1' yields slightly improved reconstruction for the 4th order tensor and two crossing fiber bundles ($m = 4, u = 2$). Figure 2 shows comparisons of 'S1' versus 'S2', and 'S2' versus 'Ico' for $m = 2, u = 1$. Our proposed sampling scheme, 'S2' is much better than 'Ico' in terms of reconstruction accuracy and robustness ($N = 21, 81$, see columns (b) and (d)). Also for a smaller number of measurements ($N = 18$), 'S1' is slightly better than 'S2'. However, as $N$ increases they show approximately the same performance (see columns (a) and (c)).

## 4.3    Discussion

We acknowledge that our results are based on simulations. It is noteworthy, however, that [3,5,9,13] found that the GEF results correlate with that of real brain data (RBD). We are not aware of publications to the contrary. This would suggest that our results should similarly hold for RBD. Indeed this will be the subject of future investigation. It should be noted that the quality of the results on RBD ultimately depends on the achievable SNR that in turn depends on the magnetic field strength and spatial resolution [8]. Thus such results must be complemented with simulation results. Given that the two proposed schemes outperform existing schemes on synthetic data, a similar conclusion is anticipated for RBD based on the above reasoning. Even if this were not the case, this would provide new insight/caution to the diffusion MRI community with respect to its use of the GEF.

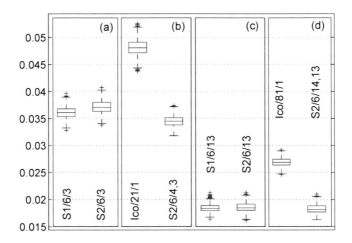

**Fig. 2.** 'S1' versus 'S2' (columns (a) and (c)) and 'S2' versus 'Ico' (columns (b) and (d)) for $u = 1, m = 2$. Our proposed 'S2' outperforms 'Ico' in terms of accuracy and robustness.

## 5    Conclusion

We proposed two new sampling schemes for diffusion tensor imaging. The first scheme utilizes repeated measurements along the directions prescribed by the icosahedral scheme in the conventional estimation framework. The second scheme uses repeated measurements of a new sampling scheme in a new estimation framework. These two schemes were evaluated and compared with known optimal sampling schemes using Monte Carlo computer simulations. Our results demonstrate that the two proposed schemes are superior in terms of accuracy and robustness. Although preliminary, these results suggest that this approach may have a significant impact on DWI acquisition protocols. Future work includes validating these results using real human brain data.

# References

1. Jones, D.K., Horsfield, M.A., Simmons, A.: Optimal strategies for measuring diffusion in anisotropic systems by magnetic resonance imaging. Magnetic Resonance in Medicine 42, 515–525 (1999)
2. Jones, D.K.: Diffusion MRI theory, methods, and applications. Oxford University Press (2011)
3. Skare, S., Hedehus, M., Moseley, M., Li, T.: Condition number as a measure of noise performance of diffusion tensor data acquisition schemes with MRI. J. Magn. Reson. 147(2), 340–352 (2000)
4. Batchelor, P., Atkinson, D., Hill, D., Calamante, F., Connelly, A.: Anisotropic noise propagation in diffusion tensor MRI sampling schemes. Magn. Reson. Med. 49(6), 1143–1151 (2003)
5. Hasan, K.M., Parker, D.L., Alexander, A.L.: Magnetic resonance water self-diffusion tensor encoding optimization methods for full brain acquisition. Image Analysis and Stereology 21(2), 87–96 (2002)
6. Mang, S.C., Gembris, D., Grodd, W., Klose, U.: Comparison of gradient encoding directions for higher order tensor diffusion data. Magnetic Resonance in Medicine 61(2), 335–343 (2009)
7. Jones, D.K.: The effect of gradient sampling schemes on measures derived from diffusion tensor MRI: A Monte Carlo study. Magnetic Resonance in Medicine 51, 807–815 (2004)
8. Zhan, L., et al.: How does angular resolution affect diffusion imaging measures? NeuroImage 49(2), 1357–1371 (2010)
9. Skare, S., Li, T.Q., Nordell, B., Ingvar, M.: Noise considerations in the determination of diffusion tensor anisotropy. Magnetic Resonance Imaging 18(6), 659–669 (2000)
10. Stejskal, E., Tanner, J.: Spin diffusion measurements: Spin echoes in the presence of a time-dependent field gradient. Journal of Chemical Physics 42(1), 288–292 (1965)
11. Gudbjartsson, H., Patz, S.: The rician distribution of noisy MRI data. Magn. Reson. Med. 34(6), 910–914 (1995)
12. Jiao, F., Gur, Y., Johnson, C.R., Joshi, S.: Detection of crossing white matter fibers with high-order tensors and rank-$k$ decompositions. In: Székely, G., Hahn, H.K. (eds.) IPMI 2011. LNCS, vol. 6801, pp. 538–549. Springer, Heidelberg (2011)
13. Barmpoutis, A., Vemuri, B.C.: A unified framework for estimating diffusion tensors of any order with symmetric positive-definite constraints. In: Proc. IEEE Int. Symp. Biomed. Imaging, pp. 1385–1388 (2010)
14. Eberhart, R.C., Shi, Y.: Comparing inertia weights and constriction factors in particle swarm optimization 1, 84–88 (2000)
15. Jansons, K., Alexander, D.: Persistent angular structure: new insights from diffusion magnetic resonance imaging data. Inverse Problems 19, 1031–1046 (2003)

# Estimation of a Multi-fascicle Model from Single B-Value Data with a Population-Informed Prior*

Maxime Taquet[1,2], Benoît Scherrer[1], Nicolas Boumal[2],
Benoît Macq[2], and Simon K. Warfield[1]

[1] Computational Radiology Laboratory, Harvard Medical School, Boston, USA
[2] ICTEAM Institute, Université catholique de Louvain, Louvain-la-Neuve, Belgium

**Abstract.** Diffusion tensor imaging cannot represent heterogeneous fascicle orientations in one voxel. Various models propose to overcome this limitation. Among them, multi-fascicle models are of great interest to characterize and compare white matter properties. However, existing methods fail to estimate their parameters from conventional diffusion sequences with the desired accuracy. In this paper, we provide a geometric explanation to this problem. We demonstrate that there is a manifold of indistinguishable multi-fascicle models for single-shell data, and that the manifolds for different b-values intersect tangentially at the true underlying model making the estimation very sensitive to noise. To regularize it, we propose to learn a prior over the model parameters from data acquired at several b-values in an external population of subjects. We show that this population-informed prior enables for the first time accurate estimation of multi-fascicle models from single-shell data as commonly acquired in clinical context. The approach is validated on synthetic and in vivo data of healthy subjects and patients with autism. We apply it in population studies of the white matter microstructure in autism spectrum disorder. This approach enables novel investigations from large existing DWI datasets in normal development and in disease.

**Keywords:** Diffusion, Single-Shell, Generative Models, Estimation.

## 1 Introduction

Diffusion tensor imaging is unable to represent the signal arising from crossing fascicles. Various approaches have been proposed to overcome this limitation. Among them, generative models such as multi-tensor models [2,3] seek to represent the signal contribution from different populations of water molecules. Based on biological modelling, they are of great interest to characterize and compare white-matter properties. However, estimating their parameters from conventional diffusion data has proven inefficient.

Recent works have suggested that part of this inaccuracy is explained by the ill-posedness of the problem and not only by the imaging nuisance [3,4]. To

* MT and NB are research fellows of the F.R.S.-FNRS. MT is also research fellow of the B.A.E.F. This work was supported in part by NIH grants 1U01NS082320, R01 EB008015, R03 EB008680, R01 LM010033, R01 EB013248, P30 HD018655, BCH TRP, R42 MH086984 and UL1 TR000170.

K. Mori et al. (Eds.): MICCAI 2013, Part I, LNCS 8149, pp. 695–702, 2013.

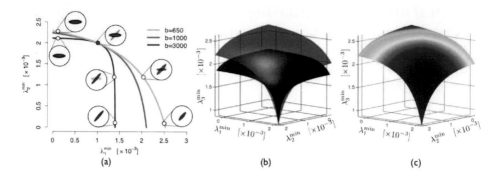

**Fig. 1.** (a) Infinitely many models produce the same diffusion signal at a given b-value and form a manifold. The manifolds for different b-values intersect at the true underlying model. (b) For $N$-fascicle models (here $N$=3), manifolds are $(N-1)$-dimensional hypersurfaces that intersect tangentially, making the estimation sensitive to noise. (c) The population-informed prior assigns different probabilities to models on the manifold.

regularize the estimation of models with a single anisotropic tensor, elaborate spatial priors have been proposed [2], and it was shown that acquiring additional b-values improves the analysis of isotropic fraction [1]. For $N$-tensors, it was proposed to fix the tensor eigenvalues [4], solving the ill-posedness problem but reducing the amount of microstructural information contained in the model. No method has proposed to regularize the estimation of an $N$-fascicle model while keeping all its degrees of freedom. Furthermore, there is a strong need for a strategy to estimate multi-fascicle models from conventional single-shell data due to their wide availability in clinical setting. Section 2 analyzes the estimation problem from a geometric point of view. Section 3 develops an estimator based on a prior informed by an external population of subjects. Section 4 presents results and Section 5 concludes. Conclusions about estimating an $N$-tensor model can be applied to all generative models that include a multi-tensor as part thereof.

## 2    Manifolds of Equivalent Models at a Given B-value

A multi-fascicle model is represented as a mixture of single fascicle models. In the multi-tensor formalism, the generative model for the formation of the diffusion signal $S$ for a b-value $b$ and a gradient direction $\boldsymbol{g}$ is:

$$S = S_0 \sum_{i=1}^{N} f_i e^{-b\boldsymbol{g}^T \boldsymbol{D}_i \boldsymbol{g}}, \tag{1}$$

where $\boldsymbol{D}_i$ and $f_i$ are the tensor and the volumetric fraction of fascicle $i$. Since $\gamma_i e^{-\log \gamma_i} = 1$, all multi-fascicle models with fractions $\gamma_i f_i$ and tensors $\boldsymbol{D}_i + \frac{\log \gamma_i}{b} \boldsymbol{I}$ produce the same signal:

$$S = S_0 \sum_{i=1}^{N} \gamma_i f_i e^{-b\boldsymbol{g}^T \left(\boldsymbol{D}_i + \frac{\log \gamma_i}{b} \boldsymbol{I}\right)\boldsymbol{g}}, \quad \text{with the constraint} \quad \sum_{i=1}^{N} \gamma_i f_i = 1. \tag{2}$$

The tensors remain positive definite as long as $\gamma_i > e^{-b\lambda_i^{\min}}$, where $\lambda_i^{\min}$ is the lowest eigenvalue of $\boldsymbol{D}_i$. Each of these models is uniquely identified by its vector $(\lambda_1^{\min}, \ldots, \lambda_N^{\min})$. The set of all models respecting Equation (2) is a manifold of dimension $(N-1)$ defined by the implicit equations (we let $\lambda_i := \lambda_i^{\min}$):

$$\begin{cases} \lambda_i = \lambda_i^{\text{true}} + \frac{1}{b}\log\left(\gamma_i\right) & \text{for } i = 1, \ldots, N \\[2mm] \sum_{i=1}^{N} \gamma_i f_i = 1, \end{cases} \qquad (3)$$

where $(\lambda_1^{\text{true}}, \ldots, \lambda_N^{\text{true}})$ is the true unknown model (Fig. 1(a)). Since these equations depend on $b$, so will the manifold. Acquiring diffusion images at different b-values amounts to defining different such manifolds. Let us investigate how those manifolds intersect at the point of interest $\lambda_i = \lambda_i^{\text{true}}$. The explicit equation of the hypersurface $\lambda_N(\lambda_1, \ldots, \lambda_{N-1})$ obtained by eliminating the $\gamma$'s between equations (3) is:

$$\lambda_N(\lambda_1, \ldots, \lambda_{N-1}) = \lambda_N^{\text{true}} + \frac{1}{b}\log\left(\frac{1 - \sum_{i=1}^{N-1} f_i e^{b(\lambda_i - \lambda_i^{\text{true}})}}{f_N}\right). \qquad (4)$$

The normal vector to the hypersurface is $\boldsymbol{\eta} = \left(\frac{\partial \lambda_N}{\partial \lambda_1}, \ldots, \frac{\partial \lambda_N}{\partial \lambda_{N-1}}, -1\right)$. Its $k$-th component evaluated at the true model is:

$$\eta_k\bigg|_{\lambda_i = \lambda_i^{\text{true}}, \forall i} = \frac{\partial \lambda_N}{\partial \lambda_k}\bigg|_{\lambda_i = \lambda_i^{\text{true}}, \forall i} = \frac{-f_k}{f_N}. \qquad (5)$$

Remarkably, this normal vector (and thereby the tangent hyperplane) does not depend on $b$ at the point of interest. In other words, at the first-order approximation, the manifolds at all b-values coincide locally, explaining the high sensitivity to noise encountered when optimizing the parameters of a multi-fascicle model (Fig. 1(b)).

At the second-order approximation, the manifold is characterized by the Hessian matrix of $\lambda_N(\lambda_1, \ldots, \lambda_{N-1})$:

$$\boldsymbol{H}\bigg|_{\lambda_i = \lambda_i^{\text{true}}} = \frac{-b}{f_N^2}\left(\tilde{f}\tilde{f}^T + f_N \text{diag}(\tilde{f})\right),$$

where $\tilde{f} = [f_1, \ldots, f_{N-1}]^T$. The difference between the Hessian matrices at two different b-values, $b$ and $b' > b$, is positive definite since, for all $x \neq 0$, we have

$$x^T\left(\boldsymbol{H}(b) - \boldsymbol{H}(b')\right)x = \frac{b' - b}{f_N^2}\left((\tilde{f}^T x)^2 + f_N x^T \text{diag}(\tilde{f})x\right) > 0. \qquad (6)$$

Therefore, there exists no direction $x$ along which the two manifolds have the same curvature. Consequently, the true model is locally the only intersection of all manifolds. Given the difference (6), it appears that a wider range of b-values leads to a larger difference between their manifolds, which should in turn improve the accuracy of the estimation (ignoring the potential impact of $b$ on noise).

When an isotropic compartment $f_{\text{iso}}e^{-bD_{\text{iso}}}$ is added to the model, one can show that the above development remains valid with an unchanged $N$ if $D_{\text{iso}}$ is known and considering an $(N+1)$-fascicle model if $D_{\text{iso}}$ needs also be optimized.

## 3   Posterior Predictive Distribution of the Parameters

While all models of (3) are equally compatible with the observed DWI at a given b-value, they are not all as likely from a biological point of view. This knowledge can be learnt from available observations at several b-values of a fascicle $i$ in $m_i$ subjects $\mathcal{F}_i = \{f_i^0, \ldots, f_i^{m_i}\}$, $\mathcal{D}_i = \{D_i^0, \ldots, D_i^{m_i}\}$, and incorporated in the estimation as a prior over the parameters $(f_i, \mathbf{D}_i)$ (Fig. 1(c)). If the effect of the fascicle properties on partial voluming is negligible, and if the properties of one fascicle are independent of those of another, then the prior can be expressed as:

$$P_{f,\mathbf{D}}(\boldsymbol{f}, \boldsymbol{D}; \boldsymbol{\theta}) = P_f(\boldsymbol{f}; \boldsymbol{\theta}_f) \prod_{i=1}^{N} P_{\mathbf{D}_i}(\boldsymbol{D}_i; \boldsymbol{\theta}_i). \tag{7}$$

The fractions are not independent since they sum to 1. However, we assume that any fraction $f_i$ is independent of the relative proportions of others $f_j/(1 - f_i)$. This *neutral vector* assumption naturally leads to the Dirichlet distribution:

$$P_f(\boldsymbol{f}; \boldsymbol{\alpha}) = \frac{\mathbb{1}_{f \in \mathcal{S}}}{B(\boldsymbol{\alpha})} \prod_{i=1}^{N} f_i^{\alpha_i - 1}, \text{ where } \mathcal{S} = \left\{ \boldsymbol{x} \in \mathbb{R}^N : x_i > 0, \sum_{i=1}^{N} x_i = 1 \right\}. \tag{8}$$

To prevent negative eigenvalues of the tensors, the prior knowledge about $\mathbf{D}_i$ can be described as a multivariate Gaussian distribution over their logarithm [5]:

$$\mathbf{L}_i = \log \mathbf{D}_i \sim \mathcal{N}(\mathbf{M}_i, \boldsymbol{\Sigma}_i). \tag{9}$$

In general, $\boldsymbol{\Sigma}_i$ has 21 free parameters, which may overfit the usually small training dataset. For DTI, it is suggested in [5] to constrain $\boldsymbol{\Sigma}_i$ to be orthogonally invariant, imposing the following structure that depends only on $\sigma_i$ and $\tau_i$:

$$\boldsymbol{\Sigma}_i = \sigma_i^2 \begin{pmatrix} I_3 + \frac{\tau_i}{1 - 3\tau_i} \mathbb{1}_3 & \mathbf{0} \\ \mathbf{0} & I_3 \end{pmatrix} \triangleq B(\sigma_i, \tau_i).$$

This structure yields a closed-form solution for the maximum likelihood [5]:

$$\hat{M}_i = \bar{L}_i = \frac{1}{m_i} \sum_{k=1}^{m_i} L_i^k \text{ and } \hat{\Sigma}_i = B(\hat{\sigma}_i, \hat{\tau}_i), \tag{10}$$

$$\text{with } \hat{\tau}_i = \frac{-\sum_{i=1}^{m_i} \|L_i^k - \bar{L}_i\|_2^2}{5 \sum_{i=1}^{m_i} \left[ \text{Tr}(L_i^k - \bar{L}_i) \right]^2} \text{ and } \hat{\sigma}_i^2 = \frac{1}{6m_i} \sum_{i=1}^{m_i} \|L_i^k - \bar{L}_i\|_{\hat{\tau}_i}^2, \tag{11}$$

where $\|.\|_t^2$ is defined by $\langle A, B \rangle_t = \text{Tr}(AB) - t\,\text{Tr}(A)\text{Tr}(B)$. The ML estimator may be unreliable for compartments with only a few observations. This uncertainty is accounted for by replacing point estimates of $\boldsymbol{\theta}$ by posterior distributions and integrating over all possible $\boldsymbol{\theta}$. This yields the *posterior predictive distribution* (PPD) which contains all the knowledge about new observations that we learn from previous observations. Its derivation requires the definition of hyperpriors over $\boldsymbol{\theta}$ and is closed-form if we select conjugate hyperpriors.

$\mathbf{M}_i \sim \mathcal{N}(\mathbf{M}_0, \mathbf{\Lambda}_0)$ is a conjugate hyperprior for the tensor part of (7) assuming a deterministic $\mathbf{\Sigma}_i = \hat{\mathbf{\Sigma}}_i$. We set $\mathbf{\Lambda}_0 = \mathbf{B}(1, 0)$ and $\mathbf{M}_0 = \log \mathbf{D}_{\text{iso}}$ to keep it weakly informative (this hyperprior merely encodes the order of magnitude of diffusivity at $37°C$). The PPD over the tensors is $\mathbf{D}_i | \mathcal{D}_i \sim \mathcal{N}(\mathbf{M}_i^{m_i}, \mathbf{\Lambda}_i^{m_i})$ with

$$\mathbf{\Lambda}_i^{m_i} = \hat{\mathbf{\Sigma}}_i + \left(\mathbf{\Lambda}_0^{-1} + m_i \hat{\mathbf{\Sigma}}_i^{-1}\right)^{-1} \triangleq \mathbf{B}(\tilde{\sigma}_i, \tilde{\tau}_i), \tag{12}$$

$$\text{and } \mathbf{M}_i^{m_i} = \left(\mathbf{\Lambda}_0^{-1} + m_i \hat{\mathbf{\Sigma}}_i^{-1}\right)^{-1} \left(\mathbf{\Lambda}_0^{-1} \mathbf{M}_0 + m_i \hat{\mathbf{\Sigma}}_i^{-1} \bar{L}_i\right). \tag{13}$$

For the parameters $\alpha_i$, a conjugate hyperprior is the Dirichlet distribution. We set all its parameters to 1, making it uniform over the simplex $\mathcal{S}$. The resulting PPD is a Dirichlet with parameters $1 + \sum_{k=1}^{m_i} f_i^k$. In this expression, we consider $f_i^k$ as frequency counts since they are samples of $\mathsf{f}_i$ rather than samples from a multinomial parameterized by $f_i$. The complete PPD is (with $C_{\mathcal{F},\mathcal{D}}$ constant):

$$P_{\mathsf{f},\mathsf{D}}(\boldsymbol{f}, \boldsymbol{D} | \mathcal{F}, \mathcal{D}) = C_{\mathcal{F},\mathcal{D}} \mathbb{1}_{\boldsymbol{f} \in \mathcal{S}} \prod_{i=1}^{N} f_i^{\sum_{k=1}^{m_i} f_i^k} \prod_{i=1}^{N} \exp\left\{-\frac{\|L_i - M_i^{m_i}\|_{\tilde{\tau}_i}^2}{2\tilde{\sigma}_i^2}\right\}. \tag{14}$$

We incorporate this PPD as a prior in the estimation. We assume Gaussian noise on the DWI measurements $y_k$ since they are acquired on a single shell typically at $b=1000$ for which noise is approximately Gaussian. The maximum a posteriori estimator at each voxel amounts to maximizing the following for $\boldsymbol{f}$ and $\boldsymbol{D}$:

$$L = \log(\mathbb{1}_{\boldsymbol{f} \in \mathcal{S}}) + \sum_{i=1}^{N} \sum_{k=1}^{m_i} f_i^k f_i - \sum_{i=1}^{N} \frac{\|L_i - M_i^{m_i}\|_{\tilde{\tau}_i}^2}{2\tilde{\sigma}_i^2} - \sum_{k=1}^{K} \frac{(S_k(\boldsymbol{f}, \boldsymbol{D}) - y_k)^2}{2\sigma_k^2}. \tag{15}$$

The influence of the noise $\sigma_k^2$ is analyzed in the next section. In practice, the prior is built from data acquired in completely different subjects at several b-values. All these subjects are registered to a multi-fascicle atlas as in [7]. Following alignment, tensors from all subjects at each voxel are clustered in $N$ compartments as in [6]. Each cluster represents the sets $\mathcal{F}_i$ and $\mathcal{D}_i$ of available observations. The prior is then aligned with an initial estimate (without prior) of the multi-fascicle model. To evaluate (14), all assignments of compartments to tensors are considered and the highest prior value is recorded. BOBYQA algorithm is used to maximize (15) and the number of fascicles is estimated by an F-test as in [3].

## 4    Results

We compare the models estimated by our method to a ground truth $\{g_i, \boldsymbol{G}_i\}$ with five root mean square metrics, $\Delta_{\text{FA}}, \Delta_{\text{MD}}, \text{Fro}, \Delta_{\text{F}}$ and $\Delta_{\text{iso}}$ defined by:

$$\Delta_{\text{FA}}^2 = \sum_{i=1}^{N} \frac{f_i + g_i}{2} (\text{FA}(\boldsymbol{F}_i) - \text{FA}(\boldsymbol{G}_i))^2, \quad \Delta_{\text{MD}}^2 = \sum_{i=1}^{N} \frac{f_i + g_i}{2} (\text{MD}(\boldsymbol{F}_i) - \text{MD}(\boldsymbol{G}_i))^2$$

$$\text{Fro}^2 = \sum_{i=1}^{N} \frac{f_i + g_i}{2} \|\boldsymbol{D}_i - \boldsymbol{G}_i\|_F, \quad \Delta_{\text{F}}^2 = \sum_{i=1}^{N} (f_i - g_i)^2 \quad \text{and} \quad \Delta_{\text{iso}}^2 = (f_{\text{iso}} - g_{\text{iso}})^2.$$

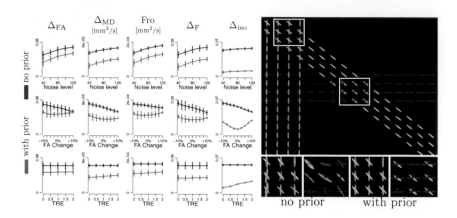

**Fig. 2.** (Left) Incorporating the prior in the estimation significantly improves the accuracy of the estimated model under the three simulated scenarios and for all five comparison metrics (distributions are shown for 20 datasets simulated for each set of parameters).(Right) The better accuracy mostly affects the diffusion properties of tensors (other than their directions), as predicted by Equation (3).

**Synthetic Phantom Experiment.** DWI were simulated under Rician noise from a phantom containing an isotropic compartment and 0 to 3 tensors of various properties with $S_0$=400. The prior was built from 20 datasets of 90 DWI at $b$=1000, 2000 and 3000. The accuracy was evaluated with 20 datasets of 30 DWI at $b$=1000 in three scenarios. First, the noise variance increased from 40 to 120. Second, the FA of the phantom was offset by $-10\%$ to $+10\%$ without changing the prior to simulate patient's data with a prior built from healthy subjects. Third, random deformations of 0 to 2 voxels were applied to the prior to simulate registration errors. In the last two scenarios, the noise variance was 80. In all scenarios and for all metrics, incorporating the prior significantly improved the accuracy of the estimation (one-tail paired t-test: $p < 10^{-6}$) (Fig. 2)

***In Vivo* Data Experiment.** Eighteen healthy subjects and 10 subjects with autism were imaged to test the method and an extra 13 healthy subjects were imaged to build the prior. For all subjects, DWI at resolution $1.7 \times 1.7 \times 2$mm$^3$ were acquired with a Siemens 3T Trio with a 32 channel head coil using the CUSP-45 sequence [3]. This includes 30 gradients on a single-shell at $b = 1000$ and 15 gradients with b-values up to 3000. For each test subject, all 45 DWI were first used to estimate a multi-fascicle model considered as a ground truth. Estimations using the single-shell subset only were then compared to it. Four strategies were compared: estimation without prior, estimation by fixing all tensors to a globally optimized value, and estimation with the prior assuming a noise level $\sigma_k^2$ of 20 and 500. Results in Fig. 3 show that estimations which incorporate a prior outperform other strategies. Estimations with $\sigma_k^2 = 500$ are significantly better than estimations without prior for all metrics and, remarkably, for both healthy controls and ASD patients (one-tail paired t-test: $p < 10^{-6}$). The true

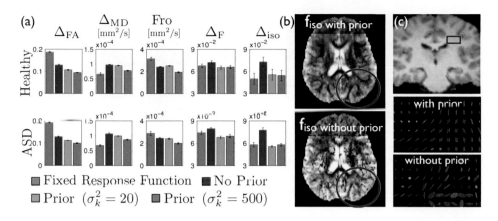

**Fig. 3.** (a) Incorporating prior knowledge significantly improves the quality of the model estimation for all five metrics and for both healthy controls and ASD patients. This improvement implies that (b) the extracellular water fraction can be visualized with more contrast and less noise in smaller details of the white matter up to its boundary with the grey matter, and (c) properties of the fascicles in crossing areas (shown is the corona radiata) are better represented and do not suffer the arbitrary choice of a model from Equation (3).

noise level of DWI is arguably closer to 500 than 20. However, estimations with $\sigma_k^2 = 20$ remain more accurate than estimations without prior, indicating that the population-informed prior improves the model accuracy even for crude estimates of the noise level. Empirical estimates of this noise level is kept for future work. Finally, fixing the fascicle response results in accuracies that strongly vary among quality metrics and, furthermore, only provides average information about the brain microstructure, which is not suitable in most studies.

**Application to Population Studies.** One could be concerned that the improved accuracy brought by the prior would come with a severe shrinkage of the estimated parameters towards the mean of the population. This would prevent its use in population studies. To address this concern, we conducted two population studies of autism spectrum disorder (ASD) using the proposed estimator. The first one focused on fascicle properties in the left arcuate fasciculus by analyzing the FA along the median tract. The second study investigated whether an increased extracellular volume fraction $f_{\mathrm{iso}}$ is observed in ASD. Less restricted diffusion may be related to the presence of edema, thinner axons, and neuroinflammation [1]. The latter has been proposed as a possible cause of autism. Corrections for multiple comparisons were based on cluster-size statistics in 1000 permutations with a threshold on t-scores of 3. As presented in Fig. 4, the first study revealed decreased FA integrity in the arcuate fasciculus of patients with ASD, in line with most recent studies of autism. The second study revealed one clusters of significantly increased unrestricted diffusion (permutation test: $p < 0.003$). Without the prior, none of these findings were observed ($p > 0.1$).

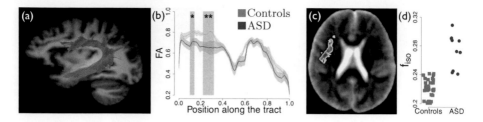

**Fig. 4.** The population-informed prior enables population studies of multi-fascicle models from single-shell HARDI data. (a-b) The first study reveals significantly decreased FA related to autism in the left arcuate fasciculus (*p<.05,**p<.01). (c-d) The second study reveals a cluster of significantly higher $f_{iso}$. (d) Average $f_{iso}$ in the cluster.

These studies show that the use of a prior in the estimation preserves contrasts of diffusion properties between groups, so that single-shell HARDI data can be used in large population studies based on multi-fascicle models.

## 5   Conclusion

Multi-fascicle models cannot be estimated from conventional single-shell HARDI data because a manifold of models produce the same diffusion signals. However, we showed that a posterior predictive distribution over the model parameters can be learnt from data acquired at several b-values in an external population. By incorporating this population-informed prior in the maximum a posteriori estimator of the parameters, we are able to estimate accurate multi-fascicle models from data at a single b-value. This method thus opens new opportunities for population studies with the large number of available clinical diffusion images.

## References

1. Pasternak, O., Shenton, M.E., Westin, C.-F.: Estimation of extracellular volume from regularized multi-shell diffusion MRI. In: Ayache, N., Delingette, H., Golland, P., Mori, K. (eds.) MICCAI 2012, Part II. LNCS, vol. 7511, pp. 305–312. Springer, Heidelberg (2012)
2. Pasternak, O., Sochen, N., Gur, Y., Intrator, N., Assaf, Y.: Free water elimination and mapping from diffusion MRI. Magnet. Reson. Med. 62(3), 717–730 (2009)
3. Scherrer, B., Warfield, S.K.: Parametric representation of multiple white matter fascicles from cube and sphere diffusion MRI. PLoS one 7(11) e48232 (2012)
4. Schultz, T., Westin, C.-F., Kindlmann, G.: Multi-diffusion-tensor fitting via spherical deconvolution: a unifying framework. In: Jiang, T., Navab, N., Pluim, J.P.W., Viergever, M.A. (eds.) MICCAI 2010, Part I. LNCS, vol. 6361, pp. 674–681. Springer, Heidelberg (2010)
5. Schwartzman, A., Mascarenhas, W.F., Taylor, J.E.: Inference for eigenvalues and eigenvectors of gaussian symmetric matrices. Ann. Stat., 2886–2919 (2008)
6. Taquet, M., Scherrer, B., Benjamin, C., Prabhu, S., Macq, B., Warfield, S.: Interpolating multi-fiber models by gaussian mixture simplification. In: IEEE ISBI, pp. 928–931 (2012)
7. Taquet, M., Scherrer, B., Commowick, O., Peters, J., Sahin, M., Macq, B., Warfield, S.K.: Registration and analysis of white matter group differences with a multi-fiber model. In: Ayache, N., Delingette, H., Golland, P., Mori, K. (eds.) MICCAI 2012, Part III. LNCS, vol. 7512, pp. 313–320. Springer, Heidelberg (2012)

# Integration of Sparse Multi-modality Representation and Geometrical Constraint for Isointense Infant Brain Segmentation

Li Wang[1], Feng Shi[1], Gang Li[1], Weili Lin[1], John H. Gilmore[2], and Dinggang Shen[1]

[1] Department of Radiology and BRIC, University of North Carolina at Chapel Hill, NC, USA
[2] Department of Psychiatry, University of North Carolina at Chapel Hill, NC, USA

**Abstract.** Segmentation of infant brain MR images is challenging due to insufficient image quality, severe partial volume effect, and ongoing maturation and myelination process. During the first year of life, the signal contrast between white matter (WM) and gray matter (GM) in MR images undergoes inverse changes. In particular, the inversion of WM/GM signal contrast appears around 6-8 months of age, where brain tissues appear isointense and hence exhibit extremely low tissue contrast, posing significant challenges for automated segmentation. In this paper, we propose a novel segmentation method to address the above-mentioned challenge based on the sparse representation of the complementary tissue distribution information from T1, T2 and diffusion-weighted images. Specifically, we first derive an initial segmentation from a library of aligned multi-modality images with ground-truth segmentations by using sparse representation in a patch-based fashion. The segmentation is further refined by the integration of the geometrical constraint information. The proposed method was evaluated on 22 6-month-old training subjects using leave-one-out cross-validation, as well as 10 additional infant testing subjects, showing superior results in comparison to other state-of-the-art methods.

## 1 Introduction

The first year of life is the most dynamic phase of the postnatal human brain development, with the rapid tissue growth and development of a wide range of cognitive and motor functions. Accurate tissue segmentation of infant brain MR images into white matter (WM), gray matter (GM) and cerebrospinal fluid (CSF) in this stage is of great importance in studying the normal and abnormal early brain development. It is well-known that segmentation of infant brain MRI is considerably more difficult than that of the adult, due to the reduced tissue contrast [1], increased noise, severe partial volume effect [2], and ongoing WM myelination [1, 3] in the infant images. Actually, there are three distinct stages in the first year brain MR images, with each stage having quite different white-gray matter contrast patterns (in chronological order) [4]: (1) the infantile stage ($\leq$ 5 months), in which the GM shows a higher signal intensity than the WM in T1 images; (2) the isointense stage (6-12 months), in which the signal intensity of the WM is increasing during the development due to the myelination and

K. Mori et al. (Eds.): MICCAI 2013, Part I, LNCS 8149, pp. 703–710, 2013.

maturation process; in this stage, the GM has the lowest signal differentiation with the WM in both T1 and T2 images; (3) the early adult-like stage (>12 months), where the GM intensity is much lower than that of the WM in T1 images, and this pattern is similar with that of the adult MR images. As an illustration, the first two images in the first row of Fig. 1 show examples of T1 and T2 images around 6 months. It can be observed that the WM and GM exhibit almost the same intensity level (especially in the cortical regions), resulting in the lowest image contrast and hence significant difficulties for tissue segmentation.

Although many methods have been proposed for infant brain image segmentation, most of them focused either on segmentation of the neonatal images (<= 3 months) or infant images (>12 months) using a single T1 or T2 modality [2, 3, 5, 6], which demonstrates a relatively good contrast between the WM and GM. Few studies have addressed the difficulties in segmentation of the isointense infant images. Shi et al. [7] first proposed a 4D joint registration and segmentation framework for the segmentation of infant MR images in the first year of life. In this method, longitudinal images in both infantile and early adult-like stages were used to guide the segmentation of images in the isointense stage. A similar strategy was later adopted in [8]. The major limitation of these methods is that they fully depend on the availability of longitudinal datasets [9]. Due to the fact that the majority of infant images are single time-point, a standalone method working for cross-sectional single-time point image is mostly desired. Kim et al. [9] proposed an adaptive prior and spatial temporal intensity change estimation to overcome the low contrast. However, their work was only evaluated on the images acquired around 12 months. Moreover, none of these methods takes advantages from the geometrical information that the WM/GM and GM/CSF surfaces should be free of geometrical defects. For example, WM surfaces obtained by these methods are normally discontinuous, corrupted by holes (or handles, which are topologically equivalent) and "sharp breaks" in cortical gyri, which could be improved by imposing the geometrical constraint [10].

Motivated by the fact that many classes of signals, such as audio and images, have naturally sparse representations with respect to each other, sparse representation has been widely and successfully used in many fields, i.e., for visual tracking, compressive sensing, image de-noising, and face recognition [11, 12]. In this paper, we propose to employ the sparse representation technique for effective utilization of multi-modality information to address the isointense infant brain segmentation. Multimodality information comes from T1, T2 and fractional anisotropy (FA) images (the first row of Fig. 1), which provide rich information of major WM bundles [13], to deal with the problem of insufficient tissue contrast [4]. Specifically, we first construct a library consisting of a set of multi-modality images from the training subjects and their corresponding ground-truth segmentations. Then we employ a patch-based method [14] to represent each patch of the testing multi-modality images by using a sparse set of library patches. The initial segmentation is thus obtained based on the majority label of library patches. By utilizing the geometrical constraint, the initial segmentation will be iteratively refined with further consideration of the patch similarities between the segmented testing image and the ground-truth segmentation in the library images.

# 2     Method

This study has been proved by institute IRB and the written informed consent forms were obtained from parents. A total of 22 healthy infant subjects (12 males/10 females) were recruited, and scanned at 27±0.9 postnatal weeks. T1, T2 and FA images were acquired for each subject. T2 and FA images were then linearly aligned onto their corresponding T1 images. Image preprocessing includes resampling to 1×1×1 mm$^3$, bias correction, skull stripping, and cerebellum removal. To generate the ground truth segmentation, we took a practical approach by first generating an initial segmentation using a publicly available software iBEAT (www.nitrc.org/projects/ibeat). Manual editing was then performed by experienced raters to correct segmentation errors and geometric defects by using ITK-SNAP (www.itksnap.org) with the help of surface rendering, e.g., filling the holes.

## 2.1     Deriving Initial Segmentation from the Library by Sparse Representation

To segment a testing image $I = \{I_{T1}, I_{T2}, I_{FA}\}$, $N$ template images $I^i = \{I_{T1}^i, I_{T2}^i, I_{FA}^i\}$ and their corresponding segmentation maps $L^i$ $(i = 1, \cdots, N)$ are first nonlinearly aligned onto the space of the testing image using Diffeomorphic Demons [15], based on T1 images. Then, for each voxel $x$ in each modality image of the testing image $I$, its intensity patch (taken from $w \times w \times w$ neighborhood) can be represented as a $w \times w \times w$ dimensional column vector. By taking the T1 image as an example, the T1 intensity patch can be denoted as $\boldsymbol{m}_{T1}(x)$. Furthermore, its patch dictionary can be adaptively built from all $N$ aligned templates as follows. First, let $\mathcal{N}^i(x)$ be the neighborhood of voxel $x$ in the $i$-th template image $I_{T1}^i$, with the neighborhood size as $w_p \times w_p \times w_p$. Then, for each voxel $y \in \mathcal{N}^i(x)$, we can obtain its corresponding patch from the $i$-th template, i.e., a $w \times w \times w$ dimensional column vector $\boldsymbol{m}_{T1}^i(y)$. By gathering all these patches from $w_p \times w_p \times w_p$ neighborhoods of all $N$ aligned templates, we can build a dictionary matrix $\boldsymbol{D}_{T1}$, where each patch is represented by a column vector. In the same manner, we can also extract T2 intensity patch $\boldsymbol{m}_{T2}(x)$ and FA intensity patch $\boldsymbol{m}_{FA}(x)$ and further build their respective dictionary matrices $\boldsymbol{D}_{T2}$ and $\boldsymbol{D}_{FA}$. Let $M(x) = [\boldsymbol{m}_{T1}(x); \boldsymbol{m}_{T2}(x); \boldsymbol{m}_{FA}(x)]$ be the testing multi-modality patch and $M^i(y) = [\boldsymbol{m}_{T1}^i(y); \boldsymbol{m}_{T2}^i(y); \boldsymbol{m}_{FA}^i(y)]$ be the template multi-modality patch in the dictionary. To represent the patch $M(x)$ by the dictionaries $\boldsymbol{D}_{T1}$, $\boldsymbol{D}_{T2}$ and $\boldsymbol{D}_{FA}$, its coefficients vector $\boldsymbol{\alpha}$ could be estimated by many coding schemes, such as sparse coding [11, 16] and locality-constrained linear coding [17]. Here, we employ sparse coding scheme [11, 16], which is robust to the noise and outlier, to estimate the coefficient vector $\boldsymbol{\alpha}$ by minimizing a non-negative Elastic-Net problem [18] ,

$$\min_{\alpha \geq 0} \sum_k \|D_k \alpha - \boldsymbol{m}_k(x)\|_2^2 + \lambda_1 \|\alpha\|_1 + \lambda_2 \|\alpha\|_2^2 \qquad (1)$$

where $k \in \{T1, T2, FA\}$. In the above Elastic-Net problem, the first term is the data fitting term based on the intensity patch similarity, and the second term is the $\ell1$ regularization term which is used to enforce the sparsity constraint on the reconstruction coefficients $\alpha$, and the last term is the $\ell 2$ smoothness term to enforce the coefficients to be similar for the similar patches. Each element of the sparse coefficient vector $\alpha$, i.e., $\alpha^i(y)$, reflects the similarity between the target patch $M(x)$ and the patch $M^i(y)$ in the patch dictionary. Based on the assumption that similar patches should share similar labels, we use the sparse coefficients $\alpha$ to estimate the probability belonging to the $j$-th tissue, i.e., $P_j(x) = \sum_i \sum_{y \in N^i(x)} \alpha^i(y) \delta_j(L^i(y))$, where $L^i(y)$ is the segmentation label (WM, GM, or CSF) for voxel $y$ in the $i$-th template image, and $\delta_j(L^i(y))=1$ if

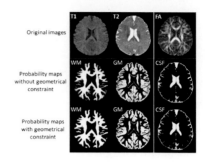

**Fig. 1.** Tissue probability maps estimated by the proposed method without and with the geometrical constraint

$L^i(y) = j$; otherwise $\delta_j(L^i(y)) = 0$. Finally, $P_j(x)$ is normalized to ensure $\sum_j P_j(x) = 1$. The second row of Fig. 1 shows an example of the estimated probability maps for a testing image, with the original T1, T2 and FA images shown in the first row. To convert from the soft probability map to the hard segmentation, the label of the voxel $x$ is determined using the *maximum a posteriori* (MAP) rule.

## 2.2    Imposing Geometrical Constraints into the Segmentation

The tissue probability maps derived in the Section 2.2 are purely based on the intensity patch similarity using the sparse representation technique. However, due to the low tissue contrast, the reliability of the patch similarity could be limited, which may result in considerable artificial geometrical errors in the tissue probability maps. A typical example is shown in Fig. 4(a), where we can observe many undesired holes (green rectangles), incorrect connections (red rectangles), and inaccurate segmentations (blue rectangles). In this section, we further address these problems by considering the geometrical constraint. As ground-truth segmentation results of template images in the library are almost free of the geometrical errors, we could expect the combination of these segmentation results will largely reduce the possible geometrical errors. Specifically, we can extract the patch $m_{seg}(x)$ from the tentative segmentation result of the testing image and also construct the segmentation patch dictionary $D_{seg}$ from all the aligned segmented images in the library. Based on Eq. (1), we further incorporate the geometrical constraint to derive the tissue probability maps:

$$\min_{\alpha \geq 0} \sum_k \|D_k \alpha - m_k(x)\|_2^2 + v\|D_{seg}\alpha - m_{seg}(x)\|_2^2 + \lambda_1 \|\alpha\|_1 + \lambda_2 \|\alpha\|_2^2 \quad (2)$$

where $k \in \{T1, T2, FA\}$ and $v$ is the weight parameters. In the same way, we can use the derived sparse coefficient vector $\alpha$ to estimate new tissue probabilities, which will be iteratively refined by using Eq. (2) until converged. An example of the probabilities derived with the geometrical constraint is shown in the third row of Fig. 1. Compared with the probability maps without the geometrical constraint (the second row), the new probability maps are more accurate.

## 3    Experimental Results and Analysis

The parameters used in this paper were determined via cross validation on a set of training images. We finally chose the following parameters for all experiments below: the weight for $\ell 1$-norm term $\lambda_1 = 0.2$, the weight for $\ell 2$-norm term $\lambda_2 = 0.01$, the patch size $w = 5$, the neighborhood size $w_p = 5$, and the weight for the geometrical constraint term $v = 1$.

**Leave-One-Out Cross-Validation.** To evaluate the performance of the proposed method, we adopted the leave-one-out cross-validation. Fig. 2(a) demonstrates the segmentation results of different methods for one typical subject. We choose to compare with the coupled level sets (CLS) method [19] provided by publicly available software iBEAT, in which multi-modality images from T1, T2 and FA were also employed. We also make comparison with the majority voting (MV) and conventional patch-based (CPB) method [14]. There are 7 different combinations for three modalities. The following rows only show the results by the proposed method with three representative combinations of three modalities (Eq. (1)). The last row shows the result by the proposed method on multi-modality images with the geometrical constraint (Eq. (2)).   To better compare the results by different methods, the label differences compared with the ground-truth segmentation were also presented, which qualitatively demonstrate the advantage of the proposed method. We then quantitatively evaluate the performance of different methods by employing Dice ratio. The average Dice ratios of different methods on 22 subjects are shown Fig. 2(b). Besides the Dice ratio, we also measure the mean surface distance error between the generated WM/GM (GM/CSF) surfaces and the ground-truth surfaces, which are plotted in Fig. 2(b) and further demonstrate the accuracy of the proposed method. It is worth noting that any combination of these different modalities generally produce more accurate results than any single modality in terms of both Dice ratios and surface distance errors.

**Results on 10 New Testing Subjects with Manual Segmentations.** Instead of using the leave-one-out cross-validation fashion, we further validated our proposed method on 10 additional subjects, which were not included in the library. The manual segmentations by experts were referred to as our golden standard. The Dice ratios and surface distance errors on 10 subjects by different methods are shown in the Fig. 3, which again demonstrates the advantage of our proposed method.

**Importance of the Geometrical Constraint.** To further demonstrate the benefit of incorporating the geometrical constraint into the proposed method, we take the WM/GM surfaces as an example to compare the results by the proposed method without and with the geometrical constraint in Fig. 4. Fig. 4(a) shows the result without the geometrical constraint. It can be observed that there are many geometrical defects such as incorrect connections indicated by the red rectangle, inaccurate "zigzag" segmentations indicated by the blue rectangle and holes indicated by the green rectangle. The intermediate and final results by the geometrical constraint are shown in Fig. 4(b) and (c). It can be observed the incorrect connections and inaccurate "zigzag" segmentations are gradually corrected. Although the proposed method cannot guarantee the topological correctness of the final WM/GM (GM/CSF) surface, the topological errors are largely reduced. By referring to the ground-truth segmentation shown in Fig. 4(d), the result with the geometrical constraint is much more accurate and reasonable than the result without the geometrical constraint, which can also be demonstrated by the quantitative evaluation results with the Dice ratios and surface distance errors as shown in Fig. 2(b).

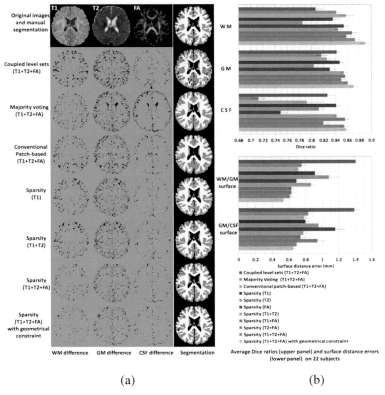

(a)                                                (b)

**Fig. 2.** (a) Comparison with the coupled level sets method [19], majority voting, conventional patch-based method [14] on T1+T2+FA images and the proposed sparsity method with different combinations of 3 modalities. In each label difference map, dark red colors indicate false negatives and the dark blue colors indicate false positives. (b) Average Dice ratios and surface distance errors on 22 subjects are shown in the right panel.

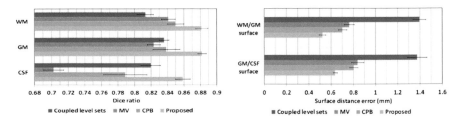

**Fig. 3.** The Dice ratios and surface distance errors on 10 subjects

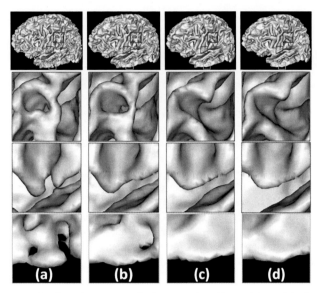

**Fig. 4.** Importance of using the geometrical constraint. From (a) to (c) shows the surface evolution from the initial stage to the final stage with the geometrical constraint. (d) is ground truth.

## 4    Discussion and Conclusion

In this paper, we have proposed a novel patch-based method for isointense infant brain MR image segmentation by utilizing the sparse multi-modality information. The segmentation is initially obtained based on the intensity patch similarity and then further refined with the geometrical constraint. The proposed method has been extensively evaluated on 22 training subjects using leave-one-out cross-validation, and also on 10 additional testing subjects. It is worth noting that our framework can also be directly applied to the segmentation of images in infantile and adult-like stages, for obtaining higher Dice ratios (compared with the isointense stage) due to their better contrast.

FA images provide rich information of major fiber bundles, especially in the subcortical regions where GM and WM are hardly distinguishable in the T1/T2 images. Therefore, FA images play a more important role in the WM/GM differentiation than GM/CSF differentiation, as demonstrated in Fig. 2.

In our experiment, we found that increasing the number of templates would generally improve the segmentation accuracy. However, more templates would also bring in more computational cost. In our test, when the number reached 20, the improvement rate of segmentation accuracies converged.

In our current method, the contributions of different modalities are equally weighted. In the future, we will further investigate to assign different weights to different modalities in different brain regions and validate on more datasets. In addition, our current library consists of only healthy subjects; therefore, it may not work well in pathological subjects. This will be our future work as well.

# References

1. Weisenfeld, N.I., Warfield, S.K.: Automatic segmentation of newborn brain MRI. Neuroimage 47, 564–572 (2009)
2. Xue, H., Srinivasan, L., Jiang, S., Rutherford, M., et al.: Automatic segmentation and reconstruction of the cortex from neonatal MRI. Neuroimage (2007)
3. Gui, L., Lisowski, R., Faundez, T., Hüppi, P.S., et al.: Morphology-driven automatic segmentation of MR images of the neonatal brain. Med. Image. Anal. 16, 1565–1579 (2012)
4. Paus, T., Collins, D.L., Evans, A.C., Leonard, G., et al.: Maturation of white matter in the human brain: a review of magnetic resonance studies. Brain Research Bulletin 54, 255–266 (2001)
5. Prastawa, M., Gilmore, J.H., Lin, W., Gerig, G.: Automatic segmentation of MR images of the developing newborn brain. Med. Image Anal. 9, 457–466 (2005)
6. Warfield, S.K., Kaus, M., Jolesz, F.A., Kikinis, R.: Adaptive, template moderated, spatially varying statistical classification. Med. Image Anal. 4, 43–55 (2000)
7. Shi, F., Yap, P.-T., Gilmore, J.H., Lin, W., et al.: Spatial-temporal constraint for segmentation of serial infant brain MR images. MIAR (2010)
8. Wang, L., Shi, F., Yap, P.-T., Gilmore, J.H., et al.: 4D Multi-Modality Tissue Segmentation of Serial Infant Images. PLoS ONE 7, e44596 (2012)
9. Kim, S.H., Fonov, V.S., Dietrich, C., Vachet, C., et al.: Adaptive prior probability and spatial temporal intensity change estimation for segmentation of the one-year-old human brain. Journal of Neuroscience Methods 212, 43–55 (2013)
10. Segonne, F., Pacheco, J., Fischl, B.: Geometrically Accurate Topology-Correction of Cortical Surfaces Using Nonseparating Loops. IEEE Trans. Med. Imaging 26, 518–529 (2007)
11. Wright, J., Yang, A.Y., Ganesh, A., Sastry, S.S., et al.: Robust Face Recognition via Sparse Representation. IEEE Trans. Pattern Anal. Mach. Intell. 31, 210–227 (2009)
12. Tong, T., Wolz, R., Hajnal, J.V., Rueckert, D.: Segmentation of brain MR images via sparse patch representation. In: MICCAI Workshop on Sparsity Techniques in Medical Imaging (STMI) (2012)
13. Liu, T., Li, H., Wong, K., Tarokh, A., et al.: Brain tissue segmentation based on DTI data. Neuroimage 38, 114–123 (2007)
14. Coupé, P., Manjón, J., Fonov, V., Pruessner, J., et al.: Patch-based segmentation using expert priors: Application to hippocampus and ventricle segmentation. Neuroimage 54, 940–954 (2011)
15. Vercauteren, T., Pennec, X., Perchant, A., Ayache, N.: Diffeomorphic demons: Efficient non-parametric image registration. Neuroimage 45, S61–S72 (2009)
16. Yang, J., Yu, K., Gong, Y., Huang, T.: Linear spatial pyramid matching using sparse coding for image classification. In: CVPR, pp. 1794–1801 (2009)
17. Wang, J., Yang, J., Yu, K., Lv, F., et al.: Locality-constrained Linear Coding for image classification. In: CVPR, pp. 3360–3367 (2010)
18. Zou, H., Hastie, T.: Regularization and variable selection via the Elastic Net. Journal of the Royal Statistical Society, Series B 67, 301–320 (2005)
19. Wang, L., Shi, F., Lin, W., Gilmore, J.H., et al.: Automatic segmentation of neonatal images using convex optimization and coupled level sets. Neuroimage 58, 805–817 (2011)

# Groupwise Segmentation with Multi-atlas Joint Label Fusion

Hongzhi Wang and Paul A. Yushkevich*

Department of Radiology, University of Pennsylvania

**Abstract.** Groupwise segmentation that simultaneously segments a set of images and ensures that the segmentations for the same structure of interest from different images are consistent usually can achieve better performance than segmenting each image independently. Our main contribution is that we adopt the groupwise segmentation framework to improve the performance of multi-atlas label fusion. We develop a novel statistical model to allow this extension. Comparing to previous atlas propagation and groupwise segmentation work, one key novelty of our method is that the error produced during label propagation is explicitly addressed in the joint label fusion framework. Experiments on hippocampus segmentation in magnetic resonance images show the effectiveness of the new groupwise segmentation technique.

## 1 Introduction

As a primary mechanism for quantifying the properties of anatomical structures and pathological formations from imaging data, image segmentation is an important task in medical image analysis. Typically, a segmentation algorithm is applied to segment one image at a time, i.e. segmenting one image is independent from segmenting other images. However, different segmentation tasks may not be independent, especially when images share common structures and similar appearances. When some images share similarities, one may expect that their segmentations should be related as well. By enforcing consistency in the segmentations produced for them, one may improve the robustness of automatic segmentation against random effects.

The idea of incorporating region coherence of same or similar objects across different images to reduce segmentation errors was initially addressed in the joint registration and segmentation framework, e.g. [2,7,10], motivated by the observation that image registration and image segmentation are highly correlated tasks. Improving one can help improve the other. By registering multiple images into a common space, appearance models of the same structure of interest from all images can be collected and re-enforced to ensure similar appearances for the segmented structures from different images. The estimated segmentations can then be used to improve registration such that segmentation alignments

---

* This work was supported by NIH awards AG037376, EB014346.

K. Mori et al. (Eds.): MICCAI 2013, Part I, LNCS 8149, pp. 711–718, 2013.

after registration are improved. With registrations between testing images, both appearance and shape consistencies can be enforced in groupwise segmentation.

Since the groupwise segmentation idea can be implemented with any non-groupwise segmentation algorithms, to directly improve upon the state of the art medical image segmentation techniques, we adopt the groupwise segmentation framework to improve the performance of multi-atlas label fusion (MALF). Through establishing one-to-one correspondence between a target image and a pre-labeled image, i.e. *atlas*, by image-based deformable registration, MALF transfers segmentation labels from the atlas to the target image and uses label fusion to combine solutions produced by different atlases. The highly competitive performance over many challenging applications, e.g. [5,13,15], show that the example-based knowledge representation and registration-based knowledge transfer model employed by MALF can produce highly accurate segmentation for medical applications.

Since pairwise or groupwise registration among testing images are often required in groupwise segmentation, it is a natural extension to apply techniques developed in MALF for groupwise segmentation. Our first contribution is to realize this extension through a novel statistical model for groupwise segmentation. Similar to the atlas propagation work [15] and the recent groupwise segmentation work [6], in our approach, each testing image and its estimated segmentation is applied as an additional atlas to help improve the segmentation accuracy for other testing images. However, when a testing image is applied as an atlas, due to the errors in producing its automatic segmentation, it is expected to be less reliable than the original atlases. Our second contribution is to extend the joint label fusion technique [14] to address this limitation. For validation, we apply our approach to segment the hippocampus from MRI and show significant performance improvements over MALF and other label propagation work.

## 2   Methods

Image segmentation can be addressed via estimating the conditional probability $p(T_S|T_F, \mathcal{D})$, where $T_F$ is the image to be segmented, $T_S$ is a segmentation for $T_F$ and $\mathcal{D}$ is the training data, which, for example, may include some images and their gold standard segmentations. The conditional probability can be estimated through various methods, e.g. discriminative learning or MALF.

In the MALF framework, $\mathcal{D}$ contains all atlases. The conditional probability is estimated in the form $p(l|x, T_F, \mathcal{D})$ through warping each atlas to the target image, followed by label fusion, where $l$ indexes through all labels and $x$ indexes through all voxels in $T_F$. This technique is described in detail below. With accurate conditional probabilities, the true segmentation can be estimated by $T_S(x) = \mathrm{argmax}_l p(l|x, T_F, \mathcal{D})$.

### 2.1   Multi-atlas Label Fusion

Since our work is based on MALF, we briefly describe the technique. Let $\mathcal{D} = \{A^1 = (A_F^1, A_S^1), ..., A^n = (A_F^n, A_S^n)\}$ be $n$ atlases, warped to the space of a target image by deformable registration. $A_F^i$ and $A_S^i$ denote the $i_{th}$ warped atlas image and manual segmentation.

One simple and powerful label fusion technique is weighted voting, where each atlas contributes to the final solution according to a weight. Among the weighted voting approaches, similarity-weighted voting strategies with spatially varying weight distributions have been particularly successful [1,13,14]. The consensus votes received by label $l$ are:

$$\hat{p}(l|x, T_F, \mathcal{D}) = \sum_{i-1}^{n} w_x^i p(l|x, A^i) \tag{1}$$

where $\hat{p}(l|x, T_F, \mathcal{D})$ is the estimated probability of label $l$ for the target image. $p(l|x, A^i)$ is the probability that $A^i$ votes for label $l$ at $x$, with $\sum_{l \in \{1,...,L\}} p(l|x, A^i) = 1$. Typically, for deterministic atlases that have one unique label for every location, $p(l|x, A^i)$ is 1 if $l = A_S^i(x)$ and 0 otherwise. $w_x^i$ is the voting weight for the $i_{th}$ atlas, with $\sum_{i=1}^{n} w_x^i = 1$.

To estimate voting weights, similarity metrics employed by image-based registration such as sum of squared distance and normalized cross correlation can be applied such that atlases with more similar appearance to the target image at location $x$ receives higher votes. One limitation of this approach is that the voting weights for each atlas is estimated independently from other atlases, ignoring potential correlations among the atlases. To address this problem, the joint label fusion algorithm estimates voting weights by simultaneously considering pairwise atlas correlations. As shown in [14], joint label fusion performed better than label fusion with independent weight estimation.

In the joint label fusion approach, segmentation errors produced by one atlas are modeled as $T_{S,l}(x) = A_{S,l}^i(x) + \delta^i(x)$. $T_{S,l}(x), A_{S,l}^i(x) \in \{0,1\}$ are the observed votes for label $l$ produced by the target image and the $i_{th}$ warped atlas, respectively. Hence, $\delta^i(x) \in \{-1, 0, 1\}$ is the observed label error. Note that both $T_{S,l}$ and $\delta^i(x)$ are unknown. The probability that different atlases produce the same label error at location $x$ are captured by a dependency matrix $M_x$, with $M_x(i,j) = p(\delta^i(x)\delta^j(x) = 1 \mid T_F, A_F^i, A_F^j)$ measuring the correlation between $i_{th}$ and $j_{th}$ atlases. In [14], the pairwise atlas correlation is estimated by appearance correlation as $M_x(i,j) \sim \left[\sum_{y \in \mathcal{N}(x)} |A_F^i(y) - T_F(y)||A_F^j(y) - T_F(y)|\right]^\beta$, where $\mathcal{N}(x)$ defines a neighborhood around $x$ and $\beta$ is a model parameter. The expected label difference between the combined solution and the target segmentation is:

$$E\left[(T_{S,l}(x) - \sum_{i=1}^{n} \mathbf{w}_x^i A_{S,l}^i(x))^2 \mid F_T, F_1, ..., F_n\right] = \mathbf{w}_x^t M_x \mathbf{w}_x \tag{2}$$

where $t$ stands for transpose. To minimize the expected label difference, the voting weights are solved by $\mathbf{w}_x = \frac{M_x^{-1} 1_n}{1_n^t M_x^{-1} 1_n}$, where $1_n = [1; 1; ...; 1]$ is a vector of size $n$.

## 2.2   Formulation for Groupwise Segmentation

Let $\mathcal{T}_F = \{T_F^1, ..., T_F^m\}$ be $m$ testing images to be segmented. Groupwise segmentation can be formulated as jointly segmenting all testing images using the training set $\mathcal{D}$ and can be solved via estimating the joint conditional probability $p(\mathcal{T}_S = \{T_S^1, ..., T_S^m\}|\mathcal{T}_F, \mathcal{D})$, where $T_S^1, ..., T_S^m$ are the estimated segmentations for $T_F^1, ..., T_F^m$, respectively. Since it is difficult to directly estimate the joint probability, we apply the pseudolikelihood approximation technique [3] and estimate the joint probability by: $p(\mathcal{T}_S|\mathcal{T}_F, \mathcal{D}) =$

$$\prod_{k=1}^{m} p(T_S^k|\mathcal{D}, \mathcal{T}_F, \mathcal{T}_S\backslash\{T_S^k\}) = \prod_{k=1}^{m} \prod_{x} p(l^k(x)|x, \mathcal{D}, \mathcal{T}_F, \mathcal{T}_S\backslash\{T_S^k\}) \qquad (3)$$

where $l^k(x) = \text{argmax}_l p(l|x, \mathcal{D}, \mathcal{T}_F, \mathcal{T}_S\backslash\{T_S^k\})$ is the estimated label for the $k_{th}$ testing image. In this model, we assume that the label probability for each voxel is conditionally independent given the images and segmentations in (3). Note that the segmentation of each testing image is estimated by both the original atlases and the remaining testing images. Hence, the correlations between testing images are explicitly considered to make their solutions compatible.

Like the pseudolikelihood approach, the segmentations for all testing images are computed through iterative estimation. First, the segmentation of each testing image is independently estimated with MALF only using the atlases. In each of the following iterations, the estimated segmentation for each testing image is updated one at a time to maximize the joint probability (3). Using weighted voting based label fusion, we estimate the label probability for one testing image $T_F^k$ by:

$$p(l|x, \mathcal{D}, \mathcal{T}_F, \mathcal{T}_S\backslash\{T_S^k\}) = \sum_{i=1}^{n} \mathbf{w}^i A_{S,l}^i + \sum_{j=1,j\neq k}^{m} \mathbf{w}^{a^j} a_{S,l}^j \qquad (4)$$

where $a^j$ is the candidate segmentation produced by warping the segmentation produced for the $j_{th}$ testing image to $T_F^k$. $\mathbf{w}^{a^j}$ is the voting weight assigned to it, with $\sum_{i=1}^{n} \mathbf{w}^i + \sum_{j=1,j\neq k}^{m} \mathbf{w}^{a^j} = 1$. Note that, for a simpler notation, the parametrization by $x$ is implicit.

*Potential risk in using testing images as atlases.* Due to registration and label fusion errors, it is reasonable to expect that the segmentation produced for each testing image is less accurate than those of the original atlases. Hence, when applying a testing image as an atlas to segment other testing images, in addition to the errors produced by image-based deformable registration, segmentation errors produced for the testing image are also propagated to other testing images. This potential risk may result in overall less accurate candidate segmentations produced by warping a testing image than by directly warping an original atlas.

Image similarity based label fusion is effective for detecting and reducing segmentation errors caused by registration errors. However, it can not detect whether the atlas contains errors in its segmentation. To address the unreliability of using testing images as additional atlases, we propose a solution based on the following observation. If an atlas produces more segmentation errors than other atlases, it is expected that its voting weight should be smaller than other atlases in the optimal solution. We propose to incorporate such prior knowledge in similarity-based weighted voting for more robust label fusion. To this end, we explicitly control the contribution from testing images in (4). Following the joint label fusion technique, we estimate the label probability for each testing image by solving the following optimization problem:

$$E\left[(T_{S,l}^k - \sum_{i=1}^n \mathbf{w}^i A_{S,l}^i - \sum_{j=1,j\neq k}^m \mathbf{w}^{a^j} a_{S,l}^j)^2 \mid \mathcal{D}, \mathcal{T}_F\right] = [\mathbf{w}; \mathbf{w}^a]^t M[\mathbf{w}; \mathbf{w}^a]$$

$$\text{subject to } \sum_{i=1}^n \mathbf{w}^i = 1 - \lambda, \qquad \sum_{j=1,j\neq k}^m \mathbf{w}^{a^j} = \lambda \quad (5)$$

For segmenting one testing image, the contribution from the remaining testing images is controlled by the total weight assigned to them, $0 \leq \lambda < 1$. Typically, when the atlases cannot produce reliable segmentation, one may expect more contribution from testing images to regularize the results and vice versa.

Applying Lagrange multipliers, we can solve (5) in closed form by:

$$[\mathbf{w}; \mathbf{w}^a]^t = M^{-1} (\mu_c c + \mu_d d) \qquad (6)$$

where $c = [1; ...; 1; 0; ...; 0], d = [0; ...; 0; 1; ...; 1]$. Only the first $n$ entries in $c$ and the last $m-1$ entries in $d$ are non-zero. $\begin{bmatrix} \mu_c \\ \mu_d \end{bmatrix} = \begin{bmatrix} c^t M^{-1} c, \ c^t M^{-1} d \\ d^t M^{-1} c, \ d^t M^{-1} d \end{bmatrix}^{-1} [1-\lambda; \lambda]$.

## 3   Experiments

*Imaging data and Experiment setup.* Our study is conducted using 1.5 T baseline MR images from the Alzheimer's Disease Neuroimaging Initiative (ADNI). Among these images, 57 are normal controls, 84 are patients with mild cognitive impairment (MCI) and 41 are patients with AD. Manual segmentations of the hippocampus are provided by ADNI as well. For cross-validation evaluation, we randomly selected 10 images to be the training images, i.e. the atlases, and another 50 images for testing. The cross-validation experiment was repeated for five times. In each experiment, a different set of atlases and testing images were randomly selected. The results reported below are averaged over the five experiments. To examine the performance with respect to the number of atlases used for producing the initial segmentation, in each cross-validation experiment, we also tested with different numbers of atlases, varying from 1 to 10.

For label fusion, we applied a $5 \times 5 \times 5$ neighborhood for $\mathcal{N}$. In our experiments, we fixed $\beta = 2$ for computing the atlas correlation matrix, which is shown to be optimal in [14] for hippocampus segmentation. For groupwise segmentation, we fixed $\lambda = 0.5$. Hence, the expected contribution from each testing image is significantly smaller than the contribution from each atlas.

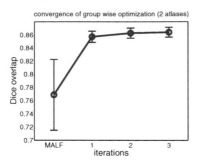
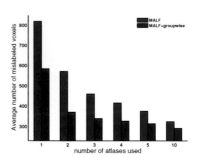

**Fig. 1.** Left: Segmentation accuracy (in terms of Dice similarity coefficient $\frac{2|A \cap B|}{|A|+|B|}$) of our groupwise segmentation algorithm at each iteration. The results are averaged over 5 cross-validation experiments. Error bar is at 0.25 standard deviation. The segmentation produced by MALF used two atlases; Right: Segmentation performance in terms of average number of mislabeled voxels per hippocampus.

*Results.* As shown in Fig. 1, our iterative optimization usually converges within a few iterations, with the first iteration producing the maximal performance improvement and dramatic diminishing performance gains in later iterations. In our experiment, we set the maximal iteration number to be 3. Fig. 1 also shows the performance produced by applying MALF alone and our groupwise segmentation method (MALF+groupwise). The results are shown in terms of average number of mislabeled voxels produced for each hippocampus. Fig. 2 shows some results produced by the two methods. As expected, the performance of MALF increases as the number of atlases increases. Our groupwise method produced consistently better results than applying MALF alone. The error reduction rates caused by groupwise segmentation vary from ~10% to ~30%.

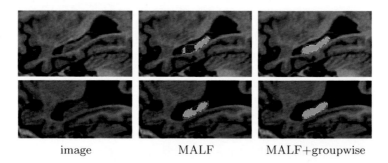

image                    MALF                MALF+groupwise

**Fig. 2.** Sagittal views of hippocampus segmentation. Red: manual segmentation; Blue: automatic segmentation; Green: overlap between manual and automatic segmentation

Fig. 3 (left) shows the Dice similarity coefficient (DSC)($\frac{2|A \cap B|}{|A|+|B|}$) for controls, patients with MCI and AD, respectively. When only one or two atlases were used by MALF to produce initial segmentations, the improvement by our groupwise method is about 10 % DSC. Our results using one atlas are better than

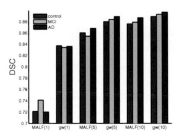 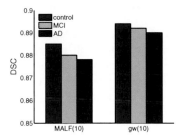

**Fig. 3.** Segmentation accuracy produced by using randomly selected atlases (left) and normal control atlases (right). The number of atlases used by MALF and our groupwise method (gw) is given in parentheses. Results are averaged over 5 cross validations.

the hippocampus segmentation results, ~0.76, reported in [12], which also performed groupwise segmentation using one training image. When 5 and 10 atlases were used, the improvements caused by our groupwise approach are >2% and >1% DSC, respectively. To further test the generalization performance, we also repeated 5 cross-validation experiments, each with randomly selected 10 normal controls as atlases and 50 randomly selected subjects as testing images. As shown in Fig. 3 (right), our groupwise segmentation method produced an average DSC of 0.892, 1 % improvement over applying MALF alone. All improvements are statistically significant, with $p<0.01$ on the paired Students t-test for each cross-validation experiment. Our results also compare well to the state-of-the-art hippocampus segmentation performance, as summarized in Table 1[1]. Overall, our results compare favorably over the state-of-the-art but we used many fewer atlases than the competing works.

**Table 1.** Hippocampus segmentation performance in the recent literature

| method : number of atlases used | Dice | JI | Tested Cohort |
|---|---|---|---|
| [13] : 38 atlases | 0.87 | - | normal control, AD |
| [4] : 79 atlases | 0.887 | - | normal control |
| [11]: 30 atlases | 0.880 | - | normal control |
| [8] : 55 atlases | | 0.80/0.81 | normal control/MCI |
| [15] : 30 atlases | <0.85 | - | normal control/MCI/AD |
| [14] : 20 atlases | 0.892 | - | normal control/MCI |
| [9] : 17 atlases | 0.870 | 0.771 | - |
| Our method : 10 atlases | 0.893 | 0.805 | normal control/MCI/AD |

---

[1] Due to the differences in the images and manual segmentations used in different studies, quantitative comparisons across different publications may not be fair.

# 4   Conclusions and Discussion

We extended the powerful MALF technique to perform groupwise segmentation and validated our method in a hippocampus segmentation task. One drawback of groupwise segmentation is the additional computational cost for registrations among the testing images. However, this added cost is justified by the performance gain. For applications, where manually labeled atlases are limited and testing images are abundant, this technique will be more suitable to be applied.

# References

1. Artaechevarria, X., Munoz-Barrutia, A., de Solorzano, C.O.: Combination strategies in multi-atlas image segmentation: Application to brain MR data. IEEE TMI 28(8), 1266–1277 (2009)
2. Bansal, R., Staib, L.H., Chen, Z., Rangarajan, A., Knisely, J.P.S., Nath, R., Duncan, J.S.: Entropy-based, multiple-portal-to-3D CT registration for prostate radiotherapy using iteratively estimated segmentation. In: Taylor, C., Colchester, A. (eds.) MICCAI 1999. LNCS, vol. 1679, pp. 567–578. Springer, Heidelberg (1999)
3. Besag, J.: Statistical analysis of non-lattice data. J. R. Statist. Soc. B 24(3), 179–195 (1975)
4. Collins, D., Pruessner, J.: Towards accurate, automatic segmentation of the hippocampus and amygdala from MRI by augmenting ANIMAL with a template library and label fusion. Neuroimage 52(4), 1355–1366 (2010)
5. Heckemann, R., Hajnal, J., Aljabar, P., Rueckert, D., Hammers, A.: Automatic anatomical brain MRI segmentation combining label propagation and decision fusion. Neuroimage 33, 115–126 (2006)
6. Jia, H., Yap, P., Shen, D.: Iterative multi-atlas-based multi-image segmentation with tree-based registration. Neuroimage 59(1), 422–430 (2012)
7. Kapur, T., Yezzi, L., Zollei, L.: A variational framework for joint segmentation and registration. In: IEEE CVPR - MMBIA, pp. 44–51 (2001)
8. Leung, K., Barnes, J., Ridgway, G., Bartlett, J., Clarkson, M., Macdonald, K., Schuff, N., Fox, N., Ourselin, S.: Automated cross-sectional and longitudinal hippocampal volume measurement in mild cognitive impairment and Alzheimer's Disease. Neuroimage 51, 1345–1359 (2010)
9. van der Lijn, F., de Bruijne, M., Klein, S., den Heijer, T., Hoogendam, Y.Y., van der Lugt, A., Breteler, M.M., Niessen, W.J.: Automated brain structure segmentation based on atlas registration and appearance models. IEEE Transactions on Medical Imaging 31(2), 276–286 (2012)
10. Lord, N.A., Ho, J., Vemuri, B.C.: Ussr: A unified framework for simultaneous smoothing, segmentation, and registration of multiple images. In: ICCV (2007)
11. Lotjonen, J., Wolz, R., Koikkalainen, J., Thurfjell, L., Waldemar, G., Soininen, H., Rueckert, D.: Fast and robust multi-atlas segmentation of brain magnetic resonance images. Neuroimage 49(3), 2352–2365 (2010)
12. Raviv, T.R., Leemput, K.V., Menze, B., Wells, W.M., Golland, P.: Joint segmentation of image ensembles via latent atlases. MedIA 14, 654–665 (2010)
13. Sabuncu, M., Yeo, B., Leemput, K.V., Fischl, B., Golland, P.: A generative model for image segmentation based on label fusion. IEEE TMI 29(10), 1714–1720 (2010)
14. Wang, H., Suh, J.W., Das, S., Pluta, J., Craige, C., Yushkevich, P.: Multi-atlas segmentation with joint label fusion. IEEE Trans. on PAMI 35(3), 611–623 (2013)
15. Wolz, R., Aljabar, P., Hajnal, J., Hammers, A., Rueckert, D.: Leap: Learning embeddings for atlas propagation. Neuroimage 49(2), 1316–1325 (2010)

# Higher-Order CRF Tumor Segmentation with Discriminant Manifold Potentials

Samuel Kadoury[1], Nadine Abi-Jaoudeh[2], and Pablo A. Valdes[3]

[1] MEDICAL, École Polytechnique de Montréal, Montréal, Canada
[2] Rad. and Imaging Sciences, National Institutes of Health, Bethesda, MD, USA
[3] Dartmouth College, Hanover, New Hampshire, USA

**Abstract.** The delineation of tumor boundaries in medical images is an essential task for the early detection, diagnosis and follow-up of cancer. However accurate segmentation remains challenging due to presence of noise, inhomogeneity and high appearance variability of malignant tissue. In this paper, we propose an automatic segmentation approach using fully-connected higher-order conditional random fields (HOCRF) where potentials are computed within a discriminant Grassmannian manifold. First, the framework learns within-class and between-class similarity distributions from a training set of images to discover the optimal manifold discrimination between normal and pathological tissues. Second, the conditional optimization scheme computes non-local pairwise as well as pattern-based higher-order potentials from the manifold subspace to recognize regions with similar labelings and incorporate global consistency in the inference process. Our HOCRF framework is applied in the context of metastatic liver tumor segmentation in CT images. Compared to state of the art methods, our method achieves better performance on a group of 30 liver tumors and can deal with highly pathological cases.

## 1 Introduction

Fast and accurate segmentation of tumors in medical images is an important yet challenging task in many clinical applications, such as radiotherapy or neurosurgery, where follow-up of the tumor size is done with predefined criterions to measure the progression. In various approaches, discrete Markov Random Fields (MRFs; [1]) and Conditional Random Fields (CRFs; [2]) were used to represent complex dependencies among data instances, giving them higher segmentation accuracy than independent and identically distributed (iid) classifiers such as Support Vector Machines (SVM). But despite significant intra- and inter-rater variabilities and the large time consumption of manual segmentation, very few of these automatic approaches are currently used in clinical practice.

State of the art tumor segmentation methods combine efficient classification techniques with low level segmentation methods. From such perspective, tumor detection is addressed as a classification problem where one aims at separating healthy from diseased tissues at the voxel level, while imposing smoothness in the process. In [3], SVM classification using multispectral intensities and

K. Mori et al. (Eds.): MICCAI 2013, Part I, LNCS 8149, pp. 719–726, 2013.
© Springer-Verlag Berlin Heidelberg 2013

textures is combined with hierarchical CRFs to segment brain tumors in MR images. In [4], a semi-automatic segmentation of liver tumors is presented using hidden Markov measure fields and non-parametric distribution estimation which are defined locally. Alternatively, allowing fully-connected pairwise models can increase expressivity over typical 4 or 8-connected MRF models. Still, the inability to handle higher-order terms is a disadvantage. Higher-order information was shown to enforce labelling consistency over homogeneous regions, as demonstrated with Pn-Potts models [5]. Co-occurrence relations between image classes have also been shown to provide important priors for segmentation [6].

A major drawback from these methods is that conditional probabilities are obtained directly from the high-dimensional image space, which is not ideal as they fail to express the underlying representation of the dataset and assimilates all measures to Euclidean distances [7]. They also assume linear discrimination (SVMs) when in most cases, sets are not linearly separable in the image space. In contrast, manifold learning techniques intrinsically consider the nonlinear distribution of the data, and allow relevant comparison of test cases to the learned population through the use of a mapping distance. Recently, various approaches have used manifolds to track organ motion or discover regional variations within images [8]. However, techniques such as Laplacian eigenmaps are sensitive to outliers and unable to cope with pathological or abnormal tissues. To the best of our knowledge, prior information captured by a discriminant embedding has yet to be exploited in a fully automatic CRF segmentation framework. We propose a segmentation approach for tumors using fully-connected higher-order conditional random field (HOCRF) which maximizes the full potential of high-level graphical models and manifold embeddings. Our contributions are two-fold. First, a discriminant graph-embedding with Grassmannian kernels is generated from prior data to learn the nonlinear intensity distributions of normal and diseased tissue. Second, we suggest to employ a recently proposed mean-field CRF inference approach where potentials are computed directly from the low-dimensional embedding, capturing the underlying structure. Unary and pairwise potentials assess the proximity to manifold regions and the dissimilarity between pairs of segments, respectively. Higher-order potentials ensure regional consistency to efficiently discriminate tumors from healthy tissue. We use the manifold constrained HOCRF segmentation method on metastatic liver tumors in CT images and show the potential of the approach on high-grade gliomas in MRI.

## 2   Learning the Discriminant Grassmannian Manifold

Manifold learning algorithms are based on the premise that data are often of artificially high dimension and can be embedded in a lower dimensional space. However the presence of outliers and multi-class information can adversely affect the discrimination and/or generalization ability of the manifold. We propose to first learn the optimal separation between normal and pathological tissue by using a discriminant graph-embedding based on Grassmannian manifolds in the segmentation process. Each sample point $x_i$ (pixel or segment) on a Grassmannian manifold can be viewed as the set of $m$-dimensional subspaces of $\mathbb{R}^D$ and represented by orthonormal matrices, each with a size of $D \times m$. Two points on a Grassmannian manifold are equivalent if one can be mapped into the other one by a $m \times m$ orthogonal matrix. In this work, similarity between two points $(x_i, x_j)$ on the manifold is measured as a combination of projection and canonical correlation Grassmannian kernels $\mathbb{K}_{i,j}$ defined in the Hilbert Space. With each kernel describing different features of the tumor and normal regions, $\mathbb{K}_{i,j}$ covers a wide spectrum of feature distributions and improves discriminatory accuracy.

In order to effectively discover the low-dimensional embedding, it is necessary to maintain the local structure of the data in the new embedding. The structure $G = (V, W)$ is an undirected similarity graph, with a collection of nodes $V$ connected by edges, and the symmetric matrix $W$ with elements describing the relationships between the nodes. The diagonal matrix $D$ and the Laplacian matrix $L$ are defined as $L = D - W$, with $D(i, i) = \sum_{j \neq i} W_{ij} \forall i$. Here, $N$ labelled points $\mathbb{X} = \{(x_i, c_i)\}_{i=1}^{N}$ are generated from the underlying manifold $\mathcal{M}$, where $c_i$ denotes the label (lesion or non-lesion). The task at hand is to maximize a measure of discriminatory power by mapping the underlying data into a vector space, while preserving similarities between data points in the high-dimensional space. Discriminant graph-embedding based on locally linear embedding (LLE) [7] uses graph-preserving criterions to maintain these similarities, which are included in a sparse and symmetric $N \times N$ matrix, denoted as $M$.

**Within and between Similarity Graphs:** In our work, the geometrical structure of $\mathcal{M}$ can be modeled by building a within-class similarity graph $W_w$ for tissues of same type and a between-class similarity graph $W_b$, to separate normal and tumor tissue. When constructing the discriminant LLE graph, elements are partitioned into $W_w$ and $W_b$ classes. The intrinsic graph $G$ is first created by assigning edges only to vertices of the same class (lesion or non-lesion). The local reconstruction coefficient matrix $M(i, j)$ is obtained by minimizing:

$$\min_{M} \sum_{j \in \mathcal{N}_w(i)} \|x_i - M(i, j)x_j\|^2 \quad \sum_{j \in \mathcal{N}_w(i)} M(i, j) = 1 \;\; \forall i \tag{1}$$

with $\mathcal{N}_w(i)$ as the neighborhood of size $k_1$, within the same region as point $i$ (e.g. tumor region). Each sample is therefore reconstructed only from images of the same region. The local reconstruction coefficients are incorporated in the within-class similarity graph, such that the matrix $W_w$ is defined as:

$$W_w(i, j) = \begin{cases} (M + M^T - M^T M)_{ij}, & \text{if } x_i \in \mathcal{N}_w(x_j) \text{ or } x_j \in \mathcal{N}_w(x_i) \\ 0, & \text{otherwise.} \end{cases} \tag{2}$$

Conversely, the between-class similarity matrix $W_b$ depicts the statistical properties to be avoided in the optimization process and used as a high-order constraint. Distances between healthy and pathological samples are computed as:

$$W_b(i, j) = \begin{cases} 1/k_2, & \text{if } x_i \in \mathcal{N}_b(x_j) \text{ or } x_j \in \mathcal{N}_b(x_i) \\ 0, & \text{otherwise} \end{cases} \tag{3}$$

with $\mathcal{N}_b$ containing $k_2$ neighbors having different class labels from the $i$th sample. The objective is to transform points to a new manifold $\mathcal{M}$ of dimensionality $d$, i.e. $x_i \rightarrow y_i$, by mapping connected healthy or tumor samples in $\boldsymbol{W}_w$ as close as possible to the class cluster, while moving tumor and healthy areas of $\boldsymbol{W}_b$ as far away from one another. This results in optimizing the objective functions:

$$f_1 = \min \frac{1}{2} \sum_{i,j} (y_i - y_j)^2 W_w(i,j) \qquad f_2 = \max \frac{1}{2} \sum_{i,j} (y_i - y_j)^2 W_b(i,j) \qquad (4)$$

**Supervised Manifold Learning:** The optimal projection matrix, mapping new points to the manifold, is obtained by simultaneously maximizing class separability and preserving interclass manifold property, as described by the objective functions in Eq.(4). Assuming points on the manifold are known as similarity measures given by the Grassmannian kernel $\mathbb{K}_{i,j}$, a linear solution can be defined, i.e., $y_i = (\langle \alpha_1, x_i \rangle, \dots, \langle \alpha_r, x_i \rangle)^T$ for the $r$ largest eigenvectors with $\alpha_i = \sum_{j=1}^N a_{ij} x_j$. Defining the coefficient $\boldsymbol{A}_l = (a_{l1}, \dots, a_{lN})^T$ and kernel $\boldsymbol{K}_i = (k_{i1}, \dots, k_{iN})^T$ vectors, the output can be described as $y_i = \langle \alpha_l, x_i \rangle = \boldsymbol{A}_l^T \boldsymbol{K}_i$. By replacing the linear solution in the minimization and maximization of the between- and within-class graphs, the optimal projection matrix $\mathbb{A}$ is acquired from the optimization of the function as proposed by Harandi [9]. The proposed algorithm uses the points on the Grassmannian manifold implicitly (i.e., via measuring similarities through a kernel) to obtain a mapping $\mathbb{A}$. The matrix maximizes a quotient similar to discriminant analysis, while retaining the overall geometrical structure. Hence for any test point $x_q$, a manifold representation $v_q = \mathbb{A}^T \boldsymbol{K}_q$ is obtained using the kernel function based on $x_q$ and mapping $\mathbb{A}$.

## 3   Fully-Connected Higher-Order CRF Segmentation

Once the Grassmannian manifolds are obtained from the training phase, the segmentation problem is performed on a higher-order CRF model where potentials of the energy function are inferred from the low-dimensional embeddings. Random variables $\mathcal{X}$ denotes whether labels belong to the object of interest (lesion or not), $\mathcal{E}$ denotes edges connecting pairs of nodes and $\mathcal{S}$ denotes the set of segments. The CRF model defines the energy function based on the sum of unary $\psi$ and pairwise potentials $\phi$, as well as higher-order functions $\theta$, minimized by:

$$E(\mathcal{C}|\mathcal{X}) = \sum_{v_i \in \mathcal{X}} \psi(c_i|v_i) + \sum_{(v_i,v_j) \in \mathcal{E}} \phi(c_i, c_j|v_i, v_j) + \sum_{s \in \mathcal{S}} \theta_s(c_s|\mathbf{v}_s) \qquad (5)$$

where $v_i$ denotes the manifold projection of data point $x_i$ and $c_i$ is the label (lesion or non-lesion) of node $v_i$. The nodes in the CRF model corresponds to the manifold embedded segments of $x_i$. Here, image segments $x_i$ are obtained by a normalized-cut segmentation method, followed by an iterative k-means clustering to create an image parcelled in equal-sized patches [10]. Then, segments are mapped using the projection matrix such that $v_i = \mathbb{A}^T \boldsymbol{K}_i$. Features are selected implicitly by the manifold from the low-dimensional space to obtain the best discrimination between the classes. Here, we employ a fully-connected CRF model using a mean-field approximation of the original CRF such that the distribution is composed of a set of independent marginals minimizing KL-divergence.

**Manifold-Based Potentials:** *Unary potentials* in the CRF model are defined based on the probability of the classifier $\psi(c_i|v_i) = -\log(P(c_i|v_i))$. *Pairwise potentials* are expressed as non-parametric manifold dissimilarities, extending the Gaussian kernel formulation in feature space which uses mean-field approximations of fully-connected CRF models [11]. Instead of forcing Euclidean features to fulfill this task, pairwise potentials are conditioned on the input data such that $\phi(v_i, v_j) = \mu(v_i, v_j)\exp(-\mathrm{d}(i, i, \mathcal{X}, \mathcal{M}))$, where $\mu$ is the label compatibility function between nodes $v_i$ and $v_j$. The distance between points $i$ and $j$, under label $l$, is the conditional distribution of the label $l$, with $\exp(-\mathrm{d}(i, i, \mathcal{X}, \mathcal{M})) = P(v_j = l|v_i = l, \mathcal{X}, \mathcal{M})$. Assuming the Frobenius distance $F$ in manifold space can offer a non-parametric estimation of the dissimilarity measure, the pairwise potential can be defined by imposing a range $\sigma_f$ over which valuable information can be inferred when applying a Gaussian window:

$$\phi(c_i, c_j|v_i, v_j) = w \exp\left(\frac{\|v_i - v_j\|_F^2}{2\sigma_f^2}\right) \tag{6}$$

with the parameter $w$ weighting the pairwise relations. Finally, quality sensitive *higher-order potentials* define the label inconsistency in regions (different labels are assigned to a set of neighboring segments) by adding edges between nodes that are not immediate neighbours. We use a strategy where for a given clique $\mathbf{v}_s$ grouping $t$ segments, $t$ different embeddings are generated with $\mathbb{A}$. We then use the variance of the embedded coordinates of $v_s$ for all $t$ data points, using it as a quality measure $G(s) : s \to \mathbb{R}$ for all consistent segments in $\mathbf{v}_s$. The higher-order potential is defined as:

$$\theta_s(\mathbf{v}_s) = \begin{cases} N(\mathbf{v}_s)\frac{1}{Q}\gamma_{\max} & \text{if } N(\mathbf{v}_s) \leq Q \\ \gamma_{\max} & \text{otherwise} \end{cases} \tag{7}$$

where $N(\mathbf{v}_s)$ is the number of segments in $\mathbf{v}_s$ not taking the dominant label, $\gamma_{\max}$ assigns the cost based on $G(s)$ and $Q$ is the truncation parameter. This potential avoids breaking a *good* segment and penalizes other *bad* segments.

**Energy Minimization:** The higher-order function is solved with $\alpha$-expansion and $\alpha\beta$-swap move making algorithms as proposed by Kholi [12]. In order to determine the optimal moves for the algorithm, higher-order move functions are minimized by transforming the function to quadratic submodular functions which add auxiliary binary variables. The solution corresponds to the energy minima yielding the optimal labeling at each segment, generating tumor and non-tumor segmentation. The optimal labeling of the HOCRF is recovered using Fast-PD based on linear programming.

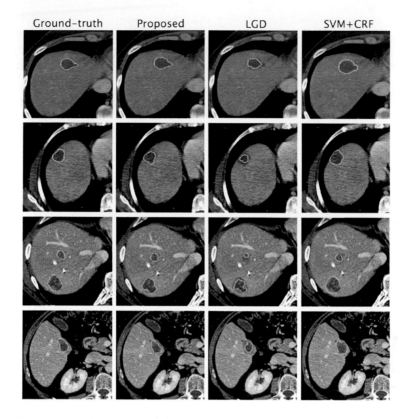

**Fig. 1.** Segmentation results of metastatic liver tumors in CT images

## 4    Experimental Validation

We validated our algorithm with the segmentation of metastatic liver tumors in CT images. Datasets from 30 liver tumors were acquired with a 64-slice CT scanner with 1mm slice thickness and in-plane resolution of 0.6mm. Tumors covered only metastasis pathologies. Contrast agent was administered in 12 cases. Tumors were manually segmented by an experimented radiologist and validated by another radiologist. The following measures were computed for each segmentation based on the 2008 liver tumor segmentation challenge: volumetric overlap error (%), average symmetric surface distance (mm), RMS symmetric surface distance (mm) and maximum symmetry surface distance (mm). The Grassmannian manifold was trained with 10 datasets and the optimal dimensionality was found at $d = 5$, when the trend of the nonlinear residual reconstruction error curve stabilized for the entire training set. Table 1 shows the performance of the method with 10 training and 20 test cases. Results were compared to an active contours approach with local Gaussian distributions [13] and to a texture classification method [3]. The average and RMS surface distances ($0.6 \pm 0.2$ and $1.4 \pm 0.2$mm) of the proposed method were significantly lower ($p \leq 0.05$) to

**Table 1.** Error metrics from the CT liver tumor segmentations. We present results using only unary and pairwise ($\psi+\phi$) and unary, pairwise higher-order terms ($\psi+\phi+\theta$).

| | Overlap error (%) | Vol. Diff. (%) | Avg. Surf. Dist. (mm) | RMS Surf. Dist. (mm) | Max. Surf. Dist. (mm) |
|---|---|---|---|---|---|
| LGD [13] | 28.2 ± 3.4 | 19.6 ± 5.3 | 1.4 ± 0.3 | 1.9 ± 0.7 | 8.1 ± 2.1 |
| SVM+CRF [3] | 26.4 ± 2.9 | 16.0 ± 4.5 | 1.1 ± 0.3 | 1.8 ± 0.5 | 7.8 ± 2.0 |
| HOCRF Training (n=10) | 2.1 ± 0.5 | 0.1 ± 0.1 | 0.1 ± 0.1 | 0.4 ± 0.2 | 1.1 ± 0.9 |
| HOCRF Test $\psi + \phi$ (n=20) | 18.5 ± 1.8 | 12.3 ± 2.9 | 0.8 ± 0.2 | 1.5 ± 0.3 | 6.6 ± 1.7 |
| HOCRF Test $\psi + \phi + \theta$ (n=20) | **16.2 ±1.6** | **9.8 ± 2.2** | **0.6 ± 0.2** | **1.4 ± 0.2** | **5.9 ± 1.4** |

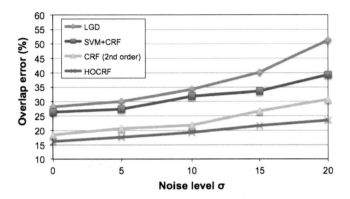

**Fig. 2.** Evolution of overlap error with increasing Gaussian noise levels added to images

distances generated by [13] and [3]. Typical problems occurred in the periphery of the tumors and in cases of rim-enhancing liver metastases. These cases offer a density which was not observed in the training set, but could be compensated with additional data in the manifold. Fig. 1 shows some segmentation results.

By assessing the gain in accuracy when adding the higher-order terms in the energy formulation, the overlap error is reduced by 2.3%, which is a statistically significant difference ($p \leq 0.05$) to the second-order MRF model. In order to evaluate the robustness of the method, we performed additional experiments by measuring segmentation accuracy with 4 different levels of Gaussian noise added to the input images. Fig. 2 demonstrates that the proposed methodology possesses increased tolerance to noise compared to the other methods.

## 5  Conclusion

We proposed a new, efficient and adaptable method for tumor segmentation. This was achieved through a higher-order fully-connected graphical model that was optimized using potential functions defined in a discriminant Grassmannian manifold. This increased the ability to isolate diseased from healthy tissue as compared to state of the art CRF or SVM techniques. Validation concerning

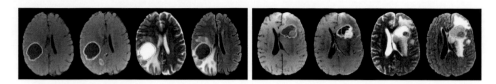

**Fig. 3.** Sample high-grade tumor segmentations in brain MRI for 2 glioma cases

the case of metastatic liver tumors was considered to evaluate the performance of the method, leading to very promising results. The approach can also be extended to other pathologies such as for example glioblastoma multiforme by segmenting high-grade gliomas in MRI. In this case, the manifold potentials could be trained to characterize different necrotic, active and edema regions in the tumor, and help to automatically discriminate between normal and diseased brain tissue. Preliminary segmentation results for high-grade glioma cases are shown in Fig. 3 . Encoding prior knowledge relating to shape representation is a natural extension of the proposed formulation. Future work will focus on a more extensive validation of the segmentation process for gliomas in brain MRI.

## References

1. Li, S.Z.: Markov Random Field Modeling in Image Analysis. Springer (2009)
2. Lafferty, J., Pereira, F., McCallum, A.: Conditional random fields: Probabilistic models for segmenting and labeling sequence data. In: ICML, pp. 282–289 (2001)
3. Bauer, S., Nolte, L.-P., Reyes, M.: Fully Automatic Segmentation of Brain Tumor Images Using Support Vector Machine Classification in Combination with Hierarchical Conditional Random Field Regularization. In: Fichtinger, G., Martel, A., Peters, T. (eds.) MICCAI 2011, Part III. LNCS, vol. 6893, pp. 354–361. Springer, Heidelberg (2011)
4. Hame, Y., Pollari, M.: Semi-automatic liver tumor segmentation with HMM field model and non-parametric distribution estimation. Med. I. Ana. 16, 140–149 (2012)
5. Sabuncu, M., Yeo, B., Leemput, K., et al.: A Generative Model for Image Segmentation Based on Label Fusion. IEEE Trans. Med. Imag. 29, 1714–1728 (2010)
6. Vineet, V., Warrell, J., Torr, P.H.S.: Filter-based mean-field inference for random fields with higher-order terms and product label-spaces. In: Fitzgibbon, A., Lazebnik, S., Perona, P., Sato, Y., Schmid, C. (eds.) ECCV 2012, Part V. LNCS, vol. 7576, pp. 31–44. Springer, Heidelberg (2012)
7. Roweis, S., Saul, L.: Nonlinear dimensionality reduction by locally linear embedding. Science 290, 2323–2326 (2000)
8. Bhatia, K.K., Rao, A., Price, A.N., Wolz, R., Hajnal, J., Rueckert, D.: Hierarchical manifold learning. In: Ayache, N., Delingette, H., Golland, P., Mori, K. (eds.) MICCAI 2012, Part I. LNCS, vol. 7510, pp. 512–519. Springer, Heidelberg (2012)
9. Harandi, M., Sanderson, C., et al.: Graph embedding discriminant analysis on grassmannian manifolds for improved image set matching. In: CVPR, p. 2705 (2011)
10. Mori, G.: Guiding model search using segmentation. In: ICCV, pp. 1417–1423 (2005)
11. Krähenbühl, P., Koltun, V.: Efficient Inference in Fully Connected CRFs with Gaussian Edge Potentials. In: NIPS, vol. 24, pp. 109–117 (2011)
12. Kohli, P., Ladicky, L., Torr, P.: Robust higher order potentials for enforcing label consistency. IJCV 82, 302–324 (2009)
13. Wang, L., He, L., Mishra, A., Li, C.: Active contours driven by local gaussian distribution fitting energy. Signal Process. 89, 2435–2447 (2009)

# Fast, Sequence Adaptive Parcellation of Brain MR Using Parametric Models

Oula Puonti[1], Juan Eugenio Iglesias[2], and Koen Van Leemput[1,2,3]

[1] Department of Applied Mathematics and Computer Science,
Technical University of Denmark, Denmark
[2] Martinos Center for Biomedical Imaging, MGH, Harvard Medical School, USA
[3] Departments of Information and Computer Science and of Biomedical Engineering
and Computational Science, Aalto University, Finland

**Abstract.** In this paper we propose a method for whole brain parcellation using the type of generative parametric models typically used in tissue classification. Compared to the non-parametric, multi-atlas segmentation techniques that have become popular in recent years, our method obtains state-of-the-art segmentation performance in both cortical and subcortical structures, while retaining all the benefits of generative parametric models, including high computational speed, automatic adaptiveness to changes in image contrast when different scanner platforms and pulse sequences are used, and the ability to handle multi-contrast (vector-valued intensities) MR data. We have validated our method by comparing its segmentations to manual delineations both within and across scanner platforms and pulse sequences, and show preliminary results on multi-contrast test-retest scans, demonstrating the feasibility of the approach.

## 1 Introduction

Computational methods for automatically segmenting magnetic resonance (MR) images of the brain have seen tremendous advances in recent years. So-called *tissue classification* methods, which aim at extracting the white matter, gray matter, and cerebrospinal fluid, are now well established. In their simplest form, these methods classify voxels independently based on their intensity alone, although state-of-the-art methods often incorporate a probabilistic atlas – a parametric representation of prior neuroanatomical knowledge that is learned from manually annotated training data – as well as explicit models of MR imaging artifacts [1–3]. Tissue classification techniques have a number of attractive properties, including their computational speed and their ability to automatically adapt to changes in image contrast when different scanner platforms and pulse sequences are used. Furthermore, they can readily handle the multi-contrast (vector-valued intensities) MR scans that are acquired in clinical imaging, and can include models of pathology such as white matter lesions and brain tumors.

Despite these strengths, attempts at expanding the scope of tissue classification techniques to also segment dozens of subcortical structures have been less successful [4]. In that area, better results have been obtained with so-called

K. Mori et al. (Eds.): MICCAI 2013, Part I, LNCS 8149, pp. 727–734, 2013.

*multi-atlas* techniques – non-parametric methods in which a collection of manually annotated images are deformed onto the target image using pair-wise registration, and the resulting atlases are fused to obtain a final segmentation [4, 5]. Although early methods used a simple majority voting rule, recent developments have concentrated on exploiting local intensity information to guide the atlas fusion process, which is particularly helpful in cortical areas for which accurate inter-subject registration is challenging [6, 7].

Although multi-atlas techniques have been shown to provide excellent segmentation results, they do come with a number of distinct disadvantages compared to tissue classification techniques. Specifically, their non-parametric nature entails a significant computational burden because of the large number of pair-wise registrations that is required for each new segmentation. Furthermore, their applicability across scanner platforms and pulse sequences is seldom addressed, and it remains unclear how multi-contrast MR and especially pathology can be handled with these methods.

In this paper, we revisit tissue classification modeling techniques and demonstrate that it is possible to obtain cortical and subcortical segmentation accuracies that are on par with the current state-of-the-art in multi-atlas segmentation, while being dramatically faster. Following a modeling approach similar to [1, 3] for tissue classification, but with a carefully computed probabilistic atlas of 41 brain substructures, we show excellent performance both within and across scanner platforms and pulse sequences. Compared to other methods aiming at sequence adaptive whole brain segmentation, we do not require specific MR sequences for which a physical forward model is available [8], and we segment many more structures without a priori defined contrast-specific initializations as in [2].

## 2    Modeling Framework

We use a Bayesian modeling approach, in which a generative probabilistic image model is constructed and subsequently "inverted" to obtain automated segmentations. We first describe our generative model, and subsequently explain how we use it to obtain automated segmentations. Because of space constraints, we only describe the uni-contrast case here (i.e., a scalar intensity value for each voxel); the generalization to multi-contrast data is straightforward [3].

### 2.1    Generative Model

Our model consists of a prior distribution that predicts where anatomical labels typically occur throughout brain images, and a likelihood distribution that links the resulting labels to MR intensities. As a segmentation prior we use a recently proposed tetrahedral mesh-based probabilistic atlas [9], where each mesh node contains a probability vector containing the probabilities for the $K$ different brain structures under consideration. The resolution of the mesh is locally adaptive, being sparse in large uniform regions and dense around the structure borders.

The positions of the mesh nodes, denoted by $\boldsymbol{\theta}_l$, can move according to a deformation prior $p(\boldsymbol{\theta}_l)$ that prevents the mesh from tearing or folding onto itself. The prior probability of label $l_i \in \{1, ..., K\}$ in voxel $i$ is denoted by $p_i(l_i|\boldsymbol{\theta}_l)$, which is computed by interpolating the probability vectors in the vertices of the deformed mesh. Assuming conditional independence of the labels between voxels given the mesh node positions, the prior probability of a segmentation is then given by $p(\mathbf{l}|\boldsymbol{\theta}_l) = \prod_i^I p_i(l_i|\boldsymbol{\theta}_l)$, where $\mathbf{l} = (l_1, ..., l_I)^T$ denotes a complete segmentation of an image with $I$ voxels.

For the likelihood distribution, we associate a mixture of Gaussian distributions with each neuroanatomical label to model the relationship between segmentation labels and image intensities [1]. To account for the smoothly varying intensity inhomogeneities that typically corrupt MR scans, we model such bias fields as a linear combination of spatially smooth basis functions [3]. Letting $\mathbf{d} = (d_1, ..., d_I)^T$ denote a vector containing the image intensities in all voxels, and $\boldsymbol{\theta}_d$ a vector collecting all bias field and Gaussian mixture parameters, the likelihood distribution then takes the form $p(\mathbf{d}|\mathbf{l}, \boldsymbol{\theta}_d) = \prod_{i=1}^I p_i(d_i|l_i, \boldsymbol{\theta}_d)$, where

$$p_i(d|l, \boldsymbol{\theta}_d) = \sum_{g=1}^{G_l} \mathcal{N}\left(d - \sum_{p=1}^{P} c_p \phi_p^i \,\middle|\, \mu_{lg}, \sigma_{lg}^2\right) w_{lg}$$

and $\mathcal{N}(d|\mu, \sigma^2) = \frac{1}{\sqrt{2\pi\sigma^2}} \exp\left(-\frac{(d-\mu)^2}{2\sigma^2}\right)$. Here $G_l$ is the number of Gaussian distributions associated with label $l$; and $\mu_{lg}$, $\sigma_{lg}^2$, and $w_{lg}$ are the mean, variance, and weight of component $g$ in the mixture model of label $l$. Furthermore, $P$ denotes the number of bias field basis functions, $\phi_p^i$ is the basis function $p$ evaluated at voxel $i$, and $c_p$ its coefficient. To complete the model, we assume a flat prior on $\boldsymbol{\theta}_d$: $p(\boldsymbol{\theta}_d) \propto 1$.

## 2.2   Inference

Using the model described above, the most probable segmentation for a given MR scan is obtained as $\hat{\mathbf{l}} = \arg\max_{\mathbf{l}} p(\mathbf{l}|\mathbf{d}) = \arg\max_{\mathbf{l}} \int p(\mathbf{l}|\mathbf{d}, \boldsymbol{\theta}) p(\boldsymbol{\theta}|\mathbf{d}) d\boldsymbol{\theta}$, where $\boldsymbol{\theta} = (\boldsymbol{\theta}_d, \boldsymbol{\theta}_l)^T$ collects all the model parameters. This requires an integration over all possible parameter values, each weighed according to its posterior $p(\boldsymbol{\theta}|\mathbf{d})$. Since this integration is intractable we approximate it by estimating the parameters with maximum weight $\hat{\boldsymbol{\theta}} = \arg\max_{\boldsymbol{\theta}} p(\boldsymbol{\theta}|\mathbf{d})$, and using the contribution of those parameters only:

$$\hat{\mathbf{l}} = \arg\max_{\mathbf{l}} p(\mathbf{l}|\mathbf{d}) \approx \arg\max_{\mathbf{l}} p(\mathbf{l}|\mathbf{d}, \hat{\boldsymbol{\theta}}) = \arg\max_{\{l_1, ... l_I\}} \prod_{i=1}^I p_i(l_i|d_i, \hat{\boldsymbol{\theta}}). \quad (1)$$

The optimization of eq. (1) is tractable because it involves maximizing $p_i(l_i|d_i, \hat{\boldsymbol{\theta}}) \propto p_i(d_i|l_i, \hat{\boldsymbol{\theta}}_d) p_i(l_i|\hat{\boldsymbol{\theta}}_l)$ in each voxel independently.

To find the optimal parameters we maximize

$$p(\boldsymbol{\theta}|\mathbf{d}) \propto p(\mathbf{d}|\boldsymbol{\theta}) p(\boldsymbol{\theta}) \propto \left(\prod_{i=1}^I \sum_{l=1}^K p_i(d_i|l, \boldsymbol{\theta}_d) p_i(l|\boldsymbol{\theta}_l)\right) p(\boldsymbol{\theta}_l) \quad (2)$$

by iteratively keeping the mesh positions $\boldsymbol{\theta}_l$ fixed at their current values and updating the remaining parameters $\boldsymbol{\theta}_d$, and vice versa, until convergence. For the mesh node position optimization we use a a standard conjugate gradient optimizer, and for the remaining parameters a dedicated generalized expectation-maximization (GEM) algorithm similar to [3]. In particular, the GEM optimization involves iteratively computing the following "soft" assignments in all voxels $i \in \{1, \ldots, I\}$:

$$q_i^{lg} = \frac{w_{lg} \mathcal{N}\big(d_i - \sum_{p=1}^{P} c_p \phi_p^i \,\big|\, \mu_{lg}, \sigma_{lg}^2\big) p_i(l|\boldsymbol{\theta}_l)}{\sum_{k=1}^{K} p_i(d_i|k, \boldsymbol{\theta}_d) p_i(k|\boldsymbol{\theta}_l)}, \quad \forall l \in \{1, \ldots, K\}, \forall g \in \{1, \ldots, G_l\}$$

based on the current parameter estimates, and subsequently updating the parameters accordingly:

$$\mu_{lg} \leftarrow \frac{\sum_{i=1}^{I} q_i^{lg}\big(d_i - \sum_{p=1}^{P} c_p \phi_p^i\big)}{\sum_{i=1}^{I} q_i^{lg}}, \quad \sigma_{lg}^2 \leftarrow \frac{\sum_{i=1}^{I} q_i^{lg}\big(d_i - \mu_{lg} - \sum_{p=1}^{P} c_p \phi_p^i\big)^2}{\sum_{i=1}^{I} q_i^{lg}},$$

$$w_{lg} \leftarrow \frac{\sum_{i=1}^{I} q_i^{lg}}{\sum_{g=1}^{G_l} \sum_{i=1}^{I} q_i^{lg}}, \quad (c_1, \ldots, c_P)^T \leftarrow \big(\mathbf{A}^T \mathbf{S} \mathbf{A}\big)^{-1} \mathbf{A}^T \mathbf{S} \mathbf{r},$$

where

$$\mathbf{A} = \begin{pmatrix} \phi_1^1 & \cdots & \phi_P^1 \\ \vdots & \ddots & \vdots \\ \phi_1^I & \cdots & \phi_P^I \end{pmatrix}, \quad \mathbf{S} = diag(s_i), \quad s_i = \sum_{l=1}^{K} \sum_{g=1}^{G_l} \frac{q_i^{lg}}{\sigma_{lg}^2},$$

$$\mathbf{r} = (r_1, .., r_I)^T, \quad r_i = d_i - \tilde{d}_i, \quad \tilde{d}_i = \frac{\sum_{l=1}^{K} \sum_{g=1}^{G_l} s_i^{lg} \mu_{lg}}{\sum_{l=1}^{K} \sum_{g=1}^{G_l} s_i^{lg}}.$$

## 3   Implementation

We used a training dataset of 39 T1-weighted scans and corresponding expert delineations of 41 brain structures to build our mesh-based atlas and to run pilot experiments to tune the settings of our algorithm. The scans were acquired on a 1.5T Siemens Vision scanner using a magnetisation prepared, rapid acquisition gradient-echo (MPRAGE) sequence (voxel size $1.0 \times 1.0 \times 1.0$ mm$^3$). The 39 subjects are a mix of young, middle-aged, and old healthy subjects, as well as patients with either questionable or probable Alzheimer's disease [6].

We used 15 randomly picked subjects out of the available 39 to build our probabilistic atlas. The remaining subjects were used to find suitable settings for our algorithm. After experimenting, we decided to restrict sub-structures with similar intensity properties to having the same GMM parameters, e.g., left and right hemisphere white matter are modeled as having the same intensity properties. Further, we experimentally set a suitable value for the number of Gaussians for each label (variable $G_l$): three for gray matter structures, cerebro-spinal fluid, and non-brain tissues; and two for white matter structures, thalamus, putamen, and pallidum.

To initialize the algorithm, we co-register our atlas to the target image using an affine transformation. For this purpose we use the method described in [10], which uses atlas probabilities, rather than an intensity template, to drive the registration process. As is common in the literature, the MR intensities are log-transformed because of the additive bias field model that is employed [3].

## 4    Experiments

To validate the proposed algorithm, we performed experiments on two datasets of T1-weighted images that were manually labeled using the same protocol as the training data, each acquired on a different scanner platform and with a different pulse sequence. We also show preliminary results on a third dataset that consists of test-retest scans of multi-contrast (T1- and T2-weighted) images without manual annotations. We emphasize that we ran our method on all three datasets using the exact same settings.

Although our method segments 41 structures in total, some of the structures are not typically validated (e.g., left/right choroid plexus, left/right vessels), thus we here report quantitative results for a subset of 23 structures: cerebral white matter (WM), cerebellum white matter (CWM), cerebral cortex (CT), cerebellum cortex (CCT), lateral ventricle (LV), hippocampus (HP), thalamus (TH), caudate (CA), putamen (PU), pallidum (PA) and amygdala (AM), for both the left and the right side, along with brainstem (BS). In order to gauge the performance of our method with respect to the current state-of-the-art in the field, we also report results for the well-known FreeSurfer package [11] and two multi-atlas segmentation methods: BrainFuse [6], which uses a Gaussian kernel to perform local intensity-based atlas weighing, and Majority Voting [5], which weighs each atlas equally. We note that all three competing methods used the same training data described in section 3, ensuring a fair comparison: FreeSurfer to build its label and intensity models; and the multi-atlas methods to perform the pair-wise atlas propagations and to tune optimal parameter settings. All three competing methods apply the same preprocessing stages to skull-strip the images, remove bias field artifacts, and perform intensity normalization as described in [11]. The proposed method works directly on the input data itself without preprocessing. For our implementation of Majority Voting, we used the pair-wise registrations computed by BrainFuse.

Figure 1(a) shows the Dice scores (averaged across left and right) between the automated and manual segmentations for the four methods on our first dataset, which consists of T1-weighted images of 13 subjects acquired with the same Siemens scanner and MPRAGE pulse sequence as the training data. Note that FreeSurfer, BrainFuse, and Majority Voting are specifically trained for this type of data, whereas the proposed method is not. It can be seen that each method gives quite accurate and comparable segmentations, except for majority voting, which clearly trails the other methods. The mean Dice score across these structures is 0.859 for the suggested method, 0.864 for BrainFuse, 0.853 for FreeSurfer, and 0.793 for Majority Voting. Table 1 shows the execution times for the methods. The experiments were run on a cluster where each node has two quad-core Xeon 5472 3.0GHz CPUs and 32GB of RAM. Only one core was used for the experiments. The multi-atlas methods require computationally heavy pair-wise registrations and thus have the longest run times, followed by FreeSurfer which is somewhat faster. The suggested method is clearly the fastest of the four, being approximately 26 times faster than BrainFuse or Majority Voting and 15 times faster than FreeSurfer. We note that our method is implemented using Matlab with the atlas deformation parts wrapped in C++, and in no way optimized for speed. To conclude our experiments on this dataset, table 2 shows how the number of training subjects in the atlas affects the mean segmentation accuracy of the proposed method, indicating that the method benefits from the availability of more training data.

Figure 1(b) shows the Dice scores on our second dataset, which consists of 14 T1-weighted MR scans that were acquired with a 1.5T GE Signa scanner using a spoiled gradient recalled (SPGR) sequence (voxel size $0.9375 \times 0.9375 \times 1.5$ mm$^3$). The overall segmentation accuracy of each method is decreased compared to the Siemens data, which is likely due to poorer image contrast as a result of the different pulse sequence and a slightly lower image resolution. Both FreeSurfer and our method are able to sustain an overall accuracy of 0.798, while the accuracies of BrainFuse and Majority Voting decrease to 0.746 and 0.70 respectively. The relatively good performance of FreeSurfer, which is trained specifically on the Siemens image contrast, can be explained by its in-built renormalization procedure for T1 acquisitions, which applies a multi-linear atlas-image registration and a histogram matching step to update the class-conditional densities for each structure [12]. The multi-atlas methods, in contrast, directly incorporate the Siemens contrast in the segmentation process, and would likely benefit from a retuning of their parameters for this specific application. Note that the proposed method requires no renormalization or retuning to perform well.

As a preliminary demonstration of the multi-contrast segmentation abilities of our method, figure 1(c) shows a measurement of volume differences between both uni-contrast (T1) and multi-contrast (T1 + T2) repeat scans of five individuals. For each subject, a multi-contrast scan was acquired with an identical Siemens 3T Tim Trio scanner at two different facilities, with a interval between the two scan sessions of maximum 3 months. The scans consist of a very fast (under 5 min total acquisition time) T1-weighted and bandwidth-matched T2-weighted image (multi-echo MPRAGE sequence for T1 and 3D T2-SPACE sequence for T2, voxel size $1.2 \times 1.2 \times 1.2$ mm$^3$). The volume difference in a structure was computed as the absolute difference between the volumes estimated at the two time points, normalized by the average of the volumes, both when only the T1-weighted image was used, and when T1 and T2 were used. The figure shows that our method seems to work as well on multi-contrast as on uni-contrast data, opening possibilities for simultaneous brain lesion segmentation in the future. An example segmentation of one of the multi-contrast scans is shown in figure 2.

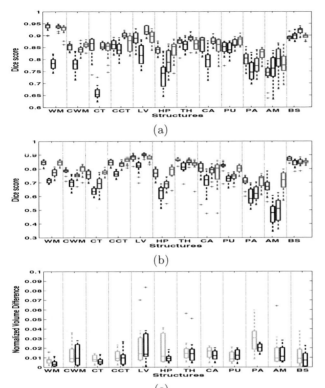

(a)

(b)

(c)

**Fig. 1.** (a) Dice scores of the first dataset (Siemens). FreeSurfer is red, BrainFuse blue, Majority Voting black, and the suggested method green. (b) Dice scores of the second data set (GE). (c) Normalized volume differences: multi-contrast data is cyan, and T1-only black. On each box, the central mark is the median, the edges of the box are the 25th and 75th percentiles, and outliers are marked with a '+'.

**Table 1.** Computational times for the four different methods

| Method | Comp. time(h) |
|---|---|
| BrainFuse | ∼ 17 |
| Majority voting | ∼ 16 |
| FreeSurfer | ∼ 9.5 |
| Suggested method | ∼ 0.6 |

**Table 2.** Average Dice score across all structures for the first (Siemens) dataset vs. number of training subjects

| Number of subjects | Mean Dice score |
|---|---|
| 5 | 0.820 |
| 9 | 0.843 |
| 15 | 0.859 |

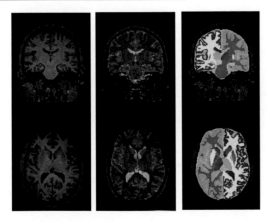

**Fig. 2.** An example of a multi-contrast segmentation generated by the proposed method

# 5    Discussion

In this paper we proposed a method for whole brain parcellation using the type of generative parametric models typically used in tissue classification techniques. Comparisons with current state-of-the-art methods demonstrated excellent performance both within and across scanner platforms and pulse sequences, as well as a large computational advantage. Future work will concentrate on a more thorough validation of the method's multi-contrast segmentation performance. We also plan to use other validation metrics beyond the mere spatial overlap used in this paper, such as volumetric and boundary distance measures.

**Acknowledgements.**    This research was supported by NIH NCRR (P41-RR14075), NIBIB (R01EB013565), Academy of Finland (133611), TEKES (Com-Brain), and financial contributions from the Technical University of Denmark.

# References

1. Ashburner, J., Friston, K.: Unified segmentation. Neuroimage 26, 839–885 (2005)
2. Bazin, P.L., Pham, D.L.: Homeomorphic brain image segmentation with topological and statistical atlases. Medical Image Analysis 12(5), 616–625 (2008)
3. Van Leemput, K., Maes, F., Vandermeulen, D., Suetens, P.: Automated model-based bias field correction of MR images of the brain. IEEE Transactions on Medical Imaging 18(10), 885–896 (1999)
4. Babalola, K.O., Patenaude, B., Aljabar, P., Schnabel, J., Kennedy, D., Crum, W., Smith, S., Cootes, T., Jenkinson, M., Rueckert, D.: An evaluation of four automatic methods of segmenting the subcortical structures in the brain. Neuroimage 47(4), 1435–1447 (2009)
5. Heckemann, R., Hajnal, J., Aljabar, P., Rueckert, D., Hammers, A.: Automatic anatomical brain MRI segmentation combining label propagation and decision fusion. Neuroimage 33, 115–126 (2006)
6. Sabuncu, M.R., Yeo, B., Van Leemput, K., Fischl, B., Golland, P.: A generative model for image segmentation based on label fusion. IEEE Transactions on Medical Imaging 29(10), 1714–1729 (2010)
7. Ledig, C., Wolz, R., Aljabar, P., Lotjonen, J., Heckemann, R.A., Hammers, A., Rueckert, D.: Multi-class brain segmentation using atlas propagation and EM-based refinement. In: 9th IEEE International Symposium on Biomedical Imaging (ISBI), pp. 896–899 (2012)
8. Fischl, B., Salat, D.H., van der Kouwe, A.J., Makris, N., Ségonne, F., Quinn, B.T., Dale, A.M.: Sequence-independent segmentation of magnetic resonance images. Neuroimage 23, S69–S84 (2004)
9. Van Leemput, K.: Encoding probabilistic brain atlases using Bayesian inference. IEEE Transactions on Medical Imaging 28(6), 822–837 (2009)
10. D'Agostino, E., Maes, F., Vandermeulen, D., Suetens, P.: Non-rigid atlas-to-image registration by minimization of class-conditional image entropy. In: Barillot, C., Haynor, D.R., Hellier, P. (eds.) MICCAI 2004. LNCS, vol. 3216, pp. 745–753. Springer, Heidelberg (2004)
11. Dale, A., Fischl, B., Sereno, M.: Cortical surface-based analysis I: Segmentation and surface reconstruction. Neuroimage 9, 179–194 (1999)
12. Han, X., Fischl, B.: Atlas renormalization for improved brain MR image segmentation across scanner platforms. IEEE Transactions on Medical Imaging 26(4), 479–486 (2007)

# Multiple Sclerosis Lesion Segmentation Using Dictionary Learning and Sparse Coding

Nick Weiss[1], Daniel Rueckert[2], and Anil Rao[2]

[1] University of Lübeck, Lübeck, Germany
[2] Imperial College London, London, UK

**Abstract.** The segmentation of lesions in the brain during the development of Multiple Sclerosis is part of the diagnostic assessment for this disease and gives information on its current severity. This laborious process is still carried out in a manual or semiautomatic fashion by clinicians because published automatic approaches have not been universal enough to be widely employed in clinical practice. Thus Multiple Sclerosis lesion segmentation remains an open problem. In this paper we present a new unsupervised approach addressing this problem with dictionary learning and sparse coding methods. We show its general applicability to the problem of lesion segmentation by evaluating our approach on synthetic and clinical image data and comparing it to state-of-the-art methods. Furthermore the potential of using dictionary learning and sparse coding for such segmentation tasks is investigated and various possibilities for further experiments are discussed.

## 1   Introduction

Multiple Sclerosis (MS) is an autoimmune demyelinating disease occurring in the central nervous system (CNS). It is chronic, inflammatory and currently incurable. The underlying cause for the spontaneous degeneration of the myelin and subsequently the axons is still unknown and the lesions can appear at various locations within the brain causing a wide range of symptoms such as numbness, weakness, visual impairment or loss of balance. Approved medications and therapies present a symptomatic treatment to decrease the severity, occurrence and duration of certain symptoms [2].

Magnetic resonance imaging (MRI) significantly contributes to the evaluation of new therapies during clinical trials, as it is very sensitive to most of the lesions appearing in the white matter (WM) of the brain [7]. Lesions are visible as hyperintense areas in T2-weighted (T2w) and often hypointense in T1-weighted (T1w) MR images. Counting these white matter lesions (WML) and determining their total lesion load (TLL) are key criteria for quantifying the progression of MS and the current diagnosis criteria for MS (McDonald Criteria) [12]. In clinical practice the detection and segmentation of WML is still done in a manual or semiautomatic fashion by most clinicians. This is a time consuming task that suffers from a large intra- and interexpert variability [9]. Thus an automatic approach is highly desirable.

K. Mori et al. (Eds.): MICCAI 2013, Part I, LNCS 8149, pp. 735–742, 2013.
© Springer-Verlag Berlin Heidelberg 2013

Over the last two decades several automatic methods have been proposed. The conclusion of two recent reviews [10,5] was that MS lesion and segmentation remains an open problem. No automatic method has been widely employed in clinical practice as they are too specific to deal with the heterogeneity in location and texture of lesions, and the differences in MRI acquisition. While supervised methods rely on images with previously segmented lesions, unsupervised methods do not require labeled data [5]. Unsupervised methods often try to model the intensity distribution of the healthy brain tissues, namely WM, grey matter (GM) and cerebrospinal fluid (CSF). Voxels that cannot be explained by this model are called outliers and labeled as lesions. Van Leemput et al. [19] developed a well-known method based on such a model.

We create an unsupervised approach that also segments the lesions as outliers with respect to healthy brain tissue. It introduces dictionary learning and sparse coding for the segmentation of MS lesions, which is new to our knowledge. Many areas of image processing have already benefited from this methodology [17,3]. The principal idea is to learn a dictionary primarily from healthy brain image tissue and then try to sparsely reconstruct image patches using the dictionary. Image patches containing lesions have a higher reconstruction error and thresholding this reconstruction error for every voxel then provides a lesion segmentation. In this paper we describe our new approach and evaluate it by using synthetic and clinical brain images with a ground truth segmentation. Finally we compare the results with other methods and outline the potential of this new approach.

## 2    Material and Methods

As stated in Fig. 1 our method can be divided into three different parts. The first part is preprocessing and includes brain extraction, image patch extraction and patch normalization. The second part focuses on learning a dictionary from these image patches and trying to reconstruct them using sparse coding. The last part shows how we provide a relative reconstruction error map and get the threshold for the final WML segmentation. In the remaining subsections we give information about the synthetic image data, clinical image data, the evaluation and the implementation.

### 2.1    Preprocessing

Since we want to segment lesions from the brain tissue, we require a brain mask that excludes the skull and all non-brain tissue. For the synthetic image data used in this paper a brain mask is provided along with the images. For the clinical image data, a brain mask is created using the brain extraction tool (BET) [13] and a bias correction is performed [18].

The $m$ image patches lying within the brain mask ($m \approx 1.5*10^6$ for a voxel size of $1\ mm^3$) are extracted and realigned to one-dimensional vectors $x_1, ..., x_m \in \mathbb{R}^k$ with $k = 27$ for a three-dimensional image patch of size $3 \times 3 \times 3$. Each patch is

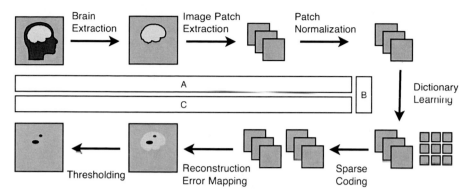

**Fig. 1.** A brief overview of the presented method. (A) Preprocessing including brain extraction, patch extraction and patch normalization. (B) Dictionary learning and sparse coding reconstruction of the image patches. (C) Mapping of the reconstruction error and finding a threshold for the final segmentation.

then divided by the value of the highest $L_1$-norm of all patches and its square root is taken so that each patch fulfills $\|x_i\|_2^2 \leq 1$. To combine image patches of different modalities the vectors can easily be concatenated after the described patch normalization. A multiplication by the weight $\sqrt{1/z}$ where $z$ is the number of available image sequences (e.g. T1/T2/FLAIR/etc.) ensures that the condition $\|x_i\|_2^2 \leq 1$ with $x_i \in \mathbb{R}^{zk}$ is still satisfied.

## 2.2 Dictionary Learning and Sparse Coding

A dictionary $D \in C = \{D \in \mathbb{R}^{k \times l} \ s.t. \ \forall j : \ \|d_j\|_2^2 \leq 1\}$ with $l$ atoms $d_j$ is learned from these image patches so that it solves the optimization problem

$$\min_{D} \sum_{i=1}^{m} \frac{1}{2} \|x_i - D\alpha_i\|_2^2 \ s.t. \ \|\alpha_i\|_1 \leq \lambda_1. \tag{1}$$

Dictionary learning searches for a basis $D$ that satisfies $x_i \approx D\alpha_i$ for most image patches. Although the image patches with lesions are included in this learning process they do not impair the dictionary's ability to only represent the healthy brain image patches well. The reason for this is that just a small percentage of the patches include lesions.

The $L_1$-norm constraint in (1) introduces sparsity to its solution so that only a few atoms of the dictionary should be used to represent an image patch [11]. It has been shown that learning a dictionary like this leads to a very precise image reconstruction [3]. If we try to reconstruct the image patches in a second optimization step

$$\min_{\alpha_i} \ \|x_i - D\alpha_i\|_2^2 \ s.t. \ \|\alpha_i\|_1 \leq \lambda_2 \tag{2}$$

we will obtain a reconstruction error for each image patch depending on the sparsity constraint. An appropriately chosen parameter $\lambda_2$ shows that healthy brain tissue can be easily reconstructed with a few atoms while the image patches containing lesions produce a higher error using the same amount of atoms.

## 2.3  Reconstruction Error and Thresholding

The relative reconstruction error of each image patch

$$err(x_i, \alpha_i) = \frac{\|x_i - D\alpha_i\|_2}{\|x_i\|_2} \tag{3}$$

can now be obtained and mapped at the position of the centered voxel within the patch. The result is an error map throughout the whole brain.

Finally a threshold is applied to obtain the segmentation of the WML from the combined error map. We do this by creating a smoothed histogram of the error map for a randomly chosen subject, and search for a point where the histogram derivative magnitude is close to zero that separates the lesion and non-lesion voxels for this subject. This derivative magnitude threshold is applied to the histograms of all subjects in the data set. Since we only use one subject during this process, this may still be considered a largely unsupervised procedure.

## 2.4  Synthetic Image Data

As suggested by Garcia-Lorenzo et al. [5] the freely available BrainWeb image data is a good first evaluation step to show a proof of concept and to test the method's robustness towards noise and intensity inhomogeneity [1]. Furthermore it allows us to compare our results to others as many authors evaluate their methods with this data.

It is possible to create T1w, T2w images with different levels of noise (3%, 5%, 7%, 9%) and intensity inhomogeneity (0%, 40%) in an online MRI simulator. The ground truth segmentation is available for all these WML as well as the brain segmentation. The images are simulated with an isotropic resolution of $1 \ mm^3$ and have a size of $181 \times 217 \times 181$.

## 2.5  Clinical Image Data

The evaluation with synthetic image data is limited since we only have one phantom and images with simulated lesions are much easier to segment [5]. Furthermore we could not consider other MRI sequences like fluid attenuated inversion recovery (FLAIR) which is known to produce images predestinated for lesion segmentation.

We therefore further validate our framework using clinical data provided by the MS lesion segmentation challenge which was introduced as a workshop at MICCAI 2008 and still available [15]. In this paper, we focus on the 20 available training cases, which we downsample from the original resolution of 0.5 $mm^3$ isotropic to 1 $mm^3$ isotropic. The resulting images are then of size $256 \times 256 \times 256$

voxels. The data comes from the Children's Hospital Boston (CHB) and the University of North Carolina (UNC).

For the synthetic data we used both T1w and T2w images, since using the T2w alone cannot discriminate between CSF and lesions. Inclusion of the T1w patches gives the CSF its own footprint, thereby reducing the number of false positives segmented as lesion. In the clinical data, we use just the FLAIR sequence since the CSF appears as hypointense and the lesions as hyperintense in these images, so T1w images are not required.

## 2.6  Evaluation

The most common validation measure in the context of segmentation is the Dice Similarity Coefficient $DSC = \frac{2 \times TP}{FP + FN + 2 \times TP}$ with the number of true positive ($TP$), false positive ($FP$) and false negative ($FN$) voxels. The DSC rewards a method for its ability to detect lesions and to reject healthy tissue. It is used to evaluate the synthetic image data as it is used by the other authors.

For the clinical image data, we also calculate the true positive rate $TPR = \frac{TP}{TP+FN}$, and the positive predictive value $PPV = \frac{TP}{TP+FP}$. This allows us to compare our results with those of Geremia et al. [8].

## 2.7  Implementation

Our approach was implemented using MATLAB and the SPArse Modeling Software (SPAMS) [11]. SPAMS was used to solve the optimization problems (1) and (2). Different parameters have been tested for this method. A good result is provided by an image patch size of $3 \times 3 \times 3$ and a dictionary $D$ with $l = 100$ atoms. The following sparsity constraints were also determined empirically: $\lambda_1 = 0.9$ and $\lambda_2 = 0.8$. The whole segmentation took approximate 5 minutes and was carried out using an Intel Core 2 Duo processor at 2.4 GHz with 4 GB of RAM.

# 3  Results and Discussion

The proposed method is evaluated first using the synthetic BrainWeb image data, using different levels of noise and intensity inhomogeneity. We compared the results with four other unsupervised methods whose authors provided the DSC for all the different cases and are considered as state-of-the-art methods for segmentation of MS lesions [19,6,4,16].

Our method gives DSC measures that are highly competitive with those of the other approaches. The mean DSC is 71 for 0 % intensity non-uniformity (INU) and 63 for 40 % INU. Though at the lower noise levels (3 %, 5 %) and independent of the intensity non-uniformity (0 %, 40 %) the results are lower with up to 16 percentage points (pps) compared to the best methods. The intensity non-uniformity of 40 % slightly decreased the DSC for most of the methods. It is noticeable that our approach is robust to the presence of noise across all experiments, despite there being no explicit noise-reducing step. The dictionary

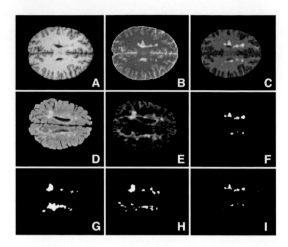

**Fig. 2.** Synthetic T1w (A) and T2w (B) images with lesions and their error map (C) after reconstruction. The final lesion segmentation (F) of the synthetic data compared with the ground truth (I). Clinical FLAIR image (D), its error map (E) after reconstruction, final lesion segmentation (H) and ground truth (G).

obviously adapts itself as it is learned with noisy image patches. This is a clear advantage of our method compared to the others.

As expected the clinical data is much more challenging (see figure 2 and Table 1). The TLL varies heavily from 105 $mm^3$ (UNC05) to 22542 $mm^3$ (CHB1) across all subjects while the TLL for the synthetic image data is constant with 3512 $mm^3$. The created brain masks also have a big impact on the results although we try to provide a good individual brain mask for each subject by varying the parameters of BET and using morphological operators. Different threshold values are provided for the synthetic data, the UNC and the CHB data as the raters show a high inter-expert variability and seem to have slightly different definitions of lesions. Across the whole clinical data, the proposed method achieved a mean (standard deviation) TPR of 33% (19) and a PPV of 37% (20). This is higher than the TPR of 21% (14) and PPV of 30% (17) provided by Souplet [14], another unsupervised approach and the MS lesion segmentation challenge winner in 2008. The method by Geremia [8] reaches a TPR of 40% (18) and a PPV of 40% (20) which is slightly higher than our results but within the reach. Other than ours their method is supervised, which therefore requires training data. This data can be expensive to obtain. However we can further extend our method to include some supervision which may improve our results. Importantly, the TPR and PPV values for the subject with the largest lesion load, CHB01, are competitive with those of the rival methods. This demonstrates that, even in the presence of larger lesion loads, the sparsity constraints in the dictionary learning and reconstruction phases enable the identification of lesions as outliers with respect to healthy tissue. Indeed, even extremely high lesion loads $\approx 60000$ $mm^3$ only represent less than 5% of the total brain volume, so their detection should still be possible.

**Table 1.** TPR/PPV/DSC results (%) on clinical brain image data. Our method is compared to two state-of-the-art rival methods (2008: Souplet [14], 2010: Geremia [8]). Note that DSC measures were not provided by the authors for those methods.

| Patient | Souplet TPR | PPV | Geremia TPR | PPV | Our Method TPR | PPV | Dice | Patient | Souplet TPR | PPV | Geremia TPR | PPV | Our Method TPR | PPV | Dice |
|---|---|---|---|---|---|---|---|---|---|---|---|---|---|---|---|
| UNC01 | 1 | 1 | 2 | 1 | 33 | 29 | 31 | CHB01 | 22 | 41 | 49 | 64 | 60 | 58 | 59 |
| UNC02 | 37 | 39 | 48 | 36 | 54 | 51 | 53 | CHB02 | 18 | 29 | 44 | 63 | 27 | 45 | 34 |
| UNC03 | 12 | 16 | 24 | 35 | 64 | 27 | 38 | CHB03 | 17 | 21 | 22 | 57 | 24 | 56 | 34 |
| UNC04 | 38 | 54 | 54 | 38 | 40 | 51 | 45 | CHB04 | 12 | 55 | 31 | 78 | 27 | 66 | 38 |
| UNC05 | 38 | 8 | 56 | 19 | 25 | 10 | 16 | CHB05 | 22 | 42 | 40 | 52 | 29 | 33 | 31 |
| UNC06 | 57 | 9 | 15 | 8 | 13 | 55 | 20 | CHB06 | 13 | 46 | 32 | 52 | 10 | 36 | 16 |
| UNC07 | 27 | 18 | 76 | 16 | 44 | 23 | 30 | CHB07 | 13 | 39 | 40 | 54 | 14 | 48 | 22 |
| UNC08 | 27 | 20 | 52 | 32 | 43 | 13 | 20 | CHB08 | 13 | 55 | 46 | 65 | 21 | 73 | 32 |
| UNC09 | 16 | 43 | 67 | 36 | 69 | 6 | 11 | CHB09 | 3 | 18 | 23 | 28 | 5 | 22 | 8 |
| UNC10 | 22 | 28 | 53 | 34 | 43 | 23 | 30 | CHB10 | 5 | 18 | 23 | 39 | 15 | 12 | 13 |

# 4    Conclusions

We have evaluated our method using dictionary learning for MS lesion segmentation with synthetic and clinical image data. The results were competitive with state-of-the-art methods and displayed the robustness of our method towards noise. There are many potential ways of extending the presented framework. One idea is to use the combined intensities from different MRI sequences to learn separate dictionaries for WM, GM and CSF. An outlier or lesion is then identified if it cannot be well reconstructed from any of the dictionaries. Alternatively, we could use the reconstruction coefficients $\alpha$ across the dictionaries to identify lesions. We could also introduce supervision into our method by learning a dictionary specific to lesions in addition to dictionaries for WM, GM and CSF. Patch size is another important factor to consider: While we have empirically found that a 3x3x3 patch works best, it would be interesting to incorporate larger patches into the framework, which may potentially capture more texture information and further improve results.

# References

1. Cocosco, C., Kollokian, V., Kwan, K., Pike, G.B.: BrainWeb: Online Interface to a 3D MRI Simulated Brain Database - Abstract - Europe PubMed Central. Neuroimage 5, 425 (1997)
2. Compston, A., Coles, A.: Multiple sclerosis. The Lancet 372(9648), 1502–1517 (2008)
3. Elad, M.: Sparse and Redundant Representations. From Theory to Applications in Signal and Image Processing. Springer (2010)
4. Forbes, F., Doyle, S., García-Lorenzo, D., Barillot, C., Dojat, M.: A Weighted Multi-Sequence Markov Model For Brain Lesion Segmentation. In: 13th International Conference on Artificial Intelligence and Statistics, AISTATS 2010, vol. 9, pp. 225–232 (2010)
5. García-Lorenzo, D., Francis, S., Narayanan, S., Arnold, D.L., Collins, D.L.: Review of automatic segmentation methods of multiple sclerosis white matter lesions on conventional magnetic resonance imaging. Medical Image Analysis 17(1), 1–18 (2013)

6. García-Lorenzo, D., Lecoeur, J., Arnold, D.L., Collins, D.L., Barillot, C.: Multiple sclerosis lesion segmentation using an automatic multimodal graph cuts. In: Yang, G.-Z., Hawkes, D., Rueckert, D., Noble, A., Taylor, C. (eds.) MICCAI 2009, Part II. LNCS, vol. 5762, pp. 584–591. Springer, Heidelberg (2009)

7. Ge, Y.: Multiple sclerosis: the role of MR imaging. AJNR. American Journal of Neuroradiology 27(6), 1165–1176 (2006)

8. Geremia, E., Menze, B.H., Clatz, O., Konukoglu, E., Criminisi, A., Ayache, N.: Spatial decision forests for MS lesion segmentation in multi-channel MR images. In: Jiang, T., Navab, N., Pluim, J.P.W., Viergever, M.A. (eds.) MICCAI 2010, Part I. LNCS, vol. 6361, pp. 111–118. Springer, Heidelberg (2010)

9. Grimaud, J., Lai, M., Thorpe, J., Adeleine, P., Wang, L., Barker, G.J., Plummer, D.L., Tofts, P.S., McDonald, W.I., Miller, D.H.: Quantification of MRI lesion load in multiple sclerosis: a comparison of three computer-assisted techniques. Magnetic Resonance Imaging 14(5), 495–505 (1996)

10. Lladó, X., Oliver, A., Cabezas, M., Freixenet, J., Vilanova, J.C., Quiles, A., Valls, L., Ramió-Torrentà, L., Rovira, À.: Segmentation of multiple sclerosis lesions in brain MRI: A review of automated approaches. Information Sciences 186(1), 164–185 (2012)

11. Mairal, J., Bach, F., Ponce, J., Sapiro, G.: Online dictionary learning for sparse coding. In: Proceedings of the 26th Annual International Conference on Machine Learning, pp. 689–696 (2009)

12. Polman, C.H., et al.: Diagnostic criteria for multiple sclerosis: 2010 revisions to the McDonald criteria. Annals of Neurology 69(2), 292–302 (2011)

13. Smith, S.M.: Fast robust automated brain extraction. Human Brain Mapping 17(3), 143–155 (2002)

14. Souplet, J.C., Lebrun, C., Ayache, N., Malandain, G.: An automatic segmentation of T2-FLAIR multiple sclerosis lesions. In: Grand Challenge Work.: Mult. Scler. Lesion Segm. Challenge, pp. 1–11 (2008)

15. Styner, M., Lee, J., Chin, B., Chin, M., Commowick, O., Tran, H., Markovic-Plese, S., Jewells, V., Warfield, S.: 3D segmentation in the clinic: A grand challenge II: MS lesion segmentation. MIDAS Journal, 1–5 (2008)

16. Tomas-Fernandez, X., Warfield, S.K.: Population intensity outliers or a new model for brain WM abnormalities. In: Proceedings of 9th IEEE International Symposium on Biomedical Imaging: From Nano to Macro, pp. 1543–1546 (2012)

17. Tošić, I., Frossard, P.: Dictionary learning. IEEE Signal Processing Magazine 28(2), 27–38 (2011)

18. Tustison, N.J., Avants, B.B., Cook, P.A., Zheng, Y., Egan, A., Yushkevich, P.A., Gee, J.C.: N4ITK: improved N3 bias correction. IEEE Transactions on Medical Imaging 29(6), 1310–1320 (2010)

19. Van Leemput, K., Maes, F., Vandermeulen, D., Colchester, A., Suetens, P.: Automated segmentation of multiple sclerosis lesions by model outlier detection. IEEE Transactions on Medical Imaging 20(8), 677–688 (2001)

# Deformable Atlas for Multi-structure Segmentation

Xiaofeng Liu*, Albert Montillo, Ek. T. Tan, John F. Schenck, and Paulo
Mendonca

General Electric Global Research Center, Niskayuna, NY USA
xiaofeng.liu@ge.com

**Abstract.** We develop a novel deformable atlas method for multi-
structure segmentation that seamlessly combines the advantages of
image-based and atlas-based methods. The method formulates a probabilistic framework that combines prior anatomical knowledge with image-
based cues that are specific to the subject's anatomy, and solves it using
expectation-maximization method. It improves the segmentation over
conventional label fusion methods especially around the structure boundaries, and is robust to large anatomical variation. The proposed method
was applied to segment multiple structures in both normal and diseased brains and was shown to significantly improve results especially in
diseased brains.

**Keywords:** Segmentation, deformable atlas, label fusion, MLE, GVF.

## 1 Introduction

Segmenting multiple structures from medical images remains a difficult task due
to the large variability of structure shape, their appearance in images, and the
lack of contrast between neighboring structures. One can roughly divide existing
segmentation methods into two categories: image-based approaches and atlas-
based approaches.

Image-based approaches are based on image cues, e.g., intensity, gradient,
texture. Among them deformable models, i.e., active contour [1] and level set
methods [2], have been widely adopted and shown success on many applications.
Atlas-based approaches [3, 4] rely largely on the prior knowledge about the spatial arrangement of structures. They are generally performed by first registering
atlas images to the subject image, called target, so that the manual segmentations on the atlases are propagated and fused to segment the target. Compared
to image-based approaches, these methods incorporate prior anatomical knowledge, but they do not explicitly consider images cues and thus are limited by
large anatomical variation and imperfect registration. Recently methods were
developed to incorporate image information into atlas-based approach[5–7], but
image cues other than intensity were not exploited. To the best of our knowledge,

---

* Corresponding author.

K. Mori et al. (Eds.): MICCAI 2013, Part I, LNCS 8149, pp. 743–750, 2013.

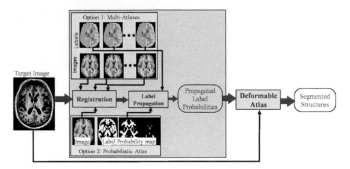

**Fig. 1.** Multi-structure segmentation using deformable atlas approach

the only work that attempted to close the gap between image-based and atlas-based methods is spectral label fusion [8]. However the method is region-based and it is difficult to extend to multiple structures especially when the boundaries between neighboring structures are weak.

In this paper we develop a novel multi-structure segmentation method, called *deformable atlas*, that seamlessly combines the advantages of image-based and atlas-based methods. The method formulates and solves a probabilistic framework that incorporates prior anatomical knowledge with image cues that are specific to the target images, including structure intensity profiles and boundaries. Significant improvements were demonstrated over common label fusion methods on the multi-structure segmentation of both normal and diseased brains.

## 2  Methods

Fig. 1 shows the flowchart of multi-structure segmentation using deformable atlas (DA) method. DA accepts as inputs the target image and spatial priors about the structures. The spatial priors can be generated using either a multi-atlas approach or a spatial probabilistic atlas. After that, DA segments the multi structures simultaneously. Consider a target image $\mathbf{I}$, where $I_j$ is the intensity at voxel $j$ with $j \in \{1, 2, ..., J\}$. Let $K$ be the number of structures or labels. The true label is represented by $\mathbf{z}_j = [z_{j1}, ..., z_{jK}]$, where $z_{jk} = 1$ if $j$ belongs to structure $k$, and 0 otherwise. The label spatial prior is $f(\mathbf{z}_j) = \mathbf{p}_j = [p_{j1}, ..., p_{jK}]$. In a multi-atlas approach, $p_{jk} = \frac{1}{N} \sum_{n=1}^{N} L_{jk}^n$ with $L_{jk}^n$ being the propagated label at $j$ from the $n^{th}$ atlas and $N$ being the number of atlases. In a probabilistic atlas approach, $\mathbf{p}_j$ is the propagated spatial prior after registration. Let $\boldsymbol{\theta} = \{\boldsymbol{\rho}, \boldsymbol{\pi}\}$ be the set of unknown parameters, where $\boldsymbol{\rho} = \{\rho_1, ...\rho_K\}$ are the intensity distribution functions for the $K$ structures, and $\boldsymbol{\pi} = \{\pi_{jk}\}$ with $\pi_{jk}$ being the probability that voxel $j$ belongs to structure $k$ and $\sum_{k=1}^{K} \pi_{jk} = 1$ for all $j$.

The deformable atlas method employs a maximum likelihood estimation (MLE) framework that combines label spatial prior knowledge with image-based cues, i.e., intensities and edges to improve the multi-structure segmentation. Using Bayes' law, the likelihood function is expressed as $f(\mathbf{Z}, \mathbf{I}|\boldsymbol{\theta}) =$

$$f(\mathbf{I}|\mathbf{Z}, \boldsymbol{\theta})f(\mathbf{Z}|\boldsymbol{\theta}) \propto f(\mathbf{I}|\mathbf{Z}, \boldsymbol{\rho})f(\mathbf{I}|\mathbf{Z}, \boldsymbol{\pi})f(\mathbf{Z}|\boldsymbol{\theta}) \propto f(\mathbf{I}|\mathbf{Z}, \boldsymbol{\rho})f(\boldsymbol{\pi}|\mathbf{I})f(\mathbf{Z}|\boldsymbol{\pi}) \quad (1)$$

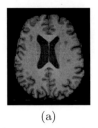
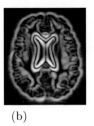

(a)                               (b)

**Fig. 2.** Example of the speed function. (a) A skull-striped brain T1 MR image, and (b) the magnitude of GVF.

with the assumptions that $\rho$ and $\pi$ are independent, $\mathbf{Z}$ and $\rho$ are independent, and $\mathbf{I}$ and $\mathbf{Z}$ are conditionally independent given $\pi$. The term $f(\mathbf{I}|\mathbf{Z},\rho)$ is based on the structure intensity profiles in the target image, while $f(\pi|\mathbf{I})$ models the distribution of $\pi$ given $\mathbf{I}$ and is defined based on structure boundaries (described below). We then develop an Expectation-Maximization(EM) algorithm to solve for $\theta$, which iterates between the E-step and the M-step.

### 2.1   The Probability $f(\pi|\mathbf{I})$

While most label fusion approaches do not explicitly explore structure boundary information, image-based methods have shown that structure boundaries are crucial for accurate segmentation. Here we conceptually define the log probability as

$$\log f(\pi|\mathbf{I}) = \log Ce^{-\gamma \sum_{k=1}^{K} F_{\mathbf{I}}(\mathbf{S_k})} = \log C - \gamma \sum_{k=1}^{K} F_{\mathbf{I}}(\mathbf{S_k}), \qquad (2)$$

where $F_{\mathbf{I}}(\mathbf{S}_k)$ is a potential energy function defined on the boundaries $\mathbf{S}_k$ of the $k^{th}$ structure segmented based on $\pi$, which typically takes local minimum at edges along structure contours. $C$ is a normalization constant.

In classic deformable models $F_{\mathbf{I}}(\mathbf{S}_k)$ often does not have an analytical form and minimizing it does not lead to a closed-form solution. Instead, it is optimized iteratively by either guiding the contour deformation using force fields in active contours [1], or evolving the level set function using speed functions in level set methods [9]. Inspired by that, we define pseudo level set functions $\phi_{jk} = \pi_{jk} - \sum_{i \neq k} \pi_{ji}$, which are similar to standard level set functions except their values are constrained to $[-1, 1]$. $\phi_{jk} \in (0, 1]$ when $i$ is inside structure $k$, and $\phi_{jk} \in [-1, 0)$ if $i$ is outside structure $k$. As in level set methods, the evolution of $\phi(j)$ to maximize Eqn. (2) can be expressed as $\phi_{jk}^{s+1} - \phi_{jk}^{s} = -\gamma \mathbf{v}_j \cdot \nabla \phi_{jk}$, with $\mathbf{v}_j$ being a speed function, and $s$ being the evolution step. It is equivalent to

$$\pi_{jk}^{s+1} - \pi_{jk}^{s} = -\gamma \mathbf{v}_j \cdot \nabla \pi_{kj} \qquad (3)$$

under the condition that $\sum_{k=1}^{K} \pi_{jk} = 1$. We use the gradient vector flow (GVF) [10] as the speed function, because it has been shown to be more flexible and provide stronger constraints than many other forces or speed functions [10].

Here we compute it from the magnitude of target image gradient $\|\nabla_{\mathbf{x}}\mathbf{I}\|$ instead of binary edge map, i.e., $\mathbf{v}_j = GVF\{\nabla\|\nabla_{\mathbf{x}}I_j\|\}$ An example is shown in Fig. 2.

A notable advantage of this formulation is $\pi_{jk}$ only evolves in regions where their labels are ambiguous based on spatial priors. For regions with definite labels, the term $\nabla\pi_{kj}$ in Eqn. (3) equals 0 and thus $\pi_{jk}$ does not evolve.

## 2.2   The E-Step

In the E-step, the conditional expectation of the log likelihood function is computed. Let $\boldsymbol{\theta}^{(t)}$ be the set of estimated parameters at iteration $t$. As in standard EM algorithm, the conditional expectation is

$$Q(\boldsymbol{\theta}|\boldsymbol{\theta}^{(t)}) = E\{\log f(\mathbf{I}|\mathbf{Z},\rho)f(\mathbf{Z}|\boldsymbol{\pi})\} + \log f(\boldsymbol{\pi}|\mathbf{I}) \tag{4}$$
$$= \sum_{\mathbf{Z}} [\log f(\mathbf{I}|\mathbf{Z},\rho)f(\mathbf{Z}|\boldsymbol{\pi})]\, f(\mathbf{Z}|\mathbf{I},\boldsymbol{\theta}^{(t)}) + \log f(\boldsymbol{\pi}|\mathbf{I})$$

Using Bayes' law and assuming the labels and intensities at voxels are independently distributed we have

$$f(\mathbf{Z}|\mathbf{I},\boldsymbol{\theta}^{(t)}) = \frac{f(\mathbf{I}|\mathbf{Z},\boldsymbol{\theta}^{(t)})f(\mathbf{Z})}{\sum_{\mathbf{Z}'} f(\mathbf{I}|\mathbf{Z}',\boldsymbol{\theta}^{(t)})f(\mathbf{Z}')} = \frac{\prod_j \prod_k [f(I_j|z_{jk},\boldsymbol{\theta}^{(t)})p_{jk}]^{z_{jk}}}{\sum_{\mathbf{Z}'} \prod_j \prod_k [f(I_j|z'_{jk},\boldsymbol{\theta}^{(t)})p_{jk}]^{z'_{jk}}}. \tag{5}$$

Thus at each voxel $j$ we have

$$w_{jk}^{(t)} = f(z_{jk} = 1|I,\boldsymbol{\theta}^{(t)}) = \frac{f(I_j|z_{jk} = 1,\boldsymbol{\theta}^{(t)})p_{jk}}{\sum_{k'=1}^{K} f(I_j|z_{jk'} = 1,\boldsymbol{\theta}^{(t)})p_{jk'}}, \tag{6}$$

and $w_{jk}$ is referred as the weighting variable. $\rho_k^{(t)}(I_j) = f(I_j|z_{jk} = 1,\boldsymbol{\theta}^{(t)})$ is the intensity distribution for structure $k$. Eqn. (4) can be expressed as

$$Q(\boldsymbol{\theta}|\boldsymbol{\theta}^{(t)}) = \sum_j \sum_k [\log f(I_j|z_{jk} = 1,\rho_k)f(z_{jk} = 1|\pi_{jk})]\, w_{jk}^{(t)} + \log f(\boldsymbol{\pi}|\mathbf{I})$$
$$= \sum_j \sum_k w_{jk}^{(t)} \log \rho_k(I_j) + \sum_j \sum_k w_{jk}^{(t)} \log \pi_{jk} + \log f(\boldsymbol{\pi}|\mathbf{I}). \tag{7}$$

## 2.3   The M-Step

In the M-step, the parameters $\boldsymbol{\theta}^{(t+1)}$ are computed by maximizing $Q(\boldsymbol{\theta}|\boldsymbol{\theta}^{(t)})$.

To estimate $\rho$, we model the intensity distribution using Parzen window method, i.e., $\rho_k(x) = \sum_j a_{kj}G(x; I_j,\sigma)$, where $G(\cdot; I_j,\sigma)$ is the Gaussian kernel with mean $I_m$ and standard deviation $\sigma$. $a_{kj}$ are the coefficients such that $\sum_j a_{kj} = 1$. By maximizing Eqn. (7) it is derived that

$$\rho_k^{(t+1)} = \arg\max_{\rho_k} \sum_j w_{jk}^{(t)} \log \rho_k(I_j) = \frac{1}{\sum_{j'} w_{j'k}^{(t)}} \sum_j w_{jk}^{(t)} G(x; I_j,\sigma), \tag{8}$$

or $a_{kj}^{(t+1)} = w_{jk}^{(t)} / \sum_{j'k} w_{j'k}^{(t)}$.

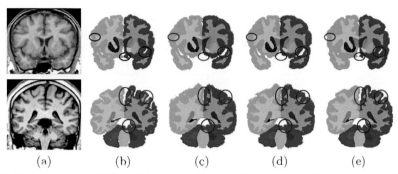

**Fig. 3.** Results on two IBSR subjects. (a) T1-weighted coronal slices, (b) ground truth, the results of (c) MV, (d) IWV, and (e) DA methods. The improvements of DA are highlighted using circles.

To etimate $\boldsymbol{\pi}$, based on Eqn. (7) we have

$$\boldsymbol{\pi}^{(t+1)} = \arg\max_{\boldsymbol{\pi}} \sum_j \sum_k w_{jk}^{(t)} \log \pi_{jk} + \log f(\boldsymbol{\pi}|\mathbf{I}) \tag{9}$$

with the constraints $\sum_k \pi_{jk} = 1$ for all $j$, or $c_j(\pi_{j1}, ..., \pi_{jK}) = 1 - \sum_k \pi_{jk} = 0$. As defined earlier, the term $\log f(\boldsymbol{\pi}|\mathbf{I})$ does not have an analytical form and thus Eqn. (9) does not have a closed-form solution. Instead we solve it iteratively using extended gradient descent method [11]. Let $\boldsymbol{\pi}_j = [\pi_{j1}, ..., \pi_{jK}]^T$, and we denote the gradient as $\mathbf{g}(\boldsymbol{\pi}_j) = \nabla_{\boldsymbol{\pi}_j} Q(\boldsymbol{\theta}|\boldsymbol{\theta}^{(t)}) = [g(\pi_{j1}), ..., g(\pi_{jK})]^T$, such that

$$g(\pi_{jk}) = \frac{\partial Q(\boldsymbol{\theta}|\boldsymbol{\theta}^{(t)})}{\partial \pi_{jk}} = \frac{w_{jk}^{(t)}}{\pi_{jk}} - \gamma \mathbf{v}_j \cdot \nabla \pi_{kj} . \tag{10}$$

Because of the constraints, $g(\pi_{jk})$ needs to be projected onto the constrained space [11], i.e., $\mathbf{g}_N(\boldsymbol{\pi}_k) = \mathbf{g}(\boldsymbol{\pi}_k) - \frac{\nabla c_j \cdot \mathbf{g}(\boldsymbol{\pi}_k)}{||\mathbf{g}(\boldsymbol{\pi}_k)||^2} \nabla c_j$, or equivalently,

$$g_N(\pi_{jk}) = g(\pi_{jk}) - \sum_{k=1}^{K} g(\pi_{jk})/K . \tag{11}$$

At iteration $s$, $\pi_{jk}^{(t+1)s+1}$ is updated as

$$\pi_{jk}^{(t+1)s+1} - \pi_{jk}^{(t+1)s} = \delta \, g_N(\pi_{jk}^{(t+1)s}) , \tag{12}$$

where $\delta$ is the small step size, and $\pi_{jk}^{(t+1)0} = \pi_{jk}^{(t)}$. After that $\pi_{jk}^{(t+1)s+1}$ is normalized to satisfy the constraint that $\sum_k \pi_{jk}^{(t+1)s+1} = 1$.

The complete deformable atlas algorithm is summarized in Algorithm 1.

## 3   Experiments and Results

Experiments were first performed using the Internet Brain Segmentation Repository (IBSR) data set[1]. It contains 18 healthy subjects with T1 weighted images,

---

[1] Provided by the Center for Morphometric Analysis at Massachusetts General Hospital and available at http://www.cma.mgh.harvard.edu/ibsr/

**Data**: Target image $\mathbf{I}$, prior spatial probability $\mathbf{p}_j$
**Initialization**: Set maximum iterations $T$ and $S$, set $t = 0$, $w_{jk}^{(0)} = \pi_{jk}^{(0)} = p_{jk}$ ;
Compute $\mathbf{v}_j$ using GVF and $\rho_k^{(0)}$ using Eqn. (8) ;
**repeat**

     **The E-Step**: compute $w_{jk}^{(t)}$ as in Eqn. (6);

     **The M-Step**: compute $\rho_k^{(t+1)}$ using (8), set s=0, $\pi_{jk}^{(t+1)0} = w_{jk}^{(t)}$;

     **repeat**

         Compute $\pi_{jk}^{(t+1)s+1}$ using Eqn. (12) ;

         Normalize $\pi_{jk}^{(t+1)s+1} = \pi_{jk}^{(t+1)s+1} / \sum_{k'=1}^{K} \pi_{jk'}^{(t+1)s+1}$;

         s=s+1;

     **until** *it converges or $s > S$*;

     $z_{jk} = 1$ if $\pi_{jk}^{(t+1)} > \pi_{ji}^{(t+1)}$ for all $i \neq k$, otherwise $z_{jk} = 0$ ;

     t=t+1 ;

**until** *the algorithm converges or $t > T$*;

**Algorithm 1.** The deformable atlas algorithm

and 32 brain structures were manually delineated on each image by experts. We also tested on Alzheimer's disease brains using the Australian Imaging, Biomarkers and Lifestyle (AIBL) data sets. For comparison, experiments were performed using three methods: majority voting (MV), intensity weighted voting (IWV), and DA. For MV, the segmentation was determined by fusing propagated label maps without considering image cues [3], i.e., j was labeled as $k$ if $p_{jk} > p_{ji}$ for $\forall i \neq k$. IWV improves MV by considering structure-specific intensity profiles, i.e., the intensity weighting $f(\mathbf{I}|\mathbf{Z}, \rho)$ in Eqn. (1) was applied but the term for structure boundary $f(\pi|\mathbf{I})$ was ignored. For DA, both the intensity weighting and the structure boundary term were applied. The parameters were empirically selected: $\gamma = 0.5$ and $\delta = 0.05$. $\sigma$ in Eqn. (8) was chosen as the intensity standard deviation of all voxels in each structure. In all experiments, the image registration was performed using SyN method [12].

For IBSR data, 18 leave-one-out experiments were performed using a multi-atlas approach. The segmentation results were compared to the manual segmentation and evaluated using the Dice coefficient, i.e., $D = \frac{2|X \cap Y|}{|X \cup Y|}$ where $X$ and $y$ are the voxel sets of manual labeling and automated segmentation result, respectively, and $|\cdot|$ is the set cardinality. Fig. 3 shows the qualitative results on two data sets, and Fig. 4 shows the quantitative results for all structures. Left and right structures are combined for clarity, and results on vessels were not shown. It was observed that IWV performed much better than MV in most structures, which demonstrated the effectiveness of incorporating intensity into the voting strategy. DA further improved the results especially in the ventricles and the cortex, and worked sightly better or similarly on other structures. The DA results are comparable to or better than state-of-the-art brain segmentation algorithms as shown in [13].

We also tested the methods on 45 AIBL images on Alzheimer's disease using the multi-atlas approach with the 18 IBSR data as the atlases, and the results were visually inspected. Fig. 5 shows the results on three selected subjects.

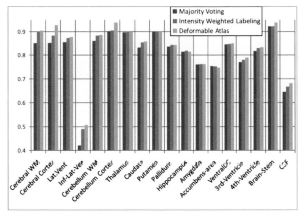

**Fig. 4.** The mean Dice coefficients of the three methods on different brain structures

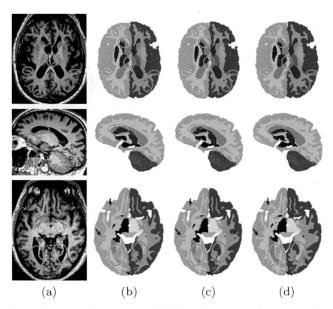

(a)          (b)          (c)          (d)

**Fig. 5.** Results on three AIBL images. (a) The T1-weighted images, the results of (b) MV, (c) IWV, and (d) DA methods. The major differences are highlighted using circles and arrows.

It was found that DA consistently worked much better than MV and IWV. This was because the diseased brains have large anatomical changes as compared to normal brains, e.g., brain tissue shrinkage and ventricle enlargement. Since the atlas images were all on normal brains, these pathological differences were not captured by the registration algorithm and resulted in failure of MV and IWV on certain parts of the brain (circled regions in Fig. 5). DA worked very well despite the anatomical changes thanks to the edge-based deformation. These results showed that deformable atlas could be successfully applied to brains with large deformation that could not be handled by voting based methods.

## 4  Discussions

We developed a deformable atlas method for multi-structure segmentation that combines the benefits of atlas-based and image-based approaches, and applied it to segment both normal brains and brains with Alzheimer's disease. Results showed that the method performed very well especially for diseased brain in spite of large anatomical deformation while other segmentation methods failed. The method can be readily extended to other applications of atlas-based segmentation, e.g., prostate and heart. Though only demonstrated using a multi-atlas approach, the method can equally be applied to probabilistic atlas approaches. Part of our future work is to include other speed functions, including curvature-based terms for smoothness, to get better segmentation results.

## References

1. Kass, M., Witkin, A., Terzopoulos, D.: Snakes: Active contour models. Int. J. Comp. Vis. 1(4), 321–331 (1988)
2. Malladi, R., Sethian, J.A., Vemuri, B.C.: Shape modeling with front propagation: a level set approach. IEEE Trans. Patt. Anal. Mach. Intell. 17(2), 158–175 (1995)
3. Heckemann, R., Hajnal, J., Aljabar, P., Rueckert, D., Hammers, A.: Automatic anatomical brain MRI segmentation combining label propagation and decision fusion. Neuroimage 33(1), 115–126 (2006)
4. Warfield, S., Zou, K., Wells, W.: Simultaneous truth and performance level estimation (STAPLE): An algorithm for the validation of image segmentation. IEEE Trans. Med. Imag. 23(7), 903–930 (2004)
5. Artaechevarria, X., Munoz-Barrutia, A., de Solorzano, C.O.: Combination strategies in multi-atlas image segmentation: Application to brain MR data. IEEE Trans. Med. Imag. 28(8), 1266–1277 (2009)
6. Sabuncu, M.R., Yeo, B.T.T., Leemput, K.V., Fischl, B., Golland, P.: A generative model for image segmentation based on label fusion. IEEE Trans. Med. Imag. 29(10), 1714–1729 (2010)
7. Shiee, N., Bazin, P.L., Cuzzocreo, J.L., Blitz, A., Pham, D.L.: Segmentation of brain images using adaptive atlases with application to ventriculomegaly. Inf. Process. Med. Imag., 1–22 (2011)
8. Wachinger, C., Golland, P.: Spectral label fusion. In: Ayache, N., Delingette, H., Golland, P., Mori, K. (eds.) MICCAI 2012, Part III. LNCS, vol. 7512, pp. 410–417. Springer, Heidelberg (2012)
9. Xu, C., Yezzi, A., Prince, J.: A summary of geometric level-set analogues for a general class of parametric active contour and surface models. In: Workshop on Variational and Level Set Methods in Computer Vision, pp. 104–111 (2001)
10. Xu, C., Pham, D.L., Prince, J.L.: Medical Image Segmentation Using Deformable Models. In: SPIE Handbook on Medical Imaging. Medical Image Analysis, vol. III, SPIE (2000)
11. Rosen, J.B.: The gradient projection method for nonlinear programming: Part II, nonlinear constraints. J. Soc. Indust. Appl. Math. 9(4), 514–532 (1961)
12. Avants, B.B., Epstein, C.L., Grossman, M., Gee, J.C.: Symmetric diffeomorphic image registration with cross-correlation: Evaluating automated labeling of elderly and neurodegenerative brain. Med. Image Anal. 12(1), 26–41 (2008)
13. Rousseau, F., Habas, P., Studholme, C.: A supervised patched-based approach for human brain labeling. IEEE Trans. Med. Imag. 30(10), 1852–1862 (2011)

# Hierarchical Probabilistic Gabor and MRF Segmentation of Brain Tumours in MRI Volumes

Nagesh K. Subbanna[1], Doina Precup[2], D. Louis Collins[3], and Tal Arbel[1]

[1] Centre for Intelligent Machines, McGill University, Canada
[2] School of Computer Science, McGill University, Canada
[3] McConnell Brain Imaging Centre, McGill University, Canada

**Abstract.** In this paper, we present a fully automated hierarchical probabilistic framework for segmenting brain tumours from multispectral human brain magnetic resonance images (MRIs) using multiwindow Gabor filters and an adapted Markov Random Field (MRF) framework. In the first stage, a customised Gabor decomposition is developed, based on the combined-space characteristics of the two classes (tumour and non-tumour) in multispectral brain MRIs in order to optimally separate tumour (including edema) from healthy brain tissues. A Bayesian framework then provides a coarse probabilistic texture-based segmentation of tumours (including edema) whose boundaries are then refined at the voxel level through a modified MRF framework that carefully separates the edema from the main tumour. This customised MRF is not only built on the voxel intensities and class labels as in traditional MRFs, but also models the intensity differences between neighbouring voxels in the likelihood model, along with employing a prior based on local tissue class transition probabilities. The second inference stage is shown to resolve local inhomogeneities and impose a smoothing constraint, while also maintaining the appropriate boundaries as supported by the local intensity difference observations. The method was trained and tested on the publicly available MICCAI 2012 Brain Tumour Segmentation Challenge (BRATS) Database [1] on both synthetic and clinical volumes (low grade and high grade tumours). Our method performs well compared to state-of-the-art techniques, outperforming the results of the top methods in cases of clinical high grade and low grade tumour core segmentation by 40% and 45% respectively.

## 1 Introduction

Worldwide, it is estimated that roughly 238,000 cases of brain tumours are diagnosed every year [2]. One of the primary diagnostic evaluation tools for brain tumours is magnetic resonance imaging (MRI) of the brain to evaluate the size of the tumour and its proximity to critical structures of the brain. Brain tumours present significant challenges to traditional segmentation techniques due to the wide variability in their appearance in terms of shape, size, position within the brain, their intensity variability and heterogeneity caused by swelling (edema), the presence of cysts, tumour type, etc. Moreover, the image acquisition parameters, scanner type, imaging artefacts, and pre-processing steps also greatly affect the appearance of tumours in MRI. The tumour boundaries appear differently in different MRI contrasts (e.g. T1w, T2w, or FLAIR images) commonly used in clinical contexts leading to non-trivial ambiguities both in terms of the

K. Mori et al. (Eds.): MICCAI 2013, Part I, LNCS 8149, pp. 751–758, 2013.

modelling and with regards to expert ground truth labelling required for training and testing. Finally, depending on the tumour type, the contrast between the boundaries and the surrounding healthy tissue can often be quite weak. These factors greatly impede the ability of generative techniques to properly model and predict tumour appearance.

Over the years, a number of techniques have been successfully devised to segment brain tumours automatically. These include atlas-based techniques [4], [5], [6], [9] which register brain tumour volumes to healthy brain atlases, and classify tumour regions as outliers. Generative techniques [3], [13] model the brain tumour intensity patterns during training and segment tumours in test images based on these models. Discriminative techniques [7], [8], [10], [11] on the other hand, avoid modelling intensity distributions and instead determine boundaries between tumour and non-tumour classes based on local intensity and/or some regional information. Overall, the literature suggests that it is advantageous to embed both local and global information into the framework in order to localise tumours and segment their boundaries correctly. Global information can be provided through position frequency techniques which offer a convenient way of coarsely detecting and locating tumours [12] based on learning texture patterns over images. Markov Random Field (MRF) approaches have been devised to model local information to segment tumours [13], however they have primarily been used to perform spatial regularisation through a class prior. The premise of this paper is that optimal tumour segmentation can be achieved through the careful design and combination of coarse Gabor texture based segmentation and a refined MRF model into a single probabilistic framework that leverages the advantages of both techniques. Preliminary work based on a similar idea was presented in [15] at MICCAI BRATS 2012, but this paper presents substantial improvements including a customised Gabor filterbank to optimally separate tumour, and non-tumour, an improved MRF to include inter-class transition probabilities, and also model intensity differences between classes.

In this paper, we develop a fully automated, hierarchical probabilistic framework for segmenting brain tumours from multimodal brain MRI. At the first stage, the goal is to coarsely segment the tumour (and associated edema) from the surrounding healthy tissue using texture based features. Here, specialised Gabor functions are developed to optimally separate the tumour class from the surrounding healthy tissues during training. A Bayesian classification framework is developed, based on the combined space Gabor decomposition, resulting in tumour/non-tumour probabilities. In the second stage, the boundaries and details of the segmentation are refined through an adapted probabilistic graphical MRF model, designed to separate the edema from the main tumour. This customised MRF differs from standard MRFs in that it is not simply a smoothing operator through a prior on class labels. In addition to taking voxel intensities and class labels into account, it also models the intensity differences between neighbouring voxels in the likelihood model and considers the likelihood of transitions between classes.

The entire proposed framework is trained and tested on the publicly available, MICCAI 2012 Brain Tumour Segmentation Challenge (BRATS) database [1]. On-line segmentation statistics (e.g. Dice overlap metrics) are provided. In comparison with other participants, our method outperforms the top methods from the competition in the cases of clinical high grade and low grade tumour core by 40% and 45% respectively, and performs roughly as well as the top methods in other categories.

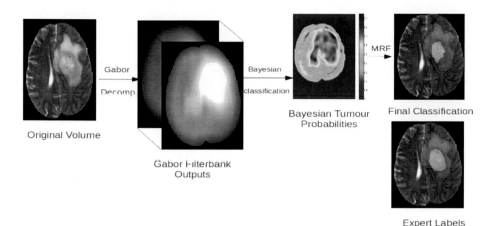

Original Volume

Gabor
Decomp.

Gabor Filterbank
Outputs

Bayesian
classification

Bayesian Tumour
Probabilities

MRF

Final Classification

Expert Labels

**Fig. 1.** Flowchart displaying the various stages of the classification technique. In the MRF classification and expert labels, red label represents edema, and green represents tumour.

## 2    Proposed Framework

We develop a hierarchical probabilistic brain tumour segmentation approach, using two stages. In the first stage, multiwindow Gabor decompositions of the multi-spectral MRI training images are used to build multivariate Gaussian models for both the healthy tissues and the tumour (including core and edema tissue). A Bayesian classification framework using these features is used to obtain initial classification results. In the second stage, Gaussian models are built for healthy tissues (i.e. grey matter (GM), white matter (WM) and cerebrospinal fluid (CSF)) as well as for tumour tissues (e.g. core tissues, edema) from intensity distributions acquired from the training dataset. A Markov Random Field is trained to classify all these types of tissues. A flowchart of the process is shown in Fig. 1. We now present in detail the two stages.

### 2.1    Stage 1: Multiwindow Gabor Bayesian Classification

**Training:** The data consists of MRI intensity volumes in different contrasts (T1, T1c (T1-post gado-contrast), T2 and FLAIR). Hence, at each voxel, we have a 4-dimensional vector containing the intensity in each contrast. Each contrast $\mathbf{f}$ of each volume is processed using multiwindow, 2D Gabor transforms of the form suggested by [16]. We use a set of $R$ window functions $g_r, r = 1 \ldots R$ of the form:

$$g_r[x, y; a, b, n_1, n_2, m_1, m_2, \sigma_{x_r}, \sigma_{y_r}] = e^{-((x-n_1a)^2/\sigma_{x_r}^2 + (y-n_2a)^2/\sigma_{y_r}^2)} e^{-j2\pi(m_1bx+m_2by)/L},$$

(1)

where $L$ is the total number of voxels in the slice under consideration, $x$ and $y$ are space coordinates within the slice, $a$ and $b$ are the magnitude of the shifts in the spatial and frequency domains respectively, $n_{1,2}$ and $m_{1,2}$ are the indices of the shifts in the position and frequency domains respectively, $\sigma_{x_r}$ and $\sigma_{y_r}$ are variance parameters of the $r$-th window. In our experiments we chose $b$ such that there are 6 equally spaced orientations between 0 and $\pi$ radians (sufficient in practice) and $a = 1$. Let $\mathbf{G}$ be the Gabor matrix whose columns are generated by picking all possible shift values for both $a$ and $b$ for all the $R$ windows with every $x$ and $y$ represented in each column. The filter bank coefficients $\mathbf{c}$ are obtained by convolving each contrast volume slice by slice with the Gabor filter bank $\mathbf{G}$. We use the same $\mathbf{G}$ matrix for all contrasts. It was proved in [18] that if both $g_r[\cdot]$ and its remapping window are positive definite[1], then any $g_r[\cdot]$ can be used and perfect reconstruction is possible. Here, both $g_r[\cdot]$ and its remapping window are Gaussian (but with different parameters), and are positive definite.

Each voxel in the training volumes belongs to one of two classes: tumour or healthy tissue. We estimate the window function parameters ($\sigma_{x_r}$ and $\sigma_{y_r}$) that will maximize the distance between the two classes. More formally, let $\{\mathbf{f}_t\}$ and $\{\mathbf{f}_h\}$ be the sets of voxels belonging to the tumour class and the healthy class respectively. The corresponding tumour coefficients $\mathbf{c}_t$ in the combined space are obtained by a convolution of the Gabor filters centred at the tumour voxels in question. Similarly, the $\mathbf{c}_h$ are obtained with Gabor filters centred at the non-tumour voxels in question. Ideally, the coefficients of the tumour and healthy class should be as different as possible. To achieve this goal, we solve the following optimisation problem:

$$(\sigma_x, \sigma_y) = \arg \max_{\sigma_x, \sigma_y} \sum_{j,k} | c_j - c_k |, \forall c_j \in \{\mathbf{c}_t\}, \forall c_k \in \{\mathbf{c}_h\} \qquad (2)$$

where $\sigma_x$ and $\sigma_y$ are the vectors containing the $R$ $\sigma_{x_r}$ and $\sigma_{y_r}$. We solve this optimisation using simulated annealing during training.

**Classification:** Each test volume is decomposed into its multiwindow Gabor filter bank outputs, $\mathbf{I}^G$, using the convolution at each voxel described above. The class of each voxel $i$, $C_i$ is then estimated using Bayesian classification:

$$P(C_i \mid \mathbf{I}_i^G) \propto P(\mathbf{I}_i^G \mid C_i)P(C_i), \qquad (3)$$

where $\mathbf{I}_i^G$ is the set of Gabor coefficients of voxel $i$.

## 2.2   Markov Random Field Classification

The main purpose of the second stage is to remove false positives, distinguish the different sub-types of tumour tissue (e.g. core vs edema), and refine the boundaries of the tumour. The proposed Markov Random Field (MRF) framework differs in several important ways from standard MRF approaches. First, the model is designed specifically to model the differences in intensity between a voxel and its neighbours probabilistically, in order to preserve the correct tumour boundaries. Our MRF uses significantly larger clique sizes than in standard models, which typically use only pairs of voxels. The prior models are conditioned on all possible class configurations within the neighbourhood. More precisely, we consider that the label of voxel $i$, $C_i$, is probabilistically inferred through an intensity vector, $\mathbf{I}_i$, and cliques involving the voxel and some of

---

[1] Positive definite windows are windows whose discrete Fourier transform is real and positive.

its adjacent voxels in the neighbourhood $N_i$. For all voxels $j$ in the neighbourhood $N_i$, $j \in N_i$, there exists a corresponding class vector $\mathbf{C}_j$ and corresponding set of intensity vectors $\mathbf{I}_j$. The energy at voxel $i$ has to be minimised to infer the optimal classification for $P(C \mid \mathbf{I})$ as follows: The energy of voxel $i$ is given by:

$$U(C_i \mid \mathbf{I}_i) = -[\log P(C_i) + \log P(\mathbf{I}_i \mid C_i) + \sum_{j \in N_i} \log P(\Delta \mathbf{I}_{i,j} \mid C_i, \mathbf{C}_j)] + \alpha m(\mathbf{C}_j, C_i),$$

(4)

where $P(C_i)$ is the prior probability of class $C_i$, $P(\mathbf{I}_i \mid C_i)$ models the likelihood of $C_i$ given the intensity of voxel $i$, $P(\Delta \mathbf{I}_{i,j} \mid C_i, \mathbf{C}_j)$ models the difference in intensity between $i$ and voxels in the $j$-th clique for classes $C_i$ and $\mathbf{C}_j$, $m(\mathbf{C}_j, C_i)$ is the potential of transitioning from $C_i$ to $\mathbf{C}_j$ and $\alpha$ ($\alpha = 1$ here) is a weighting parameter.

**Training:** During training, the volumes are non-linearly registered to a brain tissue atlas, masking out the tumour region using the experts classification labels. The registration allows us to generate separate labels for grey matter, white matter, and cerebrospinal fluid. The core and edema are superimposed from the expert labels. We consider an 8-neighbourhood around the voxel in the axial plane as well as the corresponding voxels in the slices above and below. The neighbourhood $N_i$ consists of all size 2, 3, and 4 cliques that contain voxel $i$. When only 2 tumour class labels are available for training (i.e. "Two class Gabor-MRF"), we chose to model the single voxel clique likelihood $P(\mathbf{I}_i|C_i)$ as a Gaussian mixture model (GMM) with 8 component Gaussian mixtures, for both the tumour core and edema classes due to the heterogeneity of the regions. However, when various class labels are available for the tumour core (e.g. necrotic core, enhancing tumour, solid tumour), we chose to use single multivariate Gaussian distributions for each class instead of Gaussian mixture models. The healthy classes are all modelled as multivariate Gaussians. The differences between intensities of the different classes are modelled as multivariate Gaussian distributions for all class combinations in both cases. The class transition probabilities are extracted from the frequency of co-occurrence in the training volumes.

**Classification:** The Gabor-Bayesian probabilities are used as priors for the tumour and the edema classes, with an exponential decay from the initially classified tumour regions. The tumour areas are masked out and healthy atlases are registered to the remaining regions to get the prior probabilities of healthy tissues in the non-tumour regions. Iterated conditional modes (ICM) [19] are used to minimise the total energy as the initial classification provides a good starting point for the optimisation.

## 3  Experiments and Results

The framework was trained and tested on the publicly available MICCAI 2012 Brain Tumour Segmentation Challenge datasets[1]. Here 20 high grade and 10 low grade real tumour volumes are available for training with 2 class (core and edema) and 4 class (necrotic core, enhancing tumour, solid tumour, and edema) labels. In addition, 25 high grade and 25 low grade synthetic volumes with 2 class labels are also available. The final test set consisted of 11 high grade and 4 low grade real data sets, and 10 high grade and 5 low grade synthetic volumes. The algorithm was trained on both the 2 class and 4 class labels for real glioma cases, as well as on the 2 class synthetic data, separately for both high and low grade tumours. As the system is set up to test 2 class labelling: i.e., only core and edema, for the results of the 4 class case, the 3 tumour labels were merged to create a single tumour core label. All the resulting test labels were uploaded onto the website and the statistics were provided automatically. Testing of the algorithm took slightly more than an hour per case on a Dell Optiplex 980 I7 machine.

**Qualitative Results:** Fig. 2 shows the results of our algorithm on a slice from a low grade tumour and a high grade tumour against the experts segmentation, along with the corresponding unlabelled T1c and FLAIR slices. Visually, in both cases, it can be seen that our results are comparable to the experts' labelling.

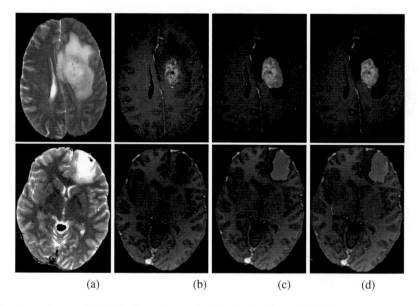

(a)                    (b)                    (c)                    (d)

**Fig. 2.** Row 1, case HG0011, Row 2, case LG0015. (a) The unlabelled FLAIR slice, (b) the unlabelled T1C slice (c) expert labelling and (d) our algorithm labels, (red = edema, green = tumour). Our algorithm's labels corresponds closely with the experts' labels.

**Quantitative Results:** Table 1 shows the results of our technique on both real glioma and synthetic tumour volumes. Dice similarity coefficient was used to compare results, as in the BRATS challenge. Our algorithm outperforms the winning algorithm by about 40% in the case of high grade (HG) tumour cores and about 45% in the case of low grade (LG) tumour cores, and has statistics comparable to the winner for edema. Table 2 shows that our statistics are comparable to the winners with Dice averages of around 0.8 overall for LG tumours (core and edema) and 0.85 for HG. The 4 class Gabor-MRF outperforms the 2 class Gabor-MRF mainly due to the heterogeneity of the tumour core. Modelling the core as a GMM with 8 modes in the 'two class case' is proven to be less effective than training on each sub-class separately, in the four class case, even with a simple model for each sub-class.

**Table 1.** Comparison of the segmentation results of the proposed method and the methods participating in the BRATS Challenge as presented on the website [1] for both edema and tumour core for clinical cases using average Dice similarity coefficient values. The final results of our method are found in the "Four class Gabor-MRF", where the method was trained and tested on the 4 class tumour labels and the 3 core labels were merged to create a single core label prior to uploading. The "Two class Gabor-MRF", where the algorithm was trained and tested on a single tumour core class, is shown for comparison. The winners of the challenge are highlighted in bold.

| Method | HG Edema | HG Tumour Core | LG Edema | LG Tumour Core |
|---|---|---|---|---|
| Shin. et. al | 0.038 | 0.144 | 0.061 | 0.232 |
| Bauer. et. al. | 0.536 | **0.512** | 0.179 | 0.332 |
| Zikic. et. al. | **0.598** | 0.476 | **0.324** | **0.339** |
| Subbanna. et. al. | 0.166 | 0.248 | 0.14 | 0.245 |
| Xiao. et. al. | 0.539 | 0.337 | 0.279 | 0.224 |
| Zhao. et. al. | 0.003 | 0.058 | 0 | 0 |
| Two class Gabor-MRF | 0.613 | 0.641 | 0.268 | 0.241 |
| Four class Gabor-MRF | 0.56 | 0.74 | 0.240 | 0.49 |

**Table 2.** Comparison of the segmentation results of the proposed method "Two class Gabor-MRF" and the methods participating in the BRATS Challenge as presented on the website [1] against the experts' labels for both the edema and the tumour core for the synthetic cases in the BRATS Challenge [1] using Dice similarity coefficient values. The winners of the challenge are highlighted in bold. As may be observed, our technique has a performance comparable to the winners of the challenge. In the case of synthetic tumour volumes, both our algorithm and the winners have Dice values of around 0.85.

| Method | HG Edema | HG Tumour Core | LG Edema | LG Tumour Core |
|---|---|---|---|---|
| Shin. et. al | 0.312 | 0.284 | 0.213 | 0.072 |
| Bauer. et. al. | 0.785 | 0.779 | 0.746 | **0.858** |
| Zikic. et. al. | **0.85** | **0.869** | **0.749** | 0.842 |
| Subbanna. et. al. | 0.696 | 0.398 | 0.645 | 0.42 |
| Xiao. et. al. | 0.343 | 0.414 | 0.1 | 0.469 |
| Zhao. et. al. | 0 | 0 | 0 | 0 |
| Two class Gabor-MRF | 0.877 | 0.841 | 0.772 | 0.832 |

## 4    Discussions, Future Work and Conclusion

The results show that our method performs very well in the task of segmenting brain tumours and edema in both synthetic and real clinical multimodal brain MRI. It outperforms other techniques in segmenting tumour cores. Its main strength is the hierarchical approach that first coarsely segments the tumour using a customised Gabor decomposition and then refines the segmentation using an adapted MRF. We hope to enhance our technique by improving the second stage to recover from any errors made during the first stage by using a more flexible hierarchical MRF. Currently, the accuracy of the second stage is dependent on obtaining a reasonable classification from the first stage. We are working on solving the optimal cluster separation analytically. Finally, although the results of the experiments on this dataset are promising, the automated approaches are all tested against the subjective ground truth labels of one set of clinicians. Further experimentation on data acquired from multiple centres would be desirable.

**Acknowledgement.** The authors wish to thank the organisers of MICCAI BRATS Challenge 2012 [1] for providing the data, tumour labels and online validation tools.

# References

1. http://www2.imm.dtu.dk/projects/BRATS2012/data.html
2. Ferlay, J., et al.: Estimates of worldside burden of cancer in 2008. In: GLOBOCAN 2008 (2008)
3. Corso, J., et al.: Efficient Multilevel Brain Tumour Segmentation with Integrated Bayesian Model Classification. IEEE Trans. Med. Imag. 27(5), 629–640 (2008)
4. Kaus, M., et al.: Adaptive Template Moderated Brain Tumour Segmentation in MRI. In: Workshop Fuer Bildverarbeitung Fur Die Medizin, pp. 102–105 (1999)
5. Prastawa, M., et al.: A brain tumor segmentation framework based on outlier detection. Med. Image Ana. 8(3), 275–283 (2004)
6. Menze, B.H., van Leemput, K., Lashkari, D., Weber, M.-A., Ayache, N., Golland, P.: A generative model for brain tumor segmentation in multi-modal images. In: Jiang, T., Navab, N., Pluim, J.P.W., Viergever, M.A. (eds.) MICCAI 2010, Part II. LNCS, vol. 6362, pp. 151–159. Springer, Heidelberg (2010)
7. Zikic, D., Glocker, B., Konukoglu, E., Criminisi, A., Demiralp, C., Shotton, J., Thomas, O.M., Das, T., Jena, R., Price, S.J.: Decision forests for tissue-specific segmentation of high-grade gliomas in multi-channel MR. In: Ayache, N., Delingette, H., Golland, P., Mori, K. (eds.) MICCAI 2012, Part III. LNCS, vol. 7512, pp. 369–376. Springer, Heidelberg (2012)
8. Wels, M., Carneiro, G., Aplas, A., Huber, M., Hornegger, J., Comaniciu, D.: A discriminative model-constrained graph-cuts approach to fully automated pediatric brain tumor segmentation in 3D MRI. In: Metaxas, D., Axel, L., Fichtinger, G., Székely, G. (eds.) MICCAI 2008, Part I. LNCS, vol. 5241, pp. 67–75. Springer, Heidelberg (2008)
9. Moon, N., et al.: Model based brain and tumor segmentation. In: ICPR, vol. 1, pp. 528–531 (2002)
10. Bauer, S., et al.: Segmentation of Brain Tumour Images Based on Integrated Hierarchical Classification and Regularisation. In: BRATS MICCAI (2012)
11. Parisot, S.: Graph-based Detection, Segmentation and Characterisation of Brain Tumours. In: CVPR, pp. 988–995 (2012)
12. Mishra, R.: MRI based brain tumor detection using wavelet packet feature and Artificial Neural Networks. In: Int. Conf. and Work. on Emerging Trends in Tech., pp. 656–659 (2010)
13. Bauer, S., et al.: Atlas-Based Segmentation of Brain Tumor Images Using a Markov Random Field-Based Tumor Growth Model and Non-Rigid Registration. In: IEEE EMBS, pp. 4080–4083 (2010)
14. Farias, G., et al.: Brain Tumour Diagnosis with Wavelets and Support Vector Machines. In: Int. Conf. Intell. Systems and Knowledge Engg., pp. 1453–1459 (2008)
15. Subbanna, N., et al.: Probabilistic Gabor and Markov Random Fields Segmentation of Brain Tumours in MRI Volumes. In: BRATS MICCAI (2012)
16. Zibulski, M.: Discrete multiwindow Gabor-type transforms. IEEE Trans. Sig. Proc. 45(6), 1428–1442 (1997)
17. Jain, A., et al.: Unsupervised Texture segmentation using Gabor filters. Patt. Rcgn. 24(12), 1167–1186 (1991)
18. Subbanna, N., et al.: Existence Conditions for Non-Canonical Discrete Multiwindow Gabor Frames. IEEE Trans. Sig. Proc. 55(10), 5113–5117 (2007)
19. Duda, R., et al.: Pattern Classification. John Wiley and Sons (2000)

# Robust GM/WM Segmentation of the Spinal Cord with Iterative Non-local Statistical Fusion

Andrew J. Asman[1], Seth A. Smith[2], Daniel S. Reich[3], and Bennett A. Landman[1,2]

[1] Electrical Engineering, Vanderbilt University, Nashville, TN, USA 37235
[2] Institute of Imaging Science, Vanderbilt University, Nashville, TN, USA 37235
[3] Translational Neuroradiology Unit, National Institutes of Health, Bethesda, MD, USA 37235
{andrew.j.asman,seth.smith,bennett.landman}@vanderbilt.edu,
daniel.reich@nih.gov

**Abstract.** New magnetic resonance imaging (MRI) sequences are enabling clinical study of the *in vivo* spinal cord's internal structure. Yet, low contrast-to-noise ratio, artifacts, and imaging distortions have limited the applicability of tissue segmentation techniques pioneered elsewhere in the central nervous system. Recently, methods have been presented for cord/non-cord segmentation on MRI and the feasibility of gray matter/white matter tissue segmentation has been evaluated. To date, no automated algorithms have been presented. Herein, we present a non-local multi-atlas framework that robustly identifies the spinal cord and segments its internal structure with submillimetric accuracy. The proposed algorithm couples non-local fusion with a large number of slice-based atlases (as opposed to typical volumetric ones). To improve performance, the fusion process is interwoven with registration so that segmentation information guides registration and vice versa. We demonstrate statistically significant improvement over state-of-the-art benchmarks in a study of 67 patients. The primary contributions of this work are (1) innovation in non-volumetric atlas information, (2) advancement of label fusion theory to include iterative registration/segmentation, and (3) the first fully automated segmentation algorithm for spinal cord internal structure on MRI.

**Keywords:** Spinal Cord Parcellation, Multi-Atlas Segmentation, Non-local Correspondence Models, Registration Refinement.

## 1 Introduction

The spinal cord is an essential and vulnerable component of the central nervous system [1, 2]. Differentiating and localizing pathology/degeneration of the gray matter (GM) and white matter (WM) plays a critical role in assessing therapeutic impacts and determining prognoses [3, 4]. Automated methods have localized the cord [5] and semi-automated segmentation has been used for internal segmentation [6]. Yet, automated GM/WM delineation has not been reported. Increased automation is necessary for routine volumetric assessment of the cord structures. Given the small size and artifacts of spinal cord MRI, the feasibility of an approach has only recently come to light using magnetization transfer (MT) MRI of the spinal cord *in vivo* [2].

K. Mori et al. (Eds.): MICCAI 2013, Part I, LNCS 8149, pp. 759–767, 2013.
© Springer-Verlag Berlin Heidelberg 2013

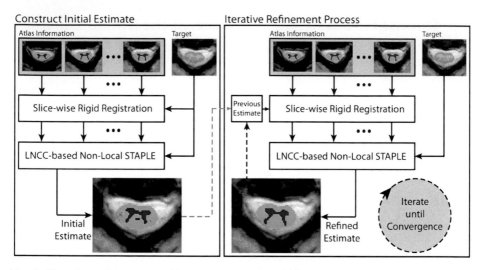

**Fig. 1.** Flowchart of the proposed iterative Non-Local STAPLE (iNLS) multi-atlas framework. Using an iterative atlas-target registration refinement framework, we expand the range of anatomical variability that can be reliably segmented.

Over the past decade, multi-atlas segmentation has come to prominence for its ability to rapidly and robustly generalize from labeled examples (i.e., atlases) [7, 8]. Unfortunately, as medical imaging researchers move out of the cranial vault towards more highly variable anatomical structures, the traditional registration followed by label fusion multi-atlas model [9-13] becomes increasingly problematic, as we are dependent upon reasonable atlas-target registrations.

Herein, we present the first fully-automated approach for GM/WM segmentation of the spinal cord through extension of a recently proposed non-local statistical fusion algorithm (Non-Local STAPLE – NLS [14]). We demonstrate submillimetric accuracy and show statistical improvement over other state-of-the-art approaches. The primary theoretical contributions of this work are: (1) we apply slice-based — as opposed to volumetric — atlases; (2) we adapt the NLS non-local correspondence model to use the locally normalized correlation coefficient (LNCC) to reduce the need for accurate intensity normalization [9]; and (3) we apply iterative registration refinement to lessens the impact of registration failures (**Figure 1**).

## 2    Theory

First, we describe the theoretical basis for the iterative non-local STAPLE (iNLS) framework and how it differs from the original NLS. Consider a target gray-level image represented as a vector, $I \in \mathbb{R}^{N \times 1}$. Let $T \in L^{N \times 1}$ be the latent representation of the true target segmentation, where $L = \{0, \dots, L - 1\}$ is the set of possible labels. Consider a collection of $R$ registered atlases with associated intensity values, $A \in \mathbb{R}^{N \times R}$, and label decisions, $D \in L^{N \times R}$. Let $\theta \in \mathbb{R}^{R \times L \times L}$ parameterize the raters (registered atlases) performance level. Each element of $\theta$, $\theta_{js's}$, represents the probability that rater $j$ observes label $s'$ given that the true label is $s$ at a given target voxel and the *corresponding* voxel on the associated atlas —

i.e., $\theta_{js's} \equiv p(D_{i^*j} = s', A|T_i = s, I)$, where $i^*$ is the voxel on atlas $j$ that corresponds to target voxel $i$. Throughout, the index variables $i$, $i^*$ and $i'$ will be used to iterate over the voxels, $s$ and $s'$ over the labels, and $j$ over the registered atlases.

Building upon the seminal Simultaneous Truth And Performance Level Estimation (STAPLE) algorithm [11], NLS reformulates the statistical fusion framework from a non-local means perspective. The goal of any non-local correspondence model is to estimate $f(A_{i'j}|I_i)$ – the probability that voxel $i'$ on atlas $j$ directly corresponds to the target image at voxel $i$. Originally, NLS used a Gaussian difference model [10, 12, 13] which has been shown to be highly successful for whole-brain segmentation [10, 12, 14]. Herein, we modify this correspondence model to be:

$$f(A_{i'j}|I_i) \equiv \alpha_{ji'i} = \frac{1}{Z_\alpha} \exp\left(\frac{LNCC_{\mathcal{N}_p}(A_{i'j}, I_i)}{\epsilon}\right) \exp\left(-\frac{\mathcal{E}_{ii'}^2}{2\sigma_d^2}\right) \tag{1}$$

where the first distribution is the intensity similarity model governed by locally normalized correlation coefficient between a patch on atlas $j$ centered at voxel $i'$ and the target image centered at voxel $i$, the second distribution is the spatial compatibility model, and $Z_\alpha$ is the partition function. In the intensity similarity model, we use the notation $LNCC_{\mathcal{N}_p}(\cdot,\cdot)$ to indicate the locally normalized coefficient using a patch window defined by $\mathcal{N}_p$, and $\epsilon$ is the weight factor for the exponential similarity. In the spatial compatibility model, $\mathcal{E}_{ii'}$ is the Euclidean distance between voxels $i$ and $i'$ in image space, and $\sigma_d$ is the corresponding standard deviation. The partition function $Z_\alpha$ enforces the constraint that $\sum_{i' \in \mathcal{N}_s(i)} \alpha_{ji'i} = 1$, where $\mathcal{N}_s(i)$ is the set of voxels in the *search neighborhood* of a given target voxel. Through this constraint, $\alpha_{ji'i}$ can be directly interpreted as the probability that voxel $i'$ on atlas $j$ is the latent corresponding voxel, $i^*$, to a given target voxel, $i$.

Using Eq. 1, we can estimate the latent performance level parameters based upon the assumed lack of atlas-target correspondence. By taking the expected value across the search neighborhood, $\mathcal{N}_s(i)$, and assuming conditional independence between the intensity-label relationships, the performance level parameters can be approximated as

$$f(D_{i^*j} = s', A_j|T_i = s, I_i, \theta_{js's}^{(k)}) \approx E[f(D_j|T_i = s, \theta_{js}^{(k)})f(A_j|I_i)]$$
$$= \sum_{i' \in \mathcal{N}_s(i)} \alpha_{ji'i}\theta_{js's}^{(k)} \tag{2}$$

We can then integrate the approximation provided in Eq. 2, directly into the Expectation-Maximization (EM) algorithm governing the statistical fusion framework. First, in the E-step, we estimate $W \in \mathbb{R}^{L \times N}$, where $W_{si}$ represents the probability that the true label associated with voxel $i$ is label $s$, given the provided information. Using a Bayesian expansion and conditional independence between the atlases, the solution for $W$ on iteration $k$ is

$$W_{si}^{(k)} \equiv f(T_i = s|D, A, I, \theta^{(k)})$$
$$= \frac{f(T_i = s) \prod_j \sum_{i' \in \mathcal{N}_s(i)} \alpha_{ji'i}\theta_{js's}^{(k)}}{\sum_n f(T_i = n) \prod_j \sum_{i' \in \mathcal{N}_s(i)} \alpha_{ji'i}\theta_{js'n}^{(k)}} \tag{3}$$

Finally, the resulting performance level parameters (M-step) are obtained by maximizing the expected value of the conditional log likelihood function.

$$\theta_{js's}^{(k+1)} = \frac{\sum_i \left( \sum_{i' \in N_s(i):D_{i'j}=s'} \alpha_{ji'i} \right) W_{si}^{(k)}}{\sum_i W_{si}^{(k)}}. \tag{4}$$

### 2.1    Iterative Global Refinement Using the Previously Estimated Segmentation

In the first iteration of iNLS, registration is based on normalized correlation between the atlas and target image intensity using a 3 degree-of-freedom rigid body transform. For subsequent iterations, we iteratively refine the registration by maximizing overlap between the atlas segmentation and the current segmentation estimation. Specifically,

$$\Phi_j^R = \arg \max_{\Phi_j^R} \sum_i \delta \left( D_{\Phi_j^R(i)j}, \Psi_i \right) \tag{5}$$

where $\Phi_j^R$ represent the parameters associated with the rigid transformation (i.e., translation and rotation) between the current estimated segmentation, $\Psi_i$, and the transformed atlas labels, $D_{\Phi_j^R(i)j}$, and $\delta(\cdot,\cdot)$ is the kronecker delta function.

### 2.2    Initialization and Convergence

For all experiments, iNLS was initialized using a 2mm isotropic search neighborhood, a 1mm isotropic patch neighborhood, and the weight factor, $\epsilon$, was set to 0.2. These parameter values were obtained by performing leave-one-out cross-validation using the provided atlases. The remaining parameters remain identical to the original NLS approach [14]. For the iterative global refinement procedure, convergence was detected when the rigid transformation parameters ceased to change across the atlases (less than 5 iterations for all presented results).

## 3    Methods and Results

### 3.1    Experimental Design

We study a dataset consisting of 67 MR images of the cervical spinal cord. All data were obtained on a 3T Philips Achieva (Philips Medical Systems, Best, The Netherlands) using a single channel body coil for transmission and a 16 channel neurovascular coil for signal reception. The center of the imaging volume was aligned to the space between the 3rd and 4th cervical levels. T2*w data were obtained using a 3D gradient echo (TR/TE/a = 121/12ms/9°) with a 3-shot EPI covering a field of view of 190 x 224 x 90 mm$^3$ with nominal resolution of 0.6 x 0.6 x 3 mm$^3$. Fat saturation was implemented by using a 1331 binomial excitation (ProSet), 2 signal averages, and a SENSE factor of 2. This acquisition was a part of an MT experiment where the same parameters would be performed with the addition of an MT prepulse.

Due to the highly variable nature of the spinal cord and the difficulty in performing consistent high degree-of-freedom registration [15], all multi-atlas segmentations were performed on a slice-by-slice basis. A collection of 85 slice atlases were randomly selected from the 2,010 (67 volumes × 30 slices) available slices. Note that atlas slices from the volume of interest were excluded during the leave-one-out segmentation to prevent biasing the results.

As benchmarks, we compare iNLS to a majority vote (MV) [8], an LNCC-weighted locally weighted vote (LWV) [9], STAPLE [11], non-local voting (NLV) [13], and a single iteration of NLS. For STAPLE, NLS and iNLS, "consensus voxels" (i.e., voxels where all registered atlases agree) were ignored. For fairness of comparison, the same non-local correspondence model was used for NLV, NLS, and iNLS. For all benchmarks, the presented results use all available atlases (up to 85) with a pairwise rigid 3 degree-of-freedom alignment using FLIRT [16]. Quantitative accuracy of each of the benchmarks was assessed on a volumetric basis using the Dice Similarity Coefficient (DSC), bi-directional mean surface distance error (MSDE), the bi-directional Hausdorff distance error (HDE).

## 3.2 Experimental Results

iNLS demonstrated statistically significant improvement over each of the considered benchmarks in terms of DSC, MSDE, and HDE for both gray matter and white matter segmentation (**Figure 2**). Importantly, iNLS is the only algorithm that provides a MSDE of less than 0.5 mm for all 67 subjects. In addition, iNLS results in a substantial decrease in outliers – particularly for the surface distance based metrics.

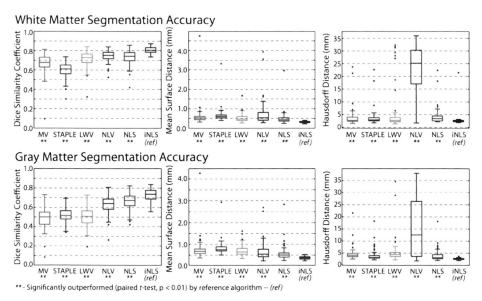

**Fig. 2.** Quantitative analysis on GM/WM segmentation of the spinal cord. iNLS provides significant improvement over all of all considered benchmarks.

As an aside, despite highly competitive results in terms of DSC and MSDE, NLV results in highly sub-optimal HDE values due to its susceptibility to outliers in the estimation process (i.e., outlier registrations result in "speckle noise" in the background of the estimate).

Qualitative results in terms of slice-wise accuracy (**Figure 3**) and volumetric surface distance error (**Figure 4**) support the quantitative improvement. iNLS provides visual (along with numeric) improvements over the initial NLS estimate. These can be appreciated in the precision with which the convoluted shape of the GM/WM boundary within the spinal cord. In **Figure 4**, it is evident that only iNLS provides estimates that are consistently less than 2mm on a voxelwise basis.

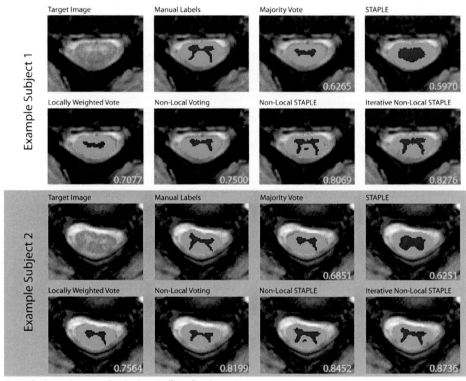

Note: Inlay shows white matter Dice Similarity Coefficient for subject volume.

**Fig. 3.** Slice-wise qualitative analysis of GM/WM segmentation of the spinal cord. Due to the lack of non-rigid registration, all of the non-local methods provide valuable accuracy improvements. However, only the proposed method, iNLS, is able to consistently maintain the complex shape of the GM/WM structures within the spinal cord.

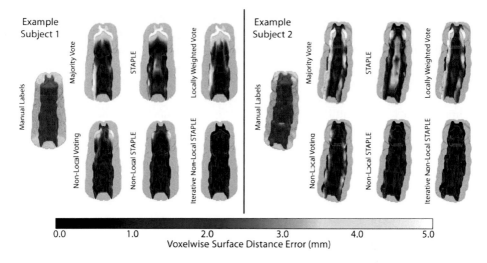

**Fig. 4.** Voxelwise surface distance error for spinal cord GM segmentation accuracy. The proposed iterative Non-Local STAPLE algorithm provides consistent volumetric improvement over the considered benchmarks in terms of voxelwise surface distance error.

## 4    Discussion

Accurate GM/WM delineation of the spinal cord plays a critical role in understanding the pathophysiological nature of spinal cord disease and assessing therapeutic interventions. Herein, we demonstrate an effective segmentation framework specifically targeting spinal cord GM/WM. We extend the recently proposed NLS algorithm with two critical advancements that enable robust GM/WM segmentation of the spinal cord. First, we reformulate the non-local correspondence model using the LNCC similarity metric to limit the need for accurate intensity normalization and to minimize the impact of imaging artifacts (e.g., intensity inhomogeneity). Second, we describe a new iterative atlas-target registration refinement process. Together, these advancements dramatically reduce the impact of initial registration failures, and, thus, significantly increase the robustness and accuracy of the resulting segmentation. We assessed the accuracy of the proposed iNLS framework against several of the current state-of-the-art benchmark algorithms and demonstrated statistically significant improvement in terms of DSC, MSDE, and HDE (**Figure 2**). Additionally, we provide both slice-wise (**Figure 3**) and volume-wise (**Figure 4**) qualitative examples that demonstrate the type of improvement exhibited by the proposed framework.

While the proposed framework is not the first algorithm to use the LNCC similarity metric (e.g., [9]) or the first approach to use segmentation-based registration refinement (e.g., [17, 18]), the provided joint-framework is novel. For example, [18] used iterative segmentation/registration to form group-wise consistent atlas representations while [17] used segmentation information in a deformable registration cost function. A fortunate consequence of moving to slice-wise registration is the speed of the individual registrations (i.e., seconds per slice as opposed to minutes/hours per volume); hence, many more simple registrations were evaluated in the iNLS framework than would have been pragmatic in a volumetric one. In fact, we evaluated the use of high degree-of-freedom registration tools, but these consistently resulted in catastrophic failures (i.e., no label overlap) when applied to the raw MRI of the spinal column (data not shown). In conclusion, our efforts demonstrate that we can achieve submillimetric segmentation accuracy in spite of the severe distortion, inhomogeneity, low-contrast, and small-scales involved in spinal cord MRI.

**Acknowledgemants.** Supported in part by NIH 1R21NS064534, 1R03EB012461, 2R01EB006136, R01EB006193, and the NIH/NINDS Intramural Research Program.

# References

1. Dietz, V., Curt, A.: Neurological aspects of spinal-cord repair: promises and challenges. The Lancet Neurology 5, 688–694 (2006)
2. Yiannakas, M., et al.: Feasibility of Grey Matter and White Matter Segmentation of the Upper Cervical Cord In Vivo: A pilot study with application to Magnetisation Transfer Measurements. Neuroimage 63, 1054–1059 (2012)
3. Gilmore, C.P., et al.: Spinal cord gray matter demyelination in multiple sclerosis—a novel pattern of residual plaque morphology. Brain Pathol. 16, 202–208 (2006)
4. Jarius, S., Wildemann, B.: AQP4 antibodies in neuromyelitis optica: diagnostic and pathogenetic relevance. Nature Reviews Neurology 6, 383–392 (2010)
5. Chen, M., et al.: Topology preserving automatic segmentation of the spinal cord in magnetic resonance images. In: 2011 IEEE International Symposium on Biomedical Imaging: From Nano to Macro, pp. 1737–1740. IEEE (2011)
6. Horsfield, M.A., et al.: Rapid semi-automatic segmentation of the spinal cord from magnetic resonance images: Application in multiple sclerosis. Neuroimage 50, 446–455 (2010)
7. Rohlfing, T., et al.: Performance-based classifier combination in atlas-based image segmentation using expectation-maximization parameter estimation. IEEE Transactions on Medical Imaging 23, 983–994 (2004)
8. Heckemann, R.A., et al.: Automatic anatomical brain MRI segmentation combining label propagation and decision fusion. Neuroimage 33, 115–126 (2006)
9. Artaechevarria, X., et al.: Combination strategies in multi-atlas image segmentation: Application to brain MR data. IEEE Trans. Med. Imaging 28, 1266–1277 (2009)
10. Sabuncu, M.R., et al.: A generative model for image segmentation based on label fusion. IEEE Transactions on Medical Imaging 29, 1714–1729 (2010)
11. Warfield, S.K., et al.: Simultaneous truth and performance level estimation (STAPLE): an algorithm for the validation of image segmentation. IEEE Transactions on Medical Imaging 23, 903–921 (2004)
12. Wang, H., et al.: Multi-Atlas Segmentation with Joint Label Fusion. IEEE Transactions on Pattern Analysis and Machine Intelligence 35, 611–623 (2012)
13. Coupé, P., et al.: Patch-based segmentation using expert priors: Application to hippocampus and ventricle segmentation. Neuroimage 54, 940–954 (2011)
14. Asman, A.J., Landman, B.A.: Non-Local STAPLE: An Intensity-Driven Multi-Atlas Rater Model. In: Ayache, N., Delingette, H., Golland, P., Mori, K. (eds.) MICCAI 2012, Part III. LNCS, vol. 7512, pp. 426–434. Springer, Heidelberg (2012)

15. Commowick, O., Wiest-Daesslé, N., Prima, S.: Automated diffeomorphic registration of anatomical structures with rigid parts: Application to dynamic cervical MRI. In: Ayache, N., Delingette, H., Golland, P., Mori, K. (eds.) MICCAI 2012, Part II. LNCS, vol. 7511, pp. 163–170. Springer, Heidelberg (2012)
16. Jenkinson, M., Smith, S.: A global optimisation method for robust affine registration of brain images. Medical Image Analysis 5, 143–156 (2001)
17. Heckemann, R.A., et al.: Improving intersubject image registration using tissue-class information benefits robustness and accuracy of multi-atlas based anatomical segmentation. Neuroimage 51, 221 (2010)
18. Jia, H., et al.: Iterative multi-atlas-based multi-image segmentation with tree-based registration. Neuroimage 59, 422–430 (2012)

# Author Index